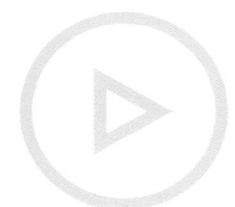

IMPORTANT:

HERE IS YOUR REGISTRATION CODE TO ACCESS
YOUR PREMIUM McGRAW-HILL ONLINE RESOURCES

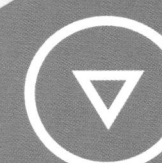

For key premium online resources you need **THIS CODE** to gain access. Once the code is entered, you will be able to use the Web resources for the length of your course.

If your course is using WebCT **or** Blackboard, **you'll be able to use this code to access the McGraw-Hill content within your instructor's online course.**

Access is provided if you have purchased a new book. If the registration code is missing from this book, the registration screen on our Website, and within your WebCT or Blackboard course, will tell you how to obtain your new code.

Registering for McGraw-Hill Online Resources

TO gain access to your McGraw-Hill web resources simply follow the steps below:

1. USE YOUR WEB BROWSER TO GO TO: **http://www.mhhe.com/wardlawcont5/**

2. CLICK ON **FIRST TIME USER**.

3. ENTER THE REGISTRATION CODE* PRINTED ON THE TEAR-OFF BOOKMARK ON THE RIGHT.

4. AFTER YOU HAVE ENTERED YOUR REGISTRATION CODE, CLICK **REGISTER**.

5. FOLLOW THE INSTRUCTIONS TO SET-UP YOUR PERSONAL UserID AND PASSWORD.

6. WRITE YOUR UserID AND PASSWORD DOWN FOR FUTURE REFERENCE.
   KEEP IT IN A SAFE PLACE.

TO GAIN ACCESS to the McGraw-Hill content in your instructor's **WebCT** or **Blackboard** course simply log in to the course with the UserID and Password provided by your instructor. Enter the registration code exactly as it appears in the box to the right when prompted by the system. You will only need to use the code the first time you click on McGraw-Hill content.

Thank you, and welcome to your McGraw-Hill online Resources!

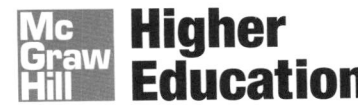

*YOUR REGISTRATION CODE CAN BE USED ONLY ONCE TO ESTABLISH ACCESS. IT IS NOT TRANSFERABLE.

0-07-290041-5 WARDLAW: CONTEMPORARY NUTRITION, 5/E.

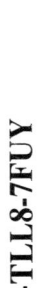

REGISTRATION CODE

V2ZO-ME5Q-SP2I-TLL8-7FUY

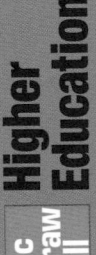

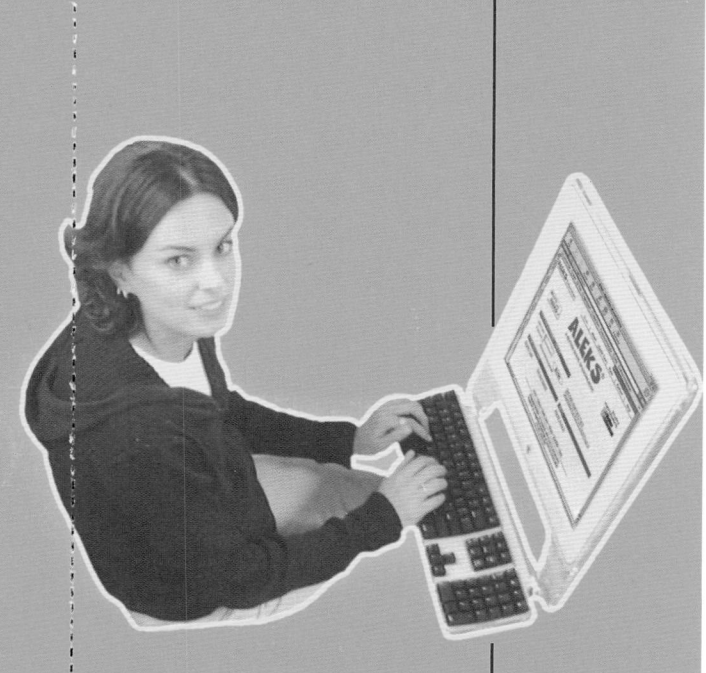
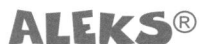

Dietary Reference Intakes (DRIs): Recommended Intakes for Individuals, Elements
Food and Nutrition Board, Institute of Medicine, National Academies

Life Stage Group	Calcium (mg/d)	Chromium (μg/d)	Copper (μg/d)	Fluoride (mg/d)	Iodine (μg/d)	Iron (mg/d)	Magnesium (mg/d)	Manganese (mg/d)	Molybdenum (μg/d)	Phosphorus (mg/d)	Selenium (μg/d)	Zinc (mg/d)
Infants												
0–6 mo	210*	0.2*	200*	0.01*	110*	0.27*	30*	0.003*	2*	100*	15*	2*
7–12 mo	270*	5.5*	220*	0.5*	130*	11	75*	0.6*	3*	275*	20*	3
Children												
1–3 y	500*	11*	340	0.7*	90	7	80	1.2*	17	460	20	3
4–8 y	800*	15*	440	1*	90	10	130	1.5*	22	500	30	5
Males												
9–13 y	1,300*	25*	700	2*	120	8	240	1.9*	34	1,250	40	8
14–18 y	1,300*	35*	890	3*	150	11	410	2.2*	43	1,250	55	11
19–30 y	1,000*	35*	900	4*	150	8	400	2.3*	45	700	55	11
31–50 y	1,000*	35*	900	4*	150	8	420	2.3*	45	700	55	11
51–70 y	1,200*	30*	900	4*	150	8	420	2.3*	45	700	55	11
>70 y	1,200*	30*	900	4*	150	8	420	2.3*	45	700	55	11
Females												
9–13 y	1,300*	21*	700	2*	120	8	240	1.6*	34	1,250	40	8
14–18 y	1,300*	24*	890	3*	150	15	360	1.6*	43	1,250	55	9
19–30 y	1,000*	25*	900	3*	150	18	310	1.8*	45	700	55	8
31–50 y	1,000*	25*	900	3*	150	18	320	1.8*	45	700	55	8
51–70 y	1,200*	20*	900	3*	150	8	320	1.8*	45	700	55	8
>70 y	1,200*	20*	900	3*	150	8	320	1.8*	45	700	55	8
Pregnancy												
≤18 y	1,300*	29*	1,000	3*	220	27	400	2.0*	50	1,250	60	13
19–30 y	1,000*	30*	1,000	3*	220	27	350	2.0*	50	700	60	11
31–50 y	1,000*	30*	1,000	3*	220	27	360	2.0*	50	700	60	11
Lactation												
≤18 y	1,300*	44*	1,300	3*	290	10	360	2.6*	50	1,250	70	14
19–30 y	1,000*	45*	1,300	3*	290	9	310	2.6*	50	700	70	12
31–50 y	1,000*	45*	1,300	3*	290	9	320	2.6*	50	700	70	12

NOTE: This table presents Recommended Dietary Allowances (RDAs) in bold type and Adequate Intakes (AIs) in ordinary type followed by an asterisk (*). RDAs and AIs may both be used as goals for individual intake. RDAs are set to meet the needs of almost all (97 to 98 percent) individuals in a group. For healthy breastfed infants, the AI is the mean intake. The AI for other life stage and gender groups is believed to cover needs of all individuals in the group, but lack of data or uncertainty in the data prevent being able to specify with confidence the percentage of individuals covered by this intake.

SOURCES: Dietary Reference Intakes for Calcium, Phosphorous, Magnesium, Vitamin D, and Fluoride (1997); Dietary Reference Intakes for Thiamin, Riboflavin, Niacin, Vitamin B6, Folate, Vitamin B12, Pantothenic Acid, Biotin, and Choline (1998); Dietary Reference Intakes for Vitamin C, Vitamin E, Selenium, and Carotenoids (2000); and Dietary Reference Intakes for Vitamin A, Vitamin K, Arsenic, Boron, Chromium, Copper, Iodine, Iron, Manganese, Molybdenum, Nickel, Silicon, Vanadium, and Zinc (2001). These reports may be accessed via www.nap.edu.

About the Author

Gordon M. Wardlaw, Ph.D., R.D., L.D., C.N.S.D., teaches nutrition to students both in the Division of Medical Dietetics, School of Allied Medical Professions and the Department of Human Nutrition at The Ohio State University. Dr. Wardlaw is the author of many articles that have appeared in prominent nutrition, biology, physiology, and biochemistry journals and was the 1985 recipient of the American Dietetic Association's Mary P. Huddleson award. Dr. Wardlaw is a full member of the prestigious American Institute of Nutrition and is certified as a Specialist in Human Nutrition by the American Board of Nutrition.

Contemporary *Nutrition*
Issues and Insights
Fifth Edition

Gordon M. Wardlaw
PH.D., R.D., L.D., C.N.S.D.

Division of Medical Dietetics
School of Allied Medical Professions *and*
Department of Human Nutrition,
College of Human Ecology
The Ohio State University

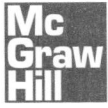

Mc
Graw
Hill

Boston   Burr Ridge, IL   Dubuque, IA   Madison, WI   New York   San Francisco   St. Louis
Bangkok   Bogotá   Caracas   Kuala Lumpur   Lisbon   London   Madrid   Mexico City
Milan   Montreal   New Delhi   Santiago   Seoul   Singapore   Sydney   Taipei   Toronto

McGraw-Hill Higher Education 🪐

A Division of The **McGraw-Hill** *Companies*

CONTEMPORARY NUTRITION: ISSUES AND INSIGHTS
FIFTH EDITION

Published by McGraw-Hill, a business unit of The McGraw-Hill Companies, Inc., 1221 Avenue of the Americas, New York, NY 10020. Copyright © 2003, 2000, 1997, 1994, 1991 by The McGraw-Hill Companies, Inc. All rights reserved. No part of this publication may be reproduced or distributed in any form or by any means, or stored in a database or retrieval system, without the prior written consent of The McGraw-Hill Companies, Inc., including, but not limited to, in any network or other electronic storage or transmission, or broadcast for distance learning.

Some ancillaries including electronic and print components may not be available to customers outside the Unied States.

 This book is printed on recycled, acid-free paper containing 10% postconsumer waste.

International   1 2 3 4 5 6 7 8 9 0 QPD/QPD 0 9 8 7 6 5 4 3 2
Domestic   4 5 6 7 8 9 0 QPD/QPD 0 9 8 7 6 5 4

ISBN 0–07–286530–X
ISBN 0–07–119908–X (ISE)

Publishers: *Colin H. Wheatley, Martin J. Lange*
Senior developmental editor: *Lynne M. Meyers*
Marketing manager: *Tami Petsche*
Senior project manager: *Joyce M. Berendes*
Lead production supervisor: *Sandra Hahn*
Design manager: *Stuart Paterson*
Cover/interior designer: *Ellen Pettengell*
Cover images: *Center photo Anne Dowie, small detail photos PhotoDisc*
Senior photo research coordinator: *John C. Leland*
Photo research: *LouAnn K. Wilson*
Supplement producer: *Brenda A. Ernzen*
Senior media project manager: *Tammy Juran*
Media technology senior producer: *Barbara R. Block*
Compositor: *GAC—Indianapolis*
Typeface: *10/12 Giovanni Book*
Printer: *Quebecor World Dubuque, IA*

The credits section for this book begins on page C1 and is considered an extension of the copyright page.

Library of Congress Cataloging-in-Publication Data

Wardlaw, Gordon M.
    Contemporary nutrition: issues and insights / Gordon M. Wardlaw.—5th ed.
      p.   cm.
    Includes bibliographical references and index.
    ISBN 0–07–286530–X—ISBN 0–07–119908–X (ISE)
    1. Nutrition.   I. Title.

QP141.W378   2003
613.2—dc21   2002022659
                                                        CIP

INTERNATIONAL EDITION ISBN 0–07–119908–X
Copyright © 2003. Exclusive rights by The McGraw-Hill Companies, Inc., for manufacture and export. This book cannot be re-exported from the country to which it is sold by McGraw-Hill. The International Edition is not available in North America.

Brief Contents

Contents

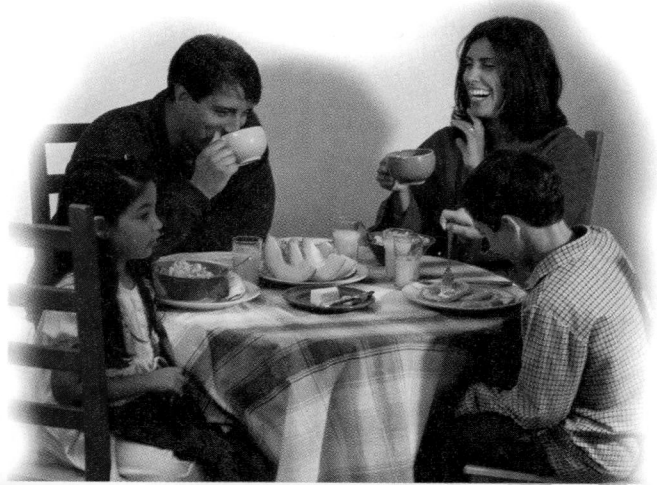

3 The Human Body: A Nutrition Perspective 71

Part Two   The Energy-Yielding Nutrients and Alcohol 109

4 Carbohydrates 109

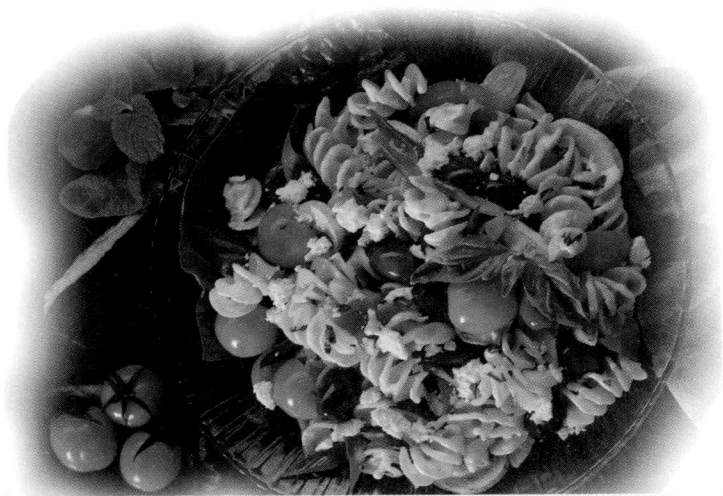

Part Three   Vitamins and Minerals 239

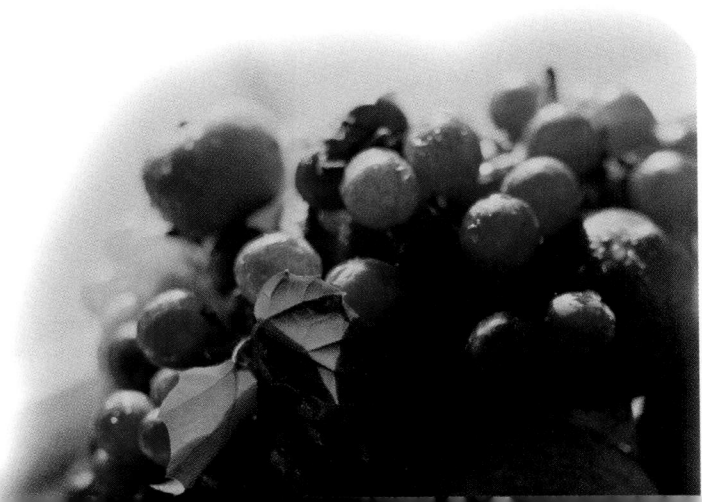

Part Four Energy: Balance and Imbalance 339

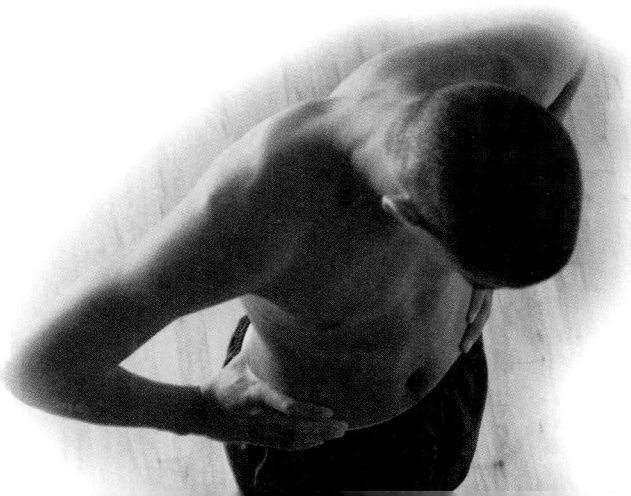

Part Five Nutrition: A Focus on Life Stages 443

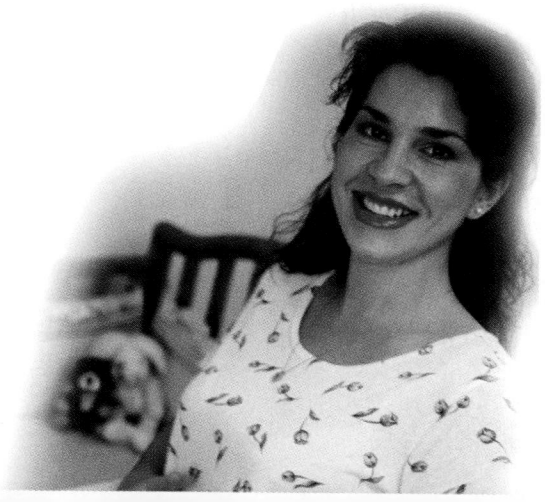

Part Six   Nutrition: Beyond the Nutrients 539

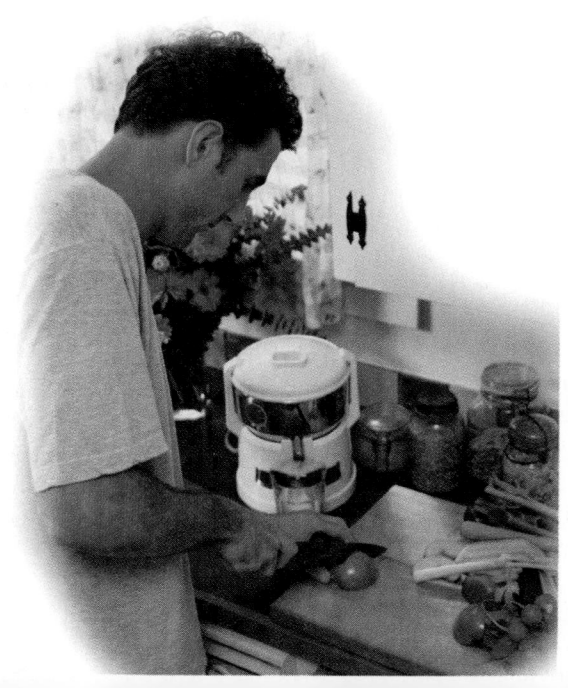

If you teach nutrition, you undoubtedly already find it a fascinating subject. However, nutrition can also be quite frustrating to teach. Claims and counterclaims abound regarding the need for certain constituents in our diets. Sodium is a good example. One group of researchers promotes a low-sodium diet for the general population as an effective measure against hypertension. Other groups state that this much less of a concern compared to other habits, such as inactivity and adult weight gain. How does an instructor adequately convey seemingly conflicting messages to introductory students?

As an author and teacher, I too am aware of conflicting opinions in our field and thus draw on as many sources as possible in the continual updating of this textbook, now in its fifth edition. I have incorporated much new material, especially from recently published articles in major nutrition and medical journals; the 9th edition of *Modern Nutrition in Health and Disease*, edited by Shils, Olson, Shike; and *Present Knowledge in Nutrition*, edited by Bowman and Russell. In addition, available information on the latest Dietary Reference Intake revisions to the 1989 RDA is incorporated where appropriate.

Personalizing Nutrition

One prominent theme in nutrition research today is *individuality*. Not all of us, for example, find that saturated fat in our diets raises our blood cholesterol values above recommended standards. Each person responds differently, often idiosyncratically, to nutrients, and I try to reinforce this point throughout the book.

Moreover even at this basic level, the text's discussions do not assume that all nutrition students are alike. Chapter content and features, such as Rate Your Plate, repeatedly ask students to learn more about themselves and their health status and to use their new knowledge to improve their health. After reading this textbook, students should be better equipped to understand how the nutrition information on the evening news, on cereal boxes, in popular magazines, and by government agencies applies to them. My goal is for students to understand that their knowledge of nutrition will allow them to evaluate and personalize nutrition information, rather than follow every guideline issued for an entire population. After all, a population by definition consists of individuals with varying genetic and cultural backgrounds, and these individuals have varying responses to diet.

As a final note on helping students bring nutrition down to a personal level, the book covers important questions students often bring to class, concerning topics such as ethnic diets, eating disorders, supplements, alternative therapies, vegetarianism, diets for athletes, and fad diets. Regardless of topic, the overall emphasis remains the same—the importance of understanding one's food choices and modifying one's diet to best meet personal needs.

Audience

Contemporary Nutrition: Issues and Insights is designed for a non-majors audience, particularly those students with little or no background in college-level chemistry, physiology, or human biology. Those topics have, for the most part, been kept to a minimum and explained in a simple, straightforward manner wherever necessary. I have been careful to include the basic scientific foundation needed to adequately comprehend certain topics in nutrition, such as a basic discussion of protein synthesis in Chapter 6.

Because of the flexible chapter organization and pedagogical features, this book can be used with students of diverse educational backgrounds and interests. Real-life examples have been incorporated to appeal to the interest of college students in general.

Organization

This book is organized into six parts that reflect the major topics typically covered in an introduction to the study of nutrition:

Part One   Nutrition: A Key to Health
Part Two   The Energy-Yielding Nutrients and Alcohol
Part Three Vitamins and Minerals
Part Four   Energy: Balance and Imbalance
Part Five   Nutrition: A Focus on Life Stages
Part Six   Nutrition: Beyond the Nutrients

The Table of Contents also reflects the inclusion of two chapters not typically found in introductory textbooks: Chapter 7, Alcohol and Chapter 12, Eating Disorders. The expanded discussion of these topics is the result of feedback from instructors who felt it was important to provide their students with a thorough, balanced discussion of these relevant topics.

Although most frequently used in semester-long courses, the text's organization allows instructors to omit Parts or Chapters to fit the needs of quarter-length courses. I have also tried as much as possible to make each chapter function independently so that instructors can cover the material in the order that best fits their particular course needs.

New to This Edition

Each edition of *Contemporary Nutrition: Issues and Insights* witnesses a profusion of new and rapidly changing information from the world of nutrition science. To give students an accurate picture of nutrition today, it is important to provide them with the most up-to-date information available. With the help of colleagues, reviewers, and my own students, I continually scour the latest research and update the text accordingly. I also carefully consider the feedback of instructors using this text to refine the content to better meets the needs of today's students. The following list highlights just some of the changes and updates that you will find in the fifth edition of *Contemporary Nutrition: Issues and Insights.*

▪ Chapter 1, What You Eat and Why

- More examples of the metric system in everyday life
- The important influence of one's psychological state on satiety and a practical result of that relationship
- The growing use of 'energy' bars by adults

▪ Chapter 2, Tools for Designing a Healthy Diet

- Current attention to energy density in the diet
- Pyramids promoted by the Mayo Clinic and the new book by Dr. Walter Willett
- New figure showing graphic representation of appropriate serving sizes

▪ Chapter 3, The Human Body: A Nutrition Perspective

- Expanded coverage of the cell and its various organelles
- Expanded coverage of the nervous system
- Expanded coverage of the cardiovascular system
- Expanded coverage of the urinary system

▪ Chapter 4, Carbohydrates

- The new sugar replacement sucralose (Splenda)
- A table to estimate fiber intake
- The glycemic index of foods is developed in detail

▪ Chapter 5, Lipids

- Latest dietary advice from the American Heart Association and the National Cholesterol Education Program

- An example of a diet containing 40% of calories from fat as advocated by Dr. Walter Willett and for those people with Syndrome X (also called metabolic syndrome)
- Practical use of the new margarines with plant sterols

▪ Chapter 6, Proteins

- New Nutrition Insight on soy protein
- Simple discussion and new figure on protein synthesis
- Vegetarian pyramid from Oldways Preservation & Trust

▪ Chapter 7, Alcohol

- New chapter is an expanded version of a Nutrition Issue in the previous edition
- Expanded look at the benefits and risks of use of alcohol
- Risks of binge drinking
- Figure showing the relationship of alcohol intake and blood-alcohol concentration

▪ Chapter 8, Vitamins

- Grouping of photos showing the clinical results of various vitamin and mineral deficiencies
- The latest vitamin recommendations from the Food and Nutrition Board
- Expanded list of rich sources of vitamins

▪ Chapter 9, Water and Minerals

- The latest recommendations for minerals from The Food and Nutrition Board
- Expanded list of rich sources of minerals
- Table to estimate calcium intake

▪ Chapter 10, Energy Balance and Weight Control

- Latest statistics regarding the growing problem of overweight and obesity in North America
- New websites for students to explore
- New annotated readings for further study

▪ Chapter 11, Nutrition: Fitness and Sports

- Growing use of 'energy' bars and gels
- Latest fluid replacement guidelines
- Expanded list of popular ergogenic aids in the Nutrition Issue

▪ Chapter 12, Eating Disorders: Anorexia Nervosa, Bulimia Nervosa, and Other Conditions

- Expanded discussion of disordered eating now begins the chapter
- Latest guidelines for diagnosis and treatment of eating disorders published by the American Psychiatric Association

Contemporary Nutrition *Online Learning Center* www.mhhe.com/wardlawcont5

A variety of study resources, conveniently correlated to each chapter, are readily available on the *Contemporary Nutrition Online Learning Center.* You'll find study quizzes with automatic feedback, crossword puzzles, flashcards, links to useful websites, animations, and much more to help you master course content!

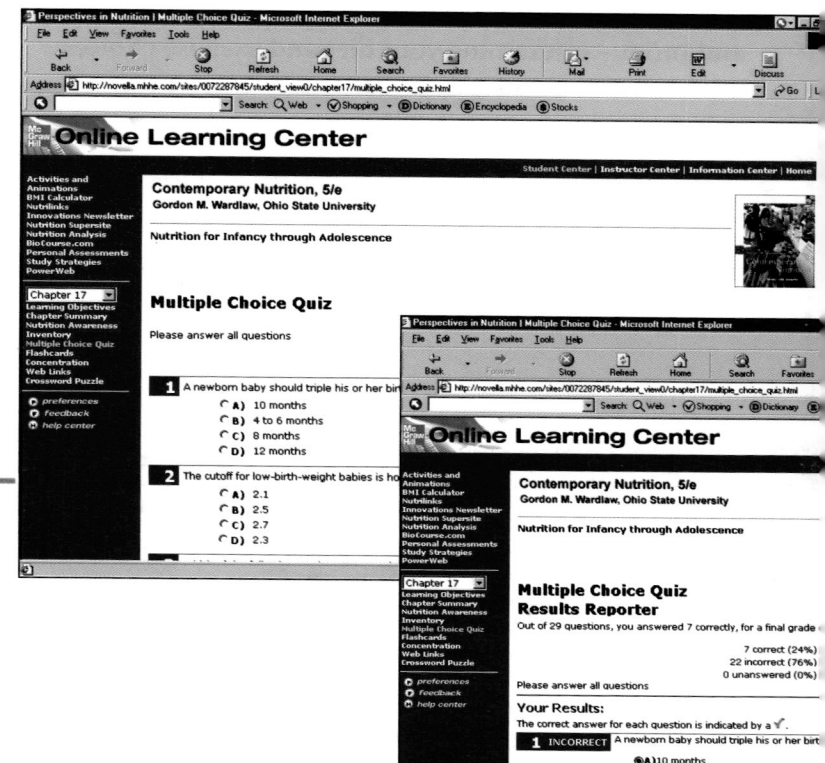

Take a Quiz

Make the most of your study time by taking an online chapter quiz. The quizzes are self-grading and provide feedback for incorrect answers. Great preparation for exams!

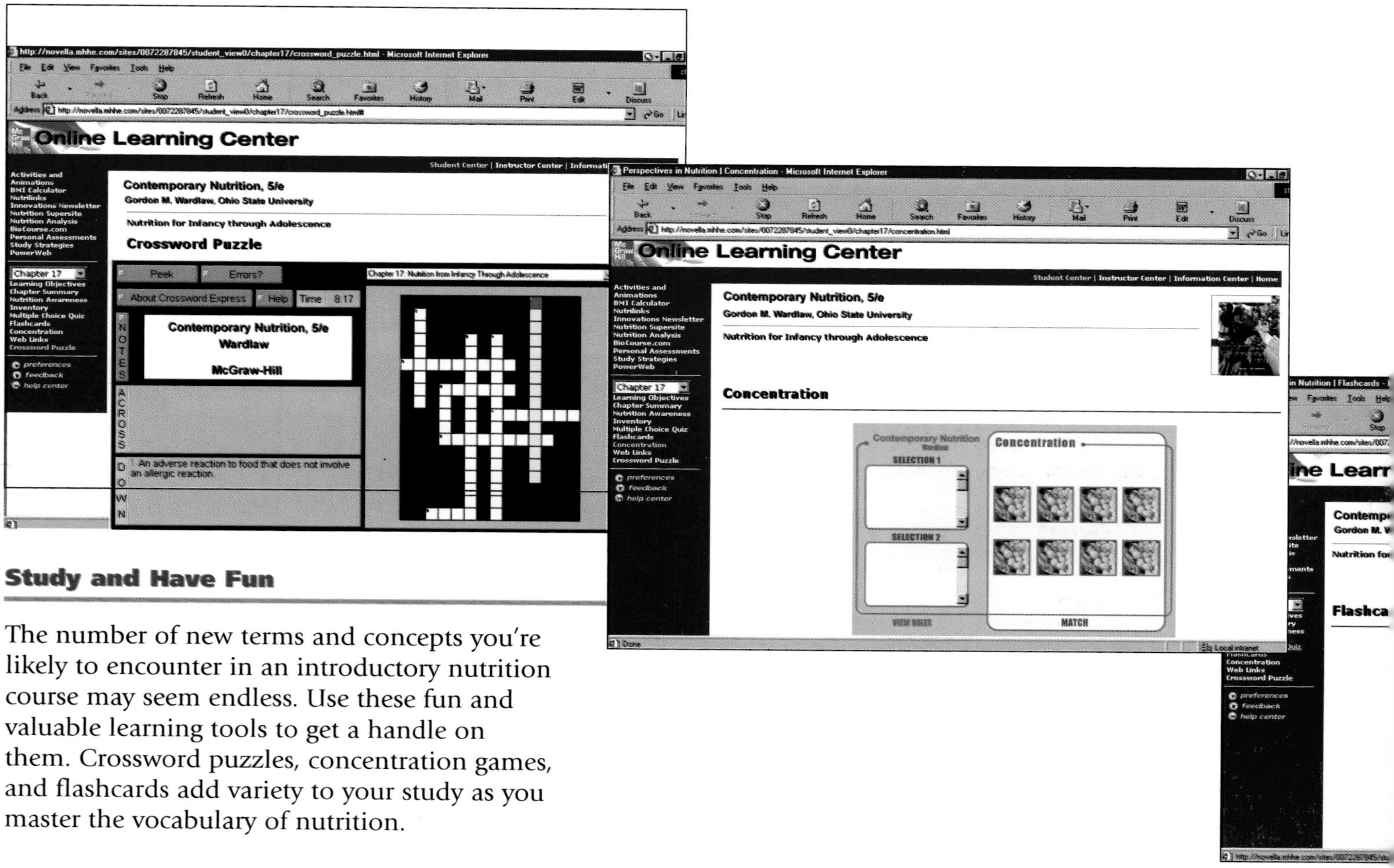

Study and Have Fun

The number of new terms and concepts you're likely to encounter in an introductory nutrition course may seem endless. Use these fun and valuable learning tools to get a handle on them. Crossword puzzles, concentration games, and flashcards add variety to your study as you master the vocabulary of nutrition.

Incorporate Annual Editions

You are probably already aware that the field of nutrition knowledge is a rapidly changing one. One way to sort out worthwhile information from the suspect is *PowerWeb: Nutrition*. This vital online resource is a wealth of up-to-date nutrition articles, representing the best of the field. The *Annual Editions* articles are supported by study questions and daily news updates.

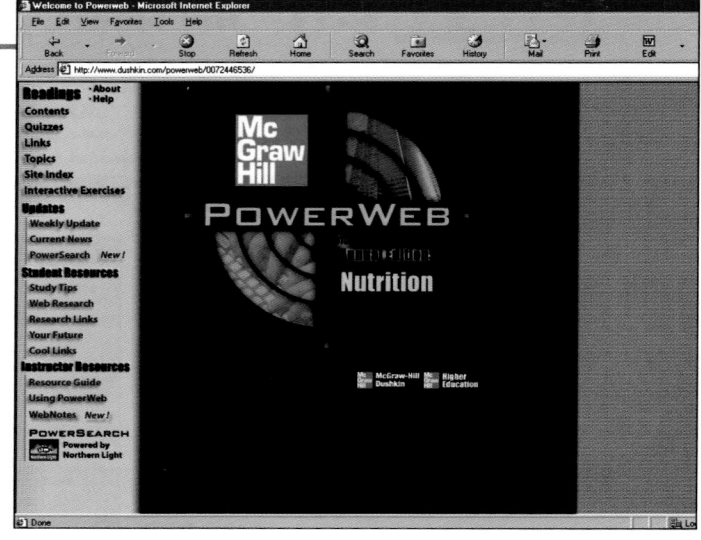

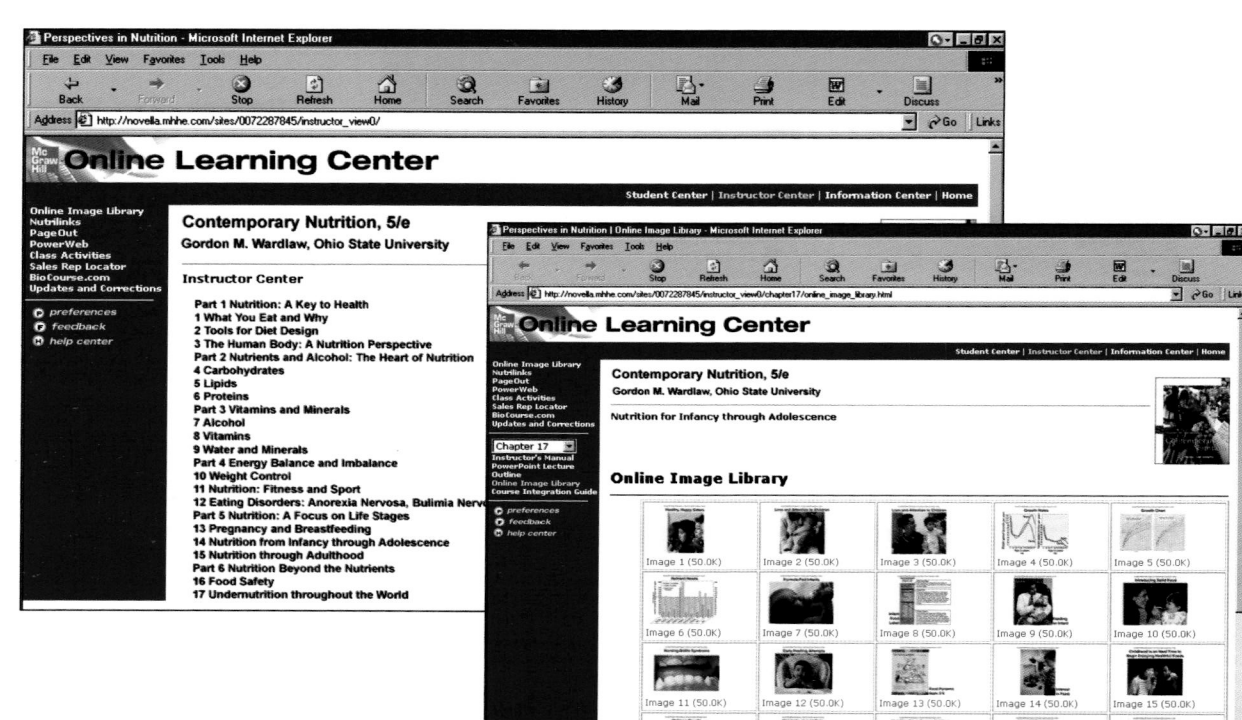

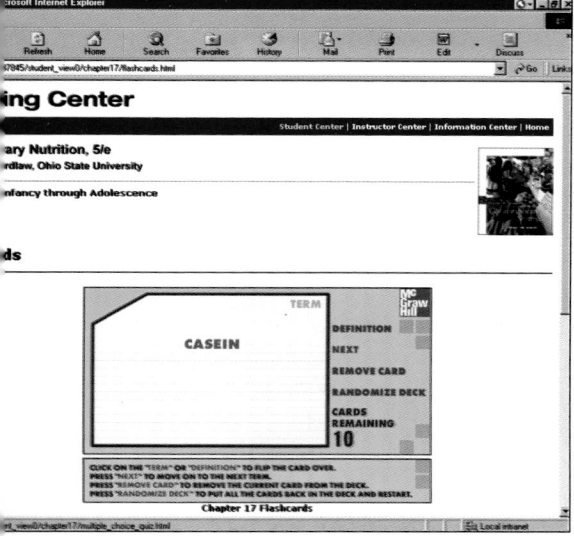

Access Instructor Tools

The *Instructor's Section of the Online Learning Center* contains a variety of supplementary materials to facilitate your teaching of introductory nutrition. This password-protected site provides lecture-enhancement resources, as well as a comprehensive *Instructor's Manual and Course Integration Guide* to alert you to the supplementary materials available for each chapter.

■ **Chapter 13, Pregnancy and Breastfeeding**

- Expanded discussion of the problems of children born small-for-gestational age
- More advantages of breastfeeding for the infant and mother

■ **Chapter 14, Nutrition From Infancy through Adolescence**

- The latest growth charts
- Implications of the growing problem of type 2 diabetes in childhood
- Use of food labels to identify potential food allergens

■ **Chapter 15, Nutrition during Adulthood**

- New Table summarizes the discussion of the effects of aging

- Tufts University pyramid for older adults
- Nutrition Issue now discusses complementary and alternative medicine practices

■ **Chapter 16, Food Safety**

- Expanded list of agents that cause food-borne illness
- Updated discussion of the risks and benefits of caffeine use
- New Tables summarize the discussion of food additives and environmental contaminants

■ **Chapter 17, Undernutrition Throughout the World**

- Update on U.S. welfare reform and it's relation to hunger
- Expanded discussion of biotechnology and use of genetically modified organisms

Special Acknowledgments

I would like to thank Susan Allerding, Brian Noble, and Andrea Pratt for their help with this revision. My editor, Lynne Meyers, supported and assisted me through every step of the revision, and facilitated the difficult decisions that frequently arose.

Joyce Berendes and Sue Dillon did excellent and careful production work and copyediting. All these individuals contributed key expertise to the project.

Thank You to Reviewers

As with the earlier editions, my goal is provide the most accurate, up-to-date, and useful textbook possible. These ambitious goals would not be possible without the meticulous, professional assistance of my colleagues who have served as reviewers of this manuscript and previous editions. I, along with my editors, would like to recognize and sincerely thank those people whose suggestions and insights did so much to guide the direction of this fifth edition:

Reviewers

Becky Alejandre
American River College

Sara Long Anderson
Southern Illinois University Carbondale

Liz Applegate
University of California Davis

Stokes S. Baker
University of Detroit Mercy

Bobby R. Baldridge
Asbury College

Cindy Beck
The Evergreen State College

Anne K. Black
Austin Peay State University

Barbara A. Brehm
Smith College

Georgia R. Brown
Southern University

Kathleen T. Brown
GMC-Augusta Community College

Judith A. Butkus

John R. Capeheart
University of Houston-Downtown

Sai Chidambaram
Canisius College

Linda S. Crawshaw
Mansfield University

Marie Dunford
Nutrition Consultant

Jeannette Endres
Southern Illinois University-Carbondale

Bernard Frye
University of Texas at Arlington

Ann Garvin
University of Wisconsin, Whitewater

Leonard E. Gerber
University of Rhode Island

Art Gilbert
University of California-Santa Barbara

Jeffrey S. Hampl
Arizona State University

Charlene G. Harkins
University of Minnesota Duluth

Nancy G. Harris
East Carolina University

Rebecca J. Hobson
College of the Sequoias

Thunder Jalili
University of Utah

Lisa Kersh
Wayland Baptist University

Zaheer Ali Kirmani
Sam Houston State University

Beth Lulinski
Northern Illinois University

Richard H. Machemer, Jr.
St. John Fisher College

Marcia Magnus
Florida International University

Barbara Mayfield
Purdue University

Karen E. McConnell
Pacific Lutheran University

Lola McGourty
Bossier Parish Community College

Janet Tompkins McMahon
Pennsylvania College of Technology

Glen F. McNeil
Fort Hays State University

Alexandria Miller
Northeastern State University

Marilyn Mook
Michigan State University

Cherie Moore
Cuesta College

Pamela Morris
Ozarks Technical Community College

Steven Nizielski
Grand Valley State University

Heather Perdue-Smith
Olivet Nazarene University

Ruth A. Reilly
University of New Hampshire

Lisa Ritchie
Harding University

Melissa Shock
University of Central Arkansas

L. E. Smith
Northwestern Michigan College

LuAnn Soliah
Baylor University

Diana-Marie Spillman
Miami University

Stasinos Stavrianeas
Willamette University

Leeann S. Sticker
Northwestern State University

Sue G. Thacker
Wytheville Community College

Danielle M. Torisky
James Madison University

Pamela S. Vande Voort
Central College

Julie Walton
Calvin College

Dana Wu Wassmer
Cosumnes River College

Kathleen Welch
Cabrillo College

H. Garrison Wilkes
University of Massachusetts-Boston

Marissa A. Winters
Mercer County Community College

Focus Group Participants

Becky Alejandre
American River College

Patricia Brown
Cuesta College

Donna V. Handley
University of Rhode Island

Madge N. Hanson
University of Minnesota

Charlene G. Harkins
University of Minnesota Duluth

Rebecca J. Hobson
College of the Sequoias

David H. Holben
Ohio University

Clarie Hollenbeck
San Jose State University

Melody Kyzer
University of North Carolina-Wilmington

Peggy Ramsey
Fullerton College

Brent J. Shriver
Texas Tech University

Dana Wu Wassmer
Cosumnes River College

Symposium Participants

Raga M. Bakhit
Virginia Tech

Mary Beck
Owens Community College

Beverly A. Benes
University of Nebraska-Lincoln

Art Gilbert
University of California-Santa Barbara

Betty Brown Joynes
Camden County College

Dorothy Klimis-Zacas
University of Maine

Barbara R. MacBriar
University of Wisconsin-Eau Claire

Marilyn Mook
Michigan State University

Ruth A. Reilly
University of New Hampshire

Matthew Christopher Schmidt
Southern Utah University

Sarah Short
Syracuse University

Frederick H. Wolfe
University of Arizona

Daniel Wulff
State University of New York at Albany

▎A Request to Those Who Use This Textbook

The first edition of this book began with a dream. Each new edition is fostered by the excitement that improvements bring, and ends with the satisfaction of knowing that we have produced an innovative textbook that will benefit students beginning their study of nutrition.

As you might imagine, it is difficult to range across the vast areas of nutrition science, following all the various controversies and new developments. I try my best but realize that sometimes I miss a side of an argument that deserves attention. If as you read this book you find content that you question or believe warrants a more detailed or broader look, feel free to contact me.

Gordon M. Wardlaw, Ph.D., R.D., L.D., C.N.S.D.
Department of Human Nutrition
347 Campbell Hall
1787 Neil Avenue, Columbus, OH 43210
Phone: (614) 688-8656
Fax: (614) 292-8880
e-mail: wardlaw.1@osu.edu
website: hec.osu.edu/people/gwardlaw

Instructor Supplements

Nutrition science is constantly evolving, and the classroom and students of today place new expectations on instructors. To help you meet these challenges, McGraw-Hill has created a suite of supplements tailored to *Contemporary Nutrition: Issues and Insights* that are intended to help you maximize your time in and out of the classroom.

Computerized Testing CD

Powerful new test generating software a gives you greater flexibility in creating a wide variety of exam types and includes over 1,500 questions based upon the chapter content in *Contemporary Nutrition: Issues and Insights*.

Online Learning Center

(www.mhhe.com/wardlawcont5)

In addition to a wealth of student-oriented study materials, the Online Learning Center for *Contemporary Nutrition: Issues and Insights* offers instructors an array of useful online teaching aids, such as chapter outlines, suggested activities, www links, and a correlation guide that coordinates all available supplement materials by chapter.

Digital Content Manager CD

If you're looking for illustrations, photographs, tables, and animations to incorporate into your lecture presentations, handouts, or quizzes, this easy-to-use CD contains hundreds of digital assets from *Contemporary Nutrition: Issues and Insights*, as well as other McGraw-Hill nutrition textbooks. Simply click on the appropriate chapter folder and select the type of image you are looking for (e.g., table), and you're ready to import the image into the application of your choice. It's that easy.

PageOut®

Create a custom course website with **PageOut**, free to instructors using a McGraw-Hill textbook.

To learn more, contact your McGraw-Hill publisher's representative or visit www.mhhe.com/solutions.

PageOut

PageOut is a course website development center that allows you to create your course web site. No need to learn special coding; simply fill in templates and you can create or modify content to fit your precise course needs. Contact your local McGraw-Hill representative for more information.

If you have questions about *Contemporary Nutrition: Issues and Insights* or the supplements that accompany it, please contact your local McGraw-Hill representative. To find out how to contact your local representative, check out *www.mhhe.com/catalogs/rep*

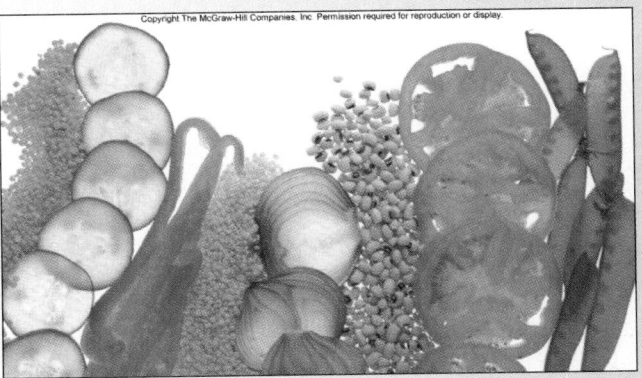

More than 200 illustrations and tables from *Contemporary Nutrition: Issues and Insights,* as well as other McGraw-Hill Nutrition texts, are available to support your classroom presentations. Artwork and labels have been enlarged to aid in classroom viewing.

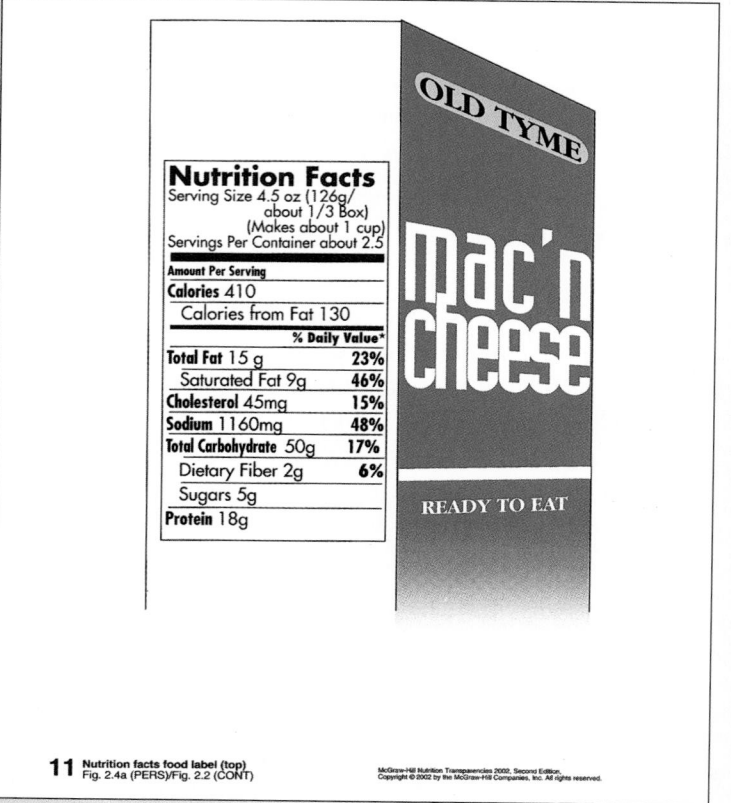

11 Nutrition facts food label (top)
Fig. 2.4a (PERS)/Fig. 2.2 (CONT)

McGraw-Hill Nutrition Transparencies 2002, Second Edition.
Copyright © 2002 by the McGraw-Hill Companies, Inc. All rights reserved.

Accessible from either the Online Learning Center or the Digital Content Manager CD, a complete PowerPoint lecture outline with illustrations from the textbook is available for every chapter. Use the outline as is or modify it to match your specific course needs.

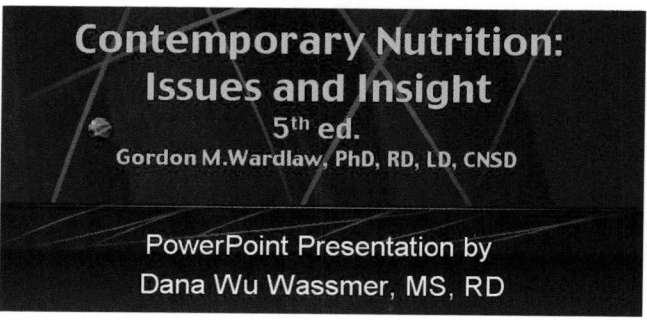

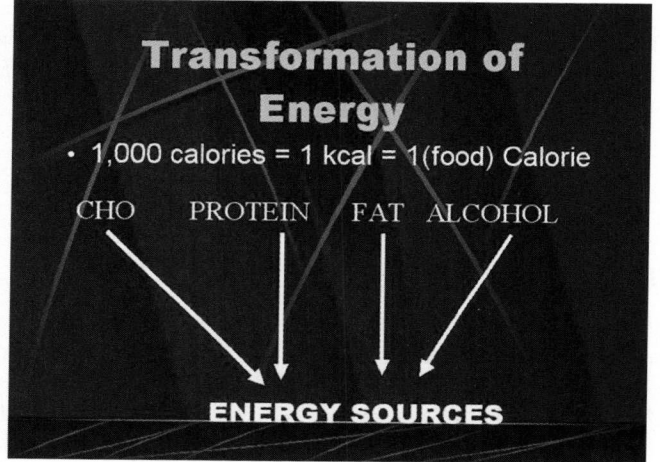

Learning and Study Aids

Because of the vast array of new terms and unfamiliar concepts introductory students will encounter in their study of nutrition, it is important that a textbook help students focus their study. In the textbook I attempt to guide students through the material by stressing the real-life relevance and by providing pedagogical support that can enhance their study habits. The sample pages below highlight a variety of features designed to make the material more accessible to students. In addition each diagram and photograph was carefully scrutinized to help students create mental images of key content.

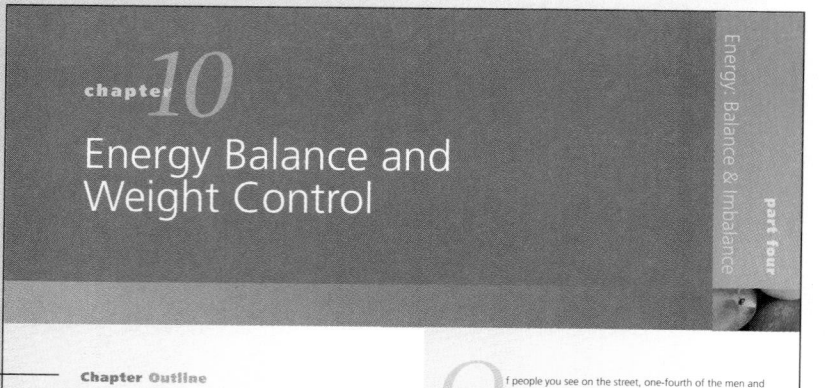

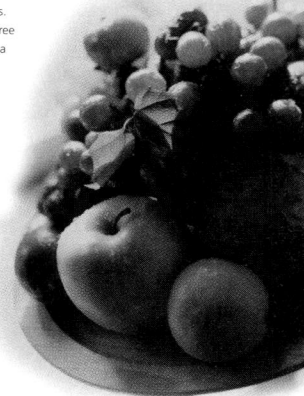

Overview

Each chapter opens with an **Overview** that conveys the significance of the nutrition concepts about to covered.

Real Life Scenario

Brief **Real Life Scenarios** at the beginning of each chapter engage students by asking them to consider the nutritional implications of a real-life situation.

Chapter Outline

The **Outline** provides a detailed preview of the material to be covered in the chapter and helps students mentally organize the concepts.

Chapter Objectives

The **Chapter Objectives** serve as guideposts to alert students to the knowledge they should expect to gain from carefully studying the chapter.

Refresh Your Memory

To reinforce their understanding, students can turn to the **Refresh Your Memory** section for related topics covered in earlier chapters.

Top-Notch Artwork

Many of the illustrations and photographs are new in this edition. They have been carefully selected and beautifully rendered to visually support the textual content.

Concept Check

At key points, brief **Concept Checks** allow students to mentally summarize what they have learned before proceeding to the next topic in the chapter.

Protein Digestion and Absorption

As with carbohydrates, cooking food can be viewed as a first step in protein digestion. Cooking unfolds (denatures) proteins and softens tough connective tissue in meat. Cooking also makes many protein-rich foods easier to chew, swallow, and break down during later digestion and absorption. As you will see in Chapter 16, cooking also makes many protein-rich foods, such as meats, eggs, fish, and poultry, much safer to eat.

Digestion

The enzymatic digestion of protein begins in the stomach. When proteins are denatured by stomach acid, **pepsin**, a major enzyme for proteins, goes to work (Fig. 6.6). Pepsin attacks the denatured proteins and breaks them down into shorter chains of amino acids. Pepsin does not completely separate proteins into amino acids because it can break only a few of the many peptide bonds found in these large molecules.

The release of pepsin is controlled by the hormone gastrin (review Table 3.3 in Chapter 3). Thinking about food or chewing food stimulates gastrin-producing cells in the stomach to release the hormone. Gastrin also strongly stimulates the stomach to produce acid.

pepsin A protein-digesting enzyme produced by the stomach.

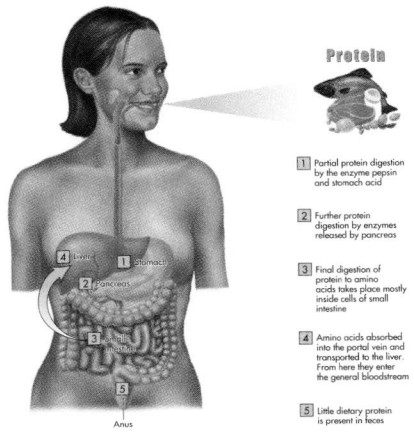

Protein

1. Partial protein digestion by the enzyme pepsin and stomach acid

2. Further protein digestion by enzymes released by pancreas

3. Final digestion of protein to amino acids takes place mostly inside cells of small intestine

4. Amino acids absorbed into the portal vein and transported to the liver. From here they enter the general bloodstream

5. Little dietary protein is present in feces

Anus

6.6 A summary of protein and absorption. Enzymatic digestion begins in the stomach where any remaining short of amino acids are broken down amino acids. Stomach acid and contribute to protein digestion. on from the intestinal lumen into ptive cells requires energy input.

Fluid and electrolyte (i.e., sodium and potassium) intake is also an essential component of an athlete's recovery diet. This helps replenish body fluids as quickly as possible. This is especially important if two workouts a day are followed and if the environment is hot and humid. If food and fluid intake is sufficient to restore weight loss, it generally will also supply enough electrolytes to meet needs during recovery from endurance activities.

Concept Check

All athletes would do well to plan a diet following the Food Guide Pyramid. High-carbohydrate foods should be emphasized, and these should dominate in pre-event meals. Protein intake above twice the RDA is not needed in most cases. Most athletes easily consume enough protein from typical food choices. If nutrient supplements are used, dosages generally should not exceed the Upper Level set for each nutrient. Fluid should be consumed as liberally as possible before, during, and after an event. Carbohydrate and electrolytes in the fluid are especially helpful when exercise duration is expected to exceed 60 minutes to help delay fatigue and maintain electrolyte balance.

Scenario *Follow-Up*

Marcella is correct in following a high-carbohydrate diet. However, in her effort to minimize her fat intake, she is probably not consuming enough calories to support her training routine. Her diet is also low in protein. She has fallen into the bagel, pasta, and pretzel routine that sports nutritionists warn is not conducive to peak performance. Marcella would be smart to have a high-protein source at each meal. She could include milk with breakfast and possibly some low-fat yogurt or low-fat cheese at lunch. She should have a carbohydrate/protein snack before her workout, such as a half a sandwich and fruit and some water. The sandwich fruit will help provide her with fuel to support her vigorous training. During her work could consume a sports drink to meet fluid needs and supply some carbohydrate, or consume water, along with a few fig cookies or other high-carbohydrate food. In the evenings, she could substitute oil and vinegar dressing for the fat-free dressing on h and cheese and crackers for the pretzels to improve protein intake. Overall, it is imp Marcella to fuel her body before, during, and after workouts.

Summary

1. A gradual increase in regular physical activity is recommended for all healthy persons. A minimum plan includes at least a total of 30 minutes of physical activity on most (or all) days. A more intense program lasting about 60 minutes should begin with warm-up exercises to increase blood flow and warm the muscles, and end with cooldown exercises. Regular resistance activities and stretching add further benefits.
2. Human metabolic pathways extract chemical energy from food and transform it into ATP, the compound that provides energy for body functions.
3. In carbohydrate fuel use, glucose is broken down into the three-carbon compound pyruvic acid, yielding some ATP. This is metabolized further via the aerobic pathway to form carbon dioxide (CO_2) and water (H_2O) or via the anaerobic pathway to form lactic acid.
4. At rest, muscle cells mainly use fat for fuel. During more intense exercise of short duration, muscles mostly use phosphocreatine (PCr) for energy. During more sustained intense activity, muscle glycogen

breaks down to lactic acid, providing a small amou endurance exercise, both fat and carbohydrate are u carbohydrate is used increasingly as activity intensifi tein is used to fuel muscles.
5. Anyone who exercises regularly should consume a di energy needs and is moderate to high in carbohydrat and adequate in other nutrients such as iron and calc
6. Athletes should consume enough fluid to both min body weight and ultimately restore preexercise w drinks aid fluid, electrolyte, and carbohydrate replac use especially should be considered when continuous beyond 60 minutes.
7. High-glycemic-index carbohydrates should be cons athlete within 2 hours after a workout to begin restora cle glycogen stores. Some protein in the meal is also use of low-glycemic-index carbohydrates in the pre-eve help some endurance athletes.

Critical Thinking

Joe is a wrestler who qualified for the 125 pound weight classification in his annual high school competition. After a few matches, Joe began to feel dizzy and faint. He was disqualified because he was unable to continue the match. Later, the coach found out that Joe had spent 2 hours in the sauna before weighing in, which had made him dehydrated. What are the consequences of dehydration? What can you suggest as an alternative way to lose weight?

To prevent such deaths in the future, the National Collegiate Athletic Association has begun requiring that a minimum safe weight be set by a physician or an athletic trainer for each wrestler at the start of the season. Several states also have adopted this practice. If athletes, such as wrestlers, wish to compete in a lower-body-weight class and have enough extra fat stores, they should begin a gradual, sustained reduction in food-energy intake long before the competitive season starts. In so doing, the athlete attains a healthier body composition (less fat) while avoiding the potentially harmful and certainly misery-creating effects of severe dehydration. Athletes who have no extra body fat should not attempt to compete at a lower-body-weight class. Coaches and trainers should be aware of the decreased performance and serious side effects of severe dehydration to wrestlers.

Carbohydrate Needs

Anyone who exercises vigorously, especially for more than 1 hour per day on a regular basis, needs to consume a diet that includes moderate to high amounts of carbohydrates. The diet should include a variety of foods, such as those recommended by the Food Guide Pyramid. Numerous servings of grains, starchy vegetables, and fruits provide enough carbohydrate to maintain adequate liver and muscle glycogen stores, especially for replacing glycogen losses from workouts on the previous day. Relatively low carbohydrate/high-protein diets, such as *The Zone Diet*, are not recommended (recall that Chapter 10 discussed the Zone Diet. The carbohydrate content of this diet is only 40% of calories, rather than 50% or more that is typically recommended for athletes).

Carbohydrate intake should be at least 5 grams per kilogram body weight. People engaged in aerobic training and endurance athletes (duration >60 minutes per day) may need as much as 6 to 10 grams per kilogram body weight. In other words, triathletes and marathoners should consider eating close to 500 to 600 grams of carbohydrates daily, and even more if necessary, to (1) prevent chronic fatigue and (2) load the muscles and liver with glycogen. This is especially important when performing multiple training bouts in a day, such as in swim practices, or heavy training on successive days, as in cross-country running. Depletion of carbohydrate ranks just behind depletion of fluid and electrolytes as a major cause of fatigue. Table 11.3 shows sample menus, based on the Food Guide Pyramid, for diets providing food energy ranging from 1500 to 5000 kcal per day. In addition, the Exchange System described in Appendix C is a very useful tool for planning all types of diets, including high-carbohydrate diets for athletes.

Note that one does not have to give up any specific food when planning a high-carbohydrate diet. The focus is to include more high-carbohydrate foods and moderation with concentrated fat sources. Sports nutritionists emphasize the difference between a high-carbohydrate meal and a high-carbohydrate/high-fat meal. Before endurance events, such as marathons or triathlons, some athletes seek to increase their carbohydrate reserves by eating potato chips, French fries, banana cream pie, and pastries. Although such foods contain carbohydrate, they also contain a lot of fat. Better high-carbohydrate food choices include pasta, rice, potatoes, bread, fruit and fruit juices, and many breakfast cereals (check the label for carbohydrate content) (Fig. 11.4). Sport drinks appropriate for carbohydrate loading, such as GatorLode and UltraFuel, can also help. Consuming a moderate amount of dietary fiber during the final day of training is a good precaution to reduce the chances of bloating and intestinal gas during the next day's event.

As a general rule, athletes should obtain at least 60% of their total energy needs from carbohydrate, rather than the 50% typical of most North American diets, especially if exercise duration is expected to exceed 2 hours and total caloric intake is about 3000 kcal per day or less. Diets containing 4000 to 5000 kcal per day can be as low as 50% carbohydrate, as these will still provide sufficient carbohydrate (500–600 grams per day).

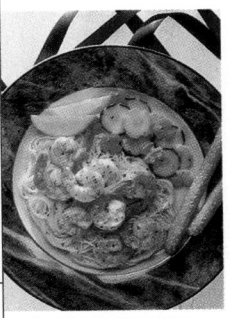

The athlete's plate should be about two-thirds grains and vegetables to provide ample carbohydrates.

Critical Thinking Questions

As students read the text, **Critical Thinking Questions** challenge them to apply their newly acquired knowledge in the context of real-life circumstances. Answers to these can be found at the end of the book.

Attractive New Design

The fifth edition of *Contemporary Nutrition: Issues and Insights* features a beautiful and functional new design. Its clean, uncluttered look skillfully integrates the dynamic features of the textbook.

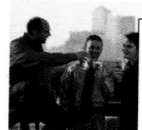

Nutrition Issue

Binge Drinking

College students are drinking more heavily and more frequently than ever before. Excessive alcohol consumption is an even bigger problem than illicit drug use on college campuses today. Many college students consider drinking alcohol to be a "rite of passage" into adulthood. The heaviest drinking population in North America is young, Caucasian college students. Bars near campus typically promote heavy drinking. Alcohol producers frequently target college students with advertising and other marketing efforts. Adding to the overall problem is typically half of all college students are not of legal drinking age. In fact, the annual overall costs related to alcohol use by those under 21 is estimated at more than $58 billion dollars. This estimate includes costs associated with violent crime, traffic accidents, treatment, and alcohol poisonings, among other variables.

Binge drinking is also common among college students. Young athletes are more likely to abuse alcohol in such a way than their nonathlete peers. Drunken athletes are more likely to drive while drinking, fight, experience memory loss, and be in academic trouble. This binging is defined as four or more drinks in a row for women and five or more for men. **Acute alcohol intoxication** is a major cause of suicide and hazing deaths related to binge drinking. Regular binge drinking also often leads to academic failure. About 50% of college students practice binge drinking.

Another Bite

*I*n 2000, a student at the University of Michigan rapidly drank 20 shots to celebrate his 21st birthday and died shortly after with a blood alcohol concentration of 0.39 percent. A student at Old Dominion University choked to death on his own vomit during a pledge-week drinking binge. A student at Ohio State University on the diving team became so intoxicated he dove head-first while "mud-diving." He is lucky to be alive but is paralyzed from the neck down. Still other students have drowned while intoxicated, even though they knew how to swim.

Binge drinking has a variety of contraindications. It can lead to unplanned sexual activity, damaged property, injury to oneself or others, and death. Death due to alcohol misuse can result, for example, from inhalation of vomit. In other cases, the body systems slowly shut down due to alcohol's overpowering depressant effect (Table 7.5). Other injuries can occur, resulting in paralysis or other lifelong medical problems.

Many problems associated with binge drinking can affect all aspects of life. Binge drinkers are more likely to miss class, damage property, and experience impaired academic performance than are students who are light drinkers or abstainers. Students that live around binge drinkers experience more unwanted sexual advances, assaults, and insults/humiliations. Bingers often do not think they have a problem because binge drinking has become so acceptable on college campuses.

According to U.S. law, one must be 21 years old to drink in all 50 states. In Canada, one must be age 18 or 19, depending on the province. However, alcohol use often begins in adolescence. For example, 31% of 12th-graders in the United States reported frequent drinking during 1999. Premature alcohol use is often seen in conjunction with athletics, as older, highly visible role models advertise products or are seen consuming alcohol. Peer pressure at school and on sports teams can cause many adolescents to drink. These habits become dangerous when young adults choose to drive drunk or ride with friends who are intoxicated. They are also creating habits that may continue and worsen throughout their lives. Education and prevention strategies should focus on behavioral and psychosocial consequences because athletic performance typically does not suffer yet.

continued

acute alcohol intoxication A temporary deterioration in mental function, accompanied by muscular incoordination and partial paralysis as a result of drinking alcoholic beverages too rapidly.

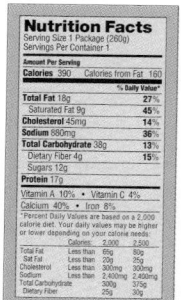

*H*ealthy People 2010 *recommends an important goal regarding binge drinking: Reduce by at least one-half the number of high school and college students engaging in binge drinking* (currently estimated at 32% and 40%, respectively).

Alcohol use often begins in adulthood and is carried in

Nutrition Issue

As a capstone to each chapter, the **Nutrition Issue** provides an in-depth look at important nutritional issues, such as Ergogenic Aids and Binge Drinking.

Margin Definitions

Definitions of key concepts and terms are found in the margin as they are first introduced in the text. All appear in the Glossary at the end of the book.

Another Bite

Short asides, called **Another Bite**, give students a bit more depth on topics of personal interest.

Rate Your Plate

Each chapter concludes with two **Rate Your Plate** activities that help students internalize nutrition concepts to their own lives.

Part IV
Food Guide Pyramid

Using the same food-intake record used in Part I or II, place each food item in the appropriate group of the Food Guide Pyramid chart in Appendix E. That is, for each food item, indicate how many servings it contributes to each group based on the amount you ate (see Table 2.6 for serving sizes). Note that many of your food choices may contribute to more than one group. For example, toast with margarine contributes to two categories: (1) the breads, cereals, rice, and pasta group; and (2) fats, oils, and sweets. After entering all the values, add the number of servings consumed in each group. Finally, compare your total in each food group with the recommended number of servings shown in Figure 2.3. Enter a minus sign (−) if your total falls below the recommendation or a plus sign (+) if it equals or exceeds the recommendation.

Part V
Further Diet Evaluation

Do the weaknesses, if any, suggested in your nutrient analysis (see Part III) correspond to missing servings in the Food Guide Pyramid chart? If so, consider changing your food choices based on the Food Guide Pyramid to help improve your nutrient profile. Finally, indicate whether your day's diet did or did not conform to the following items in the Dietary Guidelines:

Yes   No

Aim for Fitness

- Aim for a healthy weight.
- Be physically active each day.

Build a Healthy Base

- Let the pyramid guide your food choices.
- Choose a variety of grains daily, especially whole grains.
- Choose a variety of fruits and vegetables daily.
- Keep foods safe to eat.

Choose Sensibly

- Choose a diet that is a low in saturated fat and cholesterol and moderate in total fat.
- Choose beverages and foods to moderate your intake of sugars.
- Choose and prepare foods with less salt.
- If you drink alcoholic beverages, do so in moderation.

If your diet comes up short on any of these evaluations, take appropriate action to improve your eating patterns.

II. Applying the Nutrition Facts Label to Your Daily Food Choices

Imagine that you are at the supermarket looking for a quick meal before a busy evening. In the frozen food section, you find two brands of frozen cheese manicotti (see labels a and b). Which of the two brands would you choose? What information on the Nutrition Facts label in the figure contributed to this decision?

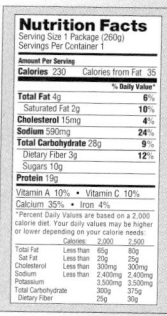

(a)   (b)

Rate Your Plate

63

Cholesterol, sports drinks, food labeling, bulimia nervosa, alternative sweeteners, vegetarianism, *Salmonella* food-borne illness and genetically-engineered foods—we suspect you have heard about these topics. Which topics are important enough to be a consideration in your life or in the life of someone you know?

North Americans pride themselves on their individuality. Nutritional advice should be given accordingly. For example, not all of us have high blood cholesterol and other significant risk factors for developing premature cardiovascular disease. The need to tailor dietary advice to each person's individual nature is the basic approach of this book. First, you are given a brief introduction to the study of nutrition; then, how to be a knowledgeable consumer is discussed. With so much information available—both accurate and inaccurate—you should know how to make informed decisions about your nutritional well-being. Second, you are encouraged to learn the basic principles of nutrition and to discover how to apply the concepts in this book that pertain specifically to you.

The text discusses some of the most interesting and important elements of nutrition and food consumption to help you understand both how your body works and how your food choices affect your health.

Features

Planning a New Way of Eating

Early in the text, many of the basic guidelines for planning a healthy diet are presented, including a description of the USDA Food Guide Pyramid, in Chapter 2. Later, in Chapter 10, the steps involved in setting nutritional goals and designing a diet plan to attain those goals are reviewed.

Understanding the World Around Us

In a college environment, it is often difficult to envision how real the problem of world hunger is. Chapter 17 examines the tragedy of undernutrition and the conditions that create it. The chapter allows you to explore possible solutions that offer hope for the future of our world.

Pedagogy

The fifth edition of *Contemporary Nutrition: Issues and Insights* incorporates some important tools to help you learn the nutrition concepts in this text. Following is a guide to those tools:

1. Each chapter after Chapter 1 begins with a Refresh Your Memory box reminding you of previous chapter content that will be helpful to know for understanding the current chapter. Following this is a real life scenario, which allows you to apply knowledge gained from the chapter in a real-life setting. An answer to each scenario is provided in the chapter at the point at which the specific content needed to answer the case scenario is covered.

2. **Chapter Objectives** then help you focus your attention on key ideas in the chapter, as well as the Nutrition Connection comic.

3. Throughout each chapter are **boldfaced key terms,** many of which are defined in the margin. All boldfaced terms appear with their definitions and pronunciations in the glossary at the end of the text.

4. Also throughout each chapter are **margin notes,** which further explain ideas, provide references to other chapters. Some URLs to nutrition-related web sites are in these margin notes, as well as in the text itself.

5. The numerous **tables** throughout the text present major points.

6. The **Concept Checks,** which follow the major sections within each chapter, summarize key points. If you are having trouble understanding the material in the Concept Check, you should reread the preceding section.

7. Each chapter ends with a **summary,** which conveys the main ideas in the chapter, and **study questions**—both provide a review of chapter material.

8. **Further Readings** with annotations are provided to back up material presented in the chapter. If you are preparing a research paper for your class, or would just like more information on specific topics, consult these sources.

9. Also at the end of each chapter are **Rate Your Plate** boxes, which make major concepts presented in the chapter relevant to daily life. For example, you may be asked to look more carefully at your own diet, examine your family history, or apply information you've learned to friends or family.

10. **Nutrition Insight boxes** allow you to explore current topics that your instructor may not have time to cover but that may be of interest to you.

11. **Critical Thinking questions** ask you to apply information as you learn it. This fosters understanding of the material.

12. **Nutrition Issue** essays at the end of each chapter develop current topics in nutrition, often covered earlier in the chapter, in greater detail.
13. A variety of supplements to this text, including a *FoodWise* dietary analysis software, are available to you. These instructional aids are designed to help you learn the major concepts developed in the text and prepare for class examinations.
14. The website www.mhhe.com/wardlawcont5 contains an **online learning center,** with quizzes, flash cards, other activities, and web links designed to further help you learn about nutrition. This is organized according to each chapter in the book.

FoodWise—Dietary Analysis Software

This user-friendly dietary analysis program provides a variety of useful features, which allow you to track daily food intake, energy expenditure, and establish weight or body mass index (BMI) goals. Several different reports and pie charts allow you to see how calories from a specific food, meal, day, or daily average break out. For example, you can click on the fat pie chart to see what percentage of calories from saturated, monounsaturated, or polyunsaturated fat were in this morning's breakfast.

Features

- *FoodWise* has a database of over 7,500 foods; the database allows you to accurately record your intake, and to analyze a specific food, meal, day, or average.

- *FoodWise* calculates recommended daily calories and body mass index (BMI) based on height, weight, and other personal information entered into the program.
- You can track your daily activities—from sleeping to jogging—and *FoodWise* will calculate daily energy expenditure.
- You can view a "personalized" food label in standard food label format for a given food.
- This colorful program is intuitively designed, making it easy to maneuver from one screen to another.
- Additional features include an easily accessible "Help" function, the ability to add your own foods to the database, and a link to the Nutrition Analysis web site.

A Request to Students Who Use This Book

I try my best but realize that sometimes I miss a side of an argument that deserves attention or do not make something perfectly clear. If as you read this book you find content that you question or needs a clearer explanation, feel free to contact me by mail, fax, or e-mail.

Gordon M. Wardlaw, Ph.D., R.D., L.D., C.N.S.D.
Department of Human Nutrition
347 Campbell Hall
1787 Neil Avenue
Columbus, OH 43210
Phone: (614) 688-8656
Fax: (614) 292-8880
e-mail: wardlaw.1@osu.edu
website: hec.osu.edu/people/gwardlaw

chapter 1

What You Eat and Why

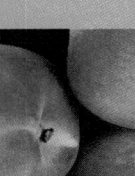

Chapter Outline

*D*o you need to take vitamin and mineral supplements? Are you eating too much fat and cholesterol? Is much of what you eat unsafe? Are some foods actually *junk foods?* Should you become a vegetarian? If you're confused about what you should eat, you are not alone. This chapter will help you sort out some of these issues as you are introduced to the science of nutrition.

And, as you begin this study of nutrition, keep in mind what nutrition expert Dr. Irwin Rosenberg has written as his "bottom line" for a healthy lifestyle: "Research has shown no better way to slow or even reverse the progress of aging itself and of all the age-related degenerative conditions than through the combination of aerobic and strength-building exercise and a balanced, nutritious diet." Overall, it is clear that the nutritional lifestyles of some (but not all) North Americans are out of balance with their physiology. And, since we live longer than our ancestors, preventing the age-related diseases that develop later in life is a more important focus today than in the past.

By optimizing dietary choices, we can strive to bring the goal of a long, healthy life within reach. This is the primary theme not just in this chapter but throughout this entire book.

Check out the **Contemporary Nutrition: Issues and Insights Online Learning Center** www.mhhe.com/wardlawcont5 *for quizzes, flash cards, other activities, and web links designed to further help you learn about what you eat and why.*

Chapter Objectives

Chapter 1 is designed to allow you to:

1. Define the terms *nutrition, carbohydrate, protein, lipid (fat), alcohol, vitamin, mineral, water, kilocalorie (kcal),* and *dietary fiber.*

2. Use the caloric values of energy-yielding nutrients to determine the total calories (kcal) in a food or diet.

3. Outline the basic units of the metric system used in nutrition and calculate a percentage value, such as percent of calories from fat in a diet.

4. List the major characteristics of the North American diet and the food habits that often need improvement.

5. Describe how various factors affect our food habits: body physiological processes, meal size and composition, early experiences, ethnic customs, health concerns, advertising, social class, and economics.

6. List various attributes of a healthful lifestyle that are also consistent with *Healthy People 2010* goals.

7. Identify diet and lifestyle factors that contribute to the 10 leading causes of death in North America.

8. Understand the basis of the scientific method as it is used in developing hypotheses and theories in the field of nutrition.

9. Identify reliable sources of nutrition information.

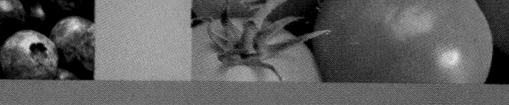

Real Life Scenario

Brendon listens to talk radio as he commutes to school each morning. He hears numerous advertisements for nutrient supplements. Commentators also warn about the dangers of certain lifestyle practices. News briefs discuss the latest breakthroughs, touting new findings regarding both positive and negative health practices. Typical terms he hears are *cardiovascular disease,* (also called *heart disease*), *diabetes, cancer, obesity, vitamin E, omega-3 fatty acids, cholesterol,* and *creatine.* All of these topics are generally covered in an introductory nutrition class. One advantage of Brendon taking such a class is to be able to decipher the health news that he reads in newspapers, hears on the radio, and is exposed to via television.

Start your exploration of nutrition by looking up these terms in the glossary at the back of this book. You will likely find this an interesting task, one that will heighten your awareness of nutrition and help you in your study of nutrition. Also consider adding a few other words you are curious about and look those up as well in the glossary, or use the index if the glossary does not contain the word.

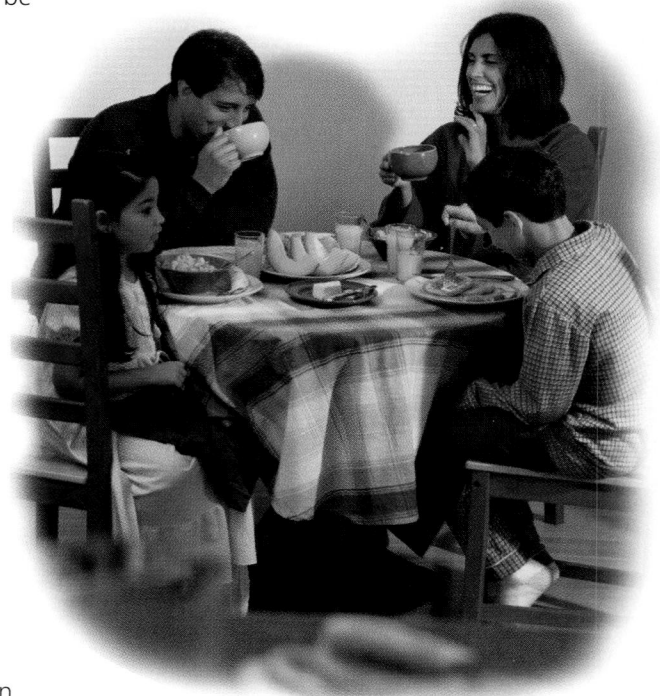

Nutrition Connection

FOR BETTER OR FOR WORSE / By Lynn Johnston

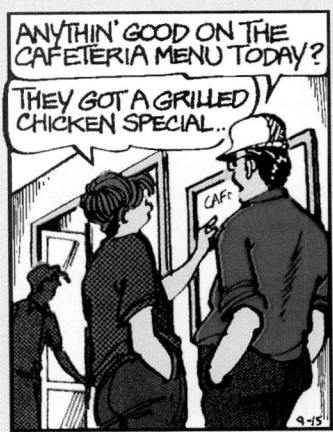 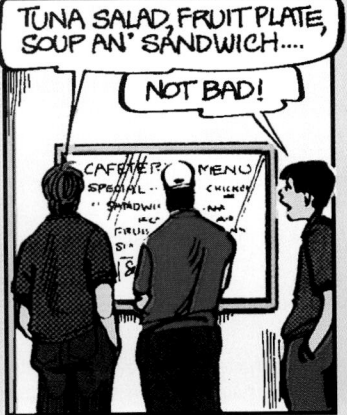 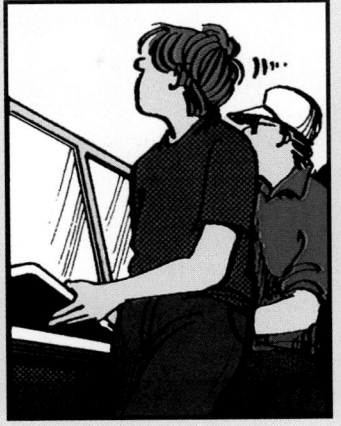 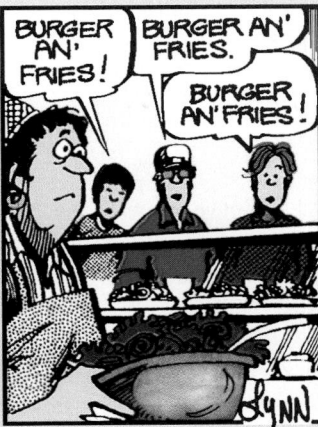

What influences daily food choices? How important is taste? Appearance? Nutrition? Convenience? Cost (Value)? Do these daily food choices go on to influence long-term health? If so, to what extent? This chapter provides some answers.

FOR BETTER OR FOR WORSE ©Lynn Johnston Productions, Inc./Dist. By United Features Syndicate, Inc. Reprinted by Permission.

Nutrition and Your Health

In your lifetime, you will eat about 70,000 meals and 60 tons of food. This opening chapter will take a close look at the general classes of nutrients supplied by this food intake, the role research plays in sorting out which food components are essential for the maintenance of health, and the powerful effect of dietary habits in determining both nutrition-related and overall health.

What Actually Is Nutrition?

The Council on Food and Nutrition of the American Medical Association defines *nutrition* as "The science of food, the nutrients and the substances therein, their action, interaction, and balance in relation to health and disease, and the process by which the [human] organism ingests, digests, absorbs, transports, utilizes, and excretes food substances."

Nutrients Come from Food

What is the difference among food, **nutrients,** and nutrition? Food provides both the energy and the materials needed to build and maintain all body cells. Nutrients are the nourishing substances we, for the most part, must obtain from food. These substances are vital for growth and maintenance of a healthy body throughout life. For a nutrient to be considered an **essential nutrient,** three characteristics are needed. First, its omission from the diet must lead to a decline in certain aspects of human health, such as function of the nervous system. Second, if the omitted nutrient is restored to the diet before permanent damage occurs, those aspects of human health hampered by its absence should regain normal function. Third, a specific biological function in the body must be identified.

*S*ome nutrients that perform life-sustaining functions can be produced by the body if they are missing from the diet. The essential nature of such nutrients sometimes is not clear-cut. For example, the body requires vitamin D, but the skin is capable of synthesizing its own vitamin D upon receiving sunlight. This reduces the need from dietary sources among people who experience regular sun exposure (see Chapter 8).

Table 1.1 Glossary Terms to Aid Your Introduction to Nutrition*

anemia Generally refers to a decreased oxygen-carrying capacity of the blood. This can be caused by many factors, such as iron deficiency or blood loss.

body mass index (BMI) Weight (in kilograms) divided by height (in meters) squared. A value of 25 or greater indicates a higher risk for body weight–related health disorders if one is also overfat.

cancer A condition characterized by uncontrolled growth of abnormal cells.

cardiovascular (heart) disease A disease characterized by the deposition of fatty material in the blood vessels that serve the heart, often called hardening of the arteries. These deposits restrict blood flow through the heart, which in turn can lead to heart damage and death. Also termed *coronary heart disease* (CHD), as the vessels of the heart are the primary site of disease. The term cardiovascular disease (CVD) is typically used, since in addition to the heart, the arteries that serve the rest of the body can experience the same deterioration.

cholesterol A waxy lipid found in all body cells; it has a structure containing multiple chemical rings (steroid structure). Cholesterol is found only in foods that contain animal products.

chronic Long-standing, developing over time. When referring to disease, this term indicates that the disease process, once developed, is slow and tends to remain; a good example is cardiovascular disease.

cirrhosis A loss of functioning liver cells, which are replaced by nonfunctioning connective tissue. Any substance that poisons liver cells can lead to cirrhosis. The most common cause is a chronic, excessive alcohol intake.

diabetes A disease characterized by high blood glucose, resulting from either insufficient or no release of the hormone insulin by the pancreas or general inability of insulin to act on certain body cells, such as muscle cells. The two major forms are type 1 (requires daily insulin therapy) and type 2 (may or may not require insulin therapy).

essential nutrient In nutritional terms, a substance that, when left out of a diet, leads to signs of poor health. The body either can't produce this nutrient or can't produce it fast enough to meet its needs. Then, if added back to a diet before permanent damage occurs, the affected aspects of health are restored.

hypertension A condition in which blood pressure remains persistently elevated. Obesity, inactivity, alcohol intake, and excess salt intake all can contribute to the problem.

kilocalorie (kcal) The heat energy needed to raise the temperature of 1000 grams (1 liter) of water 1 degree Celsius. Also written as Calories, with a capital C.

nutrients Chemical substances in food that contribute to health, many of which are essential parts of a diet. Nutrients nourish us by providing energy, materials for building body parts, and factors to regulate necessary chemical processes in the body. With only a few exceptions, the body either can't make these nutrients or can't make them in sufficient amounts for its needs.

obesity A condition characterized by excess body fat, typically defined in clinical settings as a body mass index (BMI) of 30 or above.

osteoporosis Decreased bone mass where no obvious causes can be found. This bone loss is related to the effects of aging, genetic background, poor diet, and hormonal effects of postmenopausal status in women.

risk factor A term used frequently when discussing diseases and the factors contributing to their development. A risk factor is an aspect of our lives—such as heredity, lifestyle choices (i.e., smoking), or nutritional habits—that may make us more likely to develop a disease.

stroke The loss of body function that results from a blood clot or other change in arteries in the brain that affects blood flow. This in turn causes the death of brain tissue. Also called a *cerebrovascular accident.*

*All bold terms in the book are defined in a glossary, which follows Chapter 17. Many bold terms are also defined in the chapter margin.

■ Why Study Nutrition?

Nutrition is one key to developing and maintaining a state of health that is optimal for you. In addition, a poor diet coupled with a sedentary lifestyle are known to be **risk factors** for life-threatening **chronic** diseases and deaths: **cardiovascular (heart) disease, stroke, hypertension, diabetes,** and some forms of **cancer** (Table 1.1). Together, these disorders account for two-thirds of all deaths in North America. (Table 1.2). Not meeting **nutrient** needs in younger years also makes us more likely to suffer health consequences of poor nutrition habits in later years, such as bone fractures from the disease **osteoporosis.** Iron-deficiency **anemia** is another possibility. At the same time, taking too much of a nutrient supplement—such as vitamin A, vitamin D, vitamin B-6, calcium, or copper—can be harmful. Another dietary problem, drinking too much alcohol, is associated with **cirrhosis** of the liver, some forms of cancer, accidents, and suicides.

Table 1.2 Ten Leading Causes of Death in the United States

Rank	Cause of Death	Percent of Total Deaths
	All causes	100
1	Heart disease (primarily heart attack)*‡#	31
2	Cancer*‡	23
3	Cerebrovascular diseases (stroke)*‡#	7
4	Chronic obstructive pulmonary diseases and allied conditions (lung diseases)‡	5
5	Pneumonia and influenza	4
6	Accidents and adverse effects†	4
	• Motor vehicle accidents	(2)
	• All other accidents and adverse effects	(2)
7	Diabetes*	3
8	Suicide†	1
9	Kidney disease*‡	1
10	Liver disease†	1

From Centers for Disease Control and Prevention, National Vital Statistics Report, accessed January 18, 2001. Note that recent Canadian statistics are quite similar.

*Causes of death in which diet plays a part

†Causes of death in which excessive alcohol consumption plays a part

‡Causes of death in which tobacco use plays a part

#Heart disease and cerebrovascular disease are included in the more global term "cardiovascular disease."

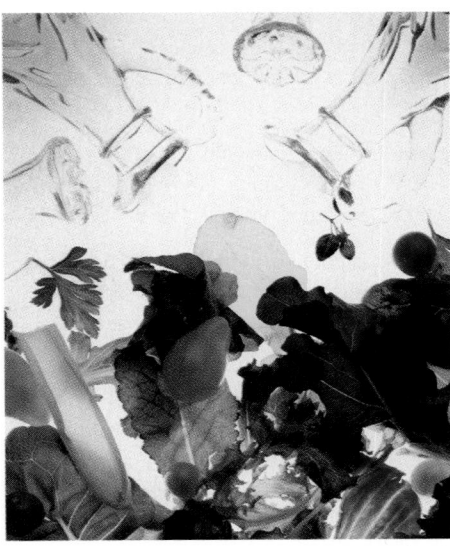

Increasing vegetable intake, such as a daily salad, is one strategy to combat development of many chronic diseases.

All of these consequences of modern living are partly an "affliction of affluence." Note, however, that these diseases are often preventable. Age fast or age slowly: It is partly your choice. U.S. government scientists have calculated that a poor diet combined with a lack of sufficient physical activity accounts for 300,000 fatal cases of cardiovascular disease, cancer, and diabetes each year among Americans. Thus, the combination of poor diet and too little physical activity is indirectly the second leading cause of death in the United States. In addition, **obesity** is considered the second leading cause of preventable death in the United States and the rest of North America (smoking is the first). Despite this relationship, the number of obese people in North America has continued to increase each year in the last decade.

As you gain understanding about your nutritional habits and increase your knowledge about nutrition, you have the opportunity to dramatically reduce your risk for many common health problems. To help, the U.S. federal government provides two websites that can link to many sites providing health and nutrition information (www.healthfinder.gov and www.nutrition.gov).

Classes and Sources of Nutrients

To begin the study of nutrition, let's start with an overview of the six various classes of nutrients. You are probably already familiar with the terms **carbohydrates, lipids** (fats and oils), **proteins, vitamins,** and **minerals** (Fig. 1.1). These, plus **water,** make up the six classes of nutrients found in food.

Nutrients can then be assigned to three functional categories: (1) those that primarily provide us with energy (typically expressed in **kilocalories [kcal]**); (2) those that are important for growth and development; and (3) those that act to keep body

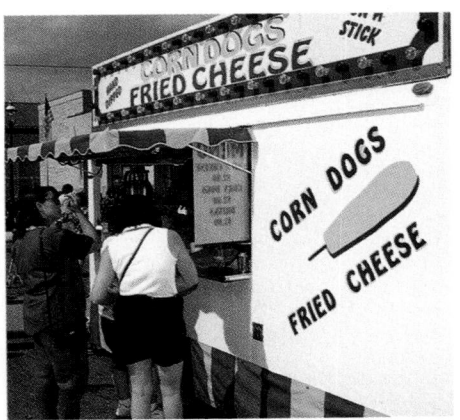

Many major health problems in North America are largely caused by a poor diet, excessive energy intake, and not enough physical activity.

carbohydrate A compound containing carbon, hydrogen, and oxygen atoms. Most are known as *sugars, starches,* and *dietary fibers.*

atom Smallest combining unit of an element, such as iron or calcium. Atoms consist of protons, neutrons, and electrons.

lipid A compound containing much carbon and hydrogen, little oxygen, and sometimes other atoms. Lipids dissolve in ether or benzene, but not in water, and include fats, oils, and cholesterol.

protein Food and body components made of amino acids; proteins contain carbon, hydrogen, oxygen, nitrogen, and sometimes other atoms, in a specific configuration. Proteins contain the form of nitrogen most easily used by the human body.

vitamins Compounds needed in very small amounts in the diet to help regulate and support chemical reactions in the body.

minerals Elements used in the body to promote chemical reactions and to form body structures.

water The universal solvent; chemically, H_2O. The body is composed of about 60% water. Water (fluid) needs are about 8 cups per day; needs are greater if one exercises heavily (see Chapter 9).

Carbohydrate

Starch
Storage form of carbohydrate in foods

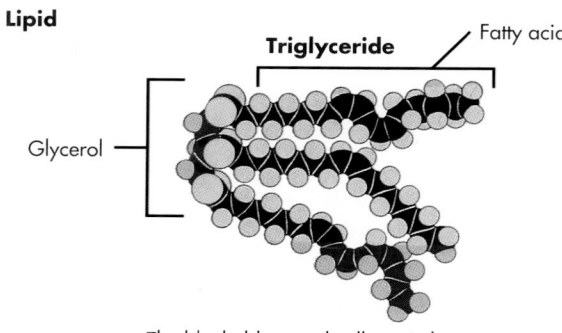

Each green circle represents one glucose molecule.

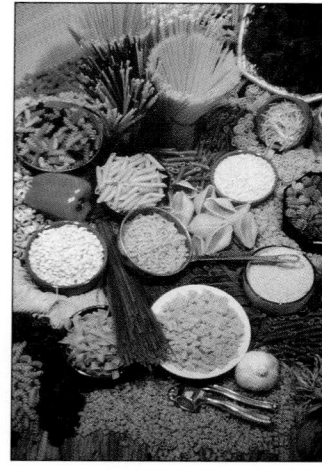

Lipid

Triglyceride   Fatty acid

Glycerol

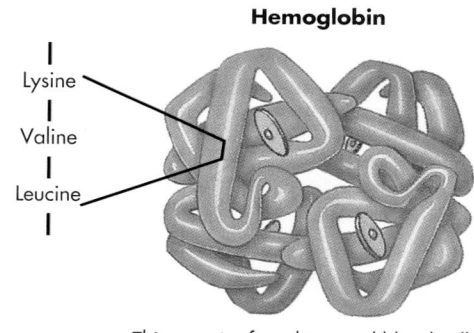

The black, blue, and yellow circles represent carbon, hydrogen, and oxygen atoms, respectively, in the triglyceride molecule.

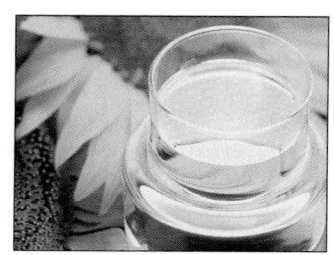

Protein

Hemoglobin

Lysine

Valine

Leucine

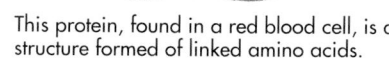

This protein, found in a red blood cell, is a structure formed of linked amino acids.

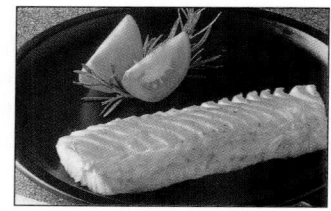

Figure 1.1 Two views of carbohydrates, lipids, and proteins—chemical and dietary perspectives. *Illustrations by William Ober.*

itamins and minerals are needed in such small amounts in the diet that they are called micronutrients. Because carbohydrates, proteins, lipids, and water are needed in much larger amounts, they are called macronutrients.

functions running smoothly. Some overlap exists among these groupings. The energy-yielding nutrients make up a major portion of most foods.

Provide Energy	**Promote Growth and Development**	**Regulate Body Processes**
Carbohydrates	Proteins	Proteins
Proteins	Lipids	Lipids
Lipids	Vitamins	Vitamins
	Minerals	Minerals
	Water	Water

Table 1.3 Essential Nutrients in the Human Diet and Their Classes*

Energy-Yielding Nutrients			
Carbohydrate	**Lipids†**	**Protein (Amino Acids)**	**Water**
Glucose† (or a carbohydrate that yields glucose)	Linoleic acid (omega-6) α-Linolenic acid (omega-3)	Histidine Isoleucine Leucine Lysine Methionine Phenylalanine Threonine Tryptophan Valine	Water

Vitamins		Minerals		
Water-Soluble	**Fat-Soluble**	**Major**	**Trace**	**Some Questionable Varieties**
Thiamin	A	Calcium	Chromium	Arsenic
Riboflavin	D§	Chloride	Copper	Boron
Niacin	E	Magnesium	Fluoride‖	Nickel
Panthothenic acid	K	Phosphorus	Iodide	Silicon
Biotin		Potassium	Iron	Vanadium
B-6		Sodium	Manganese	
B-12		Sulfur	Molybdenum	
Folate			Selenium	
C			Zinc	

*This table includes nutrients that the current *Dietary Reference Intakes* and related publications list for humans. Some disagreement exists over the questionable varieties, and certain other minerals not listed. Dietary fiber could be added to the list of essential substances, but it is not a nutrient (See Chapter 4). Alcohol is a source of calories but is not a nutrient per se.

†The lipids listed are needed only in small amounts, about 2% of total energy needs (see Chapter 5).

‡To prevent ketosis and thus the muscle loss that would occur if protein were used to synthesize carbohydrate (see Chapter 4)

§Sunshine on the skin also allows the body to make vitamin D for itself (see Chapter 8).

‖Primarily for dental health (see Chapter 9)

The vitamin-like compound choline plays essential roles in the body but is not listed under the vitamin category at this time. Rough estimates of human needs for this water-soluble compound recently have been set (see the inside cover of the text). Note, however, that body synthesis suffices during many stages of life (see Chapter 8 for details).

Let's now look more closely at these six classes of nutrients (Table 1.3).

∎ Carbohydrates

Carbohydrates are composed mainly of the **elements** carbon, hydrogen, and oxygen. Carbohydrates provide a major source of fuel for the body, on average 4 kcal per gram. Carbohydrates can exist as simple sugars and complex carbohydrates. **Simple sugars,** sometimes referred to simply as *sugars,* are relatively small molecules. The smallest simple sugars are called monosaccharides. They consist of a single sugar unit. The sugar in your blood, **glucose** (also known as *blood sugar* or *dextrose*), is an example of a monosaccharide. Other simple sugars are made by joining two monosaccharides together to form a **disaccharide.** Table sugar, sucrose, is an example of a disaccharide because it is formed from fructose and glucose (both monosaccharides). Carbohydrates are stored as large molecules, called **complex carbohydrates** or **polysaccharides.** Joining together many monosaccharides—often as a repeating unit—forms polysaccharides. For example, plants form the polysaccharide **starch** by joining hundreds of glucose molecules together as a repeating unit (review Fig. 1.1).

element A substance that cannot be separated into simpler substances by chemical processes. Common elements in nutrition include carbon, oxygen, hydrogen, nitrogen, calcium, phosphorus, and iron.

glucose A six-carbon carbohydrate found in blood and in table sugar bound to fructose; also known as *dextrose,* it is one of the simple sugars.

bond A sharing of electrons, or attractions linking two atoms.

dietary fiber Substances in plant foods that are not digested by the processes that take place in the stomach or small intestine. These add bulk to feces.

fatty acid Major part of most lipids; composed of a chain of carbons flanked by hydrogen with an acid group

$$\begin{array}{c} O \\ \| \end{array}$$

(—C—OH) at one end and a methyl group (—CH$_3$) at the other (see Chapter 5).

triglyceride The major form of lipid in the body and in food. It is composed of three fatty acids bonded to glycerol, an alcohol.

saturated fatty acid A fatty acid containing no carbon-carbon double bonds.

unsaturated fatty acid A fatty acid containing one or more carbon-carbon double bonds.

cholesterol A waxy lipid found in all body cells; it has a structure containing multiple chemical rings. Cholesterol is found only in foods that contain animal products.

Much attention has been given to saturated fat in the past few years. This is because saturated fat bears a great deal of the responsibility for raising blood **cholesterol.** *High blood cholesterol leads to clogged arteries and, so, can eventually lead to cardiovascular disease (see Chapter 6).*

enzyme A compound that speeds the rate of a chemical process but is not altered by the process. Almost all enzymes are proteins (some are made of genetic material).

Aside from enjoying their taste, we need sugars and other carbohydrates in our diets primarily to satisfy the energy needs of our body cells. Glucose, which the body can produce from most carbohydrates, is a major source of energy in most cells. When not enough carbohydrate is consumed to supply sufficient glucose, the body is forced to make glucose from proteins.

Digestion of some dietary starch begins in the mouth. The digestive process continues in the small intestine until starches break down into single sugar molecules (such as glucose), which are absorbed via the small intestine into the bloodstream (see Chapter 3 for more on digestion). However, the **bonds** between the sugar molecules in certain complex carbohydrates cannot be broken down by human digestive processes. These carbohydrates are part of what is called **dietary fiber.** Such dietary fiber passes through the small intestine undigested to provide bulk for the stool (feces), which is formed in the large intestine (colon). Chapter 4 focuses on carbohydrates.

■ Lipids

Lipids (mostly fats and oils) are composed of the elements carbon and hydrogen; they contain fewer oxygen atoms than do carbohydrates. Because of this difference in composition, lipids yield more energy per gram than do carbohydrates—on the average, 9 kcal per gram. Lipids dissolve in organic solvents (e.g., ether and benzene) but not in water.

The basic structure of most lipids is the three-carbon glycerol molecule with a **fatty acid** attached to each of the three carbons (review Fig. 1.1). This form of lipid is generally called a **triglyceride.** Triglycerides are a key energy source for the body and the major form of fat in foods. They are also the major form for energy storage in the body.

In this book, the more familiar term, *fats* or *fats and oils,* will generally be used, rather than *lipids* or *triglycerides.* Roughly speaking, fats are lipids that are solid at room temperature, and oils are lipids that are liquid at room temperature.

Most lipids can be separated into two basic types—saturated fat and unsaturated fat—based on the chemical structure of their dominant fatty acids. This property determines whether such a lipid is solid or liquid at room temperature. Plant oils tend to contain many **unsaturated fatty acids,** which makes them liquid. Animal fats are often rich in **saturated fatty acids,** which makes them solid. Almost all foods contain a variety of saturated and unsaturated fatty acids.

Certain unsaturated fatty acids are essential nutrients. Each must come from our diet. These key fatty acids that the body can't produce, called essential fatty acids, perform several important functions in the body: they help regulate blood pressure and play a role in the synthesis and repair of vital cell parts. However, we need only about 1 tablespoon of a common vegetable oil (such as the canola or soybean oil found in supermarkets) each day to supply the essential fatty acids. The average North American diet supplies about three times the amount of essential fatty acids needed daily. Adding a serving of fatty fish such as salmon or tuna to a diet at least twice a week adds to this benefit derived from the inclusion of vegetable oil. The unique fatty acids in these fish complement the healthy aspects of vegetable oil. This will be explained in greater detail in Chapter 5, which focuses on lipids.

■ Proteins

Like carbohydrates and fats, proteins are composed of the elements carbon, oxygen, and hydrogen. But, unlike the other energy-yielding nutrients, all proteins also contain much nitrogen. Proteins are the main structural material in the body (review Fig. 1.1). For example, proteins constitute a major part of bone and muscle; they are also important components in blood, body cells, **enzymes,** and immune factors. Furthermore, proteins can also provide energy for the body—on average, 4 kcal per gram. Typically, however, the body uses little protein for that purpose of meeting daily energy needs. Proteins are formed by the linking of **amino acids.** Twenty common amino acids are found in food; nine of these are essential nutrients for adults, and one additional amino acid is essential for infants.

Most North Americans eat about one and a half to two times more protein than the body needs to maintain health. In a healthy person (i.e., no evidence of cardiovascular disease, osteoporosis, kidney disease, or diabetes or family history of colon cancer or kidney stones), this amount of extra protein in the diet is generally not harmful— it simply reflects the standard of living and the dietary habits of most North Americans. The excess is used for fuel or converted into fat or carbohydrate. Chapter 6 focuses on proteins.

Three other classes of nutrients are vitamins, minerals, and water. Although vitamins and minerals are vital to good health, they are needed only in small amounts in the diet and provide no direct source of energy for the body.

■ Vitamins

Vitamins exhibit a wide variety of chemical structures and can contain the elements carbon, hydrogen, nitrogen, oxygen, phosphorus, sulfur, and others. The main function of vitamins is to enable many **chemical reactions** to occur in the body. Some of these reactions help release the energy trapped in carbohydrates, lipids, and proteins. Remember, however, that vitamins themselves provide no usable energy for the body.

The 13 vitamins are divided into two groups: four that are **fat soluble** (vitamins A, D, E, and K) and nine that are **water soluble** (vitamin C and the B vitamins). The two groups of vitamins often act quite differently. For example, cooking destroys water-soluble vitamins much more readily than it does fat-soluble vitamins. Water-soluble vitamins are also excreted from the body much more readily than are fat-soluble vitamins. Thus, the fat-soluble vitamins, especially vitamins A and D, are much more likely to accumulate in excessive amounts in the body, which then can lead to toxicity. Vitamins are the focus of Chapter 8.

■ Minerals

All of the nutrients discussed so far are **organic** compounds, whereas minerals are structurally very simple, **inorganic** substances, which exist as groups of one or more of the same atoms. These terms, *organic* and *inorganic,* have nothing to do with gardening but are based on simple chemistry concepts (see Chapter 2 for use of the term organic on food labels).

Minerals typically function as such in the body (Na^+, K^+), or as parts of simple mineral combinations, such as bone mineral [$Ca_{10}(PO_4)_6 OH_2$]. Because of their simple structure, minerals are not destroyed during cooking, but they can still be lost if they leach into the water used for cooking and then are discarded if that water is not consumed. Although minerals themselves yield no energy as such for the body, they are critical players in nervous system functioning, other cellular processes, water balance, and structural (e.g., skeletal) systems.

The amounts of the 16 or more essential minerals that are required in the diet for good health vary enormously. Thus, they are divided into two groups: **major minerals** and **trace minerals,** based on dietary needs. If daily needs are less than 100 milligrams, the mineral is put in the trace mineral class, otherwise, it is a major mineral. The actual dietary requirement for some trace minerals has yet to be determined. Minerals are the focus of Chapter 9.

■ Water

Water is the sixth class of nutrients. Although sometimes overlooked as a nutrient, water (chemically, H_2O) has numerous vital functions in the body. It acts as a **solvent** and lubricant, as a medium for transporting nutrients and waste, and as a medium for temperature regulation and chemical processes. For these reasons, and

amino acid The building block for proteins containing a central carbon atom with a nitrogen atom and other atoms attached.

chemical reaction An interaction between two chemicals that changes both participants.

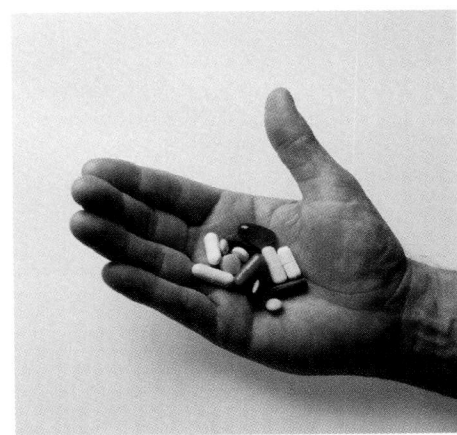

Taking a daily multivitamin and mineral supplement is generally safe. Some nutrition experts even recommend the practice. However, taking numerous nutrient supplements can lead to health problems (see Chapter 8 for details).

organic Any substance that contains carbon atoms bonded to hydrogen atoms in the chemical structure.

inorganic Any substance lacking carbon atoms bonded to hydrogen atoms in the chemical structure.

solvent A substance that other substances dissolve in.

metabolism Chemical processes in the body by which energy is provided in useful forms and vital activities are sustained.

because the human body is approximately 60% water, the average person requires about 2 liters—equivalent to 2000 grams or 8 cups—of water and/or fluids containing water every day.

Water is not only available from the obvious sources, but it is also the major component in some foods, such as many fruits and vegetables (e.g., lettuce, grapes, and melons). The body even makes some water as a by-product of **metabolism**. Water is examined in detail in Chapter 9.

Critical Thinking

Believing that supplements provide the nutrition her body needs, Janice regularly takes numerous supplements while paying relatively little attention to daily food choices. How would you explain to her that this practice may lead to health problems?

For suggested answers to the Critical Thinking questions in this and every chapter, turn to the back of the book.

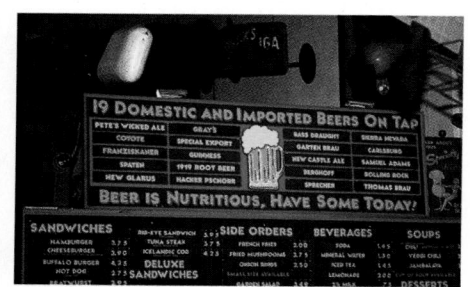

Alcoholic beverages are calorie-rich, but alcohol is not a nutrient per se.

cell A minute structure; the living basis of plant and animal organization. In animals it is bounded by a cell membrane. Cells contain both genetic material and systems for synthesizing energy-yielding compounds. Cells have the ability to take up compounds from and excrete compounds into their surroundings.

genes The hereditary material on chromosomes. Genes provide the blueprints for the production of cell proteins.

alcohol Ethyl alcohol (CH_3CH_2OH).

ion An atom with an unequal number of electrons and protons. Negative ions have more electrons than protons; positive ions have more protons than electrons.

Nutrient Composition of Diets and the Human Body

The quantities of the various nutrients that people consume vary widely, and the nutrient amounts present in different foods also vary a great deal. The total daily intake of protein, fat, and carbohydrate amounts to about 500 grams. In contrast, the typical daily mineral intake totals about 20 grams, and the daily vitamin intake totals less than 300 milligrams. Although each day we require nearly a gram of some minerals, such as calcium and phosphorus, we need only a few milligrams or less of other minerals. For example, we need about 10 milligrams of zinc per day, which is just a few specks of the mineral.

Figure 1.2 contrasts the relative concentrations of all the major classes of nutrients in a lean man and a lean woman with the composition of both a cooked steak and French fries. Note how the nutrient composition of the body differs from the nutritional profiles of the foods we eat. This is because growth, development, and later maintenance of the human body are directed by the genetic material inside body **cells.** This genetic blueprint determines how each cell uses the essential nutrients to perform body functions. These nutrients can come from a variety of sources. Cells are not concerned whether available amino acids come from animal or plant sources. The carbohydrate glucose can come from sugars or starches. Thus, you really aren't what you eat. Rather, what you eat provides cells with basic materials to function according to the directions supplied by the genetic material (**genes**) housed in body cells (see the Nutrition Insight in Chapter 3).

Energy Sources and Uses

Humans obtain the energy we need to perform body functions and do work from carbohydrates, fats, and proteins. Foods generally provide more than one energy source. Vegetable oil is an exception; it is 100% fat.

Alcohol is also a source of energy for some of us, supplying about 7 kcal per gram. It is not considered an essential nutrient, however, because it has no required function. Still, alcoholic beverages, such as beer—generally also rich in carbohydrate—are typically a contributor of energy to the diet of adults.

The body transforms the energy trapped in carbohydrate, protein, and fat (and alcohol) into other forms of energy in order to

- Build new **compounds**
- Perform muscular movements
- Promote nerve transmissions
- Maintain **ion** balance within cells

Chapter 11 describes how that energy is released from chemical bonds and then used by body cells to support the processes just described.

Composition (percent of weight)					
Nutrient	**French fries**	**Steak**		**Healthy man**	**Healthy woman**
Carbohydrate	37%	0%		<1%	<1%
Protein	4%	27%		16%	13%
Fat	17%	18%		16%	25%
Minerals	1%	1%		6%	5%
Water	41%	54%		62%	57%

Figure 1.2 You aren't what you eat. The proportions of nutrients in the healthy human body do not match those found in typical foods—animal or vegetable.

You have likely noticed on food labels that the energy in food is often expressed in terms of calories. Technically, a calorie is the amount of heat energy it takes to raise the temperature of 1 gram of water 1 degree **Celsius** (1°C, centigrade scale). (Chapter 10 has a diagram of the instrument used to measure calories in foods [bomb calorimeter].) Because a calorie is such a tiny measure of heat, food energy is more accurately expressed in terms of the kilocalorie (kcal), which equals 1000 calories. (If the "c" in calories is capitalized, this also signifies kilocalories.) A kcal is the amount of heat energy it takes to raise the temperature of 1000 grams (1 liter) of water 1°C. The term *kilocalorie* and its abbreviation *kcal* are used throughout this book. In everyday life, the word *calorie* is often used loosely to mean *kilocalorie* unless the "c" is capitalized. (In this latter case, it is an accurate use of the term.) Any values given on food labels in calories are actually in kilocalories (Fig. 1.3). A suggested intake of 2000 calories per day on a food label is really 2000 kcal.

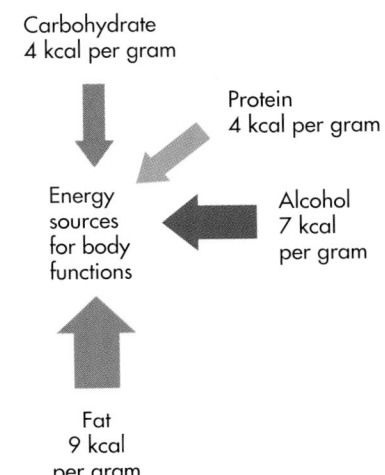

Carbohydrate
4 kcal per gram

Protein
4 kcal per gram

Energy
sources
for body
functions

Alcohol
7 kcal
per gram

Fat
9 kcal
per gram

Another Bite

Use the 4-9-4 estimates for the energy contributions of carbohydrate, fat, and protein introduced over the last few pages to determine energy content of a food. Consider a typical deluxe hamburger sandwich:

Carbohydrate	39 grams × 4 = 156 kcal
Fat	32 grams × 9 = 288 kcal
Protein	30 grams × 4 = 120 kcal
Total	564 kcal

You can also use the 4-9-4 estimates to determine what portion of total energy intake is contributed by the various energy-yielding nutrients. Assume that one day you consume 290 grams of carbohydrates, 60 grams of fat, and 70 grams of protein. This consumption yields a total of 1980 kcal ([290 × 4] + [60 × 9] + [70 × 4] = 1980). The percentage of your total energy intake derived from each nutrient can then be determined:

% of kcal as carbohydrate = (290 × 4) ÷ 1980 = 0.586 (× 100 = 59%)
% of kcal as fat = (60 × 9) ÷ 1980 = 0.273 (× 100 = 27%)
% of kcal as protein = (70 × 4) ÷ 1980 = 0.141 (× 100 = 14%)

Check your calculations by adding the percentages together. Do they total 100?

| **Nutrition** | | **Facts** | | *Percent Daily Values (DV) are based on a 2,000 calorie diet. Your daily values may be higher or lower depending on your calorie needs: | | | INGREDIENTS: WHOLE WHEAT, WATER, ENRICHED WHEAT FLOUR [FLOUR, MALTED BARLEY, NIACIN, REDUCED IRON, THIAMINE MONONITRATE (VITAMIN B1) AND RIBOFLAVIN (VITAMIN B2)], CORN SYRUP, PART-IALLY HYDROGENATED COT-TONSEED, OIL, SALT, YEAST. |

Nutrition Facts label:

Nutrition Facts
Serving Size 1 slice (36g)   Servings Per Container 19

Amount Per Serving
Calories 80   Calories from Fat 10

	% Daily Value*			% Daily Value*
Total Fat 1g	2%	**Total Carbohydrate** 15g		5%
Saturated Fat 0g	0%	Dietary Fiber 2g		8%
Cholesterol 0mg	0%	Sugars less than 1g		
Sodium 200mg	8%	**Protein** 3g		
Vitamin A 0%	Vitamin C 0%	Calcium 0%		Iron 4%

HONEY WHEAT BREAD

*Percent Daily Values (DV) are based on a 2,000 calorie diet. Your daily values may be higher or lower depending on your calorie needs:

		Calories:	2,000	2,500
Total Fat	Less than		65g	80g
Sat Fat	Less than		20g	25g
Cholesterol	Less than		300mg	300mg
Sodium	Less than		2,400mg	2,400mg
Total Carbohydrate			300g	375g
Dietary Fiber			25g	30g

Figure 1.3 Use the nutrient values on the Nutrition Facts label to calculate energy content of a food. A serving of this food contains 81 kcal ($[15 \times 4] + [3 \times 4] + [1 \times 9] = 81$). The label lists 80, suggesting that the energy value was rounded down.

Concept Check

Nutrition is the study of food and nutrients—their digestion, absorption, and metabolism, and their effect on health and disease. Food contains the vital nutrients that are essential for good health: carbohydrates, lipids (fats and oils), proteins, vitamins, minerals, and water. Nutrients have three general functions in the body: (1) to provide materials for building and maintaining the body; (2) to act as regulators for key metabolic reactions; and (3) to participate in metabolic reactions that provide the energy necessary to sustain life. A common unit of measurement for this energy is the kilocalorie (kcal). On average, carbohydrates and protein provide 4 kcal per gram of energy to the body, while lipids provide 9 kcal per gram. Alcohol provides about 7 kcal per gram. The other classes of nutrients do not supply energy but are essential for proper body functioning.

In the fifth century B.C., Hippocrates said "Let food be your medicine and medicine be your food."

The National Cholesterol Education Program also includes a strict limit on saturated fat and cholesterol intake when putting their diet guidelines into place (see Chapter 6).

Current State of the North American Diet and Overall Health

If we ignore alcohol, North American adults consume about 16% of their kcal as proteins, 50% as carbohydrates, and 33% as fats. These percentages are estimates and vary slightly from year to year and from person to person. This pattern is close to the 15%, 50% to 60%, and 25% to 35% distribution of calories from protein, carbohydrate, and fat, respectively, advocated by the latest advice from the National Cholesterol Education Program in the United States (see Chapter 6). Note that recommendations for different distributions of calories among protein, carbohydrate, and fat come and go in the popular press. The pros and cons of these patterns—such as the 45%, 15%, and 40% pattern for carbohydrate, protein, and fat calories in the book *Syndrome X*, authored by Dr. Gerald Reaven and colleagues—will be reviewed in future chapters.

Animal sources supply about two-thirds of protein intake for most North Americans; plant sources supply only about one-third. In many other parts of the world, it is just the opposite: plant proteins—from rice, beans, corn, and other vegetables—dominate protein intake. About half the carbohydrate in North American diets comes from simple sugars; the other half comes from starches (such as in pastas, breads, and potatoes). About 60% of dietary fat comes from animal sources and 40% from plant sources.

Math Tools for Nutrition

Y ou will use a few mathematical concepts in studying nutrition. Besides performing addition, subtraction, multiplication, and division, you need to know how to calculate percentages and convert English units of measurement to metric units.

Percentages

The term *percent* (%) refers to a part of the total when the total represents 100 parts. For example, if you earn 80% on your first nutrition examination, you will have answered the equivalent of 80 out of 100 questions correctly. This equivalent could be 8 correct answers out of 10; 80% also describes 16 of 20 (16/20 = 0.80 or 80%). The best way to master this concept is to calculate some percentages. Some examples follow:

Question	Answer
What is 6% of 45?	$0.06 \times 45 = 2.7$
What is 32% of 8?	$0.32 \times 8 = 2.6$
What percent of 16 is 6?	$^{6}/_{16} = 0.375$ or 37.5%
What percent of 99 is 3?	$^{3}/_{99} = 0.03$ or 3%

Joe ate 15% of the adult Recommended Dietary Allowance (RDA) for iron at lunch. How many milligrams did he eat? (RDA = 8 milligrams)

0.15×8 milligrams = 1.2 milligrams

It is difficult to succeed in a nutrition course unless you know what a percentage means and how to calculate one. Percentages are used frequently when referring to menus and nutrient composition.

The Metric System

The basic units of the metric system are the meter, which indicates length; the gram, which indicates weight; and the liter, which indicates volume. Appendix J in this textbook lists conversions from the metric system to the English system (pounds, feet, cups) and vice versa. Here is a brief summary:

One meter (m) is 39.4 inches long, or about 3 inches longer than 1 yard (3 feet).
A meter can be divided into 100 units of centimeters, or into 1000 units of millimeters.
A millimeter (mm) is about the thickness of a dime.
There are 2.54 centimeters (cm) in 1 inch and about 30 centimeters in 1 foot.

A person 6 feet tall is equivalent to 183 centimeters tall.
A gram (g) is about 1/30 of an ounce (28 grams to the ounce).
5 grams of sugar or salt is about 1 tea-spoon.
A pound (lb) weighs 454 grams.
A kilogram (kg) is 1000 grams, equivalent to 2.2 pounds.
To convert your weight to kilograms, divide it by 2.2.
A 154-pound man weighs 70 kilograms (154/2.2 = 70).
A gram can be divided into 1000 milligrams (mg) or 1,000,000 micrograms (μg or mcg).
10 milligrams of zinc (approximately adult needs) would be a few grains of zinc oxide.
Liters are divided into 1000 units called milliliters (ml).
One teaspoon equals about 5 milliliters (ml), 1 cup is about 240 milliliters, and 1 quart (4 cups) equals almost 1 liter (L) (0.946 liter to be exact).

If you plan to work in any scientific field, you will need to learn the metric system. **For now, remember that a kilogram equals 2.2 pounds, an ounce weighs 28 grams, 2.54 centimeters equals 1 inch, and a liter is almost the same as a quart.** In addition, know what the prefixes micro (1/1,000,000), milli (1/1000), centi (1/100), and kilo (1000) represent.

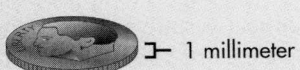

1 millimeter

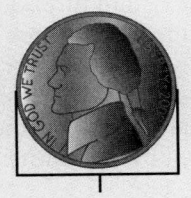

2 centimeters

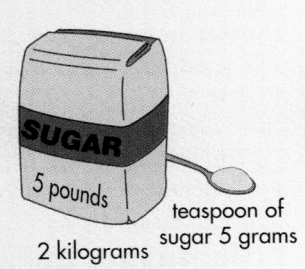

2 kilograms   teaspoon of sugar 5 grams

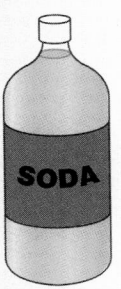

2 liter

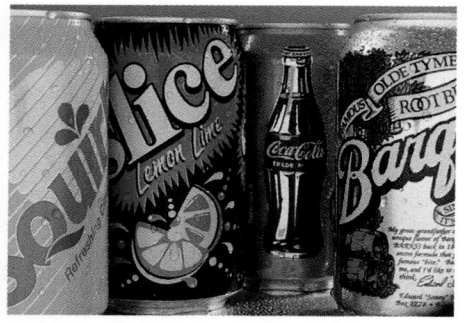

Today, soft drinks are more popular than milk, but not as beneficial to the diet. Soft drinks account for about 10% of the energy intake of teenagers in North America, and in turn contribute to generally poor calcium intakes seen in this age group.

salt Generally refers to a compound of sodium and chloride in a 40:60 ratio.

■ Assessing the Current North American Diet

Information about the North American diet comes from large surveys designed to find out what and when people eat. The primary methods the U.S. federal government uses to collect data about food and nutrient consumption, and the relationship between diet and health, are two survey programs: the Continuing Survey of Food Intakes by Individuals (CSFII) conducted by the U.S. Department of Agriculture (USDA) and the National Health and Nutrition Examination Survey (NHANES) administered by the U.S. Department of Health and Human Services. CSFII, as the name implies, is an ongoing program that collects data on America's eating habits. The NHANES is an examination of the health status of Americans as related to their nutrient intake. In Canada, this information is gathered by Health Canada in conjunction with Agriculture and Agrifood Canada. Results from these surveys and other studies show that North Americans consume a wide variety of foods. Some people are meeting their nutrient needs; some are not. Chapter 2 will look at this situation in more detail. For now, note that studies show that some of us should choose more foods that are rich in iron, calcium, vitamin A, various B vitamins, vitamin C, vitamin D, vitamin E, zinc, and dietary fiber. Daily intake of a multivitamin and mineral supplement to meet these nutrient needs is also a strategy, but does not make up for a poor diet in all respects (see Chapter 8). Routinely, experts also recommend that we pay more attention to balancing energy intake with need. An excess intake of energy is usually tied to an overindulgence in sugar, fat, and alcoholic beverages. African-Americans may need to pay special attention to the amount of **salt** (a mixture of sodium and chloride) and alcohol in their diets. This is because they have a greater chance of developing hypertension than do other ethnic groups in North America, and these substances are two of the many factors linked to that health problem. Actually, a careful look at salt and alcohol intake—along with saturated fat and total energy intake—is a recommended practice for all adults.

Many North Americans would benefit from a more helpful balance of foods in their diets—greater moderation in the intake of some foods is needed, such as sugared soft drinks and fried foods, while increasing the variety of other foods, such as fruits and vegetables. Few adults currently meet the "5-a-day" minimum recommendation for total servings of vegetables and fruits, even though, when interviewed, 70% of the people in the United States recently said these are an important part of a healthy diet.

Health Objectives for the United States for the Year 2010 Include Numerous Nutrition Objectives

Health promotion and disease prevention have been public health strategies in North America since the late 1970s. One part of this strategy is *Healthy People 2010,* a report issued in 2000 by the U.S. Department of Health and Human Services' Public Health Service. This report consists of health promotion and disease prevention objectives for the nation for the year 2010 and assigns each of the objectives to appropriate U.S. federal agencies to address. Many nutrition-related objectives are part of the overall plan (Table 1.4). The main objectives of *Healthy People 2010* are to promote healthful lifestyles and to reduce preventable death and disability.

The following Internet site provides more details on the *Healthy People* program: www.health.gov/healthypeople.

■ Improving Overall Health

Overall, how you act now is important to your later health. Successful aging is a result of wise nutrition and lifestyle choices. As noted in the introduction to this chapter, age quickly or age slowly—you have some choice in the matter.

Table 1.4 A Sample of Nutrition-Related Objectives from *Healthy People 2010*

	Target	Current Estimate
Increase the proportion of adults who are at a healthy weight (defined as a body mass index between 18.5 and 25).	60%	39%
Reduce the proportion of adults who are obese (body mass index of 30 or more).	15%	23%
Reduce the proportion of children and adolescents who are overweight or obese.	5%	10%
Increase the proportion of persons age 2 years and older who consume at least 2 daily servings of fruit.	75%	28%
Increase the proportion of persons age 2 years and older who consume at least 3 daily servings of vegetables, with at least one-third being dark green or deep yellow vegetables.	50%	3%
Increase the proportion of persons age 2 years and older who consume at least 6 daily servings of grain products, with at least 3 being whole grains (e.g., whole wheat bread and oatmeal).	50%	7%
Increase the proportion of persons age 2 years and older who consume less than 10% of calories from saturated fat.	75%	36%
Increase the proportion of persons age 2 years and older who consume no more than 30% of calories from fat.	75%	33%
Increase the proportion of persons age 2 years and older who consume 6 grams or less of salt (2400 milligrams or less of sodium) daily.	65%	21%
Increase the proportion of persons age 2 years and older who meet dietary recommendations for calcium (see inside cover of this book).	75%	46%
Reduce iron deficiency among young children and females of childbearing age.	6%	10%

Note: Related objectives include those addressing osteoporosis, various forms of cancer, diabetes prevention and treatment, food allergies, cardiovascular disease, low birth weight, nutrition during pregnancy, breastfeeding, eating disorders, physical activity, and alcohol use (see later chapters).

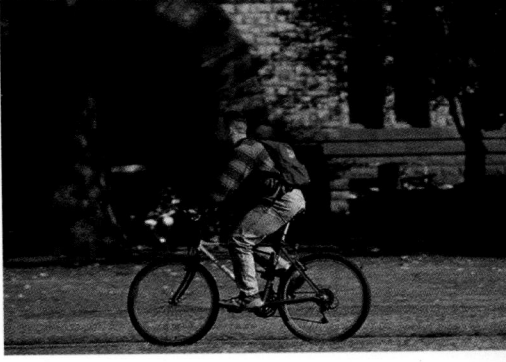

Regular physical activity complements a healthy diet; practice both each day.

One way to promote your health and prevent chronic diseases in the future is to observe the recommendations listed in Table 1.5. In total, these contribute to maximal health and prevention of disease.

Concept Check

Surveys in the United States and Canada show that we generally have a variety of foods available to us. However, some of us could improve our diets by focusing on rich food sources of various vitamins, minerals, and dietary fiber. In addition, many of us should reduce our consumption of energy, sugar, protein, fat, salt, and alcoholic beverages. These recommendations are consistent with an overall goal to attain and maintain good health.

Why Am I So Hungry?

Understanding what drives us to eat and what affects food choice will help put your study of nutrition into greater focus. This especially helps you understand the complexity of factors that influence eating, especially the effects of ethnicity and societal

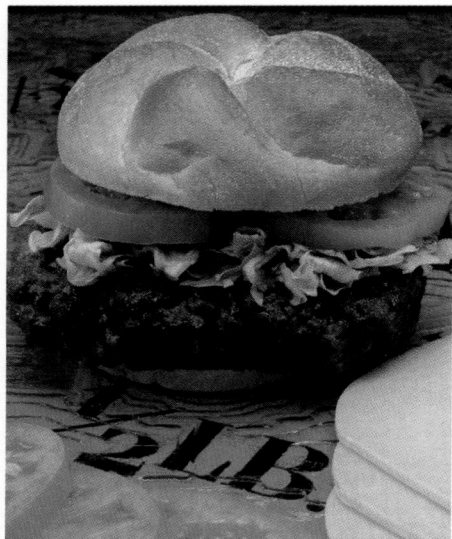

Probably the worst food-related trend in North America is super-sized servings of foods, especially in restaurants. Consumers might see these as a bargain, but few need the extra calories supplied by the increased serving sizes.

Table 1.5 Recommendations for Health Promotion and Disease Prevention: What Can Adults Expect from Adequate Nutrition and Good Health Habits?

Diet

Consuming enough essential nutrients, including dietary fiber, while moderating calorie, saturated fat, cholesterol, and alcohol intake (if used) can result in:

- Reduced risk for deficiency diseases, such as cretinism (lack of iodide), scurvy (lack of vitamin C), and anemia (lack of iron, folate, or other nutrients)
- Increased bone mass during childhood and adolescence
- Prevention of some adult bone loss and osteoporosis, especially in older adults
- Fewer dental caries
- Prevention of digestive problems, such as constipation
- Decreased susceptibility to some cancers
- Decreased degradation of the retina (intake of green and orange vegetables in particular)
- Lower risk of obesity and related diseases, such as type 2 diabetes
- Lower risk of cardiovascular diseases

Physical Activity

Adequate, regular physical activity (a minimum of 30 minutes on most or all days) helps prevent:

- Obesity
- Type 2 diabetes
- Cardiovascular disease
- Some adult bone loss and loss of muscle tone
- Premature aging

Lifestyle

Minimizing alcohol intake (no more than two drinks per day for men and one drink for both women and all adults age 65 years and older) helps prevent:

- Liver disease
- Fetal alcohol syndrome
- Accidents

Not smoking cigarettes or cigars helps prevent:

- Lung cancer, other lung disease, kidney disease, cardiovascular disease, and degenerative eye diseases

In addition, minimum use of medication, no illicit drug use, adequate sleep (7–8 hours), adequate fluid intake (about 8 cups per day), and a reduction in stress (practice better time management, relax, listen to music, have a massage, and stay physically active) provide a more complete approach to good nutrition and health. Add to this maintaining close relationships with others and a positive outlook on life. Finally, consultation with health-care professionals on a regular basis is important. This is because early diagnosis is especially useful for controlling the damaging effects of many diseases. Overall, prevention of disease is an important investment of your time, including during one's college years.

hunger The primarily physiological (internal) drive to find and eat food, mostly regulated by innate cues to eating.

appetite The primarily psychological (external) influences that encourage us to find and eat food, often in the absence of obvious hunger.

change. You can then see why foods may have different meanings to different people and, in turn, this allows for greater appreciation of food habits that differ from yours.

Two drives influence our desire to eat and thus take in food energy: **hunger** and **appetite.** These differ dramatically. Hunger, our primarily physical biological drive to eat, is controlled by internal body mechanisms. For example, as nutrients are processed by the stomach and small intestine, these organs communicate with the liver and brain, reducing further food intake. The liver then uses its direct nerve pathways to the brain to do the same.

Appetite, our primarily psychological drive to eat, is affected by external food choice mechanisms, such as seeing a tempting dessert. Fulfilling either or both drives by eating sufficient food normally brings a state of **satiety,** temporarily halting our desire to continue eating.

▮ The Hypothalamus Contributes to Satiety Regulation

The **hypothalamus,** a portion of the brain, helps regulate satiety. When stimulated, cells in the feeding centers of the hypothalamus signal us to eat. As we eat, hunger decreases. Eventually, we stop eating as cells in the satiety centers of the hypothalamus are stimulated. The amount of blood glucose probably stimulates both the feeding and satiety centers. When blood glucose drops, we eat. When it eventually rises after a meal, we no longer have a strong desire to seek food.

Certain chemicals, surgery, and some cancers can destroy both groups of centers in the hypothalamus. Without satiety-center activity, laboratory animals (and humans) eat their way to obesity. Without feeding-center activity, animals eat little and eventually lose weight.

Overall, this entire system depends on the hypothalamus to process the signals generated by nerves responding to the various mediators of food intake. However, this concept of separate satiety and feeding centers is too simplistic to fully describe hunger regulation. We know that the hypothalamus has over 40 regions criss-crossed with a huge amount of nerves that are constantly receiving and passing on information about the body's nutritional state.

▮ Meal Size and Composition Affect Satiety

The effects of stomach expansion from food intake combined with the later intestinal absorption of nutrients during a meal reduces our desire to eat more food. These actions of the **gastrointestinal (GI) tract** contribute to a feeling of satiety. In fact, a meal is generally terminated before significant amounts of nutrients are made available for metabolism and storage. Putting this information into practice, researchers have recently shown that bulky meals produce much more satiety than do more concentrated meals (see the discussion on energy density in Chapter 2). As the dietary fiber and water content of the foods increase, humans experience increased satiety and thus do not seek another meal as quickly. Consider how you would feel if you ate five pieces of whole fruit versus one regular serving of French fries (each yielding about 380 kcals).

▮ Hormones Affect Satiety

Hormones and hormone-like compounds in our body prod us to eat. Those that increase hunger include **endorphins, cortisol,** and **neuropeptide Y.** Those that cause satiety include **leptin** (working in conjunction with the hormone insulin), **serotonin,** and **cholecystokinin (CCK).** Research is underway to produce medications that will increase the action of satiety-inducing hormones. Researchers currently suspect that many overweight individuals may have defective leptin utilization, causing satiety to be inhibited. This inhibition is because one effect of leptin is to decrease neuropeptide Y production in the hypothalamus. Preliminary studies show that daily leptin injections can contribute to success in weight loss in some overweight people, especially by lessening weight regain, because as fat stores fall, so does leptin output by **adipose tissue.** Leptin injections (current forms must be injected) help compensate for this result of weight loss.

▮ Does Appetite Affect What We Eat?

Various feeding and satiety messages from body cells do not single-handedly determine what we eat. Almost everyone has encountered a mouthwatering dessert and

satiety State in which there is no longer a desire to eat; a feeling of satisfaction.

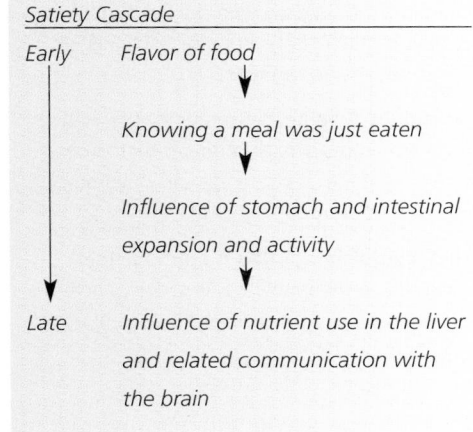

Satiety Cascade

Early — Flavor of food
↓
Knowing a meal was just eaten
↓
Influence of stomach and intestinal expansion and activity
↓
Late — Influence of nutrient use in the liver and related communication with the brain

gastrointestinal (GI) tract The main sites in the body used for digestion and absorption of nutrients. It consists of the mouth, esophagus, stomach, small intestine, large intestine, rectum, and anus.

hormone A compound secreted into the bloodstream by one type of cells that acts to control the function of another type of cells. For example, certain cells in the pancreas produce insulin, which in turn acts on muscle and other types of cells. Protein forms for the most part must be injected if used as therapy since they would be broken down if taken orally.

endorphins Natural body tranquilizers that may be involved in the feeding response.

cortisol A hormone made by the adrenal gland that, among other functions, stimulates the production of glucose from amino acids and increases the desire to eat.

adipose tissue A group of fat storing cells.

neuropeptide Y A chemical substance made in the hypothalamus that stimulates food intake. The hormone leptin inhibits neuropeptide Y production.

leptin A hormone made by adipose tissue in proportion to total fat stores in the body that influences long-term regulation of fat mass. Leptin also influences reproductive functions, as well as other body processes, such as release of the hormone insulin.

serotonin A neurotransmitter synthesized from the amino acid tryptophan that appears to decrease the desire to eat carbohydrates and to induce sleep.

cholecystokinin (CCK) A hormone that stimulates enzyme release from the pancreas, bile release from the gallbladder, and hunger regulation.

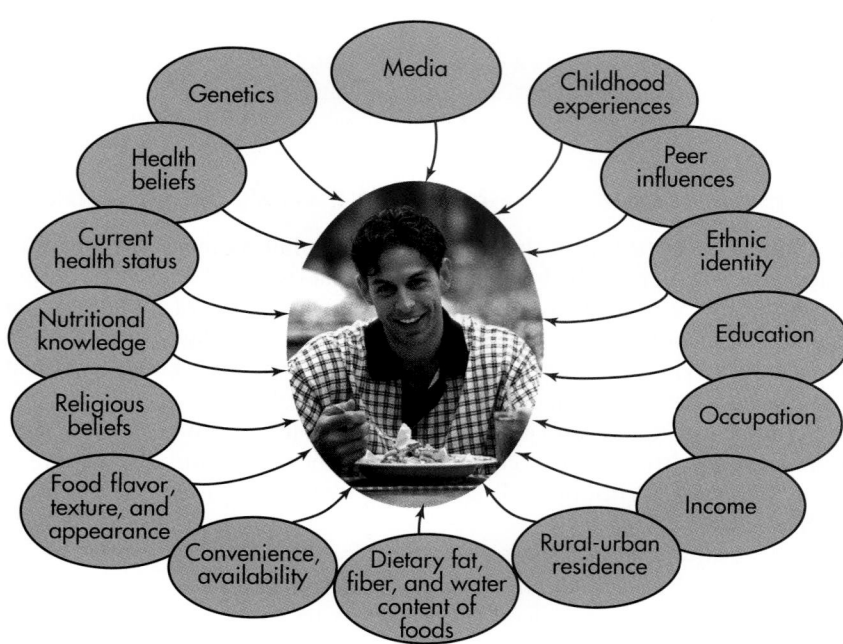

Figure 1.4 Food behavior is influenced by many sources. Which are important in your life?

Scientists suspect we are born with a taste for sweets and over time acquire a taste for fat.

devoured it, even on a full stomach. Appetite can be affected by a great variety of external forces, such as environmental and psychological factors as well as social customs (Fig. 1.4).

We often eat because food confronts us. It smells good, tastes good, and looks good. We might eat because it is the right time of day, we are celebrating, or we are trying to overcome the blues. After a meal, memories of pleasant tastes and feelings reinforce appetite. If stress or depression sends you to the refrigerator, you are mostly seeking comfort, not food energy. Appetite may not be a biological process, but it does influence food intake. Table 1.6 lists additional social and other related factors that influence food choices.

Another Bite

*S*atiety associated with consuming a meal may actually reside primarily in our psychological frame of mind. We become accustomed to a certain amount of food at a meal. Providing less than that amount leaves us wanting more. One way to put this observation into practice for weight-control purposes is to train the eye to expect less food by slowly decreasing serving sizes. Our appetites then readjust as we expect less food.

■ Putting Hunger and Appetite into Perspective

The next time you pick up a candy bar or ask for second helpings, remember the physical influences on eating behavior. Body cells (brain, stomach, small intestine, liver, and other organs), hormones (like leptin and cortisol), brain chemicals (like serotonin and neuropeptide Y), and social customs all influence food intake. When food is ample, appetite—not hunger—mostly triggers eating. Keep track of what triggers your eating for a few days. Is it primarily hunger or appetite? Note as well that satiety regulation is not perfect; body weight can fluctuate.

Table 1.6 What Else Influences Our Food Choices?

We eat primarily for nourishment, but food means far more to us than that. Food symbolizes much of what we think about ourselves. Throughout our lives, we spend 13 to 15 years eating. Beyond simple hunger and emotions, why do we choose to eat what we eat?

- Flavor and texture are the two most important aspects of our food choices. Creating more flavorful foods that are both healthy and profitable is a major focus of the food industry.

- Early influences that expose us to various people, places, and situations influence our lifelong food choices. Many aspects of ethnic diet patterns (discussed more fully in Chapter 2) begin as we are introduced to foods as children.

- Routines and habits are tied to some food choices. Most of us eat from a core group of foods: About 100 basic items account for about 75% of an individual's total food intake. Food habits and food availability strongly influence choices.

- Nutrition, or what we think of as "healthy foods," influences our food purchases. North Americans who tend to make health-related food choices are often well-educated, middle-class professionals. These same people are generally health oriented, have active lifestyles, and focus on weight control.

- Advertising is a major media tool for capturing the food interest of the consumer. The food industry in the United States alone spends well over $6 billion annually on advertising and another $26 billion on packaging. Some of this advertising is helpful, as it promotes the importance of calcium and fiber in our diets. However, the food industry also advertises highly sweetened cereals, cookies, cakes, and pastries because they often reap high profits.

- Restaurants have long been a growth industry in North America. Today, about 40% of all food dollars is spent on meals outside of home. This food is often very calorie-dense, and of poorer nutritional quality compared to foods made at home. However, over the past 10 years, restaurants have placed healthier items on their menus.

- Social changes are leading to a general "time famine" for many of us. This creates the need for convenience. Supermarkets now supply already-prepared meals, microwave entrees, and various quick-prep frozen products.

- Economics plays a minor role in food choices. The average North American spends only about 12% of after-tax income on food (compared to 50% in India). However, as income increases, so do meals eaten away from home.

Overall, daily food intake is a complicated mix of social and biological influences.

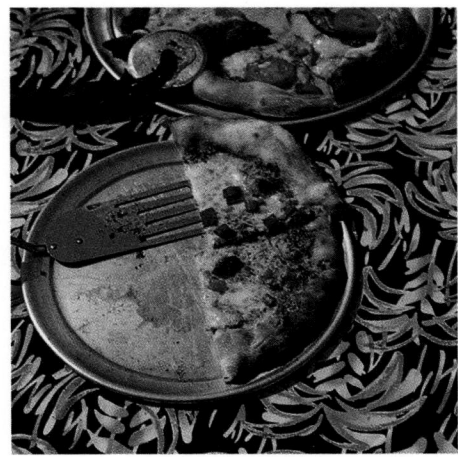

A market research firm surveyed the eating habits of people in 2000 United States households. The top meal choice was pizza, followed by ham sandwich, hot dog, peanut butter and jelly sandwich, steak, macaroni and cheese, turkey sandwich, cheese sandwich, hamburger on a bun, and spaghetti.

Concept Check

*H*unger is the primarily physical or internal desire to find and eat food. Appeasing it creates satiety—no further desire to eat exists. Satiety is influenced by hunger-related (internal) forces in the brain, gastrointestinal tract, liver, and other organs, and dietary fiber and water content of the foods in the meal. Various hormones and hormone-like compounds participate. Food intake is also affected by appetite-related (external) forces like social custom, time of day, flavor and texture, and presence of others. Recently, factors such as health concerns, economics, convenience, and social changes are also becoming important dietary determinants. North Americans probably respond more to external, appetite-related forces than to hunger-related ones in choosing when and what to eat.

Improving Our Diets

As discussed, while more efforts by the general public are needed to lower saturated fat intake and to improve variety in our diets, our cultural diversity, varied cuisines, and generally high nutritional status should be points of pride for North Americans. Today we can choose from a tremendous variety of food products, the result of continual innovation by food manufacturers.

Critical Thinking

Sarah is majoring in nutrition and is well aware of the importance of a healthy diet. She has recently been analyzing her own diet and is confused. She notices that she eats a great deal of high-fat foods, and few fruits, vegetables, and whole grains. She also has developed quite a "sweet tooth." What three factors may be influencing Sarah's food choices? What advice would you give her on how to have her diet match her needs?

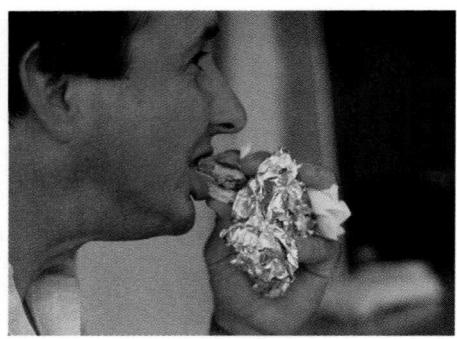

The fast-paced life for some of us requires eating on the run. What we choose should be as important as how fast it is served.

We are eating more breakfast cereals, pizza, pasta entrees, stir-fried meat and vegetables served on rice, salads, tacos, burritos, and fajitas than ever before. Sales of whole milk are down, while in the same time period sales of nonfat and 1% low-fat milk have increased. Consumption of frozen vegetables, rather than canned vegetables, is also on the rise.

Another Bite

One recent trend by food manufacturers has been to promote meal replacement bars (also called "energy" bars). These bars typically contain about 180–250 kcal, with a protein:carbohydrate:fat ratio typical of common diets. However, some bars replace much of the carbohydrate with protein. All of the bars are fortified with vitamins and minerals in amounts ranging from about 25% to 100% of typical human needs. Some people find these bars provide a convenient way to consume a meal (or snack) on the run, while also focusing on certain nutrients they may underconsume, such as the vitamin folate or the mineral calcium. These bars generally cost $1 to $2. Critics suggest these products are really just the nutritional equivalent of a low-fat yogurt and piece of fruit. Typical brands are Ensure bar, Balance bar, Gatorade Energy bar, Slim-Fast bar, Genisoy bar, Luna bar, Cliff bar, PowerBar, and Viactiv Hearty Energy bar.

Confusing and conflicting health messages also hinder diet change. Nutrition science does not have all the answers, but enough is known to (1) help you set a path to good health and (2) put diet-related recommendations you hear in the future into perspective. See Chapter 2 for details.

A dietary objective that deserves more attention is to try to eat with others more often. Mealtime is a key social time of the day. The Japanese are ahead of us in recognizing that food's powers go beyond the realm of nutrition. Their national dietary guidelines, which like ours stress the importance of eating a variety of foods, maintaining healthy weight, and moderating fat in the diet, also advise people to make all activities pertaining to food and eating pleasurable.

Today, North Americans live longer than ever before and enjoy better general health. Many also have more money, more diverse food and lifestyle choices to consider, and more time to relax and enjoy life. The nutritional consequences of these trends are not fully known. Deaths from various forms of cardiovascular disease, for example, have dropped dramatically since the late 1960s, partly because of better medical care and diets. Still, if affluence leads to sedentary lifestyles and high intakes of saturated fat, salt, and alcohol, this lifestyle pattern can lead to problems such as hypertension and obesity. Because of better technology and greater choices, we can have a much better diet today than ever before—if we know what choices to make.

The goal of this book is to help you find the best path to good nutrition. There are no "good" or "bad" (i.e., "junk") foods, but some foods provide relatively few nutrients in comparison to energy content and thus contribute to less nutritious food behaviors. One's overall diet is the proper focus in a nutritional evaluation. Chapter 2 will emphasize this point and show you how to balance your diet. As you reexamine your nutritional habits, remember your health is partly your responsibility. Your body has a natural ability to heal itself. Offer it what it needs, and it will serve you well. In addition, eating a healthy diet is one way to affirm that you care about your health.

Concept Check

Healthy food habits developed and strengthened throughout life can provide many benefits. Many of us should pay more attention to this observation.

Summary

1. Nutrition is the study of the food substances vital for health and the study of how the body uses these substances to promote and support growth, maintenance, and reproduction of cells.
2. Nutrients in foods fall into six classes: (1) carbohydrates, (2) lipids (mostly fats and oils), (3) proteins, (4) vitamins, (5) minerals, and (6) water. The first three, along with alcohol, provide energy for the body to use.
3. The body transforms the energy contained in carbohydrate, protein, and fat into other forms of energy, which allow the body to function. Fat provides, on average, 9 kcal per gram, whereas protein and carbohydrate each provides, on average, 4 kcal per gram. Vitamins, minerals, and water do not supply energy to the body but are essential for proper body function.
4. A basic plan for health promotion and disease prevention includes eating a varied diet, performing regular physical activity, not smoking, not abusing nutrient supplements (if used), getting adequate fluid and sleep, limiting alcohol intake (if consumed), and limiting or coping with stress.
5. The focus of nutrition planning should be on food, not primarily on dietary supplements. The focus on foods to supply nutrient needs avoids the possibility of severe nutrient imbalances.
6. Results from large nutrition surveys in the United States and Canada suggest that some of us need to concentrate on consuming foods that supply more of certain vitamins, minerals, and dietary fiber. Use of a daily multivitamin and mineral supplement is another strategy.
7. Groups of cells in the hypothalamus and other regions in the brain affect hunger, the primarily internal desire to find and eat food. These cells monitor hormonal and nerve signals from digestive organs and nutrients and other substances in the blood to control satiety.
8. A variety of external (appetite-related) forces affect satiety. Hunger cues combine with appetite cues, such as easy availability of food, to promote food intake.
9. The flavor and texture of foods primarily influence our food choices. Several other factors also help determine food habits and choices: our upbringing, various social and cultural factors, the image we want to project to others, economics, and concerns about health.
10. There are no true "good" or "bad" foods. The focus should be on balancing a total diet by choosing many nutritious foods.

Study Questions

1. Name one chronic disease associated with poor nutrition habits. Now list a few corresponding risk factors.
2. Explain the concept of energy as it relates to foods. What are the fuel (energy) values used for a gram of carbohydrate, fat, protein, and alcohol?
3. Identify three ways that water is used in the body.
4. Wendy's Big Bacon Classic contains 44 grams carbohydrate, 36 grams fat, and 37 grams protein. Calculate the percentage of energy derived from fat.
5. Describe two types of fat and explain why the differences are important in terms of overall health.
6. According to national nutrition surveys, which nutrients tend to be underconsumed by many North Americans? Why do you think this is the case?
7. List four health objectives for the United States for the year 2010. How would you rate yourself in each area? Why?
8. Describe the various organs and hormones that control hunger and satiety in the body. List other factors that influence our food patterns.
9. Describe how your own food preferences have been shaped by the following factors:
   a. Exposure to foods at an early age
   b. Advertising (what is the newest food you have tried?)
   c. Eating out
   d. Peer pressure
   e. Economic factors
10. What products in your supermarket reflect the consumer demand for healthier foods? For convenience?

Further Readings

1. Blumenthal SJ: A top woman doctor tells how to get past the hype to the truth. *American Health*, p. 36, January/February 1998.
The assistant U.S. surgeon general provides advice on how to interpret research findings that appear in the media, such as who paid for the study and whether the findings are supported by previous studies.

2. Breslow L: From disease prevention to health promotion. *Journal of the American Medical Association* 281:1030, 1999.
Current concepts of health promotion are discussed, including goals such as increasing moderate daily physical activity and reducing excessive alcohol use as important health preventive measures.

3. Checkup for the new millennium. *Consumer Reports on Health*, p. 1, December 1999.
A checklist of both healthy habits and not-so-healthy habits is given, along with suggested changes in habits to maximize wellness. The focus is on a balanced diet, maintaining a healthy weight, and performing regular physical activity.

4. Glanz K and others: Why Americans eat what they do: Taste, nutrition, cost, convenience, and weight control concerns as influences on food consumption. *Journal of the American Dietetic Association* 98:1118, 1998.
Nutrition concerns are, unfortunately, less relevant to most people than taste and cost when it comes to food choice. One implication is that nutrition education programs should promote nutritious diets that are tasty and inexpensive.

5. *Healthy People 2010* targets healthy diet and healthy weight as critical goals. *Journal of the American Dietetic Association* 100:300, 2000.
Many of the nutrition goals included in Healthy People 2010 are enumerated. Two key goals are to reduce obesity and inactivity in the American population.

6. Kant AK and others: A prospective study of diet quality and mortality in women. *Journal of the American Medical Association* 283:2109, 2000.
Women whose diets included plenty of fruits, vegetables, whole grains, and low-fat meats and dairy products showed a 30% reduction in death, compared with those who ate the most unhealthy diets.

7. Liebman B: Defensive eating: Staying lean in a fattening world. *Nutrition Action Healthletter*, p. 1, December 2001.
Food in North America is widely available and generally inexpensive, and the number of opportunities to eat has risen dramatically—drugstores, gas stations, and shopping malls to name a few. In response, one strategy for weight control is to fill your plate with salad greens and vegetables and use calorie-dense foods as condiments. Also watch portion size—the bigger the portion, the more people eat.

8. Liebman B, Schardt D: Diet and health: Ten megatrends. *Nutrition Action Healthletter*, p. 1, January/February 2001.
Both positive and negative trends in the American diet in the past 30 years are shown in graphic form, demonstrating that improvements have been made in deaths from cardiovascular disease, but obesity is increasingly becoming a problem. Large restaurant serving sizes are one contributor to this problem.

9. Lifestyle and aging. *Mayo Clinic Health Letter*, p. 4, July 1999.
Mayo Clinic physicians provide their advice for a healthy lifestyle, such as getting regular exercise, opting for many whole-grain choices, and drinking alcohol in moderation, if at all.

10. McBean LD: Nutrition research: What can studies tell us? *Dairy Council Digest* 72(6): 31, 2001.
Different types of nutrition research studies vary in their strengths and weaknesses. Rarely can a single study provide evidence of cause and effect between diet and disease. This cause and effect relationship becomes more probable when data from several different types of studies are consistent.

11. Rosenbaum M, Leibel RL: Role of leptin in human physiology. *The New England Journal of Medicine* 341:913, 1999.
During times of reduced energy intake, the fall in leptin production results in the preferential storage of ingested calories as fat, increased food intake, reduced metabolism (in rodents), and decreased fertility. Although leptin administration does not always produce effortless weight loss, such treatment might have clinical value in making compliance with a low-calorie diet easier and in maintaining reduced body weight by lessening the fall in both metabolism and hunger that accompanies weight loss.

12. Tippet KS and others: Food consumption surveys in the U.S. Dept. of Agriculture. *Nutrition Today* 34:33, 1999.
The variety of food consumption surveys conducted over the past 80 years by the U.S. Department of Agriculture are described, including studies currently underway. These indicate few adults consume the recommended amounts of fruits and vegetables each day.

13. Wellness guide to preventive care. *UC Berkeley Wellness Letter*, p. 4, November 2001.
Important habits that contribute to wellness are: maintaining a healthy weight; performing regular exercise; choosing a diet low in animal fat and sodium and rich in fruits, vegetables, whole grains, and low-fat or nonfat dairy products; eating at least two servings of fish a week; and moderating alcohol consumption if used.

14. Wetter AC and others: How and why do individuals make food and physical activity choices? *Nutrition Reviews* 59(3):S11–S20, 2001.
Health habits are influenced by a number of factors: beliefs, values, life experiences, socioeconomic status, educational attainment, interpersonal relationships, life stage, and social roles. Each decision made regarding health practices depends on input from these and other factors.

I. Examine Your Eating Habits More Closely

Choose one day of the week that is typical of your eating pattern. Using the first table found in Appendix E, list all foods and drinks you consumed for 24 hours. In addition, write down the approximate amounts of food you ate in units, such as cups, ounces, teaspoons, and tablespoons. Check the food composition table in Appendix A for examples of appropriate serving units for different types of foods, such as meat and vegetables. After completing this activity, you will use this list of foods for future assignments.

After you record the amount of each food and drink consumed, indicate in the table why you chose to consume the item. Use the following symbols to indicate your reasons. Place the corresponding abbreviation in the space provided to indicate why you picked that food or drink.

FLVR	Flavor/texture	ADV	Advertisement	PEER	Peers
CONV	Convenience	WTCL	Weight control	NUTR	Nutritive value
EMO	Emotions	HUNG	Hunger	$	Cost
AVA	Availability	FAM	Family/cultural	HLTH	Health

There can be more than one reason for choosing a particular food or drink.

Application

Now ask yourself what your most frequent reason is for eating or drinking. To what degree is health a reason for your food choices? *HIGH* Should you make it a higher priority? *NO*

II. Observe the Supermarket Explosion

Today's supermarkets carry up to 60,000 items, compared to 20,000 items 10 years ago. Think about your last grocery shopping trip and the items you purchased to eat. Following is a list of 20 newer food products added to supermarket shelves. Check the items that you have tried. Then use the Key from Part I of the Rate Your Plate exercise to identify why you might have chosen these products.

___X___ Prepackaged salad greens (variety packs other than iceberg lettuce) *CONV, HLTH*

_____ Gourmet salad oils (i.e., walnut, almond, olive, or sesame oil) _____

_____ Gourmet vinegars (i.e., balsamic or rice) _____

_____ Prepackaged lunch products (i.e., nacho, pizza, taco, and tortilla Lunchables) _____

_____ Precooked frozen turkey patties _____

_____ Bean soup mixes (i.e., lentil, black bean, combination bean soups) _____

_____ Microwaveable sandwiches (i.e., Hotpockets, frozen sandwiches) _____

___X___ Refrigerated, precooked pasta (i.e., tortellini, fettucini) and accompanying sauces (i.e., pesto, tomato basil) *CONV, FLVR*

_____ Imported grain products (i.e., risotto, farfalline, gnocchi, fusilli) _____

___X___ Frozen dinners (list your favorite of any of the wide variety) *BOSTON MARKET, CONV, FLVR*

_____ Imported sauces for food preparation (i.e., hoisin or brown bean sauce, mandarin marinade, sesame, curry, or fire oils) _____

_____ Bottled waters (flavored or unflavored) _____

_____ Trendy juices (i.e., draft apple cider, hurricane punch) _____

_____ Roasted and/or flavored coffees (i.e., beans, ground, or instant) _____

_____ Gourmet jelly beans and candies (i.e., gummi coca-colas or imported chocolates) _____

_____ Instant hot cereal in a bowl (add water and go!) _____

_____ "Fast-shake" pancake mix (add water, shake, and ready to cook) _____

_____ Breakfast bars (i.e., granola or fruit-flavored bars) _____

___X___ Meal replacement/fitness products (i.e., "energy" bars, high-protein bars, sports drinks) *POWER BARS, HLTH*

Finally, identify three new food products that are not on this list that you have seen in the past year. Discuss the appeal of these products to the North American consumer.

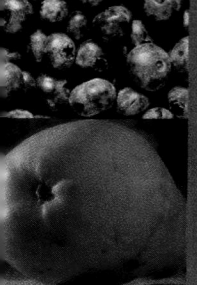

Using Scientific Research to Determine Nutrient Needs

hypotheses "Educated guesses" by a scientist to explain a phenomenon.

pellagra A disease characterized by inflammation of the skin, diarrhea, and eventual mental incapacity; results from an insufficient amount of the vitamin niacin in the diet.

experiments Tests made to examine the validity of a hypothesis.

theory An explanation for a phenomenon that has numerous lines of evidence to support it.

ulcer Erosion of the tissue lining, usually in the stomach (gastric ulcer) or the upper small intestine (duodenal ulcer). These are generally referred to as peptic ulcers.

How do we know what we know about nutrition? How has this knowledge been gained? In a word, research. Like other sciences, the research that sets the foundation for nutrition knowledge has developed through the use of the *scientific method,* a procedure for testing designed to detect and eliminate error. The first step is the observation of a natural phenomenon. Scientists then suggest possible explanations, called **hypotheses,** about its cause. Distinguishing a true cause-and-effect relationship from mere coincidence can be difficult. For instance, earlier in the twentieth century, many patients in mental hospitals in the southern United States suffered from the disease **pellagra**, which suggested a possible relationship between the climate in that region (and, in particular, the mosquitoes that thrived in the climate) and this disease. In time, it became clear that this supposed connection was simply coincidental; the real culprit was the poor diet common to rural people at that time (see Chapter 8 for details).

To test hypotheses and eliminate coincidental explanations, scientists perform controlled scientific **experiments.** The data gathered from these experiments may either support or refute each hypothesis. If the results of many experiments support a hypothesis, the hypothesis becomes generally accepted by scientists and can be called a **theory** (such as the theory of gravity). Very often, the results from one experiment suggest a new set of questions to be answered (Fig. 1.5).

The scientific method requires a skeptical attitude. Scientists must not accept proposed hypotheses and theories until they are supported by considerable evidence, and they must reject those that fail to pass critical analyses. Likewise, students should adopt a healthy skepticism and be critical of many current ideas about nutrition.

A recent example of this need for skepticism involves stomach **ulcers.** Not so many years ago, "everyone knew" that stomach ulcers were caused by a stressful lifestyle and a poor diet. Then, in 1983, an Australian physician, Dr. Barry Marshall, reported in a respected medical journal that ulcers are usually caused by a common microorganism called *Helicobacter pylori.* Furthermore, he stated that a cure is possible using antibiotics. At first, other physicians were skeptical about this finding and continued to prescribe medications that reduce stomach acid. But, as more studies were published, and patients were cured of ulcers using antibiotics, the medical profession eventually accepted the findings, and today, ulcers are managed for the most part by medications that destroy the pathogen. Overall, we can expect that scientific discoveries will always be subject to challenge and change.

In sum, scientific research requires that:

1. Questions are asked
2. Hypotheses are generated
3. Research is conducted (experiments)
4. Incorrect explanations are rejected
5. The most likely explanation for an observation is proposed
6. The research results are subjected to review by other scientists and published in a scientific journal
7. The research results are confirmed by more experiments

■ Asking Questions and Generating Hypotheses

Historical events have provided clues to important relationships in nutrition science. In the fifteenth and sixteenth centuries, for example, many European sailors on the long voyages to the Americas developed the disease scurvy. The sailors ate few fruits and vegetables, and eventually

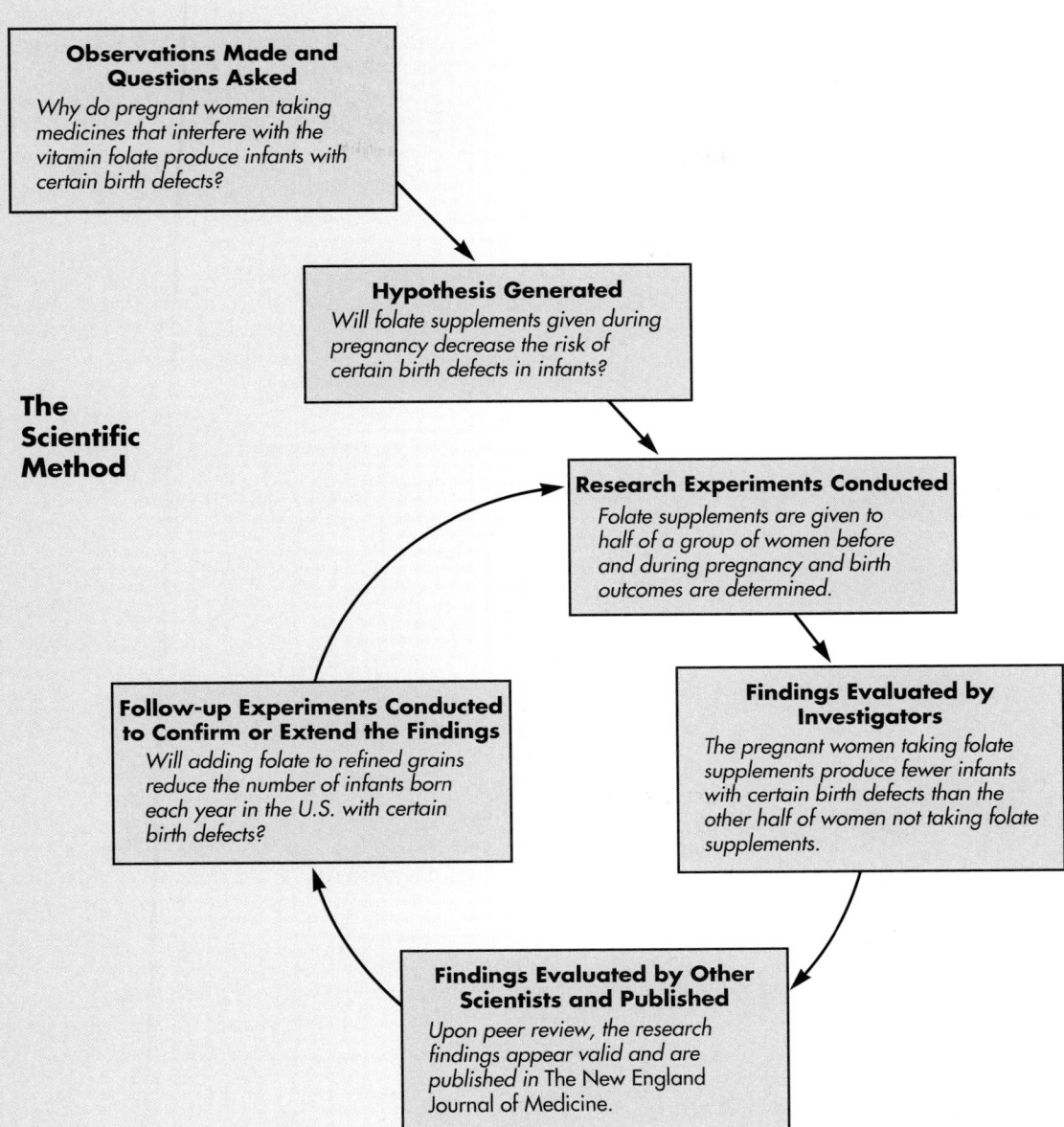

The Scientific Method

Observations Made and Questions Asked
Why do pregnant women taking medicines that interfere with the vitamin folate produce infants with certain birth defects?

Hypothesis Generated
Will folate supplements given during pregnancy decrease the risk of certain birth defects in infants?

Research Experiments Conducted
Folate supplements are given to half of a group of women before and during pregnancy and birth outcomes are determined.

Findings Evaluated by Investigators
The pregnant women taking folate supplements produce fewer infants with certain birth defects than the other half of women not taking folate supplements.

Findings Evaluated by Other Scientists and Published
Upon peer review, the research findings appear valid and are published in The New England Journal of Medicine.

Follow-up Experiments Conducted to Confirm or Extend the Findings
Will adding folate to refined grains reduce the number of infants born each year in the U.S. with certain birth defects?

Figure 1.5 Implementing the scientific method using the vitamin folate as an example. Scientists consistently follow these steps in conducting scientific research. It is important not to embrace a nutrition or other scientific concept until it has been thoroughly tested using the scientific method. Incidentally, the answer to the follow-up experiment question regarding folate was *yes* (see Chapter 8 for details).

a British naval surgeon, Dr. James Lind, discovered that lime juice prevents or cures the **scurvy.** After this, sailors were given a ration of lime juice, earning them the nickname "limeys." This simple practice ensured a healthy workforce for the British navy and helped it dominate the seas worldwide. About 200 years later, scientists identified vitamin C, the nutrient present in fruits and vegetables that prevents scurvy.

In a related approach to using historical observation, scientists establish nutritional hypotheses by studying the dietary and disease patterns among various populations in today's world. If one group tends to develop a certain disease but another group does not, scientists can speculate about the role diet plays in this difference. The study of diseases in populations is called **epidemiology,** and ultimately forms the bases for many laboratory studies.

scurvy The deficiency disease that results after a few weeks to months of consuming a diet that lacks vitamin C; pinpoint sites of bleeding are an early sign.

epidemiology The study of how disease rates vary among different population groups. For example, the rate of stomach cancer in Japan could be compared with that in Germany.

continued

infectious disease Any disease caused by invasion of the body by microorganisms, such as bacteria, fungi, or viruses.

incidence The number of new cases of a disease in a defined population over a specific period of time, such as 1 year.

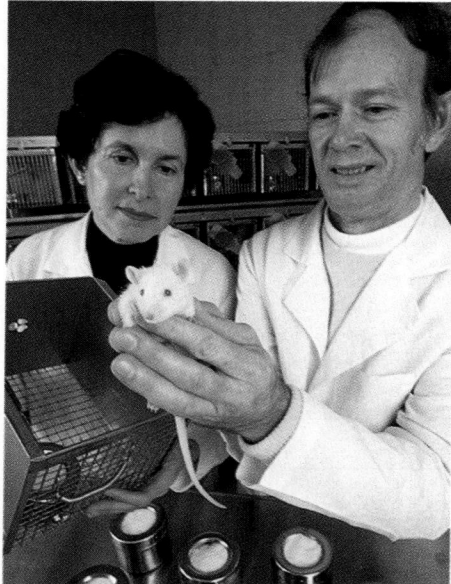

Research using laboratory animals contributes to our nutrition knowledge.

animal model Study of disease in animals that duplicates human disease. This can be used to understand more about human disease.

double-blind study An experimental design in which neither the participants nor the researchers are aware of each participant's assignment (test or placebo) or the outcome of the study until it is completed. An independent third party holds the code and the data until the study has been completed.

control group Participants in an experiment who are not given the treatment being tested.

An example of this approach occurred in the 1920s, in the United States, when a physician, Dr. Joseph Goldberger, noticed that prisoners in jail—but not their jailers—suffered from the disease pellagra discussed earlier. He reasoned that, if pellagra were an **infectious disease,** both populations would suffer from it. Since this was not the case, he concluded that pellagra is probably caused by a dietary deficiency.

Historical and epidemiological findings can suggest hypotheses about the role of diet in various health problems. To prove the role of particular dietary components, however, requires controlled experiments. For instance, once the high **incidence** of pellagra in mental institutions during the 1920s was linked to poor diet, various foods were given to patients who had the disease. These experiments showed that yeast and high-protein foods could cure these patients if the disease was not in its final stage, indicating that pellagra results from a deficiency of some nutrient present in these foods. Eventually, this nutrient was found to be the B vitamin called niacin.

■ Laboratory Animal Experiments

When scientists cannot test their hypotheses by experiments with humans, they often use animals. Much of what we know about human nutritional needs and functions has been generated from animal experiments. Still human experiments are the most convincing to scientists. In the 1930s, scientists showed that a pellagra-like disease seen in dogs, called *blacktongue,* is cured by nicotinic acid. Only when nicotinic acid actually cured the disease in humans were scientists convinced that nicotinic acid, later identified as the vitamin niacin, was the critical dietary factor.

Today, we know that low doses of the mineral fluoride can stimulate growth in rats. However, we still do not know whether this is true for humans, because it is not practical to control the fluoride intake of humans accurately enough to answer the question. Thus, fluoride might stimulate growth in humans, but real proof is lacking.

In addition, the use of humans in certain types of experiments is considered unethical. Although some people argue that animal experiments are also unethical, most people believe that the careful, humane use of animals is an acceptable alternative to using human subjects. For example, most people would think it is reasonable to feed rats a low-copper diet to study the importance of this mineral in the formation of blood vessels. Almost universally, however, people would object to a similar study in infants.

The use of animal experiments to study the role of nutrition in certain human diseases depends on the availability of an **animal model**—a disease in laboratory animals that closely mimics a particular human disease. If no animal model is available and human experiments are ruled out, scientific knowledge often cannot advance beyond what can be learned from epidemiological studies.

■ Human Experiments

Various experimental approaches are used to test research hypotheses in humans, including case-control and double-blind studies.

Case-Control Study

In a **case-control study,** individuals who have the condition in question, such as lung cancer, are compared with individuals who do not have the condition. Comparisons are made only between groups that are matched for other major characteristics (e.g., age, race, and gender) not under study. This type of study may identify factors other than the disease in question, such as fruit and vegetable intake, that differ between the two groups, thus providing researchers with clues about the cause, progression, and prevention of the disease, but no specific evidence of cause and effect.

Double-Blind Study

An important approach for more definitive testing of hypotheses is the **double-blind study,** in which a group of participants—the experimental group—follows a specific protocol (e.g., consuming a certain food or nutrient), and participants in a corresponding **control group** conform to their normal habits. People are randomly assigned to each group, such as by the flip of a coin.

Scientists then observe the experimental group over time to see if there is any effect that is not found in the control group. Sometimes individuals are used as their own control: First they are observed for a period of time, and then they are treated and their responses noted.

Two features of a double-blind study help reduce the introduction of bias (prejudice), which can easily affect the outcome of an experiment. First, neither the participants nor the researchers know which individuals are in the experimental group and which are in the control group. Second, the expected effects of the experimental protocol are not disclosed to the participants or researchers until after the entire study is completed. This approach reduces the possibility that researchers may see the change they want to see in the participants to prove a certain "pet" hypothesis, even though such a change did not actually occur. This approach also reduces the chance that the persons participating begin to feel better simply because they are involved in a research study or are receiving a new treatment, a phenomenon called the *placebo effect*.

Derived from the Latin word **placebo** meaning "I shall please," the placebo effect cannot be explained by pharmacological or other direct physical action. It may instead be linked to a simple reduction in stress and anxiety. Overall, it is critical to make allowances for the placebo effect in research studies.

In a double-blind experiment, the control group often receives a sugar pill or other placebo to camouflage who is in which group and thereby eliminate the bias introduced by the placebo effect. During the course of the experiment, neither the researchers nor the participants know who is getting the real treatment and who is getting a placebo. Sometimes only a single-blind protocol is possible, in which either the participants or the researchers are kept in the dark. Either way, now it is up to the experimental treatment—not just the practice of both groups taking a pill—to show an effect, if one is possible.

Drug studies lend themselves to double-blind protocols because it is often easy to substitute a placebo for the drug. However, food studies often cannot be placebo controlled. For example, disguising a diet high in fruits and vegetables from one low in them is difficult. In such a study, the experimenters should try to ensure that the results from blood assays or other measurements are not revealed until the end of the study. In addition, the results should be kept from the participants until the end of the study. These precautions can eliminate much potential bias. The more bias that is controlled in an experiment, the more confidence we can have in the results.

A recent example illustrates the need to test hypotheses based on epidemiological observations in double-blind studies. Epidemiologists using primarily case-control studies found that smokers who regularly consumed fruits and vegetables had a lower risk for lung cancer than smokers who ate few fruits and vegetables. Some scientists proposed that beta-carotene, a pigment present in many fruits and vegetables, could reduce the damage that tobacco smoke creates in the lungs. This hypothesis helped fuel sales of supplements of beta-carotene.

However, in double-blind studies involving heavy smokers, the risk of lung cancer was found to be higher for those who took beta-carotene than for those who did not. Some investigators criticized this research, arguing that the beta-carotene was given too late in the smokers' lives to be of much use, but even these critics did not suspect that the substance would increase cancer risk. Soon after these results were reported, the U.S. federal agency supporting two other large ongoing studies that employed beta-carotene supplements called a halt to the research, stating that these supplements are ineffective in preventing both lung cancer and cardiovascular disease.

Overall, health and nutrition advice provided by grandparents, parents, friends, and other well-meaning individuals can't be verified unless it is put to the ultimate scientific test—blinded studies. Until that is done, we can't be sure that the substance or procedure in question is truly effective. One reason for this is the influence of the placebo effect. In addition, many common symptoms, such as sneezing, lower back pain, and headache, go away within a month or so without any treatment, reflecting the natural course of the underlying diseases. When people say, "I get fewer colds now that I take vitamin C," they overlook the fact that many cold symptoms disappear quickly with no treatment; the apparent curative effect of vitamin C or any other remedy is often coincidental rather than causal to the natural healing process.

continued

placebo Generally a fake medicine used to disguise the roles of participants in an experiment; if fake surgery is performed, it is called a *sham operation*.

Critical Thinking

For thousands of years, early humans consumed a diet rich in vegetable products and low in animal products. These diets were generally lower in fat and higher in dietary fiber than modern diets. Do the differences in human diets throughout history necessarily tell us which diet is better—that of early humans or of modern humans? If not, what is a more reliable way to pursue this question of potential diet superiority?

All consumers need to become more sophisticated about science, its accepted standards of evidence, and its current limitations. Failure to do so leads many to a frantic pursuit of fraudulent remedies. To ignore science is to follow an inferior path—the road of hard knocks. Those who follow this road learn about the dangers of various health practices primarily from the experiences of being harmed by them. Medical science does not ignore novel approaches to disease prevention and cure. Anecdotes and personal experiences are important clues to fruitful experimentation, but they are not credible evidence.

■ Peer Review of Experimental Results

Once an experiment is complete, scientists summarize the findings and publish the results in scientific journals. Generally, before articles are published in scientific journals, they are critically reviewed by other scientists familiar with the subject. The objective of this peer review is to ensure that only high-quality research findings are published. This is an important step because most scientific research in this country is funded by the federal government, nonprofit foundations, drug companies, and other private industries. All of these funding sources can have strong expectations about the research outcomes. In theory, the scientists conducting these research studies will be fair in evaluating their results and will not be influenced by the funding agency. Peer review helps ensure that the researchers are as objective as possible. This then helps ensure that results published in **peer-reviewed journals,** such as the *American Journal of Clinical Nutrition, The New England Journal of Medicine,* and the *Journal of the American Dietetic Association,* are much more reliable than those found in popular magazines or promoted on television talk shows. Unfortunately, reputable journals are not the main sources for the information presented in the popular media, and claims are seldom scrutinized by competent researchers for accuracy and scientific validity.

■ Follow-Up Studies

Even if an acceptable protocol has been followed and the results of a study have been accepted by the scientific community, one experiment is never enough to prove a particular hypothesis or provide a basis for nutritional recommendations. Rather, the results obtained in one laboratory must be confirmed by experiments conducted in other laboratories. Only then can we really trust and use the results. The more lines of evidence available to support an idea, the more likely it is to be true (Fig. 1.6). It is important to avoid rushing to accept new ideas as fact or incorporating them into your health habits until they are proved by several lines of evidence.

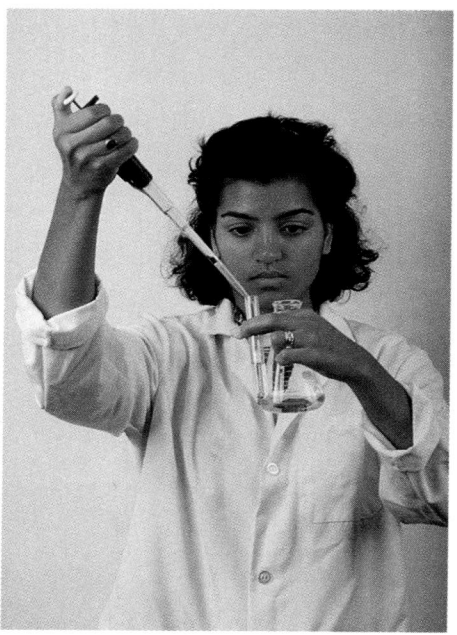

Careful research contributes to nutrition knowledge, more so than personal experience.

How to Use This Knowledge to Evaluate Nutrition Claims and Advice

Based on what has been covered so far, the following suggestions should help you make healthful and logical nutrition decisions:
1. Apply the basic principles of nutrition as outlined in this chapter (and the Food Guide Pyramid and related resources in Chapter 2) to any nutrition claim. Do you note any inconsistencies? Do reliable references support the claims? Beware of the following:
   • Testimonials about personal experience
   • Disreputable publication sources
   • Dramatic results (rarely true)
   • Lack of evidence from supporting studies made by other scientists
2. Examine the background and scientific credentials of the individual, organizations, or publication making the nutritional claim. Usually, a reputable author is one whose educational background or present affiliation is with a nationally recognized university or medical center that offers programs or courses in the field of nutrition, medicine, or a closely allied specialty.
3. Be wary if the answer is "Yes" to any of the following questions about a health-related nutrition claim:
   • Are only advantages discussed and possible disadvantages ignored?

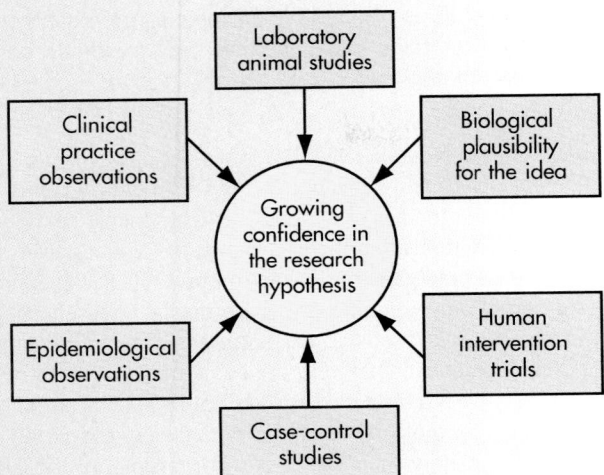

Figure 1.6 Data from a variety of sources can come together to support a research hypothesis. For example, epidemiological studies show that type 2 diabetes is characteristically found in obese populations, compared with leaner populations. Physicians notice in clinical practice that type 2 diabetes is much more likely in their obese patients, compared with their leaner patients. Laboratory animal studies show that overfeeding that eventually leads to obesity often leads to the development of type 2 diabetes. Case-control studies show that obese patients are much more likely to have type 2 diabetes than the learner comparison group that is matched for other characteristics. Finally, human intervention trials show that weight loss can correct type 2 diabetes in many people. Laboratory researchers also show that the enlarged adipose cells associated with excess fat deposition and obesity are much less responsive to the hormonal signals involved in blood glucose regulation (see Chapter 4). All of these lines of data come together with biological plausibility from various laboratory studies to support the research hypothesis that obesity can lead to type 2 diabetes.

- Are claims made about "curing" disease? Do they sound too good to be true?
- Is extreme bias against the medical community or traditional medical treatments evident? Physicians as a group strive to cure diseases in their patients, using what proven techniques are available. They do not ignore reliable cures.
- Is the claim touted as a new or secret scientific breakthrough?

4. Note the size and duration of any study cited in support of a nutrition claim. The larger it is and the longer it went on, the more dependable its findings. Also consider the type of study: epidemiology versus case-control versus double-blind. Check out the group studied; a study of men or women in Sweden may be less relevant than one of men or women of Southern European, African, or Hispanic descent, for example. Keep in mind that "contributes to," "is linked to," or "is associated with" does not mean "causes."

5. Beware of press conferences and other hype regarding the latest findings. Much of this will not survive more detailed scientific evaluation.

6. When you meet with a nutrition professional, you should expect that he or she will do the following:
   - Ask questions about your medical history, lifestyle, and current eating habits.
   - Formulate a diet plan tailored to your needs, as opposed to simply tearing a form from a tablet that could apply to almost anyone.
   - Schedule follow-up visits to track your progress, answer any questions, and help keep you motivated.
   - Involve family members in the diet plan, when appropriate.
   - Consult directly with your physician and readily refer you back to your physician for those health problems a nutrition professional is not trained to treat.

7. Avoid practitioners who prescribe **megadoses** of vitamin and mineral supplements for every-one or sell them in connection with their practice.

continued

*R*ecently major nutrition organizations put together 10 red flags that they consider signals for poor nutrition advice:

1. Recommendations that promise a quick fix
2. Dire warnings of dangers from a single product or regimen
3. Claims that sound too good to be true
4. Simplistic conclusions drawn from a complex study
5. Recommendations based on a single study
6. Dramatic statements that are refuted by reputable scientific organizations
7. Lists of "good" and "bad" foods
8. Recommendations made to help sell a product
9. Recommendations based on studies published without peer review
10. Recommendations from studies that ignore differences among individuals or groups

megadose Generally, an intake of a nutrient in excess of 10 times human need.

8. Examine product labels carefully. Be skeptical of any product promotion not clearly stated on the label. A product is not likely to do something that is not specifically claimed on its label or package insert (legally part of the label).

This cautious approach to nutrition-related advice and products is even more important today because of sweeping changes in federal law in the United States passed in 1994.

The Dietary Supplement Health and Education Act (DSHEA) of 1994 classified vitamins, minerals, amino acids, and herbal remedies as "foods," effectively restraining the U.S. Food and Drug Administration (FDA) from regulating them as heavily as food additives and drugs. According to this act, rather than the manufacturer having to prove a nutritional product is safe, FDA must prove it is unsafe before preventing its sale. In contrast, the safety of food additives and drugs must be demonstrated to FDA's satisfaction before they are marketed.

Currently, a dietary supplement (or herbal product) can be marketed in the United States without FDA approval if (1) there is a history of its use or other evidence that it is expected to be reasonably safe when used under the conditions recommended or suggested in its labeling, and (2) the product is labeled as a dietary supplement. It is permissible for the labels on such products to claim a benefit related to a classic nutrient-deficiency disease, describe how a nutrient affects human body structure or function (called structure/function claims; see the section on nutrition labeling in Chapter 2 for details), and claim that general well-being results from consumption of the ingredient(s). Examples could be "maintains bone health" or "improves blood circulation." However, the label of products bearing such claims also must prominently display in boldface type the following disclaimer: "This statement has not been evaluated by the Food and Drug Administration. This product is not intended to diagnose, treat, cure, or prevent any disease." Despite this warning, when consumers find these products on the shelves of supermarkets, health-food stores, and pharmacies, they may mistakenly assume FDA has carefully evaluated the products. (The effectiveness and safety of many herbal and related products is discussed in more detail in the Nutrition Issue in Chapter 15.)

The fact remains that many of us are willing to try untested nutrition products and believe in their miraculous actions. Popular products claim to increase muscle growth, enhance sexuality, boost energy, reduce body fat, increase strength, supply missing nutrients, increase longevity, and even improve brain function. Clearly, many nutritional products commonly found in stores are not strictly regulated in terms of effectiveness. Few have been thoroughly evaluated by reputable scientists. If you embark on a self-cure by means of such products, you will probably waste money and possibly risk ill health. A better approach is to consult a physician or registered dietitian first. You can find a registered dietitian in North America by consulting the Yellow pages in the telephone directory, contacting the local dietetic association, or calling the dietary department of a local hospital. Make sure the person has the credentials "R.D." after his/her name ("R.D.N." is also used in Canada). This indicates the person has completed rigorous classroom and clinical training in nutrition and participates in continuing education. Appendix I also lists many reputable sources of nutrition advice for your use. Finally, the following websites can help you evaluate ongoing nutrition and health claims:

www.acsh.org
www.quackwatch.com
www.ncahf.org
dietary-supplements.info.nih.gov
www.fda.gov
navigator.tufts.edu.

The sites are maintained by groups or individuals committed to providing reasoned and authoritative nutrition and health advice to consumers. If you would like a daily email on the latest in nutrition research, contact subscribe@NutritionNewsFocus.com and leave a blank message. Overall, nutrition is a rapidly advancing field and there are always new findings.

The American Dietetic Association has a toll-free hotline (800) 366-1655 that provides dietitian referrals through the Nationwide Nutrition Network and nutrition messages in English and Spanish. You can also find out more about nutrition on their website   In Canada, use   to find dietetic professionals.

www.eatright.org.
www.dietitians.ca

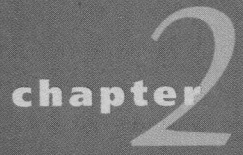

chapter 2

Tools for Designing a Healthy Diet

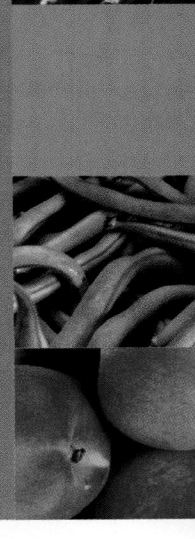

Chapter Outline

*H*ow many times have you heard wild claims about how healthful certain foods are for you? As consumers focus more and more on diet and disease, food manufacturers are asserting that their products have all sorts of health benefits. Supermarket shelves have begun to look like an 1800s medicine show. "Take fish oil capsules to avoid a heart attack." "Eat more olive oil and oat bran to lower blood cholesterol." Hearing these claims, you would think that food manufacturers have solutions to all of our health problems.

Advertising aside, nutrient intakes out of balance with our needs—such as excess energy, saturated fat, salt, alcohol, and sugar intake—are linked to many leading causes of death in North America, including obesity, hypertension, cardiovascular disease, cancer, liver disease, and type 2 diabetes. In Chapter 2, you will explore the components of a healthy diet—a diet that will minimize your risks of developing nutrition-related diseases. The goal is to provide you with a firm understanding of basic diet-planning concepts before you study the nutrients in detail.

Check out the **Contemporary Nutrition: Issues and Insights Online Learning Center at** www.mhhe.com/wardlawcont5 *for quizzes, flash cards, other activities, and web links designed to further help you learn about various tools for diet planning.*

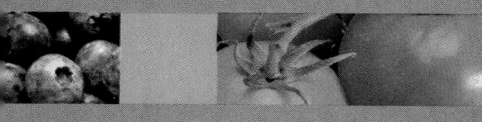
Real Life Scenario

Andy is like many other college students. He grew up on a quick bowl of cereal and milk for breakfast and a hamburger, French fries, and cola for lunch, either in the school cafeteria or at a local fast-food restaurant. At dinner, he generally avoided eating any of his salad or vegetables, and by 9 o'clock he was deep into bags of chips and cookies. Andy has taken most of these habits to college. He prefers coffee for breakfast and possibly a chocolate bar. Lunch is still mainly a hamburger, French fries, and cola, but pizza and tacos now alternate more frequently than when he was in high school. One thing Andy really likes about the restaurants surrounding campus is that, for just about half a dollar more, he can *supersize* his meal. This helps him stretch his food dollar; searching out value meals for lunch and dinner now has become part of a typical day.

Provide some dietary advice for Andy. Start with his positive habits and then provide some constructive criticism, based on what you now know.

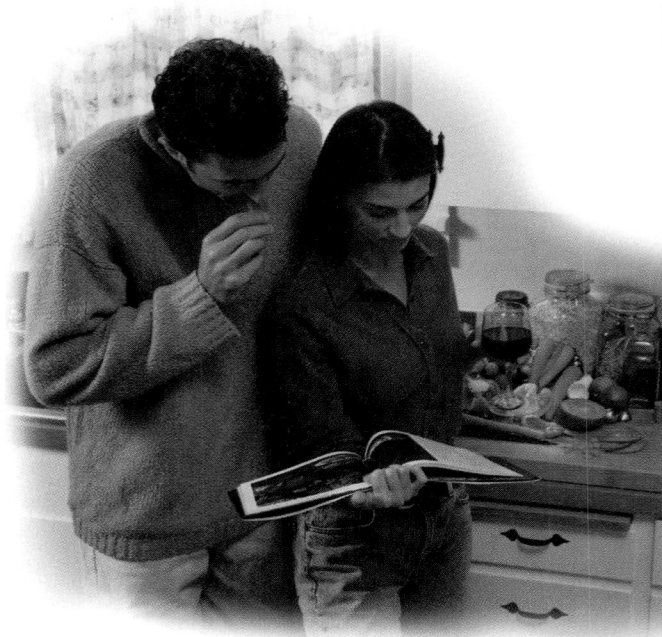

Nutrition Connection

BEETLE BAILEY

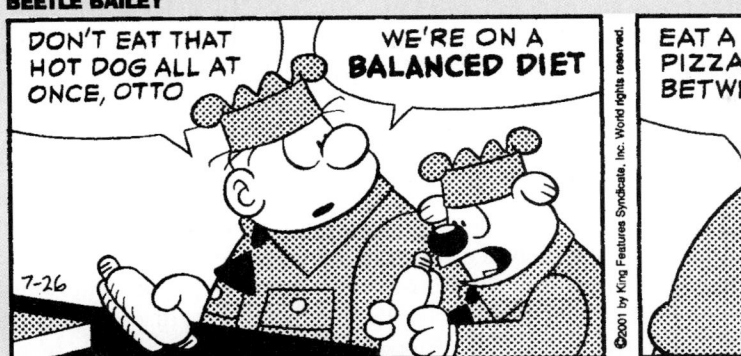
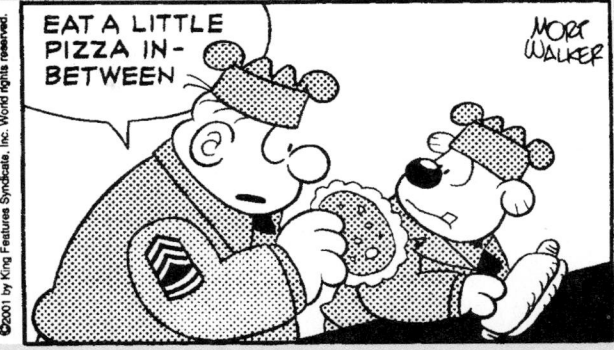

On what do nutrition experts generally agree regarding a balanced diet? Why is a diet rich in dietary fiber that includes some fish and is low in fried foods and animal fat emphasized, along with at least 30 minutes of physical activity on most or all days of the week? Are North Americans generally following this plan? What are the potential consequences for those who do not? This chapter provides some answers.

BEETLE BAILEY *Reprinted with special permission of King Features Syndicate.*

A Food Philosophy That Works

You may be surprised to learn that what you should eat to minimize the risk of developing the common nutrition-related diseases seen in North America is exactly what you've heard many times before: *Consume a variety of foods balanced by a moderate intake of each food.* A variety of foods is best because no one food meets all your nutrient needs. Human milk comes close to meeting all of an infant's needs, except that it provides only limited amounts of iron, vitamin D, and fluoride. Cow's milk contains very little iron; neither form of milk provides dietary fiber. Meat provides protein but little calcium. Eggs have no vitamin C and provide little calcium because the calcium is mostly in the shell. Thus, you need variety in your diet because the required nutrients are scattered among many different foods.

Health professionals have recommended the same basic diet and health plan for the past 30 years: Watch how much you eat, focus on the major food groups, and stay physically active. Whole grains, fruits, and vegetables have always been among the foods emphasized for our diet for the past 30 years.

It is disappointing, however, that according to a recent survey conducted by The American Dietetic Association, two of five people in the United States believe that following a healthful diet means giving up foods they enjoy. To the contrary, a healthful diet requires only some simple planning and doesn't have to mean deprivation and misery. Besides, eliminating favorite foods typically doesn't work for "dieters" in the long run. The best plan consists of learning the basics of a healthful diet—a variety and balance of foods from all food groups and moderate consumption of all foods. Let's now fine-tune this advice by focusing on variety, balance, moderation, nutrient density, and energy density.

Some people might like to live on pizza alone. What are pizza's nutrient strengths and inadequacies? Check the food composition table in Appendix A for the vitamin C content of cheese pizza. How many slices would you need to eat to yield the vitamin C RDA of 75–95 milligrams? (Answer: 30–40 slices)

phytochemical A chemical found in plants. Some phytochemicals may contribute to a reduced risk of cancer or cardiovascular disease in people who consume them regularly.

Some research suggests that increasing variety in a diet can lead to overeating. Thus, as one incorporates a wide variety of foods in a diet, attention to total calorie intake is also important to consider.

■ Variety Contributes to Diet Adequacy

Variety in your diet means choosing a number of different foods within any given food group rather than eating the "same old thing" day after day. Variety makes meals more interesting and helps ensure that a diet contains sufficient nutrients. For example, carrots may be your favorite vegetable; however, if you choose carrots every day as your only vegetable source, you may miss out on the vitamin folate. Other vegetables, such as broccoli and asparagus, are rich sources of this nutrient. This concept is true of all classes of foods: fruits, vegetables, grains, and so on. Different foods within each class vary somewhat in the nutrients they contain, but they generally provide similar types of nutrients.

An added bonus of variety in the diet, especially within the fruit and vegetable groups, is the inclusion of a rich supply of what scientists call **phytochemicals.** These substances are not absolutely required elements of the diet. Still, many of these substances provide significant health benefits. Considerable research attention is focused on various phytochemicals in reducing the risk for certain diseases such as cancer. Because current multivitamin and mineral supplements contain few or none of these beneficial substances, they generally are available only from food.

Numerous population studies show reduced cancer among people who regularly consume fruits and vegetables. This is true for cancer of the gastrointestinal (GI) tract, breast, lung, and bladder. Researchers surmise that some phytochemicals present in the fruits and vegetables block the cancer process. The cancer process is described in the Nutrition Issue in Chapter 8. For now, realize that cancer develops over many years via a multistep process. If an agent such as a phytochemical can block any one of the steps in this process, the chances that cancer will ultimately appear in the body are reduced. Other phytochemicals have been linked to a reduced risk of cardiovascular disease. Could it be that, because humans evolved on a wide variety of plant-based foods, the body developed with a need for these phytochemicals, along with the various nutrients present, to maintain optimal health?

It will likely take many years for scientists to unravel the important effects of the myriad of phytochemicals in foods, and it is unlikely that all will ever be available in supplement form. For this reason, leading cardiovascular disease and cancer researchers suggest that a diet rich in fruits, vegetables, and whole grains is the most reliable way to obtain the potential benefits of phytochemicals. Table 2.1 lists some phytochemicals under study, with their common food sources. Table 2.2 provides a number of suggestions for including more phytochemicals in your diet—especially more fruits and vegetables—as does the website www.5aday.com.

■ Balance Means Not Overconsuming Any One Food

One way to balance your diet as you consume a variety of foods is to select foods from the five major food groups every day:

- Milk, yogurt, and cheese
- Meat, poultry, fish, dry beans, eggs, and nuts
- Vegetables
- Fruit
- Bread, cereal, rice, and pasta

A lunch consisting of a bean burrito with tomatoes accompanied by a glass of milk and an apple covers all groups. Fats, oils, and sweets can also be added to your diet in moderation to increase its flavor and help deliver certain nutrients, such as vitamin E and essential fatty acids.

■ Moderation Refers Mostly to Portion Size

Although moderating portion size is a good practice, eating moderately also requires planning your entire day's diet so that you don't overconsume nutrient sources. For

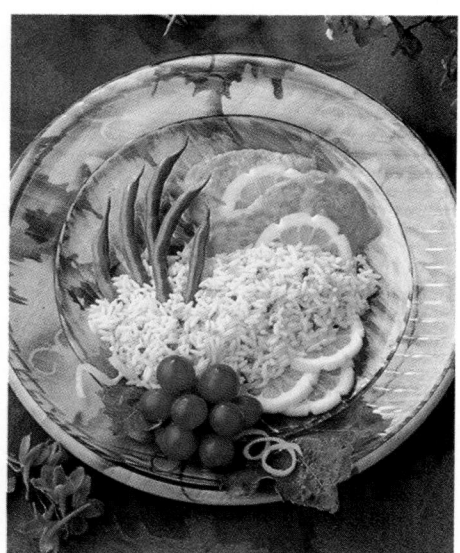

Focus on nutrient-rich foods as you strive to meet your nutrient needs.

Table 2.1 Some Phytochemical Compounds Under Study

Phytochemical	Food Sources
Allyl sulfides/organosulfurs	Garlic, onions, leeks
Saponins	Garlic, onions, licorice, legumes
Phenolic acids	All plants
Protease inhibitors	Soybeans and all other plants
Carotenoids	Orange, red, yellow fruits and vegetables (egg yolks are a source as well)
Monoterpenes	Oranges, lemons, grapefruit
Capsaicin	Chili peppers
Lignans	Flaxseed, berries, whole grains
Triterpenoids	Citrus fruit, mushrooms
Indoles	Cruciferous vegetables (broccoli, cabbage, kale)
Isothiocyanates	Cruciferous vegetables, especially broccoli
Phytosterols	Soybeans, other legumes, cucumbers, other fruits and vegetables
Flavonoids	Citrus fruit, onions, apples, grapes, red wine, tea, chocolate
Isoflavones	Soybeans, other legumes
Catechins	Tea
Ellagic acid	Strawberries, raspberries, grapes, apples, bananas
Anthocyanosides	Red, blue, and purple plants (eggplant, blueberries)
Curcumin	Turmeric
Dithiolthiones	Carrots
Fructooligosaccharides	Onions, bananas, oranges

Some related compounds under study are found in animal products, such as sphingolipids (meat and dairy products) and conjugated linoleic acid (meat and cheese). These are not phytochemicals per se because they are not from plant sources, but they have been shown to have health benefits.

A term has been coined to refer to foods rich in phytochemicals—*functional foods.* This term indicates that the food provides health benefits beyond those supplied by the traditional nutrients it contains. Since a tomato contains the phytochemical lycopene, it can be called a functional food. The food industry especially has begun to use this term.

example, if you eat something relatively high in fat, sugar, or energy, such as a bacon cheeseburger with a regular soft drink at a fast-food (quick-service) restaurant, you should eat other foods that are less concentrated sources of the same nutrients, such as fruits and salad greens that same day. This helps balance one's diet. If you prefer whole milk to low-fat or nonfat milk, reduce the fat elsewhere in your meals. Try low-fat salad dressings, or use jam rather than butter or margarine on toast. Overall, strive to simply moderate—rather than eliminate—intake of some foods.

Although there are no "good" or "bad" foods as such, many North Americans have diets overloaded with foods high in saturated fat (e.g., whole milk, doughnuts, French fries, hot dogs), white bread and related refined wheat products, and sugared soft drinks. Such diets lack the foundations of a healthy food plan—variety, balance, and moderation—and pose substantial risks for nutrition-related diseases.

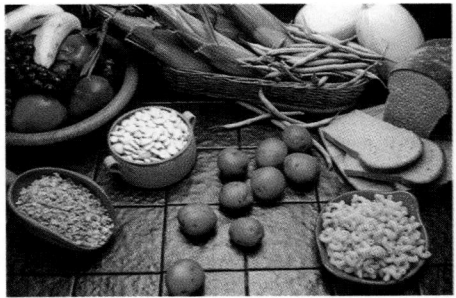

Fruits, vegetables, beans, and whole grains are typically rich in phytochemicals.

■ Nutrient Density Can Also Help Guide Food Choice

Nutrient density has gained acceptance in recent years for assessing the nutritional quality of an individual food. To determine the nutrient density of a food, simply compare its vitamin or mineral content with the amount of energy it provides. A food is said to be nutrient dense if it provides a large amount of a nutrient for a relatively small amount of calories (compared with other food sources). The higher a food's nutrient density, the better it is as a nutrient source. Comparing the nutrient density of different foods is an easy way to estimate their relative nutritional quality. Generally, nutrient density is assessed with respect to individual nutrients. For example, many

nutrient density The ratio derived by dividing a food's contribution to nutrient needs by its contribution to energy needs. When its contribution to nutrient needs exceeds its energy contribution, the food is considered to have a favorable nutrient density.

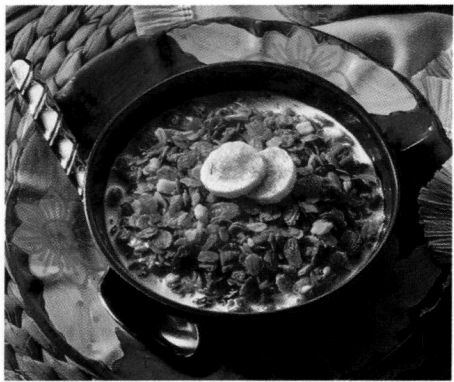

Choosing whole-grain cereals is an excellent way to increase the nutrient value of a diet. Ideally, the cereal should have at least 3 grams of dietary fiber per serving.

Critical Thinking

Andy, described in the Real Life Scenario, would benefit from more variety in his diet. What are some practical tips he can use to increase his fruit and vegetable intake?

Table 2.2 Tips for Including Foods Rich in Phytochemicals in a Diet

- Include vegetables in main and side dishes. Add these to rice, omelets, potato salad, tuna salad, and pastas. Try broccoli or cauliflower florets, mushrooms, peas, carrots, corn, or peppers.
- Look for quick-fixing grain side dishes in the supermarket. Pilafs, couscous, rice mixes, and tabbouleh are just a few that you'll find.
- Choose fruit-filled cookies, such as fig bars, instead of sugar-rich cookies. Use fresh or canned fruit as a topping for puddings, hot or cold cereal, pancakes, and frozen desserts.
- Put raisins, grapes, apple chunks, pineapples, grated carrots, zucchini, or cucumber into coleslaw, chicken salad, or tuna salad.
- Be creative at the salad bar: Try fresh spinach, leaf lettuce, red cabbage, zucchini, yellow squash, cauliflower, peas, mushrooms, or red or yellow peppers.
- Pack fresh or dried fruit for snacks away from home instead of grabbing a candy bar or going hungry.
- Add slices of cucumber, zucchini, spinach, or carrot slivers to the lettuce and tomato on your sandwiches.
- Try one or two vegetarian meals per week, such as beans and rice or pasta; Chinese vegetable stir fry; or spaghetti, squash, and tomato sauce.
- When daily protein intake more than meets recommended amounts, reduce the meat, fish, or poultry in casseroles, stews, and soups by one-third to one-half and add more vegetables and legumes.
- Keep a bowl of fresh vegetables in the refrigerator for snacks.
- Choose fruit or vegetable juices instead of soft drinks, and preferably 100% varieties.
- Substitute tea for coffee or soft drinks on a regular basis.
- Have a bowl of fruit on hand.
- Switch from crisphead lettuce to leaf lettuce, such as romaine.
- Use salsa as a dip for chips in place of creamy dips.
- Choose whole-grain breakfast cereals, breads, and crackers.
- Flavor food with plenty of herbs and spices, including ginger, rosemary, basil, thyme, garlic, parsley, and chives in place of salt.
- Experiment with soy products, such as tofu, soy milk, soy protein isolate, and roasted soybeans (see Chapter 6).

fruits and vegetables have a high content of vitamin C compared with their modest energy content: That is, they are nutrient-dense foods for vitamin C. Moreover, as Figure 2.1 shows, nonfat milk is much more nutrient dense than sugared soft drinks for many nutrients.

As noted previously, menu planning focuses mainly on the total diet—not on the selection of one critical food as key to an adequate diet. Nonetheless, nutrient-dense foods—such as nonfat and low-fat milk, lean meats, beans, oranges, carrots, broccoli, whole-wheat bread, and whole-grain breakfast cereals—do help balance less nutrient-dense foods—such as cookies and potato chips—which many people like to eat. The latter are often called empty-calorie foods because they tend to supply much energy as sugar and/or fat but few other nutrients.

Searching for nutrient-dense foods is especially important in some cases. For example, this strategy can aid diet planning for people who tend to consume little food energy, including some older people and those following weight-loss diets.

▊ Energy (kcal) Density Especially Influences Energy Intake

energy density A comparison of the energy (kcal) content of a food with the weight of the food. An energy-dense food is high in calories but weighs very little (e.g., many fried foods), whereas a food low in energy density has few calories but weight a lot, such as an orange.

Energy density is a concept that has captured the attention of nutrition scientists in recent years. Energy density of a food is determined by comparing energy (kcal)

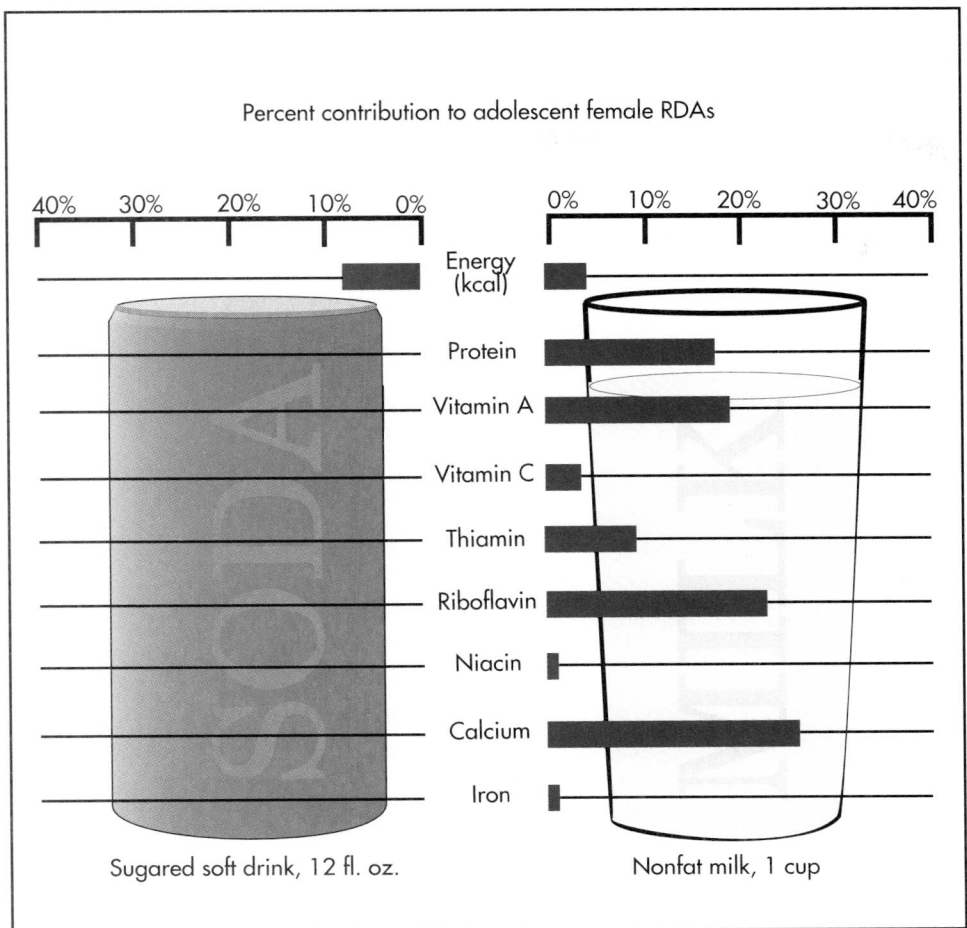

Figure 2.1 Comparison of the nutrient density of a sugared soft drink with that of nonfat milk. Choosing a glass of nonfat milk makes a significantly greater contribution to nutrient intake in comparison with a sugared soft drink. An easy way to determine nutrient density is to see how many of the nutrient bars are longer than the kcal bar. The soft drink has no longer nutrient bars. Nonfat milk has longer nutrient bars for protein, vitamin A, thiamin, riboflavin, and calcium. Including many nutrient-dense foods in your diet aids in meeting nutrient needs.

content with the weight of food. A food that is rich in calories but weights relatively very little is considered energy dense. Examples include nuts, cookies, fried foods in general, and fat-free snacks, such as fat-free pretzels. Foods with low energy density include fruits, vegetables, and any food that incorporates lots of water during cooking, such as oatmeal (Table 2.3).

Researchers have shown that having low-energy-density foods in a meal contributes to satiety without contributing many calories. This is because we probably consume a constant weight of food at a meal, rather than a constant number of calories. How this constant weight of food is regulated is not known, but careful laboratory studies show that people consume fewer calories in a meal if the food choices tend to be low in energy density, compared with foods high in energy density. Following (or maintaining) such a diet low in energy density can aid in losing weight.

Overall, foods with lots of water and dietary fiber provide a low-energy-density contribution to a meal and help one feel full, whereas foods with high energy density—especially those high in fat—must be eaten in greater amounts in order to contribute to fullness. This is one more reason to support a diet rich in fruits, vegetables, and whole grains, a pattern that also is typical of many ethnic diets throughout the world (see the Nutrition Issue at the end of this chapter). Still, favorite foods, even if

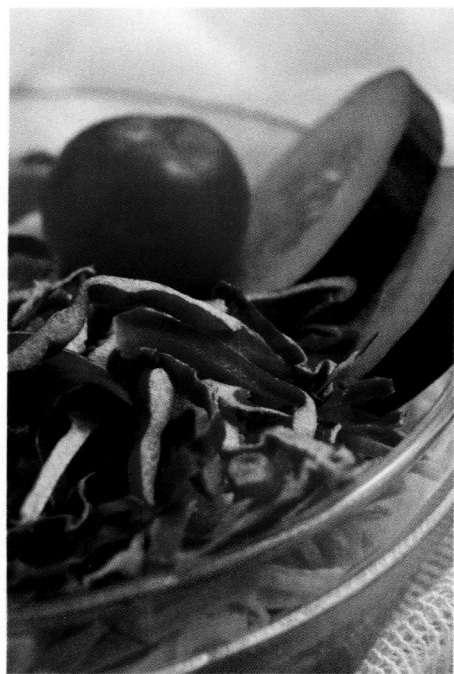

Salads are low in energy density if we limit additional calories from salad dressing, and especially minimize bacon bits, cheese crumbles or cubes, and croutons.

Table 2.3 Energy Density of Common Foods (Listed in Relative Order)

Very Low Energy Density (<0.6 kcal per gram)	Low Energy Density (0.6 to 1.5 kcal per gram)
Lettuce	Whole milk
Tomatoes	Oatmeal
Strawberries	Cottage cheese
Broccoli	Beans
Salsa	Bananas
Grapefruit	Broiled fish
Nonfat milk	Fat-free yogurt
Carrots	Ready-to-eat breakfast cereals with 1% low-fat milk
Vegetable soup	Plain baked potato
	Cooked rice
	Spaghetti noodles

Medium Energy Density (1.5 to 4 kcal per gram)	High Energy Density (>4 kcal per gram)
Eggs	Graham crackers
Ham	Fat-free sandwich cookies
Pumpkin pie	Chocolate
Whole-wheat bread	Chocolate chip cookies
Bagels	Tortilla chips
White bread	Bacon
Raisins	Potato chips
Cream cheese	Peanuts
Cake with frosting	Peanut butter
Pretzels	Mayonnaise
Rice cakes	Butter or margarine
	Vegetable oils

Data adapted from Rolls B, Barnett RA: *Volumetrics.* New York: HarperCollins, 2000.

they are high in energy density, can have a place in your dietary pattern, but you will have to plan for them. For example, chocolate is a very energy-dense food, but a small portion at the end of a meal can supply a satisfying finale. In addition, foods with high energy density can help people with poor appetites, such as some older people, to maintain or gain weight.

The following sections of the chapter describe various states of nutritional health and provide tools and nutrient guidelines for planning healthy diets to support overall health.

Concept Check

*B*asic diet-planning concepts include consuming a variety of foods, balancing a diet by consuming foods from each of the five food groups, and moderating portion size with each food choice, so that the diet is not excessive in energy. Choosing nutrient-dense foods, such as nonfat milk, fruits, vegetables, and whole grains, helps supply a diet with many nutrients but not excessive calories. Many of these foods are also rich sources of phytochemicals, supplying an even greater health benefit to the diet. Consuming foods of low energy density, such as fruits and vegetables, may also help in weight control, in that these provide satiety for a meal because of their large volume but few calories.

Table 2.4 Categories of Nutritional States with Respect to Iron*

General Conditions	Condition with Respect to Iron
Overnutrition: nutrients consumed in excess of body needs (degree of toxicity varies for each nutrient)	Results in toxic damage to liver cells; may contribute to cardiovascular disease
Desirable nutrition: nutrients consumed to support body functions and stores of nutrients for times of increased need	Adequate liver stores of iron, adequate blood values for iron-related compounds
Undernutrition: nutrient intake does not meet nutrient needs; biochemical changes then take place	Many changes in body functions associated with a decline in iron status (e.g., iron-containing proteins and pigments in the blood drop below acceptable amounts and oxygen supply to body tissues is reduced)
Clinical symptoms; these effects eventually are seen	Pale complexion; greatly increased heart rate during activity; "spooning" of the nails in a severe deficiency; poor body temperature regulation

*This general scheme can apply to all nutrients. Iron was chosen because you are likely to be familiar with this nutrient.

States of Nutritional Health

The body's nutritional health is determined by the sum of its **nutritional state** with respect to each needed nutrient. Three general categories are recognized: desirable nutrition, undernutrition, and overnutrition. Maintaining a state of desirable nutrition is the basis for establishing human nutrient needs and the diet plans to meet those needs that are discussed later in the chapter. The common term **malnutrition** can refer to either **overnutrition** or **undernutrition.** Neither state is conducive to good health.

■ Desirable Nutrition

The nutritional state for a particular nutrient is desirable when body tissues have enough of the nutrient to support normal metabolic functions as well as surplus stores that can be used in times of increased need. A desirable nutritional state can be achieved by obtaining essential nutrients from a variety of foods.

■ Undernutrition

Undernutrition occurs when nutrient intake does not meet nutrient needs. Stores are then used up and health declines. Many nutrients are in high demand due to the constant state of cell loss and later regeneration in the body, such as in the gastrointestinal tract. For this reason, certain nutrient stores are exhausted rapidly, such as for many of the B vitamins. In turn, a regular intake is needed. In addition, some women in North America do not consume sufficient iron to meet monthly losses and eventually deplete their iron stores (Table 2.4).

Once availability of a nutrient falls sufficiently low, biochemical evidence, in which the body's metabolic processes slow or stop, appears. At this state of deficiency there are not outward symptoms, thus it is termed a **subclinical** deficiency. A subclinical deficiency can go on for some time before clinicians are able to detect its effects.

Eventually clinical **symptoms** will develop, sometimes taking many years, and may result in clinical evidence of a deficiency; perhaps in the skin, hair, nails, tongue, or eyes. Often, clinicians do not detect a problem until a deficiency produces such results, such as in a vitamin C deficiency.

nutritional state The nutritional health of a person as determined by anthropometric measurements (height, weight, circumferences, and so on), biochemical measurements of nutrients or their by-products in blood and urine, a clinical (physical) examination, a dietary analysis, and economic evaluation; also called nutritional status.

malnutrition Failing health that results from long-standing dietary practices that do not coincide with nutritional needs.

overnutrition A state in which nutritional intake greatly exceeds the body's needs.

undernutrition Failing health that results from a long-standing dietary intake that does not meet nutritional needs.

subclinical Disease or disorder that is present but not severe enough to produce symptoms that can be detected or diagnosed.

symptom A change in health status noted by the person with the problem, such as stomach pain.

Table 2.5 Conducting an Evaluation of Nutritional Health

Component	Example
Background histories	Medical history, including current diseases and past surgeries
	Medications history
	Social history (marital status, cooking facilities)
	Family history
	Economic status
	Education attainment
Nutritional parameters	Anthropometric assessment: height, weight, skinfold thickness, arm muscle circumference, and other parameters
	Biochemical (laboratory) assessment of blood and urine: enzyme activities, concentrations of nutrients or their by-products
	Clinical assessment (physical examination): general appearance of skin, eyes, and tongue; rapid hair loss; sense of touch; ability to walk
	Diet history: usual intake or record or previous days' meals

■ Overnutrition

Prolonged consumption of more nutrients than the body needs can lead to overnutrition. In the short run, for instance a week or two, overnutrition may cause only a few symptoms, such as stomach distress from excess dietary fiber or iron intake. But if kept up, some nutrients may increase to toxic amounts, which can lead to serious disease. For example, too much vitamin A can have negative effects, particularly in children and pregnant women.

The most common type of overnutrition in industrialized nations—excess intake of energy-yielding nutrients—often leads to obesity. In the long run, obesity can then lead to other serious diseases, such as certain forms of diabetes and cancer. Use the website shapeup.org to learn more about this problem.

For most vitamins and minerals, the gap between desirable intake and overnutrition is wide. Therefore, even if people take a typical multivitamin and mineral supplement daily, they probably won't receive a harmful amount of any nutrient. The gap between optimal intake and overnutrition is narrowest for vitamin A, calcium, iron, copper, and other minerals. Thus, if you take nutrient supplements, keep a close eye on your total vitamin and mineral intake both from food and from supplements to avoid toxicity (see Chapter 8 for further advice on use of nutrient supplements).

How Could Your Nutritional State Be Measured?

To find out how nutritionally fit *you* are, a nutritional assessment—either whole or in part—needs to be performed (Table 2.5). Generally, this is performed by a physician and often with the aid of a registered dietitian.

■ Analyzing Background Factors

Since family history plays an important role in determining nutritional and health status, it must be carefully recorded and critically analyzed as part of a nutritional assessment. Other related background components include (1) a medical history, especially for any disease states or treatments that could impede nutrient absorptive processes or ultimate use; and (2) economic history, to determine the ability to purchase and prepare appropriate foods needed to maintain health.

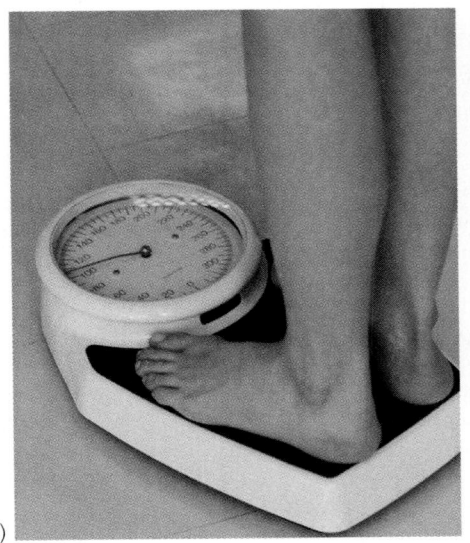
(a)

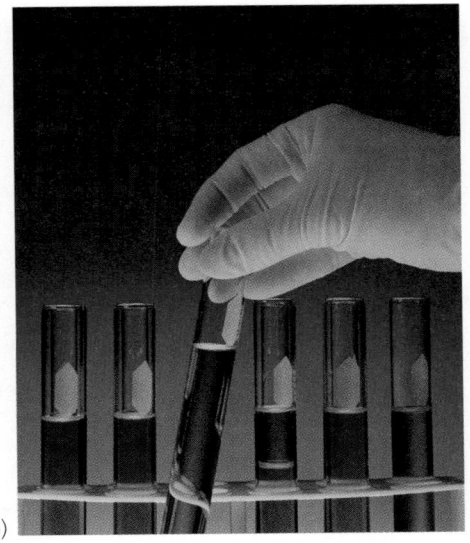
(b)

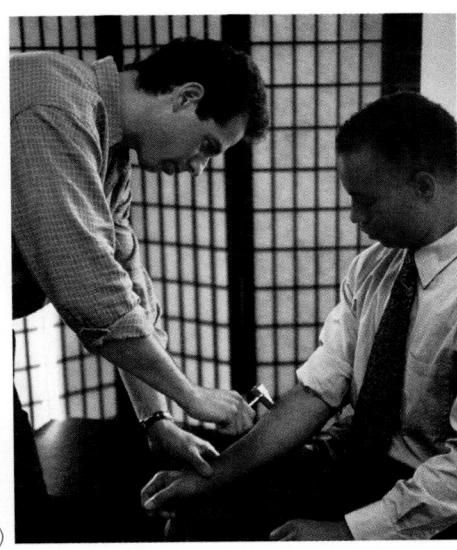
(c)

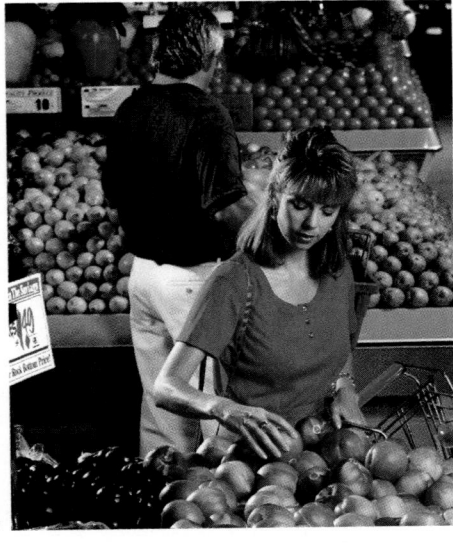
(d)

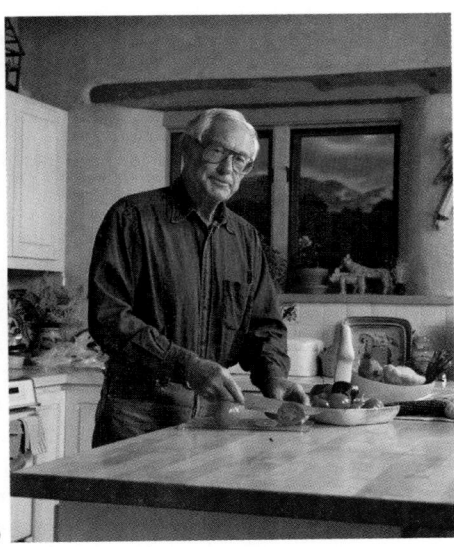
(e)

Figure 2.2   (a) **A**nthropometric, (b) **b**iochemical, (c) **c**linical, and (d) **d**ietary information helps determine a person's nutritional state. (e) **E**conomic status adds further information, rounding out the ABCDEs of nutritional assessment.

■ Evaluating the ABCDEs

Four components in combination further add to the complete nutritional picture. **Anthropometric** measurements of height, weight, body skinfolds, and body circumferences are an excellent first line of attack. They are easy to obtain and are generally reliable. However, an in-depth examination of nutritional health is impossible without the more expensive process of biochemical assessment. This involves the measurement of specific blood enzyme activities and of the concentrations of nutrients and nutrient by-products in the blood, urine, and feces.

A clinical examination would follow, during which a health professional would search for any physical evidence of diet-related diseases. Then, a diet history, documenting at least the previous few days' intake, would look into possible problem areas. Finally, current economic status discussed earlier is added to the picture, such as the ability to purchase and prepare appropriate foods needed to maintain health. Now the true nutritional state of a person emerges (Fig. 2.2). Together these activities form the ABCDEs of nutritional assessment: **a**nthropometric measurement, **b**iochemical assessment, **c**linical examination, **d**iet history, and **e**conomic status.

anthropometric Pertaining to the measurement of body weight and the lengths, circumferences, and thicknesses of parts of the body.

Another Bite

A practical example using the ABCDEs for evaluating nutritional state can be illustrated in a person who chronically abuses alcohol. Upon evaluation, the physician notes:

(a) Low weight-for-height, muscle wasting in the upper body
(b) Low amounts of the vitamins thiamin and folate in the blood
(c) Psychological confusion, facial sores, and uncoordinated movement
(d) Dietary intake of little more than alcohol-fortified wine and snack cakes for the last week
(e) Currently residing in a homeless shelter; $35.00 in wallet; unemployed

Evaluation: This person needs professional attention, including nutrient repletion.

▪ Recognizing the Limitations of Nutritional Assessment

As mentioned, a long time may elapse between the initial development of poor nutritional health and the first clinical evidence of a problem. Recall that a diet high in saturated (typically solid) fat often increases blood cholesterol concentration, but without producing any clinical evidence for years. However, when the blood vessels become sufficiently blocked by cholesterol and other materials, chest pain during physical activity or a **heart attack** may occur. Much current nutrition research aims to develop better methods for early detection of nutrition-related problems such as this.

Another example in the delay of evidence that serious consequences are occurring is with a calcium deficiency, a particularly relevant issue for adolescent females. Many young women consume well below the needed amount of calcium but often suffer no ill effects in their younger years. However, women whose bone structures do not reach full potential during the years of growth are likely to face an increased risk for osteoporosis later in life.

Furthermore, clinical evidence of nutritional deficiencies is often not very specific, such as diarrhea, an irregular walk, and facial sores. These may have different causes. Long lag times and vague evidence often make it difficult to establish a link between an individual's current diet and nutritional state.

Table 1.5 in Chapter 1 showed the close relationship of nutrition and health. The good news is that this attention to maintaining nutritional health contributes to the goal of achieving a long, vigorous life.

heart attack Rapid fall in heart function caused by reduced blood flow through the heart's blood vessels. Often part of the heart dies in the process (see Chapter 5). Technically called a myocardial infarction.

Concept Check

A desirable nutritional state results when the body has enough nutrients to function fully and contains stores to use in times of increased needs. When nutrient intake fails to meet body needs, undernutrition develops. Symptoms of such an inadequate nutrient intake can take months or years to develop. Overloading the body with nutrients, leading to overnutrition, is another potential problem to avoid. Nutritional state can be assessed by using anthropometric measurements, biochemical evidence, clinical evaluation, diet history, and economic status (ABCDEs).

Recommendations for Food Choice

The following sections of the chapter will describe various guidelines for planning healthy diets.

▪ The Food Guide Pyramid—A Menu-Planning Tool

Since the early twentieth century, researchers have worked to clarify the science of nutrition into practical terms, so that people with no special training could estimate whether their nutritional needs were being met. A seven food-group plan, based on foods traditionally eaten by people in North America, was one of the first formats designed by USDA. Daily food choices had to include items from each group. This plan had been simplified by the mid-1950s to a four food-group plan: a milk group, a meat group, a fruit and vegetable group, and a bread and cereal group. The entire plan was designed to provide a minimum foundation for a diet, and represented about 1200 to 1400 kcal per day. Other food choices were to be added to meet daily energy needs.

Today, the Food Guide Pyramid, which is designed to represent a total diet providing sufficient protein, vitamins, and minerals, is widely advocated for diet planning (Fig. 2.3). This pyramid goes beyond earlier food guides to suggest a pattern of food choices for the entire day, rather than simply a foundation diet.

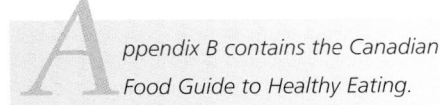
Appendix B contains the Canadian Food Guide to Healthy Eating.

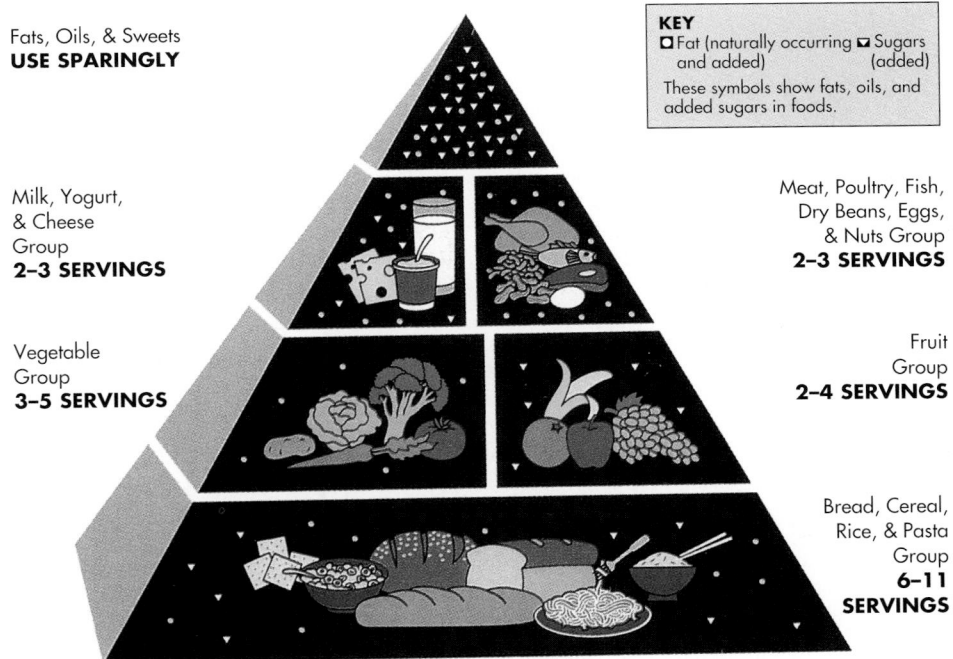

Figure 2.3 USDA's Food Guide Pyramid. The Food Guide Pyramid lists the food groups and the amount to consume from each group. Note that for children and teenagers, 3 servings should be chosen from the milk, yogurt, and cheese group. Once you have estimated your energy needs, recommended servings from the other groups with wider ranges are as follows:

Energy intake	1600 kcal	2200 kcal	2800 kcal
Grain group	6	9	11
Vegetable group	3	4	5
Fruit group	2	3	4
Meat group (ounces)	5	6	7
Total fat (grams)	53	73	93
Total added sugars (teaspoons)	6	12	18

Table 2.6 The Food Guide Pyramid—a Summary

Food Category	Major Contributions	Foods and Individual Serving Sizes[†]
Milk, yogurt, and cheese	Calcium Phosphorus Carbohydrate Protein Riboflavin Vitamin D Magnesium Zinc	1 cup milk (includes low-lactose products) 1½ oz cheese 2 oz processed cheese 1 cup yogurt 2 cups cottage cheese 1 cup soy-based beverage with added calcium
Meat, poultry, fish, dry beans, eggs, and nuts	Protein Thiamin Riboflavin Niacin Vitamin B-6 Folate[§] Vitamin B-12[‖] Phosphorus Magnesium[§] Iron Zinc	2–3 oz cooked meat, poultry, or fish 1–1½ cups cooked dry beans 4 tbsp peanut butter 2 eggs ⅔–1 cup nuts 5 oz soyburger
Fruit	Carbohydrate Vitamin A (few varieties) Vitamin C Folate Magnesium Potassium Dietary fiber	¼ cup dried fruit ½ cup cooked or canned fruit ¾ cup juice 1 whole piece of fruit 1 melon wedge (about ¼) ½ cup berries
Vegetable	Carbohydrate Vitamin A Vitamin C Folate Magnesium Potassium Dietary fiber	½ cup raw or cooked vegetables 1 cup raw leafy vegetables ¾ cup vegetable juice
Bread, cereal, rice, and pasta	Carbohydrate Thiamin Riboflavin[¶] Niacin Folate[#] Magnesium[‡] Iron[¶#] Zinc[#] Dietary fiber[‡]	1 slice of bread 1 oz (about ¾ cup) ready-to-eat cereal ½ cup cooked cereal, rice, or pasta ½ hamburger roll, bagel, or English muffin 3–4 plain crackers 1 small roll, biscuit, or muffin 1 6" tortilla
Fats, oils, and sweets	Food from this category should not replace any from the other groups. Amounts consumed should be determined by individual energy needs.	

[†]May be reduced for child servings

[§]Primarily in plant protein sources

[‖]Only in animal foods

[¶]If enriched

[#]Whole grains and some enriched/
fortified products

[‡]Whole grains

To quickly estimate serving sizes, use the following equivalents:

Thumb = 1 oz of cheese	Palm of a hand = 3 oz	Computer mouse = ½ to ¾ cups
4 stacked dice = 1 oz cheese	1 ice cream scoop = ½ cup	Ping-pong or golf ball = 2 tbsp
Thumb tip to first joint = 1 tsp	Fist or baseball = 1 cup	Yo-yo or hockey puck = 1 bagel serving
Matchbox = 1 oz meat	Handful = 1 or 2 oz of a snack food	
Bar of soap or pack of cards = 3 oz meat	Tennis ball = 1 medium fruit serving	

Components of the Food Guide Pyramid

The number of servings to consume from each food group in the current Food Guide Pyramid depends on a person's age and energy needs. Serving size is also adjusted downward for young children (see Chapter 14). Table 2.6 lists serving sizes and the recommended number of servings to consume per day for adults. The table also lists the major nutrients each food group supplies. Note the similarities and differences among the groups.

The plan for an adult over age 18 essentially consists of the following:

- 2 servings from the milk, yogurt, and cheese group
- 2 to 3 servings from the meat, poultry, fish, dry beans, eggs, and nuts group (5 to 7 ounces total)
- 3 to 5 servings from the vegetable group
- 2 to 4 servings from the fruit group
- 6 to 11 servings from the bread, cereals, rice, and pasta group

Note also that some food choices will contain servings of more than one food group (e.g., lasagna contains pasta, cheese, and tomatoes, and likely ingredients from other food groups as well).

For some population groups—children and teenagers, (including teenagers who are pregnant or breastfeeding)—three servings of the milk, yogurt, and cheese group are recommended due to higher calcium needs. The same is also true for older adults (51 years or older). Alternately, some of those servings also could be replaced with calcium-fortified foods or a calcium supplement (see Chapter 9).

Foods in a final category at the tip of the pyramid, which is not a group per se, include fats, oils, and sweets. These can be eaten to help meet individual energy needs but should not replace foods from other groups.

Menu Planning with the Food Guide Pyramid

Table 2.7 illustrates a 1-day menu based on the Food Guide Pyramid. Remember the following points when using the Food Guide Pyramid to plan daily menus:

1. The guide does not apply to infants or children under 2 years of age.
2. No one food is absolutely essential to good nutrition. Each food is deficient in at least one essential nutrient.
3. No one food group provides all essential nutrients in adequate amounts. Each food group makes an important, distinctive contribution to nutritional intake.
4. Variety is the key to success of the guide and is first guaranteed by choosing foods from all the groups. Furthermore, one should consume a variety of foods within each group, except possibly in the milk, yogurt, and cheese group.
5. The foods within a group may vary widely with respect to nutrient and energy content. For example, the energy content of 3 ounces of baked potato is 98 kcal, whereas that of 3 ounces of potato chips is 470 kcal. Compare an orange and an apple with respect to vitamin C using the food composition table in Appendix A.

Overall, the Food Guide Pyramid incorporates the foundations of a healthy diet: variety, balance, and moderation. The nutritional adequacy of diets planned using this tool, however, depends on selection of a variety of foods. In addition, to ensure enough vitamin E, vitamin B-6, magnesium, and zinc—nutrients sometimes low in diets based on this plan—consider the following advice:

1. Choose primarily low-fat and nonfat items from the milk, yogurt, and cheese group. By reducing energy intake in this way, you can select more items from other food groups. If milk causes intestinal gas and bloating, emphasize yogurt and cheese (see Chapter 4 for details on the problem of lactose maldigestion and intolerance. Milk is rich in lactose.).
2. Include plant foods that are good sources of proteins, such as beans and nuts, at least several times a week because many are rich in vitamins (such as vitamin E), minerals (such as magnesium), and dietary fiber.

*E*xperts recommend that we pay close attention to the stated serving size for each choice when following the Food Guide Pyramid. This aids in controlling total energy intake. See Figure 2.4 for a convenient guide to estimating serving size. Note that serving sizes listed for one serving in a Food Guide Pyramid group are often less than typically served in restaurants today.

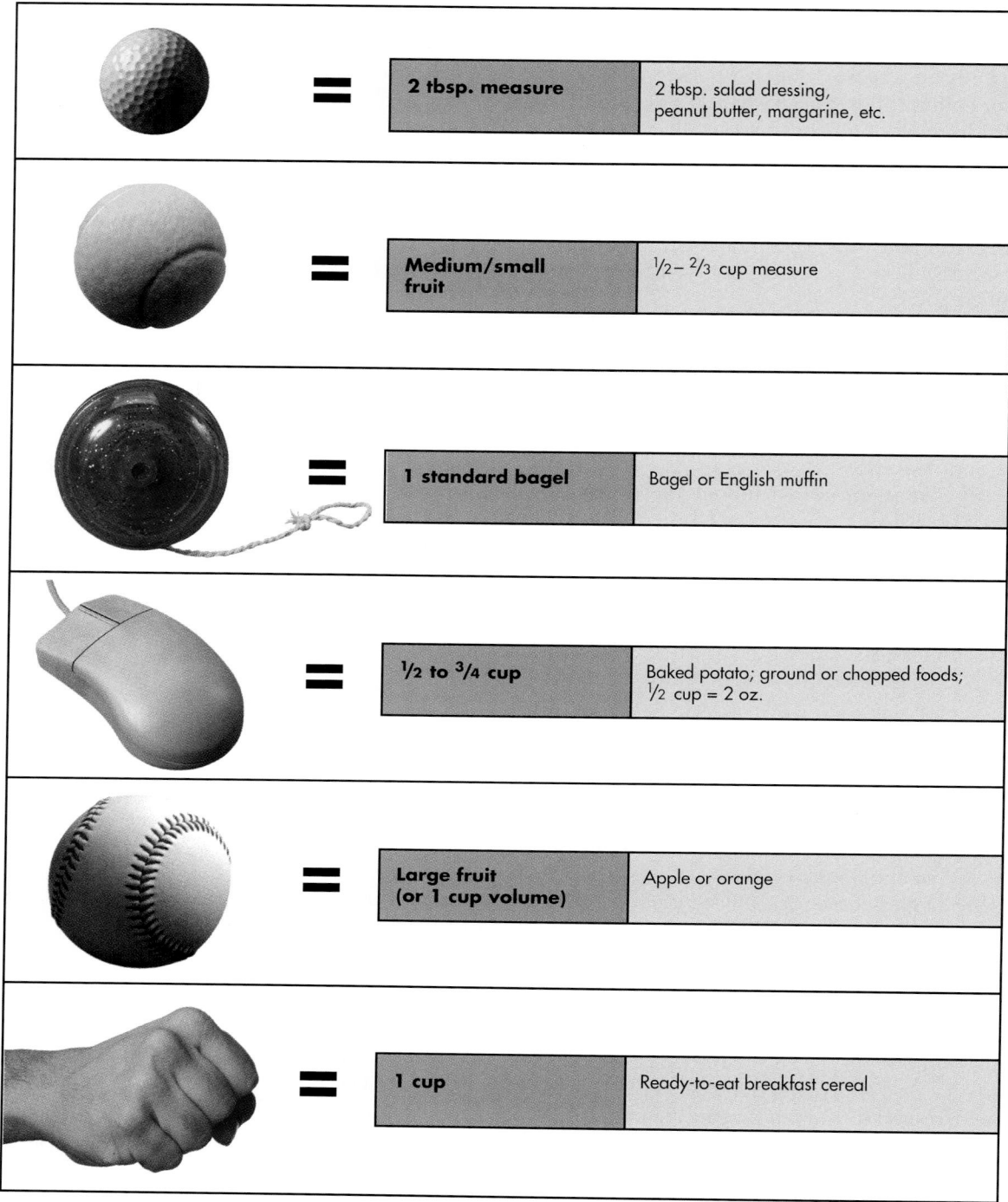

	2 tbsp. measure	2 tbsp. salad dressing, peanut butter, margarine, etc.
	Medium/small fruit	$1/2 - 2/3$ cup measure
	1 standard bagel	Bagel or English muffin
	$1/2$ to $3/4$ cup	Baked potato; ground or chopped foods; $1/2$ cup = 2 oz.
	Large fruit (or 1 cup volume)	Apple or orange
	1 cup	Ready-to-eat breakfast cereal

Figure 2.4 A golf ball, tennis ball, yo-yo, computer mouse, baseball, and fist make convenient guides to judge Food Guide Pyramid serving sizes.

3. For vegetables and fruits, try to include a dark green vegetable for vitamin A and a vitamin C–rich fruit, such as an orange, every day. Don't focus primarily on potatoes for your vegetable choices. Surveys show that only 25% of adults eat a green vegetable on any given day. Increased consumption of these foods is important because they contribute vitamins, minerals, dietary fiber, and phytochemicals.

Table 2.7 Putting the Food Guide Pyramid into Practice

Meal	Servings/Food Group*
Breakfast	
1 small, peeled orange	1 fruit
¾ cup Healthy Choice Low-fat Granola	1 bread
with ½ cup nonfat milk	½ milk
½ toasted, small raisin bagel	1 bread
with 1 tsp soft margarine	1 fat/sweet
Optional: coffee or tea	
Lunch	
Ham sandwich	
2 slices whole-wheat bread	2 bread
2 oz ham	1 meat
2 tsp mustard	
1 small apple	1 fruit
2 oatmeal-raisin cookies (small)	2 fat/sweet
Optional: diet soft drink	
3 P.M. Study Break	
6 whole wheat crackers	2 bread
1 tbsp peanut butter	¼ meat
½ cup nonfat milk	½ milk
Dinner	
Lettuce salad	
1 cup romaine lettuce	1 vegetable
½ cup sliced tomatoes	1 vegetable
1½ tbsp Italian dressing	1½ fat/sweet
½ grated carrot	1 vegetable
3 oz broiled salmon	1 meat
½ cup rice	1 bread
½ cup green beans	1 vegetable
with 1 tsp soft margarine	1 fat/sweet
Optional: coffee or tea	
Late-Night Snack	
1 cup "light" fruit yogurt	1 milk
Nutrient Breakdown	
1800 kcal	
Carbohydrate	56% of kcal
Protein	18% of kcal
Fat	26% of kcal

This menu meets nutrient needs for all vitamins and minerals for an average adult. For adolescents, teenagers, and older adults add one additional serving from the milk, yogurt, and cheese group or seek other calcium-rich sources.

*Names of food groups abbreviated as follows: milk = milk, yogurt, and cheese group; meat = meat, poultry, fish, dry beans, eggs, and nuts group; bread = bread, cereal, rice, and pasta group; fat/sweet = fats, oils, and sweets category.

4. Choose whole-grain varieties of breads, cereals, rice, and pasta often because they contribute vitamin E and dietary fiber. A plate about two-thirds covered by grains, fruits, and vegetables and one-third or less covered by protein-rich foods promotes this diet advice. As well, a daily serving of a whole-grain, ready-to-eat breakfast cereal is an excellent choice because the vitamins (such as vitamin B-6) and minerals (such as zinc) typically added to it, along with dietary fiber, help fill in the potential gaps listed earlier.

5. Include some plant oils on a daily basis, such as those in salad dressing, and eat fish at least twice a week. This supplies you with health-promoting fatty acids.

Following the Food Guide Pyramid makes it possible to create daily diets containing as few as 1600 to 1800 kcal (review Table 2.7), sufficient for a sedentary adult or an older person. Not following this advice can leave a diet 1600 to 1800 kcal short on the nutrients just mentioned. Recall that excessive consumption of any one food—even those considered "healthy"—is also undesirable and possibly risky.

If 1600 to 1800 kcal represents too much food energy for you, you should first consider becoming more physically active rather than eating less. Obtaining enough nutrients from a diet that supplies fewer than 1600 kcal per day is very difficult. If you can't increase your energy output, you can make a special attempt to choose some nutrient-fortified foods regularly (e.g., ready-to-eat breakfast cereals) or take a

There is no shortage of pyramids to choose from when planning a diet. Which pyramid looks best to you?

Another Bite

During the last few years a number of organizations and experts have proposed alternate diet plans and pyramids to replace the Food Guide Pyramid.

The American Institute for Cancer Research is promoting a plate instead of a pyramid for menu planning. The plate should be covered two-thirds or more by vegetables, fruits, and whole grains and one-third or less by meat, fish, poultry, and low-fat dairy products (www.aicr.org).

The Mayo Clinic has developed a Healthy Weight Pyramid with physical activity at the center of the pyramid. The plan allows for unlimited amounts of fruits and vegetables in the diet, 4 to 8 servings of carbohydrates (grains), 3 to 7 servings of protein/dairy products, 3 to 5 servings of fats, and very limited amounts of sweets (75 kcal/day)(www.mayo.edu/news/pyramid.jpg).

The Dietary Approaches to Stop Hypertension (DASH) Pyramid helps treat elevated blood pressure. It contains more fruit and vegetable choices (total of 8 to 10) than the Food Guide Pyramid (see the Nutrition Insight in Chapter 9).

Oldways Preservation Trust has developed Latin American, Asian, and Mediterranean pyramids to reflect traditional diets in these ethnic groups (see the Nutrition Issue in this chapter).

Oldways Preservation Trust has also developed a vegetarian pyramid (see the Nutrition Issue in Chapter 6).

Dr. Walter Willett, a well-respected nutrition scientist, has created a Healthy Eating Pyramid. The diet plan emphasizes a daily generous intake of whole grains, plant oils, and vegetables; fruits at least two to three times per day, nuts and legumes one to three times per day; fish, poultry, and eggs zero to two times per day; dairy products or calcium supplements one to two times per day; and little use of red meat, butter, white rice, white bread, potatoes, pasta, and sweets. Regular physical activity and weight control is also recommended, as is alcohol intake in moderation (if of legal age) and a multivitamin and mineral supplement for most people. Chapter 5 discusses the rationale and implications of this diet plan. To view the pyramid see www.hsph.harvard.edu/now/aug24/.

All of these plans share a common pattern of including primarily fruits, vegetables, and grains—preferably, mostly whole grains—in a diet.

balanced multivitamin and mineral supplement (see Chapter 8). In addition, for those whose diets do not include meat or other animal products, the Nutrition Issue on vegetarianism in Chapter 6 provides advice on adapting the Food Guide Pyramid to that dietary practice.

Evaluation of the Current North American Diet Using the Food Guide Pyramid

The average North American diet, based on surveys, fails to meet the serving recommendations in the Food Guide Pyramid for many food groups. For example, the average diet included only 1 to 2 fruit servings (rather than the recommended 2 to 4 servings) and only 2 to 3 vegetable servings (rather than 3 to 5 servings), and much of that comes from potatoes, not a particularly nutrient-dense vegetable choice. Overall, fruits and vegetables are the most underrepresented groups. In contrast, the fats, oils, and sweets are well represented.

How Does Your Current Diet Rate?

Regularly comparing your daily food intake with the Food Guide Pyramid recommendations is a relatively simple way to evaluate your overall diet. Strive to meet the recommendations. If that is not possible, identify the nutrients that are low in your diet based on the nutrients found in each food group (review Table 2.6). For example, if you do not consume enough servings from the milk, yogurt, and cheese group, your calcium intake is most likely too low. After completing the Rate Your Plate activity at the end of this chapter, you will be able to determine more accurately which nutrients are too low in your current diet and by how much. Armed with this knowledge, find foods that you enjoy that supply those nutrients, such as calcium-fortified orange juice. Customizing the Food Guide Pyramid to accommodate your own food habits may seem a daunting task now, but it is not difficult once you gain some additional nutrition knowledge. To learn more, see the website sponsored by USDA (www.usda.gov/cnpp). At this site, you can view the entire booklet describing the pyramid.

▌ Concept Check

The Food Guide Pyramid translates the general needs for carbohydrate, protein, fat, vitamins, and minerals into the recommended number of daily servings from each of five major food groups. It is one of many convenient and valuable tools for planning daily menus.

■ Dietary Guidelines—Another Tool for Menu Planning

Appendix B contains nutrient guidelines for Canadians.

The Food Guide Pyramid was designed to help meet nutritional needs for carbohydrate, protein, fat, vitamins, and minerals. However, most of the major chronic "killer" diseases in North America, such as cardiovascular disease, cancer, and alcoholism, are not primarily associated with deficiencies of these nutrients. Deficiency diseases such as scurvy (vitamin C deficiency) and pellagra (niacin deficiency) are no longer common. For many North Americans, the primary dietary culprit is an overconsumption of one or more of the following: energy, saturated fat, cholesterol, alcohol, and sodium (salt). Underconsumption of calcium, iron, folate and other B-vitamins, vitamin D, vitamin E, zinc, or dietary fiber is also a problem for some people, but easy to fix as the major dietary problems are addressed.

In response to concerns regarding these killer disease patterns, since 1980 the USDA and U.S. Department of Health and Human Services (DHHS) have published **Dietary Guidelines** to aid diet planning. The latest Dietary Guidelines begin with three overarching messages and then list 10 specific guidelines:

Dietary Guidelines General goals for nutrient intakes and diet composition set by the USDA and the U.S. Department of Health and Human Services.

The Alphabet Soup of Specific Nutrient Needs

Before designing a diet plan, such as the Food Guide Pyramid discussed in the previous section, we must determine what amount of each essential nutrient is needed to maintain health. The standards that have been developed for such nutrient needs, such as DRI, RDA, AI, and UL can often seem like an alphabet soup of abbreviations. However, you can more easily sift through these nutrient standards if you have a base of knowledge concerning their development and use (Table 2.8).

DRIs: RDAs and Related Standards

Most of the terms that describe nutrient standards fall under one umbrella term—**Dietary Reference Intakes (DRIs).** These apply to both U.S. and Canadian residents.

You are probably most familiar with the nutrient standard **Recommended Dietary Allowance (RDA).** An RDA represents the nutrient intake that is sufficient to meet the needs of nearly all individuals (about 97%) in an age and gender group (for specific numbers, see the inside cover of this book). The RDAs are generally set at about 20% over what is needed by an average person to balance intake with losses; this 20% increase is done in order to accommodate people who may have slightly higher nutrient needs than the average person. A person can compare his or her individual intake of specific nutrients to the RDA and evaluate whether one's diet is inadequate or ample in that nutrient. An intake slightly above or below the RDA is not of great concern since your needs do not likely fall directly on the RDA number. However, a significant deviation below (about 1/2) or above (about 3 times for some nutrients) the RDA for a

considerable length of time can eventually result in a deficiency or toxicity of nutrients, respectively.

An RDA for a nutrient can be set only if there is much information on the human needs for that particular nutrient. Today there is not enough information on nutrients such as calcium, vitamin D, fluoride, and biotin to set such a precise standard as an RDA. For these and other nutrients, the DRIs include a category called **Adequate Intake (AI).** This standard is based on observing dietary intakes of people that appear to be maintaining nutritional health. That amount of intake is assumed to be adequate, as no evidence of a nutritional deficiency is apparent. Finally, minimum requirements to maintain health are set for sodium, chloride, and potassium, and **Tolerable Upper Intake Levels (Upper Levels; ULs)** have been set for some vitamins and minerals (see Chapters 8 and 9).

How Should These Nutrient Standards Be Used?

RDAs and related standards are intended mainly for diet planning. Specifically, a diet plan should aim to meet the RDA, Adequate Intake, and minimum requirements, as appropriate, and not exceed the Upper Level on a long-term basis if one has been set. However, the Adequate Intake should not be used alone, as the RDA can be, to evaluate individual nutrient intake and needs. For these standards, individual characteristics from person to person should be more carefully considered. For example, it is recommended that the Adequate Intake be used in combination with the clinical, biochemical, and anthropometric measures of one's nutritional state, discussed earlier

in this chapter. To learn more about these nutrient standards use the web page www4.nationalacademies.org/IOM/ IOMHome.nsf/Pages/Food+and+ Nutrition+Board.

Daily Values: The Standards Used for Food Labeling

Though it is worthwhile to understand the intent behind the terms discussed in this Nutrition Insight, a nutrition standard more relevant to everyday life is **Daily Values.** These are generic standards used on food labels. The actual version used on food labels is applicable to ages 4 years old through adulthood (Table 2.9). No gender categories are used with the Daily Values, and age categories are wide, as just noted. This condensed system is essential for food labeling, since the RDAs and other nutrient standards are highly age and gender specific; there are too many categories for each nutrient for RDA and related standards to be used on food labels.

Daily Values exist for vitamins, minerals, and protein. These are mostly set at or close to the highest RDA value or related nutrient standard seen in the various age and gender categories for a specific nutrient. Daily Values are also set for dietary components that are not currently part of the DRIs, such as cholesterol, carbohydrate, fiber, and others. The values are based on dietary advice from U.S. federal agencies.

Overall, Daily Values are designed to allow consumers to compare their intake to desirable (or maximum) intakes. It is nevertheless important to understand that the nutrient standards expressed on food labels are not the same as the RDAs. Food labels will be discussed further in the following section.

Table 2.8 Putting the Alphabet Soup of Specific Nutrient Needs to Use

Recommended Dietary Allowance (RDA)—use this to evaluate your current intake for a specific nutrient. The further you stray above or below this value, the greater the chance of developing nutritional problems.

Adequate Intake (AI)—use this to evaluate your current intake of nutrients, but realize that an AI designation means that much more research is needed before scientists can establish a more definitive number.

Minimum Requirement for Health—use this as a guide for the lowest intake of sodium, chloride, and potassium that allows for health. Note that our typical intakes greatly exceed the minimum requirements for sodium and chloride.

Upper Level (UL)—use this to evaluate the highest amount of daily nutrient intake that is unlikely to cause adverse health effects in the long run in almost all people (97% to 98%) in a population. This number applies to chronic use and is set to protect even very susceptible people in the healthy general population. As intake increases above the Upper Level, the potential for adverse effects increases.

Daily Value (DV)—use this as a rough guide for comparing the nutrient content of a food to approximate human needs. Typically the Daily Value used on food labels refers to ages 4 years through adulthood. It is based on a 2000 kcal diet; Daily Values for fat, saturated fat, protein, carbohydrate, and fiber increase slightly with higher energy intakes (see Fig. 2.5b in the later section of Food Labeling).

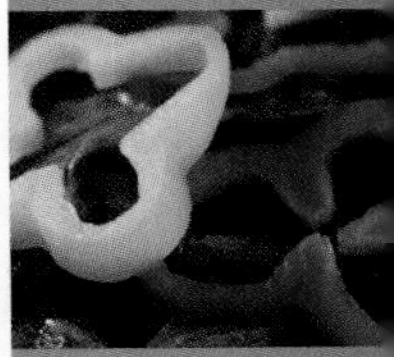

Table 2.9 Comparison of Daily Values with the latest RDAs and Other Nutrient Standards[*]

Dietary Constituent	Unit of Measure	Current Daily Values for People Over 4 Years of Age	RDA or other current dietary standard	
			Males 19 Years Old	Females 19 Years Old
Fat[‡]	grams	<65	—	—
Saturated fatty acids[‡]	"	<20	—	—
Protein[‡]	"	50	58	46
Cholesterol[§]	milligrams	<300	—	—
Carbohydrate[‡]	grams	300	—	—
Fiber	"	25	—	—
Vitamin A	micrograms Retinol Activity Equivalents	1000	900	700
Vitamin D	International Units	400	200	200
Vitamin E[§§]	"	30	22–33	22–33
Vitamin K	micrograms	80	120	90
Vitamin C	milligrams	60	90	75
Folate	micrograms	400	400	400
Thiamin	milligrams	1.5	1.20	1.10
Riboflavin	"	1.7	1.30	1.10
Niacin	"	20	16	14
Vitamin B-6	"	2	1.30	1.30
Vitamin B-12	micrograms	6	2.40	2.40
Biotin	milligrams	0.3	0.03	0.03
Pantothenic acid	"	10	5	5
Calcium	"	1000	1000	1000
Phosphorus	"	1000	700	700
Iodide	micrograms	150	150	150
Iron	milligrams	18	8	18
Magnesium	"	400	400	310
Copper	"	2	0.9	0.9
Zinc	"	15	11	8
Sodium[†]	"	<2400	500	500
Potassium[†]	"	3500	2000	2000
Chloride[†]	"	3400	750	750
Manganese	"	2	2.3	1.8
Selenium	micrograms	70	55	55
Chromium	"	120	35	25
Molybdenum	"	75	45	45

[*]Daily Values are generally set at the highest nutrient recommendation in a specific age and gender category. Many Daily Values exceed current nutrient standards. This is in part because aspects of the Daily Values were originally developed in the early 1970s using estimates of nutrient needs published in 1968. The Daily Values have yet to be updated to reflect the current state of knowledge.

[†]Sodium, potassium, and chloride values are based on the minimum requirement for health. The considerably higher Daily Values for sodium and chloride are there to allow for more diet flexibility, but the extra amounts are not needed to maintain health.

[‡]These values are based, instead, on a 2000 kcal diet, with a caloric distribution of 30% from fat (and one-third of this total from saturated fat), 60% from carbohydrate, and 10% from protein. A greater calorie intake allows more carbohydrate, fat, saturated fat, and fiber intake (see Fig. 2.5b).

[§]Based on recommendations of federal agencies.

[§§]The lower RDA value refers to vitamin E from a natural source, whereas the higher value refers to vitamin E from a synthetic source.

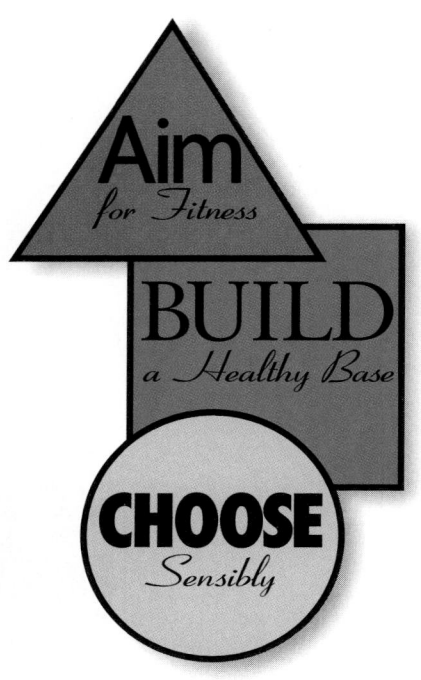

Logo for the current Dietary Guidelines.

Aim for Fitness

1. *Aim for a healthy weight*
   (body mass index of 18.5 to 24.9 and a waist circumference no more than 35 inches [88 centimeters] in women and 40 inches [102 centimeters] in men; see Chapter 10).
2. *Be physically active each day*
   (30 minutes on most or all days of the week [60 minutes per day is even better]; see Chapter 11).

Build a Healthy Base

3. *Let the pyramid guide your food choices*
   (see the previous section on the Food Guide Pyramid).
4. *Choose a variety of grains daily, especially whole grains*
   (see the Food Guide Pyramid and Chapter 4).
5. *Choose a variety of fruits and vegetables daily*
   (see the Food Guide Pyramid)
6. *Keep foods safe to eat*
   (proper cooking and refrigeration of perishable foods is especially important; see Chapter 16).

Choose Sensibly

7. *Choose a diet that is low in saturated fat and cholesterol and moderate in total fat*
   (animal fats and fast food are the chief sources; see Chapter 5).
8. *Choose beverages and foods to moderate your intake of sugars*
   (soft drinks, cookies, and candy are the chief sources; see Chapter 4).
9. *Choose and prepare foods with less salt*
   (it is easy to adjust to a lower salt intake; see Chapter 9).
10. *If you drink alcoholic beverages, do so in moderation*
    (no more than one to two drinks per day for men and one drink for women and for both men and women 65 years or older; see Chapter 7).

These guidelines are intended for healthy children (2 years and older) and adults of any age. You can view the entire Dietary Guidelines booklet at www.usda.gov/cnpp.

Practical Use of the Dietary Guidelines

The Dietary Guidelines are designed to promote adequate vitamin and mineral intake. The guidelines also emphasize changes that will reduce the risk of obesity, hypertension, cardiovascular disease, type 2 diabetes, alcoholism, and food-borne illness.

Table 2.10 Advice for Applying the Dietary Guidelines to Practical Situations

If You Usually Eat This	Eat This More Often
White bread	Whole-wheat bread (fewer nutrients lost in refinement/processing and more dietary fiber)
Sugared breakfast cereal	Low-sugar (and high-fiber) cereal (use the calories you save for a side dish of fruit)
Cheeseburger and French fries	Hamburger (hold the mayonnaise) and baked beans (for less fat and cholesterol, and the benefits of plant proteins)
Potato salad at the salad bar	Three-bean salad
Doughnut, chips, salty snack foods	Bran muffin or bagel (little or no cream cheese)
Soft drinks	Diet soft drinks (save the calories for more nutritious foods)
Boiled vegetables	Steamed vegetables (for more nutrient retention)
Canned vegetables	Frozen vegetables (fewer nutrients lost in processing)
Fried meats	Broiled meats (watch the fat drain away)
Fatty meats, such as ribs	Lean meats, such as ground round (also, eat chicken and fish often)
Whole milk and ice cream	Low-fat or nonfat milk and sherbet or frozen yogurt (to reduce saturated fat intake)
Mayonnaise or sour cream salad dressing	Oil and vinegar dressings or diet varieties (to save calories)
Cookies for a snack	Popcorn (air popped with minimal margarine or butter)
Heavily salted foods	Foods flavored primarily with herbs, spices, lemon juice

The Dietary Guidelines are not difficult to implement (Table 2.10). In addition, this overall diet approach is not especially expensive, as some people suspect. Fruits, vegetables, and low-fat and nonfat milk are no more expensive than the chips, cookies, and sugared soft drinks they should in part replace.

Note also that diet recommendations for adults have been issued by other scientific groups, such as the American Heart Association, U.S. Surgeon General, National Academy of Sciences, American Cancer Society, Canadian Ministries of Health (see Appendix B), and World Health Organization. All are consistent with the spirit of the Dietary Guidelines. These groups encourage people to modify their eating behavior in ways that are both healthful and pleasurable.

Advice from The American Dietetic Association suggests five basic principles with regard to diet and health. Be realistic, making small changes over time. Be adventurous, trying new foods regularly. Be flexible, balancing some sweet and fatty foods with physical activity. Be sensible, including favorite foods in smaller portions. Finally, be active, including physical activity in daily life.

The Dietary Guidelines and You

When using the Dietary Guidelines, you should consider your own state of health. Make specific changes and see whether they are effective. Note that results are sometimes disappointing, even when you are following a diet change very closely. Some people can eat a lot of saturated fat and still keep blood cholesterol under control. Other people, unfortunately, have high blood cholesterol even if they eat a diet low in saturated fat. Differences in genetic background are a key cause, as discussed in Chapter 3. Thus, we have individual nutritional needs and risks of developing certain diseases. One's diet should be planned with this in mind, responding to one's current health status and family history for specific diseases. However, tailoring a unique nutrition program for every North American citizen is unrealistic. The Food Guide Pyramid and the Dietary Guidelines provide typical adults with simple advice, which can be actively practiced by anyone willing to take a step toward good health.

There is no "optimal" diet. Instead, there are numerous healthful diets. The website www.ificinfo.health.org is a great source to lead you in that direction.

Critical Thinking

Athe has grown up eating the typical American diet. Having recently read and heard many news items about the relationship between nutrition and health, she is beginning to look critically at her diet and is considering making changes. However, she doesn't know where to begin. What advice would you give her?

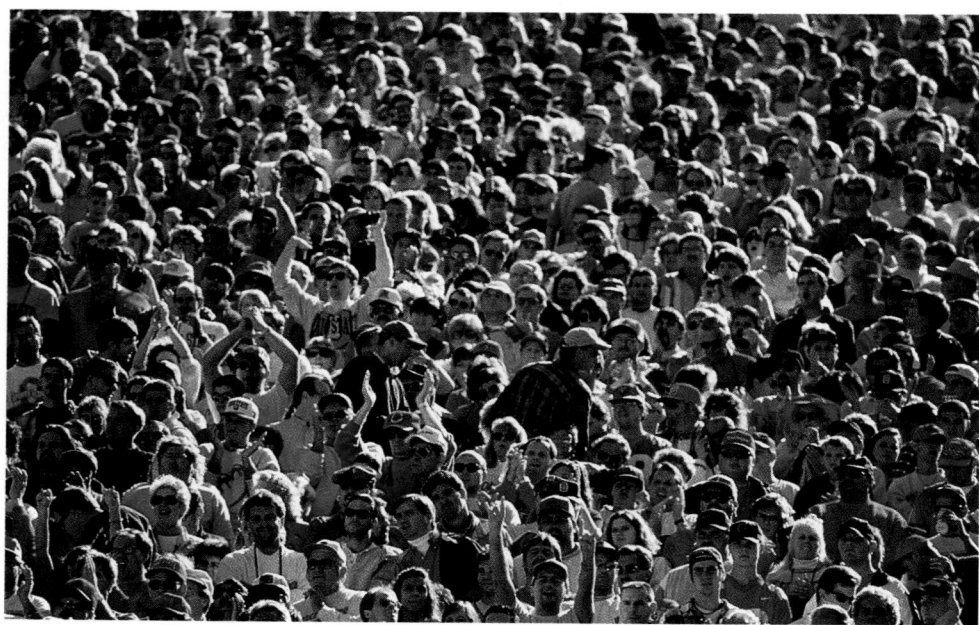

Nutrition recommendations are often made on a population-wide basis. However, in some cases, it would be more appropriate if these were made on an individual basis once a person's particular health status is known.

Concept Check

Dietary Guidelines have been set by a variety of private and government organizations. These guidelines are designed to reduce the risk of developing obesity, hypertension, type 2 diabetes, cardiovascular disease, alcoholism, and food-borne illness. To do so, they recommend eating a variety of foods, which is fostered by following the Food Guide Pyramid. They also recommend performing regular physical activity, aiming for a healthy weight, and moderating total fat, saturated fat, salt, sugar, and alcohol intake, while focusing more on fruits, vegetables, and grain products in daily menu planning. Safe food preparation and storage are also highlighted.

Scenario *Follow-Up*

The most positive aspect of Andy's diet is that it contains adequate protein, zinc, and iron because it is rich in animal protein. On the downside, his diet is low in calcium, some B-vitamins (such as folate), and vitamin C. This is because it is low in dairy products, fruits, and vegetables. It is also low in many of the phytochemical (plant-based) substances discussed at the beginning of this chapter. In addition, dietary fiber intake is low because fast-food restaurants primarily use refined grain products, rather than whole-grain products. And, since most super-sized options apply to foods rich in fat (French fries) and sugar (soft drinks), his diet is likely excessive in those two components.

He could alternate between tacos and bean burritos to gain the benefits of plant proteins in a diet. He could choose a low-fat granola bar instead of the candy bar for breakfast, or he could take the time to eat a bowl of whole-grain breakfast cereal with low-fat or nonfat milk to increase dietary fiber intake (and calcium intake in the latter case). He could also order milk at least half the time at his restaurant visits and substitute diet soft drinks for the regular variety. This would help *moderate* his sugar intake. Overall, his diet is most lacking in a variety of fruit and vegetable choices and dairy products in general because it lacks *variety* in food choice and *balance* among the five food groups.

What Do Food Labels Have to Offer in Diet Planning?

Today, nearly all foods sold in the grocery store must be labeled with the product name, name and address of the manufacturer, amount of product in the package, and ingredients listed in descending order by weight. This food and beverage labeling is monitored in North America by government agencies such as Food and Drug Administration (FDA). The listing of certain food constituents also is required—specifically, on a Nutrition Facts panel (Fig. 2.5). Use this information to learn more about what you eat. The following components must be listed: total kcal, kcal from fat, total fat, saturated fat, cholesterol, sodium, total carbohydrate, dietary fiber, sugars, protein, vitamin A, vitamin C, calcium, and iron. In addition to these required components, manufacturers can choose to list polyunsaturated and monounsaturated fat, potassium, dietary fiber, and others. Listing these components is *required*, however, if a claim is made about the health benefits of the specific nutrient (see the upcoming section in this chapter entitled "Health Claims on Food Labels") or if the food is fortified with that nutrient.

The percentage of the Daily Value (% Daily Value) is usually given for each nutrient per serving. It is important to understand that these percentages are based on a 2000 kcal diet. In other words, they are not as applicable to people who require considerably more or less than 2000 kcal per day with respect to fat and carbohydrate intake.

Serving sizes on the Nutrition Facts panel must be consistent among similar foods. This means that all brands of ice cream, for example, must use the same serving size on their label. (These serving sizes may differ from those of the Food Guide Pyramid since those of food labels are based on typical serving sizes.) In addition, food claims made on packages must follow legal definitions (Table 2.11). For example, if a product claims to be "low sodium," it must have 140 milligrams of sodium or less per serving.

Many manufacturers list the Daily Values set for dietary components such as fat, cholesterol, and carbohydrate on the Nutrition Facts panel. This can be useful as a reference point. As noted before, they are based on 2000 kcal; if the label is large enough, amounts based on 2500 kcal are listed as well for total fat, saturated fat, carbohydrate, and dietary fiber.

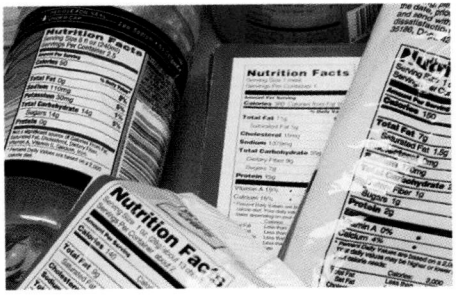

Use the Nutrition Facts label to learn more about the nutrient content of the foods you eat. Nutrient content is expressed as a percent of Daily Value. Canadian food labels have a slightly different format (review Appendix B).

Recall from Chapter 1 that the nutrition label uses the term calorie for energy values in some cases, but kilocalorie (kcal) values are actually listed.

■ Exceptions to Food Labeling

Foods such as fresh fruits and vegetables, fish, meats, and poultry currently are not required to have Nutrition Facts labels. However, many grocers and some meat packers have voluntarily chosen to provide their customers with information on these products. Nutrition Facts labels on meat products will also likely be required in the coming years. The next time you are at the grocery store, ask where you might find information on the fresh products that do not have a Nutrition Facts panel. You will likely find a poster or pamphlet near the product; often, these pamphlets contain recipes that use your favorite fruit, vegetable, or cut of meat. They may even assist you in your endeavor to improve your diet.

Because protein deficiency is not a public health concern in the United States, declaration of the % Daily Value for protein is not mandatory on foods for people over 4 years of age. If the % Daily Value is given on a label, FDA requires that the product be analyzed for protein quality. Because this procedure is expensive and time-consuming, many companies opt not to list a % Daily Value for protein rather than undergo the expense. However, labels on food for infants and children under 4 years of age must include the % Daily Value for protein, as must the labels on any food carrying a claim about protein content (see Chapter 14).

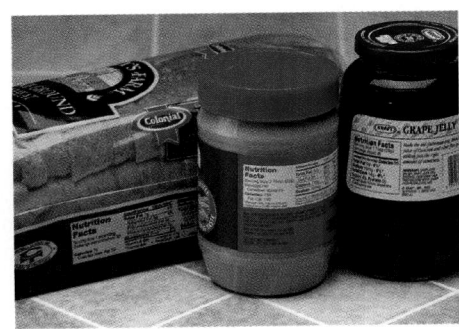

The food labels on these three products can be combined to indicate nutrient intake for a meal—a peanut butter and jelly sandwich.

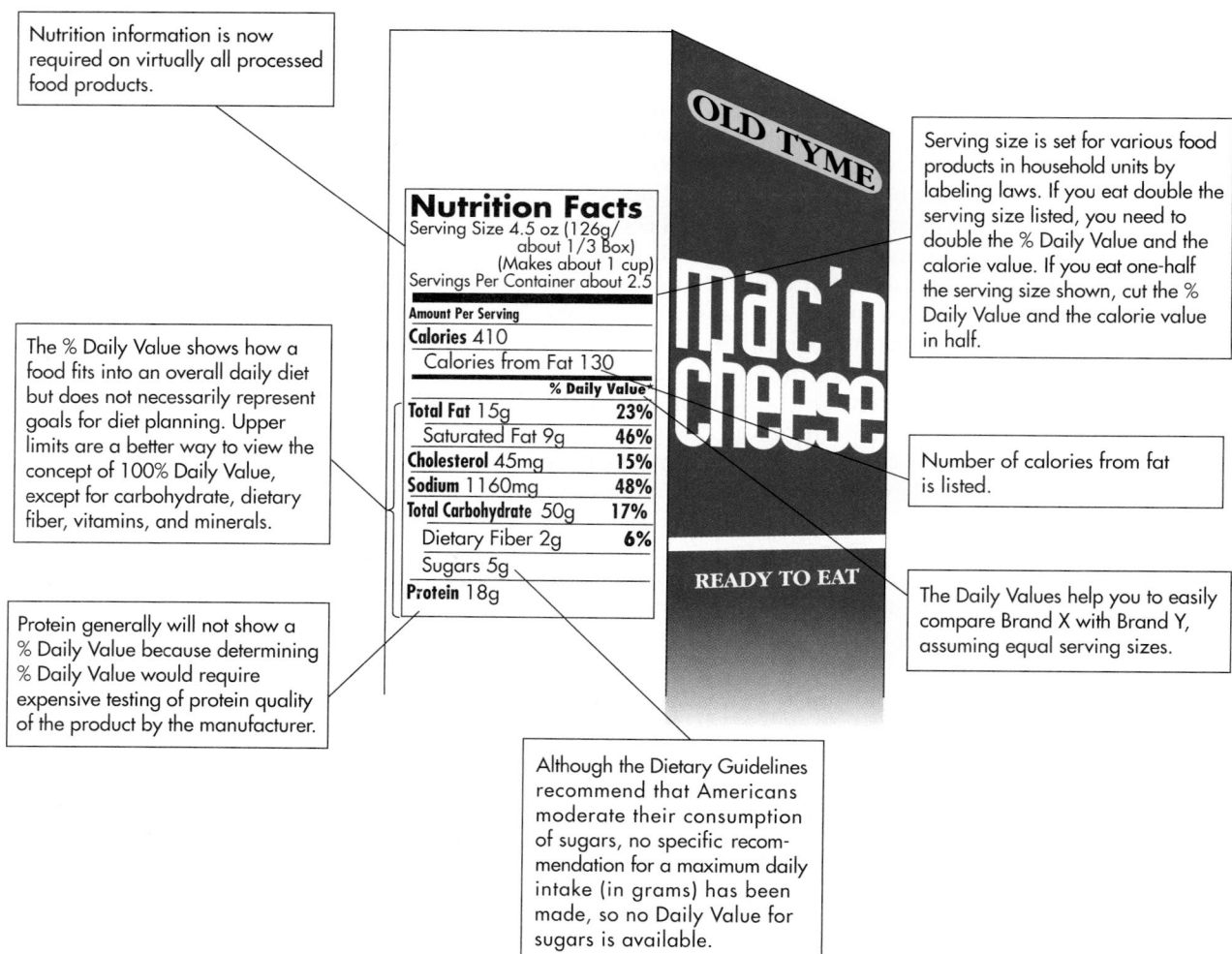

Nutrition information is now required on virtually all processed food products.

Serving size is set for various food products in household units by labeling laws. If you eat double the serving size listed, you need to double the % Daily Value and the calorie value. If you eat one-half the serving size shown, cut the % Daily Value and the calorie value in half.

The % Daily Value shows how a food fits into an overall daily diet but does not necessarily represent goals for diet planning. Upper limits are a better way to view the concept of 100% Daily Value, except for carbohydrate, dietary fiber, vitamins, and minerals.

Number of calories from fat is listed.

Protein generally will not show a % Daily Value because determining % Daily Value would require expensive testing of protein quality of the product by the manufacturer.

The Daily Values help you to easily compare Brand X with Brand Y, assuming equal serving sizes.

Although the Dietary Guidelines recommend that Americans moderate their consumption of sugars, no specific recommendation for a maximum daily intake (in grams) has been made, so no Daily Value for sugars is available.

Nutrition Facts
Serving Size 4.5 oz (126g/ about 1/3 Box) (Makes about 1 cup)
Servings Per Container about 2.5

Amount Per Serving
Calories 410
Calories from Fat 130

	% Daily Value*
Total Fat 15g	23%
Saturated Fat 9g	46%
Cholesterol 45mg	15%
Sodium 1160mg	48%
Total Carbohydrate 50g	17%
Dietary Fiber 2g	6%
Sugars 5g	
Protein 18g	

OLD TYME
mac'n cheese
READY TO EAT

Figure 2.5a The Nutrition Facts panel on a current food label. The box is broken into two parts: (a) is the top and (b) is the bottom. The % Daily Value listed on the label is the percentage of the generally accepted amount of a nutrient needed daily that is present in 1 serving of the product. You can use the % Daily Values to compare your diet with current nutrition recommendations for certain diet components. Let's consider dietary fiber. Assume that you consume 2000 kcal per day, which is the energy intake corresponding to the % Daily Values listed on labels. If the total % Daily Value for dietary fiber in all the foods you eat in one day adds up to 100%, your diet meets the recommendations for dietary fiber. Food labels also contain the name and address of the food manufacturers. This allows consumers to contact the manufacturer if they desire.

■ Health Claims on Food Labels

Nutrient and herbal supplements have a different layout with a "Supplement Facts" heading. Chapters 8 and 15 show examples of these labels.

As a marketing tool directed toward the health-conscious consumer, food manufacturers are asserting that their products have all sorts of health benefits. This campaign began in earnest in 1984, when the Kellogg Company, in conjunction with The National Cancer Institute, printed a health claim on its "high-fiber" cereals, stating that dietary fiber may help prevent certain forms of cancer. This type of label message was not allowed at the time and caused a heated debate among nutrition scientists. After reviewing hundreds of comments on the proposed rule allowing health claims, FDA, which has legal oversight over most food products, decided to permit this and other health claims with certain restrictions.

Currently, FDA limits the use of health messages to specific diseases in which there is significant scientific agreement concerning the relationship between a nutrient, food, or food constituent and the disease. The claims allowed at this time may show a link between the following:

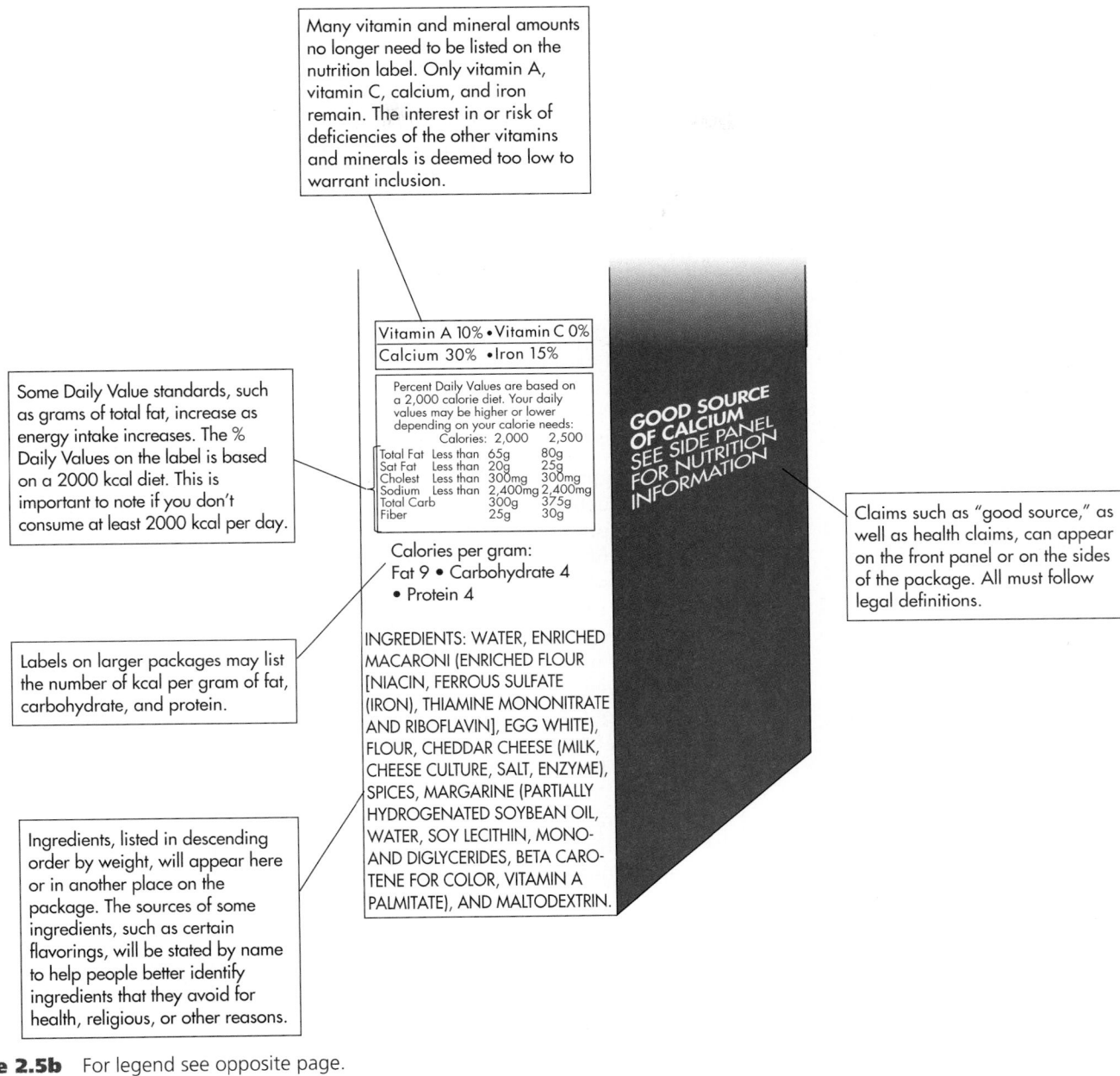

Many vitamin and mineral amounts no longer need to be listed on the nutrition label. Only vitamin A, vitamin C, calcium, and iron remain. The interest in or risk of deficiencies of the other vitamins and minerals is deemed too low to warrant inclusion.

Some Daily Value standards, such as grams of total fat, increase as energy intake increases. The % Daily Values on the label is based on a 2000 kcal diet. This is important to note if you don't consume at least 2000 kcal per day.

Labels on larger packages may list the number of kcal per gram of fat, carbohydrate, and protein.

Claims such as "good source," as well as health claims, can appear on the front panel or on the sides of the package. All must follow legal definitions.

Ingredients, listed in descending order by weight, will appear here or in another place on the package. The sources of some ingredients, such as certain flavorings, will be stated by name to help people better identify ingredients that they avoid for health, religious, or other reasons.

Vitamin A 10% • Vitamin C 0%
Calcium 30% • Iron 15%

Percent Daily Values are based on a 2,000 calorie diet. Your daily values may be higher or lower depending on your calorie needs:

	Calories:	2,000	2,500
Total Fat	Less than	65g	80g
Sat Fat	Less than	20g	25g
Cholest	Less than	300mg	300mg
Sodium	Less than	2,400mg	2,400mg
Total Carb		300g	375g
Fiber		25g	30g

Calories per gram:
Fat 9 • Carbohydrate 4 • Protein 4

INGREDIENTS: WATER, ENRICHED MACARONI (ENRICHED FLOUR [NIACIN, FERROUS SULFATE (IRON), THIAMINE MONONITRATE AND RIBOFLAVIN], EGG WHITE), FLOUR, CHEDDAR CHEESE (MILK, CHEESE CULTURE, SALT, ENZYME), SPICES, MARGARINE (PARTIALLY HYDROGENATED SOYBEAN OIL, WATER, SOY LECITHIN, MONO- AND DIGLYCERIDES, BETA CARO-TENE FOR COLOR, VITAMIN A PALMITATE), AND MALTODEXTRIN.

GOOD SOURCE OF CALCIUM SEE SIDE PANEL FOR NUTRITION INFORMATION

Figure 2.5b   For legend see opposite page.

- A diet with enough calcium and a reduced risk of osteoporosis
- A diet low in total fat and a reduced risk of some cancers
- A diet low in saturated fat and cholesterol and a reduced risk of cardiovascular disease (typically referred to as heart disease on the label)
- A diet rich in dietary fiber—containing grain products, fruits, and vegetables and a reduced risk of some cancers
- A diet low in sodium and high in potassium and a reduced risk of hypertension and stroke
- A diet rich in fruits and vegetables and a reduced risk of some cancers
- A diet adequate in the synthetic form of the vitamin folate (called folic acid) and a reduced risk of neural tube defects (a type of birth defect)
- Use of sugarless gum and a reduced risk of tooth decay, especially when compared with foods high in sugars and starches

*S*ome products make so-called "structure/function" claims, such as "improves blood circulation." These do not fall under FDA jurisdiction because of laws passed by the U.S. Congress in 1994 (see Chapter 1). View any of these non-FDA-approved claims skeptically.

- A diet rich in fruits, vegetables, and grain products that contain fiber and a reduced risk of cardiovascular disease. Oats (oatmeal, oat bran, and oat flour) and psyllium are two fiber-rich ingredients that can be singled out in reducing the risk of cardiovascular disease, as long as the statement also says the diet should also be low in saturated fat and cholesterol.
- A diet rich in whole-grain foods and other plant foods, as well as low in total fat, saturated fat, and cholesterol, and a reduced risk of cardiovascular disease and certain cancers
- A diet low in saturated fat and cholesterol that also includes 25 grams of soy protein and a reduced risk of cardiovascular disease. The statement "one serving of the (name food) provides _____ grams of soy protein" must also appear as part of the health claim.
- A diet rich in potassium and a reduced risk of stroke
- Omega-3 fatty acids from oils present in fish and a reduced risk of cardiovascular disease
- Margarines containing plant stanols and sterols and a reduced risk of cardiovascular disease (see Chapter 5 for more details on plant stanols and sterols)

A "may" or "might" qualifier must be used in the statement.

In addition, before a health claim can be made for a food product, it must meet two general requirements. First, the food must be a "good source" (before fortification) of dietary fiber, protein, vitamin A, vitamin C, calcium, or iron. The legal definition of "good source" appears in Table 2.11. Second, a single serving of the food product cannot contain more than 13 grams of fat, 4 grams of saturated fat, 60 milligrams of cholesterol, or 480 milligrams of sodium. If a food exceeds any one of these amounts, no health claim can be made for it, despite its other nutritional qualities. For example, even though whole milk is high in calcium, its label can't make the health claim about calcium and osteoporosis because whole milk contains 5 grams of saturated fat per serving.

In addition, the product must meet criteria specific to the health claim being made. For example, a health claim regarding fat and cancer can be made only if the product contains 3 grams or less of fat per serving, which is the standard for low-fat foods.

The bottom line for health claims is honesty. FDA is vigilant in controlling the claims made about foods on supermarket shelves.

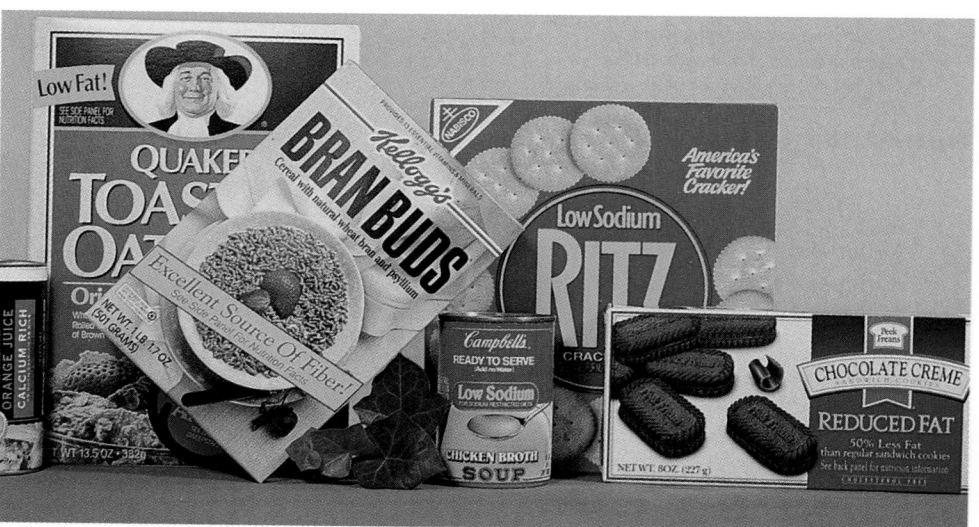

Many products prominently feature health claims.

Table 2.11 Definitions for Comparative and Absolute Nutrient Claims on Food Labels

Sugar

- *Sugar free:* less than 0.5 grams (g) per serving.
- *No added sugar; without added sugar; no sugar added:*
    - No sugars were added during processing or packing, including ingredients that contain sugars (for example, fruit juices, applesauce, or jam).
    - Processing does not increase the sugar content above the amount naturally present in the ingredients. (A functionally insignificant increase in sugars is acceptable for processes used for purposes other than increasing sugar content.)
    - The food that it resembles and for which it substitutes normally contains added sugars.
    - If the food doesn't meet the requirements for a low- or reduced-calorie food, the product bears a statement that the food is not low calorie or calorie reduced and directs consumers' attention to the nutrition panel for further information on sugars and calorie content.
- *Reduced sugar:* at least 25% less sugar per serving than reference food

Calories

- *Calorie free:* fewer than 5 kcal per serving
- *Low calorie:* 40 kcal or less per serving and, if the serving is 30 g or less or 2 tablespoons or less, per 50 g of the food
- *Reduced or fewer calories:* at least 25% fewer kcal per serving than reference food

Fiber

- *High fiber:* 5 g or more per serving. (Foods making high-fiber claims must meet the definition for low fat, or the level of total fat must appear next to the high-fiber claim.)
- *Good source of fiber:* 2.5 to 4.9 g per serving
- *More or added fiber:* at least 2.5 g more per serving than reference food

Fat

- *Fat free:* less than 0.5 g of fat per serving
- *Saturated fat free:* less than 0.5 g per serving, and the level of trans fatty acids does not exceed 0.5 g per serving

- *Low fat:* 3 g or less per serving and, if the serving is 30 g or less or 2 tablespoons or less, per 50 g of the food. 2% milk can no longer be labeled low fat, as it exceeds 3 g per serving. *Reduced fat* will be the term used instead.
- *Low saturated fat:* 1 g or less per serving and not more than 15% of kcal from saturated fatty acids
- *Reduced or less fat:* at least 25% less per serving than reference food
- *Reduced or less saturated fat:* at least 25% less per serving than reference food

Cholesterol

- *Cholesterol free:* less than 2 milligrams (mg) of cholesterol and 2 g or less of saturated fat per serving
- *Low cholesterol:* 20 mg or less cholesterol and 2 g or less of saturated fat per serving and, if the serving is 30 g or less or 2 tablespoons or less, per 50 g of the food
- *Reduced or less cholesterol:* at least 25% less cholesterol and 2 g or less of saturated fat per serving than reference food

Sodium

- *Sodium free:* less than 5 mg per serving
- *Very low sodium:* 35 mg or less per serving and, if the serving is 30 g or less or 2 tablespoons or less, per 50 g of the food
- *Low sodium:* 140 mg or less per serving and, if the serving is 30 g or less or 2 tablespoons or less, per 50 g of the food
- *Light in sodium:* at least 50% less per serving than reference food
- *Reduced or less sodium:* at least 25% less per serving than reference food

Other Terms

- **Fortified or enriched:** Vitamins and/or minerals have been added to the product in amounts in excess of at least 10% of that normally present in the usual product.
- *Healthy:* An individual food that is low fat and low saturated fat and has no more than 360 to 480 mg of sodium or 60 mg of cholesterol per serving can be labeled "healthy" if it provides at least 10% of vitamin A, vitamin C, protein, calcium, iron, or dietary fiber.
- *Light or lite:* The descriptor *light* or *lite* can mean two things: first, that a nutritionally

altered product contains one-third fewer kcal or half the fat of reference food (if the food derives 50% or more of its kcal from fat, the reduction must be 50% of the fat) and, second, that the sodium content of a low-calorie, low-fat food has been reduced by 50%. 2% milk can no longer be labeled low fat because it has more than 3 g of fat per serving. In addition, "light in sodium" may be used for foods in which the sodium content has been reduced by at least 50%. The term *light* may still be used to describe such properties as texture and color, as long as the label explains the intent—for example, "light brown sugar" and "light and fluffy."

- *Diet:* A food may be labeled with terms such as *diet, dietetic, artificially sweetened,* or *sweetened with nonnutritive sweetener* only if the claim is not false or misleading. The food can also be labeled *low calorie* or *reduced calorie.*
- *Good source:* *Good source* means that a food contains 10% to 19% of the Daily Value for a particular nutrient.
- *High:* *High* means that a food contains 20% or more of the Daily Value for a particular nutrient.
- *Organic:* Federal standards for organic foods allow claims when much of the ingredients do not use chemical fertilizers or pesticides, genetic engineering, sewage sludge, antibiotics, or irradiation in their production. At least 95% of ingredients must meet these guidelines to be labeled "organic" on the front of the package. For livestock, the animals need to be allowed to graze outdoors and as well be fed organic feed. They also cannot be exposed to antibiotics or growth hormones.
- *Natural:* The food must be free of food colors, synthetic flavors, or any other synthetic substance.

The following terms apply only to meat and poultry products regulated by USDA.

- *Extra lean:* less than 5 g of fat, 2 g of saturated fat, and 95 mg of cholesterol per serving (or 100 g of an individual food)
- *Lean:* less than 10 g of fat, 4.5 g of saturated fat, and 95 mg of cholesterol per serving (or 100 g of an individual food)

Many definitions are from FDA's *Dictionary of Terms,* as established in conjunction with the 1990 NLEA. g = grams; mg = milligrams

Concept Check

The Nutrition Facts panel on a food label provides key information for helping track one's food intake. Nutrient quantities are compared with the Daily Values and expressed on a percentage basis (% Daily Value). This information can be used to either increase or reduce intake of specific nutrients. Health claims on food labels are closely regulated by FDA. Fruits, vegetables, whole grains, soy, and rich sources of calcium are prominent among the foods that can make specific health claims.

The **Exchange System** is a final menu-planning tool. This tool organizes foods based on energy, protein, carbohydrate, and fat content. The result is a manageable framework for designing diets. For more information on the Exchange System see Appendixes C and D.

Epilogue

The tools discussed in this chapter greatly aid in menu planning. Menu planning can start with the Food Guide Pyramid. The totality of choices made within the groups can then be evaluated using the Dietary Guidelines. Individual foods that make up a diet can be examined more closely using the comparison with the Daily Values listed on the Nutrition Facts panel of the product. For the most part, these Daily Values are in line with the Recommended Dietary Allowances and related nutrient standards. The Nutrition Facts panel is especially useful in identifying nutrient-dense foods—foods that are high in a specific nutrient, such as the vitamin folate, but low in comparison with the relative amount of energy provided—as well as foods that fill you up without providing a lot of calories. The latter are described as foods with low energy density. Generally speaking, the more you learn about and use these tools, the more they will benefit your diet.

Summary

1. *Variety, balance,* and *moderation* are three watchwords of diet planning.

2. Nutrient density is a useful concept. It reflects the nutrient content of a food in relation to its energy (kcal) content. Nutrient-dense foods are relatively rich in nutrients, in comparison with energy content.

3. Energy density of a food is determined by comparing energy content with the weight of food. A food that is rich in calories but weighs relatively very little, such as nuts, cookies, fried foods in general, and fat-free snacks, is considered energy dense. Foods with low energy density include fruits, vegetables, and any food that incorporates lots of water during cooking, such as oatmeal.

4. A person's nutritional state can be categorized as *desirable nutrition,* in which the body has adequate stores for times of increased needs; *undernutrition,* which may be present with or without clinical symptoms; and *overnutrition,* which can lead to vitamin and mineral toxicities and various chronic diseases.

5. Evaluation of nutritional state involves analyzing background factors, anthropometric measurements, biochemical parameters, clinical evidence, diet history, and economic status. It is not always possible to detect nutritional inadequacies via nutrition assessment since such evidence often does not appear for many years.

6. The Food Guide Pyramid is designed to translate nutrient recommendations into a food plan that exhibits variety, balance, and moderation. The best results are obtained by using low-fat or non-fat dairy products; including some vegetable proteins in addition to animal-protein foods; including citrus fruits and dark green vegetables; and emphasizing whole-grain breads and cereals.

7. Dietary Guidelines have been issued to help reduce chronic diseases in our population. The guidelines emphasize eating a variety of foods; performing regular physical activity; maintaining or improving weight; moderating consumption of fats, cholesterol, sugar, salt, and alcohol; eating plenty of grain products, fruits, and vegetables; and safely preparing and storing foods, especially perishable foods.

8. Recommended Dietary Allowances (RDAs) are set for many nutrients. These amounts yield enough of each nutrient to meet the needs of healthy individuals within specific gender and age categories. Adequate Intake (AI) is the standard used when not enough information is available to set a revised RDA. Tolerable Upper Intake Levels (Upper Levels or ULs) for nutrient intake have been set for some vitamins and minerals. All of the many dietary standards fall under the term *Dietary Reference Intakes (DRIs).* Daily Values are used as a basis for expressing the nutrient content of foods on the Nutrition Facts panel and are based for the most part on the RDAs published in 1968.

9. Food labels are a powerful tool to track your nutrient intake and learn more about the nutritional characteristics of the foods you eat. Any health claims listed must follow specific legal criteria set by FDA.

Study Questions

1. Describe the philosophy underlying the creation of the Food Guide Pyramid. What dietary changes would you need to make to meet the Pyramid guidelines on a regular basis?
2. Trace the progression, in terms of physical results, of a person who went from an overnourished to an undernourished state.
3. How could the nutritional state of the person at each state in question 2 be evaluated?
4. Describe the intent of the Dietary Guidelines. Point out one criticism for its general application to all North American adults.
5. Based on the discussion of the Dietary Guidelines, suggest two key dietary changes the typical North American adult should consider making.
6. How do RDAs and Adequate Intakes differ from Daily Values in intention and application?
7. How would you explain the concepts of nutrient density and energy density to a fourth-grade class?
8. Nutritionists encourage all people to read labels on food packages to learn more about what they eat. What four nutrients could easily be tracked in your diet if you read the Nutrition Facts panels regularly on food products?
9. Explain why consumers can have confidence in FDA-approved health claims on food packages.
10. Relate the importance of variety in a diet, especially with regard to fruit and vegetable choices, to the discovery of various phytochemicals in foods.

Further Readings

1. ADA Reports: Position of the American Dietetic Association: Functional foods. *Journal of the American Dietetic Association,* 99:1278, 1999.
   The philosophy that food can be health promoting beyond its traditional nutritional value (i.e., phytochemical content) is gaining acceptance among scientists and health professionals. Never before have the health benefits of food had so much support.
2. American Heart Association Conference Proceedings: Unified dietary recommendations. *Circulation* 100:450, 1999.
   A variety of health-related organizations, such as the American Heart Association and American Cancer Society, provide support for the dietary pattern recommended by the Dietary Guidelines.
3. Campbell TC, Chen J: Diet and health in rural China: Lessons learned and unlearned. *Nutrition Today* 34:116, 1999.
   Studies of rural Asian subjects show that their traditional, primarily plant-based diet contributes to their low risk for chronic degenerative diseases. These findings are consistent with the observations of Asian migrants; they experience more of these diseases when they switch to a more westernized approach.
4. Clairmont MA: Nutraceuticals, phytochemicals and functional foods: A field of dreams for dietitians. *Today's Dietitian,* p. 36, April 2000.
   Growing evidence supports the role of phytochemicals in disease prevention. Phytochemical-rich foods discussed include broccoli, cabbage, tomatoes, tea, soy, whole grains, oranges, grapes, and onions.
5. de Lorgeril M and others: Mediterranean diet, traditional risk factors, and the rate of cardiovascular complications after myocardial infarction: Final report of the Lyon Diet Heart Study. *Circulation* 99:779, 1999.
   People following a Mediterranean diet plan—in this case, based on canola oil products rather than the traditional source of fat, olive oil—showed a substantial reduction in heart attack risk. This study provides further evidence of the benefits of the Mediterranean diet.
6. Hasler C and others: How to evaluate the safety, efficacy, and quality of functional foods and their ingredients. *Journal of the American Dietetic Association* 101:733, 2001.
   The term "functional food" is not yet legally defined. It is usually understood to mean any food or food ingredient that may provide a health benefit beyond the traditional nutrients it contains. The article goes on to review current health claims for foods.
7. Laudan R: Birth of the modern diet. *Scientific American,* p. 76, August 2000.
   Advances in knowledge concerning diet and nutrition have had a great effect on our diets over the last 300 years. Recognizing the importance of fruits and vegetables scores high marks for our current diet, while the central rule of fat in our diets because of the importance given to meat and fat-based sauces is blamed for the high amounts of obesity in most developed nations.
8. Rolls BJ: The role of energy density in the overconsumption of fat. *Journal of Nutrition* 130:2685, 2000.
   Eating foods that have a low energy density is one way to feel full without consuming a lot of calories. If the food is high in fat, even small portions may have a high energy content; energy-dense foods are generally consumed in larger quantities in order to feel full at the end of a meal.
9. Stampfer JM and others: Primary prevention of coronary heart disease in women through diet and lifestyle. *New England Journal of Medicine* 343:16, 2000.
   Women who consume a varied diet (one rich in fiber, includes some fish, and is low in fried foods and animal fat), avoid overweight, drink small amounts of alcohol, exercise on a daily basis for about 30 minutes, and avoid smoking reduce their risk of heart attack by over 80%, compared with women without these habits.
10. Willett WC: *Eat, drink, and be healthy,* New York: Simon & Schuster, 2001.
    The diet plan in the book emphasizes whole grains, plant oils, vegetables eaten daily; fruits at least 2–3 times per day; nuts and legumes 1–3 times per day; fish, poultry, and eggs eaten 0–2 times per day; dairy products or calcium supplements one to two times per day; and little use of red meat, butter, white rice, white bread, potatoes, pasta, and sweets. Regular physical activity and weight control is also recommended, as is alcohol intake in moderation (if of legal age) and a multivitamin and mineral supplement for most people.

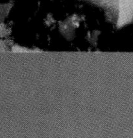

I. Does Your Diet Meet Nutrient Needs, Food Guide Pyramid Recommendations, and the Dietary Guidelines?

Complete either Part I or Part II. Then complete Parts III, IV, and V. (For help in following the instructions for this activity, see the sample assessment in Appendix E.)

Part I

Manual RDA Analysis

A. Take the information from the 1-day food-intake record you completed in Chapter 1 and record it on the blank form provided in Appendix E or by your instructor. Be sure to record the food or drink ingested and the amount (e.g., weight) consumed. Note: Your instructor may require you to keep the food record for more than 1 day.

B. Review the various nutrient standards on the inside cover of this book and choose the appropriate recommendations for your gender and age. Write the appropriate value for each nutrient on the line on the form labeled "Nutrient Need." The values for sodium and potassium from the table on the inside cover of the book are labeled "Estimated Sodium, Chloride, and Potassium Requirements of Healthy Persons."

C. Look up the foods and drinks that you listed on the form in the food composition table, Appendix A. Record on the form the amounts of each nutrient and the kcal present in them, based on the serving size and the number of servings you ate. For example, if you drank 2 cups of milk and the serving size listed in Appendix A is 1 cup, double all nutrient values as you record them. If the food is not listed, choose a substitute, such as cola for root beer.

D. For each food and drink, add the amounts in each column and record the results on the line labeled "Totals."

E. Compare the totals to your nutrient needs. Divide the total for each nutrient by the specific amount and multiply that by 100. Record the result on the line labeled "% of Nutrient Needs."

F. Keep this assessment for use in subsequent activities in other chapters.

Part II

Computer Diet Analysis

A. Load the software (shrink-wrapped with this book) into the computer.

B. Choose RDAs and related nutrient standards based on your age and gender.

C. Enter the information from the 1-day food-intake record you kept in Chapter 1. Be sure to enter each food and drink and the specific amount you ate.

D. This software program will give you the following results:

1. The appropriate RDA (or related standard) for each nutrient

2. The total amount of each nutrient and the kcal consumed for the day

3. The percentage intake compared with needs for each nutrient that you consumed

E. Keep this assessment for use in subsequent activities in other chapters.

Part III

Evaluation of Nutrient Intakes as a Percentage of Nutrient Needs

Remember that you don't necessarily need to consume your estimated nutrient needs every day. A general standard is meeting needs averaged over 5 to 8 days. It is best not to exceed the Upper Level (if set) over the long term to avoid potential toxic effects for some nutrients.

A. For which nutrients did your intakes fall below estimated nutrient needs?

B. Did you exceed the minimum requirements for sodium? To what degree?

C. For which nutrients did you exceed the Upper Level (if set)?

D. What dietary changes could you make to correct or improve your dietary profile? If you're not sure, Chapters 4 through 9 will help guide your decisions.

Part IV
Food Guide Pyramid

Using the same food-intake record used in Part I or II, place each food item in the appropriate group of the Food Guide Pyramid chart in Appendix E. That is, for each food item, indicate how many servings it contributes to each group based on the amount you ate (see Table 2.6 for serving sizes). Note that many of your food choices may contribute to more than one group. For example, toast with margarine contributes to two categories: (1) the breads, cereals, rice, and pasta group; and (2) fats, oils, and sweets. After entering all the values, add the number of servings consumed in each group. Finally, compare your total in each food group with the recommended number of servings shown in Figure 2.3. Enter a minus sign (−) if your total falls below the recommendation or a plus sign (+) if it equals or exceeds the recommendation.

Part V
Further Diet Evaluation

Do the weaknesses, if any, suggested in your nutrient analysis (see Part III) correspond to missing servings in the Food Guide Pyramid chart? If so, consider changing your food choices based on the Food Guide Pyramid to help improve your nutrient profile. Finally, indicate whether your day's diet did or did not conform to the following items in the Dietary Guidelines:

	Yes	No
Aim for Fitness		
• Aim for a healthy weight.	_____	_____
• Be physically active each day.	_____	_____
Build a Healthy Base		
• Let the pyramid guide your food choices.	_____	_____
• Choose a variety of grains daily, especially whole grains.	_____	_____
• Choose a variety of fruits and vegetables daily.	_____	_____
• Keep foods safe to eat.	_____	_____
Choose Sensibly		
• Choose a diet that is a low in saturated fat and cholesterol and moderate in total fat.	_____	_____
• Choose beverages and foods to moderate your intake of sugars.	_____	_____
• Choose and prepare foods with less salt.	_____	_____
• If you drink alcoholic beverages, do so in moderation.	_____	_____

If your diet comes up short on any of these evaluations, take appropriate action to improve your eating patterns.

II. Applying the Nutrition Facts Label to Your Daily Food Choices

Imagine that you are at the supermarket looking for a quick meal before a busy evening. In the frozen food section, you find two brands of frozen cheese manicotti (see labels a and b). Which of the two brands would you choose? What information on the Nutrition Facts label in the figure contributed to this decision?

_____

_____

_____

_____

Nutrition Facts
Serving Size 1 Package (260g)
Servings Per Container 1

Amount Per Serving
Calories 390   Calories from Fat 160

	% Daily Value*
Total Fat 18g	**27%**
Saturated Fat 9g	**45%**
Cholesterol 45mg	**14%**
Sodium 880mg	**36%**
Total Carbohydrate 38g	**13%**
Dietary Fiber 4g	**15%**
Sugars 12g	
Protein 17g	

Vitamin A 10% • Vitamin C 4%

Calcium 40% • Iron 8%

*Percent Daily Values are based on a 2,000 calorie diet. Your daily values may be higher or lower depending on your calorie needs:

	Calories:	2,000	2,500
Total Fat	Less than	65g	80g
Sat Fat	Less than	20g	25g
Cholesterol	Less than	300mg	300mg
Sodium	Less than	2,400mg	2,400mg
Total Carbohydrate		300g	375g
Dietary Fiber		25g	30g

(a)

Nutrition Facts
Serving Size 1 Package (260g)
Servings Per Container 1

Amount Per Serving
Calories 230   Calories from Fat 35

	% Daily Value*
Total Fat 4g	**6%**
Saturated Fat 2g	**10%**
Cholesterol 15mg	**4%**
Sodium 590mg	**24%**
Total Carbohydrate 28g	**9%**
Dietary Fiber 3g	**12%**
Sugars 10g	
Protein 19g	

Vitamin A 10% • Vitamin C 10%

Calcium 35% • Iron 4%

*Percent Daily Values are based on a 2,000 calorie diet. Your daily values may be higher or lower depending on your calorie needs:

	Calories:	2,000	2,500
Total Fat	Less than	65g	80g
Sat Fat	Less than	20g	25g
Cholesterol	Less than	300mg	300mg
Sodium	Less than	2,400mg	2,400mg
Potassium		3,500mg	3,500mg
Total Carbohydrate		300g	375g
Dietary Fiber		25g	30g

(b)

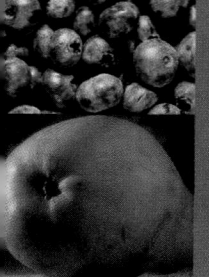

Human societies have developed under widely varying conditions. These conditions affected which foods were available (e.g., rice vs. wheat) and how long each food could be stored (e.g., tropical vs. temperate climates). This, in turn, influenced the dietary patterns of these various cultures. As these various cultures migrated to new locations, the migrants kept some traditional dietary habits, or *foodways;* changed some habits; and abandoned others. As people migrate and mingle with those of other cultures, their cuisines tend to mingle as well. Note that about 25% of all restaurants in the United States have an ethnic theme. Recent changes in affluence and technology also affect dietary habits, some for better and some for worse.

This Nutrition Issue examines how the cuisines of various cultures throughout the world have affected the North American diet. Examining the nutritional attributes of a number of ethnic diets will help you understand that no single cuisine is either completely healthful or unhealthful. The trick to finding healthful food is to evaluate individual dishes carefully. Let's look at six cuisines that contribute to food "North American style." Note that almost all North Americans sample at least one of these on a regular basis.

Native American Influences

The size and varied geography of the North American continent meant that different foods were available to people living in different locations. Some of these people were hunter-gatherers, depending on wild vegetation and wild game for subsistence. Others learned to grow vegetable crops. Depending on where they lived, Native American groups cultivated early forms of such plant foods as tomatoes, sweet potatoes, squash, vanilla, and cocoa. Their diets tended to be low in sodium and fat and high in dietary fiber. In the far north, populations subsisted on fish, sea mammals, other game, and a few plants, such as seaweed, willow leaves, and berries.

Studies have shown that the diseases that affected these societies differed significantly from the diseases common in North American society today. For example, Alaskan natives who still eat the traditional diet have cardiovascular disease rates lower than those in the general North American population. Younger generations of Alaskan natives, however, who usually do not eat the traditional diet, have developed cardiovascular disease at rates similar to North Americans in general. This is also true of the Pima Indiana tribe in Arizona. These and other studies indicate that, as societies become more uniform, so, too, do disease patterns.

Hispanic Influences

When Spanish colonists arrived in what is now called Latin America, they brought foods, flavors, and cooking techniques, which they combined with locally available foods. Several cuisines developed from those combinations, influenced also by the arrival of other groups. Thus, the Cuban cuisine combined native foods with those of both Spanish and Chinese immigrants, whereas the Puerto Rican cuisine combined native foods with Spanish and African contributions. In Mexico, the Spanish influence mingled with that of local Native American cuisines.

The Mayans, Aztecs, and other populations in Mexico grew corn, beans, and chili peppers; these were the basis of Mexican cuisine. They also grew such fruits as avocados, papayas, and pineapples. By the end of the fifteenth century, wheat, chickpeas, melons, radishes, grapes, and

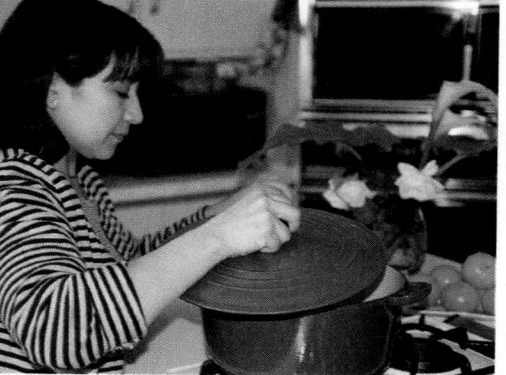

Our cooking habits often reflect our ethnic heritage.

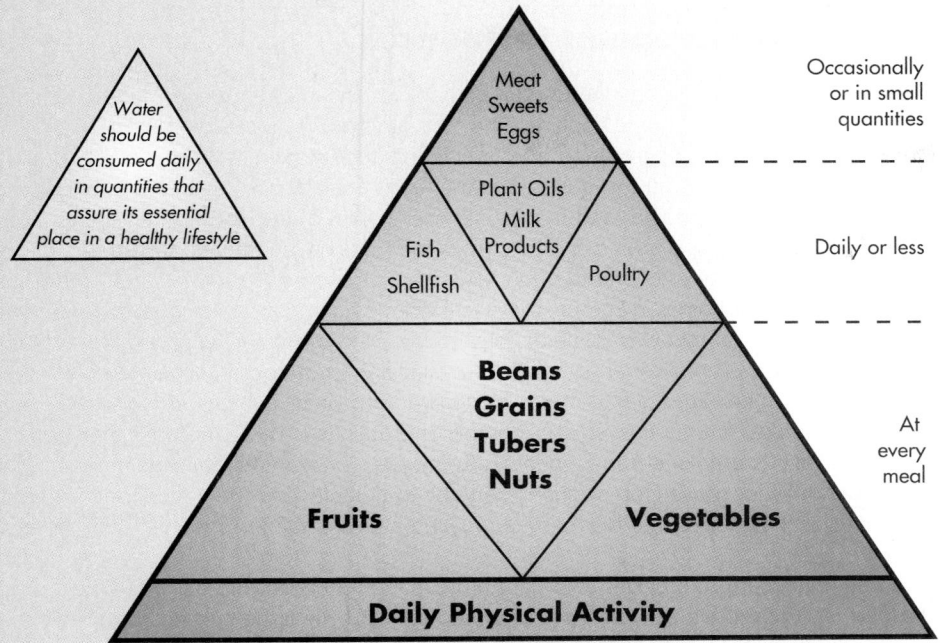

Water should be consumed daily in quantities that assure its essential place in a healthy lifestyle

Meat
Sweets
Eggs

Plant Oils
Milk
Products

Fish
Shellfish

Poultry

**Beans
Grains
Tubers
Nuts**

Fruits

Vegetables

Daily Physical Activity

Occasionally
or in small
quantities

Daily or less

At
every
meal

Alcohol may be consumed by adults in moderation and with meals, but consumption
should be avoided during pregnancy and whenever it would put the individual or others at risk.

Figure 2.6 The traditional healthy Latin American Diet Pyramid. A variety of diet pyramids have been developed by Oldways Preservation & Exchange Trust. These pyramids reflect the typical diets of rural peoples in the region, in this case Latin America. Text accompanying the Latin American Pyramid, as is true for the other Oldways ethnic pyramids, states that alcohol may be consumed with meals, but consumption should be avoided during pregnancy and whenever it would put the individual or others at risk. As you will notice throughout this Nutrition Issue, all pyramids developed by governmental or private organizations always have fruits, vegetables, and grains at the base. The Latin American Diet Pyramid then adds nuts and beans to this base; other pyramids also slightly alter the base.
Copyright 1998 Oldways Preservation & Exchange Trust

sugar cane had been brought to the New World. Rice, citrus fruits, and some kinds of nuts came soon afterward. The Spanish also introduced beef, lamb, and chicken. Native inhabitants had previously eaten mostly fish and wild game. Spices such as cinnamon, black pepper, cloves, thyme, marjoram, and bay leaves were introduced and became part of the cuisine.

Mexican cuisine today shows regional variety. In southern Mexico, savory sauces and stews and corn tortillas reflect the native heritage. The Gulf states are renowned for delicious seafood dishes prepared with tomatoes, herbs, and olives, whereas Yucatan cuisine follows Mayan tradition, with such specialties as wild turkey and fish flavored with lime juice. Fresh produce adds color, flavor, and nutrition to authentic Mexican dining. Markets in North America are beginning to offer some of these plant foods, such as chayote, squash, jicama root, plantains, and cactus leaves and fruit. Traditional Mexican cooking is healthful in that it is high in complex carbohydrates, beans, fruits, and vegetables, particularly those rich in vitamins A and C. This pattern is reflected in the Latin American Diet Pyramid issued by Oldways Preservation & Exchange Trust in 1996 (Fig. 2.6). For more information on this and other ethnic diet pyramids, see the website www.oldwayspf.org. Today, true Mexican cooking bears little resemblance to the dishes usually found in "Mexican" restaurants in North America. Usually it is neither oily nor heavy and is based primarily on rice and beans. Restaurant Mexican food tends to use larger portions of meat, as well as adding portions of high-fat sour cream, guacamole, and cheese to many dishes.

continued

Northern European Influences

Immigrants from Western Europe are responsible for the "meat-and-potatoes" presentation of traditional North American home cooking. The first large group of settlers from Europe—the English, French, and Germans—brought their traditional foodways with them. As all cooks and cultures must do, these immigrants adapted to the foods available in the regions in which they settled. Native Americans shared foods, which are now staples of the North American diet: corn and corn products, such as popcorn and hominy; some kinds of squash; and tomatoes.

However, because the immigrants often settled in regions of the "new land" that most closely resembled their homes in Europe, they were able to grow many familiar foods and retain many of their traditional foodways. One of these foodways involved the way food is presented.

A sizable portion of meat arranged with vegetables and potatoes in separate portions on a plate is the Northern European pattern, compared with other cuisines in which a mixture of starch, vegetables, and a much smaller portion of protein (such as a stir-fry) is more typical. The meat on the "North American" dinner plate may be, for example, sausage or roast beef, the potatoes may be boiled or mashed, and the vegetable may be sauerkraut or green peas. Whatever the choices, the Northern European pattern is still followed by many in North America.

This traditional pattern provides abundant protein and nutrients from dairy and meat products. However, the protein also contains saturated fat, and the large portions of protein and starch may mean that insufficient amounts of whole grains, vegetables, and fruits are eaten.

African Influences

Involuntary immigrants to the New World, people from West Africa struggled to survive under harsh conditions. Their ability to adapt familiar foodways to new conditions became a lasting influence on today's North American cuisine.

The "soul food" of African Americans is the basis of the regional cuisines of the southern United States. Many understand "soul food" to consist mainly of barbecued meat, fried chicken, sweet potatoes, and chitterlings. In fact, true soul food includes a wide range of dishes. African Americans used traditional methods and foods brought from their homelands, such as yams, okra, and peanuts, as well as what was available in the New World. African American women, cooking for their families, created dishes that they often adapted for the plantation owner's table as well, creating the basis of Southern cuisine. The combination of these foodways with Native American, Spanish, and French traditions produced the Cajun and Creole cuisines enjoyed today in Louisiana and throughout the nation.

Pork and corn products were the basis of soul food. The plantation owner ate the better parts of the pig. As with other foods, slaves learned to make the less desirable parts of the pig, such as entrails, feet, ears, and head, palatable. Corn was ground for corn bread. Unrefined yellow cornmeal was mixed with water and lard to make "hoecake," baked on a hoe blade by cooks who had neither ovens nor cooking utensils for their own use. The plantation owner probably ate white cornbread made from refined cornmeal.

Among other dishes still considered soul food staples are greens, usually cooked with a small portion of smoked pork. The greens used include collards, mustard, turnip, or dandelion greens, and kale. Black-eyed peas, first brought to the New World by slaves, are also cooked with pork. Sweet potatoes and yams were and remain basic soul foods; sweet potato pie is the soul food equivalent of pumpkin pie.

Today's traditional African American cuisine has both nutritional benefits and deficits. The variety of fruits, vegetables, and grain products used provides ample vitamins, minerals, and dietary fiber. For instance, African Americans in general consume more cruciferous vegetables, and fruits and vegetables containing vitamins A and C than do other ethnic groups in North America. However, cured pork products contribute undesirable levels of salt as well as saturated fat. Traditional reliance on frying, especially with lard, also adds saturated fat to the diet. Boiling vegetables for long periods depletes water-soluble vitamins. Dairy products may not be used enough, especially

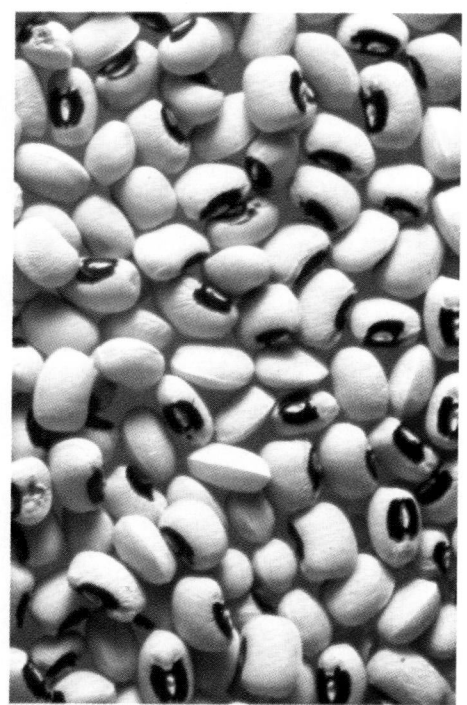

Black-eyed peas are one African contribution to the North American diet.

by older people who follow traditional dietary customs. This avoidance is based in part on the difficulty many African American adults experience in digesting lactose; see Chapter 4 for details.

To help guide African Americans toward a healthy food plan, Hebni Nutrition Consultants has developed a Soul Food Pyramid. It differs from the Food Guide Pyramid primarily by emphasizing lactose-reduced dairy products in the milk, yogurt, and cheese group and placing very-high-fat meats, such as bacon and sausage, in the fats, oils, and sweets category. To obtain a copy of the Soul Food Pyramid, call/fax (407) 345-7999.

Asian Influences

Okinawa, an island southwest of Japan, boasts some of the oldest, healthiest people in the world. Their diet of fresh vegetables, minimal amounts of meat (mainly pork and fish), and moderate fat (lower than North American diets but higher than traditional Japanese fare) has influenced the eating habits of Japan and North America alike. Studies show that the Okinawan diet of more fresh versus pickled vegetables, more fish and fiber, less salt, and a little more fat than traditional Japanese cuisine has protected them from premature death from problems such as cardiovascular disease. Since this discovery, the Japanese diet has become more like that of the Okinawans.

This idea of large portions of vegetables and grains, and small portions of meat, is becoming known in North America, but people are having difficulty complying with this more disciplined way of eating. Also influenced by Japanese cuisine is the growing popularity of soy products, such as tofu, soy milk, and miso, as well as use of flavors such as soy sauce, cilantro, and ginger.

More than 200 different vegetables are used in Chinese cuisine; bok choy and other forms of Chinese cabbage are perhaps the most widely eaten vegetables in the world. In the southeastern coastal region of China, home of the Cantonese cuisine, the number of dishes may be as high as 50,000. Rice is the core of the diet in southern China, whereas, in the temperate North, wheat is used to make noodles (China is the original home of pasta), bread, and dumplings. Popular dishes include hot pots (stews containing many ingredients) and stir-fried mixtures of vegetables and small amounts of meat or fish cooked in a lightly oiled, very hot pan.

An Asian Diet Pyramid has been proposed to reflect the Asian dietary pattern (Fig. 2.7). Like the Latin American Diet Pyramid, the bulk of the diet consists of grains, fruits, vegetables, and plant sources of protein, such as legumes, nuts, and seeds.

The Asian Pyramid does fall short in calcium but otherwise can form the basis of a healthy diet. Overall, most attention should be paid to the bottom portion of whichever pyramid you choose, and if dairy products are not included on a daily basis, other rich sources of calcium should be sought (see Chapter 9 for options).

Chinese immigration to North America began with the California gold rush in the middle of the nineteenth century. Chinese workers brought with them food-preparation methods that tend to preserve nutrients, as well as a variety of sauces and seasonings, such as gingerroot, garlic, rice wine, scallions, and sesame seeds and oil. Although many of the traditional foodways have been preserved, North American restaurant versions of Chinese cuisine, whether Cantonese, Szechwan, or Mandarin, are usually not authentic. Such food is often prepared with far more fat than in true Chinese cooking, which tends to use flavorful but fat-free sauces and seasoning. The restaurant versions of Chinese dishes also contain much larger portions of protein.

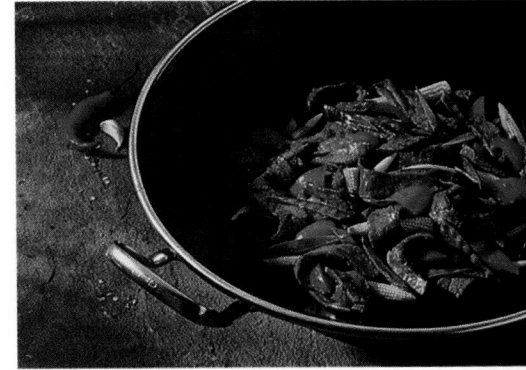

Stir-fry is commonly used in Chinese cooking.

*T*wo issues addressed by various ethnic diet pyramids developed by Oldways Preservation & Exchange Trust but not specifically included as part of the Food Guide Pyramid diagram are physical activity and alcohol intake. The ethnic diet pyramids recommend daily physical activity. Alcohol may be consumed by adults in moderation with meals, but consumption should be avoided during pregnancy and whenever it would put the individual or others at risk. The booklet accompanying the Food Guide Pyramid does address alcohol intake, suggesting that adults have no more than one drink (women and all adults age 65 years and older) to two drinks (men) per day.

Italian Influences

Authentic Italian cuisine, like Asian cuisine, is more diverse than most North Americans realize. Foods of different regions reflect Italy's varied geography and climate. Northern Italy, the more affluent part of the country, is the principal producer of meat and dairy products, such as butter and cheese. Rice dishes, such as risotto, are popular there. Fish is more important in regions near the sea, and lighter foods, such as fresh vegetables prepared with herbs, garlic, and olive oil, are characteristic. The poorer regions south of Rome, as well as the island of Sicily, have a diet rich in grains, vegetables, dried beans, and fish, with little meat or oil. Compared with northern Italians

continued

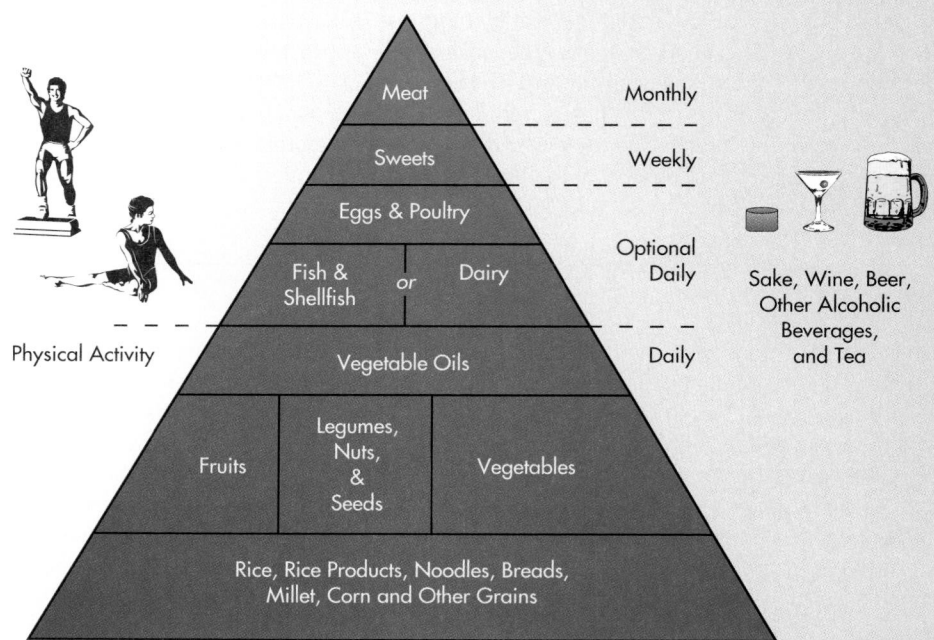

Figure 2.7 The Asian Diet Pyramid. This pyramid was inspired by the cuisines of South and East Asia, including such countries as China, Japan, South Korea, India, Thailand, Vietnam, Cambodia, Indonesia, Malaysia, Philippines, and other related Pacific Rim areas. If meat is consumed more often than monthly, it should be in small amounts. If dairy foods are consumed on a daily basis, they should be used in low to moderate amounts, and preferably low in fat. Grain products chosen should be minimally refined whenever possible.
Copyright 1998 Oldways Preservation & Exchange Trust

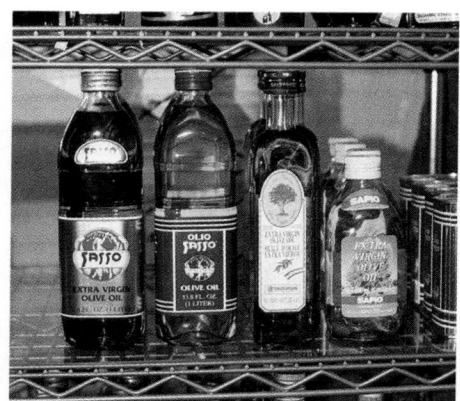

Olive oil is a principal fat source in the Mediterranean diet. Canola oil offers a similar monounsaturated fat composition at a lower price.

of the same class, southern Italians eat less beef, veal, chicken, and butter and more bread, pasta, vegetables, fruit, and fish.

Pasta is the heart of the Italian diet. Italians eat six times more of this simple wheat and water product than do North Americans, although we have also learned to enjoy this nutritious dish. Pasta in North America, however, often means spaghetti, with a tomato-based sauce that includes meatballs or sausage. In contrast, Italians eat pasta in a variety of shapes and with a variety of sauces, often excluding meat.

Most of the Italian cuisine found in restaurants offers foods more common to the north of Italy, including veal, cheese, and cream and pesto sauces for pasta. Pizza, a southern Italian dish, is the exception, and it is fast becoming the most frequently consumed food in North America. Pizza in this country is served on a variety of flour crusts topped with anything from high-fat meats, such as pepperoni, to vegetables or even fruit, combined with a variety of cheeses, tomatoes, and oregano for seasoning. Purists in Naples, however, insist that classic pizza consists only of a thin crust, tomato, basil, and mozzarella cheese.

Although some components of the Italian diet contain substantial amounts of saturated fat, nutritionists now know that other components, such as pasta, olive oil, and vegetables, contribute to healthy diets. One approach to Italian cuisine could be the Mediterranean Diet Pyramid (Fig. 2.8). This is a plan based on food choices like those traditionally found in the simple cuisines of Greece and southern Italy. The Mediterranean Diet Pyramid allows up to 35% of total calories as fat in the diet. However, it recommends consuming the type of fat consumed in the Mediterranean region: olive oil. A cheaper version, which has a similar fat profile and health benefit, is canola oil (see Chapter 5 for details).

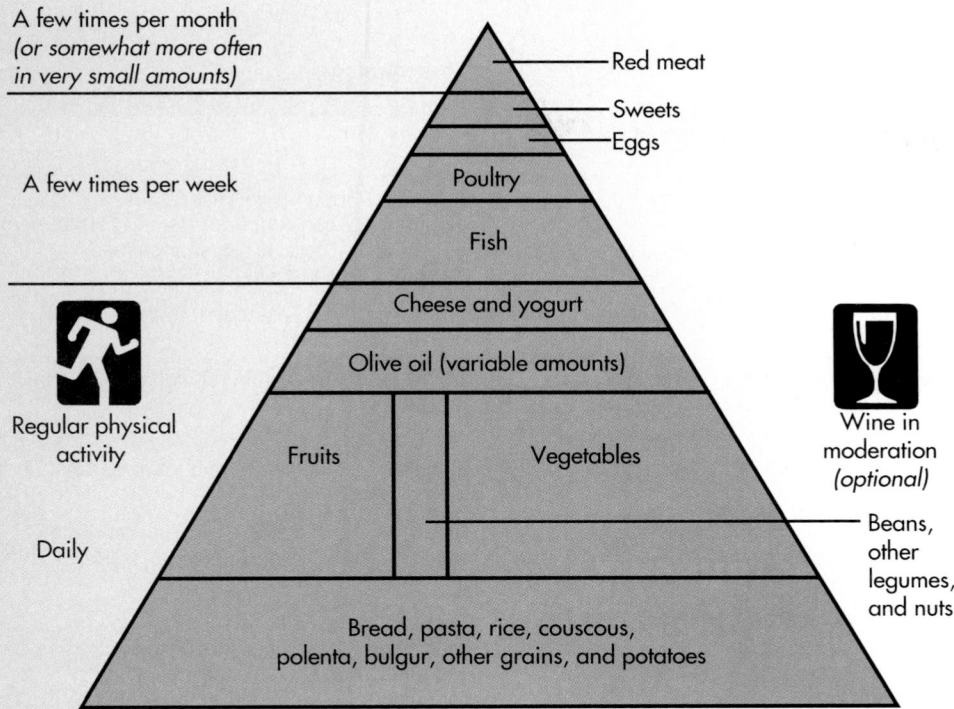

A few times per month
(or somewhat more often
in very small amounts) — Red meat

— Sweets

— Eggs

A few times per week — Poultry

— Fish

Cheese and yogurt

Olive oil (variable amounts)

Regular physical activity — Fruits — Vegetables — Wine in moderation (optional)

— Beans, other legumes, and nuts

Daily

Bread, pasta, rice, couscous,
polenta, bulgur, other grains, and potatoes

Figure 2.8 The traditional healthy Mediterranean Diet Pyramid. This plan is based on long-standing eating habits in southern Italy, Crete, and Greece. The base of the diet is bread and grains, fruits and vegetables, and beans and potatoes. Red meat is consumed sparingly— moderate amounts of fish and poultry are preferred. Most of the fat in this plan comes from olive oil. Cheese and yogurt supply some calcium. Other low-fat and nonfat milk products also can be included, if desired.
Copyright 1994 Oldways Preservation & Exchange Trust

Jewish Influences

Although Jewish immigrants arrive from all over the world, the two predominant groups are the Ashkenazic Jews, from Eastern European countries such as Russia, Germany, Poland, and Romania and from South Africa; and the Sephardic Jews from Spain, Portugal, and North Africa. Religious laws influence the dietary practices of some Jews. These Jewish laws dictate the separation of meat and milk products in a meal as well as in pots and pans used for cooking. In addition, it is important for meat to be completely drained of blood. To be sure that food laws are followed in processing, foods are labeled "kosher," meaning that a rabbi has approved food handling. Today, however, many discontinue such practices, especially as they become more integrated into North America.

Common foods for Ashkenazic Jews include dark rye bread, borscht, and herring. The Sephardic Jews eat foods that are also common in the Middle East, such as eggplant, humus, tahini, and couscous. Many of these foods have become popular in North American cuisine, including rye bread, bagels with cream cheese, corned beef, and pastrami. In Israel the food practices are similar to that of the Sephardic Jews, who traditionally ate only small amounts of meat due to economic constraints. The Ashkenazic diet is traditionally higher in fat and salt due to the consumption of foods such as high-fat meats, chicken fat, chopped liver, cream cheese, corned beef, smoked fish, sauerkraut, and pickles. Clearly, foodways of each group of Jewish immigrants have been preserved. Some are beneficial to health, while others should be practiced only occasionally.

continued

Table 2.12 The World's Fare Has Influenced the North American Diet

Diet Influences	Advantages	Shortcomings
Native American	Variety of seafood, lean wild game; early Native Americans ate many types of vegetables, berries, leaves	High fat content of some meat/seafood; low in calcium
Hispanic	Excellent variety of vegetables, legumes, fruits; high in dietary fiber	Traditional Hispanic diet may fall short in calcium; Mexican-American restaurants serve much high-fat fare, rich in sour cream, cheese, and guacamole
Northern European	Abundant sources of protein, iron, calcium from meat and dairy groups	Less variety from vegetables, fruits, legumes; high in fat
African	Good variety of vegetables; high dietary fiber; many variations, including Cajun and Creole dishes	Traditional meals high in fat; may fall short in calcium
Asian	Excellent variety of vegetables, grains; cooking methods retain nutrients in foods	Some sauces high in salt and fat; may fall short in calcium
Italian	Varies regionally—some regions provide excellent variety of seafood; overall high grain intake, good vegetable and fruit variety	Italian-American restaurants often serve many foods made with high-fat cheese, sauces, and meats, likely low in calcium
Jewish	Good variety of whole-grain products, legumes, and some types of seafood. Many traditions regarding food as an important part of Jewish culture have been retained.	Traditional Jewish foods are often high in saturated fat and salt. Limited variety from vegetables and fruits; may fall short on calcium.

This is a brief summary of healthful attributes and shortcomings of the ethnic influences covered in this Nutrition Issue.

Ethnic Diets and Present Trends

Only seven ethnic diets have been described here; see Table 2.12 for a summary of their advantages and disadvantages. Many other cuisines have also influenced the North American diet, and new arrivals continue to bring their traditions and foodways to this country. For example, social upheavals have increased the immigration of Russians and other Eastern European peoples to North America. On the other side of the world, continuing unrest in Southeast Asia has brought peoples from that area here. Restaurants serving traditional Russian or Thai fare, for instance, are offering new foodways to those willing to experiment.

Based on research also begun many years ago, still other scientists suggest that a healthful diet consists of the inexpensive traditional dishes based on grains, fruits, and vegetables that form the backbone of a number of ethnic cuisines. These are precisely the dishes that people abandon as they become affluent and seek convenience. Simple foods prepared in simple ways have fed most of humanity for virtually its entire existence. As we begin a new century, some North Americans are rediscovering the simple foods of their respective pasts, learning to enjoy a variety of cuisines and finding out how each cuisine can contribute to a healthier North American diet.

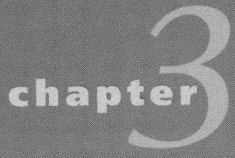
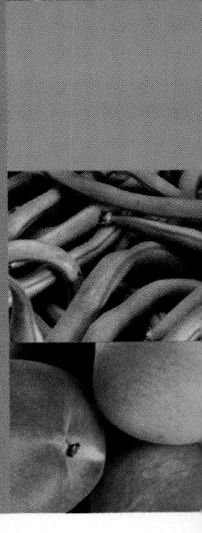

The Human Body:
A Nutrition Perspective

Chapter Outline

*M*erely eating food won't nourish you. You must first digest the food—in other words, break it down into usable forms of the essential nutrients that can be absorbed into the bloodstream. Once nutrients are taken up by the bloodstream, they can be distributed to body cells.

We rarely think about, let alone control, the digesting and absorbing of foods. Except for a few voluntary responses—such as deciding what and when to eat, how well to chew food, and when to eliminate the remains—most digestion and absorption processes control themselves. We don't consciously decide when the pancreas will secrete digestive substances into the small intestine or how quickly to propel foodstuffs down the intestinal tract. Various hormones and the nervous system mostly control these functions. Your only awareness of these involuntary responses may be a hunger pang right before lunch or a "full" feeling after eating that last slice of pizza.

Let's examine digestion and absorption as part of the study of the human physiology that supports nutritional health. In the process you will become particularly acquainted with the basic anatomy (structure) and physiology (function) that contribute to the circulatory system, nervous system, endocrine system, immune system, digestive system, urinary system, and storage capabilities of the human body.

Check out the **Contemporary Nutrition: Issues and Insights Online Learning Center** *www.mhhe.com/wardlawcont5 for quizzes, flash cards, other activities, and web links designed to further help you learn about issues surrounding human physiology.*

Chapter Objectives

Chapter 3 is designed to allow you to:

1. Identify the function of the following cellular components: cell membrane, nucleus, mitochondria, cytoplasm, endoplasmic reticulum, Golgi complex, lysosomes, and peroxisomes.

2. Define tissue, organ, and organ system.

3. List some characteristics of the 12 organ systems and outline a role for each related to nutrition, especially the cardiovascular system, endocrine system, nervous system, immune system, and urinary system.

4. Understand the role of genetic background in the development of nutrition-related diseases.

5. Outline the overall processes of digestion and absorption, including the roles played by the organs of the gastrointestinal tract and the related accessory organs: liver, gallbladder, and pancreas.

6. Become familiar with some specific enzymes and hormones that act in digestion of the various nutrient groups.

7. Identify the major nutrition-related gastrointestinal health problems and typical approaches to treatment.

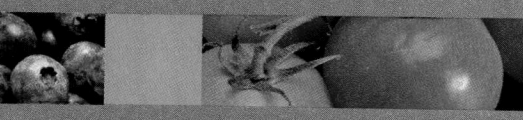

Refresh Your Memory

As you begin your study of human physiology in Chapter 3, you may want to review:

- The basic chemical composition of carbohydrates, proteins, and fat (lipids) in Chapter 1

- Cell structure and function from previous coursework in high school or university-level biology

- Also from your previous biology training, each of the body's organ systems, with special emphasis on how each system may be related to human nutrition

Real Life Scenario

Chad is a 20-year-old college sophomore. Over the last few months, he has been experiencing regular bouts of heartburn. This usually happens after a large lunch or dinner. Occasionally he has even bent down after dinner to pick up something and had some stomach contents travel back up his esophagus and into his oral cavity. This especially frightened Chad, so he visited the University Health Center.

The nurse practitioner at the Center told Chad it was good he came in for a checkup. She suspects he has a disease called gastroesophageal reflux disease (GERD). She tells Chad that this can lead to serious problems if not controlled, such as a rare form of cancer. She provides Chad with a pamphlet describing GERD and schedules an appointment with a physician for further evaluation.

What type of dietary habits likely contribute to Chad's symptoms of GERD? What types of medications have been especially useful for treating this problem? Overall, how will Chad cope with this health problem, and will it ever go away?

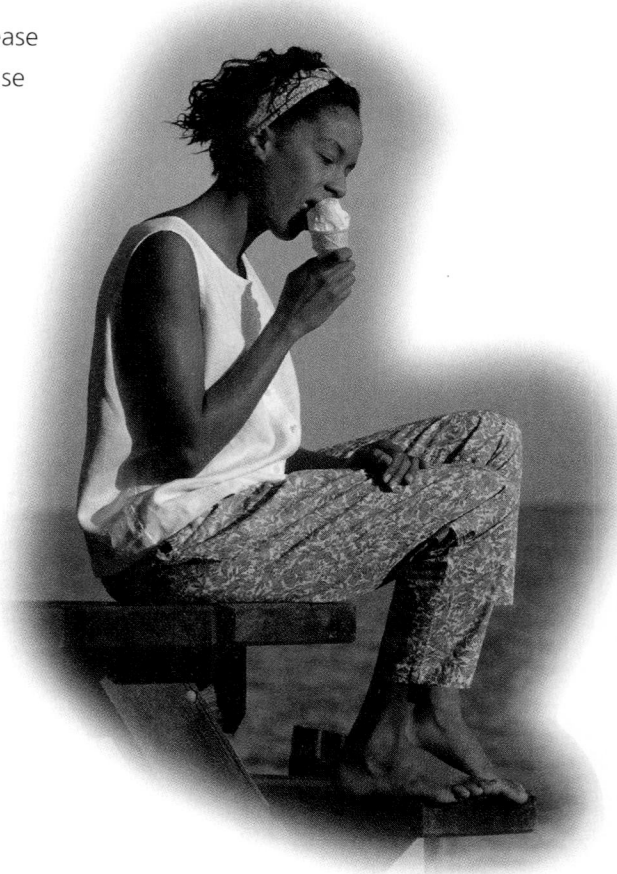

Nutrition Connection

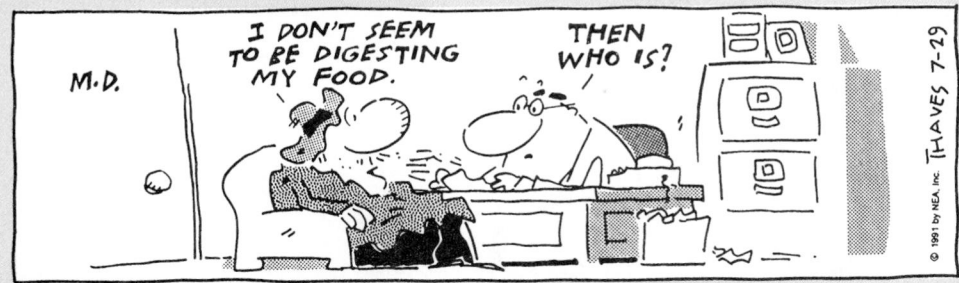

FRANK & ERNEST® by Bob Thaves

Health-food lore suggests not combining meat and potatoes in order to improve digestion; fruit should only be eaten before noon; and certain foods get stuck in the body and in turn putrefy and create toxins. Do we really need to pay so much attention to food intake in order to help out digestion? Do certain food practices actually improve digestion and subsequent absorption? This chapter provides some answers.

FRANK AND ERNEST reprinted by permission of Newspaper Enterprise Association, Inc.

Human Physiology

The body is composed of a trillion cells. Each cell is a self-contained, living entity. With the exception of red blood cells, cells of the same type join together, using intercellular substances to form **tissues,** such as muscle tissue. One, two, or more tissues combine in a particular way to form more complex structures, called **organs.** All organs contribute to nutritional health, and a person's overall nutritional state determines how well each organ functions. At a still higher level of coordination, several organs can cooperate for a common purpose to form an **organ system,** such as the digestive system. Overall, the human body is an organism made up of a coordinated unit of many highly structured organ systems (Fig. 3.1).

Chemical processes (reactions) occur constantly in every living cell: The production of new substances is balanced by the breaking down of older ones, as exemplified by the constant formation and degradation of bone. For this turnover of substances to occur, cells require a continuous supply of energy in the form of dietary carbohydrate, protein, and/or fat. Cells also need water; building supplies, especially amino acids and minerals; and chemical regulators, such as the vitamins. All of these substances enable the tissues, constituted from individual cells, to function properly.

Getting an adequate supply of all nutrients to the body's cells begins with a healthful diet. To assure optimal use of nutrients, the body's tissues, organs, and organ systems also must work efficiently.

This chapter covers subject material concerned with the anatomy and physiology of the cell and major organ systems, especially as they relate to the study of human nutrition. The information you are about to study is limited to the components of the various organ systems that are specifically influenced by the 45-plus essential nutrients discussed in this text.

tissues Collections of cells adapted to perform a specific function.

organ A group of tissues designed to perform a specific function—for example, the heart, which contains muscle tissue, nerve tissue, and so on.

organ system A collection of organs that work together to perform an overall function.

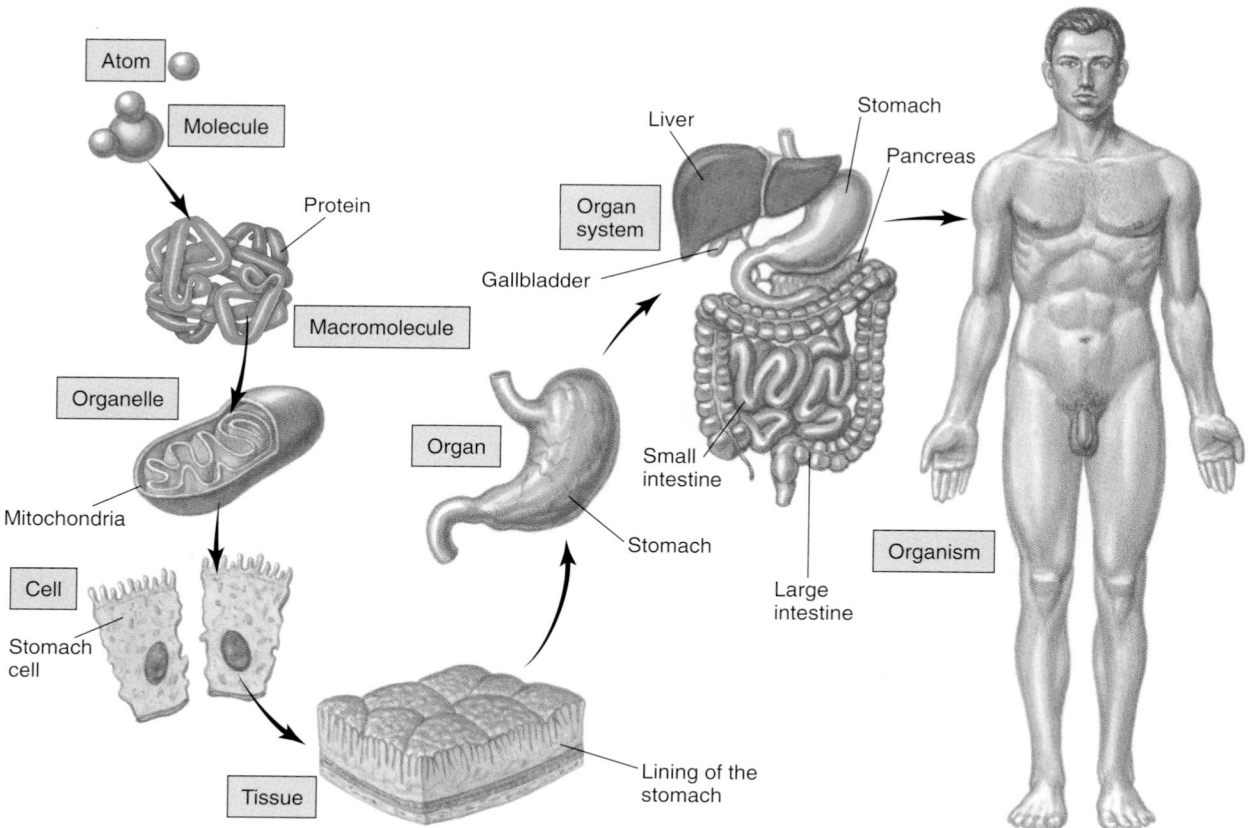

Figure 3.1 Levels of organization of the human body. Each level is more complex than the previous level. The organ system shown is the gastrointestinal (GI) tract.

The Cell: Structure and Function

The cell is the basic structural and functional component of life. Living organisms are made of many different kinds of cells specialized to perform particular functions, and nearly all cells are derived from preexisting cells. In the human body, the trillion cells all have certain basic characteristics that are alike. All cells have compartments, particles, or filaments that perform specialized functions; these structures are called **organelles** (Fig. 3.2). There are at least 15 different organelles, but this section discusses only 8. The number preceding the names of the cell structures correspond to the structures illustrated in Figure 3.2.

■ 1. Cell (Plasma) Membrane

There is an outside and inside to every cell, as defined by the cell (plasma) membrane. This membrane holds in the cellular contents and regulates the direction and flow of substances into and out of the cell. Cell-to-cell communication also occurs by way of this membrane. Some cells can even penetrate another cell membrane and so invade that cell.

The cell membrane is a lipid bilayer, (or double membrane) of **phospholipids** with their water-soluble heads facing into the interior of the cell and out to the exterior of the cell. The water-insoluble tails are tucked into the interior of the cell membrane.

Cholesterol is a fat-soluble component of the membrane, so it is embedded within the bilayer. Together with phospholipids, cholesterol keeps the membrane fluid.

There are also various proteins embedded in the membrane. Proteins provide structural support, act as transport vehicles, and function as **enzymes** that affect chemical

organelles Compartments, particles, or filaments that perform specialized functions within a cell.

phospholipid Any of a class of fat-related substances that contain phosphorus, fatty acids, and a nitrogen-containing component. Phospholipids are an essential part of every cell.

enzyme A compound that speeds the rate of a chemical process but is not altered by the chemical process. Almost all enzymes are proteins.

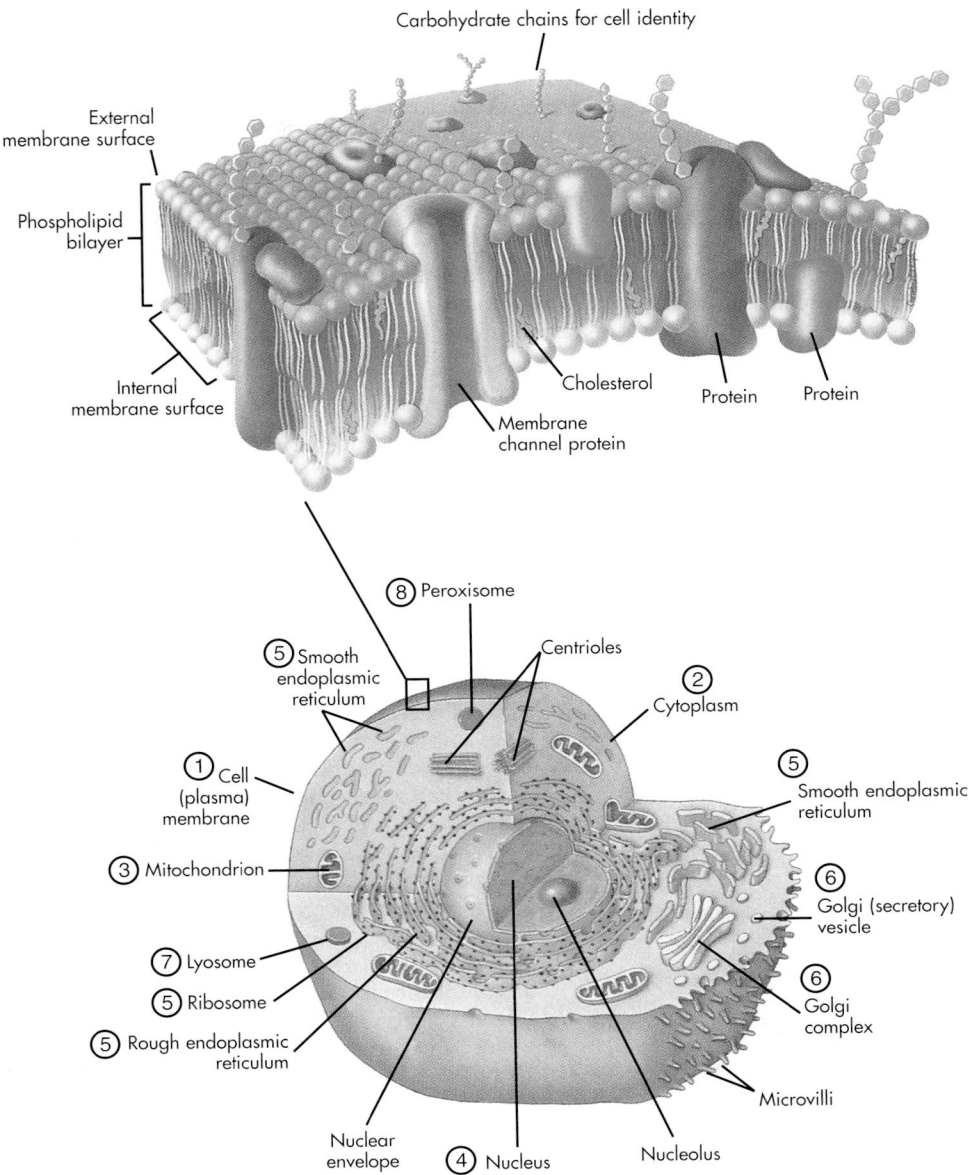

Figure 3.2 An animal cell. Almost all human cells contain these various organelles. The cell membrane is shown in greater detail. Note: Not all cells have microvilli. Shown here, but not discussed in the text, are the **nucleolus,** nuclear envelope, and centrioles. The nucleolus participates in genetic-related functions. The nuclear envelope encloses the nucleus. The centrioles participate in cell division.

processes within the membrane (see the later section on digestion for more about enzymes). Some proteins are open channels that allow water-soluble substances to pass into and out of the cell. Proteins on the outside surface of the membrane act as receptors, snagging essential substances the cell needs and drawing them into the cell. Other proteins act as gates, opening and closing to control the flow of various particles into and out of the cell.

In addition to the lipid and protein, the membrane also contains carbohydrates that mark the exterior of the cell. These carbohydrates are combined either with protein or fat and provide a delivery service for sending messages to the cell's organelles. The structures also provide distinct identification for a cell. In addition, they detect invaders and initiate defensive actions. In sum, these carbohydrates provide tags that are important to cellular identity and interaction.

cytoplasm The fluid and organelles (except the nucleus) in a cell.

anaerobic Not requiring oxygen.

mitochondria The main sites of energy production in a cell. They also contain the pathway for oxidizing fat for fuel, among other metabolic pathways.

aerobic Requiring oxygen.

cell nucleus An organelle bound by its own double membrane and containing chromosomes, the genetic information for cell protein synthesis and cell replication.

deoxyribonucleic acid (DNA) The site of hereditary information in cells; DNA directs the synthesis of cell proteins.

gene The material on chromosomes that makes up DNA. Genes provide the blueprint for the production of cell proteins.

chromosome A single, large DNA molecule and its associated proteins containing many genes; stores and transmits genetic information.

ribonucleic acid (RNA) The single-stranded nucleic acid involved in the transcription of genetic information and translation of that information into protein structure.

endoplasmic reticulum (ER) An organelle in the cytoplasm composed of a network of canals running through the cytoplasm. Rough ER contains ribosomes. Smooth ER contains no ribosomes.

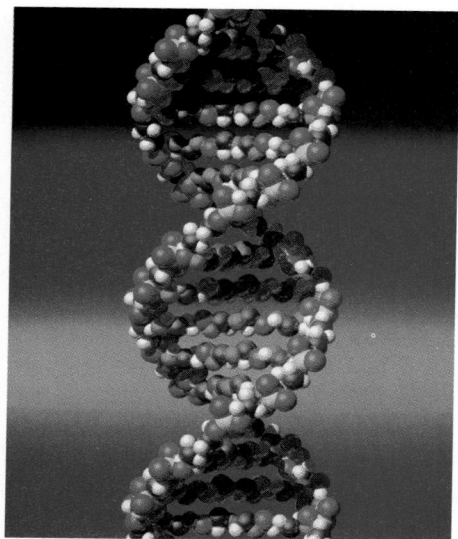

Genes are present on DNA—a double helix. The cell nucleus contains most of the DNA in the body.

Organelles

Included within the cell membrane are organelles. They carry out vital roles in cell functions.

■ 2. Cytoplasm

The **cytoplasm** is the fluid material and organelles within the cell, not including the nucleus. A small amount of energy for use by the cell can be produced by chemical processes that occur in the cytoplasm. This contributes to our survival, as it is the key process in red blood cell energy metabolism; it is called **anaerobic** metabolism because it doesn't require oxygen.

■ 3. Mitochondria

Mitochondria are sometimes called "power plants," or the powerhouse of the cell. These organelles are capable of converting the energy in our energy-yielding nutrients (carbohydrate, protein, and fat) to a form that cells can use. This is an **aerobic** process that uses the oxygen we inhale, and water, enzymes, and other compounds (see Chapter 11 for details). With the exception of red blood cells, all cells contain mitochondria; only the size, shape, and numbers vary.

■ 4. Cell Nucleus

The **cell nucleus** is bounded by its own double membrane. The nucleus controls actions that occur in the cell, using hereditary material called **deoxyribonucleic acid (DNA)**. DNA is the "code book" that contains directions for making substances the cell needs. It consists of **genes** on **chromosomes**. This "code book" remains in the nucleus of the cell, but conveys its information to other cell organelles by way of a similar molecule called **ribonucleic acid (RNA)**. The RNA has the responsibility of *transcribing* the information of the DNA and moving out through pores in the nuclear membrane to the cytoplasm. The RNA then carries the code to protein-synthesizing sites called **ribosomes**. There, the RNA code is *translated* into a specific protein (see Chapter 6 for details on protein synthesis). With the exception of the red blood cell, all cells have one or more nuclei.

DNA has the secondary task of cell replication. DNA is a double-stranded molecule, and when the cell begins to divide, each strand is separated and an identical copy of each is made. Thus, each new DNA contains one new strand of DNA and one strand from the original DNA. In this way, the genetic code is preserved from one cell generation to the next. The mitochondria contain their own DNA, so they reproduce themselves independent of action in the nucleus.

The transport of proteins, vitamins, and other material from the cytoplasm to the nucleus also occurs through pores in the nuclear membrane as just mentioned (review Fig. 6.1 in Chapter 6). These small molecules serve a variety of functions, including the activation (or inactivation) of certain parts of the DNA chain.

■ 5. Endoplasmic Reticulum (ER)

The outer membrane of the cell nucleus is continuous with a network of tubes called the **endoplasmic reticulum (ER)**. The ER is found in two types: rough and smooth. The rough endoplasmic reticulum contains the ribosomes, whereas the smooth does not. As noted earlier, ribosomes are the site where proteins are synthesized. Many of these proteins play a central role in human nutrition. The smooth ER is involved in lipid synthesis, detoxification of toxic substances, and calcium storage and release in the cell.

■ 6. Golgi Complex

The **Golgi complex** is a packaging site for proteins that are used in the cytoplasm or exported from the cell. The Golgi complex consists of sacs within the cytoplasm in which products of the rough endoplasmic reticulum are received, processed, separated according to function and destination, and "packaged" as **secretory vesicles** for secretion by the cell.

■ 7. Lysosomes

Lysosomes are the cell's digestive system. They are sacs that contain enzymes for the digestion of foreign material. Sometimes known as "suicide bags," they are responsible for digesting worn-out or damaged cells. Certain cells that are associated with immunity contain many lysosomes (see the later section on the immune system).

■ 8. Peroxisomes

Peroxisomes contain enzymes that detoxify harmful chemicals. **Hydrogen peroxide** (H_2O_2) is formed as a result of such enzyme action. Peroxisomes contain a protective enzyme called *catalase,* which prevents excessive accumulation of hydrogen peroxide in the cell, which would be very damaging. Peroxisomes also play a minor role in metabolizing one possible source of energy for cells—alcohol.

Golgi complex The cell organelle near the nucleus that processes newly synthesized protein for secretion or distribution to other organelles.

secretory vesicles Membrane-bound vesicles produced by the Golgi apparatus; contains protein and other compounds to be secreted by the cell.

lysosome A cellular organelle that contains digestive enzymes for use inside the cell for turnover of cell parts.

peroxisome A cell organelle that destroys toxic products within the cell.

hydrogen peroxide Chemically, H_2O_2.

Concept Check

*I*n Chapter 1, you learned that fat (lipids), protein, and carbohydrate function as fuels. Now you recognize that these organic nutrients also serve as structural materials in the cell membrane. This is typical of many nutrients; they can carry out multiple functions. The cell receives nutrients and other substances through the cell membrane by using various transport systems.

The basic structural unit in the body is the cell. Within the cell are a variety of organelles with unique functions to perform. Although there is no typical cell, virtually all cells have the same organelles, each performing essential tasks.

Organization of the Body

As noted earlier, when groups of similar cells work together to accomplish a specialized task, the arrangement is referred to as a tissue. Humans are composed of four primary types of tissue: **epithelial, connective, muscle,** and **nervous.** Epithelial tissue is composed of cells that cover body surfaces. These secrete important substances, absorb nutrients, and excrete waste. Connective tissue supports and protects the body, stores fat, and produces blood cells. Muscle tissue is designed for movement. Nervous tissue found in the brain and spinal cord is designed for communication. These tissues then go on to form various organs, and, ultimately, organ systems (review Fig. 3.1).

We will be particularly concerned in this chapter with the digestive system. The nutrients we consume in food are unavailable until such time as they have been processed by the digestive system using chemical and mechanical means to alter food, so that the nutrients can be released and absorbed into the body for distribution to body tissues. Table 3.1 summarizes the components and functions of the various systems.

epithelial tissue The surface cells that line the outside of the body and all external passages within it.

connective tissue Protein tissue that holds different structures in the body together. Some structures are made up of connective tissue—notably, **tendons** and **cartilages.** Connective tissue also forms part of bone and the nonmuscular structures of arteries and veins.

muscle tissue A type of tissue adapted to contract.

nervous tissue Tissue composed of highly branched, elongated cells, which transport nerve impulses from one part of the body to another.

Genetics and Nutrition

The growth, development, and maintenance of cells, and ultimately of the entire organism, are directed by genes present in the cells. The genes contain the codes that control the expression of individual traits, such as height, eye color, and susceptibility to many diseases. An individual's genetic risk for a given disease is an important factor, although often not the only factor, in determining whether he or she develops a given specific disease.

Interest in the human genetic code and its relationship to specific diseases has exploded in recent years. For example, the U.S. government sponsored a program to sequence the more than 30,000 genes present on human chromosomes. This Human Genome Project did not actually sequence the genes of just one person, but a composite genome based on the DNA contributed by a few individuals. Each gene essentially represents a recipe, noting the ingredients (specifically, amino acids) and how those ingredients should be put together. The human genome then would be the cookbook. It is likely that soon it will be relatively easy to screen a person's DNA for genes that increase the risk for specific diseases. This is a brand-new field and is about to mushroom into a significant part of medical practice, as almost every medical condition has a genetic component. Most, however, are not single gene disorders but, instead, arise from alterations in a number of genes.

Each year, new links between specific genes and diseases are reported. It is thought that the decoding of the human genome will ultimately transform the practice of medicine, allowing for the prediction of what illnesses will likely eventually develop in a person years in advance. The hope is then to replace genes that encourage diseases, such as cancer, with those that do not. Such gene therapy has shown to be effective for a few disorders, but is not generally available at this time.

Nutritional Diseases with a Genetic Link

Most chronic diseases in which nutrition plays a role are also influenced by genetics. The risks of developing cardiovascular disease, hypertension, obesity, diabetes, cancer, and osteoporosis are influenced by interactions between genetic and nutritional factors. Studies of families, including those with twins and adoptees, provide strong support for the effect of genetics in these disorders. In fact, family history is considered to be one of the important risk factors in the development of many nutrition-related diseases.

Cardiovascular Disease

About 1 of every 500 people in the North American population has a defective gene that greatly delays cholesterol removal from the bloodstream. As you will learn in Chapter 5, this and other genetic effects lead to an increased risk of developing cardiovascular disease at a young age. Diet changes can help these people, but medications and possibly surgery may be needed to address these problems.

Hypertension

An estimated 10% to 15% of the North American population is very sensitive to salt intake. When these salt-sensitive individuals consume too much salt, their blood pressure climbs above the desirable range. The fact that more of these people are of African origin suggests a genetic component. At present, the only way to determine whether individuals with hypertension are salt sensitive is to place them on a salt-restricted diet and see if their blood pressure falls. Note also that many cases of hypertension are less related to salt sensitivity, but caused by other factors (see Chapter 9).

Obesity

Most obese North Americans have at least one parent who is also obese. Findings from many human studies suggest that a variety of genes (likely 60 or more) are involved in the regulation of body weight (see Chapter 10 for more details). Little is known, however, about the specific nature of these genes in humans or how the actual changes in body metabolism (such as lower energy use in general or fat use in particular) are produced.

Still, although some individuals may be genetically predisposed to store body fat, whether they actually do so depends on how much excess energy—above energy needs—they ultimately consume. A common concept in nutrition is that nurture—how people live and the environmental factors that influence them—allows nature—each person's genetic potential—to be expressed. Although not everyone with a genetic tendency toward obesity develops this condition, he or she does have a higher lifetime risk than individuals without a genetic predisposition to obesity.

Diabetes

Both of the two common types of diabetes—type 1 and type 2—have genetic links, as revealed by family and twin studies. Only sensitive and expensive testing can determine who is at risk. The form of diabetes involved in about 90% of all cases, type 2 diabetes, also has a strong link to obesity. A genetic tendency for type 2 diabetes is expressed once a person becomes obese but often not before, again illustrating that nurture affects nature (see Chapter 4 for more details).

Cancer

A few types of cancer (e.g., some forms of colon [colon is another name for the large intestine] and breast cancer) have a strong genetic link, and genetics may play a role in others. Because obesity increases the risk of several forms of cancer, a diet with excess energy and fat is also a risk factor. And one-third of all cancers result from smoking. Again, genetics is often not enough—environment also contributes to the risk profile (see Chapter 8 for more details).

Osteoporosis

Bone mass and, in turn, bone strength, is similar in twins, as well as in mothers and their daughters. The exact relative importance of genetic versus dietary factors is unknown, but a number of genes have been shown to contribute to a person's overall risk of low bone mass. In any case, children and adolescents need to consume sufficient calcium to build strong, dense bones, thus reducing the risk of osteoporosis in later life. Adults should

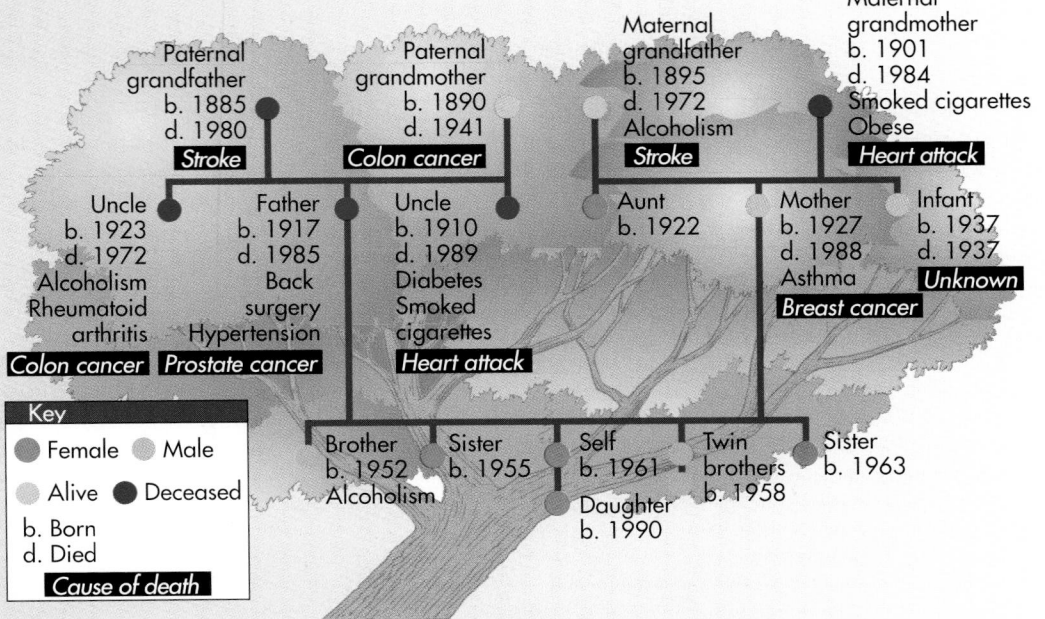

Figure 3.3 Example of a family tree. Create your family tree of frequent diseases, age, and cause of death, using the example here as a guide. Then show your tree to your physician to get a full picture of what the information means for your health.

then continue that practice. The porous bones that are a result of osteoporosis greatly increase the risk of fractures, especially in the wrist, spine, and hip. As discussed in Chapter 9, the risk of osteoporosis in women can be greatly reduced by a combination of medical and nutritional means if therapy is started at least by midlife.

Your Genetic Profile

From this discussion, you can see that a family history of certain diseases raises your risk of developing those diseases. By recognizing your potential for developing a particular disease, you can avoid behavior that contributes to it. For

Critical Thinking

Wesley notices that at family gatherings his parents, uncles, aunts, and older siblings typically drink excessive amounts of alcohol. His father has been arrested for driving while intoxicated, as has one of his aunts. Two of his uncles died before the age of 60 from alcohol abuse. As Wesley approaches the age of legal drinking, he wonders if he is destined to fall into the pattern of alcohol abuse. What advice would you give to Wesley concerning his future use of alcohol?

example, women with a family history of breast cancer should avoid becoming obese, should minimize alcohol use, and should obtain mammograms regularly. In general, the more of your relatives who had a genetically transmitted disease and the closer they are related to you, the greater your risk. One way to assess your risk is to put together a family tree of illnesses and deaths by compiling a few key facts on your primary relatives: siblings, parents, aunts and uncles, and grandparents, as suggested in the Rate Your Plate section.

Figure 3.3 shows an example of a family tree (also called a *genogram*). High-risk conditions include two or more first-degree relatives in a family with a specific disease (first-degree relatives include one's parents, siblings, and offspring). Another sign of risk of inherited disease is development of the disease in a first-degree relative before 50 to 60 years. In the family depicted in Figure 3.3, **prostate** cancer killed the man's father. This means that the son should be tested regularly for prostate cancer. His sisters should consider frequent mammograms and other preventive practices because the mother died of breast cancer. Because heart attack and stroke are also common in the family, all the children should adopt a lifestyle that minimizes the risk of

developing these conditions, such as a moderate fat and salt intake. Colon cancer is also evident in the family, so careful screening throughout life is important.

Genetic Testing

In recent years, scientists have developed ways of testing a person's genes for the likelihood of developing certain diseases. For cases such as Huntington's disease, a degenerative brain disorder, a positive gene test guarantees the eventual development of the disease. However, with diseases such as cancer, a positive gene test simply indicates a greater risk for developing the disease. In addition to the diseases mentioned, risk factors for birth defects, cystic fibrosis, certain forms of muscular dystrophy, and a host of other diseases can be detected through genetic testing.

Today in North America, newborns are routinely tested for inherited metabolic diseases that lead to mental retardation and other problems if appropriate treatment is not given. Infants found to have some of these disorders are put on a special diet, which reduces development of the disease (see Chapter 6 for one example called phenylketonuria [PKU]). In contrast, infants with genetic predispositions to many other diseases do not always develop disease.

Because genetic background does influence disease risk, certain dietary guidelines are more beneficial for some people than for others. For example, people prone to osteoporosis, as mentioned earlier, need to be more aware of calcium intake. Overall, the benefits of genetic testing include the potential for more individualized nutrition and health advice, more informed decisions by couples attempting to have children (i.e., alternatives such as adoption), increased surveillance for the disease, and the ability to plan appropriately for the future. However, it is not possible, given the resources presently allocated to medical care in North America, to identify all people at genetic risk for the major chronic diseases and other health problems. In addition, in many cases genetic susceptibility does not equate to a guarantee of development of the disease. And, in almost all cases, there is no way to cure a specific gene alteration—only the health problems that result can be treated. Thus, the wisdom of genetic testing is an open question. Perhaps preventive measures and careful scrutiny for the specific genetically linked diseases in one's family would suffice.

Researchers also are concerned that people who are found to have genetic alterations that increase disease risk may face job and insurance discrimination. Testing positive could also lead to unnecessary radical treatment. As well, a seemingly hopeless diagnosis could result in depression or withdrawal from life when a cure is out of reach.

Consider the following situations with regard to genetic testing.

- Using the family tree such as that shown in the Rate Your Plate section, you realize that colon cancer runs in your family. Knowing that the mortality rate for colon cancer is quite high, would you be tested for specific colon cancer genes (note: these genes do not guarantee colon cancer but do indicate

greater risk)? What factors would affect your decision?

- You, as a female (or a female you care about, if you are a male), carry the breast cancer gene BRCA1 or BRCA2, or you have a family history of breast cancer (see Chapter 9 for details on genes and cancer). Would you consider mastectomies to try to make sure the disease does not develop? This has been shown to be effective therapy, reducing risk of breast cancer and death by 90%. However, even some high-risk women never actually develop the disease.
- You and your (future) spouse would like to have children. You know that phenylketonuria has occurred in your family and you would like to be tested as a carrier. It turns out that both you and your spouse carry the gene for phenylketonuria. Any offspring have a 1 in 4 chance of developing the disease. How would this affect your decision to have a child?

Some experts recommend that anyone considering genetic testing should first undergo genetic counseling. Genetic counselors are trained to analyze family history and evaluate risk of developing or passing along an inherited disease. They can also help determine whether testing is worth the time and trouble, since genetic tests are primarily for people whose family history puts them at especially high risk of having a genetic defect. Genetic counselors can be found by contacting a local hospital or nearby university-affiliated hospital or medical school.

In the final analysis, would you rather know if you were at risk for a specific disease that a genetic test could point out? If so, ask your physician about the possibility and wisdom of testing you for the genetically linked diseases in your family tree. Also, be aware that throughout this book, discussions will point out how you can personalize nutrition advice based on your genetic background. In this way, you can identify

and avoid the "controllable" risk factors that would contribute to development of genetically linked diseases present in your family.

The following web links will help you gather more information about genetic conditions and testing:

www.geneticalliance.org Alliance of Genetic Support Groups.

www.kumc.edu/gec/support Information on genetic conditions and rare conditions.

cancernet.nci.nih.gov/p_genetics.html Genetics information from the National Cancer Institute.

www.nhgri.nih.gov National Human Genome Research Institute (at the NIH) home page. Describes latest research findings, and ethics issues, and provides a talking glossary.

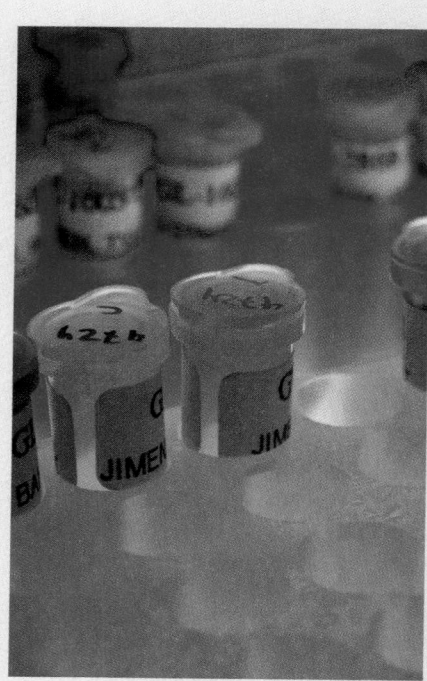

Genetic testing for disease susceptibility will be more common in the future as the genes that increase risk for various diseases are isolated and deciphered.

Table 3.1 Organ Systems of the Body

System	Major Components	Functions Related to Nutrition
Cardiovascular	Heart, blood vessels, and blood	Transports nutrients, waste products, gases, and hormones throughout the body and plays a role in the immune response and the regulation of body temperature
Lymphatic	Lymph vessels, lymph nodes, and other lymph organs	Removes foreign substances from the blood and lymph, combats disease, maintains tissue fluid balance, and aids in fat absorption
Nervous	Brain, spinal cord, nerves, and sensory receptors	A major regulatory system: detects sensation, controls movements, and controls physiological and intellectual functions
Endocrine	Endocrine glands, such as the pituitary, thyroid, and adrenal glands	A major regulatory system: participates in the regulation of metabolism, reproduction, and many other functions through the action of hormones
Immune	White blood cells, lymph vessels and nodes, spleen, thymus gland, and other lymph tissues	Provides defense against foreign invaders; formation of white blood cells
Digestive	Mouth, esophagus, stomach, intestines, and accessory structures	Performs the mechanical and chemical processes of digestion, absorption of nutrients, and elimination of wastes
Urinary	Kidneys, urinary bladder, and the ducts that carry urine	Removes waste products from the circulatory system and regulates blood acid-base balance, overall chemical balance, and water balance
Integumentary	Skin, hair, nails, and sweat glands	Protects, regulates temperature, prevents water loss, and produces a substance that converts to vitamin D
Skeletal	Bones, associated **cartilage,** and joints	Protects, supports, and allows body movement; produces blood cells; and stores minerals
Muscular	**Smooth, cardiac,** and **skeletal muscle**	Produces body movement, maintains posture, and produces body heat
Respiratory	Lungs and respiratory passages	Exchanges gases (oxygen and carbon dioxide) between the blood and the air and regulates blood acid-base (pH) balance
Reproductive	Gonads, accessory structures, and genitals of males and females	Performs the processes of reproduction and influences sexual functions and behaviors

The cardiovascular and lymphatic organ systems together make up the circulatory system, and so contribute to circulatory functions in the body. The endocrine and nervous organ systems contribute to the regulatory functions. The digestive, urinary, integumentary, and respiratory organ systems contribute to the excretory functions, while the muscular and skeletal organ systems contribute to storage functions in the body.

Sometimes organs within a system can serve another system. For example, the basic function of the digestive system is to convert the food we eat into absorbable nutrients. At the same time, the digestive system serves the immune system by preventing dangerous pathogens from invading the body and causing illness. As you study nutrition, you will note the multiple roles played by many organs (Fig. 3.4).

The overriding theme of human nutrition is to understand the actions of nutrients as they affect different cells, tissues, organs, and organ systems. Each type of organ system is impacted by nutrient intake and simultaneously determines how each nutrient is used.

Our task now is to explore the key systems in the body as they specifically relate to the study of human nutrition: circulatory (cardiovascular and lymphatic), nervous, endocrine, immune, digestive, and urinary systems. This part of the chapter will set the stage for a more detailed look at these and other organ systems in later chapters covering various aspects of human nutrition.

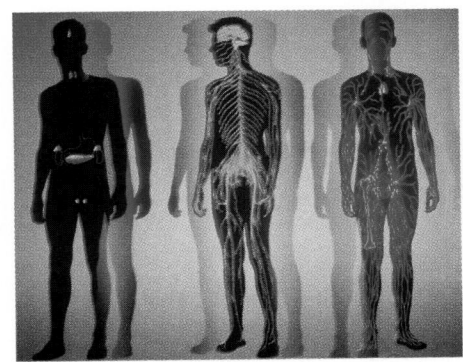

The body is made up of numerous organ systems.

■ Circulatory System: Cardiovascular System and Lymphatic System

The circulatory system is made up of two separate organ systems: the **cardiovascular system** and the **lymphatic system.** The cardiovascular system consists of the heart and blood vessels. The lymphatic system consists of lymphatic vessels and a number of lymph tissues. Blood flows through the cardiovascular system, while **lymph** flows through the lymphatic system.

cardiovascular system The body system consisting of the heart, blood vessels, and blood. This system transports nutrients, waste products, gases, and hormones throughout the body, and plays an important role in immune responses and regulation of body temperature.

Figure 3.4 Exchanges of nutrients occur between our external environment and the internal environment of the circulatory system via the digestive, respiratory, and urinary systems. Overall, the human body is a combination of 12 systems working together to support cell needs.

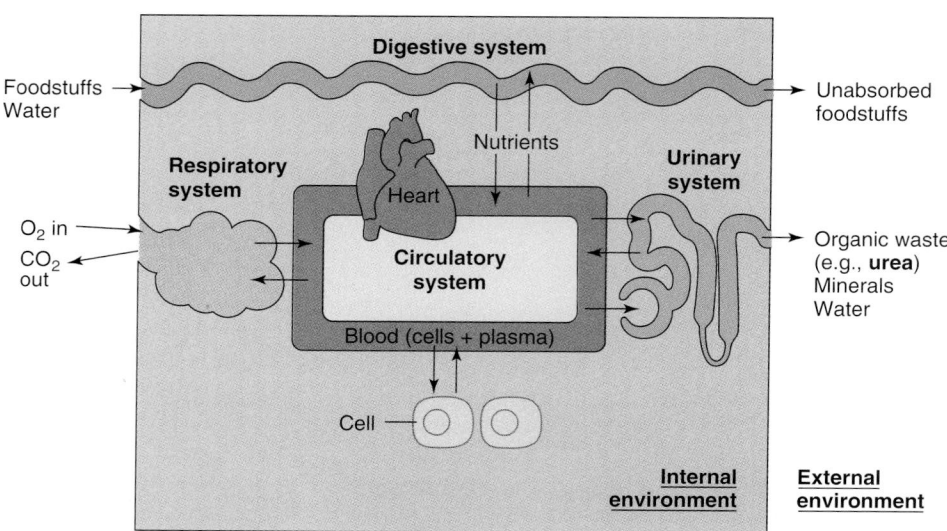

urea Nitrogenous waste product of protein metabolism; major source of nitrogen in the urine, chemically

$$H_2N-\overset{\overset{\textstyle O}{\|}}{C}-NH_2$$

lymphatic system A system of vessels that can accept fluid surrounding cells and large particles, such as products of fat absorption. This lymph fluid eventually passes into the bloodstream via the lymphatic system.

plasma The fluid, extracellular portion of the circulating blood. This includes the blood serum plus all blood-clotting factors. In contrast, serum is the fluid that results after the blood is first allowed to clot before being centrifuged; this will not contain the blood-clotting factors.

pulmonary circuit The system of blood vessels from the right side of the heart to the lungs and back to the left side of the heart.

systemic circuit The part of the circulatory system concerned with the flow of blood from the left ventricle to the body and back to the right atrium.

artery A blood vessel that carries blood away from the heart.

capillary A microscopic blood vessel that connects the smallest arteries and veins; site of nutrient, oxygen, and waste exchange between body cells and the blood.

vein A blood vessel that conveys blood to the heart.

portal circulation A process that utilizes a vein to convey blood from capillaries in the intestines and portions of the stomach to capillaries in the liver.

Cardiovascular System

The blood that flows through the cardiovascular system is composed of **plasma,** red blood cells, white blood cells, platelets, and many other substances. It travels two basic routes. In the first route, blood circulates from the right side of the heart, through the lungs, and then back to the heart (the **pulmonary circuit**). In the lungs, the blood picks up oxygen and releases carbon dioxide. In the second route, the oxygenated blood circulates between the left side of the heart and all other body cells, eventually returning back to the right side of the heart (the **systemic circuit**) (Fig. 3.5). The heart is a muscular pump that normally contracts and releases 50 to 90 times per minute when the body is at rest. This continual pumping keeps blood moving through the circuits.

In the cardiovascular system, blood leaves the heart via **arteries.** Exchange of nutrients, oxygen, and waste products between the blood and cells occurs in the **capillaries.** In the capillaries, which are made up of a network of tiny blood vessels, the exchange takes place through tiny, weblike pores. In this way, cells empty their waste products into the blood and take nutrients from it. Capillaries service every region of the body via individual capillary beds that are only one cell layer thick. The blood then returns to the heart via the **veins.**

The cardiovascular system distributes nutrients yielded from digestion and absorption, and oxygen from the air, to all body cells (review Fig. 3.4). The cardiovascular system also ensures that hormones arrive at their target cells, a constant body temperature is maintained, and white blood cells are distributed adequately to protect against pathogens as part of immune system function (see the later section on the immune system).

Portal Circulation in the Gastrointestinal Tract   Water and nutrients, once absorbed through the intestinal wall, travel one of two different routes. One pathway is **portal circulation.** Some nutrients are taken up by cells in the intestines and portions of the stomach for nourishment, but much of the nutrients from recently eaten foods are transferred into portal circulation. The actual transfer points are the capillary beds in these organs. The nutrients then pass into veins that eventually collect in a very large vein called the *portal vein.* Unlike most veins in the body—which double back to the heart—the portal vein leads directly to the liver. This enables the liver to process absorbed nutrients before they enter the general circulation of the bloodstream. Overall, this portal circulation represents a special form of circulation in the cardiovascular system.

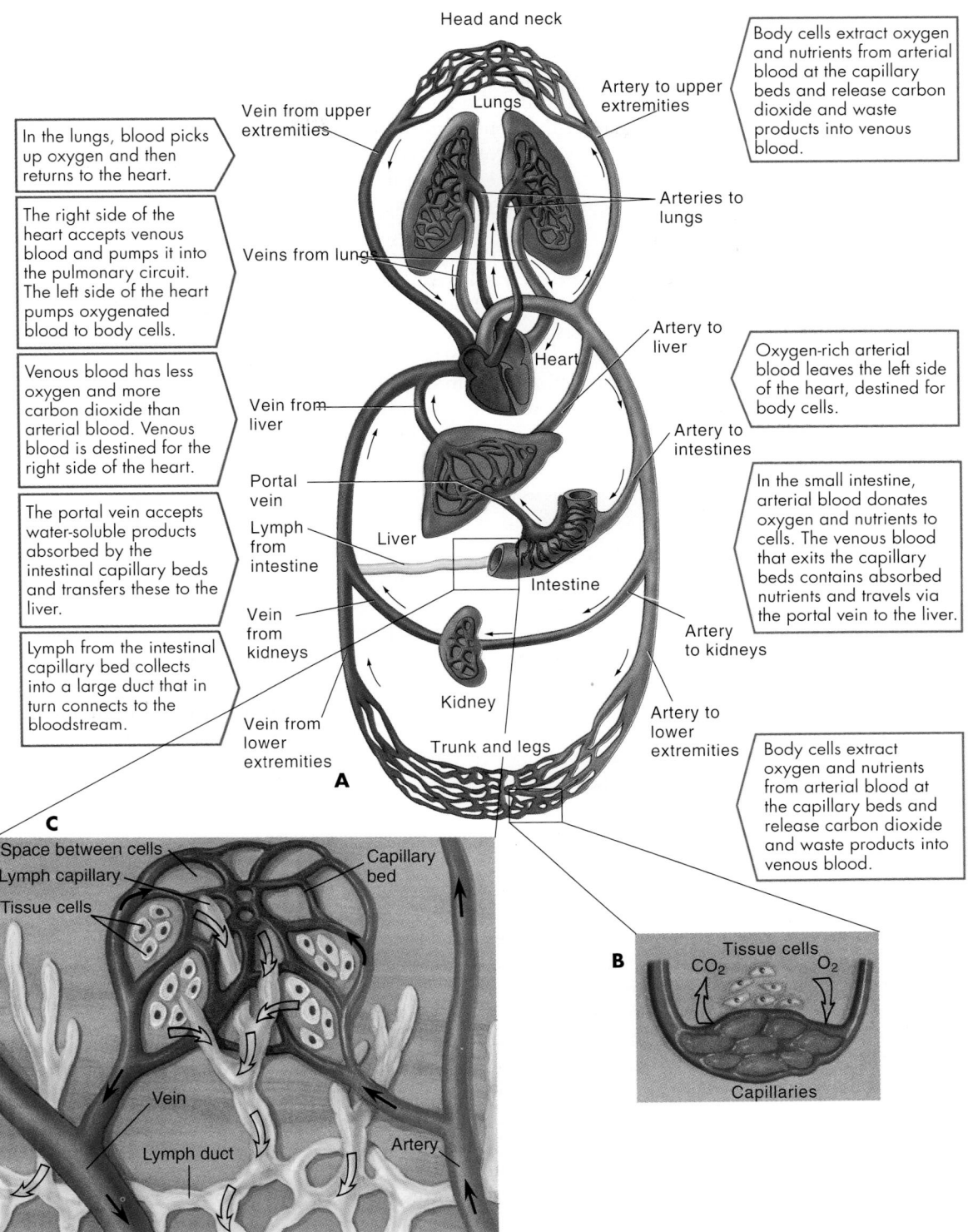

Head and neck

Lungs

Vein from upper extremities

Artery to upper extremities

Body cells extract oxygen and nutrients from arterial blood at the capillary beds and release carbon dioxide and waste products into venous blood.

In the lungs, blood picks up oxygen and then returns to the heart.

Arteries to lungs

The right side of the heart accepts venous blood and pumps it into the pulmonary circuit. The left side of the heart pumps oxygenated blood to body cells.

Veins from lungs

Heart

Artery to liver

Oxygen-rich arterial blood leaves the left side of the heart, destined for body cells.

Venous blood has less oxygen and more carbon dioxide than arterial blood. Venous blood is destined for the right side of the heart.

Vein from liver

Artery to intestines

The portal vein accepts water-soluble products absorbed by the intestinal capillary beds and transfers these to the liver.

Portal vein

Liver

In the small intestine, arterial blood donates oxygen and nutrients to cells. The venous blood that exits the capillary beds contains absorbed nutrients and travels via the portal vein to the liver.

Lymph from intestine

Intestine

Lymph from the intestinal capillary bed collects into a large duct that in turn connects to the bloodstream.

Vein from kidneys

Artery to kidneys

Kidney

Vein from lower extremities

Trunk and legs

Artery to lower extremities

A

Body cells extract oxygen and nutrients from arterial blood at the capillary beds and release carbon dioxide and waste products into venous blood.

C

Space between cells

Lymph capillary

Capillary bed

Tissue cells

Vein

Lymph duct

Artery

B

Tissue cells

CO_2 O_2

Capillaries

Figure 3.5 Blood circulation throughout the body. (a) This represents the route blood takes through the two circuits that begin and end at the heart. The red color indicates blood that is richer in oxygen; blue is for blood carrying more carbon dioxide. (b) Oxygen and nutrients are exchanged for carbon dioxide and waste products in the capillaries, the points at which the arteries and veins merge. The bottom box (c) shows a close-up of a capillary bed in the small intestine, including the location of the lymphatic vessels. This second set of circulatory vessels—part of the lymphatic system—picks up fluid that builds up between cells and large particles, such as some fats. Notice that lymphatic capillaries are blind-ended. They are, however, highly permeable, so that substances can drain into the lymphatic system. All this becomes lymph, which travels through further lymph vessels to reach the bloodstream. Lymph vessels in the intestine are also called **lacteals.** Hold this book up to your chest in order to have this figure reflect the orientation of your heart.

Lymphatic System

The **lymphatic system** is the other system of circulatory vessels that serves the body. It carries lymph, which is similar to blood but contains no platelets (clotting cells) or red blood cells. The lymph is mostly composed of a clear fluid that forms between cells. This fluid enters into tiny lymphatic vessels, composing a one-way network that funnels lymph from all over the body into large lymphatic vessels. From these vessels, the lymph fluid empties into major veins returning to the heart. The lymph moves through the lymph vessels by muscular action.

Lymphatic Circulation in the Gastrointestinal Tract   Besides contributing to the defense of the body against invading pathogens, lymphatic vessels that serve the small intestine play an important role in nutrition. These vessels pick up and transport the majority of products yielded from fat absorption. These products are too large to enter the bloodstream directly. The lymphatic vessels from the intestine drain into a large duct that connects with the bloodstream through a vein near the neck. Most of all absorbed fat products enter the bloodstream in this way.

Concept Check

*B*lood is transported from the right side of the heart to the capillaries in the lungs. Carbon dioxide is removed and oxygen is taken up by red blood cells. The oxygenated blood returns to the left side of the heart. Here it is pumped into systemic circulation. In the capillaries, oxygen is released from the red blood cells and delivered through pores in the capillaries to the surrounding cells. Nutrients also are distributed from the bloodstream via the capillaries. Carbon dioxide released from cells then travels through the capillary pores to the blood.

The lymph system serves several purposes: the transport of absorbed dietary lipids, the uptake of excess fluid that forms between cells and its return to the bloodstream, and the defense of the body against invading pathogens.

■ Nervous System

nervous system The body system consisting of the brain, spinal cord, nerves, and sensory receptors. This system detects sensations, controls movements, and controls physiological and intellectual functions.

The **nervous system** is a regulatory system that controls a variety of body functions. The nervous system can detect changes occurring in various organs and take corrective action when needed to maintain the constancy of the internal environment. The nervous system also regulates activities that change almost instantly, such as muscle contractions and perception of danger. The body is made up of many receptors that receive incoming information about what is happening within the body and what is happening in the outside environment. Specifically, these receptors represent our eyes, ears, skin, nose, and stomach. We act on that information via the nervous system.

neuron The structural and functional unit of the nervous system. Consists of a **cell body, dendrites,** and an **axon.**

The basic structural and functional unit of the nervous system is the **neuron.** These are elongated, highly branched cells. The body contains about 100 billion neurons. Neurons respond to electrical and chemical signals, conduct electrical impulses, and release chemical regulators. Overall, neurons allow us to perceive what is occurring in our environment, engage in learning, store vital information in memory, and control the body's voluntary (and involuntary) actions.

central nervous system (CNS) The brain and spinal cord part of the nervous system.

peripheral nervous system (PNS) The nerves of the nervous system that lie outside the brain and spinal cord.

The brain and spinal cord make up the **central nervous system (CNS).** The brain stores information, reacts to incoming information, solves problems, and generates thoughts. In addition, the brain plans a course of action based on the other sensory inputs. Responses to the stimuli are carried out mostly through the **peripheral nervous system (PNS)** to accommodate one's will.

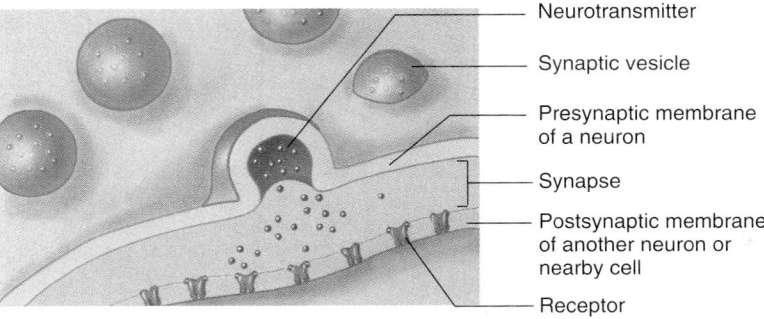

- Neurotransmitter
- Synaptic vesicle
- Presynaptic membrane of a neuron
- Synapse
- Postsynaptic membrane of another neuron or nearby cell
- Receptor

Figure 3.6 Transmission of the message from one neuron to another neuron or other cell relies on neurotransmitters. Vesicles containing neurotransmitters fuse with the membrane of the neuron and the neurotransmitter is released into the synapse. The neurotransmitter then binds to the receptors on the nearby neuron (or cell). In this way, the message is sent from one neuron to another, or to the cell that ultimately performs the action directed by the message.

Simply put, the nervous system receives information through stimulation of various receptors, processes this information, and sends out signals for an action that needs to be taken through its various branches. Actual transmission of the signal utilizes a change in the sodium and potassium concentration in the neuron. There is an influx of sodium and a loss of potassium as the message is sent. Ion concentrations are then restored to normal amounts in the neuron and it is ready to conduct another message.

When the signal must bridge a gap (**synapse**) between the branches of different neurons, the message is generally converted to a chemical signal called a **neurotransmitter.** The neurotransmitter itself is then released into the gap, thereby passing the signal from one neuron to another (Fig. 3.6). Another type of cell may also be at the receiving end of the neurotransmitter, such as a muscle cell. If the signal is sent to another neuron, this allows it to continue on to its final destination. The neurotransmitters used in this process are often made from common nutrients found in foods, such as amino acids. Examples are the amino acid tryptophan being converted to the neurotransmitter serotonin, and the amino acid tyrosine being converted to the neurotransmitters **dopamine, norepinephrone,** and **epinephrine** (see Chapter 6 for details).

Other nutrients also play a role in the nervous system. Calcium is needed for the release of neurotransmitters from neurons. Vitamin B-12 plays a role in the formation of a **myelin sheath,** which provides a form of insulation around specific parts of most neurons. Finally, a regular supply of carbohydrate in the form of glucose is important for providing for the energy needs of the brain. The brain can use other fuels, but generally relies on glucose.

synapse The space between one neuron and another neuron (or cell).

neurotransmitter A compound made by a nerve cell that allows for communication between it and other cells.

myelin sheath A combined lipid and protein (lipoprotein) that covers nerve fibers.

■ Endocrine System

The **endocrine system** plays a major role in the regulation of metabolism, reproduction, water balance, and many other functions by producing hormones in the endocrine glands of the body and subsequently releasing them into the blood. The term *hormone* comes from the Greek word for "to stir or excite." To be a true hormone, a regulatory compound must have a specific site of synthesis from which it then enters the bloodstream to reach target cells. Hormones are the messengers of the body. They can be permissive (turn on), antagonistic (turn off), or synergistic (work in cooperation with another hormone) in performing a task. Some compounds must undergo chemical changes before they can function as a hormone in the body. For example, vitamin D, synthesized in the skin and/or obtained from food, is converted into an active hormone by actions of the liver and kidneys (see Chapter 8).

The hormone **insulin,** which is synthesized in and released from the pancreas, helps control the amount of glucose in the blood. Insulin is produced when glucose in the blood rises to a certain level. At this point, insulin is released and it travels to the muscle, adipose, and liver cells of the body. In muscle and adipose cells, insulin allows for the movement of glucose from the blood into those cells. In the liver cells, insulin

endocrine system The body system consisting of the various glands and the hormones these glands secrete. This system has major regulatory functions in the body, such as reproduction and cell metabolism.

Table 3.2 Hormones of the Endocrine System

Hormone	Gland/Organ	Target	Effect	Role in Nutrition
Epinephrine, Norepinephrine	Adrenal glands	Heart, blood vessels, brain, lungs	Increased body metabolism	Release of glucose into the blood, fat mobilization
Thyroid hormones	Thyroid gland	Most organs	Increased oxygen consumption, growth, brain development, development of the nervous system	Protein synthesis, increased body metabolism
Insulin	Pancreas	Adipose (fat) and muscle cells	Decreased blood glucose	Storage of glucose as glycogen, increased fat storage, increased amino acid uptake by cells
Glucagon	Pancreas	Liver	Increased blood glucose	Release of glucose from liver stores, increased fat mobilization
Growth hormone	Pituitary gland	Most cells	Promotion of amino acid uptake by cells, increased blood glucose	Promotion of protein synthesis and growth, increased fat utilization for energy

receptor A site in a cell at which compounds (such as hormones) bind. Cells that contain receptors for a specific compound are partially controlled by that compound.

stimulates the synthesis of glycogen from glucose, thus storing glucose in those cells. Once a sufficient amount of glucose has been cleared from the blood, the production of insulin lessens. The hormones epinephrine and norepinephrine, glucagon, and growth hormone have just the opposite effect on blood glucose. They all cause an increase in blood glucose through a variety of actions (Table 3.2).

Thyroid hormones, which are synthesized in and released from the thyroid gland, help to control the body's rate of metabolism. Other hormones are especially important in regulating digestive processes, such as the hormone **gastrin,** which is produced in the stomach (see the later section on the digestive system).

Hormones are not available to all cells in the body, but only those with the correct **receptor** protein. These binding sights are highly specific for a certain hormone. They are generally found on the cell membrane. The hormone attaches to a receptor on the cell membrance. This binding activates a "second messenger" system within the cell to carry out the assigned task. This is true of insulin. A few hormones can penetrate the cell membrane and bind to receptors either in the cytoplasm (e.g., thyroid hormones) or on the DNA in the nucleus (e.g., estrogen).

Concept Check

*T*he nervous system consists of the central nervous system and the peripheral nervous system. The functional unit of the nervous system is the neuron. Communication between neurons themselves, and other types of cells, is via neurotransmitters released into the synapse between the cells.

In the endocrine system, hormones are produced by glands in response to a change in the internal environment of the body. The gland secretes the hormone into the blood, and the blood delivers it to target cells. The hormone either enters the cell to cause changes within the cell, or attaches to the cell membrane and, through the action of a second messenger system, causes changes within the cell.

■ Immune System

immune system The body system consisting of white blood cells, lymph glands and vessels, and various other body tissues. The immune system provides defense against foreign invaders, primarily due to the action of various types of white blood cells.

Many types of body cells and body components work in cooperation as part of the **immune system** to maintain a defense against infection (Fig. 3.7). The components that work as part of the immune system include the skin, intestinal cells, and white blood cells. It is easy to demonstrate the importance of nutritional health for immune function. Early humans were plagued by famine, infections, and death. Today, because of better nutrition, many of us avoid that cycle.

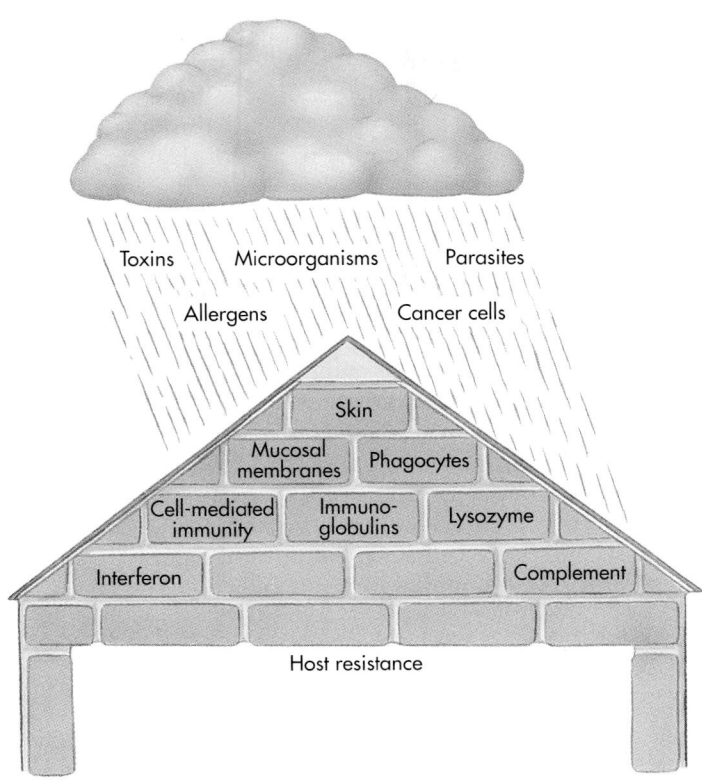

Figure 3.7 Host protective factors. The immune system has many components, all of which are affected by nutrient intake. We are born with most of these aspects of immune function; these are termed **nonspecific** (or innate). Use of the term nonspecific refers to the fact that the targets are a variety of microorganisms, rather than one specific organism, such as a specific bacterium. In contrast, white blood cells that produce immunoglobulins and those involved in cell-mediated immunity constitute the **specific** (or adaptive) aspect of immune function. Now the target is an individual microbe, such as specific bacterium. And once exposed, a memory is created such that a second exposure will produce a more vigorous and rapid attack.

Skin

The skin forms an almost continuous barrier surrounding the body. Invading microbes have difficulty penetrating the skin. However, if the skin is split by lesions, bacteria can easily penetrate this barrier. Skin health is hampered by deficiencies of such nutrients as essential fatty acids, vitamin A, niacin, and zinc. Vitamin A deficiency also decreases gland secretions in the skin—necessary cell secretions that contain the enzyme **lysozyme,** which is capable of killing bacteria. Bacterial eye infections in citizens of poorer countries are often due to vitamin A deficiency.

lysozyme A set of enzyme substances produced by a variety of cells; it can destroy bacteria by rupturing cell membranes.

Intestinal Cells

The cells of the intestines form an important barrier to invading microbes. Not only are the cells closely packed together, but specialized cells that produce immune bodies—such as **immunoglobulins**—are also scattered throughout the intestinal tract. These immune bodies bind to the invading microbes, preventing them from entering the bloodstream. This process contributes to the **mucosal membrane** aspect of immunity (see the section on the digestive system for more on mucosal membranes).

For a person in a nutritionally deficient state, the intestinal cells break down so that microbes more easily enter the body and cause infections. Two common results of undernutrition are diarrhea and bacterial infections of the bloodstream. To protect the health of the intestinal tract, an adequate nutritional intake is necessary—especially of protein, vitamin A, vitamin B-6, vitamin B-12, vitamin C, folate, and zinc.

immunoglobulins Proteins found in the blood that bind to specific **antigens;** also called *antibodies.* The five major classes of immunoglobulin play different roles in antibody-mediated immunity.

Another Bite

Although many studies show that a healthy nutritional state is associated with immune status, other studies show that an overabundance of certain nutrients can actually harm the immune system. For example, taking too much zinc also decreases immune function (see Chapter 9).

phagocytosis A process in which a cell forms an indentation, and particles or fluids entering the indentation are then engulfed by the cell.

cell-mediated immunity A process in which certain white blood cells come in actual contact with the invading cells in order to destroy them.

complement A series of blood proteins that participate in a complex reaction cascade following stimulation by an antigen-antibody complex or the surface of a bacterial cell. Various activated complement proteins can enhance phagocytosis, contribute to inflammation, and destroy bacteria.

antibody Blood protein that inactivates foreign proteins found in the body. This helps to prevent and control infections.

antigen Any substance that induces a state of sensitivity and/or resistance to microbes or toxic substances after a lag period; substance that stimulates a specific aspect of the immune system.

interferons A group of proteins released by virus-infected cells that bind to other cells, stimulating synthesis of antiviral proteins that in turn inhibit viral multiplication.

digestion The process by which large ingested molecules are mechanically and chemically broken down to produce smaller forms that can be absorbed across the wall of the GI tract.

absorption The process by which substances are taken up from the GI tract and enter the bloodstream or the lymph.

motility Generally, the ability to move spontaneously. It also refers to movement of food through the GI tract.

White Blood Cells

Once a microbe enters the bloodstream, **white blood cells** move in to attack it. A variety of types of white blood cells participate in this response and function in unique ways. For example, a class called **phagocytes** circulates throughout the circulatory system and ingests and sometimes digests microbes and foreign particles (via lysosomes present in the cells) in a process called **phagocytosis.** Other white blood cells participate in **cell-mediated immunity,** achieved when certain immune cells recognize foreign cells and directly attack and destroy them. White blood cells, along with immunoglobulins and proteins in the blood called **complement,** contribute to an **antibody-antigen** response that binds microbes and proteins that are foreign to the body and destroys them, and then creates a template (memory) that allows future recognition of the microbe or foreign protein. Recognition allows more rapid attacks in the future. **Interferons** also participate in the attack, especially against **viruses.**

Some white blood cells live only a few days. Their constant resynthesis requires steady nutrient input. The immune system needs (1) iron to produce an important killing factor, (2) copper for the synthesis of a specific type of white blood cell, and (3) adequate amounts of protein, vitamin B-6, vitamin B-12, vitamin C, and folate for general cell synthesis and, later, cell activity. Zinc and vitamin A are also needed for the overall growth and development of immune cells.

Concept Check

Many types of body cells and body components work in cooperation as part of the immune system to maintain a defense against infection. The skin forms an almost continuous barrier surrounding the body. Cell secretions contain the enzyme lysozyme. Specialized cells in the intestines and certain white blood cells secrete immunoglobulins. Phagocytes roam throughout the circulatory system and ingest and sometimes digest microbes and foreign particles. Other white blood cells participate in cell-mediated immunity. This happens when certain immune cells recognize foreign cells and directly attack them, with the aid of complement and interferons. Many nutrients are needed for the overall growth and development of immune cells.

❚ Digestive System

Before we eat a morsel of most foods, the work of **digestion**—the breakdown of foods into usable forms we can absorb—is already partially accomplished. Cooking or other preparations, such as marinating, pounding, and dicing, generally begin the process. Starch granules in foods swell as they soak up water during cooking, making them much easier to digest. Cooking also softens the tough connected tissues in meats and the fibrous tissue of plants, such as that in broccoli stocks. As a result, the food is easier to chew, swallow, and break down during later digestion. As you will see in Chapter 16, cooking also makes many foods, such as eggs, meat, fish, and poultry, much safer to eat.

The foods and beverages we consume, for the most part, must undergo extensive alteration to provide us any nutrients. The **digestive system** processes of digestion and absorption take place in a long tube, open at both ends, extending from the mouth to the anus. This is what is called the gastrointestinal (GI) tract (Fig. 3.8). Nutrients from the food we eat must pass through the walls of this tube—from the inside to the outside—to be absorbed into the bloodstream.

The GI tract promotes digestion and, later, **absorption** of nutrients through a variety of functions. It simultaneously moves and mixes food (as part of a process called **motility**). The GI tract also secretes chemical substances to promote the breakdown of foods. Finally, the GI tract eliminates wastes. The GI tract also promotes nutrient production; the bacteria living in the intestine make vitamin K and the vitamin biotin, some of which we can then use. Most of these GI tract processes are under autonomic

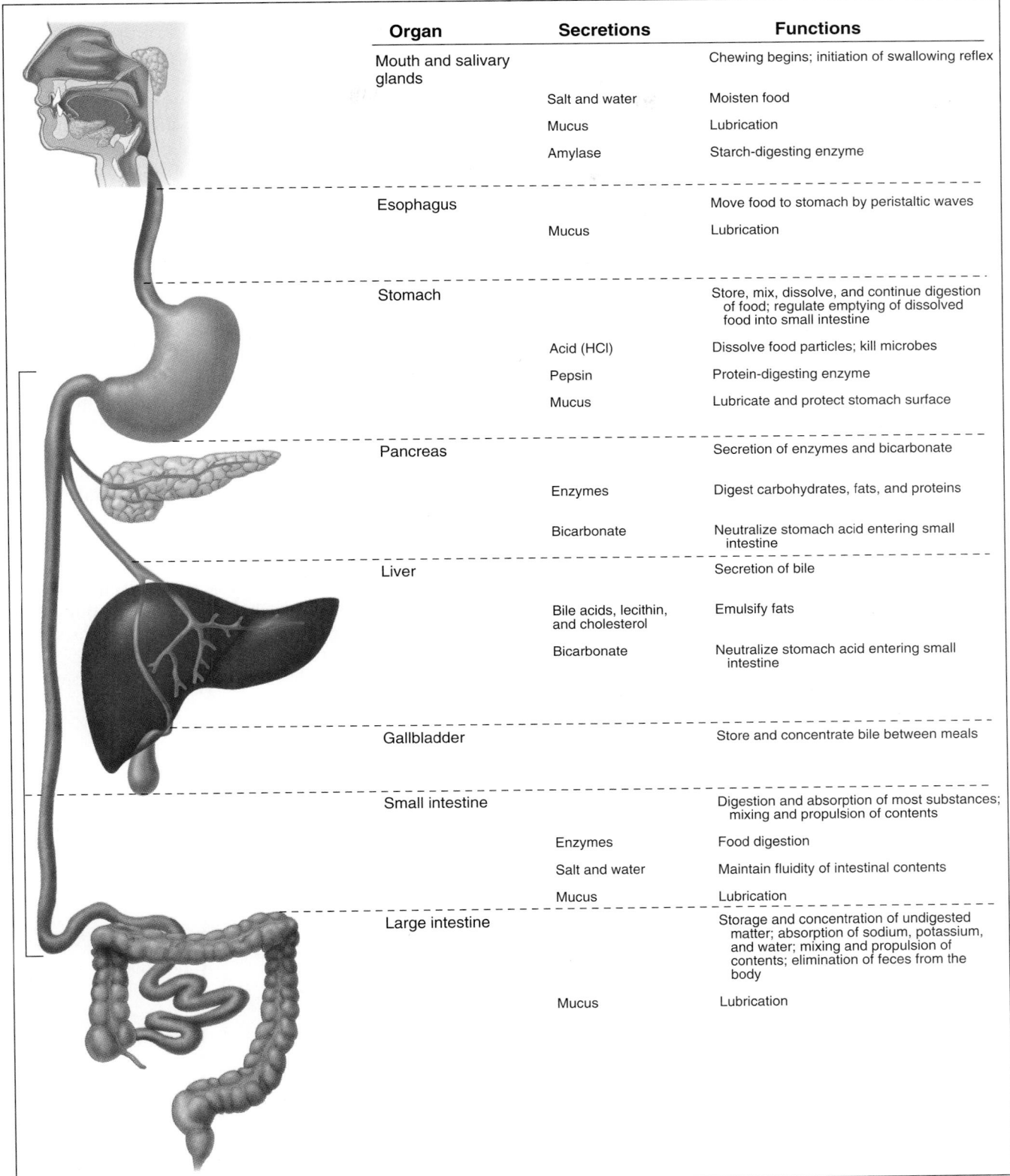

Organ	Secretions	Functions
Mouth and salivary glands		Chewing begins; initiation of swallowing reflex
	Salt and water	Moisten food
	Mucus	Lubrication
	Amylase	Starch-digesting enzyme
Esophagus		Move food to stomach by peristaltic waves
	Mucus	Lubrication
Stomach		Store, mix, dissolve, and continue digestion of food; regulate emptying of dissolved food into small intestine
	Acid (HCl)	Dissolve food particles; kill microbes
	Pepsin	Protein-digesting enzyme
	Mucus	Lubricate and protect stomach surface
Pancreas		Secretion of enzymes and bicarbonate
	Enzymes	Digest carbohydrates, fats, and proteins
	Bicarbonate	Neutralize stomach acid entering small intestine
Liver		Secretion of bile
	Bile acids, lecithin, and cholesterol	Emulsify fats
	Bicarbonate	Neutralize stomach acid entering small intestine
Gallbladder		Store and concentrate bile between meals
Small intestine		Digestion and absorption of most substances; mixing and propulsion of contents
	Enzymes	Food digestion
	Salt and water	Maintain fluidity of intestinal contents
	Mucus	Lubrication
Large intestine		Storage and concentration of undigested matter; absorption of sodium, potassium, and water; mixing and propulsion of contents; elimination of feces from the body
	Mucus	Lubrication

Figure 3.8 Physiology of the GI tract. Many organs cooperate in a regulated fashion to allow digestion and subsequent absorption of nutrients in foods.

GI Tract Flow

Mouth
↓
Esophagus (10 inches long)
↓
Stomach—4-cup (1-liter) capacity. Food remains about 2 to 3 hours. Large meals take the longest time to empty.
↓
Small intestine—duodenum (10 in long), jejunum (4 ft long), ileum (5 ft long)—about 10 ft (3.1 meters) in total length. Food remains about 3 to 10 hours.
↓
Large intestine (colon)—cecum, ascending colon, transverse colon, descending colon, sigmoid colon—3½ ft (1.1 meters) in total length. Food can remain up to 72 hours.
↓
Rectum
↓
Anus

umami A brothy, meaty, savory flavor in some foods. Monosodium glutamate enhances this flavor when added to foods.

salivary amylase A starch-digesting enzyme produced by salivary glands.

control; that is, they are involuntary. Almost all of the functions involved in digestion and absorption are controlled by hormones, hormone-like compounds, and nervous system input. Many common ailments arise from problems with GI tract function (see the Nutrition Issue).

The digestive system is composed of six separate organs; each organ performs one or more specific job(s). Let's look briefly at the role of each organ. A more complete description of the digestive process will be explained in later chapters as each nutrient is introduced.

Mouth

The mouth performs many functions in the digestion of food. Besides chewing food to reduce it to smaller particles, the mouth also senses the taste of the foods we consume. In tasting, the tongue, through the use of its taste buds, identifies foods on the basis of their specific flavor(s). Sweet, sour, salty, bitter, **umami** and, perhaps, the tastes of water and fat comprise the taste sensations we experience. Surprisingly, the nose and our sense of smell greatly contribute to our ability to sense the taste of food. When we chew a food, chemicals are released that stimulate the nasal passages. Thus, it makes perfect sense that when we are sick and our noses are stuffed up and congested, even our most favorite foods will not taste as good as they normally do.

Once we have established (or even begin to anticipate) the taste of the food in our mouth—the first step that signals the rest of the digestive system to prepare for the digestion of food—we move on to the actual digestion of food that takes place in the mouth. In the mouth, salivary glands produce saliva, which functions as a solvent so that food particles can be further separated and tasted. In addition, saliva contains a starch-digesting enzyme, **salivary amylase** (see Chapter 4 for more on starch-digesting enzymes). This and other enzymes are a key part of digestion. Overall, enzymes work to hasten certain events that take place in the body. The pancreas and the small intestine produce the most digestive enzymes; however, the mouth and the stomach also contribute their own enzymes to digestion. (Fig. 3.9).

Mucus, another component of saliva, makes it easy to swallow a mouthful of food (Table 3.3). The food then travels to the esophagus.

Table 3.3 Important Secretions and Products of the Digestive Tract

Secretion	Site of Production	Purpose
Saliva	Mouth	Contributes to starch digestion, lubrication, swallowing
Mucus	Mouth, stomach, small intestine, large intestine	Protects cells, lubricates
Enzymes **(amylases, lipases, proteases)**	Mouth, stomach, small intestine, pancreas	Promote digestion of foodstuffs into particles small enough for absorption
Acid	Stomach	Promotes digestion of protein among other functions
Bile **(bile acids, cholesterol, and lecithins)**	Liver (stored in gallbladder)	Suspends fat in water to aid fat digestion in the small intestine
Bicarbonate	Pancreas, small intestine	Neutralizes stomach acid when it reaches the small intestine
Hormones **(gastrin, secretin, cholecystokinin, gastric-inhibitory peptide)**	Stomach, small intestine	Stimulate production and/or release of acid, enzymes, bile, and bicarbonate; help regulate peristalsis and overall GI tract flow

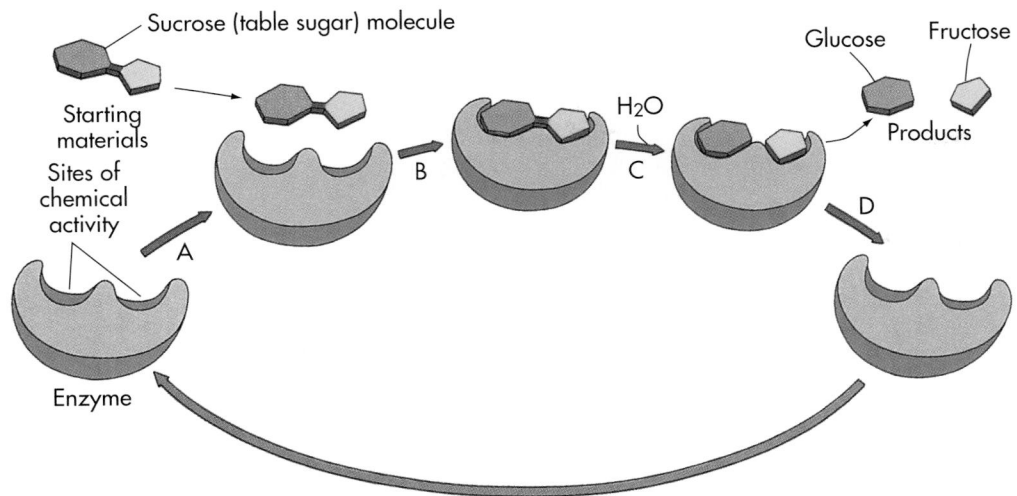

Figure 3.9 A model of enzyme action. Enzymes act as catalysts to speed chemical reactions, including those that contribute to the digestion of foodstuffs. In this example, an enzyme is contributing to the breakdown of sucrose (from *A* to *D*) into the smaller sugar forms glucose and fructose. Only these smaller sugar forms are absorbed from the small intestine to enter the bloodstream. Note that with some enzymes the action can go both ways. In addition, sometimes energy input is needed to allow the enzyme to push the reaction along.

Another Bite

*E*ach enzyme is specific to one type of chemical process. For example, enzymes that recognize and digest table sugar (sucrose) ignore milk sugar (lactose). Besides working on only particular types of chemicals, enzymes are sensitive to acidic and alkaline conditions, temperature, and the types of vitamins and minerals they require. Digestive enzymes that work in the acidic environment of the stomach do not work well in the alkaline environment of the small intestine. The body is also able to increase the production of certain digestive enzymes in response to the type of diet consumed. Because of this fine-tuning, the GI tract can respond to the nutritional makeup and amount of food consumed. Multiple enzymes attack the contents of the foods consumed in preparation for absorption. The authors of some fat diet books contend that ingestion of certain combinations of foods, such as meats and fruits together, hinders the digestive process. This does not make sense in light of our knowledge about GI tract physiology and our collective experience.

Esophagus

The **esophagus** is a long tube that connects the **pharynx** with the stomach. Near the pharynx is a flap of tissue (called the **epiglottis**) that prevents food from being swallowed into the trachea. During swallowing, food lands on a flap, folding it down to cover the opening of the trachea. Breathing also stops automatically. These responses ensure that swallowed food will only travel down the esophagus.

At the top of the esophagus, nerve fibers release signals to tell the GI tract that food has been consumed. This results in an increase in gastrointestinal muscle action, called **peristalsis.** Continual waves of muscle contractions, followed by muscle relaxation, force the food down the digestive tract from the esophagus onward (Fig. 3.10).

At the end of the esophagus is the **lower esophageal sphincter,** a muscle that constricts after food enters the stomach (Fig. 3.11). The main function of sphincters is to prevent the backflow of GI tract contents. Sphincters respond to various stimuli, such as signals from the nervous system, hormones, acidic versus alkaline conditions, and pressure that builds up around the sphincter itself. The primary function of the lower esophageal sphincter is to prevent the acidic contents of the stomach from flowing back up into the esophagus—which can cause many health problems (see the Nutrition Issue).

esophagus A tube in the GI tract that connects the pharynx with the stomach.

pharynx The organ of the digestive tract and respiratory tract located at the back of the oral and nasal cavities.

epiglottis The flap that folds down over the trachea during swallowing.

lower esophageal sphincter A circular muscle that constricts the opening of the esophagus to the stomach.

Figure 3.10 Peristalsis. Peristalsis is a progressive type of movement, propelling material from point to point along the GI tract. To begin this, a ring of contraction occurs where the GI wall is stretched, passing the food mass forward. The moving food mass triggers a ring of contraction in the next region, which pushes the food mass even farther along. The overall result is a ring of contraction that moves like a wave along the GI tract, pushing the food mass forward. In a related action, the intestinal muscles contract, causing an alternative forward-and-backward mixing movement. This process, called *segmentation,* results in little net forward movement.

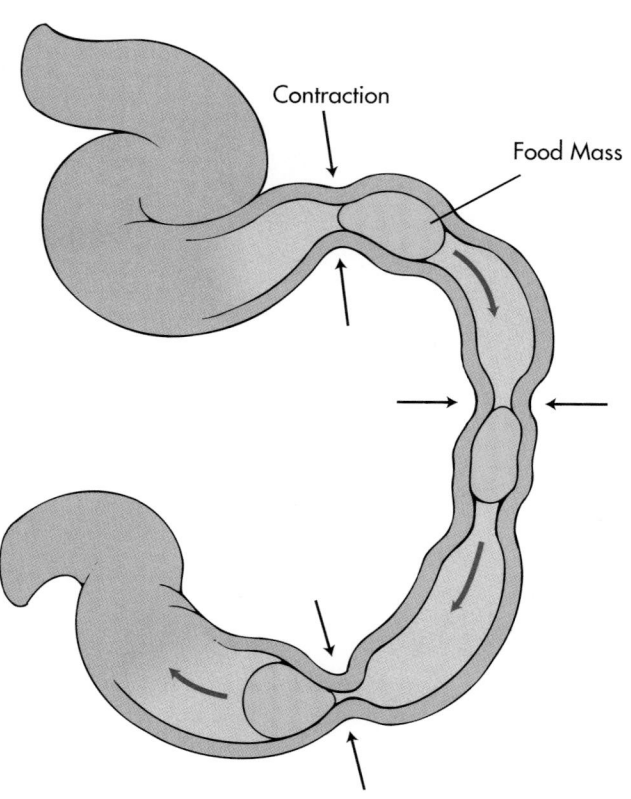

Contraction

Food Mass

chyme A mixture of stomach secretions and partially digested food.

pyloric sphincter The ring of smooth muscle between the stomach and the small intestine.

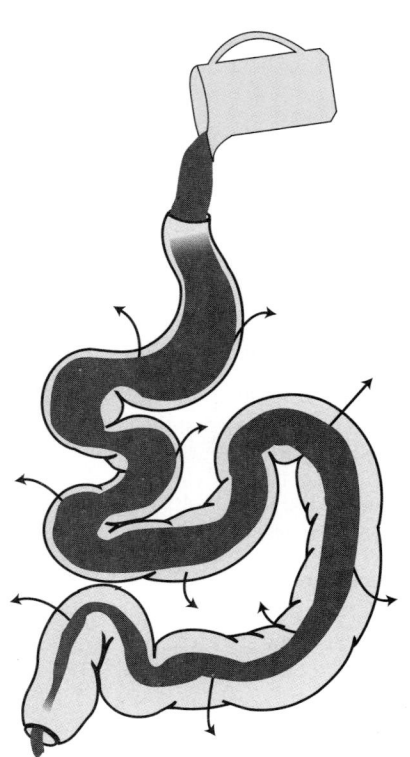

As the intestinal contents pass down the tract, nutrients are absorbed from the "hollow tube" into the body.

Stomach

The stomach is a large tank that holds up to 4 cups of food for several hours until all of the food is able to enter the small intestine. While in the stomach, the food is mixed with gastric juice, which contains water, a very strong acid, and enzymes. The acid in the gastric juice maintains the acidity of the stomach, thereby destroying the biological activity of proteins, converting inactive digestive enzymes to their active form, partially digesting food protein, and making dietary minerals soluble so that they can be absorbed. This mixing produces a watery food mixture, called **chyme,** which then leaves the stomach a teaspoon (5 milliliters) at a time and enters the small intestine.

You might wonder how the stomach protects itself from the acid and enzymes it produces. First, the stomach has a thick layer of mucus that lines and protects it from the acid and enzymes produced for digestion. The production of acid and enzymes is also tied to the release of a specific hormone (gastrin). This release happens primarily when we are thinking about eating or are actually in the process of eating. Lastly, as the concentration of acid in the stomach increases, acid production tapers off, also because of hormonal control.

The **pyloric sphincter,** located at the base of the stomach, then controls the rate at which the chyme is released into the stomach (review Fig. 3.11). There is very little absorption of nutrients in the stomach, except for some alcohol.

One other important function of the stomach is the production of a substance called **intrinsic factor.** This vital material is essential for the absorption of one of the B-vitamins, vitamin B-12 (see Chapter 8).

Small Intestine

The small intestine is about 10 feet (3 meters) long and has boundaries of the stomach on the "north" and the large intestine (colon) on the "south." (The small intestine is considered small because of its narrow (1 inch [2.5 centimeters]) diameter. Most of

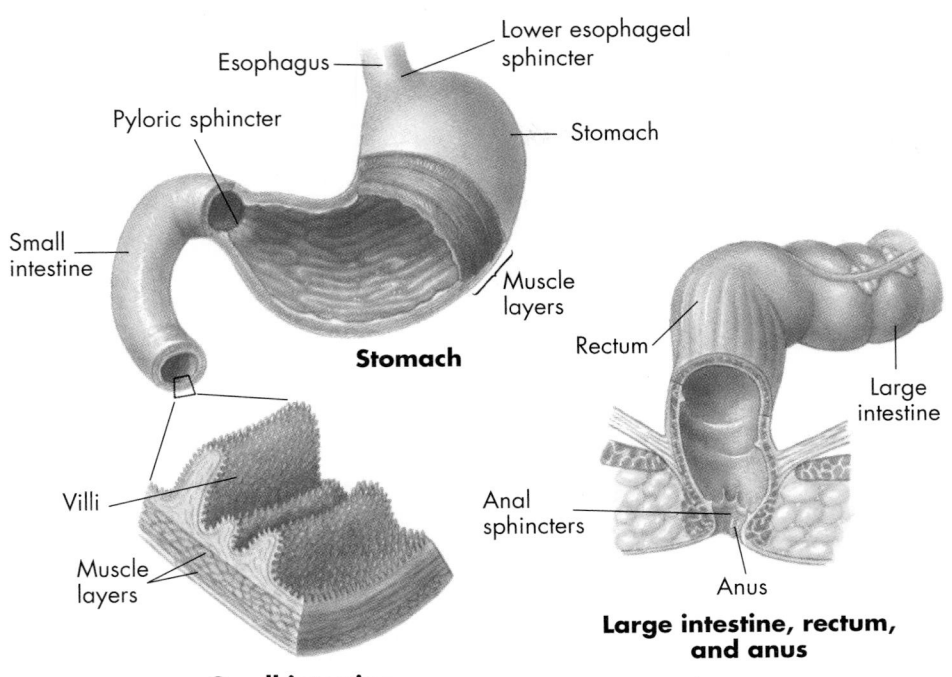

Stomach

Esophagus

Lower esophageal sphincter

Pyloric sphincter

Stomach

Small intestine

Muscle layers

Villi

Muscle layers

Small intestine

Rectum

Large intestine

Anal sphincters

Anus

Large intestine, rectum, and anus

Figure 3.11 A close-up view of the intestinal tract—muscles, sphincters, and villi. These features of the GI tract perform key roles in digestion, absorption, and elimination.

the digestion and absorption of food occurs in the small intestine. The chyme secreted from the stomach is moved through the small intestine by peristaltic contractions so that it can be well mixed with the digestive juices of the small intestine. These juices contain many enzymes that function in the digestion of carbohydrates, protein, and fat, as well as the preparation of vitamins and minerals for absorption.

The physical structure of the small intestine is very important to the body's ability to digest and absorb the nutrients it needs. The lining of the small intestine is folded many times; within these folds are fingerlike projections called **villi**. These "fingers" are constantly moving, which helps them trap food to enhance absorption. Each individual villus (singular) is made up of many absorptive cells, and each of these cells has a highly folded cap. The combined folds, villi, and caps in the small intestine increase its surface area 600 times beyond that of a simple tube (Fig. 3.12).

New **absorptive cells** are constantly produced and appear daily along the surface of each villus "finger." This is probably because absorptive cells are subjected to a harsh environment, so renewal of the intestinal lining is necessary. This rapid cell turnover leads to a high nutrient demand from the small intestine. Fortunately, many of the old cells can be broken down and the component parts reused. The health of the cells is further enhanced by various hormones and other substances that participate in or are produced as part of the digestive process.

The small intestine absorbs nutrients through the intestinal wall through various means and processes. When the nutrient concentration is higher in the inside cavity (**lumen**) of the small intestine than in the absorptive cells, the difference in nutrient concentration drives absorption because nutrients naturally move from higher concentrations to lower concentrations. This **passive absorption** allows for the absorption of fats, water, and some minerals (Fig. 3.13).

Another method of absorption uses both a carrier protein and energy input to actively pump nutrients from the lumen of the small intestine into the absorptive cells. This mechanism makes it possible for cells to take up nutrients even when they are in low concentration in the diet. Some sugars, such as glucose, follow this route of **active absorption**, as do amino acids.

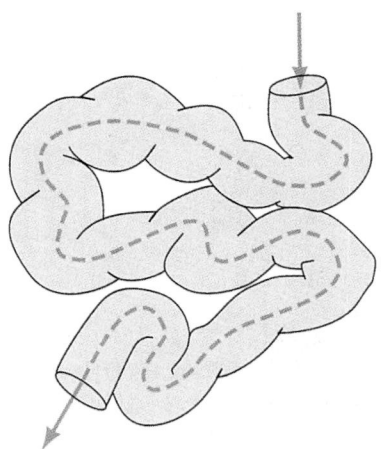

lumen The inside of a tube, such as the inside cavity of the GI tract.

villi The fingerlike protrusions into the small intestine that participate in digestion and absorption of food.

absorptive cells A class of cells, also called **enterocytes**, that line the villi; these cells participate in nutrient absorption.

Figure 3.12 Organization of the small intestine. The small intestine has several structural levels that increase the surface area for absorption up to 600 times that of a simple tube.

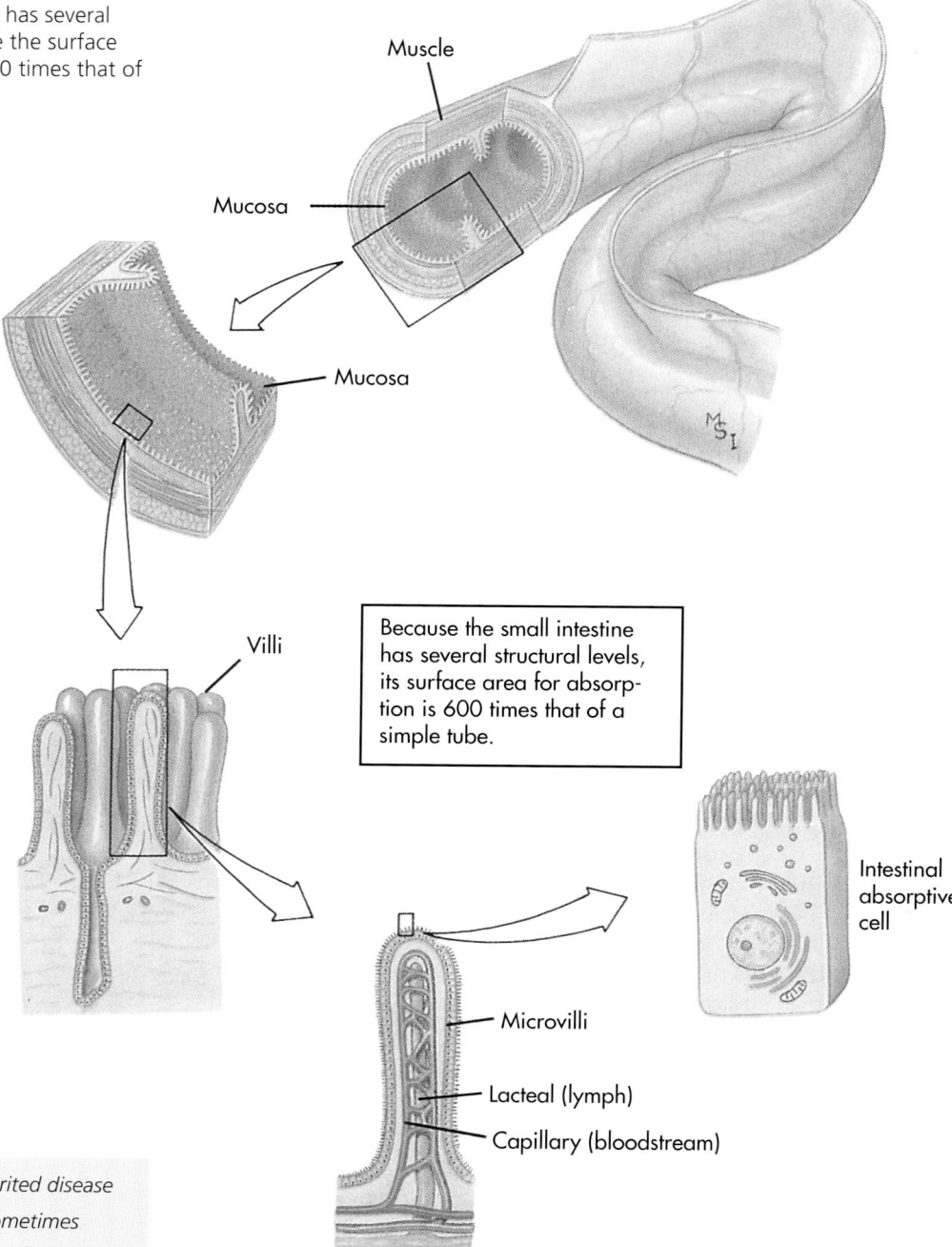

Because the small intestine has several structural levels, its surface area for absorption is 600 times that of a simple tube.

*I*n **cystic fibrosis**—an inherited disease of infants, children, and sometimes adults—the pancreas often develops thick mucus that blocks its ducts, and active cells then die. As a result, the pancreas is not able to effectively deliver its digestive enzymes into the small intestine. Digestion of carbohydrate, protein, and—most notably—fat then is impaired. Often the missing enzymes must be ingested in capsule form with meals to aid in digestion.

A further means of active absorption entails the absorptive cells literally engulfing compounds (phagocytosis) or liquids (**pinocytosis**). As described earlier, a cell membrane can form an indentation of itself so that when particles or fluids move into the indentation, the cell membrane surrounds and engulfs them. This process is used when an infant absorbs immune substances from human milk (see Chapter 13).

Once absorbed, water-soluble compounds such as glucose and amino acids go to the capillaries and then on to the portal vein. Recall that the liver is the end point of this vein. Most fats go into the lymph vessels. In doing so, they can eventually enter the bloodstream (see the earlier section on the circulatory system for details; review Fig. 3.5).

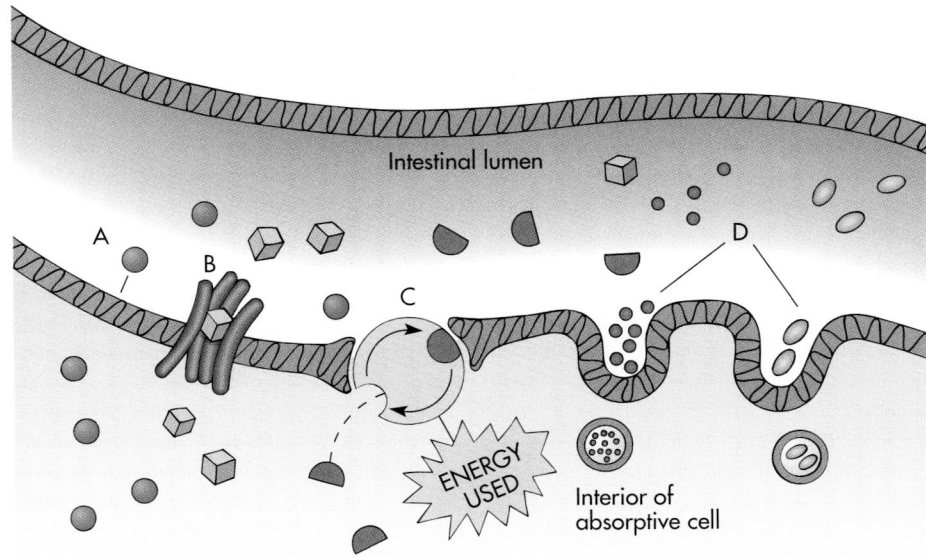

Figure 3.13 Nutrient absorption relies on these major forms of absorptive processes. (a) Passive absorption involves simple diffusion of substances across the cell membrane of absorptive cells. No energy is expended because the substances follow a favorable concentration gradient (from high to low concentrations). Water and fats are absorbed in this manner. (b) **Facilitated absorption** (not described in the chapter) uses a carrier protein or other process to aid in absorption of specific substances, such as fructose, but no energy is expended; the process is simply aided by the carrier. (c) Active absorption uses a carrier protein and expends energy in the process. The use of energy allows the absorptive cells to absorb nutrients against their concentration gradient (from low to high concentrations). Glucose and amino acids are two examples of nutrients that undergo active absorption. (d) Phagocytosis—"cell eating" involves cells taking in substances, including whole particles, by forming an indentation in the cell membrane and then surrounding the particle, with eventual incorporation into the cell. This is an active form of transport of substances. Pinocytosis—"cell drinking" involves cellular uptake of liquids in a manner similar to phagocytosis.

ileocecal sphincter The ring of smooth muscle between the end of the small intestine and the large intestine.

Any undigested food that reaches the end of the small intestine must pass through the **ileocecal sphincter** on the way to the large intestine. This sphincter prevents the contents of the large intestine from reentering the small intestine.

Large Intestine

When the contents of the small intestine enter the large intestine, little of the original food eaten remains. Only a minor amount (5%) of carbohydrate, protein, and fat have escaped absorption (Fig. 3.14).

Physiologically, the large intestine differs from the small intestine in that there are no villi or human digestive enzymes in the large intestine. This lack of villi allows for little absorption in the large intestine. However, the large intestine is able to absorb water, some vitamins, some fatty acids, and the minerals sodium and potassium. Unlike the small intestine, the large intestine has a number of mucus-producing cells. The mucus secreted by these cells helps to hold the feces together. This mucus also functions to protect the large intestine from ongoing bacterial activity in the organ. The large intestine has a large bacteria population. Note that these bacteria can even break down some of the products that enter the large intestine, such as starch and the milk sugar lactose that escapes digestion, and some components of dietary fiber. Products such as various acids can then be absorbed (Chapter 4 will discuss this further).

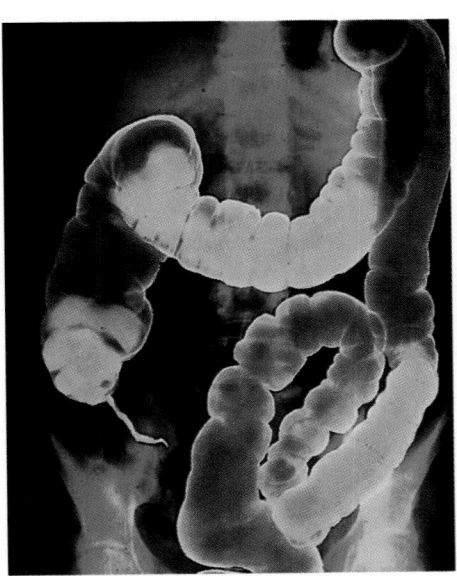

The large intestine (colon) has a large diameter and no villi.

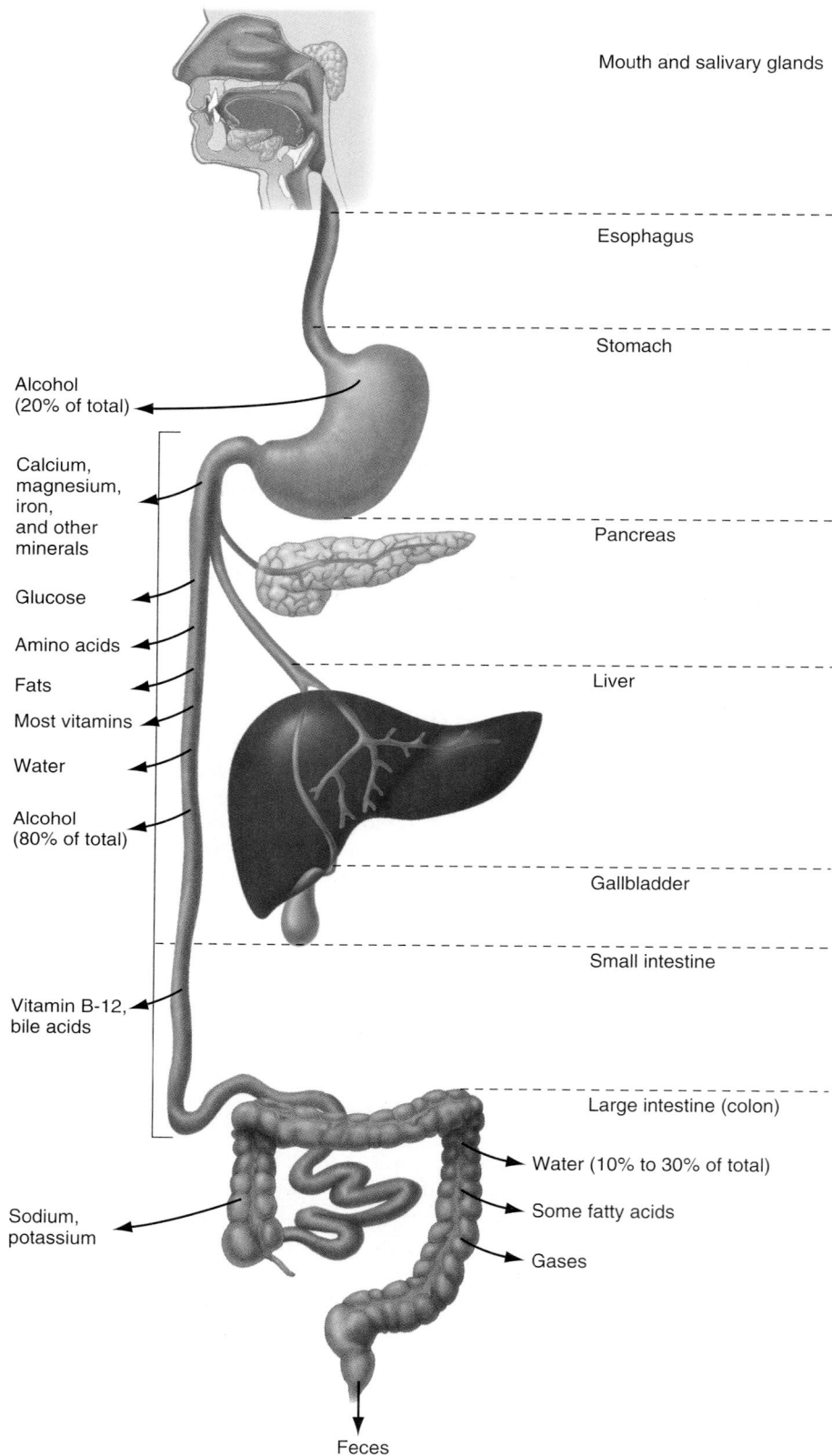

Critical Thinking

The medical history of a young girl who is greatly underweight shows that she had three-quarters of her small intestine removed after she was injured in a car accident. Explain how this accounts for her underweight condition, even though her medical chart shows that she eats well.

*N*utrient intake also directly influences nutrient absorption. *For example, vitamin C in a meal modestly increases iron absorption in the same meal because it changes iron into a more absorbable state.*

Mouth and salivary glands

Esophagus

Stomach

Alcohol (20% of total)

Calcium, magnesium, iron, and other minerals

Pancreas

Glucose

Amino acids

Fats

Liver

Most vitamins

Water

Alcohol (80% of total)

Gallbladder

Small intestine

Vitamin B-12, bile acids

Large intestine (colon)

Water (10% to 30% of total)

Sodium, potassium

Some fatty acids

Gases

Feces

Figure 3.14   Major sites of absorption along the GI tract. Note that minimal absorption of vitamin K and biotin takes place in the large intestine.

Table 3.4 A Summary of Digestion Functions, Organ-by-Organ

Organ	Functions
Mouth	Chewing of food Some digestion of starch
Esophagus	Passageway
Stomach	Food storage; acidity kills bacteria Some digestion of protein
Small intestine	Final digestion of all energy-yielding nutrients Absorption of nutrients
Large intestine	Absorption of water and some minerals; storage of nondigestible remains
Anus	Elimination of waste as feces

Some water remains in the mass found in the large intestine because the small intestine absorbs only 70% to 90% of the fluid it receives, which includes large amounts of GI-tract secretions produced during digestion. The remnants of a meal also include some minerals and some dietary fiber. The contents of the large intestine are semisolid by the time they have passed through the first two-thirds of it. What remains in the **feces,** besides water and undigested dietary fiber, is tough connective tissues (from animal foods), bacteria from the large intestine, and some body wastes, such as parts of dead intestinal cells.

Rectum

The stool remains in the last portion of the large intestine, the **rectum,** until muscular movements push it into the **anus** to be eliminated. The presence of feces in the rectum stimulates elimination. The anus contains two, final **anal sphincters** (internal and external), one of which is under voluntary control (external sphincter). Once children are toilet trained, they can generally control when the external anal sphincter will relax and when it will stay rigid. Relaxation of this sphincter allows for elimination.

Table 3.4 summarizes the major roles of each organ in digestion and absorption discussed so far.

Accessory Organs

There are other organs that play a necessary role in the process of digestion. These accessory organs do not directly participate in digestion. However, they do provide digestive fluids that enable the digestive processes to chemically change the food into absorbable components. Ducts leading from the **pancreas** and **gallbladder** merge and connect to the small intestine allowing output from the **liver** (and stored in the gallbladder) to eventually blend with pancreatic output as both are released into the small intestine for digestive purposes (review Fig. 3.8). In this way, the liver, pancreas, and gallbladder work with the GI tract. Thus, the liver, gallbladder, and pancreas are considered *accessory* organs to the process of digestion.

The liver produces a substance called **bile.** The bile is then stored in the gallbladder until it receives a hormonal signal from the digestive tract to release it. The signal itself is induced by the presence of fat in the small intestine. Once the hormonal signal is received by the gallbladder, bile is released and delivered to the small intestine via a tube called the *bile duct.*

In action, bile is very much like soap: Constituents in the bile take large portions of fat and break them into smaller portions so that they can be suspended in water (Chapter 5 will cover this process in detail). An interesting aspect of bile transport is some of the bile constituents can be reabsorbed from the small intestine, returned to the liver via the portal vein, and reused. This circuit is known as **enterohepatic circulation.**

*F*oods containing microbes such as lactobacilli are getting a lot of attention these days. The term **probiotic** is used for these microbes because once consumed, these microbes take up residence in the large intestine. Their presence in the large intestine leads to some health benefits, including improving intestinal tract health, enhancing immune function, reducing symptoms of lactose maldigestion and intolerance, and decreasing the prevalence of allergies in susceptible individuals. You can find these probiotic microbes in certain forms of fluid milk, fermented milk, and yogurt. They can even be found in pill form. Regular consumption of yogurt is one way to gain the benefits of these microbes. A related term is **prebiotic.** These are substances that increase growth of probiotic microbes. One example is fructooligosaccharides (see Table 2.1 in Chapter 2 for dietary sources).

gallbladder An organ attached to the underside of the liver and in which bile is stored and secreted.

bile A liver secretion that is stored in the gallbladder and released through the common bile duct into the duodenum. It is essential for the absorption of fat.

enterohepatic circulation The recycling of compounds between the small intestine and the liver over and over again, as happens with certain bile constituents.

Figure 3.15 Organs of the urinary system. The kidneys, bean-shaped organs located on either side of the spinal column, filter waste from the blood, which is then stored in the bladder as urine. The kidneys are connected to the urinary bladder by ureters. The urinary system of the female is shown. The male's urinary system is the same, except that the urethra extends through the penis.

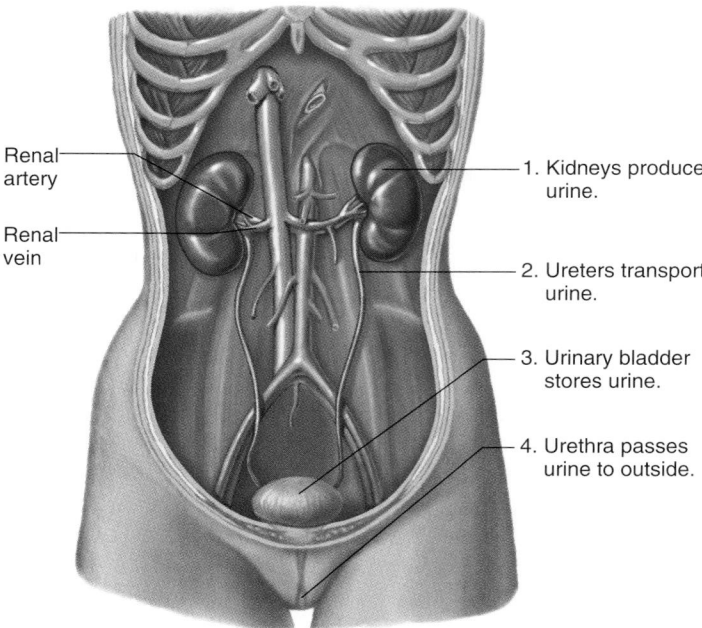

Renal artery

Renal vein

1. Kidneys produce urine.

2. Ureters transport urine.

3. Urinary bladder stores urine.

4. Urethra passes urine to outside.

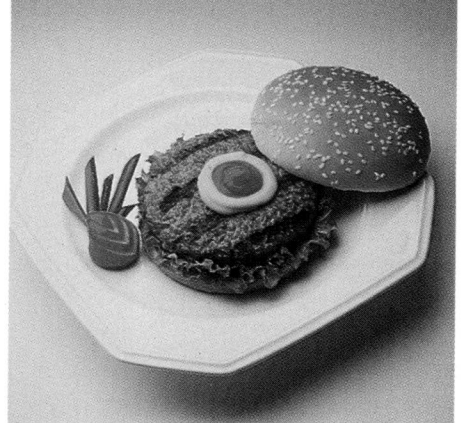

The body digests the foods presented—the order in which foods are eaten plays no role. You can eat the bun and then the burger, or both at the same time.

In addition to bile, the liver releases a number of other substances that travel with the bile to the gallbladder—eventually ending up in the small intestine. The liver functions in this manner to remove unwanted substances from the blood. After processing, by the liver, some by-products end up in the bile. (Other by-products are excreted via the urine; see the next section on the urinary system.)

The pancreas is another accessory digestive organ. It manufactures a variety of digestive enzymes capable of breaking apart carbohydrates, proteins, and fats into small fragments. In addition, the pancreas produces glucagon and insulin, two very important hormones that function in blood glucose regulation (see the earlier discussion on the endocrine system). The pancreas also secretes pancreatic juice. This digestive juice contains water, bicarbonate (a base to counteract stomach acid present in the chyme once it reaches the small intestine), and a variety of digestive enzymes. It is important that bicarbonate neutralizes the acid coming from the stomach as it enters as part of the chyme reaching the small intestine. If the acid is not neutralized, it will erode the wall of the small intestine and could quickly lead to formation of an ulcer (see the Nutrition Issue). This is because the small intestine, unlike the stomach, lacks a protective layer of mucus. This form of protection is not possible because it would impede nutrient absorption.

Concept Check

Digestion is a mechanical and chemical process controlled by enzymes and coordinated by hormones and nerves. The end products of digestion are small molecules of the original food or beverage, small enough to enter into the villi for pickup by either the blood in the capillaries or the lymph system. Any dietary component that escapes digestion by human enzymes or bacterial action in the large intestine exits the body in the feces. Whereas swallowing food and ultimate elimination of feces from the anus is voluntary, the rest of the digestive process is involuntary. The stomach initiates the process of digestion by mixing food with gastric juice and converting this partially digested food into a liquid called chyme. Absorption takes place mostly in the small intestine. The feces, or undigested material, are expelled from the body.

■ Urinary System

The **urinary system** is composed of two kidneys, one on each side of the spinal column. Each kidney is connected to the bladder by a **ureter.** The bladder is emptied by way of the **urethra** (Fig. 3.15). The main function of the kidneys is to remove waste from the body. The kidneys are constantly filtering blood to control its composition. This results in the formation of urine, which is mostly water; however, it does contain dissolved particles such as urea, **creatinine,** and excess and unneeded water-soluble vitamins and various minerals.

Together with the lungs, the kidneys also maintain the acid-base balance (**pH**) of the blood. The kidneys also convert a form of vitamin D into its active hormone form, and produce a hormone that stimulates red blood cell synthesis (**erythropoietin;** see Chapter 11 for information on misuse of this hormone by some athletes). During times of fasting, the kidneys even produce glucose from certain amino acids (see Chapter 4). Thus, the kidneys perform many important functions and are a vital component of the body.

The proper function of the kidneys is closely tied to the strength of the cardiovascular system (i.e., adequate blood pressure) and the consumption of sufficient fluids. Uncontrolled diabetes, hypertension, and drug abuse are very harmful to the kidneys.

■ Storage Capabilities

The human body must maintain reserves of nutrients. Otherwise, we would need to eat continuously. Storage capacity varies for each different nutrient. Most fat is stored at sites designed specifically for this—adipose tissue. Short-term storage of carbohydrate occurs in muscle and liver, and the blood maintains a small reserve of glucose and amino acids. Many vitamins and minerals are stored in the liver, while other nutrient stores are found in other sites in the body.

When people do not meet their nutrient needs, some nutrients are obtained by breaking down a tissue that contains high concentrations of the nutrient. Calcium is taken from bone, and protein is taken from muscle. These nutrient losses in cases of long-term deficiency harm these tissues.

Many people believe that if too much of a nutrient is obtained—for example, from a vitamin or mineral supplement—only what is needed is stored and the rest is excreted by the body. Though partially true, as with vitamin C, the large dosages found frequently in supplements such as vitamins A and D can cause harmful side effects because these are not readily excreted. This is one reason why obtaining your nutrients primarily (or exclusively) from a balanced diet is the safest means to acquire the building blocks you need to maintain the good health of all organ systems.

This review of human anatomy and physiology from a nutrition perspective sets the stage for developing a more detailed understanding of the nutrients. Chapters 4, 5, and 6 will build on this information.

Concept Check

The urinary system removes the wastes that are produced by the body and most nutrients that are ingested in excess of storage capacity and need. The kidneys maintain the chemical composition of the blood and a stable environment within the body. The kidneys help convert vitamin D to its active form and participate in red blood cell synthesis.

Nutrients are constantly present in the blood for immediate use and are stored to a greater or lesser extent in the body tissues for later use when sufficient amounts from food intake is unavailable. However, when the body suffers a nutrient deficiency caused by an inadequate diet, it breaks down vital tissues for their nutrients, which can lead to ill health. Additionally, too much of any nutrient can be detrimental. It's best to focus primarily (or exclusively) on obtaining all essential nutrients from a balanced diet.

urinary system The body system consisting of the kidneys, urinary bladder, and the ducts that carry urine. This system removes waste products from the circulatory system and regulates blood acid-base balance, overall chemical balance, and water balance in the body.

creatinine Nitrogenous waste product of the compound creatine found in muscles.

pH A measure of relative acidity or alkalinity of a solution. The pH scale is 0–14. A pH below 7 is acidic; a pH above 7 is alkaline.

erythropoietin A hormone secreted mostly by the kidneys that enhances red blood cell synthesis and stimulates red blood cell release from bone marrow.

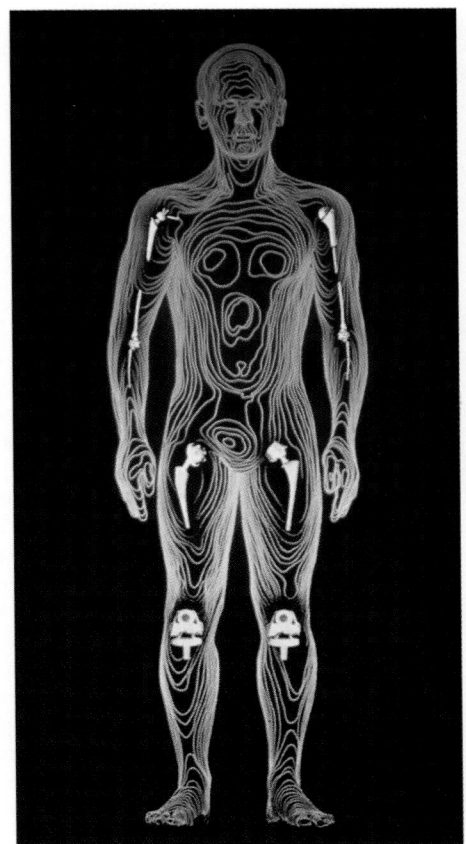

The skeletal system provides a reserve of calcium and phosphorus for day-to-day needs when dietary intake is inadequate. Long-term use of this reserve, however, reduces bone strength.

Summary

1. The basic structural unit of the human body is the cell. Although almost all cells contain the same collection of organelles (nucleus, mitochondria, endoplasmic reticulum, lysosomes, peroxisomes, and cytoplasm), their structure varies according to the type of job they must perform.
2. Cells join together to make up tissues, tissues unite to form organs, and organs work together as an organ system.
3. In the circulatory system, blood travels the pulmonary circuit, picking up oxygen at the lungs, as part of cardiovascular function. Then, via the systemic circuit, the blood delivers essential nutrients, oxygen, and water to all body cells. Nutrients and wastes are exchanged between the blood and cells across the cell membrane. This exchange occurs in the capillaries.
4. Water-soluble compounds in the villi enter the portal vein and travel to the liver. Fat-soluble compounds enter the lymphatic system, which eventually connects to the bloodstream.
5. The nervous system's neurons are the body's communication network. They control and manage all other organ systems of the body. Neurotransmitters are used to carry the message from one neuron to another (or to another cell).
6. The endocrine system produces hormones, which chemically regulate almost all other cells.
7. The immune system is responsible for protecting the body from invading pathogens. We activate immunity, such as production of antibodies, when we come in contact with a pathogen.
8. The gastrointestinal (GI) tract consists of the mouth, esophagus, stomach, small intestine, large intestine (colon), rectum, and anus.
9. Spaced along the GI tract are ringlike valves (sphincters) that regulate the flow of foodstuffs. Muscular contractions, called *peristalsis*, move the foodstuffs down the GI tract. A variety of nerves,

hormones, and other substances control the activity of sphincters and peristaltic muscles.
10. Digestive enzymes are secreted by the mouth, stomach, wall of the small intestine, and pancreas. The presence of food in the small intestine stimulates the release of pancreatic enzymes.
11. The major absorptive sites consist of fingerlike projections called *villi*, located in the small intestine. Absorptive cells cover the villi. This intestinal lining is continually renewed. Absorptive cells can perform various passive and active forms of absorption.
12. Little digestion and absorption occur in the stomach or large intestine, but some protein is digested in the stomach. Some constituents of dietary fiber and undigested starch are broken down by bacteria in the large intestine; undigested dietary fiber that remains is eliminated in the feces.
13. Final water and mineral absorption takes place in the large intestine. Products from bacterial breakdown of some dietary fibers and other substances are also absorbed here. The presence of feces in the rectum provides a strong impetus for elimination.
14. The liver, gallbladder, and pancreas participate in digestion and absorption. Products from these organs, such as enzymes and bile, enter the small intestine and play important roles in digesting protein, fat, and carbohydrate.
15. The urinary system is responsible for filtering the blood, removing body wastes, and maintaining the chemical composition of the blood.
16. Limited stores of nutrients are present in the blood for immediate use and stored to a greater or lesser extent in body tissues for later use when sufficient food is unavailable. When the body suffers a nutrient deficiency caused by a poor diet, it breaks down vital tissues for their nutrients, which can lead to ill health. Additionally, too much of any nutrient can be detrimental.

Study Questions

1. Identify at least one contribution to overall nutrition status provided by each of the 12 organ systems of the body.
2. Draw and label parts of the cell, and explain the function of each organelle discussed in the text as it relates to human nutrition.
3. What is the difference between nature and nurture? Relate these terms to the attempt to prevent three common chronic diseases.
4. Trace the flow of blood from the right side of the heart around the body and back to the same site. How is blood routed through the villi? Which class of nutrients enters the body via the blood? Via the lymph?
5. Explain why the small intestine is better suited than the other GI tract organs to carry out the absorptive process.
6. Identify the four basic tastes. Give an example of one food that exemplifies each of these basic taste sensations. Why can't you taste food when you have a cold? What is umami?

7. What is one role of acid in the process of digestion? Where is it secreted?
8. Contrast the processes of active and passive absorption of nutrients.
9. Identify the two accessory organs that empty their contents into the small intestine. How do the digestive substances made by these organs contribute to the digestion of food?
10. In which organ systems would the following substances be found?
   chyme
   plasma
   lymph
   urine

Further Readings

1. Answering your questions about immunity. *UC Berkeley Wellness Letter*, p. 4, May 2001.
   An adequate diet helps maintain the immune system. Nutrients such as protein, essential fatty acids, and certain vitamins and minerals play key roles. Moderate exercise and adequate sleep also improve immune function. Severely malnourished people are particularly vulnerable to immune dysfunction. Since many older people may not consume much food, there is evidence that they stay healthier if they take a multivitamin and mineral supplement. Still, megadoses of certain nutrients, such as zinc, can significantly harm some immune responses.

2. Collins FS, McKusick VA: Implications of the human genome project for medical science. *Journal of the American Medical Association* 285:540, 2001.
   In the coming years, genetic tests will be available for many common conditions. This will allow individuals who wish to know this information to learn more about their individual susceptibilities, and to take steps to reduce those risks for which interventions are available. These could include diet and lifestyle modifications and drug therapy. One concern is the potential for discrimination in the workplace once a person's genetic information is known. Ideally, federal legislation will outlaw that practice.

3. Constipation becomes more common with age. *Tufts University Health and Nutrition Letter* 17:7, 1999.
   Normal frequency of bowel movements ranges from three times a day to three times a week. Constipation is an aging problem that can be treated with regular exercise, decreased dosage of medications that cause constipation, increased dietary fiber, more water consumption, and avoidance of laxatives unless absolutely necessary.

4. Heartburn, don't ignore it. *Mayo Clinic Health Letter* 18:8, 2000.
   The causes of heartburn are explained. The new FDA-approved treatments for heartburn are introduced. One treatment is sewing up the lower esophageal sphincter (LES) and the other is burning a scar into the LES that tightens up the sphincter.

5. H. pylori: What's the story? *Health News.* p. 1. December 2001.
   The bacterium H. pylori is a common cause of ulcers. People that should be tested for the presence of H. pylori include those with active stomach ulcers and those with stomach cancer or a family history of stomach cancer. Therapy generally includes the use of two antibiotics plus a proton pump inhibitor. It is successful in more than 90 percent of cases.

6. Horwitz BJ, Fisher RS: Irritable bowel syndrome. *The New England Journal of Medicine* 344:1846, 2001.
   People with irritable bowel syndrome often benefit from a diet adequate in fiber (20–30 grams per day) and low in caffeine, alcohol, fatty foods, gas-forming vegetables, and products containing sorbitol, such as sugarless gum and dietetic candy. Certain medications are also helpful in treating such individuals.

7. Kopp-Hoolihan L: Prophylactic and therapeutic uses of probiotics: A review. *Journal of the American Dietetic Association* 101:229, 2001.
   Probiotic microbes in foods beneficially affect the human host. These benefits include improving intestinal tract health, enhancing immune function, synthesizing some nutrients, enhancing bioavailability of some nutrients, reducing symptoms of lactose maldigestion and intolerance, decreasing the prevalence of allergies in susceptible individuals, and reducing risk of certain cancers. Certain forms of fluid milk, fermented milk, and yogurt contain probiotic microbes, such as Lactobacillus.

8. Lewis C: Irritable bowel syndrome: A poorly understood disorder. *FDA Consumer*, p. 30, July–August 2001.
   Irritable bowel syndrome may affect up to 20 percent of people in North America, and is more common in women. Stress does not normally cause irritable bowel syndrome, although it may aggravate the symptoms. The first step in treatment is evaluation of personal history of symptoms and life stress. A low-fat diet in particular helps some people.

9. Kaynard A, Flora K: Gastroesophageal reflux disease (GERD). *Postgraduate Medicine* 110(3):42, 2001.
   Large surveys show that half of the general adult population experiences monthly heartburn. A trial of high doses of proton pump inhibitors is becoming accepted therapy for GERD. Complications of long-standing GERD include damage to the esophagus and a form of esophageal cancer.

10. Smith DV, Margolskee RF: Making sense of taste. *Scientific American*, p. 32, March 2001.
    Taste buds are scattered throughout the tongue, rather than in specific regions, as was previously thought. These taste buds sense sweet, salty, bitter, sour, and umami. When these compounds that cause these taste sensations bind to appropriate taste buds, changes in ion balance ultimately take place in the cell. This triggers the message that is sent to the nervous system.

11. Tso P, Crissinger K: Overview of digestion and absorption. In Stepanuk MH (ed.): *Biochemical and physiological aspects of human nutrition* W. B. Saunders, 2000.
    One chapter in this Human Nutrition textbook identifies the major structures and functions of the digestive tract. Control of absorption and metabolism is explained.

12. Van De Graaff KM, Fox SI: *Concepts of human anatomy & physiology.* 5th ed. Boston: WCB McGraw-Hill, 1999.
    The basis for understanding human nutrition is to comprehend the role of anatomy and physiology as they relate to the foundation for personal health. This text provides the framework for integrating modern biology into the study of scientific nutrition.

13. Wong PWK, Kadakia S: How to deal with chronic constipation. *Postgraduate Medicine* 106:199, 1999.
    The authors list the diagnostic criteria used to establish chronic constipation. Treatment includes patient education, bowel habit training, increased fluid and fiber intake, and laxative use.

14. Wulfsberg DA: The impact of genetic testing on primary care: Where's the beef? *American Family Physician* 61:971, 2000.
    Recent genetic discovery has led to a better understanding of many rare genetic disorders. However, the lack of effective interventions and public resistance suggest genetic technologies will be slow to be introduced into common medical practice. Currently, genetic testing is especially useful for people who have a family history of disorders in which the tests are applicable.

I. Are You Taking Care of Your Digestive Tract?

People need to think about the health of their digestive tracts. There are symptoms we need to notice, as well as habits we need to practice in order to protect it. The following assessment is designed to help you examine your habits and symptoms associated with the health of your digestive tract. The Nutrition Issue explains why these habits are important to examine. Put a *Y* in the blank to the left of the question to indicate yes and an *N* to indicate no.

_____ 1. Are you currently experiencing greater than normal stress and tension?

_____ 2. Do you have a family history of digestive tract problems (e.g., ulcers, hemorrhoids, recurrent heartburn, constipation)?

_____ 3. Do you experience pain in your stomach region about 2 hours after you eat?

_____ 4. Do you smoke cigarettes?

_____ 5. Do you take aspirin frequently?

_____ 6. Do you have heartburn at least once per week?

_____ 7. Do you commonly lie down after eating a large meal?

_____ 8. Do you drink alcoholic beverages more than two or three times per day?

_____ 9. Do you experience abdominal pain, bloating, and gas about 30 minutes to 2 hours after consuming milk products?

_____ 10. Do you often have to strain while having a bowel movement?

_____ 11. Do you consume less than 8 cups of a combination of water and other fluids per day?

_____ 12. Do you perform physical activity for at least 30 minutes on most or all days of the week (e.g., jog, swim, walk briskly, row, stair climb).

_____ 13. Do you eat a diet relatively low in dietary fiber (recall that significant dietary fiber is found in whole fruits, vegetables, legumes, nuts and seeds, whole-grain breads, and whole-grain cereals)?

_____ 14. Do you frequently have diarrhea?

_____ 15. Do you frequently use laxatives or antacids?

Interpretation

Add up the number of yes answers you gave and record the total in the blank to the right.   _____

If your score is from 8 to 15, your habits and symptoms put you at risk for experiencing future digestive tract problems. Take particular note of the habits to which you answered yes. Consider trying to cooperate more with your digestive tract.

II. Create Your Family Tree for Health-Related Concerns

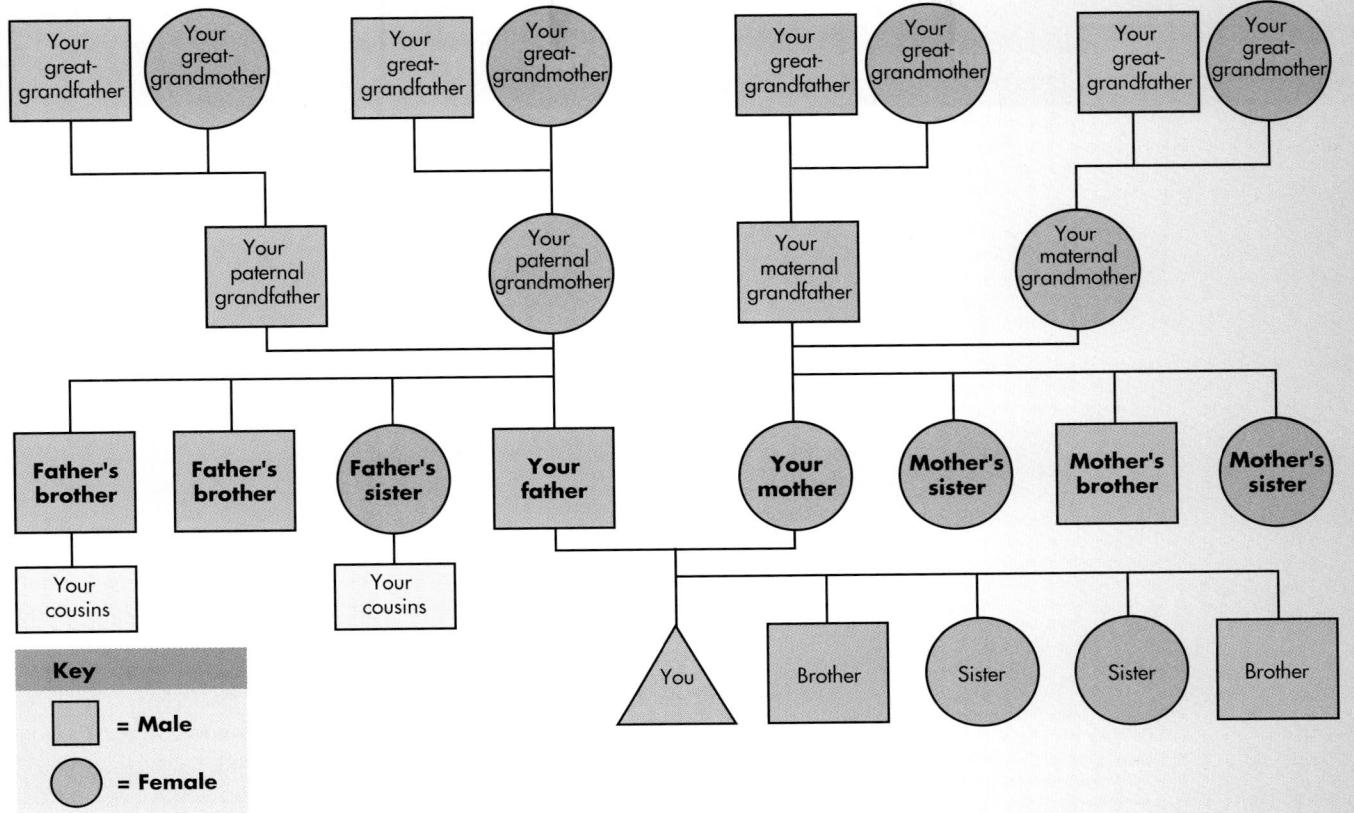

Under each heading, list year born, year died (if applicable), major diseases that developed during the person's lifetime, and cause of death (if applicable). Figure 3.3 in the Nutrition Insight provides one such example.

Note that you are likely to be at risk for any diseases listed. Creating a plan for preventing such diseases when possible, especially those that developed in your family members before age 50–60 years, is advised. Speak with your physician about any concerns arising from this exercise.

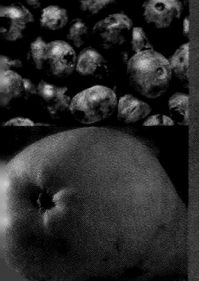

The fine-tuned organ system we call the *GI tract* can develop problems. Knowing about these common problems can help you avoid them.

Ulcers

Many adults develop ulcers each year. Millions of North Americans develop them during their lifetimes. The principal causes are an acid-resistant bacterial infection *(Helicobacter pylori [H. pylori])*, the heavy use of aspirin and related medications, and disorders that cause excessive acid production in the stomach (Fig. 3.16). And, after being out of favor for some years, stress is now regarded as a predisposing factor, albeit a minor one, for ulcers.

As the stomach lining deteriorates in ulcer development and loses its mucus layer protection, the acid erodes the stomach tissue. Acid can also erode the tissue lining of the first part of the small intestine. *Peptic ulcer* is the general term for both of these two cases. Most ulcers in young people occur in the small intestine; in older people they occur primarily in the stomach.

The typical symptom of an ulcer is pain about 2 hours after eating. Digestive acid acting on a meal irritates the ulcer after most of the meal has moved from the site of the ulcer.

The primary risk associated with an ulcer is the possibility that it will erode entirely through the stomach or intestinal wall. The GI contents could then spill into the body cavities, causing a massive infection. In addition, an ulcer may erode a blood vessel, leading to massive blood loss. For these reasons, it is important not to ignore the early warning signs of ulcer development.

In the past, milk and cream therapy—the Sippy diet—was used to help cure ulcers. Clinicians now know that milk and cream are two of the worst foods for an ulcer. The calcium in these foods stimulates stomach acid secretion and actually inhibits ulcer healing.

Today, a combination of approaches is used for ulcer therapy. People infected with *H. pylori* are given antibiotics with stomach acid-blocking medications called proton pump inhibitors (e.g., omeprazole [Prilosec]) to eradicate *H. pylori*. Note that proton is another term for the hydrogen ion that creates acidity. In many cases, there is a 90% cure rate for *H. pylori* in the first week of this treatment. Recurrence is unlikely if the infection is cured, but an incomplete cure almost certainly leads to repeated ulcer formation.

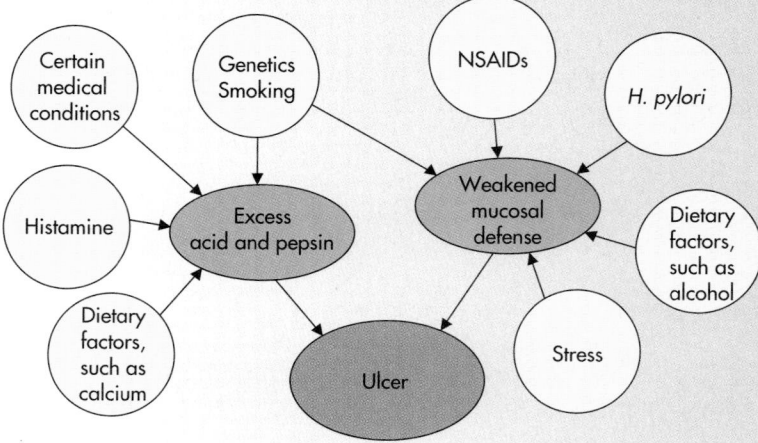

Figure 3.16 Development of a peptic ulcer. *H. pylori* bacteria and NSAIDs cause ulcers by impairing mucosal defense, especially in the stomach. In the same way, smoking, genetics, and stress can impair mucosal defense, as well as cause an increase in the release of pepsin and stomach acid. All of these factors can contribute to ulcers.

104

Table 3.5 Recommendations to Prevent Ulcers and Heartburn from Occurring or Recurring

Ulcers

1. Stop smoking, if you are now a smoker.

2. Avoid large doses of aspirin, ibuprofen, and other NSAID compounds unless a physician advises otherwise. For people who must use these medications, FDA has approved an NSAID combined with a medication to reduce gastric damage. The medication reduces gastric acid production and enhances mucus secretion.

3. Limit consumption of coffee, tea, and alcohol (especially wine), if this helps.

4. Limit consumption of pepper, chili powder, and other strong spices, if this helps.

5. Eat nutritious meals on a regular schedule; include enough dietary fiber (see Chapter 4 for sources of fiber).

6. Chew foods well.

7. Lose weight if you are currently overweight.

Heartburn

1. Wait about 2 hours after a meal before lying down.

2. Don't overeat at mealtime. Smaller meals that are low in fat are advised.

3. Try elevating the head of the bed (6-inch blocks).

4. Observe the recommendations for ulcer prevention.

5. Stop smoking cigarettes.

6. Lose excess weight.

Antacid medications may also be part of ulcer care, as is a class of medicines called **H₂ blockers.** These include cimetidine (Tagamet), ranitidine (Zantac), and famotidine (Pepcid), all of which prevent histamine-related acid secretion in the stomach. Some of these medications are now available over the counter in nonprescription doses for cases of indigestion and heartburn (see next section). Medications that coat the ulcer, such as sucralfate (Carafate), are also commonly used.

People with ulcers should also refrain from smoking and minimize the use of aspirin and related NSAIDs. These practices reduce the mucus secreted by the stomach. Medications that are used to treat arthritis pain, called "Cox-2 inhibitors" (e.g., celecoxib [Celebrex]), are less likely to cause stomach ulcers and, so, have been used as a replacement for NSAIDs. They do offer some advantages over NSAIDS, but they may not be totally safe for some people. Overall, this combination of lifestyle therapy and medical treatment has so revolutionized ulcer therapy that dietary changes are of minor importance today. Current diet-therapy approaches recommend simply avoiding foods that increase ulcer symptoms (Table 3.5).

Note also that stomach acid is not a problem for those not prone to or currently experiencing ulcers. The acid in the stomach enhances the absorption of iron, calcium, and vitamin B-12. Acid also minimizes bacterial growth in the stomach; the stomach is essentially bacteria free because of its high acid content. Bacteria in food are quickly destroyed, which reduces the risk of these bacteria forming cancer-causing agents or leading to foodborne illness (see Chapter 16). Thus, acid production by the stomach is an important part of the physiology of digestion and absorption. This means that, despite their usual presence alongside the breath mints in a convenience store, antacids should not be used excessively. If an antacid contains magnesium (and many do), magnesium toxicity is another possible result of antacid abuse.

Heartburn

About half of North American adults experience occassional heartburn. This gnawing pain in the upper chest is caused by the movement of acid from the stomach into the esophagus and, so, the more serious form of the problem is called **gastroesophageal reflux disease (GERD).**

continued

A number of over-the-counter medications are marketed for heartburn. Attention to diet and lifestyle, however, is generally a more important measure to take.

H₂ blockers Medications such as cimetidine (Tagamet) that block the increase of stomach acid production caused by histamine.

A spirin is part of the class of medications called nonsteroidal anti-inflammatory drugs (NSAIDs). Also included are ibuprofen (Motrin or Advil) and naproxen (Aleve).

gastroesophageal reflux disease (GERD) A disease that results from stomach acid backing up into the esophagus. The acid irritates the lining of the esophagus, causing pain.

Unlike the stomach, the esophagus has very little mucus lining to protect it, so acid quickly erodes the lining of the esophagus, causing pain. Symptoms may also include nausea, gagging, cough, or hoarseness. GERD is characterized by such symptoms of acid reflux two or more times per week. People who have GERD experience occasional relaxation of the sphincter. Typically it should be relaxed only during swallowing, but in individuals with GERD it is relaxed at other times as well.

Certain physical conditions can lead to heartburn. For example, both pregnancy and obesity result in increased production of estrogen and progesterone. These hormones relax the lower esophageal (cardiac) sphincter, making heartburn more likely. In the latter case, adipose tissue turns certain circulating hormones into estrogen; thus, the more adipose tissue, the more estrogen is produced.

Scenario *Follow-Up*

Chad's GERD can be treated, but currently it is a lifelong condition. Typical dietary advice includes consuming smaller, more frequent meals that are low in fat, not overeating at mealtimes, waiting about 2 hours after meals before lying down, and elevating the head of the bed about 6 inches (review Table 3.5). All of these recommendations reduce the risk of stomach contents forcing their way back up the esophagus. Other helpful advice includes stopping smoking if practiced, losing excess weight if overweight, and limiting intake of chili powder, onions, garlic, peppermint, caffeine, alcohol, and chocolate. All of these factors encourage relaxation of the sphincter and/or irritate the esophagus. If this advice doesn't control symptoms, the primary medications used to control GERD inhibit acid production in the stomach (see the earlier discussion on the ulcer medication omeprazole (Prilosec). If this and other medical therapy fails to control the problem, surgery to strengthen the lower esophageal sphincter is possible, but generally will not cure the problem. Currently, lifetime diet and lifestyle management, and most likely medications as well, will still be needed to manage the problem. Such management is important since long-standing GERD increases the risk of esophageal cancer.

Constipation and Laxatives

constipation A condition characterized by infrequent bowel movements.

Constipation, which is difficult or infrequent evacuation of the bowels, is commonly reported by adults. Slow movement of fecal material through the large intestine causes constipation. As fluid is increasingly absorbed during the extended time the feces stay in the large intestine, they become dry and hard.

Constipation can result when people regularly inhibit their normal bowel reflexes for long periods. People may ignore normal urges when it is inconvenient to interrupt occupational or social activities. Muscle spasms of an irritated large intestine can also slow the movement of feces and contribute to constipation. Medications such as antacids and calcium and iron supplements can also cause constipation.

Eating foods with plenty of dietary fiber, such as whole-grain breads and cereals, is the best method for treating typical cases of constipation. Dietary fibers stimulate peristalsis by drawing water into the large intestine and helping form a bulky, soft fecal output. People with constipation should also drink more fluids, and eating dried fruits can help stimulate the bowel. In addition, people with constipation may need to develop more regular bowel habits; allowing the same time each day for a bowel movement can help train the large intestine to respond routinely. Finally, relaxation facilitates regular bowel movements, as does regular physical activity.

laxative A medication or another substance that stimulates evacuation of the intestinal tract.

Laxatives can also lessen constipation. These work by irritating the intestinal nerve junctions to stimulate the peristaltic muscles, or by drawing water into the intestine to enlarge fecal output. The larger output stretches the peristaltic muscles, making them rebound and then constrict. Regular use of laxatives, especially irritating ones, however, can decrease muscle action in the large intestine—in time, causing more constipation. The GI tract can then actually become dependent on laxatives. Thus, it is unwise for anyone to use laxatives routinely, although people in certain circumstances—for example, those who are bedridden or quite elderly—may need periodic help from laxatives to relieve constipation.

Hemorrhoids

Hemorrhoids, also called *piles*, are swollen veins of the rectum and anus. The blood vessels in this area are subject to intense pressure, especially during bowel movements. Added stress to the vessels from pregnancy, obesity, prolonged sitting, violent coughing or sneezing, or straining during bowel movements, particularly with constipation, can lead to a hemorrhoid. Hemorrhoids can develop unnoticed until a strained bowel movement precipitates symptoms, which may include pain, itching, and bleeding.

Itching, caused by moisture in the anal canal, swelling, or other irritation, is perhaps the most common symptom. Pain, if present, is usually aching and steady. Bleeding may result from a hemorrhoid and may appear in the toilet as a bright red streak in the feces. The sensation of a mass in the anal canal after a bowel movement is symptomatic of an internal hemorrhoid that protrudes through the anus.

Anyone can develop a hemorrhoid, and about half of adults over age 50 do. Pressure from prolonged sitting or exertion is often enough to bring on symptoms, although diet, lifestyle, and possibly heredity play a role. If you think you have a hemorrhoid, you should consult your physician. Rectal bleeding, although usually caused by hemorrhoids, may also indicate other problems, such as cancer.

A physician may suggest a variety of self-care measures for hemorrhoids. Pain can be lessened by applying warm, soft compresses or sitting in a tub of warm water for 15 to 20 minutes. Dietary recommendations are the same as those for treating constipation, emphasizing the need to consume adequate dietary fiber and fluid. Over-the-counter remedies, such as Preparation H, can also offer relief of symptoms.

Irritable Bowel Syndrome

Many adults have irritable bowel syndrome, a combination of cramps, gassiness, bloating, and irregular bowel function (diarrhea, constipation, or alternating episodes of both). It is more common in women than in men.

Symptoms associated with irritable bowel syndrome include visible abdominal distension, pain relief after a bowel movement, increased stool frequency with pain onset, looser stools with pain onset, mucus in stool, and a feeling of incomplete elimination even after a bowel movement.

The cause is thought to be altered intestinal peristalsis, coupled with a decreased pain threshold for abdominal distension—in other words, a minor amount of abdominal bloating causes pain that the average person would not sense. It is also noteworthy that up to 50% of sufferers report a history of verbal or sexual abuse.

Therapy is individualized and can include a trial of high-fiber foods: elimination diets that focus on avoiding dairy products and gas-forming foods, such as legumes and certain vegetables (cabbage, beans, and broccoli) and fruits such as grapes, raisins, cherries, and cantaloupe. The patient should have only moderate caffeine intake or eliminate caffeine-containing foods/beverages altogether. Low-fat and more frequent, small meals may help the patient because large meals can trigger contractions of the large intestine. Other strategies include a reduction in stress, psychological counseling, and certain antidepressant medications.

Referral to a registered dietitian can be beneficial, as many patients experience improvement with the elimination of specific problem foods. A good patient/physician relationship is also necessary for the treatment of irritable bowel syndrome; however, before any single treatment is applauded, it is important to note that placebo response alone has been as high as 70% in this population. Although irritable bowel syndrome can be uncomfortable and upsetting, it is harmless; it carries no risk for cancer or other serious digestive problems.

continued

Perhaps you have heard that taking laxatives after overeating prevents deposition of body fat from the excess energy intake. This erroneous and dangerous premise has gained popularity among followers of numerous fad diets. You may temporarily feel less full after using a laxative because laxatives hasten emptying of the large intestine and increase fluid loss. Most laxatives, however, do not speed the passage of food through the small intestine, where digestion and most nutrient absorption take place. As a result, you can't count on laxatives to prevent fat gain from excess energy intake.

Diarrhea

Diarrhea, a GI tract disease that generally lasts only a few days, is defined as increased fluidity, frequency, or amount of bowel movements compared to a person's usual pattern. Most cases of diarrhea result from infections in the intestines, with bacteria and viruses the usual offending agents. They produce substances that cause the intestinal cells to primarily secrete fluid rather than absorb fluid. Another form of diarrhea can be caused by consumption of substances that are not readily absorbed, such as the sugar alcohol sorbitol found in sugarless gum (see Chapter 4). When consumed in large amounts the unabsorbed substance draws much water into the intestines, in turn leading to diarrhea. Treatment of diarrhea generally requires drinking lots of fluid during the affected stage; reduced intake of the poorly absorbed substance also is important if that is a cause. Prompt treatment—within 24 to 48 hours—is especially important for infants and older people, as they are more susceptible to the effects of dehydration associated with diarrhea (see Chapters 14 and 15). Diarrhea that lasts more than 7 days in adults should be investigated by a physician as it can be a symptom of more serious intestinal disease, especially if there is also blood in the stool.

A Recap

Overall, typical medical disorders of the GI tract arise from differences in anatomical features and lifestyle habits among individuals. Because of the importance of various nutrition and lifestyle habits, such as adequate dietary fiber and fluid intake, as well as not smoking or abusing NSAID medications, nutrition and lifestyle therapy is often effective in helping treat GI tract disorders.

chapter 4

Carbohydrates

Chapter Outline

What did you eat to obtain the energy you are using right now? Chapters 4, 5, and 6 will examine this question by focusing on the main nutrients the human body uses for fuel. These energy-yielding nutrients are carbohydrates (on average, 4 kcal per gram) and fats and oils (on average, 9 kcal per gram). Little of the other common fuel—protein (on average, 4 kcal per gram) is used for that purpose by the body. Most people know that potatoes have carbohydrates and steak has fat and protein, but few people know what those terms signify.

It is likely that you have recently consumed fruits, vegetables, dairy products, cereal, breads, and pasta. All of these foods supply carbohydrates. Unfortunately, the benefits of these foods are often misunderstood. Many people think carbohydrate-rich foods are fattening—they are not. Pound for pound, carbohydrates are much less fattening than fats and oils. Furthermore, carbohydrates, especially fiber-rich foods such as fruits, vegetables, whole grains, and legumes, have been promoted by many experts for the important health benefits these foods supply. Some people think sugars cause diabetes or hyperactivity—not so, according to well-designed scientific investigations. Almost all carbohydrate-rich foods, except pure sugars, provide essential nutrients and should constitute 50 to 60% of our daily energy intake. Let's take a closer look at carbohydrates.

Check out the **Contemporary Nutrition: Issues and Insights Online Learning Center** www.mhhe.com/wardlawcont5 *for quizzes, flash cards, other activities, and web links designed to further help you learn about carbohydrates.*

Chapter Objectives

Chapter 4 is designed to allow you to:

1. Identify the basic structures and food sources of the major carbohydrates—monosaccharides, disaccharides, polysaccharides (e.g., starches), and dietary fiber.

2. Describe food sources of carbohydrate and list some alternate sweeteners.

3. List the functions of carbohydrate in the body and the problems that result from not eating enough carbohydrate.

4. Describe the regulation of blood glucose and the nutrients that can become blood glucose.

5. Outline the effects of dietary fiber on the body.

6. List guidelines for carbohydrate intake.

7. Identify the consequences of lactose maldigestion and diabetes, and explain appropriate dietary measures to take to reduce these health problems.

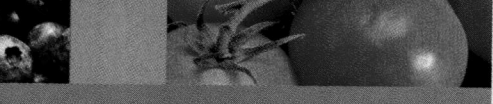

Refresh Your Memory

As you begin your study of carbohydrates in Chapter 4, you may want to review:

- The concept of energy density in Chapter 2
- The processes of digestion and absorption in Chapter 3
- The hormones that regulate blood glucose in Chapter 3

Real Life Scenario

Myeshia is a 19-year-old African-American female who recently read about the health benefits of calcium and decided to increase her intake of dairy products. To start, she drank 2 cups of 1% milk at lunch. Not long afterward, she experienced bloating, cramping, and increased gas production. She suspected that the culprit of this source of pain was the milk she consumed, especially since her parents and her sister complain of the same problem. As well, the problem first appeared when she added the 2 servings of milk. She wanted to determine if other milk products were, in fact, the cause of her gastrointestinal discomfort, so the next day she again ate 2 servings of milk products, but this time a cup of yogurt and a glass of milk, for lunch. Subsequently, she did not have any pain. What has Myeshia discovered? What component of milk is the likely culprit?

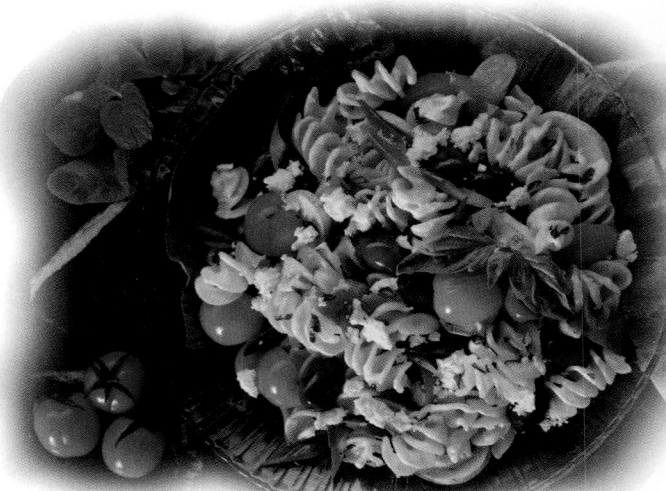

Nutrition Connection

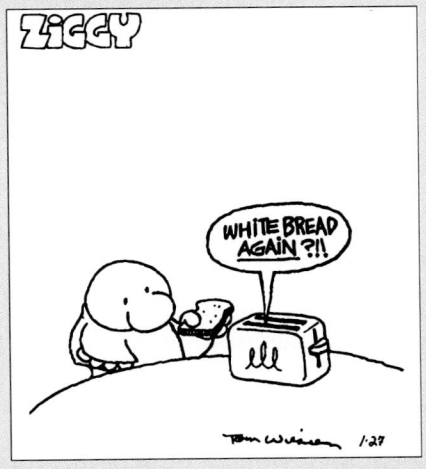

The class of carbohydrate that has gained the most attention recently is dietary fiber. Why is this so? Which health problems typically result from a limited intake of dietary fiber? Which health problems can be prevented by an adequate intake? How much dietary fiber is enough? Too much? This chapter provides some answers.

Carbohydrates—An Introduction

Carbohydrates are a primary fuel source for some cells, such as those in the nervous system and red blood cells. Muscles also rely on a dependable supply of carbohydrate in order to support intense physical activity. Yielding on average 4 kcal per gram, carbohydrates are a readily available fuel for all cells, both in the form of blood glucose and that stored in the liver and muscles as **glycogen.** The glycogen stored in the liver can even be used to maintain blood glucose availability in times when the diet does not supply enough carbohydrate. Regular intake of carbohydrate is important, because liver glycogen stores are exhausted in about 18 hours if no carbohydrate is consumed. After that point, the body is forced to produce its own carbohydrate from body and food protein; this eventually leads to health problems.

North Americans obtain about 50% of their energy intake from carbohydrate; this percentage is higher in the developing world. We humans have sensors on our tongues that recognize sweet carbohydrates. Researchers surmise that this sweetness indicated a safe energy source to early humans, and so it became an important energy source. The returning Crusaders brought **sugar** from the Holy Land to Europe. Columbus introduced sugarcane to the Americas. The French later exploited sugar beets as a source of sugar.

Primarily choosing the healthiest carbohydrate sources, while moderating intake of those that are less healthful, contributes to a well-planned diet. It is difficult to eat so little carbohydrate that body needs are not met, but it is easy to overconsume the carbohydrates that can contribute to health problems. Let's explore this concept further as we look at carbohydrates in detail.

glycogen A carbohydrate made of multiple units of glucose with a highly branched structure; sometimes known as *animal starch.* It is the storage form of glucose in humans and is synthesized (and stored) in the liver and muscles.

sugar A simple carbohydrate with the chemical composition $(CH_2O)_n$. Most sugars form a ringed structure when in solution. The primary sugar in the diet is sucrose, which is made up of glucose and fructose.

Forms of Simple Carbohydrates

Green plants create the carbohydrates in our foods. Leaves capture the sun's solar energy in their cells and transform it to chemical energy. This energy is then used to produce the carbohydrate glucose from carbon dioxide and water. This complex process is called **photosynthesis.**

photosynthesis Process by which plants use solar energy from the sun to synthesize energy-yielding compounds, such as glucose.

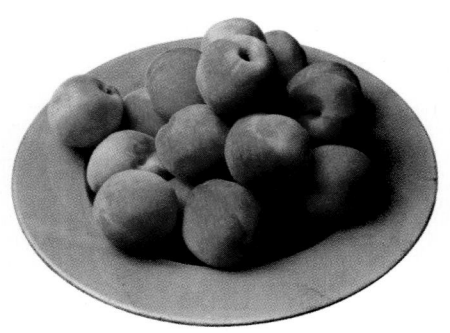

Fruits such as peaches are an excellent source of carbohydrate for a diet.

glucose A six-carbon monosaccharide that forms a six-membered ring with oxygen in the ring; found as such in blood, and in table sugar bonded to fructose; also known as *dextrose*.

sucrose Fructose bonded to another sugar glucose; table sugar.

fructose A monosaccharide with six carbons that form a five-membered or six-membered ring with oxygen in the ring; found in fruits and honey.

$$6 \text{ carbon dioxide} + 6 \text{ water} \rightarrow \text{glucose} + 6 \text{ oxygen}$$
$$(CO_2) \qquad (H_2O) \quad (C_6H_{12}O_6) \quad (O_2)$$

Translated into English, this reads: 6 molecules of carbon dioxide combine with 6 molecules of water to form one molecule of **glucose.** Trapping the solar energy from the sun and converting this into chemical bonds in the sugar is a key part of the process. Six molecules of oxygen are then released into the air.

As the name suggests, most carbohydrate molecules are composed of carbon, hydrogen, and oxygen atoms. Simple forms of carbohydrates are called *sugars.* Larger, more complex forms are primarily called either *starches* or *dietary fibers,* depending on their digestibility by human GI tract enzymes. Starches are the digestible form.

■ Monosaccharides—Glucose, Fructose, and Galactose

Monosaccharides are the simple sugar forms (*mono* means one) that serve as the basic unit of all sugar structures. The most common monosaccharides in foods are glucose, fructose, and galactose (Fig. 4.1).

Glucose is the major monosaccharide found in the body. Glucose is also known as *dextrose,* and glucose in the bloodstream may be called blood sugar. Glucose is a primary source of energy for human cells, although foods contain little of this single sugar form. Most glucose comes from starches and **sucrose** (common table sugar). The latter is made up of the monosaccharides glucose and fructose. For the most part, sugars and other carbohydrates in foods are eventually converted to glucose in the liver. This glucose then goes on to serve as a source of cellular energy.

Fructose, also called *fruit sugar,* is another common sugar. After it is consumed, fructose is absorbed by the small intestine and then transported to the liver, where it is quickly metabolized. Much is converted to glucose, and the rest goes on to form other compounds, such as fat, if fructose is consumed in high amounts. Most of the fructose as such in our diets comes from the use of **high-fructose corn syrup** in food production (see the later discussion on nutritive sweeteners). Fructose also is found in fruits, and forms half of sucrose, as previously noted.

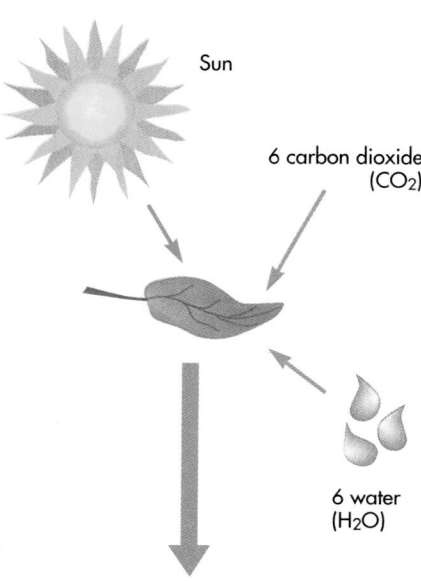

A summary of photosynthesis. Glucose is stored in the leaf, but can also undergo further metabolism.

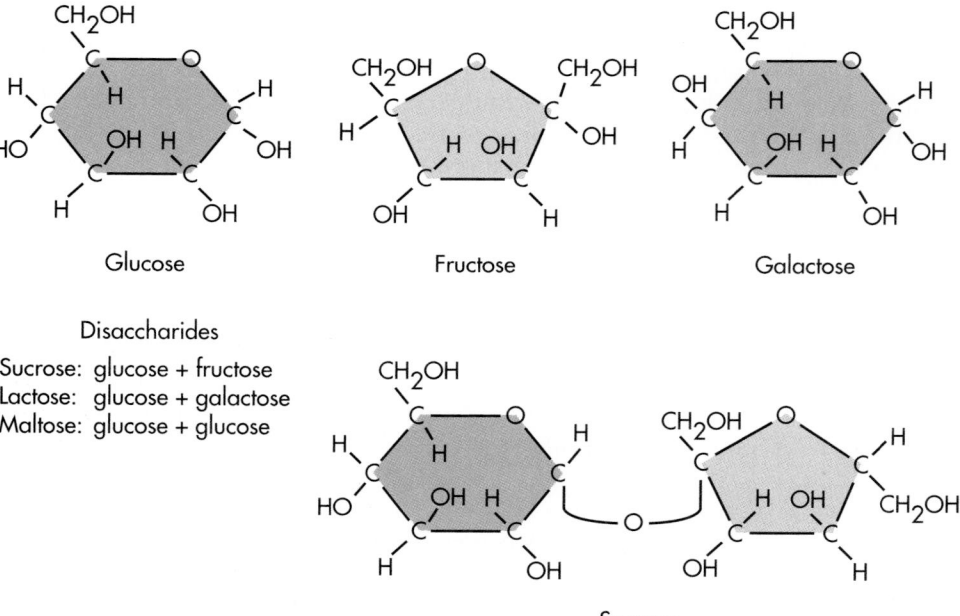

Figure 4.1 Some common sugars. Sucrose and fructose are the most common sugars in our diets.

The sugar **galactose** has nearly the same structure as glucose. Large quantities of pure galactose do not exist in nature. Instead, galactose is usually found bonded to glucose in **lactose,** a sugar found in milk and other milk products. After it is absorbed, galactose arrives in the liver. There it is either transformed into glucose per se or further metabolized into glycogen.

galactose A six-carbon monosaccharide that forms a six-membered ring with oxygen in the ring; closely related to glucose.

lactose Glucose bonded to another sugar galactose.

Another Bite

Now is a good time to begin emphasizing a key concept in nutrition: the difference between *intake* of a substance and the body's *use* of that substance. The body often does not use all nutrients in their original states. Some of these substances are broken down and later reassembled into the same or a different substance when and where necessary. For example, much of the galactose in the diet is metabolized to glucose. When later required, as in the mammary gland of a lactating female, galactose is resynthesized.

■ Disaccharides—Sucrose, Lactose, and Maltose

Disaccharides are formed when two monosaccharides combine (*di* means two). The most common disaccharides in food are sucrose, lactose, and **maltose.**

Sucrose forms when the two sugars glucose and fructose bond together. Sucrose is found in sugarcane, sugar beets, honey, and maple sugar. These products are processed to varying degrees to make brown, white, and powdered sugars. Animals do not produce sucrose, or typically much of any carbohydrate for that matter (glycogen is an exception).

Lactose forms when glucose bonds with galactose. Again, our major food source for lactose is milk products. A later section on lactose maldigestion and lactose intolerance discusses the problems that result when a person can't readily digest lactose.

Maltose forms when two glucose molecules bond together. Maltose is of nutritional interest primarily because of its role in alcohol production in the beer and liquor industry. In the production of alcoholic beverages, starches in various cereal grains are first converted to simpler carbohydrates by enzymes present in the grains. The end products of this step—maltose, glucose, and other sugars—are then mixed with yeast cells in the absence of oxygen. The yeast cells convert most of the sugars to alcohol (ethanol) and carbon dioxide, a process called **fermentation.** Little maltose remains in the final product. Few other food products and beverages contain maltose. In fact, most maltose that we ultimately digest in the small intestine is produced during the digestion of starch.

Monosaccharides and disaccharides are often referred to as *simple sugars* because they contain few sugar units. Food labels lump all of these sugars under one category, listing them as "sugars."

Simple	**Monosaccharides**
↓	*Glucose, fructose, galactose*
	Disaccharides
	Sucrose, lactose, maltose
	Polysaccharides
	Starches (amylose and amylopectin), glycogen
Complex	*Most dietary fibers*

maltose Glucose bonded to glucose.

fermentation The conversion of carbohydrates to alcohols, acids, and carbon dioxide without the use of oxygen.

Forms of the More Complex Carbohydrates

The scientific name for the large, complex carbohydrates is polysaccharides. They are often referred to as complex carbohydrates. Polysaccharides are very long carbohydrate chains composed of many monosaccharide units, mainly glucose (*poly* means many). Some polysaccharides have 3000 or more glucose units, and are found primarily in grains, vegetables, and fruits. When food labels on breakfast cereals list "Other Carbohydrates," this primarily refers to starch content.

Amylose, a long, straight chain of glucoses, forms about 20% of the starch found in vegetables, beans, breads, pasta, and rice. **Amylopectin** makes up the rest of food starch. It has many branches off its glucose backbone. These starches function as a carbohydrate storage form in plants (Fig. 4.2).

Amylopectin raises blood glucose much more readily than does amylose, since its numerous branches provide many areas for digestive enzyme activity. The enzymes

amylose A digestible straight-chain type of starch composed of glucose units.

amylopectin A digestible branched-chain type of starch composed of glucose units.

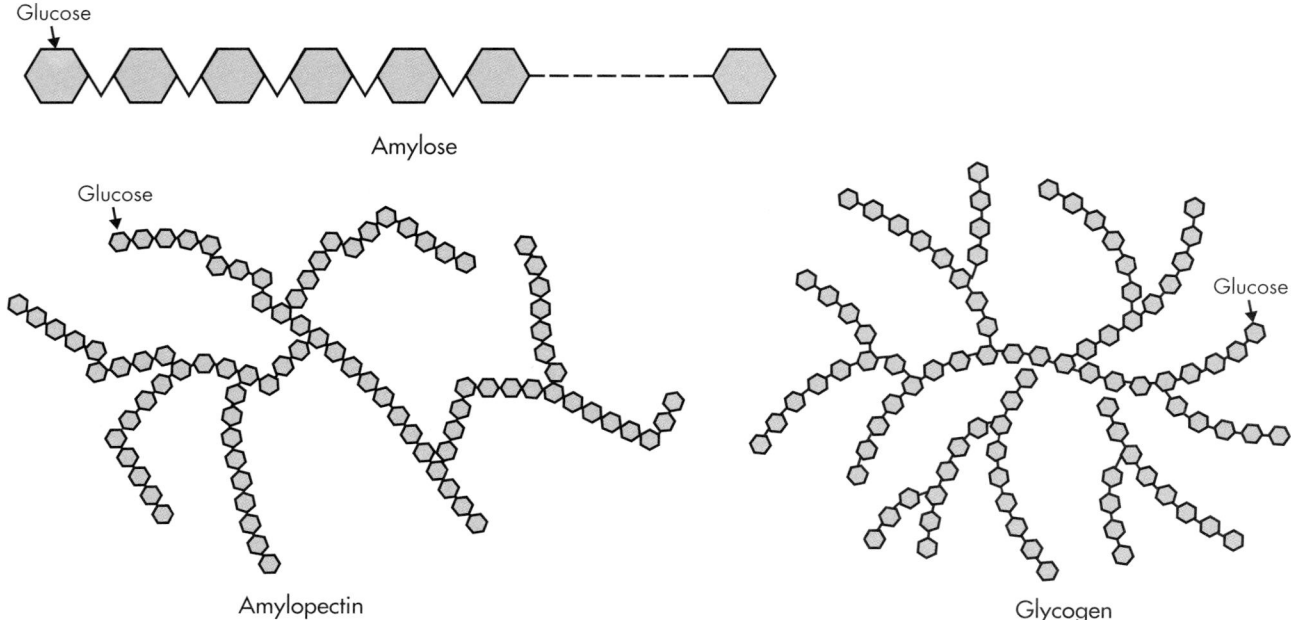

Glucose

Amylose

Glucose

Glucose

Amylopectin

Glycogen

Figure 4.2 Some common starches. We consume essentially no glycogen. All glycogen found in the body is made by our cells, primarily in the liver and muscles.

Dietary fiber is an indigestible form of polysaccharide. This means that dietary fiber passes through the small intestine without being digested. Detailed information about the forms, recommendations, and benefits of dietary fiber can be found in the Nutrition Insight in this chapter.

that break down starches to glucose and other related sugars act only at the end of the glucose chains. The more numerous the branches of this starch provide more sites (ends) for enzyme action (see the discussion of glycemic index in a later section of this chapter). As noted before, glycogen (animal starch) is made by humans and is a storage form for glucose. Like amylopectin, this polysaccharide consists of a chain of glucoses with many branches, but even more branches than present in amylopectin. The numerous branches of glycogen also provide many sites (ends) for enzyme action. Glycogen is thus an ideal form for carbohydrate storage in the body because it can be quickly broken down.

The liver and muscles are the major storage sites for glycogen. Because only about 120 kcal of glucose are available as such in body fluids, these storage sites for carbohydrate energy—amounting to about 1800 kcal—are extremely important. As noted in the introduction, the 400 kcal of liver glycogen can be turned into blood glucose, but the 1400 kcal of muscle glycogen cannot. Still, glycogen in muscles can supply glucose for muscle use, especially during high-intensity and endurance exercise. (See Chapter 11 for a detailed discussion of carbohydrate use in exercise.)

Although animals contain carbohydrate in the form of glycogen, meat, fish, and poultry are not good sources of this (or any other) carbohydrate. This is because glycogen stores quickly degrade after death of the animal.

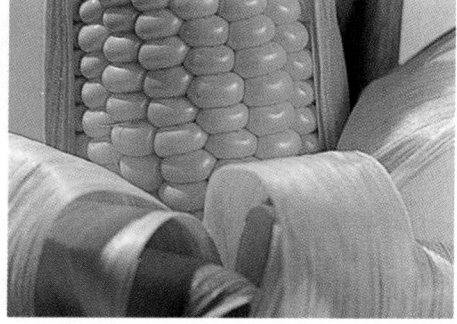

As plants mature, some sugars are turned into starch.

Concept Check

*I*mportant monosaccharides in nutrition are glucose, fructose, and galactose. Glucose is a primary energy source for body cells. Disaccharides form when two monosaccharides bond together. Important disaccharides in nutrition are the table sugar sucrose (glucose bonded to fructose), maltose (glucose bonded to glucose), and the milk sugar lactose (glucose bonded to galactose). Once digested into monosaccharide forms and absorbed, most carbohydrates are transformed into glucose by the liver.

The major digestible polysaccharides—the starches amylose and amylopectin— contain multiple glucose units bonded together. Glycogen is animal starch and acts as a storage form of glucose in the liver and muscles.

Dietary Fiber: An Often Underappreciated Class of Carbohydrates

Dietary fibers as a class are mostly made up of polysaccharides, but they differ from starches insofar as the chemical links that join individual sugar units cannot be digested by human enzymes in the GI tract. This prevents the small intestine from absorbing the sugars that make up dietary fibers. Dietary fiber is not a single substance, but a group of substances with similar characteristics (Table 4.1). The group comprises the carbohydrates **cellulose, hemicelluloses, pectins, gums,** and **mucilages,** as well as the noncarbohydrate **lignin.** In total, these constitute all the nonstarch polysaccharides in foods. Note that Nutrition Facts labels do not list these individual forms of dietary fiber.

Cellulose, hemicelluloses, and lignin form the structural parts of plants. A cotton ball is pure cellulose. Bran fiber is rich in hemicelluloses. The woody fibers in broccoli are partly lignin. Bran layers form the outer covering of all grains, so **whole grains** (i.e., unrefined) are good sources of this dietary fiber (Fig. 4.3). Because the majority of these compounds neither readily dissolve in water nor are readily metabolized by intestinal bacteria, they are called *insoluble fibers.*

Pectins, gums, and mucilages are contained around and inside plant cells. These compounds either dissolve or swell when put into water and are therefore called *soluble fibers.* They also are readily fermented by bacteria in the large intestine. These exist as gum arabic, guar gum, locust bean gum, and various pectin forms and are found in several foods, especially in salad dressings, some frozen desserts, jams, and jellies. Some forms of hemicelluloses also fall into the soluble category.

Most foods contain mixtures of soluble and insoluble fibers, but food labels do not generally distinguish between the two types. Still, manufacturers have the option to do so. Similarly, if food is listed as a good source of one type of fiber, it usually contains some of the other type of dietary fiber as well.

Dietary Fiber Provides Health Benefits

Many types of dietary fiber absorb water and hold onto it in the intestine. When enough fiber is consumed, its water-retaining property helps enlarge and soften the stool, easing elimination. Basically the larger stool size stimulates the intestinal muscles that promote peristalsis (see Chapter 3). Consequently, less pressure is needed to expel the stool.

When too little dietary fiber is eaten, the opposite can occur: the stool may be small and hard. Constipation may result, requiring strong pressures to move the stool in the large intestine during elimination. **Hemorrhoids** may then result from excessive straining. Also, the high pressures can force parts of the large intestine wall to pop out from between the surrounding bands of muscle. This forms small pouches, called **diverticula,** leading to a condition called **diverticulosis.** About 50% of older people have many of these pouches (Fig. 4.4). Diverticula rarely occur in people in developing countries, probably because of their high dietary fiber intakes. In contrast, people in Western countries often ingest much less dietary fiber in their diets.

Adequate dietary fiber promotes cardiovascular health. Soluble fibers taken in high amounts in the diet can decrease blood cholesterol. The effect is partly caused by inhibiting bile recycling in the intestinal tract. Bile, which is formed from cholesterol, is then combined with the feces for elimination. Additional mechanisms for the blood-cholesterol lowering effect may be at work as well. Other rich sources of soluble fibers include fruits and vegetables in general, soybean fiber, rice bran, and **psyllium** seeds (found in many commercial fiber laxatives).

A recent study showed that men who ate more than 25 grams of dietary fiber per

Critical Thinking

Your grandfather has diverticulosis. At a holiday party, he insists on eating popcorn and nuts even though you tell him that doing so is not good for his condition. He ignores your warning and 2 days later tells you that he has abdominal cramps and a fever. How would you explain his symptoms?

Table 4.1 Classification of Dietary Fibers

Type	Component(s)	Examples	Physiological Effects	Major Food Sources
Insoluble				
Noncarbohydrate	Lignin	Wheat bran	Increases fecal bulk; estrogen-like effects	Whole grains, flax seeds
Carbohydrate	Cellulose Hemicelluloses	Wheat products Brown rice	Increases fecal bulk Decreases intestinal transit time	All plants Wheat, rye, rice, vegetables
Soluble				
Carbohydrate	Pectins, gums, mucilages, some hemi-celluloses	Apples Bananas Oranges Carrots Barley Oats Kidney beans	Delays gastric emptying; slows glucose absorption; can lower blood cholesterol	Citrus fruits, oat products, beans, thickeners added to foods

continued

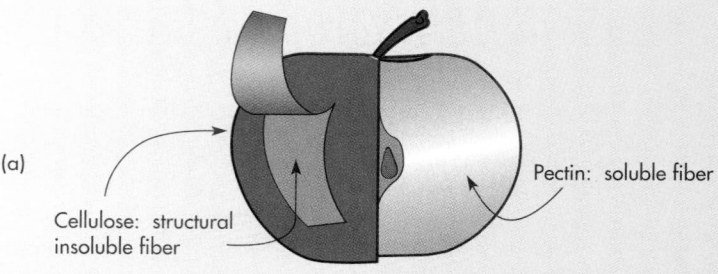

(a)

Cellulose: structural
insoluble fiber

Pectin: soluble fiber

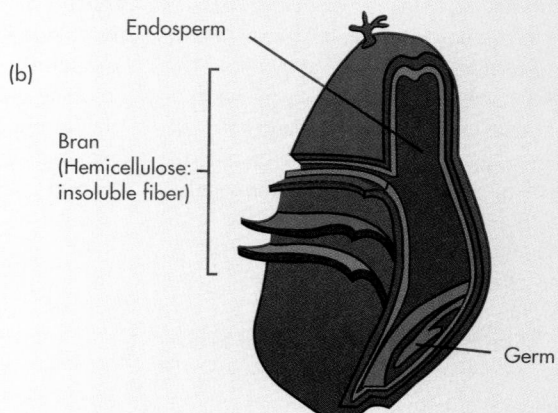

(b)

Endosperm

Bran
(Hemicellulose:
insoluble fiber)

Germ

Figure 4.3 Soluble and insoluble fiber. (a) The skin of an apple consists of the insoluble fiber cellulose, which provides structure for the fruit. The soluble fiber pectin "glues" the fruit cells together. (b) The outside layer of a wheat kernel is made of layers of bran—primarily hemicellulose, an insoluble fiber—making this whole grain a good source of fiber. Overall, fruits, vegetables, whole grains, and legumes are rich in dietary fiber.

day had a 36% lower risk of developing cardiovascular disease, and those eating 29 grams of dietary fiber per day decreased their risk by 41%. For this reason, experts recommend a 10 gram per day increase in dietary fiber above the typical 14 to 15 gram per day intake of the average North American, especially from grain sources, to prevent cardiovascular disease. A large study of women with a high intake of whole grains (about 3 servings per day) showed a 30% decreased risk for cardiovascular disease, compared with a low intake of whole grains (less than 1 serving per day). Overall, a dietary fiber-rich diet containing fruits, vegetables, beans, and whole grains (including whole-grain breakfast cereals) is advocated as part of a strategy to reduce risk for many forms of cardiovascular disease. Recall from Chapter 2 that FDA has approved the following claim: "Diets rich in whole-grain foods and other plant foods and low in total fat may decrease the risk for cardiovascular (heart) disease."

A diet high in dietary fiber may also aid weight control and reduces the risk of developing obesity. As noted in Chapter 2, the bulky nature of high-fiber foods fills us up without yielding much energy. High-fat foods tend to do just the opposite, contributing to obesity. Increasing intake of foods rich in dietary fiber is one strategy for remaining satisfied after a meal even if the fat content in a diet is low.

Finally, when consumed in large amounts, soluble fiber slows glucose absorption from the small intestine. This effect can be helpful in treatment of diabetes. In fact, women whose main carbohydrate source is low-fiber foods are 2.5 times more likely to develop diabetes than those who have high-fiber diets (see the Nutrition Issue at the end of this chapter). As well, another recent study found that 50 grams of dietary fiber per day improved blood glucose regulation in type 2 diabetes.

Can Dietary Fiber Play Other Roles in Preserving Health?

Over the past 30 years, many population studies have shown a link between increased dietary fiber intake and a decrease in colon cancer development. However, recent clinical trials have questioned the relationship between intake of dietary fiber and colon cancer development. Currently, most of the research on colon cancer focuses on the potential preventive effects of vegetable intake; regular physical activity; the use of aspirin and related pain medications; and adequate folate, selenium, and calcium intakes. Smoking, obesity in men, saturated fat, and red meat intake are under study as potential causative factors. Overall, the health benefits to the colon that stem from a high-fiber diet are probably due mostly to the nutrients that are commonly part of high-fiber foods, such as vitamins, minerals, phytochemicals, antioxidants, and essential fatty acids. Thus, it is more advisable to increase dietary fiber intake using fiber-rich foods, rather than mostly relying on fiber supplements.

Table 4.5 (later in the chapter) allows you to estimate your typical dietary fiber intake. How much dietary fiber do you eat each day?

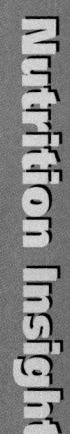
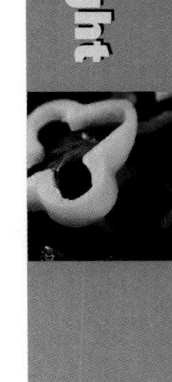

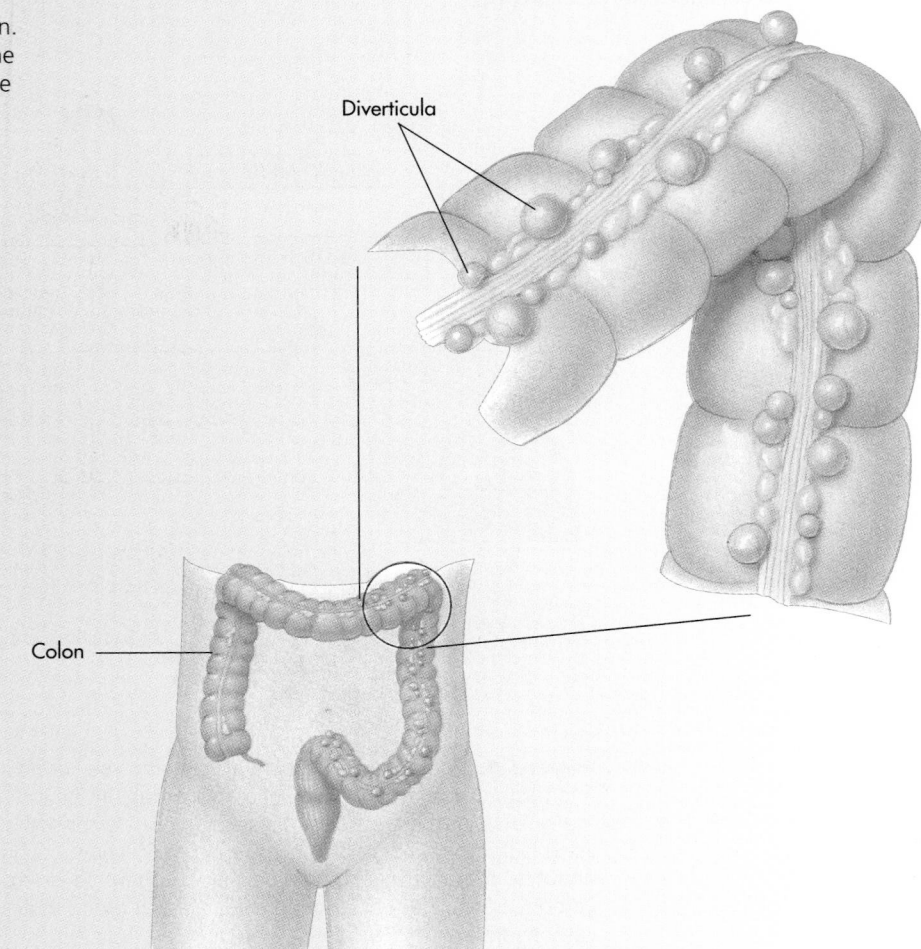

Figure 4.4 Diverticula in the colon. A diet low in dietary fiber increases the risk for their development. The disease is commonly seen in older people in Western societies.

Diverticula

Colon

Carbohydrates in Foods

The foods that yield the highest percentage of energy from carbohydrates are table sugar, honey, jam, jelly, fruit, and plain baked potatoes. These foods are rich sources of carbohydrate; carbohydrates deliver much of their food energy. Corn flakes, rice, bread, and noodles all contain at least 75% of energy as carbohydrates. Foods with moderate amounts of carbohydrate energy are peas, broccoli, oatmeal, dry beans and other legumes, cream pies, French fries, and skim milk. In these foods, the carbohydrate content is diluted either by protein, as in the case of skim milk, or by fat, as in the case of a cream pie. Foods with essentially no carbohydrates include beef, eggs, chicken, fish, vegetable oils, butter, and margarine.

Figure 4.5 shows that, in planning a high-carbohydrate diet, you need to emphasize grains, pasta, fruits, and vegetables. On the other hand, you can't create a diet high in carbohydrate energy from chocolate, potato chips, and French fries because these foods contain too much fat. The percentage of energy from carbohydrate is more important than the total amount of carbohydrate in a food when planning a high-carbohydrate diet. Currently, the top five carbohydrate sources for U.S. adults are white bread, soft drinks, cookies and cakes (including doughnuts), sugars/syrups/jams, and potatoes. Clearly many North Americans (teenagers included) should take a closer look at their main carbohydrate sources and strive to improve them from a nutritional standpoint.

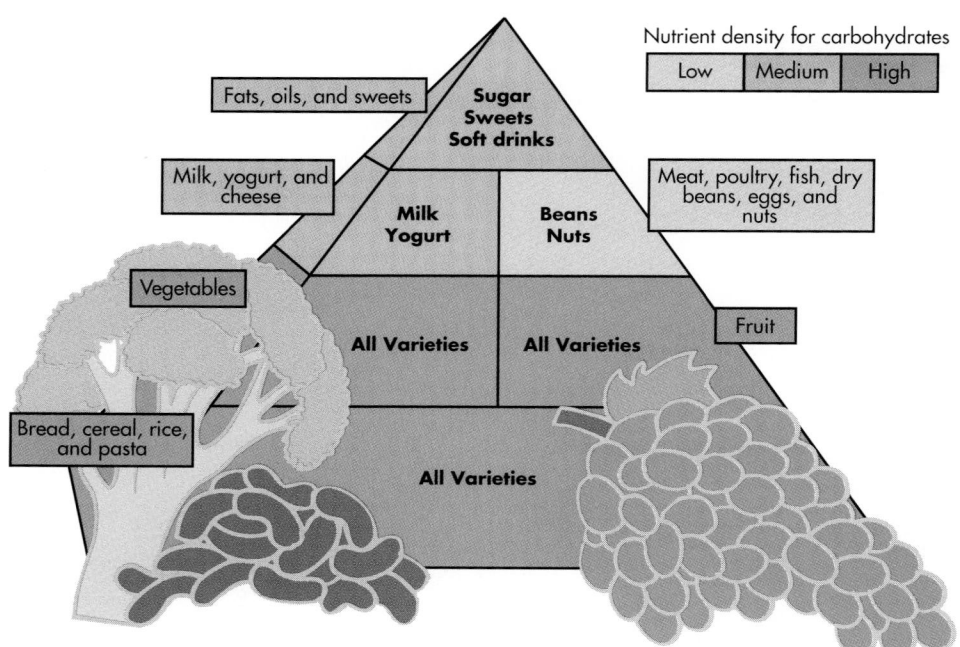

Figure 4.5 Sources of carbohydrates from the Food Guide Pyramid. The bread, cereal, rice, and pasta group, fruit group, vegetable group, and milk, yogurt, and cheese group contain many foods that are nutrient dense sources of carbohydrate. Based on serving sizes for the Food Guide Pyramid, milk and yogurt contain about 12 grams, beans about 40 grams, nuts about 20 grams, fruits and grain products about 15 grams, and vegetables about 5 grams of carbohydrates. The background color of each group indicates the average nutrient density for carbohydrate in that group.

■ A Closer Look at Sweeteners

The various substances that impart sweetness to foods fall into two broad classes: nutritive sweeteners, which can yield energy for the body; and alternative sweeteners, which, for the most part provide no food energy. As shown in Table 4.2, the alternative sweeteners are much sweeter on a per-gram basis than the nutritive sweeteners.

Nutritive Sweeteners

Both sugars and sugar alcohols provide energy along with sweetness. Sugars are found in many different food products, whereas sugar alcohols have rather limited uses.

Sugars All of the monosaccharides (glucose, fructose, and galactose) and disaccharides (sucrose, lactose, and maltose) discussed earlier are designated *nutritive sweeteners* (Table 4.3). The taste and sweetness of sucrose make it the benchmark against which all other sweeteners are measured. Consumption of table sugar (sucrose) in the United States currently ranges from 12 to 48 pounds per year for each person.

High-fructose corn syrup, which is 40% to 90% fructose, is used extensively today. High-fructose corn syrup is made by treating cornstarch with acid and enzymes. This treatment breaks down much of the starch into glucose. Then some of the glucose is converted by enzymes into fructose. The final syrup is usually as sweet as sucrose. Its major advantage is that it is cheaper than sucrose. Also, it doesn't form crystals and it has better freezing properties. High-fructose corn syrups are used in soft drinks, candies, jam, jelly, other fruit products, and desserts (e.g., packaged cookies).

In addition to sucrose and high-fructose corn syrup, brown sugar, turbinado sugar, honey, maple syrup, and other sugars are also added to foods. Turbinado sugar, a

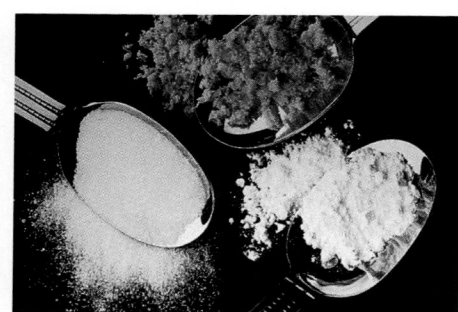

There are many forms of sugar on the market. Used in many foods, together they contribute to our daily intake of approximately 82 grams (16 teaspoons) of sugars in our diets.

Table 4.2 The Sweetness of Sugars and Alternative Sweeteners

Type of Sweetener	Relative Sweetness* (Sucrose = 1)	Typical Sources
Sugars		
Lactose	0.2	Dairy products
Maltose	0.4	Sprouted seeds
Glucose	0.7	Corn syrup
Sucrose	1.0	Table sugar, most sweets
Invert sugar†	1.3	Some candies, honey
Fructose	1.2–1.8	Fruit, honey, some soft drinks
Sugar Alcohols		
Sorbitol	0.6	Dietetic candies, sugarless gum
Mannitol	0.7	Dietetic candies
Xylitol	0.9	Sugarless gum
Alternative Sweeteners		
Cyclamate	30	Not currently in use in the United States but available in Canada
Aspartame	180	Diet soft drinks, diet fruit drinks, sugarless gum, powdered diet sweetener
Acesulfame-K	200	Sugarless gum, diet drink mixes, powdered diet sweeteners, puddings, gelatin desserts
Saccharin (sodium salt)	300	Diet soft drinks
Sucralose	600	Diet soft drinks, tabletop use, sugarless gums, jams, frozen desserts

*On a per gram basis
†Sucrose broken down into glucose and fructose
From the American Dietetic Association, 1993, and other sources.

INGREDIENTS: SORBITOL, GUM BASE, MANNITOL, GLYCEROL, HYDROGENATED GLUCOSE SYRUP, XYLITOL, ARTIFICIAL AND NATURAL FLAVORS, ASPARTAME, RED 40, YELLOW 6 AND BHT (TO MAINTAIN FRESHNESS). PHENYLKETONURICS: CONTAINS PHENYLALANINE. *NUTRASWEET IS A REGISTERED TRADEMARK OF THE NUTRASWEET CO.

Sugarless Gum

Sugar alcohols can be found in sugarless gum. Note that aspartame is also used to sweeten this product.

Table 4.3 Names of Sugars Used in Foods

Sugar	Invert sugar	Honey	Maple syrup
Sucrose	Glucose	Corn syrup or sweeteners	Dextrin
Brown sugar	Sorbitol	High-fructose corn syrup	Dextrose
Confectioner's sugar (powdered sugar)	Levulose		Fructose
	Polydextrose	Molasses	Maltose
Turbinado sugar	Lactose	Date sugar	Caramel
	Mannitol		Fruit sugar

partially refined version of raw sucrose, has a slight molasses flavor. Brown sugar is essentially sucrose containing some molasses; either the molasses is not totally removed from the sucrose during processing or it is added to the sucrose crystals.

Maple syrup is made by boiling down and concentrating the sap that runs during the late winter in sugar maple trees. Most pancake syrup sold in supermarkets is not pure maple syrup, which is quite expensive. Instead, it is primarily corn syrup and high-fructose corn syrup.

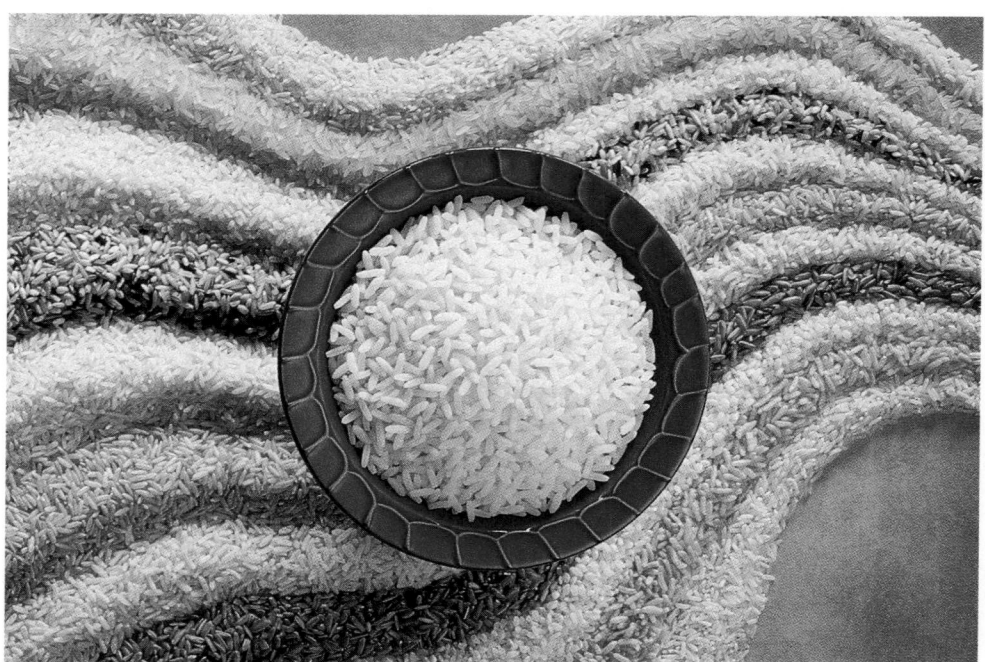

Rice is a rich source of carbohydrates.

Honey is a product of plant nectar that has been altered by bee enzymes. The enzymes break down much of the nectar's sucrose into fructose and glucose. Honey offers essentially the same nutritional value as other simple sugars—a source of energy and little else. However, honey is not safe to feed to infants because it can contain spores of the bacterium *Clostridium botulinum*. These spores can become the bacteria that cause fatal foodborne illness. Honey does not pose the same threat to adults because the acidic environment of an adult's stomach inhibits the growth of the bacteria. An infant's stomach, however, does not produce much acid, making infants susceptible to the threat that this bacterium poses (see Chapters 14 and 16).

sorbitol An alcohol derivative of glucose.

xylitol An alcohol derivative of a five-carbon monosaccharide called xylose.

Sugar Alcohols   Sugar alcohols such as **sorbitol** and **xylitol** are also used as nutritive sweeteners. Although sugar alcohols contribute energy (about 1.5 to 3 kcal per gram), they are absorbed and metabolized to glucose more slowly than are simple sugars. Still, in large quantities, these substances do not provide a significant advantage for people with diabetes because such amounts can cause diarrhea, and they are usually found primarily in diabetic candy and gum. In fact, any products whose foreseeable consumption may result in a daily ingestion of 50 grams of sorbitol or mannitol must bear this labeling statement: "Excess consumption may have a laxative effect."

Sugar alcohols must be listed on labels, and if only one sugar alcohol is used in a product, it must be distinguished; however, if two or more are used in one product, they are grouped together under the heading "sugar alcohols." The actual caloric value is calculated, taking in account each sugar alcohol, so that when one reads the total amount of calories a product provides, it includes the sugar alcohols in the overall amount.

dental caries Erosions in the surface of a tooth caused by acids made by bacteria as they metabolize sugars.

Sorbitol and xylitol are used in sugarless gum, breath mints, and candy. These are not readily metabolized by bacteria in the mouth and thus do not promote **dental caries** nearly so readily as do simple sugars such as sucrose (see the later section on problems linked to carbohydrate intake). Recall from Chapter 2 that such a health claim can be made on these products.

Alternative Sweeteners

Often called artificial sweeteners, alternative sweeteners include **saccharin,** cyclamate, **aspartame, acesulfame-K,** and **sucralose.** From 1971 to 1991, intake nearly quintupled for low-calorie sweeteners in the United States, from 5 pounds per person to 24 pounds. Alternative sweeteners yield little or no energy when consumed in amounts typically used in food products. Four are currently available in the United States: saccharin, aspartame, acesulfame-K, and sucralose. Cyclamate was banned for use in the United States in 1970, although it has never been conclusively proved to cause health problems when used appropriately. Cyclamate is used in Canada as a sweetener in medicines and as a tabletop sweetener.

Saccharin   The oldest alternative sweetener, saccharin, was first produced in 1879 and is currently approved for use in more than 90 countries. It represents about half of the alternative sweetener market in North America. Saccharin was once thought to pose a risk of bladder cancer based on laboratory animal studies, but it is no longer listed as a potential cause of cancer in humans, due to the failure of population studies to support that assumption.

Aspartame   In 1981, the alternative sweetener aspartame became available. Its trade name is NutraSweet® when added to foods and Equal® when sold as a powder. Aspartame is in widespread use throughout the world. It has been approved for use by more than 90 countries, and its use has been endorsed by the World Health Organization, the American Medical Association, the American Diabetes Association, and the American Academy of Pediatrics Committee on Nutrition.

The components of aspartame are the amino acids phenylalanine and aspartic acid, along with methanol. Recall that amino acids are the building blocks of proteins, so aspartame is more of a protein than a carbohydrate. Aspartame yields about 4 kcal per gram, but it is 180 times sweeter than sucrose. Thus, only a small amount of aspartame is needed to obtain the desired sweetness, so the amount of energy added is insignificant unless the product is abused. Aspartame is used in beverages, gelatin desserts, chewing gum, toppings and fillings in precooked bakery goods, and cookies. Aspartame does not cause tooth decay. Like other proteins, however, aspartame is damaged when heated for a long time and thus cannot be widely used in products requiring cooking.

To date, about 7000 complaints have been filed with FDA by people claiming to have had adverse reactions to aspartame: headaches, dizziness, seizures, nausea, and other side effects. It is important for people who are sensitive to aspartame to avoid it. But the percentage of sensitive people is likely to be extremely small. The relatively limited number of complaints about aspartame, considering its wide use in food products, means that most people can use it.

The acceptable daily intake of aspartame set by FDA is 50 milligrams per kilogram of body weight per day. This is equivalent to about 14 cans of diet soft drink for an adult or about 80 packets of Equal®. Aspartame appears to be safe for pregnant women and children, but some scientists suggest cautious use by these groups, especially young children, who need ample food energy to grow.

Persons with a rare disease called phenylketonuria (PKU), which interferes with the metabolism of phenylalanine, should avoid aspartame because of its high phenylalanine content. (PKU is discussed further in Chapter 6.)

Acesulfame-K   The alternative sweetener acesulfame-K (Sunette; the *K* stands for potassium) was approved by FDA in July 1988. It is approved for use in more than 40 countries and has been in use in Europe since 1983. Acesulfame-K is 200 times sweeter than sucrose. It contributes no energy to the diet because it is not digested by the body, and does not cause dental caries.

Unlike aspartame, acesulfame-K can be used in baking because it does not lose its sweetness when heated. In the United States, it is currently approved for use in chewing gum, powdered drink mixes, gelatins, puddings, baked goods, tabletop

---

saccharin An alternative sweetener that yields no energy to the body; it is 300 times sweeter than sucrose.

aspartame An alternative sweetener made from two amino acids and methanol; it is 200 times sweeter than sucrose.

acesulfame-K An alternative sweetener that yields no energy to the body; it is 200 times sweeter than sucrose.

sucralose An alternative sweetener that has chlorines in place of three hydroxyl (—OH) groups on sucrose. It is 600 times sweeter than sucrose.

CONTAINS: CARBONATED WATER, ORANGE JUICE, CITRIC ACID, NUTRASWEET* BRAND OF ASPARTAME**, POTASSIUM BENZOATE (A PRESERVATIVE), CITRUS PECTIN, POTASSIUM CITRATE, CAFFEINE, MALTODEXTRIN, GUM ARABIC, NATURAL FLAVORS, BROMINATED VEGETABLE OIL, YELLOW #5 AND ERYTHORBIC ACID (TO PROTECT FLAVOR). *NUTRASWEET® AND THE NUTRASWEET SYMBOL ARE REGISTERED TRADEMARKS OF THE NUTRASWEET COMPANY. PHENYLKETONURICS: CONTAINS PHENYLALANINE.

Note the warning for people with PKU that this diet soft drink with aspartame contains phenylalanine.

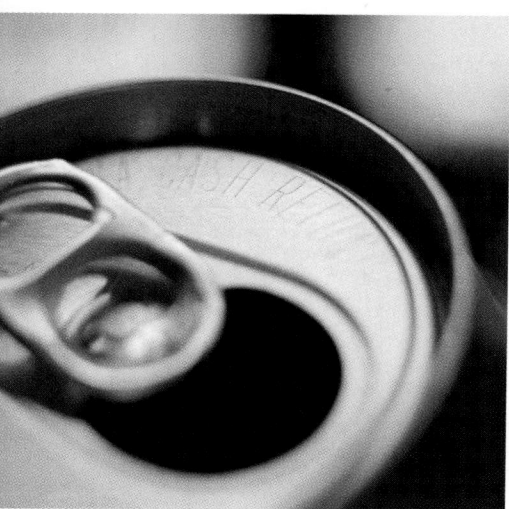

Diet soft drinks take advantage of the alternative sweeteners saccharin, aspartame, and acesulfame-K.

sweeteners, candy, throat lozenges, yogurt, and nondairy creamers; additional uses may soon be approved. One recent trend is to combine it with aspartame in soft drinks.

A product called Diabetisweet® uses a combination of acesulfame-K and Isomalt (a sweetener made of sugar alcohols) to produce a product that completely replaces sugar in baking and cooking. This product allows people with diabetes to decrease sugar intake, but it is very expensive in comparison with sugar.

Sucralose Sucralose (Splenda) is 600 times sweeter than sucrose. It is made by substituting three chlorines for three hydroxyl groups (—OH) on sucrose. FDA approved use of sucralose in 1998 as an additive to foods such as soda, gum, baked goods, syrups, gelatins, frozen dairy desserts such as ice cream, jams, and processed fruits and fruit juices and for tabletop use. Sucralose doesn't break down under high heat conditions and can be used in cooking and baking. It is also excreted as such in the feces. The little that is absorbed is excreted in the urine. Because of such recent introduction, it is not clear whether the public will embrace this product. Canadians had access to sucralose before its U.S. introduction.

Overall, alternative sweeteners enable people with diabetes to enjoy the flavor of sweetness while controlling sugars in their diets; they also provide noncaloric or very-low-calorie sugar substitutes for persons trying to lose (or control) body weight.

Concept Check

Dietary fiber is essentially the portion of ingested food that remains undigested as it enters the large intestine. Dietary fiber components include cellulose, hemicelluloses, lignins, pectins, gums, and mucilages. Dietary fiber forms a vital part of the diet by adding mass to the stool, which eases elimination. It also helps in weight control and reduces the risk of developing obesity and cardiovascular disease. Soluble fibers can also be useful for controlling blood glucose in patients with diabetes and in lowering blood cholesterol. Whole grains, vegetables, beans, and fruits are excellent sources of dietary fiber.

Table sugar, honey, jam, fruit, and plain baked potatoes contain the highest percentage of energy from carbohydrates. Foods such as cream pies, potato chips, whole milk, and oatmeal contain moderate amounts of carbohydrate. Common nutritive sweeteners added to foods include sucrose, maple sugar, honey, brown sugar, and high-fructose corn syrup. For people who want to limit sugar intake, alternative sweeteners are available and include the sugar alcohols, saccharin, aspartame, acesulfame-K, and sucralose. Of these, aspartame is the most common alternative sweetener in use.

Making Carbohydrates Available for Body Use

As discussed in Chapter 3, simply eating a food does not supply nutrients to body cells. Digestion and absorption must occur first.

■ Digestion of Starches and Disaccharides

Food preparation can be viewed as the start of carbohydrate digestion because cooking softens tough connective tissues in the fibrous tissue of plants, such as broccoli stalks. When starches are heated, the starch granules swell as they soak up water, making them much easier to digest. All of these effects of cooking generally make these foods easier to chew, swallow, and break down during digestion.

The enzymatic digestion of starch begins in the mouth, when the saliva, which contains an enzyme called salivary **amylase**, mixes with the starchy products during the chewing of the food. This amylase breaks down starch into many smaller units (e.g., disaccharides, such as maltose) (Fig. 4.6). You can observe this conversion while chewing a saltine cracker. Prolonged chewing of the cracker causes it to taste sweeter

amylase Starch-digesting enzyme from the salivary glands or pancreas.

Figure 4.6 Carbohydrate digestion and absorption. Enzymes made by the mouth, pancreas, and small intestine participate in the process of digestion. Most carbohydrate digestion and absorption take place in the small intestine. Note that Chapter 3 covered the physiology of digestion and absorption in detail.

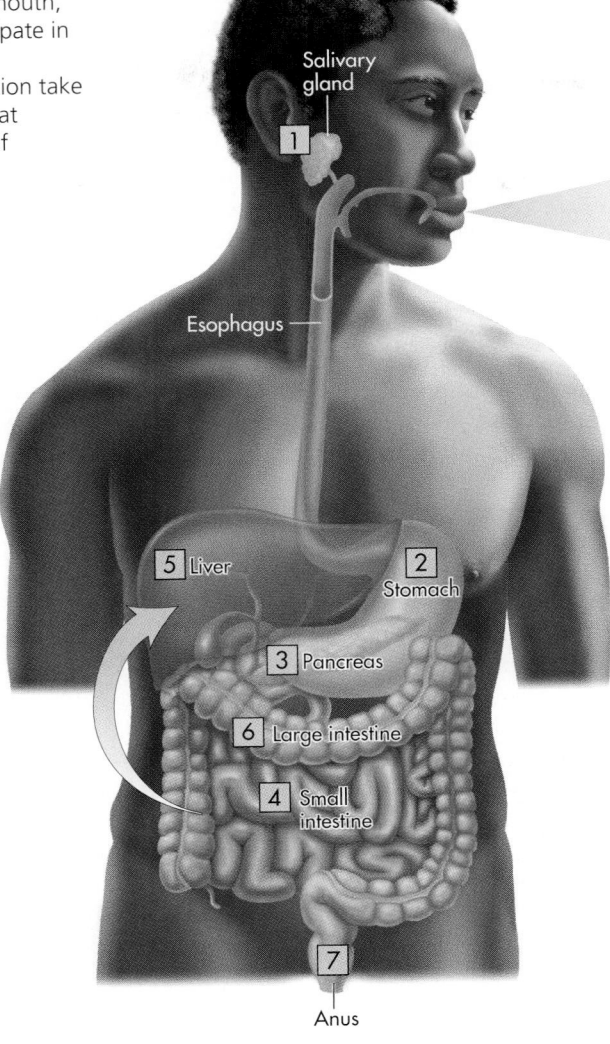

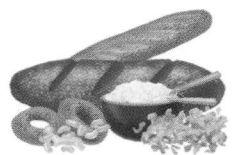

Carbohydrates

1 Some starch is broken down by salivary amylase to maltose

2 Salivary amylase is inactivated by strong acid

3 Enzymes (amylase) from pancreas break down starch into maltose

4 Enzymes in wall of the small intestine break down disaccharides sucrose, lactose, and maltose into monosaccharides glucose, fructose, and galactose

5 Absorption of glucose, fructose, and galactose into blood to be taken to the liver

6 Some soluble fiber is fermented into various acid and gases by bacteria in the large intestine

7 Insoluble fiber is excreted in feces, but little other dietary carbohydrate is present

as some starch breaks down into the sweeter sugars, such as maltose. Still, food is in the mouth for such a short amount of time that this phase of digestion is negligible. In addition, once the food moves down the esophagus and reaches the stomach, the acidic environment inactivates salivary amylase.

After the carbohydrates have reached the small intestine—which has a more alkaline environment and thus is well suited for further carbohydrate digestion—the pancreas releases enzymes, such as pancreatic amylase. This is the last stage of starch digestion. After amylase action, the original carbohydrates in a food are now present in the small intestine as monosaccharides (mostly any glucose and fructose present as such in food), disaccharides (maltose from starch breakdown, lactose mainly from dairy products, and sucrose from food and that added at the table).

The disaccharides are digested to their monosaccharide units once they reach the wall of the small intestine, where the specialized enzymes on the mucosal cells digest each disaccharide into the monosaccharide components. The enzyme **maltase** acts on maltose to produce two glucose molecules. **Sucrase** acts on sucrose to produce glucose and fructose. **Lactase** acts on lactose to produce glucose and galactose.

When considering carbohydrate digestion, you should remember that the key digestive enzymes come from the pancreas and the cells of the intestinal wall. Intestinal

maltase An enzyme made by absorptive cells of the small intestine; this enzyme digests maltose to two glucose molecules.

sucrase An enzyme made by absorptive cells of the small intestine; this enzyme digests sucrose to glucose and fructose molecules.

lactase An enzyme made by absorptive cells of the small intestine; this enzyme digests lactose to glucose and galactose molecules.

diseases can interfere with the efficient digestion of the sugars maltose, lactose, and sucrose. The portion of these carbohydrates that is not fully broken down to single sugars is then not absorbed. When these unabsorbed carbohydrates eventually reach the large intestine, the bacteria there ferment the sugars to produce acids and gases (review Fig. 4.6). If produced in large amounts, these gases can cause abdominal discomfort. People recovering from intestinal disorders, such as diarrhea or bacterial infections, may need to avoid lactose for a few weeks if these symptoms of poor lactose digestion are experienced. Two weeks is sufficient time for the small intestine to resume producing enough lactase enzyme to allow for more complete lactose digestion (see the later section on moderation in lactose intake for more details).

▪ Absorption of Monosaccharides

Single sugars found naturally in foods and those formed as by-products of earlier starch digestion in the mouth and small intestine generally follow an active absorption process. Recall from Chapter 3 that this is a process that requires a specific carrier and energy input in order for the substance to be taken up by the absorptive cells in the small intestine. Glucose and its close relative, galactose, undergo active absorption. They are pumped into the absorptive cells along with sodium.

Another Bite

*F*ructose is taken up by the absorptive cells via facilitated diffusion. In this case, a carrier is used, but no energy input is needed. This absorptive process is slower than that seen with glucose or galactose. Thus, large doses of fructose are not readily absorbed and can contribute to diarrhea as this remains in the small intestine and attracts water.

Once glucose, galactose, and fructose enter the intestinal cells, some fructose is metabolized to glucose. The single sugars in the absorptive cells are then transported via the portal vein to the liver. The liver then exercises its metabolic options—transforming the monosaccharides into glucose and releasing it directly into the bloodstream for transport to organs such as the brain, muscles, kidneys, and adipose tissues; producing the storage form of the carbohydrate, glycogen; or producing fat. Of these three options, producing fat is the least likely, except when consumed in high amounts.

Only a minor amount of starch (about 5%) escapes digestion. This travels down to the large intestine and is fermented there by bacteria. Then some of the starch is absorbed in the form of acids and gases produced by bacterial metabolism, as is true for undigested lactose. Scientists suspect that some of these products actually promote the health of the large intestine by providing it with a source of energy.

*A*s bacteria in the large intestine ferment certain dietary fibers into such products as acids and gases, these in turn can cause intestinal gas (flatulence). Gas is not harmful but can be inconvenient. However, the body tends to adapt over time to a high dietary fiber intake and produce less gas.

Concept Check

*C*arbohydrate digestion is the process of breaking down larger carbohydrates into smaller units, and eventually to monosaccharide forms. The enzymatic digestion of starches begins in the mouth with salivary amylase. Enzymes made by the pancreas and small intestine complete the digestion of carbohydrates to single sugars in the small intestine. Primarily following an active absorption process, the single sugars (glucose and galactose)—either resulting from the digestive process or present in the meal—are taken up by absorptive cells in the intestine. Fructose undergoes facilitated diffusion. All of the monosaccharides then enter the portal vein and travel to the liver. The liver finally exercises its metabolic options, primarily producing glucose and glycogen from the various sugars.

Putting Simple Carbohydrates to Work in the Body

The functions of glucose in the body start with supplying energy, but that is only the beginning. Because the other sugars can generally be converted to glucose and starches are broken down to yield glucose, the functions described here apply to most carbohydrates.

■ Yielding Energy

The main function of glucose is to supply energy for the body. Certain tissues in the body, such as red blood cells, can use only glucose and other simple carbohydrate forms for energy. Most parts of the brain and central nervous system also derive energy only from simple carbohydrates, unless the diet contains almost none. In that case, much of the brain can use partial breakdown products of fat—called **ketone bodies**— for energy. Simple carbohydrates can also fuel muscle cells and other body cells, but many of these cells can also use fat for energy needs (see Chapter 11 for details on muscle metabolism).

ketone bodies Incomplete breakdown products of fat containing three or four carbons

■ Sparing Protein from Use As an Energy Source and Preventing Ketosis

The importance of carbohydrate fuel for the body cannot be overstated. As a fuel for the brain and central nervous system and red blood cells, carbohydrate is critical. If you don't eat enough carbohydrates, your body is forced to make glucose from other nutrients, mainly certain amino acids that make up proteins. When this occurs, some of the proteins from your diet can't be used to make body tissues and perform other vital functions. Under normal circumstances, digestible carbohydrates in the diet mostly end up as blood glucose to be used by the brain and central nervous system, red blood cells, and most other body cells for fuel. This then allows proteins to be saved for their normal functions, like building and maintaining muscles. Therefore, digestible carbohydrates are considered protein sparing.

During long-term starvation, proteins in the muscles, heart, liver, kidneys, and other vital organs break down into amino acids, and certain forms are turned into needed glucose. If the process occurs over weeks at a time, these organs become partially weakened. (See Chapters 6 and 17 for discussions of the specific effects of starvation.)

When you don't eat enough carbohydrates, an additional result is that fats don't break down completely in metabolism. In other words, without enough carbohydrate present, fat metabolism is hampered. Ketone bodies then form. This condition, known as **ketosis,** should be avoided because it disturbs the body's normal acid-base balance and leads to other health problems.

For now, keep in mind that eating at least 50 grams of carbohydrates per day ensures complete metabolism of fats. It also prevents the body weakness that usually results from having to use protein to compensate for an insufficient carbohydrate intake. Still, typical adults in North America need not worry. Daily carbohydrate intakes usually averages 200 to 300 grams per day.

Another Bite

The life-threatening wasting of protein that occurs during long-term fasting has prompted companies that produce medical products for rapid weight loss to include about 100 grams of carbohydrate in the formulation.* This significantly decreases protein breakdown and thereby helps protect vital tissues and organs, including the heart (see Chapter 10 for details).

*Most of these products are powders that can be mixed with different kinds of fluids, are consumed five or six times per day, and are very low in calories.

Regulating This Energy Source

Under normal circumstances, a person's blood glucose concentration is regulated within a very narrow range.

Recall from Chapter 3 that when carbohydrates are digested and taken up by the absorptive cells of the small intestine, the portal vein then transports the resulting monosaccharides to the liver. The liver is the first organ to screen the absorbed sugars. One of its roles is to guard against excess glucose entering the bloodstream after a meal.

The pancreas works with the liver to control blood glucose. As soon as eating begins, the pancreas releases small amounts of the hormone **insulin.** Once much glucose enters the bloodstream, the pancreas releases more insulin. This insulin stimulates the liver to synthesize glycogen—the storage form of glucose in the body—and stimulates muscle cells, adipose cells, and other cells to increase glucose uptake. By triggering both glucose storage in the liver and glucose movement out of the bloodstream into certain cells, insulin keeps glucose from rising too high in the blood (Fig. 4.7).

Other hormones have the opposite effect of insulin. When a person has not eaten for a few hours and blood glucose begins to fall, the pancreas releases the hormone **glucagon.** This hormone prompts the breakdown of glycogen into glucose, which is then released from the liver into the bloodstream. In this way, glucagon keeps blood glucose from falling too low.

insulin A hormone produced by the beta cells of the pancreas. Among other processes, insulin increases the synthesis of glycogen in the liver and the movement of glucose from the bloodstream into body cells.

glucagon A hormone made by the pancreas that stimulates the breakdown of glycogen in the liver into glucose; this ends up increasing blood glucose. Glucagon also performs other functions.

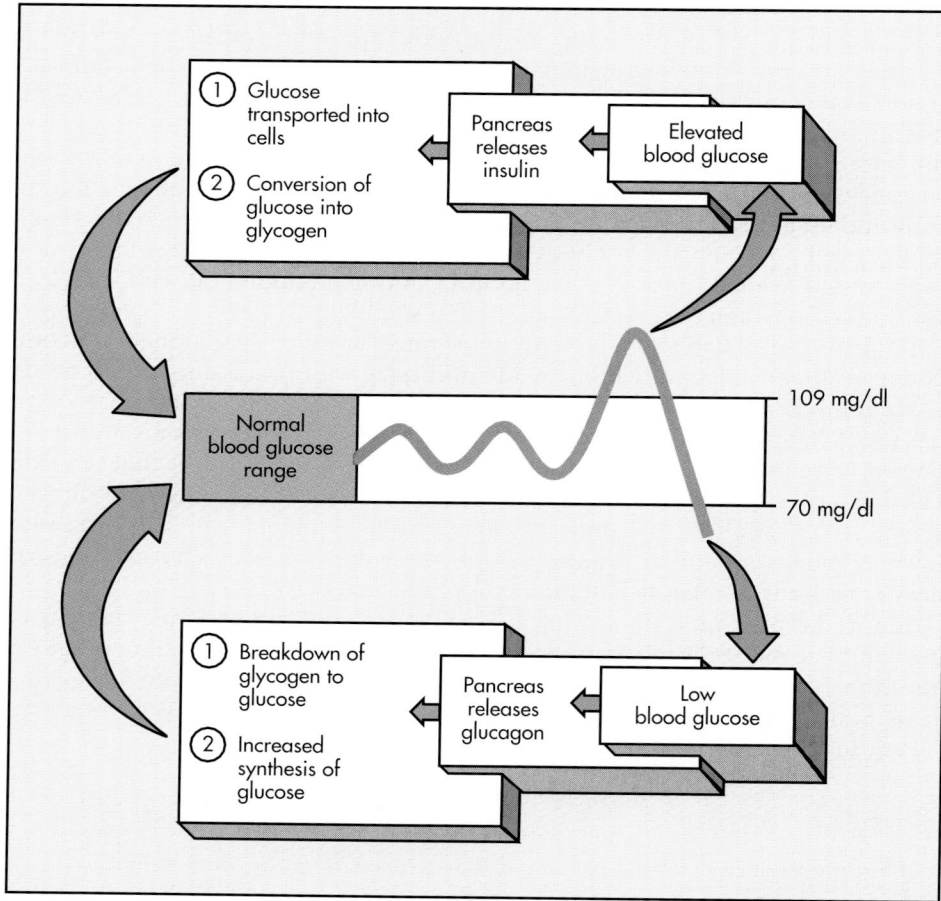

Figure 4.7 Regulation of blood glucose. Insulin and glucagon are key hormones in controlling blood glucose. Other hormones, such as epinephrine, norepinephrine, cortisol, and growth hormone, also contribute to blood glucose regulation. When we eat a meal, insulin is released to promote glucose uptake by cells, thus lowering high blood glucose. When fasting, glucagon is released to promote glucose release from liver stores (those are present in the form of glycogen). This raises blood glucose.
Illustration by William Ober.

A different mechanism increases blood glucose during times of stress. **Epinephrine** (adrenaline) is the hormone responsible for the "flight or fight" reaction. Epinephrine and a related compound are released in large amounts from the adrenal gland (located on each kidney) and various nerve endings in response to a perceived threat, such as a car approaching head-on. These cause glycogen in the liver to break down into glucose. The resulting rapid flood of glucose from the liver into the bloodstream helps promote quick mental and physical reactions.

In essence, the actions of insulin on blood glucose are balanced by the actions of glucagon, epinephrine, and other hormones. If hormonal balance is not maintained, such as during over- or under-production of insulin or glucagon, major changes in blood glucose concentrations occur.

Before we move on, let's step back and look at one of the intricacies of our body's metabolism. To maintain blood glucose within an acceptable range, the body relies on a complex regulatory system. This provides a safeguard against extremely high (**hyperglycemia**) or low (**hypoglycemia**) blood glucose if one control mechanism fails. Suppose instead there were only one mechanism for controlling blood glucose, such as a nerve connection between the brain and pancreas that when appropriately stimulated caused release of insulin. Damage to this nerve would prevent insulin release, causing extreme fluctuations in blood glucose, with dire physiological consequences. In fact, a disturbance in one of the body's control mechanisms—such as insulin release from the pancreas—can greatly influence blood glucose, but it doesn't knock out all of the other regulatory systems. The liver and adrenal glands still act to provide moderate regulation of blood glucose. This example of checks and balances is typical of how the body maintains blood and other tissue concentrations of its key constituents within fairly narrow ranges.

epinephrine A hormone also known as *adrenaline;* it is released by the adrenal gland (located on each kidney) and various nerve endings in the body. It acts to increase glycogen breakdown in the liver, among other functions.

hyperglycemia High blood glucose, above 125 milligrams per 100 milliliters of blood.

hypoglycemia Low blood glucose, below 40 to 50 milligrams per 100 milliliters of blood.

■ Flavoring and Sweetening Foods

Even a baby responds to sugars with a smile. Sensors on the tongue recognize a variety of sugars and even some noncarbohydrate substances. Sugars improve the palatability of many foods and thus enhance diets in general. For example, a small amount of sucrose on a grapefruit improves the taste of this sour fruit. Moderation in using sugars is recommended, but there is no need to avoid sugars altogether. Recall from Chapter 2 that the Food Guide Pyramid suggests the following for moderation in sugar intake from table sugar as such and sugars in food (except lactose) based on one's energy intake: 1600 kcal, 8 teaspoons; 2200 kcal, 12 teaspoons; 2800 kcal, 18 teaspoons.

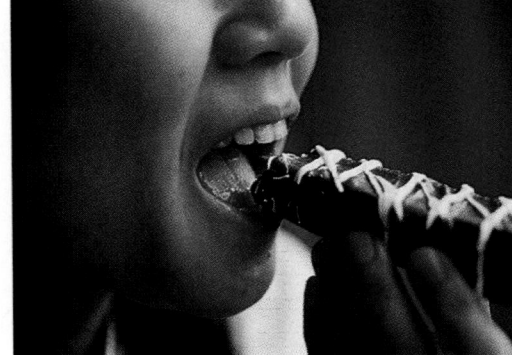

Many foods we enjoy are sweet. These should be eaten in moderation.

Concept Check

*I*n addition to providing sweetness to food, carbohydrates provide glucose for the energy needs of red blood cells and parts of the brain and central nervous system. Eating less than 50 grams of carbohydrates per day forces the body to make glucose using primarily amino acids from proteins found in vital organs. A low glucose supply in cells also inhibits efficient metabolism of fats. Ketosis can then result.

Blood glucose concentration is maintained within a very narrow range. When blood glucose rises after a meal, the hormone insulin is released in great amounts from the pancreas. Insulin acts to lower blood glucose by increasing glucose storage in the liver and glucose uptake by many body cells. If blood glucose falls during fasting, glucagon and other hormones increase the liver's release of glucose into the bloodstream to restore normal blood glucose values. In a similar way, the hormone epinephrine can make more glucose available in response to stress. This balance in hormone activity helps maintain blood glucose within a healthy range.

*A*dvice from the Dietary Guidelines regarding carbohydrates is:
- Choose a variety of grains daily, especially whole grains.
- Choose a variety of fruits and vegetables daily.
- Choose beverages and foods that limit your intake of sugars.

*H*ealthy People 2010 has the following goals related to carbohydrate intake:
- Increase the proportion of persons age 2 years and older who consume at least 6 daily servings of grain products, with at least three being whole grains.
- Increase the proportion of persons age 2 years and older who consume at least 2 daily servings of fruit.
- Increase the proportion of persons age 2 years and older who consume at least 3 daily servings of vegetables, with at least one-third being dark green or orange vegetables.

Syndrome X A condition in which the person has insulin resistance, hypertension, increased blood triglycerides, and decreased **high density lipoprotein (HDL)** cholesterol levels. This condition is usually accompanied by obesity, lack of physical activity, and a diet high in refined carbohydrates. Also called metabolic syndrome.

high-density lipoprotein (HDL) The lipoprotein in the blood that picks up cholesterol from dying cells and other sources and transfers it to the other lipoproteins in the bloodstream, as well as directly to the liver. A low blood HDL value increases the risk for cardiovascular disease.

Recommended Carbohydrate Intakes

There is currently no RDA or related dietary standard for carbohydrate, but one may become available soon. Check the website for this text for an update on this issue. It is important to consume at least 50 grams of carbohydrates per day to prevent ketosis.

It is easy to consume 50 grams of carbohydrates. Just three pieces of fruit or three slices of bread or a little more than 3 cups of milk will suffice. In fact, it is difficult to follow a diet that will produce ketosis.

In North America, carbohydrates supply about 50% of dietary energy intake for adults. The latest guidance from the National Cholesterol Education Program in the United States is that we consume 50% to 60% of our energy as carbohydrate. The Nutrition Facts panel on food labels uses 60% of calories as the standard for recommended carbohydrate intake. In addition, one recommendation on which almost all experts agree is that one's carbohydrate intake should be based primarily on fruits, vegetables, whole grains, and legumes (beans), not mostly on refined grains and sugar.

Only when a person's blood triglycerides are high is a carbohydrate-rich diet not recommended. (This will be covered further in Chapter 5 with respect to **Syndrome X.**) Actually, the chief culprits in this case are not carbohydrates as a class of nutrients, but excessively large meals full of foods rich in simple sugars and refined starches and low in dietary fiber, coupled with little physical activity. These practices should not form the basis of daily habits, but unfortunately, they do for many adults.

■ How Much Dietary Fiber Do We Need?

A reasonable goal for dietary fiber intake for the average adult is 20 to 30 grams per day (10 to 13 grams per 1000 kcal), based again on the latest advice from the National Cholesterol Education Program. The Nutrition Insight earlier in the chapter covered the many benefits of such an intake. In North America, the average whole-grain intake is less than one serving per day. This low intake is attributed to the lack of knowledge on the benefits of whole grains, as well as the lack of ability to recognize whole-grain products at the time of purchase. Thus, most of us should increase our dietary fiber intake. At least 3 servings of whole grains is recommended each day. (For children over age 2, experts recommend a dietary fiber intake of age + 5 grams per day.) Eating a high-fiber cereal (at least 3 grams of dietary fiber per serving) for breakfast is one easy way to increase dietary fiber intake (Fig. 4.8). Also, mentioned in the Nutrition Insight, whole-food sources such as cereals, not bran supplements, are preferable because foods provide a broader variety of nutrients. This is especially true for many natural high-fiber foods—whole grains, fruits, vegetables, and beans.

Table 4.4 shows a diet containing 30 grams of dietary fiber and only 1750 kcal. Table 4.5 is a handy tool for estimating your dietary fiber score.

Note that manufacturers list enriched white (refined) flour as wheat flour on food labels. Most people think that if the words "wheat bread" are on the label, they are buying a whole-wheat product. Not so. If the label does not list "whole-wheat flour" first, the product is not primarily a whole-wheat bread and thus does not contain as much dietary fiber as it could. Careful reading of labels is important in the search for more dietary fiber—look especially for whole grains as the first ingredient.

Keep in mind, however, that any nutrient can lead to health problems when consumed in excess, including carbohydrate and dietary fiber. High carbohydrate, high fiber, and low fat does not mean zero calories. Carbohydrates help moderate energy intake in comparison with fats, but the contribution of high-carbohydrate foods to total energy intake still has to be accounted for.

■ Problems with High-Fiber Diets

Very high intakes of dietary fiber—for example, 60 grams per day—can pose some health risks and require close physician supervision. A high dietary fiber intake

Nutrition Facts

Serving Size   1 cup (55g/2.0 oz.)
Servings Per Container   10

Amount Per Serving	Cereal	Cereal with ½ Cup Vitamins A & D Skim Milk
Calories	170	210
Calories from Fat	10	10
		% Daily Value**
Total Fat 1.0g*	2%	2%
Sat. Fat 0g	0%	0%
Cholesterol 0mg	0%	0%
Sodium 300mg	13%	15%
Potassium 340mg	10%	16%
Total Carbohydrate 43g	14%	16%
Dietary Fiber 7g	28%	28%
Sugars 16g		
Other Carbohydrate 20g		
Protein 4g		
Vitamin A	15%	20%
Vitamin C	20%	22%
Calcium	2%	15%
Iron	65%	65%
Vitamin D	10%	25%
Thiamin	25%	30%
Riboflavin	25%	35%
Niacin	25%	25%
Vitamin B6	25%	25%
Folate	30%	30%
Vitamin B12	25%	35%
Phosphorus	20%	30%
Magnesium	20%	25%
Zinc	25%	25%
Copper	10%	10%

*Amount in cereal. One half cup skim milk contributes an additional 40 calories, 65mg sodium, 6g total carbohydrate (6g sugars), and 4g protein.
**Percent Daily Values are based on a 2,000 calorie diet. Your daily values may be higher or lower depending on your calorie needs:

		Calories:	2,000	2,500
Total Fat	Less than		65g	80g
Sat Fat	Less than		20g	25g
Cholesterol	Less than		300mg	300mg
Sodium	Less than		2,400mg	2,400mg
Potassium			3,500mg	3,500mg
Total Carbohydrate			300g	375g
Dietary Fiber			25g	30g

Calories per gram:
Fat 9 • Carbohydrate 4 • Protein 4

Ingredients: Wheat bran with other parts of wheat, raisins, sugar, corn syrup, salt, malt flavoring, glycerin, iron, niacinamide, zinc oxide, pyridoxine hydrochloride (vitamin B₆), riboflavin (vitamin B₂), vitamin A palmitate, thiamin hydrochloride (vitamin B₁), folic acid, vitamin B₁₂, and vitamin D.

Nutrition Facts

Serving Size: ¾ Cup (30g)
Servings Per Package: About 17

Amount Per Serving	¾ Cup Cereal	Cereal With ½ Cup Skim Milk
Calories	120	160
Calories from Fat	0	5
	%Daily Value**	
Total Fat 0g*	0%	1%
Saturated Fat 0g	0%	1%
Cholesterol 0mg	0%	1%
Sodium 40mg	2%	4%
Potassium 60mg	2%	8%
Total Carbohydrate 26g	9%	11%
Dietary Fiber 1g	4%	4%
Sugars 15g		
Other Carbohydrate 10g		
Protein 2g		
Vitamin A	25%	30%
Vitamin C	0%	2%
Calcium	0%	15%
Iron	10%	10%
Vitamin D	10%	20%
Thiamin	25%	25%
Riboflavin	25%	35%
Niacin	25%	25%
Vitamin B6	25%	25%
Folate	25%	25%
Vitamin B12	25%	30%
Phosphorus	4%	15%
Magnesium	4%	8%
Zinc	10%	10%
Copper	2%	2%

*Amount in Cereal. One-half cup skim milk contributes an additional 65mg sodium, 6g total carbohydrate (6g sugars), and 4g protein.
**Percent Daily Values are based on a 2000 calorie diet. Your daily values may be higher or lower depending on your calorie needs:

		Calories:	2,000	2,500
Total Fat	Less than		65g	80g
Sat. Fat	Less than		20g	25g
Cholesterol	Less than		300mg	300mg
Sodium	Less than		2,400mg	2,400mg
Potassium			3,500mg	3,500mg
Total Carbohydrate			300g	375g
Dietary Fiber			25g	30g

Calories per gram:
Fat 9 • Carbohydrate 4 • Protein 4

Ingredients: Wheat, Sugar, Corn Syrup, Honey, Caramel Color, Partially Hydrogenated Soybean Oil, Salt, Ferric Phosphate, Niacinamide (Niacin), Zinc Oxide, Vitamin A (Palmitate), Pyridoxine Hydrochloride (Vitamin B6), Riboflavin, Thiamin Mononitrate, Folic Acid (Folate), Vitamin B12 and Vitamin D.

Figure 4.8 Reading the Nutrition Facts on food labels helps us choose more nutritious foods. Based on the information from these nutrition labels, which cereal is the better choice for breakfast? Consider the amount of dietary fiber in each cereal, based on the amount per 100 kcal. Did the ingredient lists give you any clues? (Note: Ingredients are always listed in descending order by weight on a label.) When choosing a breakfast cereal, it is generally wise to focus on those that are rich sources of dietary fiber. Sugar content can also be used for evaluation. However, sometimes this number does not reflect added sugar but simply the addition of fruits, such as raisins, complicating the evaluation.

especially requires a high fluid intake. Not consuming enough fluid with the fiber can leave the stool very hard and make it difficult and painful to eliminate. Large amounts of dietary fiber may also bind minerals, such as calcium, zinc, and iron.

High-fiber diets often contribute to intestinal gas and occasionally to the production of fiber balls, called **phytobezoars,** in the stomach. These have been found in diabetic patients and in older people who consume large amounts of dietary fiber. Phytobezoars can lead to blockage of intestinal flow. Dietary fiber may also contribute

phytobezoars Pellets of dietary fiber, characteristically found in the stomach.

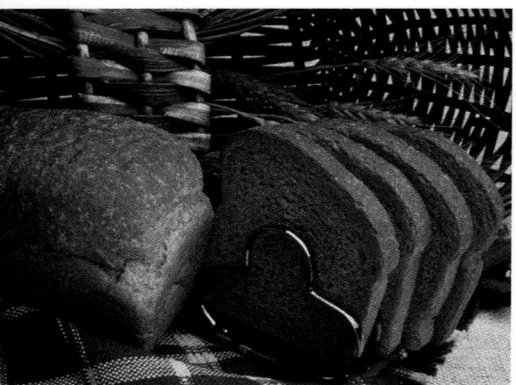

Whole grains are an excellent source of dietary fiber.

Table 4.4 Sample 1750 kcal Menu Containing 30 Grams of Dietary Fiber*

Menu	Carbohydrate Content (grams)	Fiber Content (grams)
Breakfast		
1 cup orange juice (with pulp)	28	0.5
¾ cup Wheaties	17	2
½ cup 2% milk	6	—
1 slice whole-wheat toast	13	2
1 teaspoon margarine	—	—
Coffee	1	—
Lunch		
2 ounces lean ham	—	—
2 slices whole-wheat bread	26	4
2 teaspoons mayonnaise	2	—
¼ cup lettuce	—	0.2
⅓ cup cooked white beans	15	4
1 pear (with skin)	25	4
½ cup 1% milk	6	—
Snack		
1 carrot (as carrot sticks)	8	2
Dinner		
3 ounces broiled chicken (no skin)	—	—
1 baked potato (large, with skin)	30	3
1½ teaspoons margarine	—	—
1 cup cooked green beans	10	4
½ teaspoon margarine	—	—
1 cup 1% milk	12	—
1 apple (with peel)	32	3.7
Snack		
1 raisin bagel	39	1.2
Total	270 grams	30.6 grams

*The overall diet pattern is based on the Food Guide Pyramid. Breakdown of energy content: carbohydrate, 60%; protein, 20%; fat, 20%.

to blockages in the intestine when intake is high and sufficient fluid is not consumed. Finally, large amounts of dietary fiber may add such an excess of bulk to a child's diet that energy intake is reduced; dietary fiber fills the stomach before food intake meets energy needs.

▪ Moderating Intake of Simple Sugars Is Important for Many of Us

Nutrition experts suggest that simple sugars added to foods should provide no more than about 10% of total energy intake daily. This moderate intake corresponds to a maximum of about 50 grams (or 10 teaspoons) of simple sugars per day, based on a 2000 kcal diet. On average, North Americans eat about 82 grams of added simple

Table 4.5 Estimate Your Dietary Fiber Intake

To roughly estimate your daily dietary fiber consumption, determine the number of servings of each food category listed that you consumed yesterday. Multiply the serving amount by the value listed and then add up the total amount of dietary fiber. How does your total fiber intake for yesterday compare with the general recommendation of 20 to 30 grams of dietary fiber per day?

Food	Servings	Grams
Vegetables		
(serving size: 1 cup raw leafy greens or ½ cup other vegetables)	_____ × 2	_____
Fruits		
(serving size: 1 whole fruit; ½ grapefruit; ½ cup berries or cubed fruit; ¼ cup dried fruit)	_____ × 2.5	_____
Beans, lentils, split peas		
(serving size: ½ cup cooked)	_____ × 7	_____
Nuts, seeds		
(serving size: ¼ cup; 2 tablespoons peanut butter)	_____ × 2.5	_____
Whole grains		
(serving size: 1 slice whole-wheat bread; ½ cup whole-wheat pasta, brown rice, or other whole grain; ½ each bran or whole-grain muffin)	_____ × 2.5	_____
Refined grains		
(serving size: 1 slice bread, ½ cup pasta, rice, or other processed grains; and ½ each refined bagels or muffins)	_____ × 1	_____
Breakfast cereals		
(serving size: check package for serving size and amount of fiber per serving)	_____ × grams of fiber per serving	_____
	Total grams of dietary fiber =	_____

Adapted from Fiber: Strands of protection. *Consumer Reports on Health,* p. 1, August 1999.

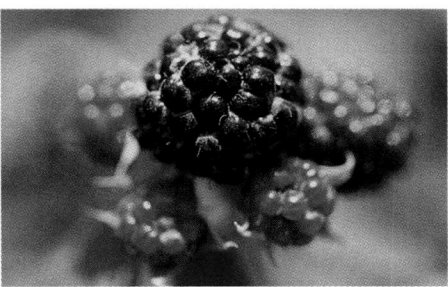

In the search for dietary fiber sources, berries may be overlooked. Just 1 cup contains up to 6 grams of dietary fiber.

sugars daily, amounting to about 16% of energy intake. Table 4.6 suggests ways to reduce intake of simple sugars. For many of us, this would be a healthful practice.

Most of the simple sugars that we eat come from foods and beverages to which sugar has been added during processing and/or manufacture. The major sources are soft drinks, candy, cakes, cookies, pies, fruitades, and dairy desserts, such as ice cream. The rest of the sugar in our diets is present naturally in foods, such as fruits, or comes from the sugar bowl.

It has been mentioned several times that milk and some dairy products contain the milk sugar lactose. This should in no way be construed to mean that milk is a food to avoid in order to limit simple-sugar consumption. In fact, low-fat and nonfat dairy products have an overall high nutrient density and would be one of the last sources of sugars to limit.

Another Bite

During food processing, the simple-sugar content is often increased. The more processed the food, generally the higher the simple-sugar content. An apple contains no added sugars, canned apples in heavy syrup contain 10 to 15 grams (2 to 3 teaspoons) of added sugars, and one-sixth of a 9-inch apple pie contains 30 grams (6 teaspoons) of added sugars. Careful label reading will suggest when a major increase in sugar content has occurred.

Table 4.6 Suggestions for Reducing Simple-Sugar Intake

At the Supermarket

- Read ingredient labels. Identify all the added sugars in a product. Select items lower in total sugar when possible.
- Buy fresh fruits or fruits packed in water, juice, or light syrup, rather than those packed in heavy syrup.
- Buy fewer foods that are high in sugar, such as prepared baked goods, candies, sugared cereals, sweet desserts, soft drinks, and fruit-flavored punches. Substitute vanilla wafers, graham crackers, bagels, English muffins, and diet soft drinks, for example.
- Buy reduced-fat microwave popcorn to replace candy for snacks.

In the Kitchen

- Reduce the sugar in foods prepared at home. Try new recipes or adjust your own. Start by reducing the sugar gradually until you've decreased it by one-third or more.
- Experiment with spices such as cinnamon, cardamom, coriander, nutmeg, ginger, and mace to enhance the flavor of foods.
- Use home-prepared items (with less sugar) instead of commercially prepared ones that are higher in sugar.

At the Table

- Use less of all sugars. This includes white and brown sugars, honey, molasses, and syrups.
- Choose fewer foods high in sugar, such as prepared baked goods, candies, and sweet desserts.
- Reach for fresh fruit instead of a sweet for dessert or between-meal snacks.
- Add less sugar to foods—coffee, tea, cereal, and fruit. Get used to using half as much; then see if you can cut back even more.
- Cut back on the number of sugared soft drinks, punches, and fruit juices you drink. Substitute water, diet soft drinks, and whole fruits rather than fruit juice.

Modified from USDA *Home and Garden Bulletin* No. 232-5, 1986.

*T*here is a widespread notion that high sugar intake by children causes hyperactivity, typically part of the syndrome called attention deficit hyperactive disorder (ADHD). *However, most researchers find that sucrose may actually have the opposite effect. A high-carbohydrate meal, if also low in protein and fat, has a calming effect and induces sleep; this effect may be linked to changes in the synthesis of certain neurotransmitters in the brain, such as serotonin (see Chapter 1). If there is a problem, it is probably the excitement or tension in situations in which sugar-rich foods are served, such as at birthday parties and on Halloween.*

■ Problems with High-Sugar Diets

The main problem with consuming an overabundant amount of sugar is that it provides empty calories; this translates to a decline in the nutritional value of a diet.

Diet Quality

Overcrowding the diet with sweet treats can leave little room for important, nutrient-dense foods, such as fruits and vegetables. Children and teenagers are at the highest risk for overconsuming empty calories in place of nutrients that are essential for growth. Many children and teenagers are drinking an excess of sugared soft drinks and other sugar-containing beverages and much less milk than ever before. Milk contains calcium and vitamin D, both of which are essential for bone health; therefore, this exchange of soft drinks for milk can compromise bone health.

Super-sizing beverages is also a growing problem; for example, in the 1950s a typical serving size of soft drink was a 6½-ounce bottle, and now a 20-ounce plastic bottle is a typical serving. This one change contributes 170 extra kcal to the diet. Filling up on sugared soft drinks in place of foods is not a healthy practice, but enjoying an occasional soft drink or limiting intake to one 12-ounce serving a day is generally fine. Switching to diet soft drinks would spare the simple sugar calories, but still lacks in nutritional value, except for the fluid.

The sugar found in cakes, cookies, and ice cream supplies many extra calories that promote weight gain, unless an individual is physically active. Today's low-fat and fat-free snack products usually contain lots of added sugar to produce a product with an acceptable taste. The result is to produce a high-calorie food that is equal to or

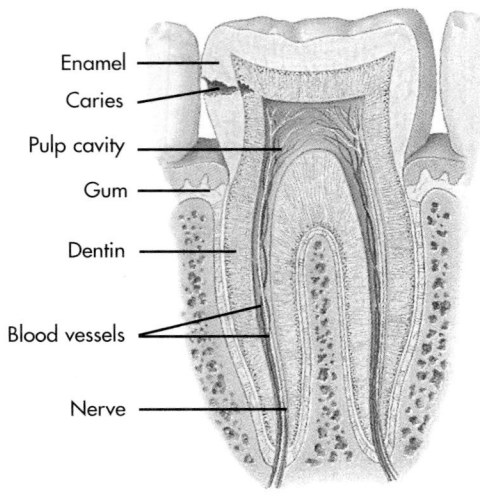

Enamel
Caries
Pulp cavity
Gum
Dentin
Blood vessels
Nerve

Figure 4.9 Dental caries. Bacteria can collect in various areas on a tooth. Using simple sugars such as sucrose, bacteria then create acids that can dissolve tooth enamel, leading to caries. If the caries process progresses and enters the pulp cavity, damage to the nerve and resulting pain are likely. The bacteria also produce plaque whereby they adhere to the tooth surface.

greater in calories than the high-fat food product it was designed to replace. Following the recommendation of having no more than 10% of added sugars is easier if sweet desserts such as cakes, cookies, and ice cream (full and reduced fat), are consumed sparingly.

Dental Caries

Sugars in the diet (and starches that are readily broken down in the mouth, such as crackers and white bread) also increase the risk of developing dental caries. Caries are formed when sugars and other carbohydrates are metabolized into acids by bacteria that live in the mouth (Fig. 4.9). These acids dissolve the tooth enamel and underlying structure. Bacteria also use the sugars to make plaque, a sticky substance that both adheres bacteria to teeth and diminishes the acid-neutralizing effect of saliva.

The worst offenders in terms of dental caries are sticky and gummy foods high in sugars, such as caramel, because they stick to the teeth and supply the bacteria with a long-lived carbohydrate source. These long-lived carbohydrates are termed **cariogenic** (*cario* means "cavity"). Although liquid sugar sources (e.g., fruit juices) are not as potent at causing dental caries as sticky and gummy foods, they still warrant consideration. Some experts caution that sports drinks may also lead to dental caries due to their acid content.

Snacking regularly on sugary foods is also likely to cause caries because it gives the bacteria on the teeth a steady source of carbohydrate from which to continually make acid. Sugared gum chewed between meals is a prime example of a poor dental habit. Still, sugar-containing foods are not the only foods that allow acid production by the bacteria in the mouth. As mentioned, if starch-containing foods (e.g., crackers and bread) are held in the mouth for a long time, they can be acted on by enzymes in the mouth that break down the starch to sugars; bacteria can then produce acid from these sugars. Overall, the sugar and starch content of a food and its retentive ability largely determine its cariogenicity.

Fluoridated water and toothpaste have contributed to fewer dental caries in North American children over the past 20 years due to the mineral's tooth-strengthening effect (see Chapter 9). Research has also indicated that certain foods—such as cheese, peanuts, and sugar-free chewing gum—can actually help reduce the amount of acid on teeth. In addition, rinsing the mouth after meals and snacks reduces the acidity in the mouth. Certainly, good nutrition, habits that do not present an overwhelming challenge to oral health (e.g., chewing sugar-free gum), and routine visits to the dentist all contribute to improved dental health.

cariogenic Literally, "caries-producing"; a substance, often carbohydrate-rich (such as caramel), that promotes dental caries.

Critical Thinking

John and Mike are identical twins who like the same games, sports, and foods. However, John likes to chew sugar-free gum and Mike doesn't. At their last dental visit, John had no cavities, but Mike had two. Mike wants to know why John, who chews gum after eating, doesn't have cavities and he does. How would you explain this to him?

Table 4.7 Glycemic Index (GI) of Common Foods

Reference food glucose = 100			**Sugars**	
Low GI foods—below 55			Honey	73
Intermediate GI foods—between 55 and 70			Sucrose	65
High GI foods—more than 70			Fructose	23
			Lactose	46
Pastas/Grains			**Breads and Muffins**	
Brown rice	55		Bagel	72
White, long grain	56		Whole-wheat bread	69
White, short grain	72		White bread	70
Spaghetti	41		Croissant	67
Vegetables			**Fruits**	
Carrots, boiled	49		Apple	38
Sweet corn	55		Banana	55
Potato, baked	85		Grapefruit	25
Potato, mashed*	73–83		Orange	44
New (red) potato, boiled	62			
Dairy Foods			**Beverages**	
Milk, whole	27		Apple juice	40
Milk, skim	32		Orange juice	46
Yogurt, low-fat	33		Gatorade	78
Ice cream	61		Coca-Cola	63
Legumes			**Snack Foods**	
Baked beans	48		Potato chips	54
Kidney beans	27		Vanilla wafers	77
Lentils	30		Chocolate	49
Navy beans	38		Jelly beans	80

*Higher value refers to instant mashed potatoes.
Adapted from Brand-Miller J, Wolever T, Colagiuri S, Foster-Powell K: *The glucose revolution—The authoritative guide to the glycemic index.* New York: Marlowe & Company, 1999.

glycemic index (GI) The blood glucose response of a given food, compared to a standard (typically, glucose or white bread). Glycemic index is influenced by starch structure, fiber content, food processing, physical structure, and macronutrients in the meal, such as fat.

low-density lipoprotein (LDL) The lipoprotein in the blood, containing primarily cholesterol; elevated LDL-cholesterol is strongly linked to cardiovascular disease risk.

High Glycemic Index

Many foods high in sugar produce a high **glycemic index (GI)** in the body. Glycemic index is defined as the blood glucose response to a given food, compared to a standard (typically, glucose) (Table 4.7). Glycemic index is influenced by starch structure, fiber content, food processing, physical structure, and macronutrients in the meal, such as fat. Foods with particularly high GI values are baking potatoes (not seen as much with red potatoes, as these are low in amylopectin), mashed potatoes (due to greater surface area exposed), short grain white rice, honey, jelly beans, and vanilla wafers.

Nutritionists are concerned about the effect of high-GI carbohydrates on blood glucose because these carbohydrates especially increase insulin output from the pancreas. Chronically high insulin output leads to many deleterious effects on the body: high blood triglycerides; smaller **low-density lipoprotein (LDL)** particles, which are more prone to lead to cardiovascular disease; increased fat deposition in adipose tissue; increased tendency for blood to clot; increased fat synthesis in the liver; and a more rapid return of hunger after a meal (insulin rapidly lowers the macronutrients in the blood as it stimulates their storage). Over time, this increase in insulin output may actually cause the muscles to become resistant to the action of insulin, creating a state of insulin resistance and, eventually, type 2 diabetes in some people.

There are many ways to address this problem of high-GI carbohydrates. The most important is to not overeat high-GI carbohydrates at any one meal, especially foods that are rich in added sugars. This greatly minimizes the effects of high-GI foods on blood glucose and the related increased insulin release. Combining a low-GI index food, such as an apple, baked beans, milk, or salad with dressing, with a high-GI index food also reduces the effect on blood glucose. In addition, maintaining a healthy body weight and performing regular physical activity further reduce the negative effects of a high GI diet.

As you will see in the Nutrition Issue at the end of the chapter, a focus on low-GI foods can help in the treatment of diabetes; Chapter 11 discusses the use of foods with different GI values in planning diets for athletes.

■ Moderation in Lactose Intake Is Important for Some People

Lactose maldigestion (when noticeable symptoms develop after lactose intake it is then called **lactose intolerance**) is a normal pattern of physiology that probably develops after early childhood. It can lead to symptoms of abdominal pain, gas, and diarrhea after consuming lactose, generally when eaten in large amounts. This *primary* form of lactose maldigestion is estimated to be present in about 75% of the world's population, although not all of these individuals experience symptoms. It is hypothesized that approximately 3000 to 5000 years ago, a genetic mutation occurred in regions that relied on milk and dairy foods as a main food source, allowing those individuals (mostly in northern Europe, pastoral tribes in Africa, and the Middle East) to retain the ability to maintain high lactase output for their entire lifetime. This was not seen in other populations in the world, and so such digestive capability was not retained.

Another form of the problem, *secondary* lactose maldigestion, is a temporary condition in which lactase production is decreased in response to an underlying disease, such as intestinal diarrhea. The bloating and gas in lactose maldigestion are caused by bacterial fermentation of lactose in the large intestine. The diarrhea is caused by undigested lactose in the large intestine as it draws water from the circulatory system into the large intestine (osmotic effect; see Chapter 9 for more on osmosis).

In North America, approximately 25% of adults show signs of decreased lactose digestion in the small intestine, many of whom are Asian Americans, African-Americans, and Hispanic Americans, especially as they age. Still, many of these individuals can consume moderate amounts of lactose with minimal or no gastrointestinal discomfort because of eventual lactose breakdown by bacteria in the large intestine, in turn reducing the osmotic effect. Thus, it is unnecessary for these people to greatly restrict their intake of lactose-containing foods. These calcium-rich food products are important in preventing osteoporosis. Obtaining enough calcium and vitamin D from the diet is much easier if milk and milk products are included.

Recent studies have shown that nearly all individuals with decreased lactase production can tolerate 1/2 to 1 cup of milk with meals, and that most individuals adapt to intestinal gas production resulting from the breakdown of lactose by bacteria in the large intestine. Combining lactose-containing foods with other foods also helps because certain properties of foods can have positive effects on rates of digestion. For example, fat in a meal slows digestion, leaving more time for lactase action. Hard cheese and yogurt also are more easily tolerated than milk. Much of the lactose is lost in the production of cheese, and the active bacteria cultures in yogurt digest the lactose when these bacteria are broken apart in the small intestine and release lactase. In addition, an array of products, such as low-lactose milk and lactase pills, are available to assist lactose maldigesters; still, few people actually need to use these products because their degree of maldigestion is moderate.

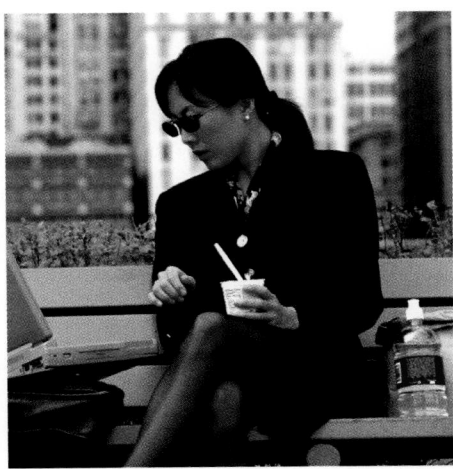

Use of yogurt helps people with lactose maldigestion meet calcium needs.

lactose maldigestion (primary and secondary) Primary lactose maldigestion occurs when lactase production declines for no apparent reason. Secondary lactose maldigestion occurs when a specific cause, such as long-standing diarrhea, results in a decline in lactase production. When noticeable symptoms develop after lactose intake, it is then called lactose intolerance.

Scenario Follow-Up

In the case scenario, Myeshia suspected she was sensitive to milk because, when she consumed 2 servings of milk during one meal, she developed bloating and gas. She tried to reproduce these symptoms by eating 2 servings of dairy foods—one being yogurt—in one meal, but to no avail. In this way she discovered that consuming yogurt in conjunction with milk during the meal did not produce any symptoms. As you just learned, yogurt is tolerated better than milk by people with lactose maldigestion because the bacteria that are present in yogurt digest much of the lactose. Her symptoms likely were also lessened because many people with lactose maldigestion can consume moderate amounts of milk with few or no symptoms.

Concept Check

The prevention of ketosis requires consuming at least 50 grams of carbohydrate per day. The typical North American diet provides 200 to 300 grams per day. A reasonable goal is to have our total carbohydrate intake make up about 50% to 60% of our energy intake. This should allow for the recommended intake of 20 to 30 grams of fiber per day. High-fiber diets must be accompanied by adequate fluid intakes to avoid constipation and phytobezoars and should be followed under a physician's guidance.

North Americans eat about 82 grams of simple sugars added to foods each day. Most of these sugars are added to foods and beverages in processing. The rest occurs naturally in foods or is added from the sugar bowl. To reduce consumption of sugars, one must reduce consumption of items with added sugars, such as some baked goods, sweetened beverages, and presweetened ready-to-eat breakfast cereals. This is one practice that can help reduce the development of dental caries and likely improve diet quality. Lactose maldigestion is a condition that results when cells of the intestine do not make sufficient lactase, the enzyme necessary to digest lactose. If symptoms such as abdominal gas, bloating, and diarrhea develop, the condition is termed lactose intolerance. Most people with lactose maldigestion can tolerate cheeses and yogurt, as well as moderate amounts of milk.

Summary

1. The monosaccharides in our diet include glucose, fructose, and galactose (the latter as part of lactose). Once absorbed via the small intestine and transported through the portal vein into the liver, much of the fructose and galactose is turned into glucose.

2. The major disaccharides are sucrose (glucose bonded to fructose), maltose (glucose bonded to glucose), and lactose (glucose bonded to galactose). When digested, these yield monosaccharide forms. Both monosaccharides and disaccharides are classified as simple sugars.

3. The major digestible polysaccharides—starches such as amylose and amylopectin—contain multiple glucose units bonded together. Glycogen is an animal starch that acts as a storage form of glucose in the liver and muscles. Under the influence of hormones, liver glycogen is readily broken down to glucose, which can enter the bloodstream.

4. Dietary fibers include the indigestible polysaccharides cellulose, hemicelluloses, pectins, gums, and mucilages, as well as the non-carbohydrate lignin. Dietary fiber, especially insoluble varieties, provide mass to the stool, thus easing elimination. Soluble fibers can help control blood glucose in diabetic people and also lower blood cholesterol.

5. Table sugar, honey, jelly, fruit, and plain baked potatoes are some of the most concentrated sources of carbohydrates. Other high-carbohydrate foods, such as pie and nonfat milk, are diluted by either fat or protein. Nutritive sweeteners in food include sucrose, high-fructose corn syrup, brown sugar, and maple syrup.

6. Some starch digestion occurs in the mouth. Carbohydrate digestion is finished in the small intestine. Some plant fibers are fermented by the bacteria present in the large intestine; undigested plant fibers end up in the feces. Single sugars mostly follow an active absorption process in the small intestine. They are then transported to the liver.

7. Carbohydrates provide energy (on average 4 kcal per gram), protect against needless metabolism of protein for energy, and add flavor and sweetness to foods. They are not necessarily fattening. Many types of carbohydrates can be metabolized to acids by bacteria on teeth. The acid can erode the tooth surface, leading to dental caries.

8. A minimal intake of 50 grams of carbohydrate per day is needed; about 50% to 60% of total energy intake is generally recommended. If carbohydrate consumption is inadequate, the body can make what sugars it needs to support cell metabolism. However, if inadequate carbohydrate intake continues for weeks at a time, the price is a loss of body protein, ketosis, and a general weakening of the body.

9. Diets high in complex forms of carbohydrates are encouraged, with an emphasis on fiber-rich foods. The foods to emphasize would be whole grains, pastas, fruits, vegetables, and legumes (beans). Sugar intake should be limited to 10% of energy intake. Moderating sugar intake, especially between meals, reduces the risk of dental caries. Other health benefits also occur, such as a reduced glycemic index (GI) for a meal or snack. Use of alternative sweeteners, such as aspartame, can help in limiting sugar intake.

10. Lactose maldigestion is a condition that results when cells of the intestine wall do not make sufficient lactase, the enzyme necessary to digest lactose. Undigested lactose travels to the large intestine, where it is fermented by bacteria. This can lead to abdominal gas, pain, and diarrhea. In such a case, the problem is called lactose intolerance. Most people with lactose maldigestion can tolerate cheese and yogurt and moderate amounts of milk.

Study Questions

1. Outline the basic steps in blood glucose regulation, including the roles of insulin and glucagon.
2. What are the three major monosaccharides and the three major disaccharides? Describe how each plays a part in the human diet.
3. Why are some foods that are high in carbohydrates, such as cookies and nonfat milk, not considered to be concentrated sources of carbohydrates?
4. Describe the digestion of the various types of carbohydrates in the body.
5. Describe the reason why some people are unable to tolerate high intakes of milk.
6. What are the important roles that dietary fiber plays in the diet?
7. What, if any, are the proven ill effects of sugar in the diet?
8. Why do we need carbohydrates in the diet? How does the body regulate the blood concentration of these carbohydrates?
9. Summarize current carbohydrate intake recommendations.
10. List three alternatives to simple sugars for adding sweetness to the diet.

Further Readings

1. Anderson JW and others: Whole grain foods and heart disease risk. *Journal of the American College of Nutrition* 19:291S, 2000.
   Foods that are rich in dietary fiber, including fruits, vegetables, legumes (beans), and whole-grain cereals, tend to be rich in vitamins, minerals, phytochemicals, antioxidants, and other micronutrients. Each of these components contributes to a reduction in cardiovascular disease risk.

2. Byers T: Diet, colorectal adenomas, and colorectal cancer. *The New England Journal of Medicine* 342:1206, 2000.
   Nutrients such as folate, selenium, and calcium are associated with a lower risk of colon cancer. Medications such as aspirin and related agents (e.g., celecobix [Celebrex]) also may reduce the risk of this disease. Some studies from around the world also have shown a lower risk of colon cancer among populations with high intakes of fruits and vegetables (especially vegetables).

3. Do you know your blood sugar level? *Consumer Reports on Health*, p. 1, July 2000.
   Even just slightly elevated blood glucose can put a person at health risk. People who should especially be tested for elevated blood glucose include those who are overweight, those with relatives with diabetes, non-Caucasians, women who had a baby weighing more than 9 pounds, and those who have hypertension, low HDL-cholesterol, or high blood triglycerides.

4. Guthrie JF, Morton JF: Food sources of added sweeteners in the diets of Americans. *Journal of the American Dietetic Association* 100:43, 2000.
   Americans older than 2 years consume the equivalent of 82 grams of carbohydrate per day from added sweeteners. This accounts for 16% of total energy intake. Adolescent males consume the most added sweeteners, averaging 20% of total energy intake. The biggest source of added sweeteners are regular soft drinks, which account for one-third of intake. Other sources are table sugars, syrups, and cakes and other sweets.

5. Henkel J: Sugar substitutes: Americans opt for sweetness and lite. *FDA Consumer*, p. 12, November/December 1999.
   FDA has approved four sugar substitutes—saccharin, aspartame, acesulfame-K, and sucralose. At least three other sweeteners are under FDA review but have not been approved at this time. FDA stands behind its approval of current sugar substitutes.

6. Morris KL, Zemel MB: Glycemic index, cardiovascular disease, and obesity. *Nutrition Reviews* 57:273, 1999.
   The glycemic index of food is influenced by starch structure (amylose vs. amylopectin), fiber content, food processing, physical structure of the food, and other macronutrients in a meal. Low-glycemic-index diets have been reported to lower blood glucose after a meal and insulin release, to improve blood lipids, and to increase insulin sensitivity.

7. Roberts K and others: Syndrome X: Medical nutrition therapy. *Nutrition Reviews* 58:154, 2000.
   Lifestyle factors such as overeating and physical inactivity play a pivotal role in Syndrome X. The typical Western diet, which is high in refined carbohydrates, low in dietary fiber, and high in saturated fat, is associated with an increased risk of obesity, leading to insulin resistance and Syndrome X.

8. Slavin JL and others: The role of whole grains in disease prevention. *Journal of the American Dietetic Association* 101:780, 2001.
   Current intakes of whole grains are about 1/3 of the recommended intake of 3 or more servings per day. This is unfortunate as an ample dietary fiber intake reduces the risk for developing cardiovascular disease and some forms of cancer. Dietary fiber also helps regulate blood glucose, and so especially is beneficial for people with diabetes.

9. Tuomilehto J and others: Prevention of type 2 diabetes mellitus by changes in lifestyle among subjects with impaired glucose tolerance. *New England Journal of Medicine* 344:1343, 2001.
   The onset of type 2 diabetes can be delayed or prevented when high-risk people make lifestyle changes that include weight reduction, increased physical activity, adequate dietary fiber intake, and moderation in total fat and saturated fat intake.

10. Vesa TH and others: Lactose intolerance. *Journal of the American College of Nutrition* 19:165S, 2000.
    Many lactose maldigestors tolerate small to moderate amounts of lactose without remarkable discomfort. Lactose-hydrolysed milk products and fermented milk products also can help people exhibiting lactose intolerance.

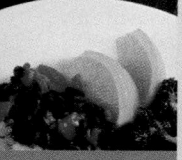
I. How Does Your Diet Rate for Carbohydrate and Dietary Fiber?

Let's reevaluate the nutritional assessment you completed at the end of Chapter 2. Here are your tasks:

1. Look at your analysis and find the total number of grams of carbohydrate you ate.

   TOTAL GRAMS OF CARBOHYDRATE _____

   a. Did you consume more than the minimum amount to avoid ketosis, at least 50 grams?

   b. Now calculate the percentage of energy in your diet from carbohydrate. You will need the total grams of carbohydrate from your assessment, as well as the total kcals you ate. Use this formula to calculate it:

   $$\frac{\text{Total grams of carbohydrate} \times 4}{\text{Total kcals consumed}} \times 100 = \% \text{ of energy intake from carbohydrate}$$

   ANSWER: _____

   Was 50% to 60% or more of your total energy intake from carbohydrate? Yes _____ No _____

   If not, list several ways you could increase your carbohydrate intake. _____

   _____

2. Look again at the list of foods you ate, including the amounts, and determine the total amount of dietary fiber you consumed. If you have a computer analysis of your diet, your dietary fiber intake is listed in the printout. Otherwise, look up the dietary fiber content of each food you ate in the food composition table in Appendix A; then calculate your total intake, taking into account the amount of each food you ate.

   TOTAL AMOUNT OF DIETARY FIBER CONSUMED _____ grams

   a. Did you eat the 20 to 30 grams suggested in this chapter?

   b. If not, what could you do to increase your dietary fiber intake? What foods could you substitute for some of the foods you ate?

   _____

3. Finally, use Table 4.6 as a guide if you need to reduce your intake of sugars, especially if you need to watch your total energy intake to maintain an appropriate weight. What three foods might you, in fact, limit in the future?

   _____

II. Can You Choose the Sandwich with the Most Dietary Fiber?

Assume the sandwiches on the blackboard are available at your local deli and sandwich shop. All of the sandwiches provide about 350 kcal. The dietary fiber content ranges from about 1 gram to about 7.5 grams. Rank the sandwiches from highest amount of dietary fiber to lowest amount; then check your answers on page 142.

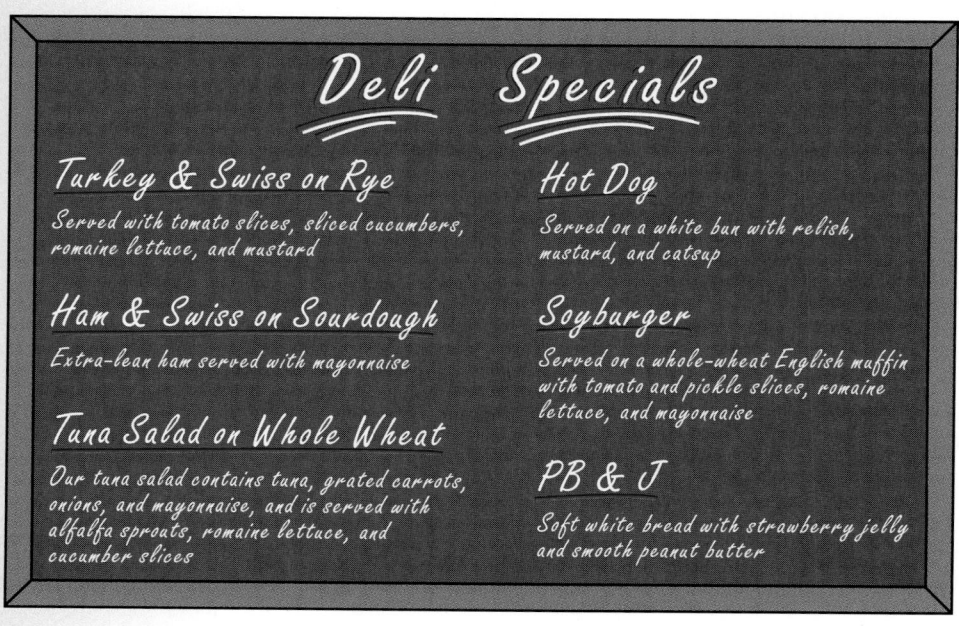

Deli Specials

Turkey & Swiss on Rye
Served with tomato slices, sliced cucumbers, romaine lettuce, and mustard

Ham & Swiss on Sourdough
Extra-lean ham served with mayonnaise

Tuna Salad on Whole Wheat
Our tuna salad contains tuna, grated carrots, onions, and mayonnaise, and is served with alfalfa sprouts, romaine lettuce, and cucumber slices

Hot Dog
Served on a white bun with relish, mustard, and catsup

Soyburger
Served on a whole-wheat English muffin with tomato and pickle slices, romaine lettuce, and mayonnaise

PB & J
Soft white bread with strawberry jelly and smooth peanut butter

When Blood Glucose Regulation Fails

Improper regulation of blood glucose results in either hyperglycemia (high blood glucose) or hypoglycemia (low blood glucose) as noted in the chapter. High blood glucose is most commonly associated with diabetes (technically, *diabetes mellitus*), a disease that affects 7% of the North American population. Of these, it is estimated one-third to one-half of these people do not know that they have the disease. Diabetes leads to about 200,000 deaths each year in North America. New recommendations promote testing fasting blood glucose in adults over age 45 every 3 years to help diagnose these missed cases. The diagnostic criteria based on fasting blood glucose is 126 milligrams per 100 milliliters of blood or greater. In contrast, low blood glucose is a much rarer condition.

Diabetes

There are two major forms of diabetes: **type 1** (formerly called insulin-dependent or juvenile-onset diabetes), and **type 2** (formerly called **non–insulin-dependent** or adult-onset **diabetes**). The change in names to type 1 and type 2 diabetes stems from the fact that many "non–insulin-dependent" diabetics eventually have to also rely on insulin injections as a part of their treatment. A third form, called gestational diabetes, occurs in pregnant women (see Chapter 13). It is usually treated with an insulin regimen and diet, and resolves after delivery of the baby. However, evidence of this problem suggests that women are at high risk for developing diabetes later in life.

Type 1 Diabetes

Type 1 diabetes often begins in late childhood, around the age of 8 to 12 years, but can occur at any age. The disease runs in certain families, indicating a clear genetic link. Children usually are admitted to the hospital with abnormally high blood glucose after eating, with ketosis.

The onset of type 1 diabetes is generally associated with decreased release of insulin from the pancreas. As insulin in the blood declines, blood glucose increases, especially after eating. When blood glucose exceeds the kidney's threshold, excess glucose spills over into the urine. Figure 4.10 shows a typical glucose tolerance curve observed in a patient with this form of diabetes.

An exciting finding regarding the cause of type 1 diabetes may help physicians treat this disease or even prevent its onset in the future. Most cases of type 1 diabetes begin with an immune system disorder, which causes destruction of the insulin-producing cells in the pancreas. Most likely, a virus or protein foreign to the body sets off the destruction. In response to their destruction, the affected pancreatic cells release other proteins, which stimulate a more furious attack. Eventually, the pancreas loses its ability to synthesize insulin, and the clinical stage of the disease begins. Consequently, early treatment to stop the immune-linked destruction in children may be important. Research on this is continuing.

Type 1 diabetes is treated primarily by insulin therapy, either with injections two to six times a day or with an insulin pump. The pump dispenses insulin at a steady rate into the body, with greater amounts delivered after each meal. Dietary measures include three regular meals and one or more snacks (including one at bedtime), having a regulated carbohydrate:protein:fat ratio to maximize insulin action and minimize swings in blood glucose. If one does not eat often enough, the injected insulin can cause severe hypoglycemia, since it acts on whatever little glucose is available. The diet should be rich in complex carbohydrates, include ample dietary fiber and polyunsaturated fat, supply an amount of energy in balance with energy needs, and be low in both animal and other solid fats, as well as moderate in high GI carbohydrates.

type 1 diabetes A form of diabetes prone to ketosis and that requires insulin therapy.

type 2 (non–insulin-dependent) diabetes A form of diabetes in which ketosis is not commonly seen. Insulin therapy can be used but is often not required. This form of the disease is often associated with obesity.

Traditional symptoms of diabetes are excessive urination, excessive thirst, and excessive hunger. No one symptom is diagnostic of diabetes, and other symptoms—such as unexplained weight loss, exhaustion, blurred vision, tingling in hands and feet, frequent infections, poor wound healing, and impotence—often accompany traditional symptoms.

continued

In both type 1 and type 2 diabetes, control of blood pressure and blood lipids are keys to long-term health (see Chapters 5 and 9 for strategies).

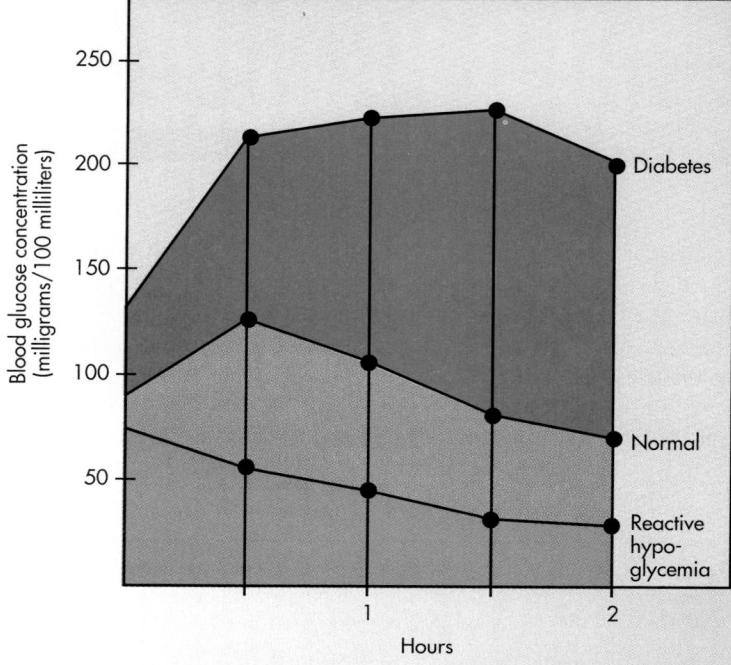

Figure 4.10 A comparison of blood glucose concentrations among diabetic, hypoglycemic, and healthy (normal) persons.

If a high carbohydrate intake raises triglyceride and cholesterol in the blood beyond desired ranges, carbohydrate intake can be reduced and replaced with unsaturated fat. This change tends to reduce blood triglycerides and cholesterol. Chapter 5 discusses how to implement such a diet. Some consumption of sugars with meals is fine, as long as blood glucose regulation is preserved and the sugars replace other carbohydrates in the meal, so that undesirable weight gain does not take place.

Because people with diabetes (type 1, as well as type 2) are at a high risk for cardiovascular disease and related heart attacks, they should take an aspirin each day if their physicians find no reason not to do so. As discussed in Chapter 5, this practice reduces the risk of heart attack. In fact, the latest evidence suggests that diabetes essentially guarantees development of cardiovascular disease. Vitamin E (200 milligrams [about 400 IU] per day) may be prescribed because of this increased risk of cardiovascular disease. However, there is conflicting information on whether this vitamin E use produces such a benefit with regard to prevention of cardiovascular disease in people with diabetes (see Chapters 5 and 8 for details on vitamin E and cardiovascular disease).

The hormone imbalances that occur in people with untreated type 1 diabetes—chiefly, not enough insulin—lead to mobilization of body fat, which is released into liver cells. Ketosis is the result because the fat is mostly converted to ketone bodies. Ketone bodies can rise excessively in the blood, eventually forcing ketone bodies into the urine. These pull sodium and potassium ions with them into the urine. This series of events can contribute to a chain reaction, which eventually leads to dehydration, ion imbalance, coma, and even death, especially in patients with poorly controlled type 1 diabetes. Treatment includes insulin, fluids, and minerals such as sodium and potassium.

Other complications of diabetes can be degenerative conditions, such as blindness, cardiovascular disease, and kidney disease; all are caused by poor blood glucose regulation. Nerves can also deteriorate, resulting in many changes that decrease proper nerve stimulation. When this occurs in the intestinal tract, intermittent diarrhea and constipation result. Because of nerve deterioration in the extremities, many people with diabetes lose the sensation of pain associated with injuries or infections. Not having as much pain, they often delay treatment of hand or foot problems. This delay, combined with a rich environment for bacterial growth (bacteria thrive on glucose) sets the stage for complications in the extremities, such as the need for amputation of feet and legs.

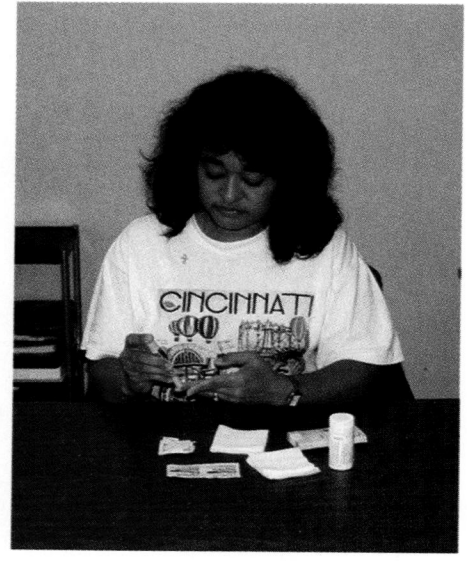

Regularly checking blood glucose is part of diabetes therapy today.

Current research, such as the Diabetes Control and Complications Trail (DCCT), has shown that the development of blood vessel and nerve complications of diabetes can be slowed with aggressive treatment directed at keeping blood glucose within the normal range. The therapy poses some risks of its own, such as hypoglycemia, so it must be implemented under the close supervision of a physician.

A person with diabetes generally must work closely with a physician and dietitian to make the correct alterations in diet and medications and to perform physical activity safely. Physical activity enhances glucose uptake by muscles independent of insulin action, which in turn can lower blood glucose. This outcome is beneficial, but people with diabetes need to be aware of their own blood glucose response to physical activity and compensate appropriately.

■ Type 2 Diabetes

Type 2 diabetes usually begins after age 40. This is the most common type of diabetes, accounting for about 90% of the cases diagnosed in North America. Minority populations such as Latino/Hispanic, African-Americans, Asian Americans, Native Americans, and Pacific Islanders are at particular risk. The overall number of people affected also is on the rise, primarily because of widespread inactivity and obesity in our population. In fact, recently there has been a substantial increase in type 2 diabetes in children, due mostly to an increase in overweight in this population (coupled with limited physical activity). This type of diabetes is also genetically linked, but the initial problem is not with the insulin-secreting cells of the pancreas. Instead, it arises with the insulin receptors on the cell surfaces of certain body tissues, especially muscle tissue. In this case, blood glucose is not readily transferred into cells, so the patient develops high blood glucose as a result of the glucose's remaining in the bloodstream. The pancreas attempts to increase insulin output to compensate, but there is a limit to its ability to do this. Thus, rather than insufficient insulin production, there is an abundance of insulin, particularly during the onset of the disease. As the disease develops, pancreatic function can fail, leading to reduced insulin output. Because of the genetic link for type 2 diabetes, those who have a family history should be careful to avoid risk factors such as obesity, a diet rich in animal and other solid fats, high GI carbohydrates, and inactivity, and as well should be tested regularly for hyperglycemia.

Many cases of type 2 diabetes (about 80%) are associated with obesity (especially fat located in the abdominal region), but high blood glucose is not directly caused by the obesity. In fact, some lean people also develop this type of diabetes. Obesity associated with oversized adipose cells simply increases the risk for insulin resistance by the body.

Type 2 diabetes linked to obesity often disappears if the obesity is corrected. Achieving a healthy weight should be a primary goal of treatment, but even limited weight loss can lead to better blood glucose regulation. Certain oral medications can also help control blood glucose. Adequate chromium intake is also important for blood glucose regulation (see Chapter 9). Supplemental vitamin E may also be prescribed, as discussed for type 1 diabetes.

Sometimes it may be necessary to provide insulin injections in type 2 diabetes because nothing else is able to control the disease. (This eventually becomes the case in about half of all cases of type 2 diabetes.) Regular physical activity also helps the muscles take up more glucose. And regular meal patterns, with an emphasis on control of energy intake, consumption of low-GI carbohydrates, with ample dietary fiber, is important therapy. Some intake of sugars is fine with meals, but again these must be substituted for other carbohydrates, not simply added to the meal plan. Distributing carbohydrates throughout the day is also important, as this helps minimize the high and low swings in blood glucose concentrations. Moderate alcohol use is fine (1 serving per day). One recent study showed that this practice substantially reduced heart attack risk in people with type 2 diabetes. Still, the person must be warned that alcohol can lead to hypoglycemia and that the person must test him- or herself regularly for this possibility.

People with type 2 diabetes who have high blood triglycerides should moderate their carbohydrate intake and increase their intake of unsaturated fat and dietary fiber, as noted earlier for people with type 1 diabetes.

Development of type 2 diabetes in those at risk and progression of type 1 diabetes can both be decreased almost 60% by participating in regular exercise and controlling body weight.

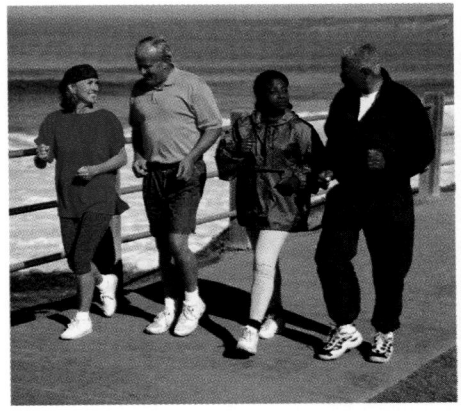

Regular exercise is a key part of a plan to prevent (and control) type 2 diabetes.

continued

*F*or more information on diabetes, consult the following websites: *www.diabetes.org* and *ndep.nih.gov*. Also, see the latest guidelines for diets in diabetes treatment in the January, 2002 issue of the Journal of the American Dietetic Association.

reactive hypoglycemia Low blood glucose that follows a meal high in simple sugars, with corresponding symptoms of irritability, headache, nervousness, sweating, and confusion; also called *postprandial hypoglycemia*.

fasting hypoglycemia Low blood glucose that follows about a day of fasting.

Although many cases of type 2 diabetes can be relieved by reducing excess adipose tissue stores, many people are not able to lose weight. They remain affected with diabetes and may experience the degenerative complications seen in the type 1 form of the disease. Ketosis, however, is not usually seen in type 2 diabetes.

Hypoglycemia

As noted earlier, diabetic people who are taking insulin sometimes have hypoglycemia if they don't eat frequently enough. Hypoglycemia can also develop in nondiabetic individuals. The two common forms of nondiabetic hypoglycemia are termed *reactive* and *fasting*.

Reactive hypoglycemia is described as irritability, nervousness, headache, sweating, and confusion 2 to 4 hours after eating a meal, especially a meal high in simple sugars. The cause of reactive hypoglycemia is unclear, but it may be overproduction of insulin by the pancreas in response to rising blood glucose. **Fasting hypoglycemia** usually is caused by pancreatic cancer, which may lead to excessive insulin secretion. In this case, blood glucose falls to low concentrations after fasting for about 8 hours to 1 day. This form of hypoglycemia is rare.

The diagnosis of hypoglycemia requires the simultaneous presence of low blood glucose and the typical hypoglycemic symptoms. Blood glucose of 40 to 50 milligrams per 100 milliliters is suggestive, but just having low blood glucose after eating is not enough evidence to make the diagnosis of hypoglycemia. Although many people think they have hypoglycemia, few actually do.

It is normal for healthy people to have some hypoglycemic symptoms, such as irritability, headache, and shakiness, if they have not eaten for a prolonged period of time. Although not diagnostic of hypoglycemia, if you sometimes have symptoms of hypoglycemia, the standard nutrition therapy is one we all could follow. You need to eat regular meals, make sure you have some protein and fat in each meal, and eat complex carbohydrates with ample soluble fiber. Avoid meals or snacks that contain little more than simple carbohydrates. If symptoms continue, try small protein-containing snacks between meals or fruits and juice. Fat, protein, and soluble fiber in the diet tend to moderate swings in blood glucose. Last, moderate caffeine and alcohol intake.

Answer Key: 1. Soyburger: 7.5 grams, 2. Tuna Salad on Whole Wheat: 7 grams, 3. Turkey & Swiss on Rye: 4 grams, 4. PB&J: 3 grams, 5. Ham & Swiss on Sourdough: 1.5 grams, 6. Hot dog: 1 gram.

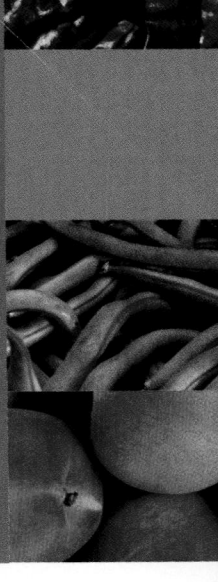

chapter 5

Lipids

Y our doctor informs you that your "triglycerides are too high." Your bill from a medical laboratory reads "Blood lipid profile—$55." A health-food advertisement suggests using cholestin, a dietary supplement, to lower blood cholesterol. Advertisers plug foods "lowest in saturated fat." All of these substances—triglycerides, saturated fat, and cholesterol—are lipids, a collective term referring to fats and oils.

Lipids contain more than twice the energy per gram (on average, 9 kcal) as proteins and carbohydrates (on average, 4 kcal each). Consumption of common saturated fatty acids also contributes to the risk of cardiovascular disease. For this reason, some concern about certain lipids is warranted, but lipids also play vital roles both in the body and in foods. Their presence in the diet is essential to good health.

Let's look at lipids in detail—their forms, functions, metabolism, and food sources. This chapter will then conclude with a look at the link between lipid intake and the major "killer" disease in North America: cardiovascular disease, which involves both the coronary arteries (coronary heart disease) and other arteries in the body.

Check out the **Contemporary Nutrition: Issues and Insights Online Learning Center** www.mhhe.com/wardlawcont5 *for quizzes, flash cards, other activities, and web links designed to further help you learn about dietary lipids.*

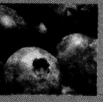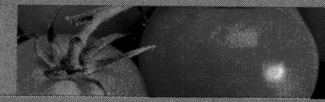

Real Life Scenario

Jackie is a 21-year-old health-conscious individual, in her third year of nursing school. She recently learned that a diet high in saturated fat can contribute to high blood cholesterol and that exercise is beneficial for the heart. Jackie now takes a brisk 30-minute walk each morning before going to class, and she has started to cut as much fat out of her diet as she can, replacing it mostly with carbohydrates. A typical daily intake for Jackie now might begin with a breakfast of a bowl of Fruity Pebbles with 1 cup of skim milk and ½ cup of apple juice. For lunch, she might pack a turkey sandwich on white bread with lettuce, tomato, and mustard; a small package of fat-free pretzels; and a handful of fat-reduced vanilla wafers. Dinner could be a large portion of pasta with some olive oil and garlic mixed in, and a small iceberg lettuce salad with lemon juice squeezed over it. Her snacks are usually baked chips, low-fat cookies, fat-free frozen yogurt, or the fat-free pretzels. She drinks diet soft drinks throughout the day as her main beverage.

Do you think this is a healthy way for Jackie to reduce fat in her diet? Point out some positive practices. What would you suggest changing in her diet to make it more heart healthy?

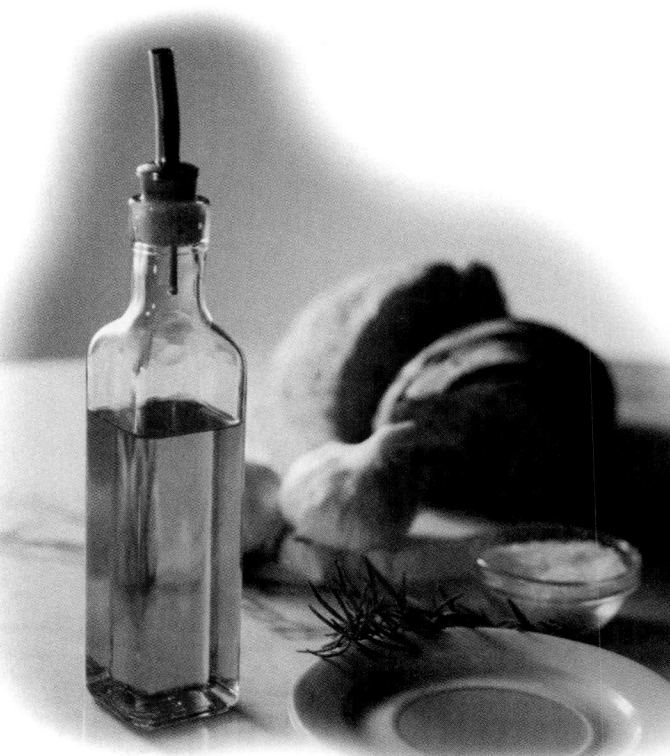

Nutrition Connection

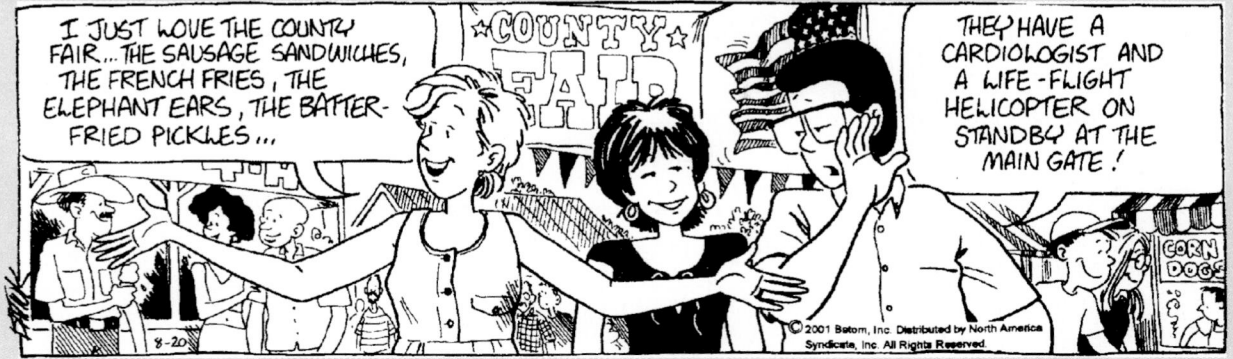

FUNKY WINKERBEAN

High fat, low fat, no fat—what is the answer? And why is there such a debate? Would it be easier just to avoid fat altogether? Doesn't a high-fat diet lead to obesity? To cardiovascular disease? Overall, which are the "best" fats, and why are French fries, doughnuts, stick margarine, and crackers getting such a bad rap? This chapter provides some answers.

Lipids: Common Properties and Main Types

Humans need very little fat in their diet to maintain health. In fact, daily consumption of a tablespoon or so of plant oil incorporated into foods and at least twice weekly consumption of fatty fish such as salmon or tuna meet the body's need for the essential fatty acids. If fish is not consumed, the essential fatty acids in canola oil and soybean oil contribute much of the same health benefit as those found in fish. Thus, one could follow a purely vegetarian diet containing about 10% of calories from fat and still maintain health. However, as long as saturated fat and partially hydrogenated fat (technically called *trans* fat) is minimized, fat intake can be considerably higher than that 10% allotment. The National Cholesterol Education Program in the United States suggests that fat intake can be as high as 25% to 35% of calories. Some experts suggest that an intake as high as 40% of calories is appropriate. After learning more about lipids—fats, oils, and related compounds—in this chapter, you can decide for yourself how much fat you want to consume, as well as how to track your daily intake.

Lipids are a diverse group of chemical compounds. They share one main characteristic: They do not readily dissolve in water. Think of an oil and vinegar salad dressing. The oil is not soluble in the water-based vinegar; on standing, the two separate into distinct layers, with oil on top and vinegar on the bottom.

The diversity of lipids is evident when you compare the structures of two common examples: a fatty acid versus cholesterol, shown in Figure 5.1. Triglycerides are the most common type of lipid found in the body and in foods. Each triglyceride molecule consists of a **glycerol** with three fatty acids bonded to it. **Phospholipids** and **sterols** are also classified as lipids, although their structures can be quite different from the structure of triglycerides (Fig. 5.2). All of these lipid compounds are described in this chapter.

As noted in Chapter 1, lipids that are solid at room temperature are called *fats,* and lipids that are liquid are called *oils.* Most people use the word *fat* to refer to all lipids

glycerol A three-carbon alcohol used to form triglycerides.

phospholipid Any of a class of fat-related substances that contain phosphorus, fatty acids, and a nitrogen-containing base. The phospholipids are an essential part of every cell.

sterol A compound containing a multiring (steroid) structure and a hydroxyl group (–OH).

*S*aturated fatty acids are linear, allowing them to pack tightly together. In contrast, unsaturated fatty acids have a kinked shape and, thus, pack together only loosely (this is depicted later in Fig. 5.10). The loose organization of unsaturated fats is more easily disrupted by heat than is the more ordered organization of saturated fats. Thus, fats high in unsaturated fatty acids melt at a lower temperature than fats high in typical saturated fatty acids.

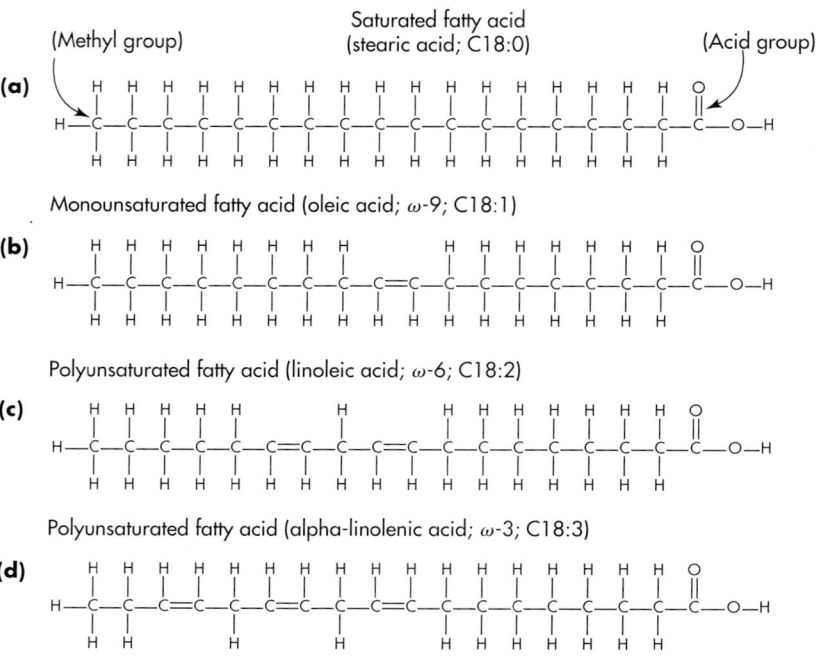

Figure 5.1 Chemical forms of saturated, monounsaturated, and polyunsaturated fatty acids. Note the shorthand notation used to describe fatty acids. The first number indicates the number of carbons; the second number lists the number of double bonds. Thus, stearic acid (structure a) is C18:0.

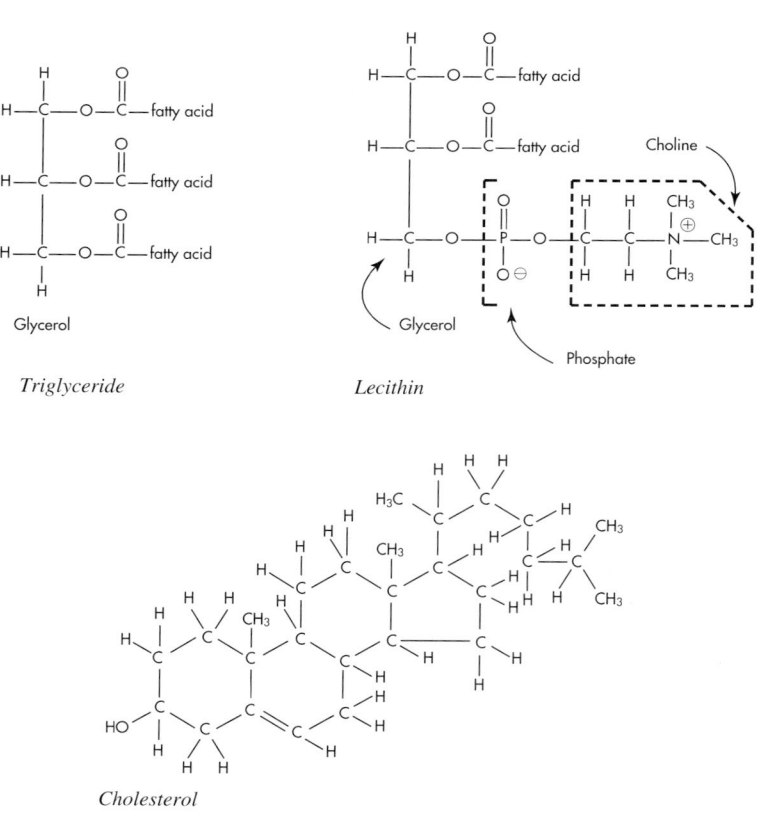

Figure 5.2 Chemical forms of triglycerides, a phospholipid (lecithin), and a sterol (cholesterol).

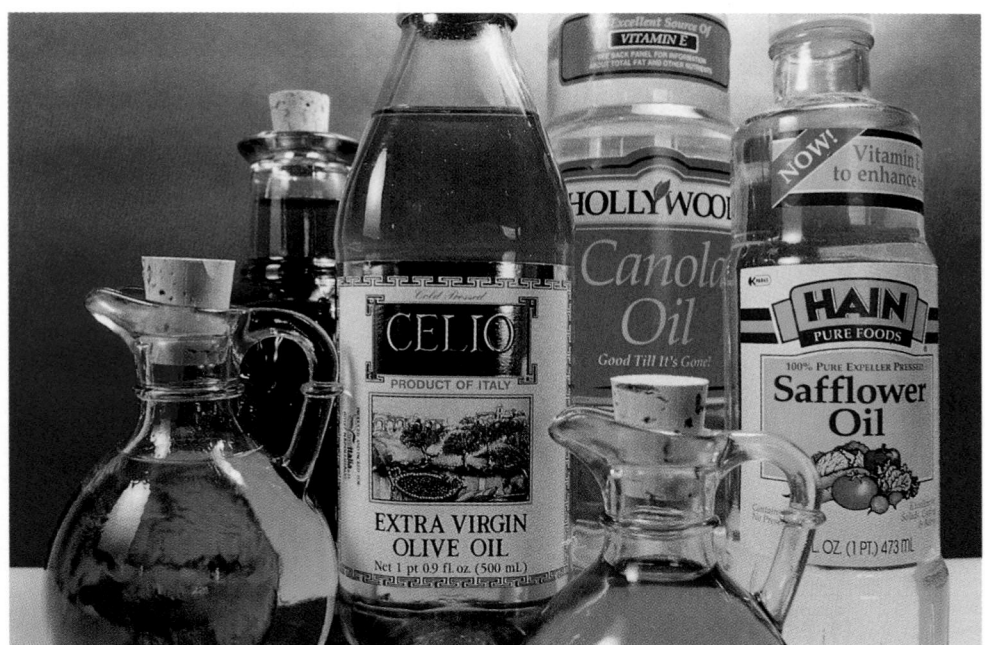

Olive and canola oils are rich in monounsaturated fat; olive oil has been awarded much attention in recent years. Canola oil, however, is a much less expensive choice for consumers. Safflower oil is rich in polyunsaturated fat.

because they don't realize there is a difference. As already covered, however, *lipid* is a generic term that includes triglycerides and many other substances. To simplify our discussion, this chapter primarily uses the term *fat*; however, as you will see later, not all the substances we call fats truly are fats. When necessary for clarity, the name of a specific lipid, such as cholesterol, will be used. This word usage is consistent with the way many people use these terms.

■ Fatty Acids: The Simplest Form of Lipids

The fatty acid is common to most lipids, both those in the body and in foods. It is basically a long chain of carbons bonded together and flanked by hydrogens. At one end of the molecule, designated the *alpha end,* is an acid

$$\begin{matrix} O \\ \parallel \end{matrix}$$

($-C-OH$) group. At the other end, called the *omega* (ω) *end,* is a methyl group ($-CH_3$) (Fig. 5.1a). In the Greek alphabet, *alpha* is the first letter and *omega* is the last.

Fats in foods are not composed of a single type or category of fatty acid. Rather, each dietary fat is a complex mixture of different fatty acids. Butterfat, for example, contains numerous different fatty acids.

If all the chemical bonds between the carbons are single connections and the carbons are filled with hydrogens, a fatty acid is said to be saturated (Fig. 5.1a). To understand this concept, picture a sponge saturated (full) with water.

As noted earlier, most fats high in saturated fatty acids, such as animal fats, remain solid at room temperature. A good example is the solid fat surrounding a piece of uncooked steak at room temperature. Chicken fat, semisolid at room temperature, contains less saturated fat. In some foods, such as whole milk, saturated fats are suspended in liquid, so the solid nature of these fats at room temperature is less apparent. Milk actually contains a combination of liquid and solid fats, as will be discussed shortly.

If a fatty acid is unsaturated, hydrogens are missing from the carbon chain—specifically, at the area of the carbon-carbon double bonds. If a fatty acid has one double bond between the carbons, it is **monounsaturated** (Fig. 5.1b). Canola and olive oils

monounsaturated fatty acid A fatty acid containing one carbon-carbon double bond.

Fats and oils high in saturated fat

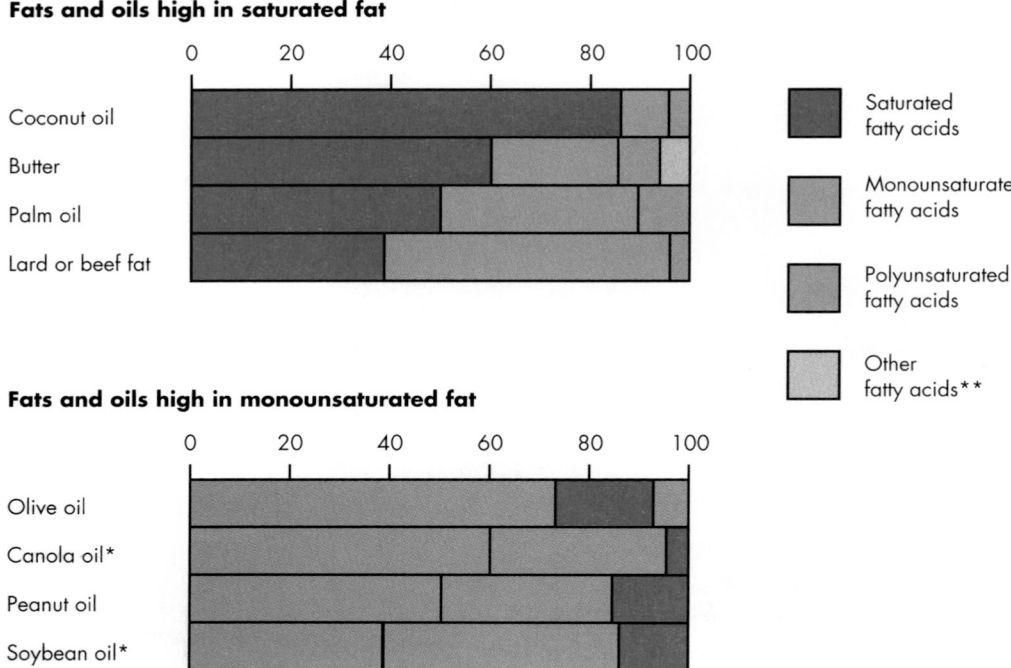

Fats and oils high in monounsaturated fat

Fats and oils high in polyunsaturated fat

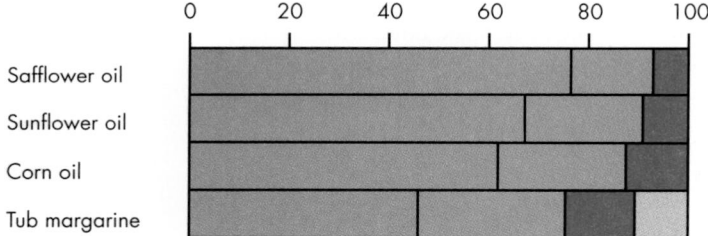

Note that animal fats are also typically rich in monounsaturated fatty acids (40% to 50% of total fatty acids).
*Rich source of the omega-3 fatty acid alpha-linolenic acid (7% and 12% of total fatty acid for soybean oil and canola oil, respectively).
**Primarily trans fatty acids (see page 164 for details on trans fatty acids).

Figure 5.3 Percentage of saturated, monounsaturated, or polyunsaturated fatty acids in common oils and fats (expressed as percent of total fatty acids in the product).

polyunsaturated fatty acid A fatty acid containing two or more carbon-carbon double bonds.

long-chain fatty acids A fatty acid that contains 12 or more carbons.

contain a high percentage of monounsaturated fatty acids. If two or more bonds between the carbons are double bonds, the fatty acid is **polyunsaturated** and, thus, even less saturated with hydrogens (Fig. 5.1c, d). Corn, soybean, sunflower, and safflower oils are rich in polyunsaturated fatty acids.

Overall, a fat or an oil is classified as saturated, monounsaturated, or polyunsaturated based on the nature of the fatty acids present in the greatest concentration (Fig. 5.3).

Fats in foods that contain primarily saturated fatty acids are solid at room temperature, especially if the fatty acids have a **long chain. Medium-chain** saturated fatty acids (6 to 10 carbons long), such as those in coconut oil, produce liquid oils at room temperature. This remains true even though coconut oil consists primarily of saturated fatty acids, because the shorter chain length overrides the effect of saturation. **Short-chain** saturated fatty acids (less than six carbons long) also form liquid oils at room temperature. Dairy fats are sources of these short-chain fatty acids. Triglycerides containing primarily polyunsaturated or monounsaturated fatty acids are also usually liquid at room temperature. These are not affected by chain length. Another important characteristic of unsaturated fatty acids is the location of the double bonds. If the first double bond starts three carbons from the methyl (omega) end of the fatty acid, it is an **omega-3 (ω-3) fatty acid** (review Fig. 5.1d). If the first double bond starts six carbons from the methyl end of the fatty acid, it is an **omega-6 (ω-6) fatty acid** (review Fig. 5.1c). Following this scheme, an omega-9 fatty acid has the first double bond starting at the ninth carbon from the methyl end (review Fig. 5.1b). In foods, **alpha-linolenic acid** is the major omega-3 fatty acid; **linoleic acid** is the major omega-6 fatty acid. These are also the **essential fatty acids** that we need to consume (see the later section on putting lipids to work in the body). **Oleic acid** is the major omega-9 fatty acid.

■ Triglycerides

Fats and oils in foods are mostly in the form of triglycerides. The same is true for fats found in body structures. Some fatty acids are found attached to proteins in the bloodstream as they are being transported, but most fatty acids do not exist in the body as such. Instead, they form into triglycerides.

As noted before, triglycerides contain a simple three-carbon alcohol, glycerol, which serves as a backbone for the three attached fatty acids (review Fig. 5.2). Removing one fatty acid from a triglyceride forms a diglyceride. Removing two fatty acids from a triglyceride forms a **monoglyceride.** Later you see that before most dietary fats are absorbed in the small intestine, the upper and lower fatty acids are typically removed from the triglyceride. This produces fatty acids and monoglycerides, which are absorbed into the intestinal cells. After absorption the fatty acids and monoglycerides are mostly re-formed into triglycerides.

■ Phospholipids

Phospholipids are another class of lipid. Like triglycerides, they are built on a backbone of glycerol. However, at least one fatty acid is replaced with a compound containing phosphorus (and often other elements, such as nitrogen) (review Fig. 5.2). Many types of phospholipids exist in the body, especially in the brain. They form important parts of cell membranes. The various forms of lecithins are common examples of phospholipids. These are found in body cells, where they participate in fat digestion in the intestine. We produce these lecithins; there is no reason to seek a dietary source of phospholipids.

■ Sterols

Sterols are the last class of lipids this chapter covers. Their characteristic multiringed structure makes them different from the other lipids already discussed (review Fig. 5.2). One example is the sterol cholesterol. This waxy substance doesn't look like a triglyceride—it doesn't have a glycerol backbone or any fatty acids. Still, because it doesn't readily dissolve in water, it is a lipid. Among other functions, cholesterol is used to form certain hormones and bile acids, and is incorporated into cell structures. The body can make all the cholesterol it needs.

omega-3 (ω-3) fatty acid An unsaturated fatty acid with the first double bond on the third carbon from the methyl end ($-CH_3$).

omega-6 (ω-6) fatty acid An unsaturated fatty acid with the first double bond on the sixth carbon from the methyl end ($-CH_3$).

alpha-linolenic acid An essential omega-3 fatty acid with 18 carbons and three double bonds (C18:3, ω-3).

linoleic acid An essential omega-6 fatty acid with 18 carbons and two double bonds (C18:2, ω-6).

essential fatty acids Fatty acids that must be supplied by the diet to maintain health. Currently, only linoleic acid and alpha-linolenic acid are classified as essential.

oleic acid An omega-9 fatty acid with 18 carbons and one double bond (C18:1, ω-9).

monoglyceride A breakdown product of a triglyceride consisting of one fatty acid attached to a glycerol backbone. A diglyceride contains two fatty acids attached to glycerol.

lecithins A group of phospholipids containing two fatty acids, a phosphate group, and a choline molecule. Lecithins are a group of compounds, since they can differ based on the types of fatty acids found on each lecithin molecule.

Concept Check

Lipids are a group of compounds that do not dissolve readily in water. They include fatty acids, triglycerides, phospholipids, and sterols. Fatty acids can differ from each other in the number of the double bonds between carbons in the carbon chain and the chain length. Saturated fatty acids contain no carbon-carbon double bonds; that is, they are fully saturated with hydrogens. Monounsaturated fatty acids contain one carbon-carbon double bond, and polyunsaturated fatty acids contain two or more carbon-carbon double bonds. Certain omega-3 and omega-6 fatty acids are the essential fatty acids needed in the human diet.

Triglyceride is the major form of fat in the body and in food. It is formed by bonding three fatty acids to a glycerol backbone. Phospholipids differ from triglycerides. Their glycerol backbone has fatty acids attached, but at least one fatty acid is replaced by another type of compound. Many phospholipids are present in cell membranes. Sterols, another class of lipids, are constructed quite differently from either triglycerides or phospholipids. Cholesterol, a sterol, forms parts of cells, some hormones, and bile acids. The body produces all the phospholipids and cholesterol needed.

Fats and Oils in Foods

The foods with the highest energy density for fats and oils are those highest in fat, such as salad oils, butter, margarine, and mayonnaise (Fig. 5.4). All of these foods contain close to 100% of energy as fat. In fat-reduced margarines, water replaces some of the fat. Typical margarines are 80% fat by weight (11 grams per tablespoon). Some fat-reduced margarines are as low as 30% fat by weight (4 grams per tablespoon). The extra water added to these margarines can cause texture and volume changes when used in recipes. Cookbooks can provide guidance for appropriate use of these products by suggesting alterations in recipes to compensate for the increased water content.

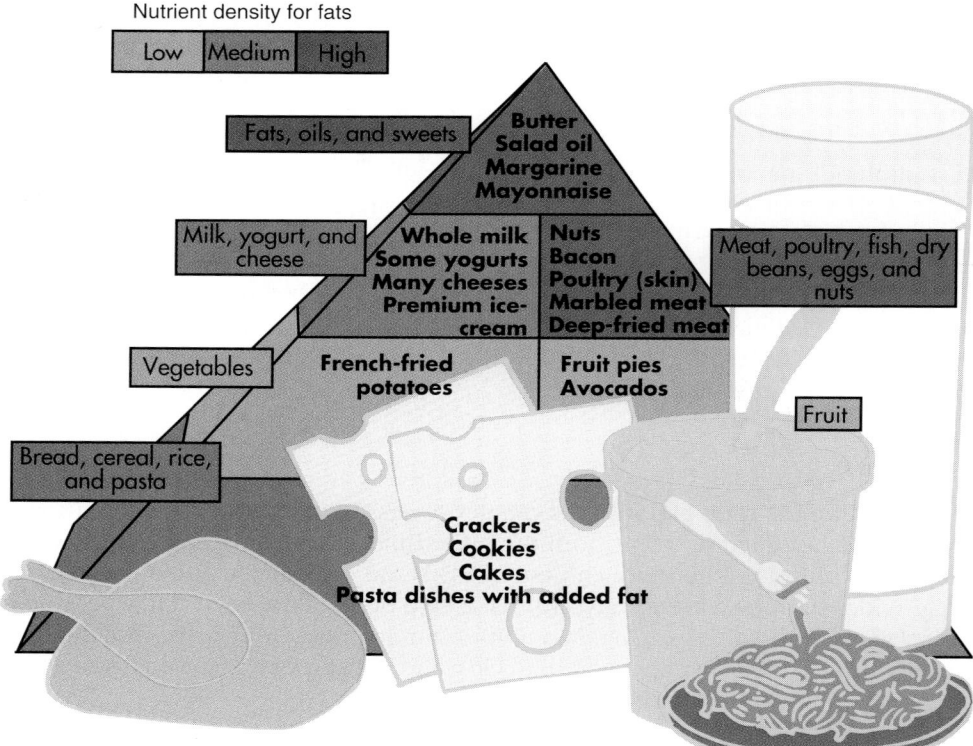

Figure 5.4 Some sources of fats in foods from the Food Guide Pyramid. The background color of each group indicates the average nutrient density for fat in that food group. The fruit group and vegetable group are generally low in fat. In the other groups, both high-fat and low-fat choices are available. Careful food label reading can help you decide which is the case. In general, any type of frying adds significant amounts of fat to a product, as with French fries and fried chicken.

Walnuts, bologna, avocados, and bacon have about 80% of energy as fat. Peanut butter and cheddar cheese have about 75%. Marbled steak and hamburgers (ground chuck) have about 60%, and chocolate bars, ice cream, doughnuts, and whole milk have about 50% of energy as fat. Eggs, pumpkin pie, and cupcakes have 35%, as do lean cuts of meat, such as top round (and ground round) and sirloin. Bread contains about 15%. Cornflakes, sugar, and nonfat milk have essentially no fat. Careful label reading is necessary to determine the true fat content of food—these are only rough guidelines.

Animal fats, which contain about 40% to 60% of total fat as saturated fatty acids, are the chief contributors of saturated fatty acids to the North American diet. Saturated fatty acids with 12, 14, and 16 carbons (lauric acid, myristic acid, and palmitic acid, respectively) are the primary contributors to elevated blood cholesterol, and so contribute to cardiovascular disease. Of these, the 14-carbon myristic acid is the main culprit. Dairy fats are rich sources of myristic acid. The saturated fatty acids with 12, 14, or 16 carbons generally constitute about 25% to 50% of the total fat in animal foods. In general, dairy fats and meat are rich in the fatty acids that raise blood cholesterol. In some plant oils, these saturated fatty acids also make up a notable percentage of the total fat—for example, cottonseed oil (27%) and coconut oil (89%). Stearic acid is the saturated fatty acid with 18 carbons. It is also thought to increase the risk of cardiovascular disease. The negative effect on the heart is probably due in part to an increase in blood clotting. You will see in the Nutrition Issue that blood clots are part of the story behind cardiovascular-related death. Stearic acid constitutes about 20% of saturated fats in meats.

Plant oils contain mostly unsaturated fatty acids, ranging from 73% to 94% of total fat. Canola oil, olive oil, and peanut oil contain moderate to high amounts of total fat as monounsaturated fatty acids (49% to 77%). Some animal fats are also good sources of monounsaturated fatty acids (30% to 47%) (review Fig. 5.3). Corn, cottonseed, sunflower, soybean, and safflower oils contain mostly polyunsaturated fatty acids (54% to 77%) in terms of total fat. These plant oils supply the majority of the linoleic acid and alpha-linolenic acid in the North American food supply. Note that plant oils vary in their content of polyunsaturated fatty acids. Oils that are similar in appearance still may vary significantly in fatty acid composition.

As noted before, egg yolks, wheat germ, peanuts, and organ meats are rich sources of phospholipids. Cholesterol is found only in the animal foods we eat (Table 5.1). An egg yolk contains about 210 milligrams of cholesterol. This is our main dietary source of cholesterol, along with meats and whole milk. Some plants contain related

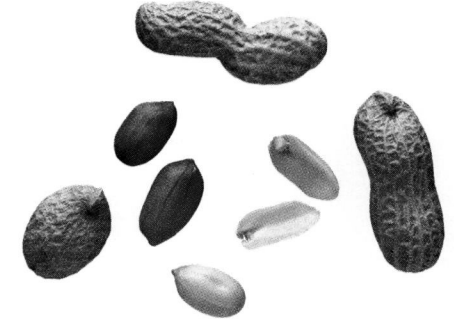

Peanuts are a source of lecithins, as are wheat germ and egg yolks.

Table 5.1 Cholesterol Content of Selected Foods in Ascending Order

Food	Amount	Cholesterol in Milligrams	Food	Amount	Cholesterol in Milligrams
Skim milk	1 cup	4	Oysters, salmon	3 ounces	40
Mayonnaise	1 tablespoon	10	Clams, halibut, tuna	3 ounces	55
Butter	1 pat	11	Chicken, turkey* (white meat)	3 ounces	70
Lard	1 tablespoon	12	Beef,* pork	3 ounces	75
Cottage cheese	½ cup	15	Lamb, crab	3 ounces	85
Low-fat milk (2%)	1 cup	22	Shrimp, lobster	3 ounces	110
Half-and-half	¼ cup	23	Heart, beef	3 ounces	165
Hot dog*	1	29	Egg (egg yolk)*†	1	210
Ice cream, ~10% fat	½ cup	30	Liver, beef	3 ounces	410
Cheese, cheddar	1 ounce	30	Kidney	3 ounces	540
Whole milk	1 cup	34	Brains	3 ounces	2640

*Leading contributors of cholesterol to the U.S. diet.
†Egg whites are cholesterol-free

Fat Replacement Strategies for Foods

Currently, five types of fat replacements are available to food manufacturers. Addition of these substances during manufacture yields products that, to varying degrees, satisfy consumers' desire for fat-reduced products that are still tasty.

Water, Starch Derivatives, and Fibers

The first and simplest fat replacement is water. The addition of water yields a product, such as diet margarine, with less fat per serving than the normal product. Starch derivatives that bind water form a second type of fat replacement. The resulting gel replaces some of the mouth feel lost by the removal of fat. Z-trim is one example. It is made from the hulls of oats, soybeans, peas, and rice or bran from corn or wheat. Other derivatives commonly used by food manufacturers include the fiber cellulose, Maltrin, Stellar, and Oatrim. These substances are used in a variety of foods, including luncheon meats, salad dressings, frozen desserts, table spreads, dips, baked goods, and candies. Most starch derivatives contain some calories, although they have at least less than half the amount that is in fat. Note that these starch derivatives cannot be used in fried foods.

Gum fiber extracted from plants can also be used to replace fat. This thickens a product and replaces some of the body that fat provides. Diet salad dressings have gums added for this reason.

Protein-Derived Fat Replacements

Still another type of fat replacement on the market consists of proteins that have been treated to produce microscopic, mistlike protein globules. Both egg and milk proteins can be used. When these substances replace fat in a food product, they feel like fat in the mouth, although the product does not contain any fatty acids. One example is Dairy-Lo, which is used in milk and other dairy products, baked goods, frostings, salad dressings, and mayonnaise-type products. Such fat replacements yield some energy—but only about 1 to 2 kcal per gram, much less than the 9 kcal per gram supplied by regular fats. They have this low energy value primarily for two reasons: Proteins contain only 4 kcal per gram and the products have a high water content.

Engineered Fats and Related Products

The last form of fat replacement is the engineered fat. This type of product is synthesized in the laboratory from various food constituents. Olestra (Olean) is a good example. It is made by chemically bonding fatty acids to sucrose (table sugar). The resulting product cannot be digested by either human digestive enzymes or bacteria that live in the intestine. Therefore, olestra yields no energy to the body.

Olestra can replace much of the fat in salad dressings and cakes and is the first fat replacement that can be used in fried foods. After almost 200 animal and human studies over a 25-year period, olestra was approved by FDA in 1996 for use in fried snack foods. It underwent such strict scrutiny because it did not exist as such in nature or arise from typical cooking procedures, as is the case for the other products mentioned.

Some problems are associated with the use of olestra. It binds the fat-soluble vitamins A, D, E, and K, thus reducing absorption. To compensate, the manufacturer adds these vitamins to olestra. Olestra also may cause abdominal cramping and loose stools in some people, because, even though it is not absorbed in the small intestine, it still may influence intestinal function. The problem is seen mostly with intakes of 20 grams at a meal. In comparison, a 1-ounce bag of chips has about 10 grams

---

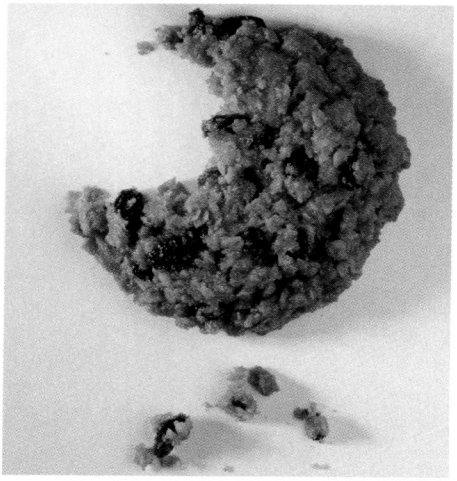

The North American diet contains many high-fat foods—including typical cookie choices. Portion control with these foods is thus important, especially if one is trying to control energy intake.

sterols, but none we typically eat contains cholesterol. Manufacturers who advertise peanut butter, vegetable shortening, margarines, and vegetable oils as containing no cholesterol are taking advantage of uninformed consumers. Peanut butter and margarine never contain cholesterol—it's not naturally present.

■ Hidden Fat

Some fat discussed so far is obvious: butter on bread, mayonnaise in potato salad, and marbling in raw meat. Fat is harder to detect in other foods that also contribute significant amounts of fat to our diets. Fat is hidden in whole milk, pastries, cookies, cake, cheese, hot dogs, crackers, French fries, and ice cream. When we try to cut down on fat intake, hidden fats need to be considered, along with the more obvious sources.

A place to begin searching for hidden fat is on the Nutrition Facts labels of foods you buy in the supermarket. Some signals that can alert you to the presence of fat are animal fats, such as bacon, beef, ham, lamb, pork, chicken, and turkey fats; lard; vegetable oils; nuts; dairy fats, such as butter and cream; egg and egg-yolk solids; and hydrogenated shortening or vegetable oil. Conveniently, the label lists ingredients by order of weight in the product. If fat is one of the first ingredients listed, you are probably looking at a high-fat product. Use food labels to learn more about the fat content of the foods you eat (Fig. 5.5). Table 2.11 in Chapter 2 listed the definitions for various fat descriptors on food labels, such as "lowfat," "fat-free," and "reduced-fat."

of olestra and has little effect. Those who experience such symptoms as a result of eating olestra should limit or avoid using products that contain this fat replacement.

The following statement is required on all products made with olestra: "This product contains olestra. Olestra may cause abdominal cramping and loose stools. Olestra inhibits the absorption of some vitamins and other nutrients. Vitamins A, D, E, and K have been added." As a condition of approval, the manufacturer must conduct studies to monitor olestra consumption and its long-term effects. FDA recently reviewed the safety of olestra and did not find enough evidence that it causes severe gastrointestinal problems. Still, the FDA committee was not convinced that consumers are knowledgeable enough about olestra to warrant taking the warnings off the products made with olestra. Canada has turned down the use of olestra in food products; this decision makes the United States the sole country that permits the use of this fat substitute in foods.

One final problem linked to olestra is its ability to bind carotenoids, the yellow, orange, or red pigments found in many fruits and vegetables. Recall from Chapter 2 the discussion of phytochemicals and their proposed contribution to overall health; one class of phytochemicals is carotenoids. Population studies have linked fruits and vegetables containing carotenoids to a reduced risk of cardiovascular disease, some forms of cancer, and certain eye disorders. There is no planned attempt to add carotenoids to olestra. This effect of olestra is most important when it is consumed in large amounts with meals rich in carotenoids. Typical projected intakes of 10 to 20 grams don't have much of an effect. Nevertheless, this ability to bind carotenoids has caused some experts to recommend that we not consume olestra. At the very least, organizations such as the American Heart Association recommend moderate intake until we know more about its long-term effects.

Food manufacturers are working on still other types of engineered fats, which either wholly or partially escape absorption by the body. One example is salatrim, which is marketed under the name Benefat and yields only about 5 kcal per gram. It is generally composed of stearic acid, which the body absorbs poorly, and short-chain fatty acids. This product has been used in reduced-fat chocolate.

Fat Replacements in Perspective

So far, fat replacements have had little impact on our diets, partly because the currently approved forms either are not very versatile or have not been used extensively by manufacturers. The public, in fact, has shown little interest in their use. In addition, fat replacements are of little use in many foods that contribute the most fat to our diets—beef, margarine, salad dressings/mayonnaise, cheese, whole and reduced-fat milk, and pastries—to name some key players. We consumers must decide to limit our intake of these fat sources; the replacements currently can't help us much.

The main benefit of fat replacements will be in helping us cut some fat and calories from our diets. The reduction in overall energy intake, however, will probably be small because we tend to make up the lost energy by increasing our intake of other foods or by eating more of fat-reduced foods than the corresponding conventional foods.

Recall that "lowfat" indicates, in most cases, that a product contains no more than 3 grams of fat per serving. Products claimed to be fatfree must have less than one-half of a gram of fat per serving. A claim of "reduced-fat" means the product has at least 25% less fat than is usually found in that food.

When there is no Nutrition Facts label to inspect, controlling portion size is a good way to control fat intake. Table 5.3 on page 169 lists many ways to help avoid eating too much total fat and saturated fat. Whether or not to choose a fat-rich food should depend on how much fat you have eaten or will eat for that particular day. So, if you plan to eat high-fat foods at your evening meal, you could reduce your fat intake at a previous meal in order to balance overall fat intake for the day.

■ Wise Use of Reduced-Fat Foods

In recent years, manufacturers have introduced reduced-fat versions of numerous food products. The fat content of these alternatives ranges from 0% in fat-free Fig Newtons to about 75% of the original fat content in other products. However, the total energy content of most fat-reduced products is not substantially lower than that of their conventional versions. Generally, when fat is removed from a product, something must be added—commonly, sugars—in its place. It is very difficult to reduce both the fat and sugar contents of a product at the same time. For this reason, many fat-reduced products (for example, cakes, cookies, and yogurt) are still very energy dense.

When many North Americans think of a low-fat diet, they include reduced-fat versions of pastries, cookies, and cakes. When health professionals refer to a low-fat diet, they often have a very different plan in mind: replacing high-fat snacks with fruits, vegetables, and whole grains. Most North Americans could benefit from this paradigm shift.

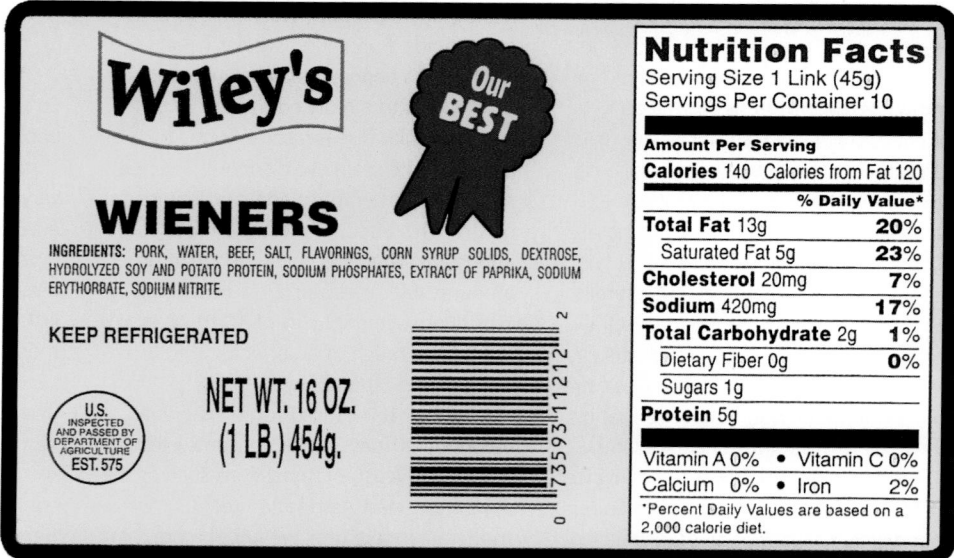

Figure 5.5 Reading labels helps locate hidden fat. Who would think that wieners (hot dogs) can contain about 85% of food energy as fat? Looking at the hot dog itself does not suggest that almost all of its food energy comes from fat, but the label shows otherwise. Let's do the math: (13 grams × 9 kcal per gram)/140 kcal = 0.84, or 84%.

Similarly, some cookbooks are modifying recipes to make them lower in fat. This is accomplished by replacing the fat with applesauce or other fruit purees. Keep in mind that these carbohydrate replacements still contain calories, but not as much as the fat that is left out. As noted in Chapter 4, don't be fooled into thinking you can eat substantially more of such foods just because some or all of the fat has been removed. "Reduced-fat" is not a license to overeat. Use the Nutrition Facts label to guide the portion size you choose.

Concept Check

*F*at-dense foods—those with more than 60% of total energy as fat—include plant oils, butter, margarine, mayonnaise, walnuts, bacon, avocados, peanut butter, cheddar cheese, steak, and hamburger. Of the foods we typically eat, cholesterol is found naturally only in those of animal origin, with eggs being a primary source. Fat is often hidden in foods such as whole milk, pastries, cookies, cake, cheese, hot dogs, crackers, French fries, ice cream, and quick-service (fast) foods. Fat free doesn't mean calorie free; moderation in the use of fat-reduced products is still important.

Making Lipids Available for Body Use

Dietary fat is digested and absorbed primarily in the small intestine.

■ Digestion

lipase Fat-digesting enzyme produced by the salivary glands, stomach, and pancreas.

In the first phase of fat digestion, the stomach (and salivary glands) secretes **lipase** enzymes that act primarily on triglycerides with fatty acids of short-chain and medium-chain lengths, such as those found in butterfat. The action of this enzyme, however, is usually dwarfed by that of a lipase enzyme released from the pancreas and active in the small intestine. In addition, triglycerides and other lipids found in common vegetable oils and meats are generally not digested until they reach the small intestine (Fig. 5.6).

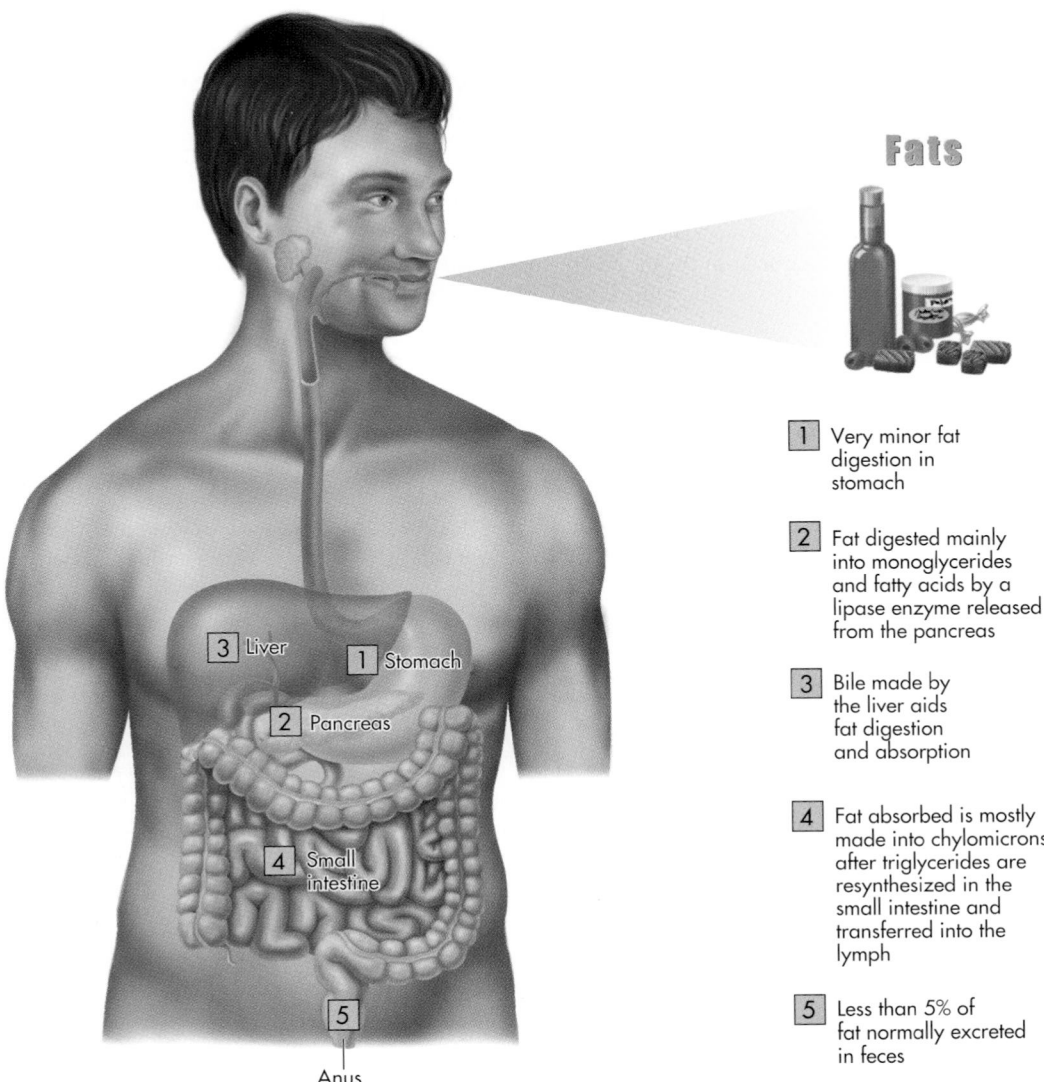

Fats

1. Very minor fat digestion in stomach

2. Fat digested mainly into monoglycerides and fatty acids by a lipase enzyme released from the pancreas

3. Bile made by the liver aids fat digestion and absorption

4. Fat absorbed is mostly made into chylomicrons after triglycerides are resynthesized in the small intestine and transferred into the lymph

5. Less than 5% of fat normally excreted in feces

3 Liver 1 Stomach

2 Pancreas

4 Small intestine

5

Anus

Figure 5.6 A summary of fat digestion and absorption. Chapter 3 covered general aspects of this process.

In the small intestine, triglycerides break down into smaller products, namely monoglycerides (glycerol backbones with a single fatty acid attached) and fatty acids. In the right circumstances, digestion is very rapid and thorough. The "right" circumstances include the presence of bile from the gallbladder. **Bile acids** present in the bile act as an **emulsifier** on the digestive products of lipase action, suspending them in the watery digestive juices. In effect, this is like dishwashing detergent breaking up oil spots in a dishwater (see Fig. 5.8 on page 163 for a depiction of emulsifier action). This emulsification improves digestion and absorption because as large fat globules are broken down into smaller ones, the total surface area for lipase action increases.

With regard to phospholipid and cholesterol digestion, certain enzymes from the pancreas and cells in the wall of the small intestine digest phospholipids. The eventual products are glycerol, fatty acids, and remaining parts such as choline. Any cholesterol with a fatty acid attached is broken down to free cholesterol and fatty acids by certain enzymes released from the pancreas.

bile acids Emulsifiers synthesized by the liver and released by the gallbladder during digestion; they have a cholesterol-like structure.

emulsifier A compound that can suspend fat in water by isolating individual fat droplets, using a shell of water molecules or other substances to prevent the fat from coalescing.

Another Bite

*D*uring meals, bile acids circulate in a path that begins in the liver, goes on to the gallbladder, and then moves to the small intestine. After participating in fat digestion, the bile acids are absorbed and end up back at the liver. Approximately 98% of the bile acids are recycled. Only 1% to 2% ends up in the large intestine to be eliminated in the feces. Using medicines and various plant sterols is one way to block some of this reabsorption of bile acids in treating high blood cholesterol. The liver takes cholesterol from the bloodstream to form replacement bile acids. Soluble fiber in the diet can produce the same effect (see the Nutrition Issue for details).

■ Absorption

Most products of fat digestion have by now been reduced to mere fatty acids and monoglycerides in the small intestine. These diffuse as such into the absorptive cells of the small intestine. One key characteristic of fatty acids and monoglycerides affects their ultimate fate after absorption. If the chain length of a fatty acid is less than 12 carbon atoms (a short-chain or medium-chain variety), it is water soluble and will therefore probably travel as such through the portal vein to the liver. If the fatty acid is long-chain variety (especially 14 or more carbon atoms), it must eventually be re-formed into a triglyceride and eventually enter circulation via the lymphatic system (see Chapter 3 for a review of this process).

Concept Check

*I*n the small intestine, a lipase enzyme released from the pancreas digests dietary triglycerides into smaller breakdown products, namely monoglycerides (glycerol backbones with single fatty acids attached) and fatty acids. The breakdown products then diffuse into the absorptive cells of the small intestine. These products are mostly resynthesized into triglycerides, using the lymphatic system to enter the bloodstream. Other lipids are prepared for absorption by different enzymes.

Carrying Lipids in the Bloodstream

As noted earlier, fat and water don't mix easily. This incompatibility presents a challenge in transporting fats through the watery media of blood and lymph systems.

■ Carrying Dietary Fats Utilizes Chylomicrons

As just reviewed, once the various dietary fats are digested and absorbed into the small intestine cells, most of the by-products of digestion—glycerol, monoglycerides, and fatty acids—are re-formed into triglycerides. They are then packaged into **lipoprotein** particles—large droplets of lipid surrounded by a thin shell of phospholipid, cholesterol, and protein (Fig. 5.7). The lipoprotein particles produced by intestinal cells are called **chylomicrons.** The shell around a chylomicron allows the lipid it is carrying to float freely in the water-based blood. Some of the proteins present also help other cells identify this particle as a chylomicron. After being assembled in intestinal cells, chylomicrons enter the lymphatic system and eventually the bloodstream (review Fig. 3.3 for a depiction of lymphatic circulation).

Once chylomicrons enter the bloodstream, the triglycerides in the chylomicrons are broken down into fatty acids and glycerol by an enzyme called **lipoprotein lipase** on the inside wall of the blood vessel. Muscle cells, adipose cells, and other cells in the vicinity then absorb most of the fatty acids. Cells can immediately use absorbed

lipoprotein A compound found in the bloodstream containing a core of lipids with a shell composed of protein, phospholipid, and cholesterol.

chylomicron Lipoprotein made of dietary fats surrounded by a shell of cholesterol, phospholipids, and protein. Chylomicrons are formed in the absorptive cells (enterocytes) of the small intestine after fat absorption and travel through the lymphatic system to the bloodstream.

lipoprotein lipase An enzyme attached to the outside of cells that line the capillaries in the blood vessels; it breaks down triglycerides into free fatty acids and glycerol.

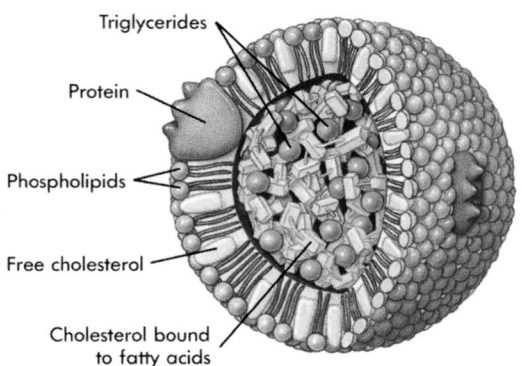

Triglycerides

Protein

Phospholipids

Free cholesterol

Cholesterol bound
to fatty acids

Figure 5.7 The structure of a lipoprotein, in this case an LDL. This structure allows fats to circulate in the water-based bloodstream. Various lipoproteins are found in the bloodstream. Chylomicrons carry fats absorbed from foods through the bloodstream to body cells. VLDLs do the same but mostly carry various lipids made by the liver. LDLs carry cholesterol to the body cells and result from breakdown of VLDLs. HDLs carry cholesterol primarily back to other lipoproteins that, in turn, are mostly taken up by the liver. HDLs also take some of their cholesterol load directly back to the liver.

fatty acids for fuel, or they can re-form them into triglycerides and store them as such. Muscle cells tend to metabolize fatty acids, whereas adipose cells tend to store them.

Another Bite

After eating a meal, the whole process of clearing chylomicrons from the blood via lipoprotein lipase activity takes about 2 to 10 hours, depending in part on fat content. After 12 to 14 hours of fasting, the chylomicrons should be totally absent from the bloodstream. People should fast for 12 to 14 hours before having certain blood tests to assure that chylomicrons, whose presence could affect the results, have been cleared.

■ Transporting Lipids Mostly Made by the Body Uses Other Lipoproteins

The liver produces more lipids than does any other body organ. It also produces cholesterol. The source of the needed carbon, hydrogen, and energy to make such substances as triglycerides and cholesterol includes the carbohydrate and protein the liver takes up from the bloodstream. Still, free fatty acids taken up from the bloodstream are the major source for triglyceride synthesis. Any alcohol consumed can also be used for triglyceride and cholesterol synthesis. The liver coats the cholesterol and triglycerides that collect with a shell of protein and lipids. This process produces what is called a **very-low-density lipoprotein (VLDL)**.

When the VLDL leaves the liver, the enzyme lipoprotein lipase on the blood vessels breaks down the triglyceride in the VLDL into fatty acids and glycerol. Again, fatty acids and glycerol are released into the bloodstream and are taken up by the body cells. Because fats are less dense than water, the VLDL becomes much heavier—proportionately denser—as triglyceride is released. Much of what eventually remains of the VLDL fraction becomes particles called low-density lipoprotein (LDL). LDL is composed primarily of cholesterol.

LDL particles are taken up from the bloodstream by receptors on cells, internalized, and broken down. Most LDL is taken up by receptors on liver cells. Diets low in

Lipoprotein	Key Role
Chylomicron	Carries dietary fat to cells
VLDL	Carries lipids made and taken up by the liver to cells
LDL	Carries cholesterol made by the liver and other sources to cells
HDL	Contributes to cholesterol removal from cells and, in turn, excretion of it from the body

very-low-density lipoprotein (VLDL) The lipoprotein created in the liver that carries cholesterol and lipids both taken up and newly synthesized by the liver.

oxidize In the most basic sense, a chemical substance that has either lost an electron or gained an oxygen. This change typically alters the shape and/or function of the substance. An oxidizing agent then is a substance capable of capturing an electron from another source. That source is then "oxidized" when it loses the electron.

plaque A cholesterol-rich substance deposited in the blood vessels; it contains various white blood cells, smooth muscle cells, various proteins, cholesterol and other lipids, and eventually calcium.

atherosclerosis Buildup of fatty material (plaque) in the arteries, including those surrounding the heart.

homocysteine An amino acid not used in protein synthesis, but instead arises during metabolism of the amino acid methionine. Homocysteine is likely toxic to many cells, such as those lining the blood vessels.

antioxidant Generally, a compound that stops the damaging effects of reactive substances seeking an electron (i.e., oxidizing agent). This prevents the breakdown **(oxidation)** of substances in food or the body, particularly lipids. Antioxidants are especially important in preventing the breakdown of polyunsaturated lipids in the membranes of cells. An antioxidant is able to donate electrons to electron-seeking compounds. This in turn reduces electron capture and, thus, breakdown of unsaturated fatty acids and other cell components by oxidizing agents. Vitamin E is one antioxidant that cells use for protection. Some compounds have antioxidant capabilities (i.e., stop oxidation) but are not electron donors per se.

carotenoids Plant pigments, some of which can yield vitamin A.

saturated fat and cholesterol encourage this process, whereas diets high in those lipids can reduce LDL uptake by the liver (see the Nutrition Issue at the end of this chapter). The cholesterol and protein parts absorbed then are transported throughout the cell. By this process, cells take up some of the building blocks necessary for cell growth and development.

A second process can also remove LDL from the circulation. This is carried out by certain "scavenger" white blood cells, which leave the bloodstream and bury themselves in blood vessels. These scavenger cells detect, alter **(oxidize)**, engulf, and digest the extra circulating LDL. Once within the scavenger cells, the oxidized LDL is prevented from reentering the bloodstream. Over time, cholesterol builds up in the scavenger cells, especially when the amount of LDL in the bloodstream is excessive.

When scavenger cells have collected and deposited cholesterol for many years at a heavy pace, cholesterol builds up on the inner blood vessel walls—especially in arteries—and **plaque** develops (see Fig. 5.12 in the Nutrition Issue at the end of this chapter). The plaque eventually mixes with various proteins and is then covered with a cap of muscle cells and calcium. **Atherosclerosis,** also referred to as *hardening of the arteries,* develops as plaque grows in the vessel. This eventually chokes off the blood supply to organs, setting the stage for a heart attack and other problems, or it breaks apart and leads to clot formation in this or another artery.

Plaque is probably first deposited to repair damage to the cells lining the arteries. The damage that starts plaque formation can be caused by smoking, diabetes, hypertension, a compound called **homocysteine** (likely, but yet to be proven), and LDL itself. Viral and bacterial infections are also implicated, as well as ongoing blood vessel inflammation (see the Nutrition Issue for details). Note also that these plaques can develop in arteries throughout the body, not just the arteries serving the heart. This explains the use of the term *cardiovascular disease* in this book to describe the general condition.

Some nutrients have **antioxidant** properties. These likely reduce LDL oxidation in the bloodstream and thus slow LDL uptake into scavenger cells. Fruits and vegetables are rich in such antioxidants as the various **carotenoids** and vitamins C and E. Eating fruits and vegetables regularly is one positive step we can take to reduce cholesterol buildup and slow the progression of cardiovascular disease. Fruits and vegetables that are rich sources of antioxidants include dried plums (prunes), raisins, various berries, plums, oranges, grapes, spinach, broccoli, red bell peppers, and onions. Consuming megadoses of antioxidant vitamins to do the same thing is controversial. Chapter 8 will discuss this controversy in detail. Currently, the American Heart Association does not support the use of antioxidant supplements, such as vitamin E, in an effort to reduce cardiovascular disease risk. Most large-scale studies (five out of six) of people with existing cardiovascular disease have generally shown no benefit from megadose vitamin E therapy. Other studies are ongoing, using people with cardiovascular disease and those with no evidence of such disease. Still, some experts suggest that megadose vitamin E use (200 milligrams [about 400 IU] per day) may be helpful, but should be taken under a physician's guidance. This caution is because, in some cases, the megadose use of antioxidant supplements can cause harm, especially if one is taking certain anticoagulant medications (these reduce blood clotting). On the other hand, an excessive intake of iron probably speeds LDL oxidation, making it unwise to take an iron supplement unless a physician prescribes it. People who experience iron storage disease and men in general should pay special attention to this warning (see Chapter 9).

A final critical participant in this extensive process of fat transport is high-density lipoprotein (HDL). Its high proportion of protein makes it the heaviest (densest) lipoprotein. The liver and intestine produce most of the HDL in the blood. It roams the bloodstream, picking up cholesterol from dying cells and other sources. HDL donates the cholesterol primarily to other lipoproteins for transport back to the liver to be excreted. Some HDL travels directly back to the liver. Another beneficial function of HDL is that it may block oxidation of LDL.

Many studies demonstrate that the amount of HDL in the bloodstream can closely predict the risk for cardiovascular disease. The risk increases with low HDL because little blood cholesterol is transported back to the liver and excreted. Women tend to have high amounts of HDL, especially before **menopause,** whereas low amounts are more common in men.

Because high amounts of HDL slows the development of cardiovascular disease, any cholesterol carried by HDL can be considered "good" cholesterol. By convention, then, cholesterol carried by LDL would be "bad" cholesterol because high amounts of LDL speeds the development of cardiovascular disease. Still, LDL is only a problem when it is too high in the bloodstream; low amounts are needed as part of routine body functions.

menopause The cessation of menses in women, usually beginning at about age 50.

Concept Check

*T*he bloodstream carries absorbed dietary fat as chylomicrons. Lipid synthesized and taken up by the liver is carried in the bloodstream as very-low-density lipoprotein (VLDL). Once a VLDL has most triglycerides removed by lipoprotein lipase, it eventually becomes low-density lipoprotein (LDL), which is rich in cholesterol. LDL is picked up by receptors on body cells, especially liver cells. Scavenger cells in the arteries may do the same, speeding the development of atherosclerosis. High-density lipoprotein (HDL) picks up cholesterol from cells and transports it primarily to other lipoproteins for eventual transport back to the liver. HDL may also decrease LDL oxidation, thereby reducing LDL uptake into atherosclerotic plaque. Elevated amounts of LDL in the bloodstream is one major risk factor associated with cardiovascular disease, as is low amounts of HDL.

*T*wo approaches have been shown to cause regression of atherosclerosis in the body. One employs a vegan diet and other lifestyle changes that are part of the Dr. Dean Ornish program. The other employs aggressive LDL-lowering with medications (see the Nutrition Issue).

Functions of Lipids

The various classes of lipids have diverse functions in the body. All are necessary for health, but, as mentioned earlier, not all are needed in our diet. Of all the classes of lipids, only certain polyunsaturated fatty acids are essential parts of a diet.

■ Essential Fatty Acids

Because we must obtain linoleic acid (omega-6) and alpha-linolenic acid (omega-3) from foods in order to maintain health, as noted before, they are called essential fatty acids. These omega-3 and omega-6 fatty acids form parts of vital body structures, perform important roles in immune system function and vision, help form cell membranes, and produce hormone-like compounds. This dietary necessity arises because cells in the human body can produce carbon-carbon double bonds in a fatty acid only after the ninth carbon numbered from the methyl end. In other words, human cells do not have the enzyme to place double bonds between the methyl end and the ninth carbon. On the other hand, omega-9 fatty acids can be synthesized in the body because the double bond falls after the ninth carbon.

Still, we need to consume only about 1% to 2% of our total energy intake from essential fatty acids. On a 2500 kcal diet, that corresponds to 1 tablespoon of plant oil each day. We easily get that much—via mayonnaise, salad dressings, and other foods—without even noticing. Barring these foods, regular consumption of whole grains and vegetables can also supply enough essential fatty acids.

Current research also suggests that we should specifically include a regular intake of alpha-linolenic acid or one of its related omega-3 fatty acids, **eicosapentaenoic acid (EPA)** and **docosahexaenoic acid (DHA).** This would almost certainly require consumption of fatty fish, such as salmon, tuna, sardines, herring, mackeral, white fish, wild trout, swordfish, and halibut at least twice a week; regular intake of canola or soybean oil; or consumption of walnuts or flax seeds. All are sources of omega-3 fatty acids. Mussels, crab, and shrimp are additional sources.

eicosapentaenoic acid (EPA) An omega-3 fatty acid with 20 carbons and five carbon-carbon double bonds (C20:5, ω-3). It is present in large amounts in fatty fish and is synthesized in the body from alpha-linolenic acid.

docosahexaenoic acid (DHA) An omega-3 fatty acid with 22 carbons and six carbon-carbon double bonds (C22:6, ω-3). It is present in large amounts in fatty fish and is synthesized in the body from alpha-linolenic acid. DHA is especially present in the retina and brain.

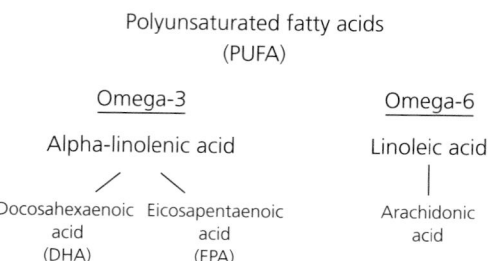

Polyunsaturated fatty acids
(PUFA)

Omega-3

Alpha-linolenic acid

Docosahexaenoic   Eicosapentaenoic
acid   acid
(DHA)   (EPA)

Omega-6

Linoleic acid

Arachidonic
acid

Essential fatty acid (EFA) family. All are available from dietary sources; linoleic acid and alpha-linolenic acid must be consumed as body synthesis does not take place. These are the essential fatty acids. The other fatty acids in this figure can be synthesized from the essential fatty acids.

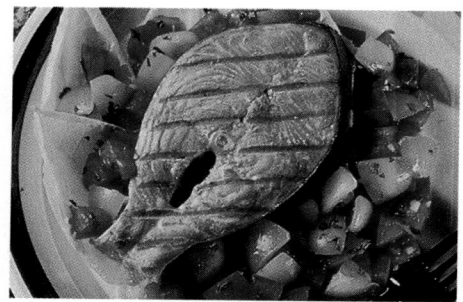

Eating fatty fish such as salmon at least twice a week makes a healthy addition to a diet as it contributes to omega-3 fatty acid intake. The American Heart Association recommends this practice.

hemorrhagic stroke Damage to part of the brain resulting from rupture of a blood vessel and subsequent bleeding within or over the internal surface of the brain.

Critical Thinking

Advertisements often claim that fats are bad. Your classmate Mike asks, "If fats are so bad for us, why do we need to have any in our diets?" How would you answer him?

rancid Containing products of decomposed fatty acids; they yield unpleasant flavors and odors.

This recommendation for consuming omega-3 fatty acids stems from the observation that compounds made from omega-3 fatty acids tend to decrease blood clotting and inflammatory processes in the body, whereas the omega-6 fatty acids generally increase these processes.

Some studies show that people who eat fish twice a week or more (total weekly intake: 8 ounces [240 grams]) run lower risks for heart attack than do people who rarely eat fish. In these cases, the omega-3 fatty acids in fish oil are probably acting to reduce blood clotting. As noted before, blood clots are part of the heart attack process. In addition, these omega-3 fatty acids have a favorable effect on heart rhythm. Consequently, the risk of heart attack decreases, especially for people already at high risk.

We need to remember, however, that blood clotting is a normal body process. Certain groups of people, such as Eskimos in Greenland, eat so much seafood that their blood-clotting ability can be impaired. An excess of omega-3 fatty acid intake can allow uncontrolled bleeding and may cause **hemorrhagic stroke**. However, the risk of stroke has not been seen in studies using moderate amounts of omega-3 fatty acids.

Studies also have shown that large amounts of omega-3 fatty acids from fish (3 to 4 grams per day; one 3-ounce serving of fatty fish has about 1.6 grams) can lower blood triglycerides in people with high triglyceride concentrations. In addition, these omega-3 fatty acids are suspected to be helpful in managing the pain of inflammation associated with rheumatoid arthritis (by suppressing immune system responses) and may help with certain behavioral disorders and depression.

In some instances, fish oil capsules can be safely substituted (under a physician's guidance) for fish consumption if a person does not like fish. Generally, about 900 milligrams of omega-3 fatty acids (about three capsules) from fish oil per day is required to experience the benefits of reduced risk of cardiovascular disease that are associated with fish consumption at least twice a week. However, individuals who have bleeding disorders, are taking anticoagulant medications, are anticipating surgery, or have uncontrolled hypertension should not be taking fish oil capsules because of the increased risk of hemorrhagic stroke.

Another Bite

*F*lax seeds are getting attention today because they are a rich vegetable source of the omega-3 alpha-linolenic acid. About 2 tablespoons per day is typically recommended if used as an omega-3 fatty acid source. Flax seeds can be purchased in many natural food stores rather inexpensively. These need to be chewed thoroughly or they will pass through the GI tract undigested. Many people find it easier to grind them in a coffee grinder before eating them. Flax seed oil is also available, but it turns **rancid** very quickly.

■ Effects of a Deficiency of Essential Fatty Acids

If humans fail to consume enough essential fatty acids, their skin becomes flaky and itchy, and diarrhea and other symptoms such as infections often are seen. Growth and wound healing may be retarded, and anemia can develop. These signs of deficiency have been seen in people fed **total parenteral nutrition** solutions containing little or no fat for 2 to 3 weeks, as well as in infants receiving formulas low in fat. However, because our bodies need the equivalent of only about 1 tablespoon of plant oils a day, even a low-fat diet will provide enough essential fatty acids if it follows a balanced plan such as the Food Guide Pyramid and includes a serving of fatty fish at least twice a week.

total parenteral nutrition The intravenous feeding of all necessary nutrients, including the most basic forms of protein, carbohydrates, lipids, vitamins, minerals, and electrolytes.

Concept Check

*B*ecause humans can't make either omega-3 or omega-6 fatty acids, which perform vital functions in the body, they are essential parts of a diet and therefore called essential fatty acids. Plant oils are generally rich in omega-6 fatty acids. Eating fatty fish at least twice a week is a good way to meet omega-3 fatty acid needs. Fish oil supplementation (about 900 milligrams per day of the related omega-3 fatty acids) is generally acceptable under a physician's guidance if a person does not like fish; however, people with certain medical conditions (e.g., taking anticoagulant medications) should not take fish oil supplements due to increased risk of hemorrhagic stroke. Essential fatty acid deficiency can occur after 2 to 3 weeks if fat is omitted from total parenteral nutrition solutions, which in turn can lead to skin disorders, diarrhea, and other health problems.

■ Broader Roles for Fatty Acids and Triglycerides

Many key functions of fat in the body require the use of fatty acids in the form of triglycerides. Triglycerides are used for energy storage, insulation, and transportation of fat-soluble vitamins.

■ Providing Energy for the Body

Triglycerides both contained in the diet and stored in adipose tissue are the main fuel for muscles while at rest and during light activity. Only in endurance exercise, such as long-distance running and cycling, or in short bursts of intense activity, such as a 200-meter run, do muscles use a lot of carbohydrate in addition to fatty acids supplied by triglycerides for fuel. Other body tissues also use fatty acids for energy. Overall, about half of the energy used by the entire body at rest and during light activity comes from fatty acids. On a whole-body basis, the use of fatty acids by skeletal and heart muscle is balanced by the use of glucose by the nervous system and red blood cells. Recall from Chapter 4 that cells also need carbohydrate to efficiently process fatty acids for fuel.

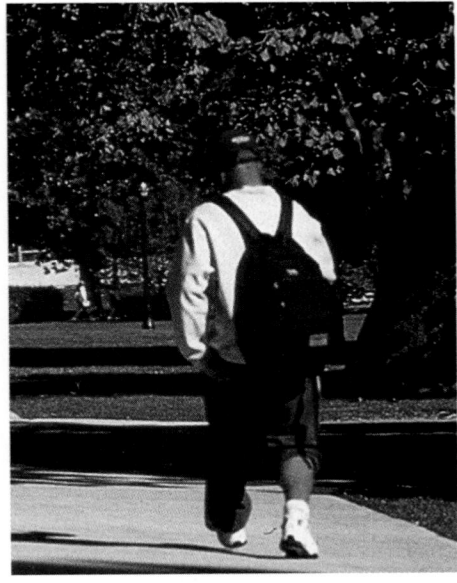

When at rest or during light activity, the body uses mostly fatty acids for fuel. Note also that brisk walking for a total of at least 30 minutes on most (or all) days has been shown to reduce cardiovascular disease risk.

■ Storing Energy for Later Use

We store energy mainly in the form of triglycerides. The body's ability to store fat is essentially limitless. Its fat storage sites, adipose cells, can increase about 50 times in weight. If the amount of fat to be stored exceeds the ability of the cells to expand, the body can form new adipose cells. (This is discussed further in Chapter 10.)

An important advantage of using triglycerides to store energy in the body is that they are energy dense. Recall that these yield, on average, 9 kcal per gram, whereas proteins and carbohydrates yield only about 4 kcal per gram. In addition, triglycerides are chemically very stable, so they are not likely to react with other cell constituents, making them a safe form for storing energy. Finally, when we store triglycerides in adipose cells, we store little else; adipose cells contain about 80% lipid and only 20% water and protein. In contrast, imagine if we were to store energy as muscle tissue, which is about 73% water. Body weight linked to energy storage would increase dramatically. The same would be true if we stored energy primarily as glycogen, as about 3 grams of water are stored for every gram of glycogen.

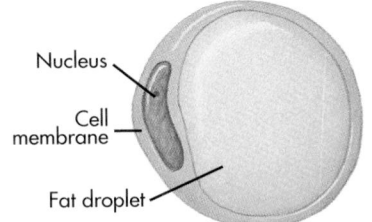

Nucleus

Cell membrane

Fat droplet

Adipose cell

anorexia nervosa An eating disorder involving a psychological loss or denial of appetite and self-starvation, related in part to a distorted body image and to various social pressures commonly associated with puberty.

lanugo Downlike hair that appears after a person has lost much body fat through semistarvation. The hair stands erect and traps air, acting as insulation for the body to compensate for the relative lack of body fat, which usually functions as insulation.

*U*nabsorbed fatty acids can bind minerals, such as calcium and magnesium, and draw them into the stool for elimination. This can harm mineral status (see Chapter 9).

■ Insulating and Protecting the Body

The insulating layer of fat just beneath the skin is made mostly of triglycerides. Fat tissue also surrounds and protects some organs—kidneys, for example—from injury. We usually don't notice the important insulating function of fat tissue, because we wear clothes and add more as needed. But a layer of insulating fat is quite apparent in animals, particularly those in cold climates. Polar bears, walruses, and whales all build a thick layer of fat tissue around themselves to insulate against cold-weather environments. The extra fat also provides energy storage for times when food is scarce.

People with **anorexia nervosa** often lose 25% or more of body weight and become about as fat free as is biologically possible. In turn, they lose the insulating property of fat storage. This poses many other health risks, such as bone loss linked to cessation of menstrual periods (see Chapter 12). In place of the layer of fat tissue under the skin, people with anorexia nervosa often develop downy hair, called **lanugo,** all over the body. These hairs insulate the body by standing up and trapping air.

■ Transporting Fat-Soluble Vitamins

Triglycerides and other fats in food carry fat-soluble vitamins to the small intestine and aid their absorption. If the small intestine is diseased, however, it may not be able to adequately digest and absorb fat from foods. When this happens, the unabsorbed fat carries the fat-soluble vitamins—A, D, E, and K—into the large intestine. From there, they are eliminated in the feces, and the body loses the benefits of the vitamins. If the disease doesn't resolve quickly, medical attention is necessary.

People who absorb fat poorly, such as those with the disease cystic fibrosis, are also at risk for deficiencies of fat-soluble vitamins, especially vitamin K. A similar risk comes from taking mineral oil as a laxative at mealtimes. Because the body cannot digest or absorb mineral oil, the undigested oil carries the fat-soluble vitamins from the meal into the feces, where they are eliminated.

■ Phospholipids in the Body

Many types of phospholipids exist in the body, especially in the brain. They form important parts of cell membranes. Recall that the various forms of lecithins (discussed earlier) are common examples of phospholipids (review Fig. 5.2). These are found in body cells, and they participate in fat digestion in the intestine.

Cell membranes are composed primarily of phospholipids. A cell membrane looks much like a sea of phospholipids with protein "islands" (review Fig. 3.2). Among their many roles, the proteins form receptors for hormones, function as enzymes, and act as transporters for nutrients. The fatty acids on the phospholipids present also serve as a source of essential fatty acids for the cell. Some cholesterol is also present in the membrane.

Some phospholipids, such as the family of compounds just mentioned, called *lecithins,* function as emulsifiers. As covered in the discussion of fat digestion, these allow fat and water to mix. By breaking fat globules into small droplets, emulsifiers enable a fat to be suspended in water. For example, when lecithins are added to an oil and water mixture, they act as bridges between the oil and water that in turn lead to the formation of tiny oil droplets surrounded by thin shells of water. In an emulsified solution, millions of tiny oil droplets are separated by shells of water (Fig. 5.8).

The body's main emulsifiers are the lecithins and bile acids, which are produced by the liver and released into the small intestine via the gallbladder during digestion.

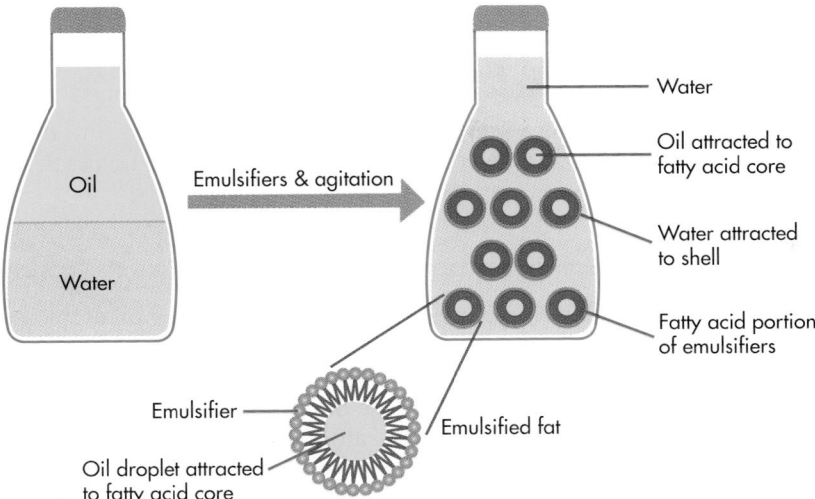

Figure 5.8 Emulsifiers in action. Emulsifiers prevent many brands of salad dressings and other condiments from separating into layers of water and fat. Emulsifiers attract fatty acids inside and have a water-attracting group on the outside. Add them to salad dressing, shake well, and they hold the oil in the dressing away from the water. Emulsification is important in both food production and fat digestion/absorption.

Cholesterol in the Body

Cholesterol forms part of some important hormones, such as estrogen, testosterone, and a form of the active vitamin D hormone. Cholesterol is also the building block of bile acids, which are needed for fat digestion. Finally, cholesterol is an essential structural component of cells and the outer layer of particles that transport lipids in the blood, as discussed in the next section. The cholesterol content of the heart, liver, kidney, and brain is quite high, reflecting its critical role in these organs.

Cholesterol is made by body cells (two-thirds of total daily body exposure) and is consumed in the diet (about one-third of total daily body exposure). Each day, our cells produce approximately 700 milligrams of cholesterol. About 10% of this cholesterol is produced by the liver. Note, however, that this small amount of cholesterol production by the liver is very important in the regulation of blood cholesterol (see the Nutrition Issue at the end of this chapter). Of the 700 milligrams, about 400 are used to make new bile acids to replenish those lost in the feces, and about 50 milligrams are used to make certain hormones. Recall that we consume about 200 to 400 milligrams of cholesterol per day from animal-derived food products (review Table 5.1). Of that, we absorb about 40% to 65%. As well, there is no need to consume cholesterol per se, as body cells can make all that they need.

Concept Check

*T*riglycerides are the major form of fat in the body. They are used for and stored as energy, they insulate and protect body organs, and they transport fat-soluble vitamins. Phospholipids are emulsifiers—compounds that can suspend fat in water. Phospholipids also form parts of cell membranes and various compounds in the body. Cholesterol, a sterol, forms part of cell membranes, hormones, and bile acids.

Exploring Another Dimension of Fat—Properties in Foods

Various fats play important roles in foods. Much ingenuity must go into the production of fat-reduced products to preserve flavor and texture. In some cases, "fat-free" also means tasteless.

■ Fat in Food Provides Some Satiety, Flavor, and Texture

Fat in foods has generally been considered to be the most satiating of all the macronutrients. However, this assumption has been called into question because recent studies show that protein probably leads to the most satiety (gram for gram). High-fat meals do provide satiety, but primarily because one consumes a lot of calories in the process. A high-fat meal is likely to be a high-calorie meal.

Fat components in foods provide important textures and carry flavors. If you've ever eaten a high-fat yellow cheese or cream cheese, you probably agree that fat melting on the tongue feels good. The fat in reduced-fat and whole milk also gives body, which nonfat milk lacks, and the most tender cuts of meat are high in fat, visible as the marbling of meat. In addition, many flavorings dissolve in fat. Heating spices in oil intensifies the flavors of an Indian curry or a Mexican dish by carrying the flavors to the sensory cells in the mouth that discriminate taste and smell. For these reasons, a person who has been following a typical North American diet will probably need some time to adjust to a lower-fat diet. For example, if one changes from the regular use of whole milk to 1% low-fat milk but then after a few weeks switches back to the whole milk, it will taste more like cream than milk. One has thus adjusted to the flavor of the low-fat milk and will likely now find the whole milk to be not as palatable. Emphasizing flavorful fruits, vegetables, and whole grains also helps one to adapt to a low-fat diet. Thus, it is certainly possible to make the change from a higher-fat diet to a lower-fat diet, but it takes some effort.

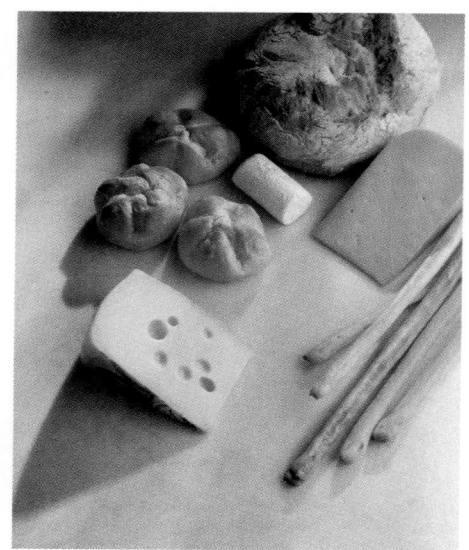

Fat is an important component of the flavor and overall appeal of cheese.

■ Hydrogenation of Fatty Acids Aids in Food Formulation But Increases Trans Fatty Acid Content

As mentioned previously, for the most part fats with long-chain saturated fatty acids are solid at room temperature, and those with unsaturated fatty acids are liquid at room temperature. In some kinds of food production, solid fats work better than liquid oils. In pie crust, for example, solid fats yield a flaky product, whereas crusts made with liquid oils tend to be greasy and more crumbly. If they are used to replace solid fats, oils with unsaturated fatty acids often must become more saturated (with hydrogen), as this solidifies the vegetable oils into shortenings and margarines. Hydrogen is added by bubbling hydrogen gas under pressure into liquid vegetable oils in a process called **hydrogenation** (Fig. 5.9). The fatty acids aren't fully hydrogenated to the saturated fatty acid form, as this would make the product too hard and brittle. Partial hydrogenation—leaving some monounsaturated fatty acids—creates a semisolid product.

In their original form, monounsaturated and polyunsaturated fatty acids are in the *cis* form (Fig. 5.10). By definition, the hydrogens in the *cis* form are on the same side of the carbon-carbon double bond. During hydrogenation, some hydrogens are transferred to opposite sides of the carbon-carbon double bond, creating the *trans* form, or a **trans fatty acid.** As seen in Figure 5.10, the *cis* bond causes the fatty acid backbone to bend, whereas the *trans* bond allows the backbone to remain straighter. This *trans* form makes it similar to the shape of a saturated fatty acid. This may be the mechanism whereby trans fatty acids raise LDL. Trans fatty acids also lower HDL. Thus, people with elevated LDL should limit intake of partially hydrogenated fat. It is less clear that this is important for the average person, as long as trans fatty acid intake is not

hydrogenation The addition of hydrogen to a carbon-carbon double bond, producing a single bond. Because hydrogenation of unsaturated fatty acids in a vegetable oil increases its hardness, this process is used to convert liquid oils into more solid fats, which are used in making margarine and shortening. Trans fatty acids are a by-product of hydrogenation of vegetable oils.

trans fatty acid A form of an unsaturated fatty acid, usually a monounsaturated one when found in food, in which the hydrogens on both carbons forming the double bond lie on opposite sides of that bond. A *cis* fatty acid has the hydrogens lying on the same side of the carbon-carbon double bond.

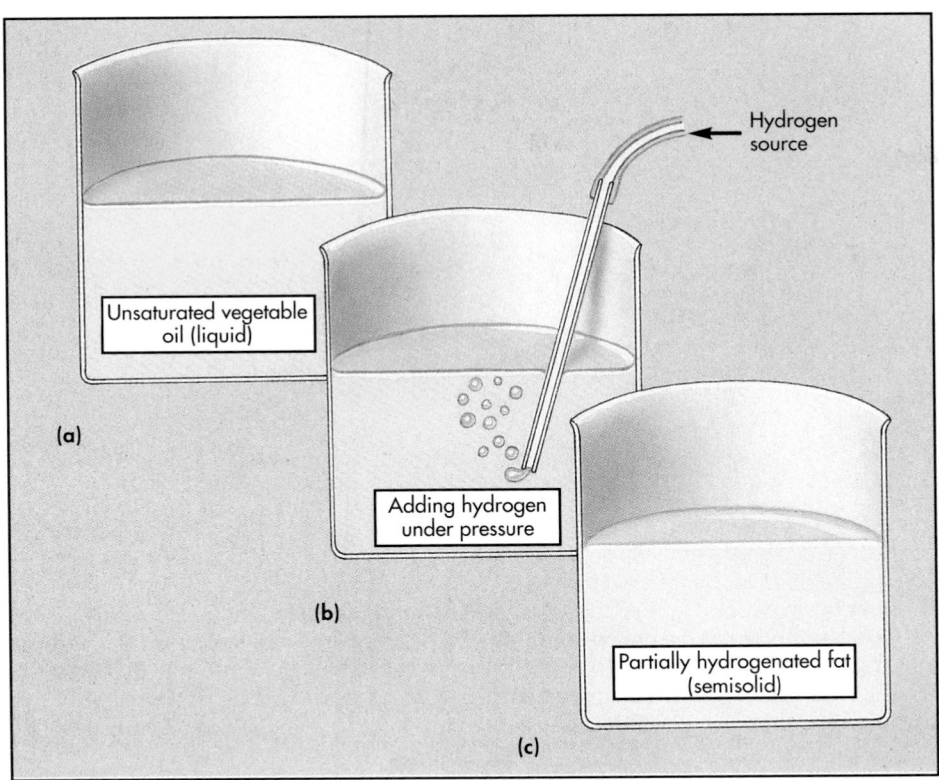

Figure 5.9 How liquid oils become solid fats. (a) Unsaturated fatty acids are present in liquid form. (b) Hydrogens are added (hydrogenation), changing some carbon-carbon double bonds to single bonds and producing some trans fatty acids. (c) The completed partially-hydrogenated product, which is likely to be used in margarine, shortening, or deep-fat frying.

excessive and the diet is adequate in polyunsaturated fat. However, since these fatty acids serve no particular role in maintaining body health, many experts concur with the latest Dietary Guidelines and advice from the American Heart Association that recommend minimal trans fatty acid intake.

As public pressure has persuaded manufacturers to eliminate the tropical oils rich in saturated fat (palm, palm olein, and coconut) from food processing, partially hydrogenated soybean oil—rich in trans fatty acids—has become the major replacement. Currently, trans fatty acid intake in North America is estimated to contribute about 3% of total calories, amounting to on average about 10 grams per day.

FDA is in the process of requiring the labeling of trans fatty acid content in foods. Currently no such labeling is present in the United States, but is so in Canada. FDA hopes to make consumers more aware of trans fatty acid intake, and as well as the negative health consequences associated with high intakes of trans fatty acids. North American companies are already responding to this issue before labeling is in place by creating products that are free of trans fatty acids. For example, Promise, Smart Beat, and some Fleischmann's margarines are now trans fatty acid–free products (less than 0.5 grams per serving). The new U.S. labeling requirements will likely combine grams of saturated fat and trans fatty acids into one category, with an asterisk after the total number, referring to a footnote at the base of the Nutrition Facts label detailing the exact amount of trans fatty acids.

This addition of listing trans fatty acids on labels will help consumers at the supermarket, but, when dining out, consumers are left in the dark as to which foods contain trans fatty acids. Currently, restaurant foods are rich not only in saturated fatty acids but also in trans fatty acids (Table 5.2). Knowing which foods are low in trans fatty acids when ordering at a restaurant is extremely difficult because the information

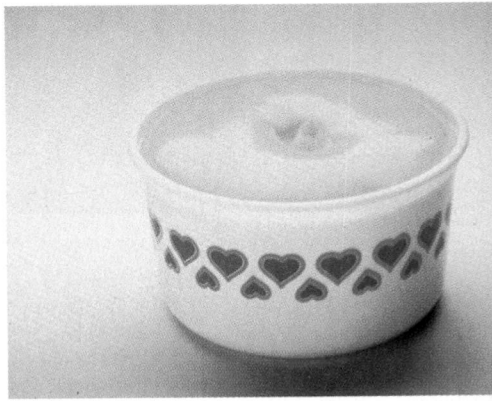

Tub margarine is much lower in trans fatty acids than stick margarine or shortenings (9%, 14%, and 26% of fatty acids respectively). Some newer brands of tub margarines are even free of trans fatty acids.

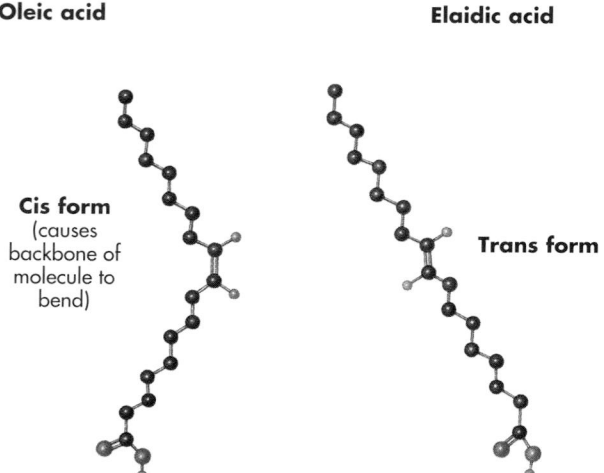

Figure 5.10 *Cis* and *trans* fatty acids. In the *cis* form at double carbon-carbon bonds in a fatty acid, the hydrogens (in blue) lie on the same side of the double bond. This causes a "kink" at that point in the fatty acid, which is typical of unsaturated fatty acids in nature. In contrast, in the *trans* form at double carbon-carbon bonds in a fatty acid, the hydrogens lie across from each other at the double bond. This causes the fatty acid to exist in a linear form, like a saturated fatty acid. *Cis* fatty acids are much more common in foods than *trans* fatty acids. The latter are primarily found in foods containing partially-hydrogenated fats, notably stick margarine, shortening, and deep-fat fried foods. *Trans* fatty acids raise LDL and lower HDL, so a generous intake is discouraged.
Illustration by William Ober.

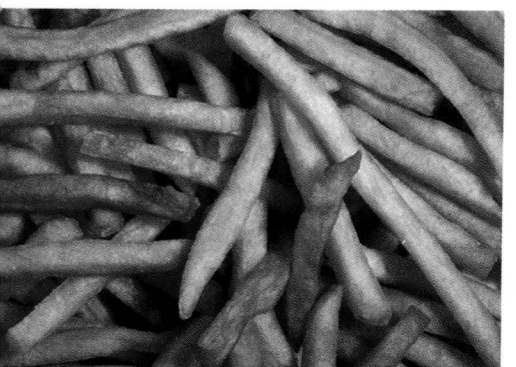

French fries are a common source of fat and trans fatty acids for many adults. For regular consumers, a small serving size is recommended if a person has elevated blood lipids, or weight control is a problem.

on how these foods are prepared or the precise fat composition is typically not available. You can follow this tip when ordering to limit trans fatty acids: Limit fried (especially deep-fat fried) food items, any pastries or flaky bread products (such as piecrusts, crackers, croissants, and biscuits), and cookies.

Until FDA approves and enforces the labeling of trans fatty acids, U.S. consumers can also make educated guesses on the trans fatty acid content of foods that have ingredients listed on the label (most foods do). If partially hydrogenated vegetable oil is one of the first three ingredients on the label, you can assume there is a significant amount of trans fatty acids in the product. Unfortunately, partially hydrogenated vegetable oil is a broad term that does not indicate the extent of hydrogenation. Although currently unavailable, this information would be helpful because, the more hydrogenated a product is, the more trans fatty acids it contains.

Limiting trans fatty acids at home is a much easier task. Most important, use little or no stick margarine or shortening; instead, substitute vegetable oils and softer tub margarines (whose labels list vegetable oil or water as the first ingredient). Avoid deep-fat frying any food in shortening. Substitute baking, pan-frying, broiling, steaming, grilling, or deep-fat frying in unhydrogenated vegetable oils. Replace nondairy creamers with reduced-fat or nonfat milk, since most nondairy creamers are rich in hydrogenated vegetable oils. Last, read all food ingredient's labels, using the tips listed on estimating trans fatty acid content.

▪ Fat Rancidity Limits Shelf Life of Foods

Decomposing oils emit a disagreeable odor and taste sour and stale. Stale potato chips are a good example. As double bonds in fatty acids break down, rancid by-products appear. Ultraviolet rays of light, oxygen, and certain procedures can break double bonds and, in turn, destroy the structure of polyunsaturated fatty acids. Saturated fats and trans fats can much more readily resist these effects. Why?

Table 5.2 Trans Fatty Acids in Restaurant Foods

Fried Foods	Calories	Total Fat (grams)	Trans Fat (grams)
Onion Rings (8 rings—6 oz)	650	47	7
Burger King French fries (king-size—6 oz)	540	24	7
McDonald's chicken nuggets (9)	510	29	3
McDonald's French fries (large—5 oz)	470	19	4
Fried mozzarella sticks (4 sticks—4 oz)	370	23	3
Fried fish (6 oz)	350	16	3
Miscellaneous Foods			
Prime rib, untrimmed (6 oz precooked weight)	480	35	3
Hamburger (5 oz)	470	26	2
Chicken pot pie (7 oz)	370	20	3
KFC biscuit (2 oz)	210	12	4
Pastries and Desserts			
Cinnabon Cinnabun (8 oz)	670	34	6
Apple pie (3.5 oz)	236	12	3

Adapted from *Nutrition Action Health Letter,* June 1999.

Rancidity is not a major problem for consumers because, although eating rancid oils can cause sickness, the odor and taste generally discourage us from eating enough to become sick. However, rancidity is a problem for manufacturers because it reduces a product's shelf life. For this reason, manufacturers often add hydrogenated plant oils to products to increase shelf life. Foods most likely to become rancid are deep-fried foods and foods with a large amount of exposed surface (such as powdered eggs or powdered milk). The fat in fish is also very susceptible to rancidity because it is highly polyunsaturated.

Vitamin E helps protect foods against rancidity because it acts as an antioxidant. It guards against the fat breakdown caused by various agents, such as metals found as impurities in vegetable oils. The vitamin E in plant oils reduces the breakdown of double bonds in fatty acids. (The role of vitamin E is explained more fully in Chapter 8.) When food manufacturers want to prevent rancidity in polyunsaturated fats, they often add **BHA** and **BHT.** (Chapter 16 discusses the safety of these and other food additives.) Look for these food additives in salad dressings, cake mixes, and other products that contain fat. They can even be added to a food's paper packaging. Vitamin C may also be added for the same reason. Manufacturers also tightly seal products and use other methods to reduce oxygen levels inside packages.

BHA, BHT Butylated hydroxyanisol and butylated hydroxytoluene—two common synthetic antioxidants added to foods.

■ Emulsifiers Improve Many Food Products

Food manufacturers add emulsifiers in the preparation of many food products, primarily to improve texture. For example, lecithins, monoglycerides and diglycerides, polysorbate 60, and other emulsifiers are added to salad dressings to keep the vegetable oil suspended in water (review Fig. 5.8). Eggs added to cake batters likewise emulsify the fat with the milk. Monoglycerides and related compounds are also good emulsifiers and, for that reason, are sometimes used in cake mixes and salad dressings. Over the next few days, examine the labels of salad dressings and cake mixes, and see how many emulsifiers are listed.

Concept Check

*F*at has a variety of roles in foods, including that of contributing to flavor and texture. Fat also provides the pleasurable mouth feel of many of our favorite foods, intensifies the taste of many spices, and tenderizes many popular cuts of meat.

Hydrogenation of unsaturated fatty acids consists of adding hydrogen to carbon-carbon double bonds to produce single bonds; some trans fatty acids are also created. Hydrogenation changes vegetable oil to solid fat. It is wise to monitor trans fatty acid intake, as this form of fat raises LDL and lowers HDL.

The carbon-carbon double bonds in polyunsaturated fatty acids are easily broken, yielding products responsible for rancidity. The presence of antioxidants, such as vitamin E in oils, naturally protects unsaturated fatty acids against oxidative destruction. Manufacturers can use hydrogenated fats and add synthetic antioxidants to reduce the likelihood of rancidity.

Manufacturers of commercial salad dressings find practical use for emulsification. Emulsifiers, such as lecithins, monoglycerides and diglycerides, and polysorbate 60 are added to salad dressings and other fat-rich products to keep the vegetable oils and other fats suspended in the water.

Trim meats before cooking to help reduce your saturated fat intake.

vegan A person who eats only plant foods.

Recommendations for Fat Intake

There is currently no RDA for fat. Standards for dietary fat and individual fatty acids (omega-3 and omega-6 fatty acids), phospholipids, and cholesterol, are under development and should be published in 2002 (see the website for this book for updates). To obtain the essential fatty acids, adults should consume about 4% of total energy intake from plant oils incorporated into foods and eat fatty fish at least twice a week. The typical North American diet derives about 7% of energy content from polyunsaturated fatty acids. An upper amount of 10% of energy intake as polyunsaturated fatty acids is often recommended, in part because the breakdown (oxidation) of those present in lipoproteins is linked to increased cholesterol deposition in the arteries, as discussed previously. Depression of immune function is also suspected to be caused by an excessive intake of polyunsaturated fats.

General consensus among nutrition experts suggests that we should limit saturated fat and trans fatty acid intake and that the diet needs to contain some omega-3 and omega-6 fatty acids. Furthermore, if fat intake exceeds 30% of calories, the extra fat should come from monounsaturated fat. No expert suggests that a diet be dominated by saturated fat or trans fat.

Dietary fat supplies about 33% of North Americans' total energy intake, in which the major sources are animal flesh, whole milk, pastries, cheese, margarine, and mayonnaise. In contrast, the major sources of fat in the Mediterranean Pyramid diet include liberal amounts of olive oil and the fat found in the small amount of animal flesh and dairy products allowed on the diet. The main sources of fat in Dr. Dean Ornish's **vegan** diet plan are a scant amount of vegetable oil used in cooking and the negligible amount found in various plant foods. Table 5.3 provides numerous tips for reducing fat intake.

Because many North Americans are at risk for developing cardiovascular disease, the American Heart Association (AHA) promotes dietary and lifestyle goals aimed at reducing this risk. One set of recommendations is made for the general public (Table 5.4). Then a more detailed list of recommendations is made for those at high risk or who currently have cardiovascular disease (Table 5.5). For high-risk individuals, the AHA recommendation is that total fat intake should not exceed 20% to 30% of total energy intake, with no more than 7% to 10% of total energy intake from saturated fat (include trans fat in the allowance). The intake of saturated fats currently averages about 13% of energy intake. Cholesterol intake should be no more than

Table 5.3 Tips for Avoiding Too Much Fat and Saturated Fat

1. Steam, boil, or bake vegetables. For a change, stir-fry in a small amount of vegetable oil. Consider buying an insert for a pot, so you can easily steam your vegetables.

2. Season vegetables with herbs and spices, rather than with sauces, butter, or margarine.

3. Try lemon juice on salad or use limited amounts of oil-based salad dressing.

4. To reduce saturated fat, use vegetable oils and tub margarine instead of butter, stick margarine, or hydrogenated shortenings in baked products.

5. Limit baked goods made with large amounts of fat, especially croissants, doughnuts, muffins, biscuits, and butter rolls.

6. Try whole-grain flours to enhance flavors when baking goods with less fat. Use applesauce and other fruit purees in place of fat when possible, such as in quick breads.

7. Replace whole milk with nonfat or reduced-fat or 1% milk in puddings, soups, and baked products and for use as a beverage.

8. Substitute plain low-fat yogurt, blender-whipped low-fat cottage cheese, or buttermilk in recipes that call for sour cream or mayonnaise.

9. Choose lean cuts of meat. Limit bacon, ribs, and high-fat ground meats.

10. Trim fat from meat before and after cooking.

11. Roast, bake, or broil meat, poultry, and fish, so that fat drains away as the food cooks.

12. Remove skin from poultry before cooking. This eliminates the temptation to eat it along with the meat.

13. Use a nonstick pan for cooking, so that added fat will be unnecessary; use a vegetable spray for frying.

14. Chill meat or poultry broth until the fat solidifies. Spoon off the fat before using the broth.

15. Eat a vegetarian main dish at least once a week. Include fish (cooked without much added fat) in the diet two times or more a week. Think about this when you make choices in a restaurant.

16. Choose fat-reduced ice cream, low-fat frozen yogurt, sorbet, and popsicles as substitutes for regular ice cream.

17. Try angel food cake, fig bars, and gingersnaps as substitutes for commercially baked goods high in saturated fat.

18. Limit high-fat cheese intake (replace with low-fat cheese if cheese is desired).

19. Read labels on commercially prepared foods to find out what type of fat or how much saturated fat they contain.

20. Use jam, jelly, or marmalade on bread and toast instead of butter or margarine.

21. Buy whole-grain breads and rolls. They have more flavor and do not need butter or margarine to taste good. The dietary fiber present is an added bonus.

22. Think about the balance of fats in the menu. If a meal contains whole milk, cheese, ice cream, a higher-fat meat, or poultry with skin, use tub margarine and unsaturated vegetable oils for your spreads and dressings. Small amounts of butter, sour cream, or cream cheese can be included if other menu items are low in saturated fat.

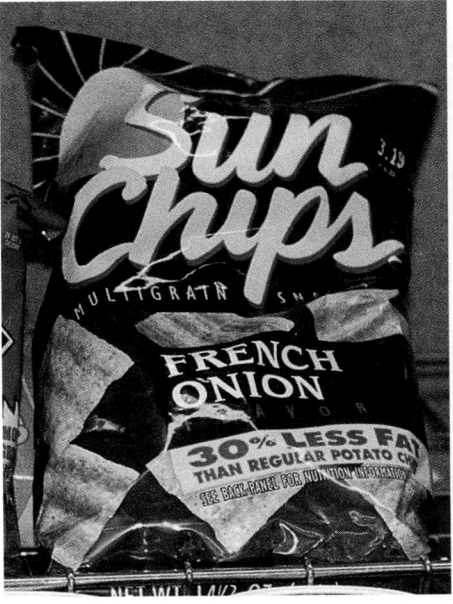

Many manufacturers offer products that are lower in fat than the traditional product. Even though these products are lower in fat, portion size and the total calories supplied still must be considered.

200–300 milligrams per day. Recall that we consume 200–400 milligrams per day, with men consuming the greater amount. Table 5.6 shows a diet that follows those guidelines. The latest guidelines from the National Cholesterol Education Program in the United States concur with this advice, except fat intake could be as high as 35% of total calories as long as saturated fat intake does not exceed 7% of calories and cholesterol intake does not exceed 200 milligrams per day. Making sure weight gain does not become a problem is also important when switching to such a high fat diet.

Current research shows that our palates can adapt to a lower fat intake over time, so we miss it less. Reducing fat intake also allows us to include more healthful foods—fruits, vegetables, and whole grains—in our diets. A good start for this type of diet is a low-fat breakfast: One option is a high-fiber cereal, reduced-fat or nonfat milk, and fruit juice.

Table 5.4 Current Dietary Guidance for the General Population (2 Years of Age and Older) from the American Heart Association

Population Goals	Major Guidelines
Overall healthy eating pattern	Include a variety of fruits, vegetables, grains, low-fat or nonfat dairy products, fish, legumes, poultry, lean meats.
Appropriate body weight	Match energy intake to overall energy needs, with appropriate changes to achieve weight loss when indicated.
Desirable blood cholesterol profile	Limit foods high in saturated fat and cholesterol; and substitute unsaturated fat from vegetables, fish, legumes, nuts.
Desirable blood pressure	Limit salt and alcohol (see Table 5.5); maintain a healthy body weight (see Table 5.5); and a diet with emphasis on vegetables, fruits, and low-fat or nonfat dairy products.

*R*ecommendations for fat intake are stated as percentages of total energy intake—usually 20% to 30%. The following table shows how many grams of fat per day are allowed with diets ranging from 1200 to 3900 kcal.

Energy Intake (kcal)	Fat Intake Grams	
	30% of Energy	20% of Energy
1200	40	27
1500	50	33
1800	60	40
2100	70	47
2400	80	53
2700	90	60
3000	100	67
3600	120	80
3900	130	87

Table 5.5 Specific Dietary Recommendations from American Heart Association, Especially for Those People at High Risk or Currently Have Cardiovascular Disease

Diet	**Consume at least:**
	5 servings of fruits and vegetables each day. Up to 9 servings per day is advised if the person has hypertension.
	6 servings of grains, including some whole grains, each day.
	At least 2 (3-ounce) servings of fish per week (or 900 milligrams of a combination of omega-3 fatty acids from fish oil supplements per day).
	25 grams of dietary fiber each day, including some sources of soluble fiber.
	Consume no more than:
	30% of calories from total fat or 20% if blood lipids are still too high.
	10% of calories as saturated fat, or 7% if blood lipids are still too high. As well, limit trans fatty acid intake (combine with saturated fat gram allowance).
	300 milligrams of cholesterol per day (on average), or 200 milligrams per day if blood lipids are still too high or the person has diabetes or cardiovascular disease.
	6 grams of salt each day (6 grams equals 2400 milligrams of sodium).
	2 alcoholic drinks per day for men and one drink for women.
	Additional advice includes:
	Specifically meeting vitamin B-6, folate, vitamin B-12, and potassium needs, limiting sugar intake, and possible use of soy protein and stanol/sterol containing margarines (see the Nutrition Issue for details). Megadose vitamin E supplements are not recommended at this time, and vitamin C and beta-carotene supplements provide no benefit.
Body Weight	Maintain a body mass index between 18.5 and 25. Waist circumference should not exceed 40 inches (102 centimeters) in men or 35 inches (88 centimeters) in women (see Chapter 10 for details).
Physical Activity	30 to 60 minutes of brisk activity on most, if not all, days of the week.

These specific recommendations apply to individuals 2 years of age and older. The latest guidelines from the National Cholesterol Education Program in the United States also concur with this advice for high-risk individuals, except that fat could be as high as 35% of total calories if saturated fat intake is 7% of calories or less and cholesterol intake does not exceed 200 milligrams per day.

Table 5.6 Daily Menu Examples Containing 2000 kcal and Various Percentages of Fat

30% of Energy As Fat		20% of Energy As Fat	
Food	Fat (grams)	Food	Fat (grams)
Breakfast			
Orange juice, 1 cup	0.5	Same	0.5
Shredded wheat, ¾ cup	0.5	Shredded wheat, 1 cup	0.7
Toasted bagel	1.1	Same	1.1
Tub margarine, 3 teaspoons	11.4	Tub margarine, 2 teaspoons	7.6
1% low-fat milk, 1 cup	2.5	Nonfat skim milk, 1 cup	0.6
Lunch			
Whole-wheat bread, 2 slices	2.4	Same	2.4
Roast beef, 2 ounces	4.9	Light turkey roll, 2 ounces	0.9
Mayonnaise, 3 teaspoons	11.0	Mayonnaise, 2 teaspoons	7.3
Lettuce	—	Same	—
Tomato	—	Same	—
Oatmeal cookie, 1	3.3	Oatmeal cookie, 2	6.6
Snack			
Apple	—	Same	—
Dinner			
Chicken tenders frozen meal	18.0	Fat-free chicken tenders	—
Dinner roll, 1	2.0	Same	2.0
Margarine, 1 teaspoon	3.8	Same	3.8
Banana	0.6	Same	0.6
1% low-fat milk, 1 cup	2.5	Non-fat skim milk, 1 cup	0.6
Snack			
Raisins, 2 teaspoons	—	Raisins, ½ cup	—
Air-popped popcorn, 3 cups	1.0	Air-popped popcorn, 6 cups	2.0
Margarine, 2 teaspoons	7.6	Same	7.6
Totals	73.1		44.3

Monitoring by a physician is important when fat is restricted to 20% of calories, as the resulting increase in carbohydrate intake can increase blood triglycerides in some people, which is not a healthful change. Over time, however, this problem of high blood triglycerides on a low-fat diet may self-correct, as has been shown in people following the Dr. Dean Ornish vegan diet for a year or more. Their blood triglycerides increased initially on the diet but, within a year, fell to normal values as long as they emphasized carbohydrate sources high in dietary fiber, controlled (or improved) body weight status, and followed a regular exercise program.

Recently some researchers have begun to question the dietary fat recommendation of 20% to 35% (or less) of total calories, stating that diet can be as high as 40% of calories from fat as long as saturated fat and trans fat intake is minimal and body weight is maintained (or improved). This change in advice is evidenced in the new book by Dr. Walter C. Willett, entitled *Eat, Drink, and Be Healthy* (2001). Dr. Willett is well respected among nutrition scientists. The diet plan in the book emphasizes whole grains, plant oils, vegetables in abundance, fruits at least two to three times per day, nuts and legumes one to three times per day, fish, poultry, and eggs zero to two times per day, dairy products one to two times per day, and little use of red meat,

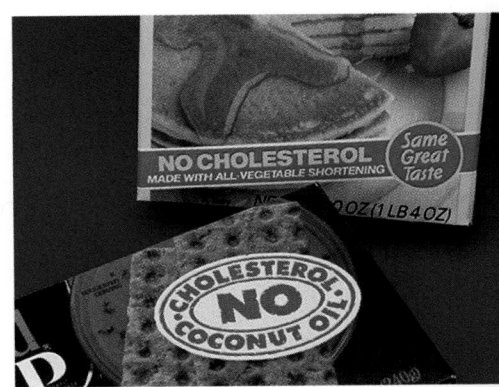

Manufacturers now offer a variety of low-cholesterol foods.

butter, white rice, white bread, potatoes, pasta, and sweets. Overall, this diet especially avoids simple sugars and refined carbohydrates because diets high in these constituents tend to raise blood triglycerides, which is not a healthful result. Diets high in these carbohydrates are discouraged, especially if a person is overweight (and so likely insulin-resistant; see Chapter 4 for details) and performs little physical activity (regular physical activity increases carbohydrate use). Table 5.7 shows a diet that contains 40% calories as fat and otherwise follows the plan indicated by Dr. Willett. This type of diet is also advocated for people who have Syndrome X (also called metabolic syndrome). Still, neither the American Heart Association nor the National Cholesterol Education Program in the United States endorses such a high fat intake.

Most people probably have no idea how much of the energy in their diets comes from fat. You've already tracked your food intake for one day. A Rate Your Plate exercise at the end of the chapter asks you to compare your fat intake with current guidelines. Using the information on food labels and recording and analyzing daily food intake also allow you to track fat intake.

Another Bite

The advice to consume 20% to 30% of energy as fat does not apply to infants and toddlers below the age of 2 years. These youngsters are forming new tissue, especially in the brain, so their intake of fat and cholesterol should not be greatly restricted.

Scenario *Follow-Up*

Jackie's approach to lowering blood cholesterol does not incorporate the best choices; she has excluded a great deal of fat in her diet by merely replacing it with refined carbohydrates. To make a shift to a more heart-healthy diet, Jackie would need to include at least 2 fruit and 3 vegetable servings a day, along with more whole-grain products (such as whole-wheat bread and a breakfast cereal that has at least 3 grams of fiber per serving). Lowering fat as drastically as she has is not really necessary, especially for a 21-year-old female who is physically active. Jackie could allow a more liberal amount of fat in her diet by including more monounsaturated fats (canola oil and olive oil, as well as fats found in nuts and avocados). These do not increase blood cholesterol. In addition to allowing more liberal fat intake from monounsaturated oils and including more fruits, vegetables, and whole grains, Jackie would benefit from including good sources of omega-3 fatty acids (fatty fish, flaxseeds, walnuts, or soybean and canola oil). One option is to use a canola oil-and-vinegar dressing on her salad, rather than lemon juice.

Concept Check

We need about 4% of total energy intake from plant oils to obtain the needed essential fatty acids. Eating fatty fish at least twice a week is also advised to supply omega-3 fatty acids. Many health-related agencies recommend a diet containing no more than 30% to 35% of energy intake as fat, with no more than 7% to 10% of energy intake as a combination of saturated fat and trans fat for the general public. Cholesterol intake should be limited to 200–300 milligrams per day. The current North American diet contains about 33% of energy content as fat, with about 13% of energy content as saturated fat and about 3% as trans fatty acids. Cholesterol intake varies from about 200–400 milligrams per day.

Table 5.7 A Diet Containing 40% of the Calories As Fat but Is Low in Saturated Fat and Trans Fat

Food	Fat (grams)	Saturated Fat (grams)
Breakfast		
¾ cup fresh orange juice	—	—
1 whole-grain bagel	2.0	—
2 teaspoons soft trans-free margarine	7.6	1.3
Snack		
1 cup raw carrots	—	—
2 celery stalks	—	—
3 tablespoons smooth trans-free peanut butter	24.5	5.0
Lunch		
¾ cup apple juice	—	—
Sandwich:		
2 slices whole-wheat bread	1.0	—
2 teaspoons mayonnaise	4.7	0.7
2 ounces light meat turkey	4.1	1.2
2 pieces lettuce	—	—
1 slice tomato	—	—
Salad:		
1½ cups tossed green salad	—	—
3 tablespoons Italian salad dressing	21.3	3.1
2 teaspoons dry sunflower seeds	3.0	0.3
1 ounce low-fat cheddar cheese	2.0	1.2
¼ cup green pepper slices	—	—
3 baby carrots	—	—
Snack		
1 cup fresh strawberries	0.6	—
½ cup plain skim yogurt	0.2	0.1
Dinner		
1 cup V8 juice	—	—
3.5 ounces broiled chicken breast	6.1	1.7
⅛ cup Italian dressing (marinade)	14.2	2.1
⅔ cup brown rice	—	—
2 teaspoons soft trans-free margarine	7.6	1.3
½ cup green beans	—	—
2 teaspoons soft trans-free margarine	7.6	1.3
1 cup grapes	0.7	—
Snack		
3 cups air-popped popcorn	1.0	—
Total	108	19

This diet contains 2400 calories and 7% of the calories as saturated fat. Whether monounsaturated fat or polyunsaturated fat would dominate depends on the type of oil used for salad dressings, such as canola oil for monounsaturated fat versus corn oil for polyunsaturated fat. Use of a vegetable oil rich in monounsaturated fat is the preferred choice. The cholesterol content is 180 milligrams. The trans fat content is less than 1% of the calories.

Summary

1. Compared with carbohydrates and proteins, lipids are a group of relatively oxygen-poor compounds that dissolve in organic solvents, such as chloroform, benzene, and ether. Saturated fatty acids contain no carbon-carbon double bonds, monounsaturated fatty acids contain one carbon-carbon double bond, and polyunsaturated fatty acids contain two or more carbon-carbon double bonds in the carbon chain. Triglycerides rich in long-chain saturated fatty acids tend to be solid at room temperature, whereas those rich in monounsaturated and polyunsaturated fatty acids are liquid at room temperature.

2. In omega-3 polyunsaturated fatty acids, the first of the carbon-carbon double bonds is located three carbons from the methyl end of the carbon chain. In omega-6 polyunsaturated fatty acids, the first carbon-carbon double bond counting from the methyl end occurs at the sixth carbon. Both omega-3 and omega-6 fatty acids are essential fatty acids; these must be included in the diet to maintain health.

3. Triglycerides are formed from a glycerol backbone with three fatty acids. Triglyceride is the major form of fat in both food and the body. It allows for efficient energy storage, protects certain organs, transports fat-soluble vitamins, and helps insulate the body. Phospholipids are derivatives of triglycerides. Phospholipids are important parts of cell membranes, and some act as efficient emulsifiers.

4. Cholesterol forms vital biological compounds, such as hormones, components of cell membranes, and bile acids. Cells in the body make cholesterol whether we eat it or not. It is not a necessary part of an adult's diet.

5. Body cells can synthesize hormone-like compounds from both omega-3 and omega-6 fatty acids. These compounds produced from omega-3 fatty acids tend to reduce blood clotting, blood pressure, and inflammatory responses in the body. Those produced from omega-6 fatty acids tend to increase blood clotting.

6. Foods rich in fat include salad oils, butter, margarine, and mayonnaise. Walnuts, bologna, avocados, and bacon are also high in fat, as are peanut butter and cheddar cheese. Steak and hamburger are moderate in fat content, as is whole milk. Many grain products, and fruits and vegetables in general, are very low in fat.

7. Fat digestion takes place primarily in the small intestine. Lipase enzyme released from the pancreas digests the long-chain triglyc-erides into smaller breakdown products—namely, monoglycerides (glycerol backbones with single fatty acids attached) and fatty acids. The breakdown products are then absorbed by the absorptive cells of the small intestine. These products are mostly resynthesized into triglycerides and combined with cholesterol, protein, and other substances to yield a chylomicron. Chylomicrons enter the lymphatic system, in turn passing into the bloodstream.

8. Lipids are carried in the bloodstream by various lipoproteins, which are particles consisting of a central triglyceride core encased in a shell of protein, cholesterol, and phospholipid. Chylomicrons are released from intestinal cells and carry lipids arising from dietary intake. Very-low-density lipoprotein (VLDL) and low-density lipoprotein (LDL) carry lipids both taken up by and synthesized in the liver. High-density lipoprotein (HDL) picks up cholesterol from cells and acts in allowing transport of it back to the liver.

9. In the blood, elevated amounts of LDL and low amounts of HDL are strong predictors of the risk for cardiovascular disease.

10. Fat adds flavor and texture to foods and can increase satiety after meals. Hydrogenation is the process of converting carbon-carbon double bonds into single bonds by adding hydrogen at the point of unsaturation. The partial hydrogenation of fatty acids in vegetable oils changes the oils to semi-solid fats and helps reduce rancidity, which results from the breakdown of fatty acids. This hydrogenation also increases the trans fatty acid content. High amounts of trans fatty acids in the diet are discouraged, as these increase LDL and reduce HDL. When fatty acids break down, food becomes rancid, emitting a foul odor and flavor. Some phospholipids are used in food as emulsifiers. These suspend fat in water.

11. There is currently no RDA for fat. We need about 4% of total energy intake from plant oils to obtain the needed essential fatty acids. Fatty fish is a rich source of omega-3 fatty acids and should be consumed at least twice a week.

12. The typical North American diet contains about 33% of total energy as fat. Many health agencies and scientific groups suggest a fat intake of no more than 30% to 35% of energy intake. Some health experts advocate an even further reduction to 20% of energy intake for some people, but such a diet requires professional guidance. If fat intake exceeds 30% of total calories, the diet should emphasize monounsaturated fat.

Study Questions

1. Describe the chemical structures of saturated and polyunsaturated fatty acids and their different effects in both food and the human body.

2. Relate the need for omega-3 fatty acids in the diet to the recommendation to consume fatty fish at least twice a week.

3. Describe the structures, origins, and roles of the four major blood lipoproteins.

4. What are the recommendations from various health-care organizations regarding fat intake? What does this mean in terms of actual food choices?

5. What are two important attributes of fat in food? How are these different from the general functions of lipids in the human body?

6. What is the significance of and possible uses for reduced-fat foods?

7. Does the total cholesterol concentration in the bloodstream tell the whole story with respect to cardiovascular disease risk?

Read the Nutrition Issue before answering the following questions:

8. List five risk factors for the development of cardiovascular disease.

9. What lifestyle factors decrease the risk of cardiovascular disease development?

10. When are medications most effective in cardiovascular disease therapy, and how in general do the various classes of medications operate to reduce risk?

Further Readings

1. de Lorgeril M and others: Mediterranean Diet: Traditional risk factors and the rate of cardiovascular complications after myocardial infarction. *Circulation* 99:779, 1999.

   People who had already suffered a heart attack and followed a Mediterranean Diet enjoyed a significantly reduced risk from suffering another heart attack. The majority of the subjects instructed on the Mediterranean Diet were compliant, suggesting that implementing this dietary style with instructions from trained individuals is not as difficult as one might think.

2. Expert Panel on Detection, Evaluation, and Treatment of High Blood Cholesterol in Adults: Executive summary of the third report of the National Cholesterol Education Program (NCEP) expert panel on detection, evaluation, and treatment of high blood cholesterol in adults (Adult Treatment Panel III). *Journal of the American Medical Association* 285:2486, 2001.

   All adults ages 20 years or older should have a fasting lipoprotein profile (total cholesterol, LDL-cholesterol, HDL-cholesterol, and triglycerides) once every 5 years. Diabetes no longer is considered just a risk factor for cardiovascular disease, but virtually guarantees the disease will develop. Other new recommendations are raising the desirable HDL-cholesterol level of 40 mg/dL or more, and using a combination of age, total cholesterol, HDL-cholesterol, blood pressure, and smoking history in a formula to determine which persons need cholesterol-lowering medications.

3. Healing broken hearts. *Nutrition Action Health Letter*, p. 1, June 1999.

   Dr. Dean Ornish reviews his diet solution to reversing atherosclerosis in people with obvious disease. The vegan diet used includes about 10% of calories from fat. Yoga, exercise, and stress-management sessions are additional lifestyle changes that are part of the diet plan.

4. Heinecke JW: Is the emperor wearing clothes? Clinical trials of vitamin E and the LDL oxidation hypothesis. *Atherosclerosis, Thrombosis, and Vascular Biology* 21:1261, 2001.

   Evidence that vitamin E supplements augment antioxidant defense mechanisms in the body is not compelling. The vitamin E doses used in the clinical trials have not been convincingly shown to inhibit development of cardiovascular disease in humans.

5. Hu FB and others: Dietary saturated fats and their food sources in relation to the risk of coronary heart disease in women. *American Journal of Clinical Nutrition* 70:1001, 1999.

   Along with other saturated fatty acids, stearic acid was found in this study to be associated with increased cardiovascular disease risk. Since saturated fats are usually found together in foods, there is no need to differentiate between them in the diet (e.g., mystric acid vs. stearic acid).

6. Hu FB and others: Types of dietary fat and risk of coronary heart disease: A critical review. *Journal of the American College of Nutrition* 20:5, 2001.

   Replacing saturated fat with unsaturated fat is more effective for lowering the risk of cardiovascular disease than simply reducing total fat consumption. There is strong evidence that a higher intake of omega-3 fatty acids from fish or plant sources lowers cardiovascular disease risk. The belief that fat is bad is widespread but is incorrect; saturated fat and trans fat should get the attention when recommending lower fat intakes.

7. Jacobs DR and others: Whole-grain intake may reduce the risk of ischemic heart disease death in postmenopausal women: The Iowa women's health study. *American Journal of Clinical Nutrition* 68:248, 1998.

   There is a clear association between a generous whole-grain intake and reduced risk of cardiovascular disease in women. The constituents of the whole grains that may be responsible for this reduced risk include phytochemicals, dietary fiber, and antioxidants.

8. Krauss RM and others: AHA Dietary Guidelines: Revision 2000: A Statement for Healthcare Professionals From the Nutrition Committee of the American Heart Association. *Circulation* 102:2284, 2000.

   This report contains the latest advice for the public regarding diet and cardiovascular disease from the American Heart Association. The revised guidelines place an increased emphasis on the need for weight control and heart-healthy diet.

9. Lichtenstein AH and others: Effects of different forms of dietary hydrogenated fats on serum lipid and cholesterol levels. *The New England Journal of Medicine* 340:1933, 1999.

   Oil that has not been hydrogenated was found to have the most favorable results on total blood cholesterol and LDL-cholesterol, whereas margarine that was high in trans fatty acids produced more negative blood cholesterol profiles.

10. Lius and others: A prospective study of dietary glycemic load, carbohydrate intake, and risk of coronary heart disease in U.S. women. *American Journal of Clinical Nutrition* 71:1455, 2000.

    A high intake of refined carbohydrates increases the risk of cardiovascular disease. The link exists primarily because these foods greatly increase insulin release and contribute to glucose intolerance.

11. Nicolosi RJ and others: Dietary effects on cardiovascular disease risk factors: Beyond saturated fat and cholesterol. *Journal of the American College of Nutrition* 20(5):4215s, 2001.

    Soy protein, soluble fiber, and plant sterols are all helpful in lowering blood cholesterol. Fruits, vegetables, and minimally processed grains are also helpful in lowering cardiovascular disease risk.

12. Stampfer M and others: Primary prevention of coronary heart disease in women through diet and lifestyle. *The New England Journal of Medicine* 343:16, 2000.

    Following a set of specific lifestyle factors, including a balanced diet with a small amount of wine each day, exercise, and abstinence from smoking, can help protect women from coronary heart disease.

13. Truan TL: Antioxidant supplements to prevent heart disease: Real hope or empty hype? *Postgraduate Medicine* 109(1):109, 2001.

    The notion that antioxidant supplements can prevent cardiovascular disease is not supported by current clinical evidence. Until conclusive evidence is available regarding the efficacy, safety, and appropriate dosage of antioxidants, the more prudent recommendation for the general public is to consume more fruits, vegetables, and whole grains.

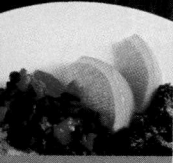

I. Are You Eating a Diet That Includes Many Saturated Fat and Trans Fatty Acid Sources?

Instructions:
Check the food you would typically select from the two choices given.

1. _____ Bacon and eggs or   _____ Ready-to-eat whole-grain breakfast cereal

2. _____ Doughnut or sweet roll or   _____ Whole-wheat (or white) roll, bagel, or bread, no margarine

3. _____ Breakfast sausage or   _____ Fruit

4. _____ Whole milk or   _____ Low-fat or nonfat milk

5. _____ Cheeseburger or   _____ Turkey sandwich, no cheese

6. _____ French fries or   _____ Plain baked potato with minimal added fat or salad with low-cal or fat-free dressing

7. _____ Meal including fried hamburger or fatty beef or   _____ Meal including broiled lean hamburger (ground round), chicken, or fish

8. _____ Creamed soup or   _____ Clear soup (could contain some meat or vegetables)

9. _____ Potato salad or   _____ Baked potato, limited added fat

10. _____ Cream/fruit pie or   _____ Graham crackers

11. _____ Ice cream or   _____ Frozen yogurt, sherbet, or fat-reduced ice cream

12. _____ Butter or stick margarine or   _____ Vegetable oils or soft margarine in a tub

Interpretation

The foods listed on the left tend to be high in saturated fat, trans fatty acids, cholesterol, and total fat. Those on the right generally are low. If you want to help reduce the risk of cardiovascular disease, choose the foods on the right more often than the foods on the left.

II. *What Is Your Current Fat and Cholesterol Intake?*

How do your food practices compare with general guidelines suggested for fat, saturated fat, and cholesterol intake? Refer to the nutritional assessment you completed at the end of Chapter 2, and compare it with the following guidelines, issued by the American Heart Association and the National Cholesterol Education Program in the United States for people at high risk for development of cardiovascular disease.

- Limit or reduce total fat intake to 20% to 35% or less of total energy intake.

- Reduce saturated fat intake to 7% to 10% of energy intake or less.

- Limit cholesterol to 200 to 300 milligrams per day.

To compare your nutritional assessment with these guidelines, first fill in the values for your intakes of the following:

TOTAL ENERGY: _____ **TOTAL FAT:** _____ **SATURATED FAT:** _____ **CHOLESTEROL:** _____

Now complete the following steps:

1. Multiply your total grams of fat by 9 (kcal per grams of fat). Then divide the result by your total energy intake. Next multiply this number by 100. This will give you the percentage of energy you consumed from fat.

   % OF ENERGY FROM FAT _____ IS IT 35% OR LESS OF TOTAL ENERGY INTAKE? YES _____ NO _____

2. Multiply your grams of saturated fat by 9 (kcal per grams of fat). Divide the result by your total energy intake. Now multiply this number by 100. This will give you the percentage of energy you consumed from saturated fat.

   % OF ENERGY FROM SATURATED FAT _____ IS IT 7% to 10% OF ENERGY INTAKE OR LESS? YES _____ NO _____

3. Look at your milligrams of cholesterol.

   IS YOUR INTAKE LESS THAN 200–300 milligrams? YES _____ NO _____

4. Look back at the foods you ate and notice the foods that contributed the most fat, saturated fat, and cholesterol. If you didn't meet one or more of the guidelines and had elevated LDL, how could you change what you ate that day to improve your diet?

5. Now take the next step. Do you know your blood lipid values? If not, have them checked soon. All adults should know whether these values are in the abnormal ranges.

6. Finally, fill in the following assessment of your risk for developing cardiovascular disease. Decide today how you could modify your diet and lifestyle, if necessary, to reduce your risk.

Do you have:	YES	NO		YES	NO
A history of smoking?	_____	_____	Diabetes?	_____	_____
Hypertension?	_____	_____	A history of physical inactivity?	_____	_____
High LDL?	_____	_____	A family history of premature cardiovascular disease (before age 60 years)?	_____	_____
Low HDL?	_____	_____	A history of obesity?	_____	_____
			A diet that lacks sufficient B vitamins, such as B-6, folate, and B-12?	_____	_____

Other factors also could be considered, as discussed in the Nutrition Issue, but this provides a good start for assessing your risk.

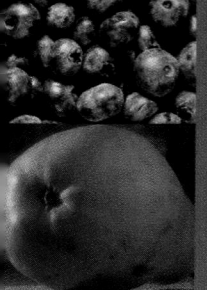
Cardiovascular disease typically involves the coronary arteries and, thus, frequently the term coronary heart disease (CHD) or coronary artery disease (CAD) is used.

A heart attack can strike with the sudden force of a sledgehammer, with pain radiating up the neck or down the arm. It can also sneak up at night, masquerading as indigestion, with slight pain or pressure in the chest. Many times, the symptoms are so subtle in women that it often is too late once she or the health professional realizes that a heart attack is taking place. If there is any suspicion at all that a heart attack is taking place, the person should first chew an aspirin (325 milligrams) thoroughly and then call 911. Aspirin helps reduce the blood clotting that leads to a heart attack. Typical warning signs are:

- Intense, prolonged chest pain or pressure, sometimes radiating to other parts of the upper body (men and women)
- Shortness of breath (men and women)
- Sweating (men and women)
- Nausea and vomiting (especially women)
- Dizziness (especially women)
- Weakness (men and women)
- Jaw, neck, and shoulder pain (especially women)
- Irregular heartbeat (men and women)

Cardiovascular disease is the major killer of North Americans. Each year about 500,000 people die of coronary heart disease in the United States alone. The figure rises to almost 1 million if strokes and other circulatory diseases are included in the global term *cardiovascular disease*. About 1.5 million people in the United States each year have a heart attack. The overall male-to-female ratio for cardiovascular disease is about 2:1. Women generally lag about 10 years behind men in developing the disease. Still, it eventually kills more women than any other disease—twice as many as does cancer. And, for each person in North America who dies of cardiovascular disease, 20 more have symptoms of the disease.

Healthy People 2010 has set a goal of reducing death from coronary heart disease by 30%, compared with today's incidence.

Worldwide, the highest incidence of cardiovascular disease occurs in the Russian Federation; in contrast, the lowest incidence occurs in Japan. The U.S. and Canadian numbers are midway between those of these two countries. This highlights the powerful influence of environment and lifestyle factors on its development.

Development of Cardiovascular Disease

The symptoms of cardiovascular disease develop over many years and often do not become obvious until old age. Nonetheless, autopsies of young adults under 20 years of age have shown that many of them had atherosclerotic plaque in their arteries. This finding indicates that plaque buildup can begin in childhood and continue throughout life, although it usually goes undetected for quite some time.

Preventing premature cardiovascular disease—that which appears before age 60 years—deserves everyone's consideration. Heart attacks at ages 40 through 60 are closely linked to the risk factors discussed later in this feature. Most people at risk can greatly improve their chance to avoid premature cardiovascular disease by making some long-term lifestyle changes, as has been clearly demonstrated in women.

The typical forms of cardiovascular disease—coronary heart disease and strokes—are associated with inadequate blood circulation in the heart and brain. Blood supplies the heart muscle and brain—and other body organs—with oxygen and nutrients. When blood flow via the coronary arteries surrounding the heart is interrupted, the heart muscle can be damaged. A heart

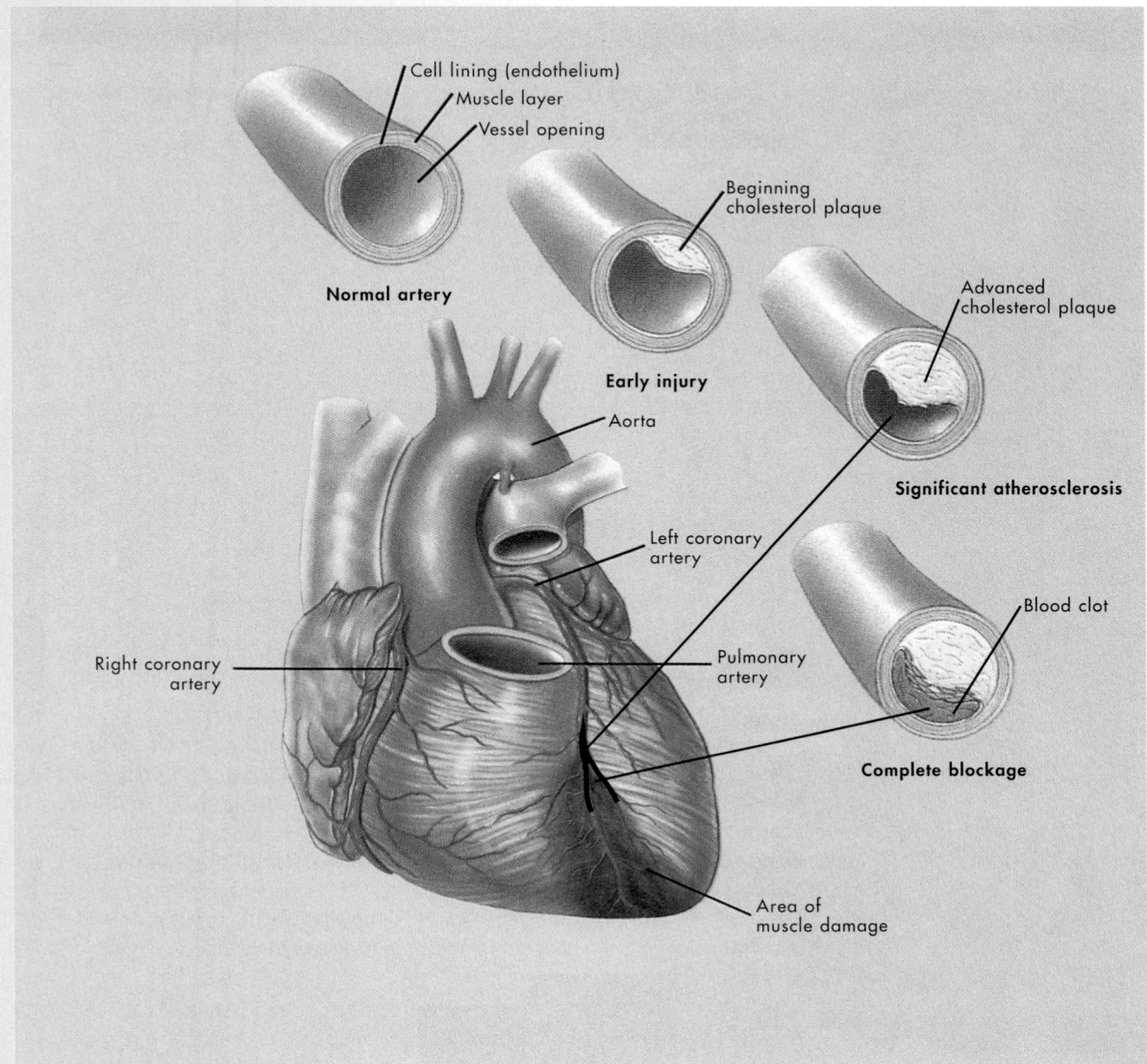

Figure 5.11 The road to a heart attack. Injury to an artery wall begins the process. This is followed by a progressive buildup of plaque in the artery walls. The heart attack represents the final phase of the process. Blockage of the left coronary artery by a blood clot is evident. The point where arteries such as these branch into small arteries is the typical site of major blockage. The heart muscle that is served by the portion of the coronary artery beyond the point of blockage lacks oxygen and nutrients; it is damaged and may die. This can lead to a significant drop in heart function and often total heart failure.

attack, or **myocardial infarction,** may result (Fig. 5.11). This may cause the heart to beat irregularly or to stop altogether. About 25% of people do not survive their first heart attack. If blood flow to parts of the brain is interrupted long enough, part of the brain dies, causing a **cerebrovascular accident,** or **stroke.** When a stroke causes loss of muscle control, death may occur.

More than 95% of all heart attacks are caused by blood clots that stop blood flow to the heart or brain. Clots form more readily where atherosclerotic plaque has built up in the arteries that serve the heart (coronary arteries) or brain (carotid arteries) (Fig. 5.12). Actually, the most dangerous lesions aren't the large, advanced ones but the smaller, unstable lesions covered by a thin, fibrous cap. In essence, heart attacks generally are caused not by total blockage of the coronary arteries by plaque but by disruption of a partial blockage, leading to eventual clot formation.

myocardial infarction Death of part of the heart muscle.

cerebrovascular accident (CVA) Death of part of the brain tissue due typically to a blood clot. Also termed a stroke.

continued

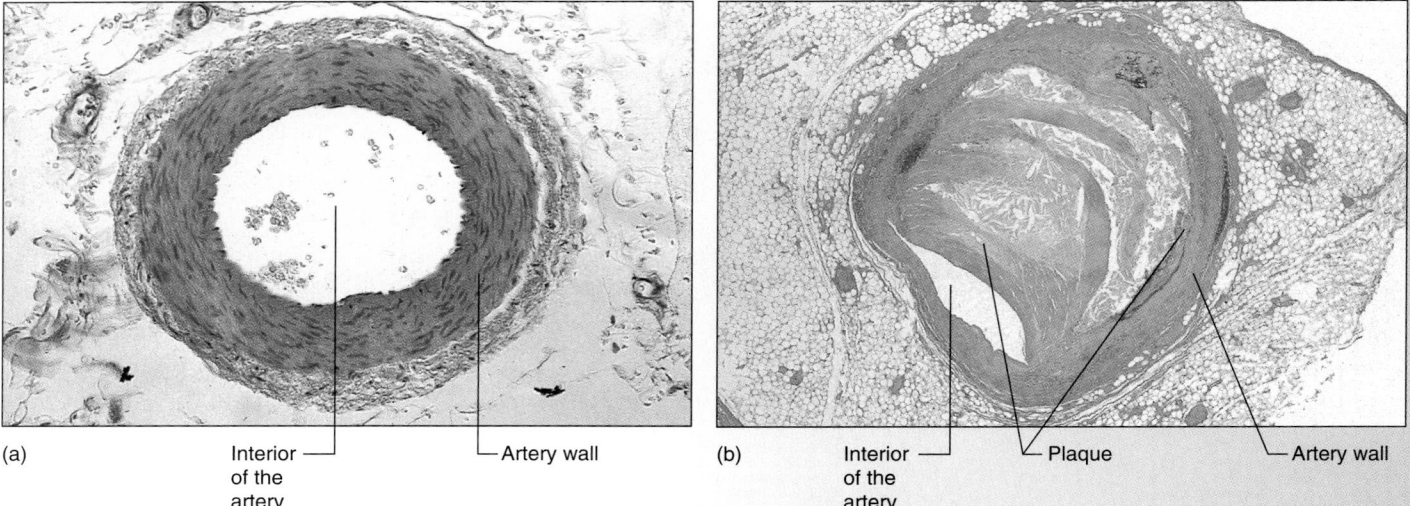

(a) Interior of the artery — Artery wall (b) Interior of the artery — Plaque — Artery wall

Figure 5.12 Atherosclerosis. (a) Cross section of a healthy coronary artery. (b) Cross section of a coronary artery with advanced atherosclerosis. The greatly reduced interior size in the diseased artery can easily be blocked by a blood clot or portion of plaque that breaks off another site and lodges in the narrowed portion of the artery. The latest research indicates, however, that these large plaques pose less of a risk than smaller plaques with a thinner fibrous cap, as the latter rupture very readily. This then leads to blood clots.

*W*hen 28-year-old gold medallist Sergei Grinkov died suddenly of a heart attack while ice skating, researchers investigated the case and discovered a protein abnormality in his blood. This abnormal protein caused Grinkov's blood to clot easier than normal. Grinkov was otherwise healthy. The only cardiovascular disease risk factor he had was that his father died of a heart attack at the age of 52. It is thought that up to 25% of North Americans may have this same protein abnormality and that the only sign is a family history of heart-related death under age 60. For this reason, it is wise for all adults to have a careful evaluation of cardiovascular disease risks conducted by a physician.

As mentioned earlier in this chapter, plaque is probably first deposited to repair injuries in a vessel lining. It develops especially at points where an artery branches into two arteries. Much stress is placed on an artery at these points from the changes in blood flow that occur at the branch point. The *athero* in *atherosclerosis* comes from the Greek and means "gruel or paste." This process of damage repair is part of the initiation phase of atherosclerosis. The rate of further plaque deposition in the next phase, called the progression phase, partly depends on the amount of LDL in the blood. The plaque thickens as layers of cholesterol (part of LDL), muscle cells, various proteins, and calcium are deposited. Arteries harden and narrow as plaque builds up, making them less elastic. They are thus unable to expand to accommodate alterations in blood pressure.

Affected arteries become further damaged as blood pumps through them and pressure increases. Finally, in the terminal phase, a clot or spasm in a plaque-clogged artery leads to a heart attack.

Factors that typically bring on a heart attack in a person at risk include dehydration, acute emotional stress (such as firing an employee), strenuous physical activity when not otherwise physically fit (shoveling snow, for example), waking during the night or getting up in the morning (linked to an abrupt increase in stress), and consuming large, high-fat meals (increases blood clotting).

Risk Factors for Cardiovascular Disease

Many of us are free of the risk factors that contribute to rapid development of atherosclerosis. If so, the advice of health experts is to simply consume a balanced diet, perform regular physical activity, have a complete fasting lipoprotein performed at age 20 or beyond, and reevaluate risk factors every 5 years.

People who face the highest risk for premature cardiovascular disease have a rare genetic defect, which substantially blocks the clearance of chylomicrons and triglycerides from the blood, reduces LDL uptake by the liver, limits synthesis of HDL, or enhances blood clotting. Other medical conditions, such as certain forms of liver and kidney disease, low concentrations of thyroid hormone, and use of certain medications to treat hypertension, can increase LDL and thus increase the risk for cardiovascular disease.

For most people, however, the most likely risk factors are

- Total cholesterol over 200 milligrams per 100 milliliters of blood (mg/dl; dl is short for 100 milliliters) especially when it is at or over 240 mg/dl and coupled with LDL-cholesterol over 130 to 160 mg/dl (130 mg/dl is used for people with two or more cardiovascular disease risk factors). The term LDL-cholesterol (and HDL-cholesterol) is used when expressing the blood concentration since it is the cholesterol content of these lipoproteins that is actually measured. The reference standard for expressing blood lipid concentrations also generally refers to the **serum** concentration. This is what remains after blood clots, and is then centrifuged to remove all red and white blood cells and clotting factors. Although *blood cholesterol* is a common term, the value actually refers to the concentration in the serum portion of the blood.
- HDL-cholesterol under 40 mg/dl, especially when the ratio of total cholesterol to HDL-cholesterol is greater than 4:1. Women often have high values for HDL-cholesterol and therefore it is important for this to be measured in women to establish cardiovascular disease risk. A value ≥60 mg/dl is especially protective.
- Age. Men over 45 years and women over 55 years.
- Family history of premature cardiovascular disease, especially before age 55 in a father or brother and 65 in a mother or sister.
- Smoking. This generally negates the female advantage of later presentation of the disease and is the main cause of about 20% of cardiovascular disease deaths. A combination of smoking and oral contraceptive use worsens matters even more. Smoking greatly increases the ultimate expression of a person's genetically linked risk for cardiovascular disease and even increases risk if one's blood lipids are low. Smoking also makes blood more likely to clot. Even secondhand smoke has been implicated.
- Hypertension. **Systolic blood pressure** over 140 (millimeters of mercury) and **diastolic blood pressure** over 90 indicate hypertension. Ideal blood pressure values are less than 120 and 80, respectively. (Treatment of hypertension is reviewed in Chapter 9.)
- Diabetes. This disease negates the female advantage. Insulin increases cholesterol synthesis in the liver, in turn increasing LDL in the bloodstream. Recently, diabetes has even been removed from the list of risk factors, stating its presence virtually guarantees development of cardiovascular disease, and so puts such a person in the high-risk group.
- Obesity (especially fat accumulation in the waist). Typical weight gain seen in adults is a chief contributor to the increase in LDL seen with aging. Obesity also typically leads to insulin resistance, creating a diabetes-like state, and ultimately the disease itself.
- Inactivity. Exercise conditions the arteries to adapt to physical stress. Regular exercise also improves insulin action in the body. The corresponding reduction in insulin output leads to a reduction in lipoprotein synthesis in the liver. Both regular aerobic exercise and resistance exercise are recommended. A person with existing cardiovascular disease should seek physician approval before starting such a program, as should older adults (see Chapter 11).

Researchers are currently trying to unravel and quantify numerous other factors that may be linked to premature cardiovascular disease, such as the connection between inadequate intake of vitamin B-6, folate, and vitamin B-12 and increased homocysteine in the blood. As noted in the chapter, homocysteine may damage the cells lining the blood vessels, in turn promoting atherosclerosis. It is likely the cause in about 10% of cases especially if the person has evidence of cardiovascular disease. Ongoing inflammation in the blood vessels is also gaining much attention.

The term *risk factor* is not intended to mean causality; nevertheless, the more of these risk factors one has, the greater the chances of ultimately developing cardiovascular disease. A good example is Syndrome X (also called metabolic syndrome). Recall from Chapter 4 that such a person would have abdominal obesity, high blood triglycerides, low HDL-cholesterol, hypertension, and evidence of insulin resistance (i.e., high fasting blood glucose) and increased blood clotting. This profile raises the risk for cardiovascular disease considerably. On a positive note, premature cardiovascular disease is rare in populations who have low LDL-cholesterol, have normal blood pressure, and do not smoke. By minimizing these three risk factors, along with following the Food Guide Pyramid (or related pyramid) and staying physically active, one will most likely reduce

Most commonly, LDL-cholesterol is not actually measured in a serum sample but is calculated using the following equation: LDL-cholesterol = total cholesterol − HDL-cholesterol − (triglycerides/5). This formula cannot be used, however, if blood triglycerides are >400 mg/dl. Recently laboratories have also implemented a test that measures LDL-cholesterol directly (without the use of this formula).

systolic blood pressure The pressure in the arterial blood vessels associated with the pumping of blood from the heart.

diastolic blood pressure The pressure in the arterial blood vessels when the heart is between beats.

Healthy People 2010 has set a goal of reducing total blood cholesterol among adults from an average of 206 mg/dl to 199 mg/dl, as well as a reduction in the percentage of adults with high blood cholesterol from 21% to 17%.

continued

Critical Thinking

As part of his annual health checkup, Juan has a blood sample drawn for the measurement of cholesterol values. The results of the test indicate that his total cholesterol is 210 mg/dl, HDL cholesterol is 65 mg/dl, and triglycerides are 100 mg/dl. Juan has read that total cholesterol should be less than 200 mg/dl to minimize cardiovascular problems. However, he is happy with the results of the blood test. How would Juan explain his satisfaction to his parents?

many of the other, less common controllable risk factors as well. In other words, develop and follow a total lifestyle plan. Still, if a person has a history of premature cardiovascular disease in the family but the usual risk factors aren't present, a rarer defect might be the cause. In this case, having a detailed physical examination for other potential causes is advised because only about 50% to 60% of one's risk for cardiovascular disease can be accounted for by the main risk factors just discussed.

Lowering LDL-cholesterol by Diet Changes

If your LDL-cholesterol is high, the first step should be a detailed examination by a physician. Some diseases (for example, a form of kidney disease) raise LDL-cholesterol, and treating the disease may remedy the LDL problem as well. If no such disease is present, diet change is advised.

Nutrition experts recommend several approaches for lowering LDL-cholesterol. Because changes that work for one person may be ineffective for another, values should be rechecked a month or so after any of the changes discussed here are implemented.

Reducing Dietary Saturated Fat and Cholesterol Intake

Reducing saturated-fat intake can lower elevated LDL. Although high total cholesterol in the blood indicates that an individual is at risk for cardiovascular disease, the most potent dietary factor associated with a high LDL-cholesterol value is overconsumption of saturated fat, not of cholesterol.

Almost everyone who minimizes saturated-fat intake can lower elevated LDL-cholesterol by about 15% to 20%, especially if the person has been eating lots of foods that are high in saturated fat. About 10% of the population has trouble decreasing LDL-cholesterol by dietary means. Genetic defects are one reason. On the other hand, about 10% can expect an even bigger drop.

About 20% of the population who eat a diet low in saturated fat find that reducing dietary cholesterol lowers LDL-cholesterol even more. Still, most authorities encourage a general limitation of cholesterol intake to less than 200–300 milligrams per day, especially for people with diabetes. Reducing cholesterol intake minimizes the cholesterol content of the chylomicrons that arise right after eating. Deposition of cholesterol from circulating chylomicrons probably contributes to atherosclerosis.

High intakes of saturated fat affect the liver's ability to clear LDL from the bloodstream, leading to increased LDL-cholesterol values. It appears that saturated fatty acids promote an increase in the amount of free cholesterol (not attached to fatty acids) in the liver, whereas unsaturated fatty acids do the opposite. As free cholesterol in the liver increases, it causes the liver to reduce cholesterol uptake from the bloodstream, contributing to elevated LDL-cholesterol. (Trans fatty acids are thought to act in the same ways as saturated fatty acids.)

The contribution of dietary saturated fat to elevated LDL-cholesterol can be minimized by eating no more than 7% to 10% of total energy as saturated fats. Finding substitutes for foods rich in animal fat, such as butter, shortening, and partially hydrogenated (solid) fats (i.e., trans fatty acids) is a must. Routinely reading food labels is also important, as saturated fats are often hidden in foods.

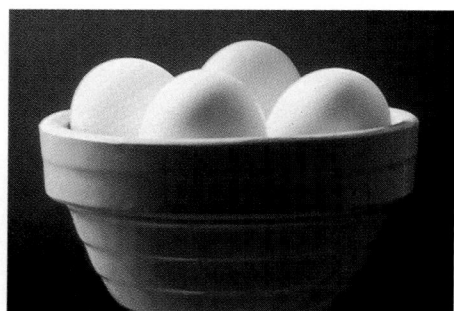

Eggs are the principal source of cholesterol in the North American diet.

Only animal and fish products contain cholesterol (review Table 5.1). Although egg whites contain no cholesterol, a single egg yolk contains about 210 milligrams of cholesterol. Thus, to meet the recommendation for cholesterol intake of no more than 300 milligrams per day, intake of egg yolks must be limited to no more than one per day. A reduction to 200 milligrams per day would essentially mean consuming egg yolks only occasionally. Many egg-containing foods (for example, pancakes, French toast, cookies, and cakes) can be prepared using egg whites rather than whole eggs. Cholesterol-free egg substitutes are also available in the grocery store. Most of these are egg whites colored yellow, to which a small amount of fat has been added to improve the flavor. Trimming the fat before and after cooking a 3- to 4-ounce serving of chicken, beef, or pork leaves roughly one-third to one-half the cholesterol content of an egg. A 10-ounce portion of meat can contain 260 milligrams of cholesterol, slightly more than the amount of one egg. If meats have a reputation for being high in cholesterol, it is mainly because of an overly generous portion size.

■ Increasing Monounsaturated and Polyunsaturated Fat Intake

Until recently, polyunsaturated fatty acids, but not monounsaturated fatty acids, were recommended as a substitute for saturated fatty acids in the diet to lower LDL-cholesterol. However, recent studies show that both monounsaturated and polyunsaturated fatty acids have this effect. In fact, monounsaturated fatty acids may be more beneficial, since LDLs containing these fatty acids are less likely to be oxidized. Recall that oxidized LDL probably contributes more to plaque formation in the arteries than does LDL itself. The key here is to replace saturated fat with monounsaturated fat, not simply to add it to the diet. This may also be beneficial for both blood triglycerides and HDL, because diets that are very low in fat and very high in carbohydrate tend to raise triglycerides and decrease HDL-cholesterol in some people, as discussed in the chapter. This can be avoided by replacing saturated fat in the diet with mostly monounsaturated fat.

However, increasing intake of monounsaturated fat is difficult for the typical North American. Foods and meals rich in monounsaturated fats are not widely available here, nor are they a big part of our cuisine. If you do much of your own cooking, using canola oil, canola oil blended with other vegetable oils, and olive oil on a regular basis will increase your intake of monounsaturated fats. A further emphasis on monounsaturated fat would probably require the counsel of a registered dietitian to design a specific meal pattern. One approach could be the Mediterranean Pyramid discussed in Chapter 2.

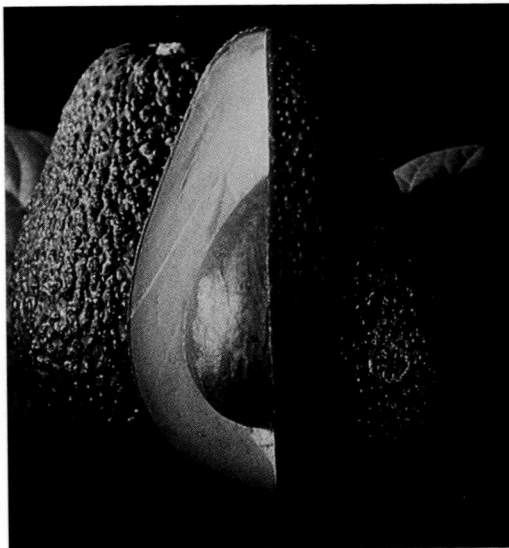

Most fruits and vegetables are low in fat; however, avocados are an exception. Most of this fat is monounsaturated.

■ Increasing Dietary Fiber Intake

Another dietary means of reducing LDL-cholesterol is increasing intake of soluble fibers, as discussed in Chapter 4. These bind bile acids and, so, reduce their reabsorption. The liver must pull cholesterol out of the bloodstream to make new bile acids. This then lowers LDL in the bloodstream. Although large amounts of fiber must be eaten to have a significant effect, any amount helps—and has other health benefits. Diets with an overall fiber content of 20 to 30 grams per day, especially those that emphasize soluble fiber, are most effective. Most people would have to change their diets extensively to achieve high intakes of soluble fiber. Instead, the focus could simply be on high-fiber foods—fruits, vegetables, beans, and whole grains. Use of the psyllium fiber found in some laxatives also helps meet this goal.

▌ Lowering Blood Triglycerides

Blood triglycerides are the most diet-responsive blood lipid. Ideally, these should be 150 mg/dl or lower when in a fasted state. Not overeating, limiting alcohol and simple-sugar intake, spreading meals throughout the day (not just one or two), and including some fatty fish in the diet on a regular basis all help. Controlling diabetes, if present, also is important, as are losing excess weight, performing regular physical activity, and not smoking.

▌ Raising HDL-cholesterol: A Difficult Task

Physical activity is one way to raise HDL-cholesterol. Exercising for at least 45 minutes four times a week can raise it by about 5 mg/dl. Sedentary people, in particular, should focus on increasing physical activity because this has other heart-healthy benefits as well. Losing excess weight (especially around the waist) and avoiding smoking also help maintain or raise HDL-cholesterol.

In addition, eating regularly (three or more balanced meals daily), balancing the amount of energy eaten with that expended, and eating less total fat often raise HDL-cholesterol because these practices lower blood triglycerides. This in turn is associated with higher HDL-cholesterol. The reason for this is not clear. Certain medications, such as high doses of the vitamin nicotinic acid and the medications gemfibrozil (Lopid) and certain "statin" drugs (see the following

continued

section on medical intervention), also lower blood triglycerides, thereby indirectly increasing HDL-cholesterol.

Consumption of alcohol is also associated with higher HDL-cholesterol and reduced blood clotting—two factors that reduce the risk of heart attack. However, excessive consumption of alcohol has many negative effects. The Dietary Guidelines indicate that most people can consume one to two drinks daily (no more) without negative health consequences. But, for people at risk for alcoholism, any alcohol may be too much (see Chapter 7).

It is unfortunate that raising HDL-cholesterol is difficult. Lowering LDL-cholesterol is much easier. Sometimes, as LDL-cholesterol falls, so does HDL-cholesterol. This often occurs with very-low-fat diets. However, if LDL-cholesterol drops to about 100 mg/dl, the fall in HDL-cholesterol is not of much concern. Researchers note that the main problem with low HDL-cholesterol is for people who have high LDL-cholesterol. In this case, the HDL fraction has not increased to compensate for the high LDL-cholesterol value. Researchers also note that people in rural Asia who eat low-fat diets generally have low LDL-cholesterol and HDL-cholesterol, but they also show low risk for cardiovascular disease.

Medical Intervention

Some people need even more aggressive therapy added to their regimen of a diet and lifestyle overhaul. The clearest indication for this more aggressive approach is in people who already have had a heart attack or have cardiovascular disease symptoms or diabetes.

Medications are the cornerstone of this more aggressive therapy. The National Cholesterol Education Program in the United States has developed a formula based on age, total blood cholesterol, HDL-cholesterol, smoking history, and blood pressure to determine who needs such medications. Check out this formula at www.nhlbi.nih.gov/guidelines/cholesterol/index/htm. Currently, medications work to lower LDL in one of two ways. Some reduce cholesterol synthesis in the liver. Such medicines are known as "statins" (e.g., atorvistatin [Lipitor]). The cost of being on one of these drugs ranges from $1000–$1800 per year, depending on the dose needed. These medications lead to problems in some people, and so require physician monitoring. The other group of medications binds bile acids in the small intestine and leads to their elimination in the feces. This requires the liver to synthesize new bile acids. The liver removes LDL from the blood to do this. These medications taste gritty and therefore are not very popular. Use of one or both of these classes of medications should ideally drive LDL down to about 100 mg/dl—the current therapeutic goal for people with (or at high risk for) cardiovascular disease.

A third group of drugs can be used to lower blood triglycerides for decreasing the triglyceride production of the liver. As mentioned, these include gemfibrozil (Lopid) and megadoses of the vitamin nicotinic acid. The use of nicotinic acid does result in pesky side effects, however, but these are typically manageable.

Other Possible Medical Therapies for Cardiovascular Disease

Cholestin comes from a strain of Chinese red yeast that has been used as a natural flavoring agent and food coloring in Chinese cooking for many years. Cholestin has an active "statin" component as do the prescription medications. Cholestin has been successful in reducing blood cholesterol in numerous studies. However, currently FDA does not regulate this product based on the limitation put on FDA by the U.S. Congress with regard to dietary supplements (see the Nutrition Issue in Chapter 1). Cholestin is labeled as a dietary supplement and can be purchased in many stores. However, to self-prescribe cholestin as a drug in the treatment of high blood cholesterol is not recommended by many physicians, due to lack of regulation by FDA. The lack of FDA oversight means that consumers cannot be sure the dietary supplement contains the active ingredient or the amount specified on the bottle. Cholestin is also very expensive. Overall, high blood cholesterol is a serious disease that requires medical supervision. In addition, if a physician does not

A s noted earlier, aspirin in small doses reduces blood clotting. It is often used under a physician's guidance to treat people at risk for heart attack or stroke, especially if one has already occurred. Studies show this with 325 milligrams of aspirin per day. One recent study suggests that only 80–160 milligrams per day may be needed for benefits. This lower amount would decrease the side effects of the aspirin, such as risk for ulcers (see Chapter 3).

follow a person, how will the person know that cholestin is actually lowering blood cholesterol? For this reason, cholestin should be used in conjunction with a physician's supervision.

FDA has approved two margarines that have positive effects on blood cholesterol levels—Benecol and Take Control. These margarines contain plant stanols/sterols, which have been researched since the 1950s for their cholesterol-lowering effects. However, it wasn't until the mid-1990s that researchers modified the plant stanols to be fat soluble and found a suitable medium for consumption. The plant stanols/sterols work by decreasing absorption of cholesterol and lowering its return to the liver through enterohepatic circulation. The liver responds by taking up more cholesterol from the blood. The studies done on the cholesterol-lowering effect of these margarines have found that 2 to 5 grams of plant stanols/sterols per day reduces total blood cholesterol by 8% to 10% and LDL-cholesterol by 9% to 14% (similar to what is seen with some cholesterol-lowering drugs).

Benecol is made from plant stanols called *sitostanols,* which are extracted from wood pulp trees. This product is sold as margarine and has been added to salad dressings. Take Control is made from plant sterols called *sitosterols,* which are isolated from soybeans. The recommended amount for both is about 2–3 grams per day as part of at least two meals; this works out to about 2 tablespoons of Take Control or 1 tablespoon of Benacol per day. Use would cost about $1.00 per day.

In people who have borderline high total blood cholesterol (between 200 and 239 mg/dl), these margarines can be helpful in avoiding future drug therapy. Even though these products exhibit significant results, it is still important to follow a balanced diet low in saturated fat and trans fatty acids, as well as to exercise on a regular basis. People with high total blood cholesterol (greater than 240 mg/dl) who plan to consume these margarines should inform their physicians because, if they are currently on cholesterol-lowering drug therapy, their doctors may be able to decrease the dosage. For healthy individuals with total blood cholesterol within normal limits, the use of these margarines is unnecessary, especially because their cholesterol-lowering effect is not needed and they are expensive.

General Strategy for Reducing Cardiovascular Disease Risk

Table 5.8 outlines a comprehensive strategy for lowering LDL-cholesterol and preventing cardiovascular disease development. Of particular interest with regard to dietary strategies is the results obtained from a Harvard study conducted on nurses. This study revealed that women who used a group of lifestyle factors had a greater than 80% lower risk for cardiovascular disease than those who did not include these advantageous lifestyle factors in their lives. The lifestyle factors that translated into such a drop in risk are a healthy body weight, moderate to vigorous activity (e.g., brisk walking) for at least 30 minutes per day, nonsmoking or quitting smoking, an average of ½ of an alcoholic drink per day, and a score in the highest intakes of the following categories on a food intake questionnaire: cereal fiber, omega-3 fatty acids, and the vitamin folate. In addition, these women had a higher intake of polyunsaturated fatty acid with low-saturated and trans fat intake and consumed a low-GI load. This study shows that combining several lifestyle factors is highly effective in protecting against cardiovascular disease in women. The bottom line for almost anyone is to combine these lifestyle factors as a comprehensive approach to reduce cardiovascular disease risk.

For more information on cardiovascular disease, see the website of the American Heart Association at *www.americanheart.org* or the heart disease section of Healthfinder at *www.healthfinder.gov/tours/heart.htm.* This is a site created by the U.S. government for consumers. In addition, visit the website *www.nhlbi.nih.gov/chd.*

continued

Table 5.8 General Diet-Related Strategies for Reducing the Risk of Cardiovascular Disease and Heart Attack

Action	Rationale
Consume less saturated fat, trans fatty acids and cholesterol, while replacing this decreased amount of fat with monounsaturated fat and some omega-3 and omega-6 fatty acid sources.	These unsaturated fatty acids have positive effects on blood cholesterol, whereas saturated fats, trans fatty acids, and cholesterol exhibit negative effects.
Eat fish rich in omega-3 fatty acids at least twice a week and include plant sources that are rich in omega-3 fatty acids in your diet. One could also consider use of a fish oil supplement (900 milligrams of omega-3 fatty acids per day).	Omega-3 fatty acids decrease blood clotting and blood triglycerides, and have a favorable effect on heart rhythm.
Eat plenty of fruits and vegetables and include some nuts and soy on a regular basis. Some experts suggest switching to a primarily or totally vegan diet (see Chapter 6).	The dietary fiber, antioxidants, and other phytochemicals present in these foods can reduce risk of cardiovascular disease.
Eat more whole grains and less refined carbohydrates, especially sugar-rich foods.	Whole grains are rich in dietary fiber, vitamins, and minerals and have been shown to decrease blood cholesterol, whereas refined carbohydrates provide little, if any, cardiovascular benefits.
Eat at least three regularly spaced meals, while combining any high-glycemic-index foods with low-glycemic-index foods.	The frequency and glycemic index of meals affects blood triglycerides. Studies show that increasing meal frequency (from three to nine per day or so) and lowering the glycemic index while controlling portion size can help reduce LDL production (see Chapter 4 for glycemic index values of various foods).
Consume moderate amounts of alcohol with food, if you can control this practice and your physician gives approval based on your age and current health.	Consumption of red wine, in particular, has been noted to reduce cardiovascular disease, but it is speculated that small amounts of any form of alcohol may have the same effect. The benefits are primarily seen in middle-aged and older adults who are otherwise at risk of cardiovascular disease. Reducing blood clotting is just one mechanism that is suspected of having protective effects, as is raising HDL-cholesterol.
Moderate coffee intake, and replace some use with tea.	Heavy coffee use, especially unfiltered coffee (espresso and French press types), increases LDL-cholesterol. Moderate intake of filtered coffee appears to be fine for most healthy individuals. And instead of drinking coffee exclusively, consider switching to some black or green tea, which contains many flavonoids and antioxidants that reduce cardiovascular disease development.
Moderate salt intake.	High intakes of salt in overweight people have been found to cause a higher risk of death from cardiovascular disease. It is a good idea for all individuals to moderate salt in the diet, since it can cause some people's blood pressure to rise too high.
Meet calcium needs (see inside cover of text).	Some studies show a fall in LDL-cholesterol when calcium intake increases from about 400 milligrams per day to 1200 milligrams per day or more. At the higher intake, calcium is likely binding fatty acids in the intestine, in turn reducing fat absorption.
Avoid excess iron intake (see inside cover of text).	Iron likely speeds oxidation of LDL, which makes LDL more atherogenic. The degree to which this takes place in the body is a subject of debate. The effect is especially prominent in people with elevated LDL-cholesterol.
Possible use of a vitamin E supplement.	A vitamin E supplement providing 200 milligrams [about 400 IU] per day is recommended by some experts, especially for high-risk individuals, but even these experts recognize there are many more studies that refute this advice than support it. Anyone taking anticoagulant or cholesterol-lowering medications should be especially cautious, as vitamin E supplements may interfere with their otherwise beneficial effects.
Minimize large, fat-rich meals, especially those high in saturated fat.	These meals cause the blood to clot more than is regularly seen.
Lose weight if needed, ideally to attain a healthy body weight (see Chapter 10).	This especially helps reduce blood triglycerides (if elevated), lowers blood pressure, and can increase HDL, especially if the fat is lost from the abdominal region.

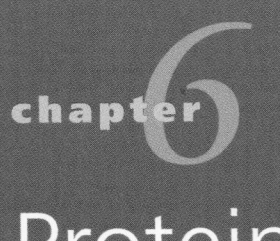

chapter 6

Proteins

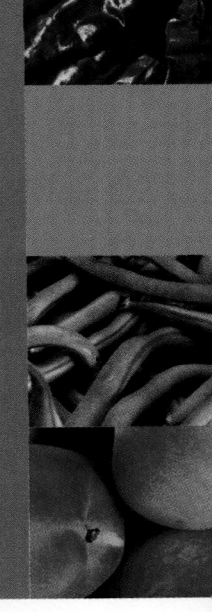

Consuming enough protein is vital for maintaining health. Proteins form important structures in the body, make up a key part of the blood, help regulate many body functions, and can fuel body cells.

North Americans eat a lot of protein—generally more than is needed to maintain health. Our daily protein intake comes mostly from meat, poultry, fish, eggs, milk, and cheese. In contrast, our Stone Age ancestors obtained a greater percentage of their protein from vegetables. They primarily picked and gathered their dietary protein, rather than hunted it. Not until *Homo erectus,* our immediate ancestors, emerged about 2.5 million years ago did meat displace other foods in a primarily vegetarian diet. Diets that are mostly vegetarian still predominate in much of Asia and areas of Africa, and many North Americans are currently adopting the practice.

Few of us wish to exchange our comfortable modern lifestyles with those of our Stone-Age ancestors, yet we could benefit from eating more plant sources of proteins. It is possible—and desirable—to incorporate the most nutritious practices of both eras and enjoy the benefits of animal and plant protein. Let's see why this is worth your attention.

Check out the **Contemporary Nutrition: Issues and Insights Online Learning Center** www.mhhe.com/wardlawcont5 *for quizzes, flash cards, other activities, and web links designed to further help you learn about proteins.*

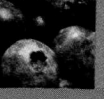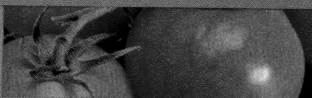

Real Life Scenario

Shannon is a freshman in college. She lives in a campus dorm and is an aerobics instructor in the afternoon. She eats two or three meals a day at the dorm cafeteria and snacks between meals. Shannon and her roommate both decided to become vegetarians because they recently read a magazine article describing the health benefits of a vegetarian diet. Yesterday her vegetarian diet consisted of a pop tart for breakfast and a tomato-pasta dish (no meat) with pretzels and a diet soft drink for lunch. In the afternoon, after her aerobics class, she had a few cookies. At dinnertime, she had a vegetarian sub sandwich with two glasses of fruit punch. In the evening, she had a bowl of popcorn.

What type of vegetarian is she? How could she improve her new diet to meet her nutritional needs?

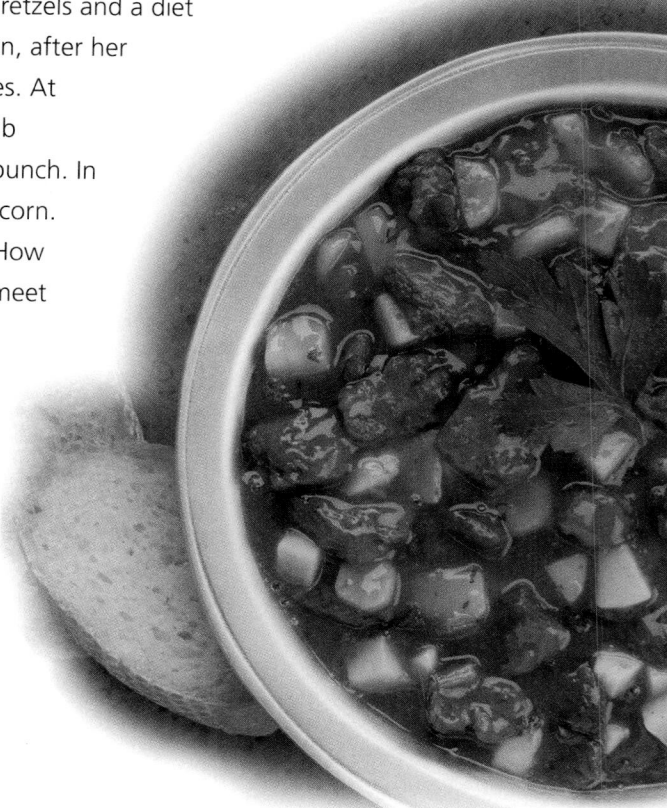

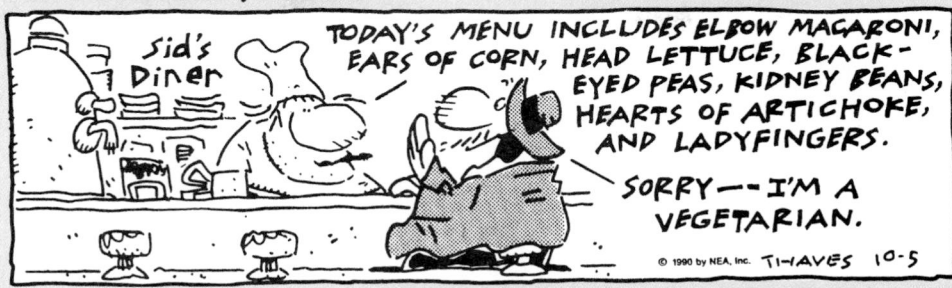

FRANK & ERNEST® by Bob Thaves

Can a vegetarian diet provide enough protein? What is prompting the growing interest in vegetarian diets? Why are plant proteins especially gaining more attention—soy being one example? Should meat-eaters abandon that dietary practice? This chapter provides some answers.

FRANK & ERNEST © United Features Syndicate. Reprinted by Permission.

Protein—An Introduction

The term *protein* comes from the Greek word *protos,* which means "to come first." In the developing world, such a primary focus on protein in diet planning is important because diets in those areas of the world can be deficient in protein. In contrast, diets in the developed world are generally rich in protein, and therefore a specific focus on eating enough protein is, for the most part, not needed.

Thousands of substances in the body are made of proteins. Aside from water, proteins form the major part of lean body tissue, totaling about 17% of body weight. Amino acids—the building blocks for proteins—contain a special form of nitrogen: essentially, carbon bonded to nitrogen. Plants combine nitrogen from soil and air with carbon and other elements to form amino acids. They then bond these amino acids together to make proteins. We get the nitrogen we need by consuming dietary proteins. Proteins are thus an essential part of a diet because they supply nitrogen in a form we can readily use—namely, amino acids. Directly using simpler forms of nitrogen is, for the most part, impossible for humans.

Proteins are crucial to the regulation and maintenance of the body. Body functions such as blood clotting, fluid balance, hormone and enzyme production, visual processes, transport of many substances in the bloodstream, and cell repair require specific proteins. The body generates proteins in many configurations and sizes so that they can serve these greatly varied functions. All of these proteins use the amino acids in the protein-containing foods we eat, plus some arising from cell synthesis. Proteins can also supply energy for the body—on average, 4 kcal per gram.

If you fail to consume an adequate amount of protein for weeks at a time, many metabolic processes slow down. This is because the body does not have enough amino acids available to build the proteins it needs. For example, the immune system no longer functions efficiently when it lacks key proteins, thereby increasing the risk of infections, disease, and eventually death.

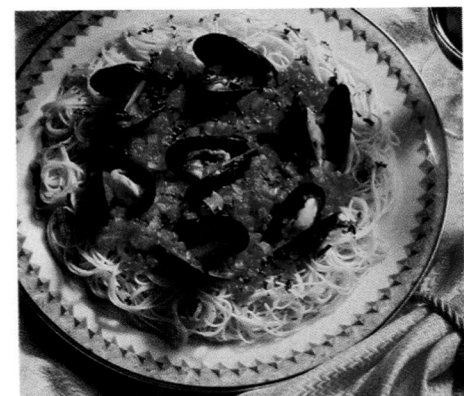

Small amounts of animal protein in a meal easily add up to meet daily protein needs.

*B*ecause two cysteine molecules can bond to form a new amino acid called cystine, the number of nonessential amino acids is sometimes listed as 12. If this form of cysteine is not counted as a unique form, then there are 11 nonessential amino acids. Our discussion will not count cystine and, thus, uses the figure of 20 amino acids in foods—9 essential and 11 nonessential.

Table 6.1 Classification of Amino Acids

Essential (Indispensable) Amino Acids	Nonessential (Dispensable) Amino Acids
Histidine	Alanine
Isoleucine*	Arginine
Leucine*	Asparagine
Lysine	Aspartic acid
Methionine	Cysteine†
Phenylalanine	(Cystine)
Threonine	Glutamic acid
Tryptophan	Glutamine
Valine*	Glycine
	Proline
	Serine
	Tyrosine†

*A branched-chain amino acid

†These amino acids are also classed as **semiessential.** This means they must be made from essential amino acids if insufficient amounts are eaten. When that occurs, the body's supply of certain essential amino acids is depleted. Researchers now suggest that some other nonessential amino acids assume a more essential status when the body cannot readily generate them. This occurs during some illnesses. Glutamine may assume an essential status in body injury, especially in the period after intestinal surgery, and arginine is essential for infants and children.

*T*he R group on some amino acids has a branched shape, like a tree. These so-called **branched-chain amino acids** are leucine, isoleucine, and valine (see Appendix F for the chemical structures of the amino acids). The branched-chain amino acids are the primary amino acids used by muscles for energy. This has implications for athletes (see Chapter 11 for details).

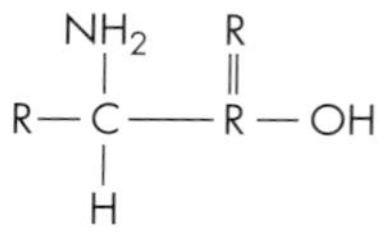

nonessential amino acids Amino acids that can be synthesized by a healthy body in sufficient amounts; there are 11 nonessential amino acids. These are also called *dispensable amino acids.*

essential amino acids The amino acids that cannot be synthesized by humans in sufficient amounts and therefore must be included in the diet; there are nine essential amino acids. These are also called *indispensable amino acids.*

■ Amino Acids

Amino acids—the building blocks of proteins—are formed mostly of carbon, hydrogen, oxygen, and nitrogen. The following diagram shows the general form of an amino acid and what a typical amino acid looks like. The amino acids used to make protein have different chemical makeups, but all are slight variations of the glutamic acid pictured (see Appendix F).

"Generic" amino acid. The R signifies another chemical group that would be present.

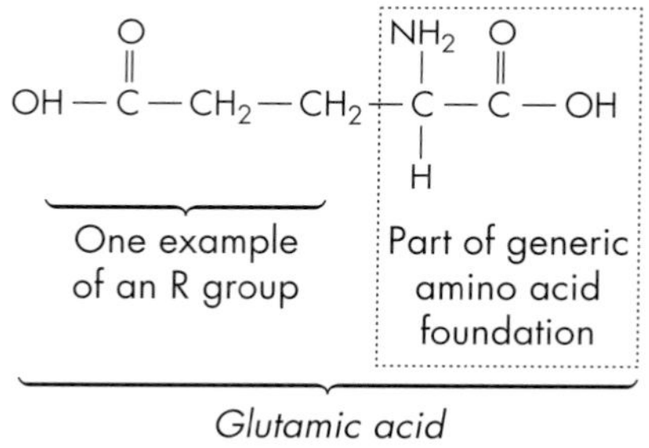

One example of an R group | Part of generic amino acid foundation

Glutamic acid

Your body needs to use 20 different types of amino acids to function (Table 6.1). Although they are all important, 11 of these amino acids are considered **nonessential** (also called *dispensable*) with respect to our diets. Human cells can produce these certain amino acids as long as the right ingredients are present—the key factor being nitrogen that is already part of another amino acid.

The nine amino acids the body cannot make are known as **essential** (also called *indispensable*)—they must be obtained from foods. This is because body cells either cannot make the needed carbon-based foundation of the amino acid, cannot put a nitrogen group on the needed carbon-based foundation, or just cannot do the whole process fast enough to meet body needs.

Both nonessential and essential amino acids are present in foods that contain protein. If you don't eat enough essential amino acids, your body first struggles to conserve what essential amino acids it can. However, eventually your body progressively slows production of new proteins until at some point you will break protein down faster than you can make it. When that happens, health deteriorates.

■ Putting Essential and Nonessential Amino Acids into Perspective

Eating a balanced diet can supply us with both the essential and nonessential amino-acid building blocks needed to maintain good health. Let's now take a more detailed look at this concept of essential amino acids, especially in relation to nonessential amino acids.

Physiological Aspects

The disease phenylketonuria (PKU) illustrates the importance of one essential amino acid. Recall from Chapter 4 that a person with PKU has a limited ability to metabolize the essential amino acid phenylalanine. Normally, the body uses an enzyme to convert much of our dietary phenylalanine intake into the nonessential amino acid tyrosine.

In PKU-diagnosed persons, the enzyme activity may be grossly or mildly insufficient in processing phenylalanine to tyrosine. When the enzymes cannot synthesize enough tyrosine, both amino acids must be derived from foods. The key point here is that both amino acids become *essential* in terms of dietary needs because the body can't produce enough tyrosine. In the treatment of PKU, consumption of phenylalanine must also be controlled by consuming a special diet (ideally throughout life) because phenylalanine and its by-products can rise to toxic concentrations in the body. These are thought to cause the severe mental retardation seen in untreated PKU cases.

Dietary Considerations

Animal and plant proteins can differ greatly in proportions of essential and nonessential amino acids. Animal proteins contain ample amounts of all nine essential amino acids. (Gelatin—made from the animal protein collagen—is an exception because it loses one essential amino acid during processing and is low in other essential amino acids.) With the exception of soybeans, plant proteins don't match our need for essential amino acids as precisely as animal proteins. Many plant proteins, especially those found in grains, are low in one or more of the nine essential amino acids.

As you might expect, human tissue composition resembles animal tissue more than it does plant tissue. The similarities enable us to use proteins from single animal sources more efficiently to support human growth and maintenance than we do those from single plant sources. For this reason, animal proteins, except gelatin, are considered **high-quality** (also called **complete**) **proteins**—they contain all the amino acids we need in sufficient amounts. Individual plant sources of proteins are considered **lower-quality** (also called **incomplete**) **proteins** because their amino-acid patterns can be quite different from ours. A single plant protein, such as corn alone, cannot easily support body growth and maintenance. To obtain a sufficient amount of amino acids, a variety of plant proteins need to be consumed because each protein lacks adequate amounts of one or more essential amino acids.

When only lower-quality protein foods are consumed, enough of the essential amino acids needed for protein synthesis may not be obtained. Therefore, a greater amount of lower-quality protein is needed to meet the needs of protein synthesis. Moreover, once any of the nine essential amino acids in the plant protein was used up, further protein synthesis would be impossible. The remaining amino acids would be used for energy or converted to fat or carbohydrate and stored as such. Because the depletion of just one of the essential amino acids prevents protein synthesis, the

Critical Thinking

Rina is 7 months pregnant and has read about various tests that her baby will undergo when he or she is born. How can you explain to Rina the purpose and significance of one of those tests, the one that screens for PKU?

high-quality (complete) proteins Dietary proteins that contain ample amounts of all nine essential amino acids.

lower-quality (incomplete) proteins Dietary proteins that are low in or lack one or more essential amino acids.

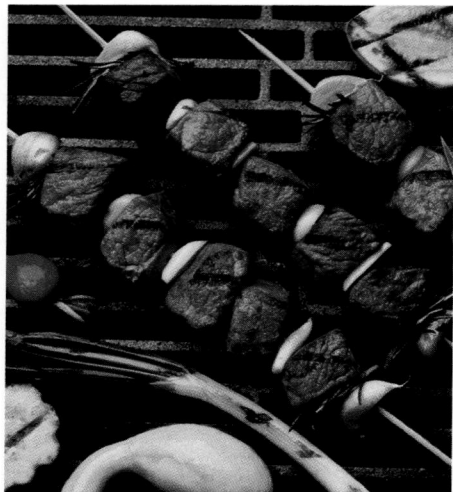

When combined with vegetables, high-protein foods such as meats also help balance the amino acid content of the diet.

Table 6.2 Limiting Amino Acids in Plant Foods

Food	Limiting Amino Acids	Good Plant Source of the Limiting Amino Acids*	Traditional Uses in Which the Proteins Complement Each Other in a Meal
Beans (legumes)	Methionine	Grains, nuts, seeds	Red beans and rice
Grains	Lysine, threonine	Legumes	Rice and red beans; lentil curry and rice
Nuts and seeds	Lysine	Legumes	Soybeans and ground sesame seeds (miso); peanuts, rice, and black-eyed peas; green peas and sunflower seeds
Vegetables	Methionine	Grains, nuts, seeds	Green beans and almonds
Corn	Tryptophan, lysine	Legumes	Corn tortillas and beans

Note: As you might suspect from the information in this table, the amino acids most likely to be low in a diet are lysine, methionine, threonine, and tryptophan. If a diet is low in an amino acid, nutrition experts recommend finding a good food source to supply it. Finding the right combinations of amino acids, such as a dish of rice and beans, is recommended. Forget about amino-acid supplements—they can lead to problems, such as decreased absorption of other, similar amino acids. Amino acids as such also have a disagreeable odor and flavor and are also much more expensive than food protein.

*Animal products in the diet serve the same purpose, such as when fish is consumed with rice.

limiting amino acid The essential amino acid in lowest concentration in a food or diet relative to body needs.

complementary proteins Two food protein sources that make up for each other's inadequate supply of specific essential amino acids; together they yield a sufficient amount of all nine and, so, provide high-quality (complete) protein for the diet.

Critical Thinking

Leon, a vegetarian, has heard of the "all-or-none principle" of protein synthesis but doesn't understand how this law applies to protein synthesis in the body. He asks you, "How important is this nutritional concept for diet planning?" How would you answer his question?

process illustrates the *all-or-none principle:* Either all essential amino acids are available or none can be used. The essential amino acid in smallest supply in a food or diet in relation to body needs becomes the limiting factor (called the **limiting amino acid**) because it limits the amount of protein the body can synthesize.

For example, assume the letters of the alphabet represent the 20 or so different amino acids we consume. If *A* represents an essential amino acid, we need four of these letters to spell the hypothetical protein *ALABAMA*. If the body had an *L*, a *B*, and an *M*, but only three *A*s, the "synthesis" of *ALABAMA* would not be possible. *A* would then be seen as the limiting amino acid.

When two or more proteins combine to compensate for deficiencies in essential amino acid content in each protein, the proteins are called **complementary proteins** (Table 6.2). Mixed diets generally provide high-quality protein because a complementary protein pattern results. Therefore, healthy adults should have little concern about balancing foods to yield the proteins needed to obtain enough of all nine essential amino acids. Even on plant-based diets, complementing proteins need not be consumed at the same meal by adults. Meeting amino-acid needs over the course of a day is a reasonable goal for adults because there is a ready supply of amino acids from those present in body cells and in the blood (review Fig. 6.7 on page 202). In addition, adults need only about 11% of their total protein requirement to be supplied by essential amino acids. Typical diets supply an average of 50% of protein as essential amino acids.

The estimated needs for essential amino acids for infants and preschool children are 30% of total protein intake; however, in later childhood the number drops to 20%. Consequently, diets for young children must be carefully planned to make sure enough proteins are present to yield high-quality protein intake. Including some animal products in the diet, such as human milk or formula for infants, or cow's milk for children, helps ensure this. Otherwise, complementary amino acids from plant proteins should be consumed in each meal or within two subsequent meals. A major health risk for infants and children occurs in famine situations in which only one type of cereal grain is available, increasing the probability that one or more of the nine essential amino acids is lacking in the total diet. This is discussed further in a later section in the chapter on protein-energy malnutrition.

Concept Check

*T*he human body uses 20 different amino acids from protein-containing foods. Because a healthy body can synthesize 11 of the amino acids, it is not necessary to obtain all amino acids from foods—only nine of these must come from the diet and are therefore termed *essential (indispensable) amino acids*. Foods that contain all nine essential amino acids in about the proportions we need are considered high-quality (complete) protein foods. Those low in one or more essential amino acids are lower-quality (incomplete) protein foods. When different lower-quality protein foods are eaten together, the total intake of amino acids generally makes up for the individual foods' shortcomings to yield a high-quality protein meal.

Proteins—Amino Acids Bonded Together

Amino acids are bonded together by chemical links—technically called **peptide bonds**—to form proteins. Although these bonds are difficult to break, acids, enzymes, and other agents are able to do so—for example, during digestion.

The body can synthesize many different proteins by bonding together the 20 types of amino acids with such peptide bonds.

■ Protein Synthesis

To begin a discussion of protein synthesis, we need to focus on DNA, which is present in the nucleus of the cell. Recall from Chapter 3 that DNA is a double-stranded molecule. DNA contains coded instructions for protein synthesis (i.e., which specific amino acids are to be placed in a protein).

Protein synthesis in a cell, however, takes place in the cytoplasm, not in the nucleus. Thus, the DNA code used for synthesis of a specific protein must be transferred to the cytoplasm to allow for such synthesis. That is the job of messenger RNA (mRNA). Enzymes in the nucleus read the code on one strand of the DNA and *transcribe* that into a single-stranded mRNA (Fig. 6.1). The segment that is read is the gene. This mRNA undergoes processing and then it is ready to leave the nucleus.

The mRNA travels to the ribosomes in the cytoplasm, present on the rough endoplasmic reticulum and floating free in the cell. The ribosomes read the code on the mRNA and *translate* those instructions so as to produce a specific protein. Amino acids are added one at a time to the **polypeptide** chain as directed by the instructions on the mRNA. Energy input from ATP is needed to add each amino acid to the growing polypeptide chain, making protein synthesis very "costly" to the body in terms of energy use. Many ribosomes can combine to simultaneously translate a large mRNA.

One other key participant in protein synthesis in the cytoplasm is transfer RNA (tRNA). These units bring specific amino acids to the ribosomes as needed during protein synthesis (review Fig. 6.1). Numerous tRNA carriers are present during protein synthesis to continually supply the ribosomes with needed amino acids.

Once synthesis of the polypeptide is completed, it is released from the ribosomes, as is the mRNA. The polypeptide may then undergo further metabolism in the cell, such as is true for the hormone insulin, or be functional as such as a specific body protein after it twists and folds into a very complex, three-dimensional structure (see the next section on protein organization for details).

The important message in this discussion is the relationship between DNA and the ultimate proteins produced by a cell. If the DNA contains errors, an incorrect mRNA will be produced. The ribosomes will then read this incorrect message and produce an incorrect polypeptide chain. As discussed in Chapter 3, ultimately we may be able to correct many gene defects in humans such that the correct DNA code can be placed in the nucleus, so that the correct protein can be made by the ribosomes.

peptide bond A chemical bond formed between amino acids in a protein. The acid group

$$\overset{\text{O}}{\underset{\|}{}}$$

($-C-OH$) from one amino acid reacts with the amino group ($-NH_2$) of another amino acid to form the peptide bond

$$\overset{\text{O}}{\underset{\|}{}}$$

($-C-NH_2-$). Water (H_2O) is a by-product of the reaction.

polypeptide A group of amino acids bonded together, from a few to 1000 or more.

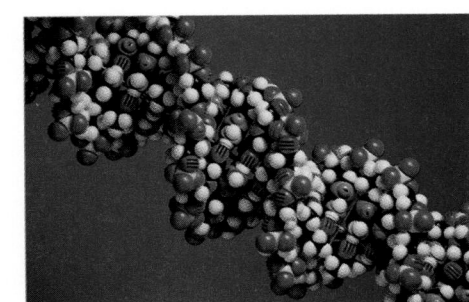

Genes are present on DNA—a double-stranded helix. The cell nucleus contains most of the DNA in the body.

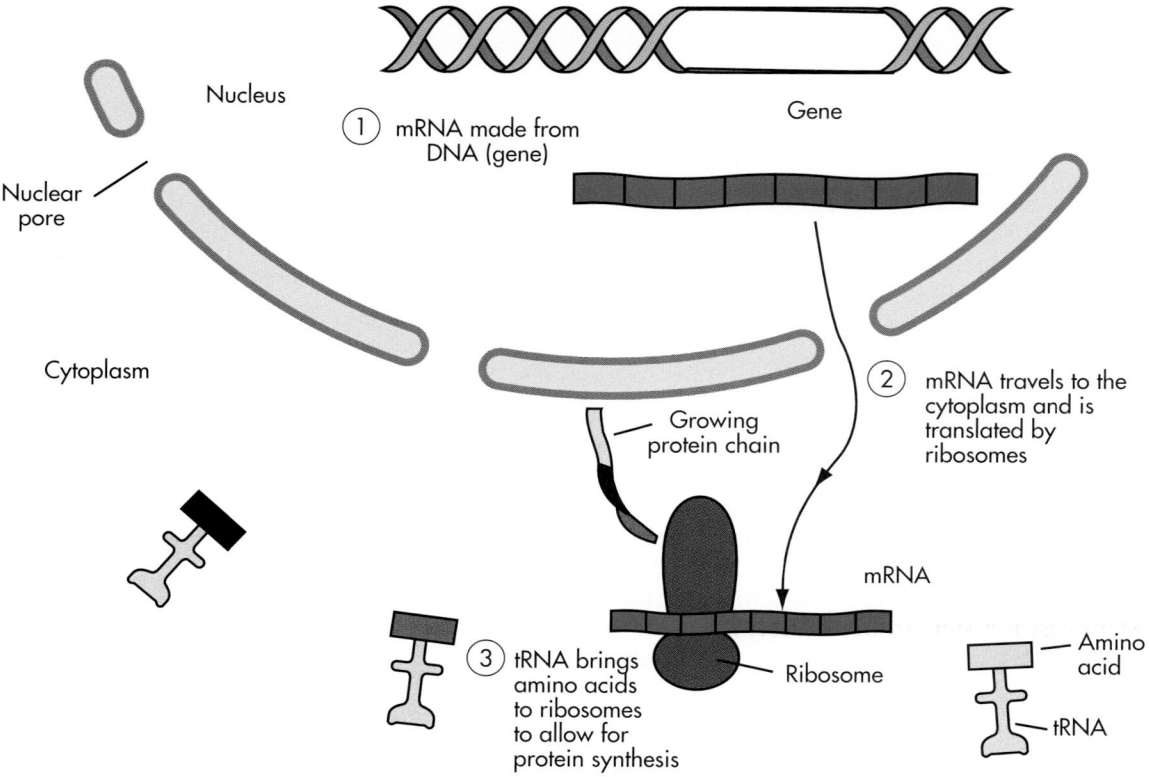

Figure 6.1 Protein synthesis (simplified). (1) DNA present in the nucleus of the cell uncoils and the code embedded in the DNA is *transcribed* into a messenger RNA (mRNA). This is processed further in the nucleus and then leaves the nucleus through nuclear pores. (2) For protein synthesis, the ribosomes in the cytoplasm and on the endoplasmic reticulum read the code on the mRNA and *translate* this into a polypeptide. The code on the mRNA dictates the order of the amino acids on the polypeptide. (3) Transfer RNA (tRNA) supplies amino acids to the ribosomes to allow for protein synthesis. Each amino acid has one or more unique tRNA molecules to use as a carrier. Once the mRNA is fully read, the polypeptide is released into the cytoplasm. It generally is then processed further to become a cell protein.

■ Protein Turnover

Cell proteins are constantly undergoing synthesis and degradation (breakdown). This process, called protein turnover, allows cells to adapt to changing circumstances. For example, when we eat more protein, the liver needs to make more enzymes to process the waste product of some of the resulting amino acid metabolism—ammonia—into urea. The amino acids needed to make the enzymes can come from the diet and from amino acids released from the breakdown of other proteins in cells. For example, the GI tract lining is constantly **sloughed** off. The digestive tract treats sloughed cells just like food particles and absorbs the amino acids released during their digestion. In fact, most protein breakdown products—amino acids—released throughout the body can be recycled and are added to the pool of amino acids available for future protein synthesis. Overall, protein turnover is a process by which a cell can respond to its changing environment and produce needed proteins, while also reducing the content of proteins not currently needed.

sloughed Shed or cast off.

During any day, an adult makes and degrades about 250–300 grams of protein; many of the amino acids are recycled. By comparing 250–300 grams with the 65–95 grams or more of protein typically consumed by adults in North America, you can see the importance of recycling amino acids in the body when possible.

■ Protein Organization

As noted before, by bonding together various combinations of the 20 types of amino acids, the body synthesizes thousands of different proteins. The sequential order of the amino acids then ultimately determines the protein's shape. The key point is that only correctly positioned amino acids can interact and fold properly to form the intended shape for the protein. The resulting unique, three-dimensional form goes on to dictate the function of each particular protein. If it lacks the appropriate configuration, a protein cannot function (Fig. 6.2).

Sickle cell disease (also called **sickle cell anemia**) illustrates what happens when amino acids are out of order on a protein. North Americans of African descent are especially prone to this genetic disease. It originates in defective production of the protein chains of hemoglobin, a compound found in red blood cells. In two of its four protein chains, a slight error in the amino-acid order occurs. This small error produces a profound change in hemoglobin structure. It can no longer form the shape needed to carry oxygen efficiently inside the red blood cell. Instead of forming normal circular disks, the red blood cells collapse into crescent shapes (Fig. 6.3). Health deteriorates, and eventually episodes of severe bone and joint pain, abdominal pain, headache, convulsions, and paralysis may occur.

These life-threatening symptoms are caused by a minute, but critical, error in the hemoglobin amino-acid order. Why does this error happen? It results from a defect in a person's genetic blueprint, DNA, which is inherited through one's parents. A defect in the DNA can dictate that a wrong amino acid will be built into the sequence of the body proteins. Many diseases stem from incorrect DNA information passed on in the body. Cancer, which is discussed in Chapter 8, is an example.

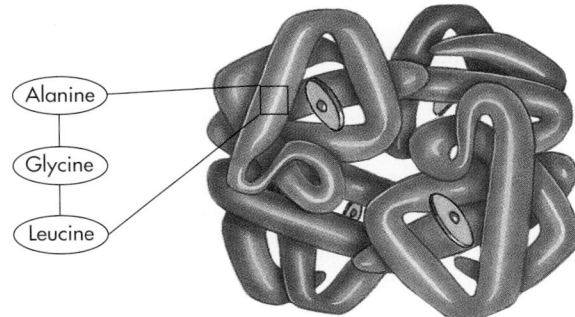

Figure 6.2 Protein organization. Proteins often form a coiled shape, as shown by this drawing of the blood protein hemoglobin. This shape is dictated by the order of the amino acids in the protein chain. To get an idea of its size, note that each teaspoon (5 milliliters) of blood contains about 10^{18} hemoglobin molecules. Note that 1 billion is 10^9.

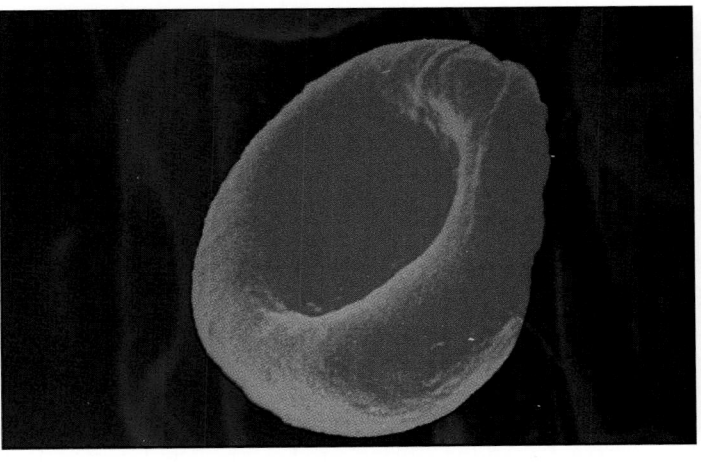

(a)

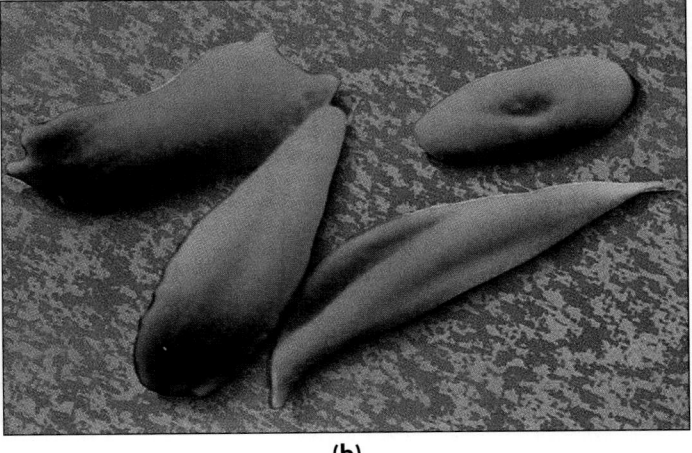

(b)

Figure 6.3 Sickle cell disease from the perspective of the red blood cell. (a) Normal red cell, (b) blood from a person with sickle cell disease. Note the abnormal crescent (sicklelike) shape of the red blood cell near the center.

denaturation Alteration of a protein's three-dimensional structure, usually because of treatment by heat, enzymes, acid or alkaline solutions, or agitation.

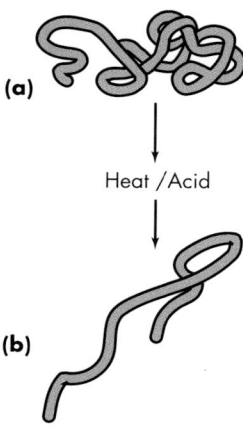

(a)

Heat /Acid

(b)

(a) Protein showing typical coiled state.
(b) Protein is now partly uncoiled. This uncoiling can reduce protein function.

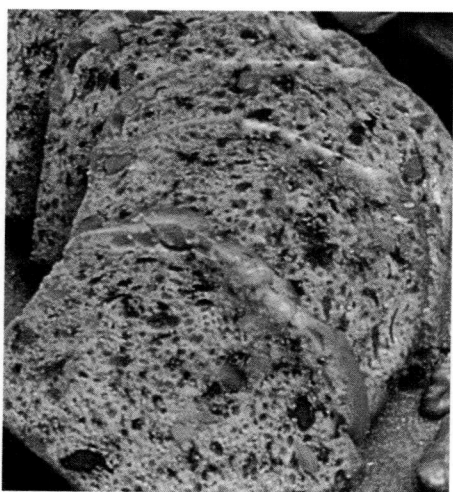

Nuts, like walnuts, can be incorporated into one's diet in numerous ways, such as adding them to banana bread.

■ Denaturation of Proteins

Treatment with acid or alkaline substances, heat, or agitation can alter a protein's structure, leaving it in a **denatured** state. The protein can no longer perform its function. For example, once the bacteria in yogurt have synthesized enough acid and enzymes to precipitate some of the milk protein, the product solidifies irreversibly. Note that denaturation does not affect the primary structure.

Unraveling a protein's shape often destroys its normal functioning, such that it loses its biological activity. That characteristic is useful for some body processes, such as digestion. The secretion of stomach acid denatures some bacteria, plant hormones, many active enzymes, and other forms of proteins in foods. The heat produced during cooking likewise denatures proteins. Both processes make foods safer to eat. Digestion is also enhanced because the unraveling increases exposure of the food to digestive enzymes. Denaturing proteins in some foods can also reduce their tendencies to cause allergic reactions.

Recall that we need proteins in the diet to supply essential amino acids—not the active proteins themselves. We dismantle the dietary proteins and use the amino acids to assemble proteins we need.

Concept Check

Amino acids are bonded together in specific sequences to form distinct proteins. Proteins in cells are in a constant state of turnover. The degradation of existing proteins and synthesis of new proteins takes place on a minute-by-minute basis, amounting to a turnover about 250–300 grams a day for the entire human body. DNA provides the directions for synthesizing these new proteins. Specifically, DNA directs the order of the amino acids on the protein. The amino acid order within a protein determines its ultimate shape and function. Destroying the shape of a protein denatures it. Acid conditions present during the body's digestive processes, heat, and other factors can denature proteins, causing them to lose their biological activity.

▌ Protein in Foods

The most nutrient-dense source of protein is water-packed tuna, which has over 80% of energy as protein. Of the typical foods we eat, about 70% of our protein comes from animal sources (Fig. 6.4). The top five contributors of protein to the North American diet are beef, poultry, milk, white bread, and cheese. In North America, meat and poultry consumption amounts to about 150 pounds per person per year. Worldwide, 35% of protein comes from animal sources. In Africa and East Asia, about 20% of the protein eaten comes from animal sources.

■ The Value of Plant Protein

Vegetable sources of proteins deserve more attention from North Americans. Many plant foods—in proportion to the amount of energy they supply—provide not only much protein but also ample magnesium and dietary fiber, along with other benefits. Proteins are used somewhat less efficiently by the body than are animal proteins (10% to 20% less), but this drop is not significant enough to influence diet planning when a variety of foods is used. The vegetable proteins we eat also contain no cholesterol and little saturated fat, unless these are added during processing. Regular use of plant proteins is a valuable addition to a diet because these supply a variety of other nutrients. Soy sources of proteins are receiving much attention today (see the Nutrition Insight).

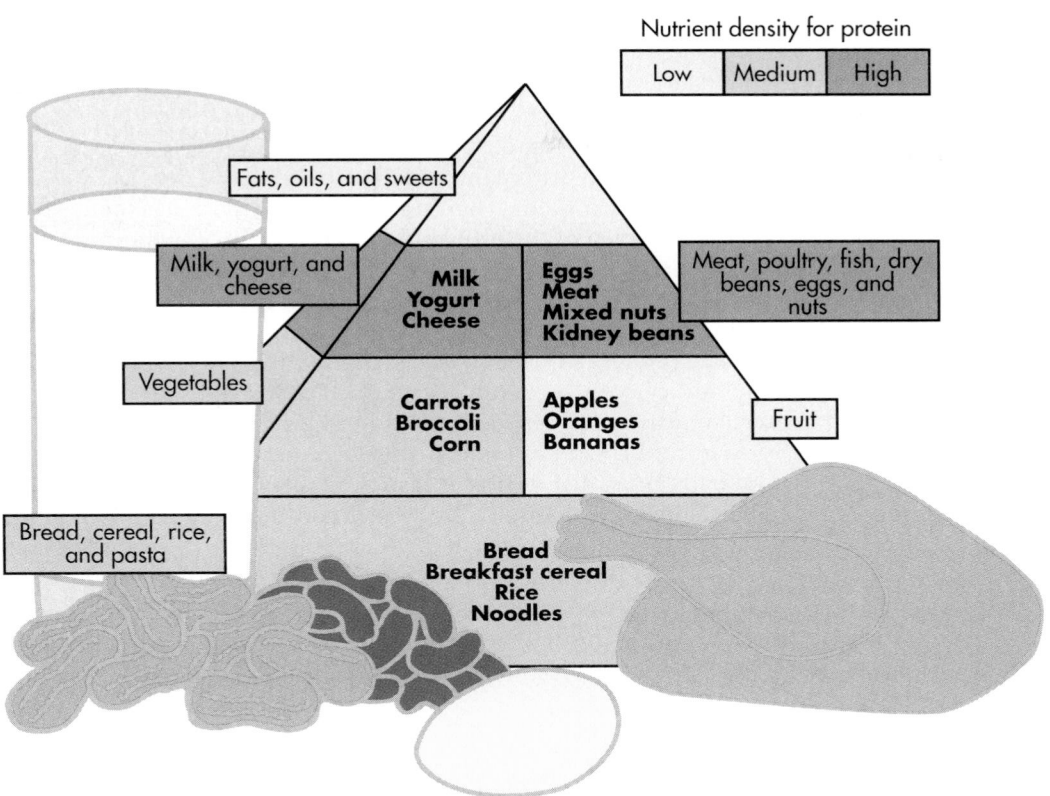

Nutrient density for protein

| Low | Medium | High |

Fats, oils, and sweets

Milk, yogurt, and cheese

Milk Yogurt Cheese

Eggs Meat Mixed nuts Kidney beans

Meat, poultry, fish, dry beans, eggs, and nuts

Vegetables

Carrots Broccoli Corn

Apples Oranges Bananas

Fruit

Bread, cereal, rice, and pasta

Bread Breakfast cereal Rice Noodles

Figure 6.4   Sources of protein in foods from the Food Guide Pyramid. Based on serving sizes listed for the Food Guide Pyramid, the fruit group, vegetable group, and fats, oils, and sweet category generally contain little protein (about 0.1 to 3 grams), whereas the other groups contain moderate to high amounts (about 8 to 10 grams for milk products, 12 grams for nuts and beans, and 7 grams per ounce for meat, fish, and poultry). The background color of each group indicates the average nutrient density for protein in that group.

Another Bite

Nuts are often overlooked as a source of plant protein. Recent studies have linked consumption of nuts to decreased blood cholesterol and blood pressure. The protective action of nuts probably stems from their lack of cholesterol and abundance of unsaturated fatty acids. These unsaturated fats do not raise blood cholesterol as does saturated fat. Of course, this benefit occurs only if nuts are used to replace saturated fats in the diet. Phytochemicals in nuts, such as flavonoids, are also thought to provide health benefits. For these reasons, a 30 grams (1 ounce) serving of nuts or 2 tablespoons of peanut butter per day provides an especially healthy source of protein. Nuts also contain vitamin E, magnesium, calcium, and fiber. However, it is important to keep in mind that nuts are very energy dense, so portion control is also important.

Legumes are a plant family with pods that contain a single row of seeds: garden and black-eyed peas; green, black, red, great northern, lima, kidney, pinto, and garbanzo beans; lentils; and soybeans. Dried varieties of the mature seeds—what we know as beans—also make an impressive contribution to the protein, vitamin, mineral, and dietary fiber content of a meal (Fig. 6.5). Regularly consuming these legume protein sources can add substantial amounts of nutrients to a diet. Moreover, as discussed in Chapter 4, legumes contain soluble fiber, which can help lower blood

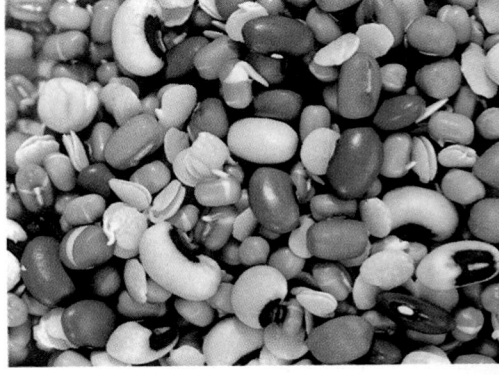

Legumes add color and many nutrients to meals.

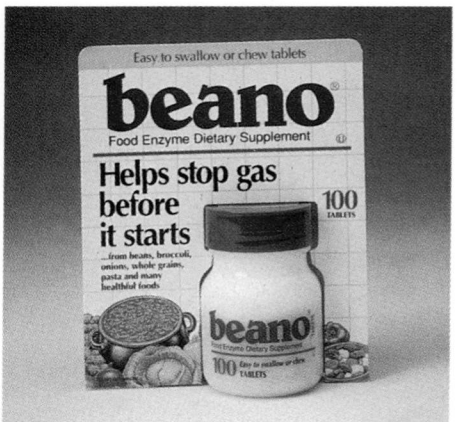

Beano® reduces intestinal gas produced by bacterial metabolism of the undigestible sugars of legumes in the large intestine. It does so by breaking down these sugars so the breakdown products (monosaccharides) can be absorbed in the small intestine.

cholesterol. In addition, the soluble fiber moderates the swings in blood glucose that occur after eating.

When you initially add legumes to your diet, they may cause intestinal gas. Split peas, limas, and lentils are less likely to cause this problem than the others, so start with them. Eat small servings at first, and give your GI tract a few weeks to adjust.

You can also reduce your risk of getting intestinal gas by cooking dry beans in boiling water for 3 minutes to soften them. Then turn off the heat and let the covered beans soak for a few hours. Much of the indigestible sugars that cause the gas (recall from Chapter 3 that this happens when certain compounds, such as sugars in beans, escape digestion in the small intestine and are fermented by the bacteria in the large intestine) will leach into the water. The water should be poured off and the beans further cooked in fresh water as desired. This practice will lead to some vitamin loss but will not affect protein or dietary fiber content. For canned beans, draining and rinsing with water is an excellent way to lower the content of gas-forming sugars.

Many people have no trouble with beans and other legumes, but it's best to be cautious. An enzyme preparation called *Beano*® is also available to ease gas symptoms. Taken right before a meal in tablet or liquid form and according to directions, it helps digest the beans' undigestible carbohydrates in the small intestine and thereby lessens the intestinal gas production in the large intestine. Because Beano® is made from mold, people sensitive to molds may have allergic reactions and should avoid this product or use it with care. For more information and/or free samples, contact the manufacturer at 1-800-257-8650.

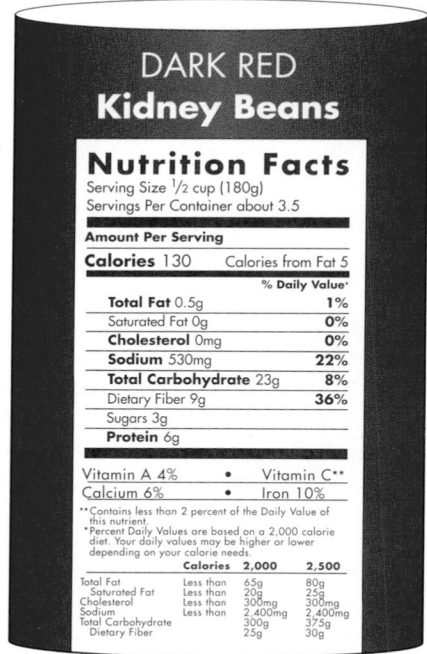

Figure 6.5 Legumes are rich sources of protein. One-half cup meets about 10% of protein needs, and at a cost of only about 5% of energy needs.

Interest in Soy Protein Is Growing

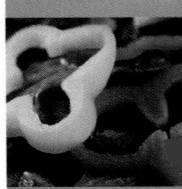

North American farmers harvest soybeans mostly to feed livestock, but lately health researchers are highlighting the health benefits of this plant. Since 1999, soy has had an FDA-approved health claim for lowering blood cholesterol. The claim is limited to foods high in soy protein, and the recommended daily intake is 25 grams to acquire the benefits. As noted in Chapter 2, qualifying for the health claim requires an individual product to have at least 6.25 grams of soy protein and less than 3 grams of fat, 1 gram of saturated fat, and 20 milligrams of cholesterol per serving. Consuming soy daily can lower blood cholesterol by about 10% or more, and as well increase the flexibility of arteries; thus reducing cardiovascular disease risk.

Some people might say that consuming 25 grams of soy protein per day would be difficult. This is true if soy is not added or mixed in dinner dishes. Overall, a daily intake of this magnitude needs a conscious effort to work soy into the diet, but can be accomplished. One suggestion is to introduce soy slowly by adding small amounts daily. Then, as the taste and texture become familiar, one can add more.

Soy is one of just a few foods that contain a source of the phytochemical class called *isoflavones*. The two primary isoflavones found in soy are genistein and diadzein. The isolation of these isoflavones is currently popular for use as supplements. However, the overall recommendation is to consume soy as a whole food. Supplements vary in the amount of isoflavones. Also, the benefits of soy do not solely exist in these two isoflavones.

Isoflavones act as plant-like estrogens, especially when the body is deficient in estrogen. Menopause is the common time for women to be deficient in estrogen. The isoflavones help compensate by acting as weak estrogens. Women have been encouraged to experiment with consuming more soy products to relieve menopausal symptoms, but the actual intake of soy protein needed to produce the benefit is still under investigation (about 40 grams per day is the typical dose used in studies). One recent study from Japan showed that women who consumed 115 grams of soy products per day (this would include the protein, carbohydrate, fat, and water in the products) had fewer menopausal symptoms (hot flashes, vaginal dryness, and so on) compared to women who consumed 45 grams per day.

Animal protein consumption in Asian countries is one-half that found in North America. In addition, the calcium intake is less than half in North America, yet Asian countries show hip fracture rates that are less than one-third of those in North America. The greater use of plant proteins in Asia, primarily soy, may be decreasing Asians' risk for osteoporosis. Regular exercise or other differences in lifestyle in Asian populations may also contribute to these statistics. Note that the bone loss from osteoporosis is very rapid during and after menopause, due to the loss of estrogen secretion (see Chapter 9 for details). The isoflavones of soy are being used in research to slow this loss, and so far such use has maintained or actually increased the bone density in some studies, but not all. Results of more studies are expected in the next few years.

In laboratory animals, the isoflavones of soy have been shown to directly slow the growth of prostate cancer cells. This adds to the ability of isoflavones to decrease a tumor's blood supply and block the action of some cancer-promoting hormones. Soy intake might be the reason why Japanese men have a lower risk of prostate cancer than North American men.

There is some interest that regular soy intake may decrease breast cancer risk by blocking estrogen action, but increasing soy in the diet is not recommended for women with breast cancer. This is because the phytoestrogens can also stimulate the growth of breast cancer cells, especially after menopause when the natural output of estrogen is dwindling. Women with breast cancer (or a family history of the disease) should talk to their physicians before consuming soy on a regular basis. People with a history of kidney stones should do the same, as regular use of soy has been linked to that problem. (See the discussion of oxalates in Chapter 9. Soy is a source.)

Common soy protein sources include tofu, soy milk, soy flour, textured soy protein, tempeh, and miso. Soy protein powders are also availabale. An explanation of these soy foods may help:

- Tofu is made from cooked, pureed soybeans that are processed into a custard-like cake. It absorbs the flavor of the food it is mixed with, such as in a stir fry or smoothie, or blended into dips as a cheese substitute. Tofu can be purchased in firm, soft, and silken textures, depending on how it is to be used.

- Soy milk is produced by grinding dehulled soybeans and mixing them with water to form a milk-like liquid. This milk can substitute in recipes for cow's milk or be consumed as a beverage. Soy milk is comparable to cow's milk in that many brands have just as much calcium, but most lack the vitamin D content of cow's milk. Soy milk is available in plain or vanilla, chocolate, and coffee flavors.

- Soy flour is created by grinding roasted soybeans into a fine powder. This flour can add protein and moisture to baked goods. Soy flour may also be used as egg substitute in these products.

- Textured soy protein is made from soy flour, which is compressed and dehydrated. It is used as a meat substitute or filler for casseroles and meatloaf.

- Tempeh is a flat cake made from fermented soybeans. It has a mild flavor and chewy texture. Tempeh can be grilled, used in sandwiches, or combined in casseroles.

- Miso is a fermented soybean paste that is used for seasoning and in soup stock.

The goal for 25 grams of soy protein may seem high, but most people eat more than 1 food serving at a meal. In addition, most of the meat alternatives found in the produce or refrigerated section of the supermarket have 8–15 grams of soy protein per serving. These include hot dogs, burgers, and ground tofu. Soy milk, soy yogurt, and soy flour are the next-highest sources of soy protein, with 6–9 grams per serving. These soy products can easily be added to foods in baking or cooking to increase daily intake. Regular tofu—firm or soft—has 4 grams of protein per ⅛-inch slice, or 1.5 ounces. Other soy protein products of interest are tempeh, with 16 grams of protein per ½ cup; soy nuts, with 19 grams per ¼ cup; and a soy protein bar, with 14 grams.

The switch to soy may be difficult at first, but as one becomes accustomed to the taste, receives more recipes, and learns the varying preparation methods, he or she will benefit from the health effects of soy. Daily soy intake certainly is worth a try to combat high blood cholesterol and to treat menopausal symptoms in women. For others, 2 to 4 servings a week of soy-based foods such as tofu and soy milk is a good target, especially as it replaces animal proteins in the diet. And again, there is a general recommendation to consume soy isoflavones from soy foods, not from supplements.

■ Protein Digestion and Absorption

As with carbohydrates, cooking food can be viewed as a first step in protein digestion. Cooking unfolds (denatures) proteins and softens tough connective tissue in meat. Cooking also makes many protein-rich foods easier to chew, swallow, and break down during later digestion and absorption. As you will see in Chapter 16, cooking also makes many protein-rich foods, such as meats, eggs, fish, and poultry, much safer to eat.

■ Digestion

pepsin A protein-digesting enzyme produced by the stomach.

The enzymatic digestion of protein begins in the stomach. When proteins are denatured by stomach acid, **pepsin**, a major enzyme for proteins, goes to work (Fig. 6.6). Pepsin attacks the denatured proteins and breaks them down into shorter chains of amino acids. Pepsin does not completely separate proteins into amino acids because it can break only a few of the many peptide bonds found in these large molecules.

The release of pepsin is controlled by the hormone gastrin (review Table 3.3 in Chapter 3). Thinking about food or chewing food stimulates gastrin-producing cells in the stomach to release the hormone. Gastrin also strongly stimulates the stomach to produce acid.

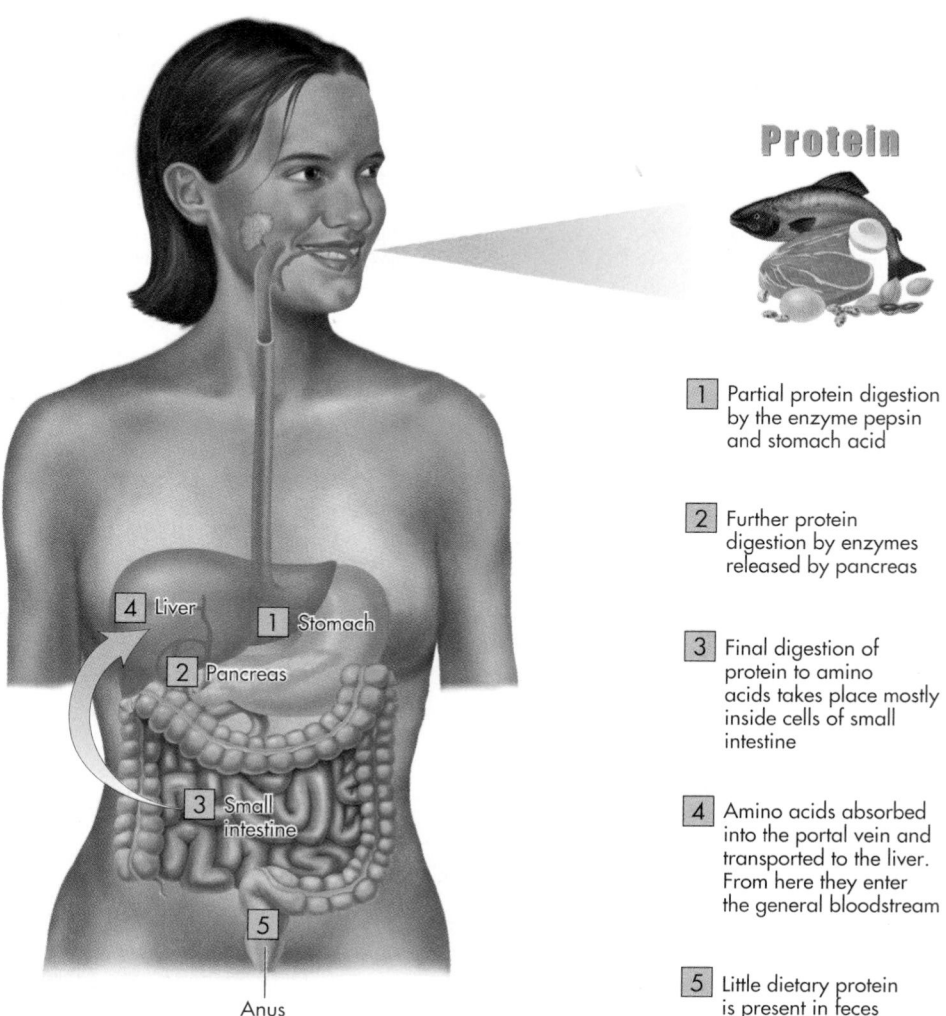

Protein

1. Partial protein digestion by the enzyme pepsin and stomach acid

2. Further protein digestion by enzymes released by pancreas

3. Final digestion of protein to amino acids takes place mostly inside cells of small intestine

4. Amino acids absorbed into the portal vein and transported to the liver. From here they enter the general bloodstream

5. Little dietary protein is present in feces

4 Liver   1 Stomach
2 Pancreas
3 Small intestine
5
Anus

Figure 6.6 A summary of protein digestion and absorption. Enzymatic protein digestion begins in the stomach and ends in the absorptive cells of the small intestine, where any remaining short groupings of amino acids are broken down into single amino acids. Stomach acid and enzymes contribute to protein digestion. Absorption from the intestinal lumen into the absorptive cells requires energy input.

The partially digested proteins move with the rest of the nutrients and other substances in a meal (chyme) from the stomach into the small intestine. Once in the small intestine, the partially digested proteins (and any fats accompanying them) trigger the release of the hormone cholecystokinin (CCK) from the walls of the small intestine. CCK, in turn, travels through the bloodstream to one of its target organs, the pancreas. This causes the pancreas to release protein-splitting enzymes, such as **trypsin**. These digestive enzymes divide the partially digested proteins into short groupings of amino acids made up of two to three amino acids and some free amino acids. Eventually, digestion of some of this mixture into amino acids occurs, using other enzymes secreted into the intestine by glands located in the small intestine.

trypsin A protein-digesting enzyme secreted by the pancreas to act in the small intestine.

■ Absorption

The short groupings of amino acids and any free amino acids in the small intestine are taken up by active absorption into the absorptive cells lining the small intestine.

Any remaining peptide bonds are eventually broken down to yield individual amino acids inside the intestinal cells. The amino acids travel via the portal vein to the liver, where they are combined into protein, converted to glucose or fat, used for energy needs, or released into the bloodstream.

Few whole proteins are absorbed. The only time that this is not true is during infancy (up to 4 to 5 months of age). Until that time, whole proteins can be absorbed by the intestines of infants. This is particularly harmful if infants are fed cow's milk or egg whites, as these may predispose the infant to food allergies (see Chapter 14 for details).

Concept Check

*E*nzymatic protein digestion begins in the stomach. In the small intestine, protein breakdown products formed in the stomach separate finally into amino acids as the breakdown products enter the absorptive cells of the small intestine. The amino acids then travel via the portal vein to the liver.

▌ Putting Proteins to Work in the Body

As you have learned, proteins function in many crucial ways in human metabolism and in the formation of body structures. We rely on foods to supply the amino acids needed to form these proteins. Note, however, that only when we also eat enough carbohydrate and fat can food proteins be used most efficiently. If we don't consume enough energy to meet energy needs, some amino acids from proteins are broken down to produce needed energy, rather than used to make needed body proteins.

■ Producing Vital Body Constituents

Every cell contains protein. Muscles, connective tissue, mucus, blood-clotting factors, transport proteins in the bloodstream, lipoproteins, enzymes, immune bodies, some hormones, visual pigments, and the support structure inside bones are mainly made of protein (Fig. 6.7). Excess protein in the diet doesn't enhance the synthesis of these body components, but eating too little can impede it.

As mentioned before, most vital body proteins are in a constant state of breakdown, rebuilding, and repair, especially in the bone marrow and the intestine. If a person habitually doesn't eat enough protein, the rebuilding and repairing process slows. Eventually, skeletal muscles, heart, liver, blood proteins, and other organs decrease in size or volume. Only the brain resists protein breakdown.

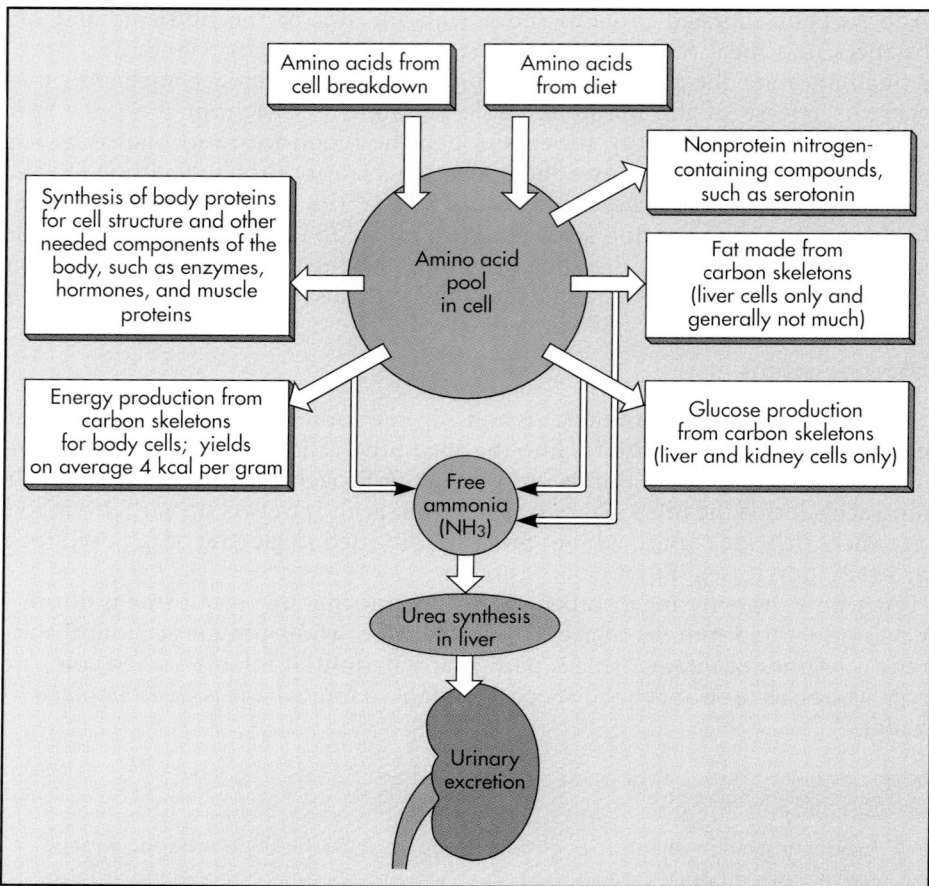

Figure 6.7 Amino acid metabolism. The amino acid **pool** in a cell can be used to form body proteins, as well as a variety of other possible products—from fat and glucose to urea. The urea is a waste product made from the nitrogen-containing ammonia (NH_3) released during amino acid breakdown.

pool The amount of a nutrient found within the body that can be mobilized when needed.

capillary bed Minute, one cell thick vessels that create a junction between arterial and venous circulation. It is here that gas and nutrient exchange occurs between body cells and the blood.

extracellular space The space outside cells.

edema The buildup of excess fluid in extracellular spaces.

■ Maintaining Fluid Balance

Blood proteins maintain body fluid balance. Blood pressure in the arteries forces blood into capillary beds. The blood fluid then enters from the **capillary beds** into the spaces between nearby cells (**extracellular spaces**) to provide nutrients to those cells (Fig. 6.8). Proteins in the bloodstream are too large to move out of the capillary beds into the tissues. The presence of these proteins in the capillary beds attracts the fluid back to the blood, partially counteracting the force of blood pressure. This is especially true in the areas of the capillary beds right next to their venous connections.

Unless enough protein is consumed, the concentration of proteins eventually decreases in the bloodstream. Excessive fluid then builds up in the surrounding tissues because the counteracting force produced by the smaller amount of blood proteins is too weak to pull much of the fluid back from the tissues into the bloodstream. As fluids pool in the tissues, the tissues swell, causing **edema.** Because edema sometimes leads to serious medical problems, the cause must be identified. An important step in diagnosing the cause is to measure the concentration of blood proteins, although many other medical problems cause edema.

■ Contributing to Acid-Base Balance

Proteins help regulate acid-base balance in the blood. Proteins located in cell membranes pump chemical ions in and out of cells. The pumping action, among other

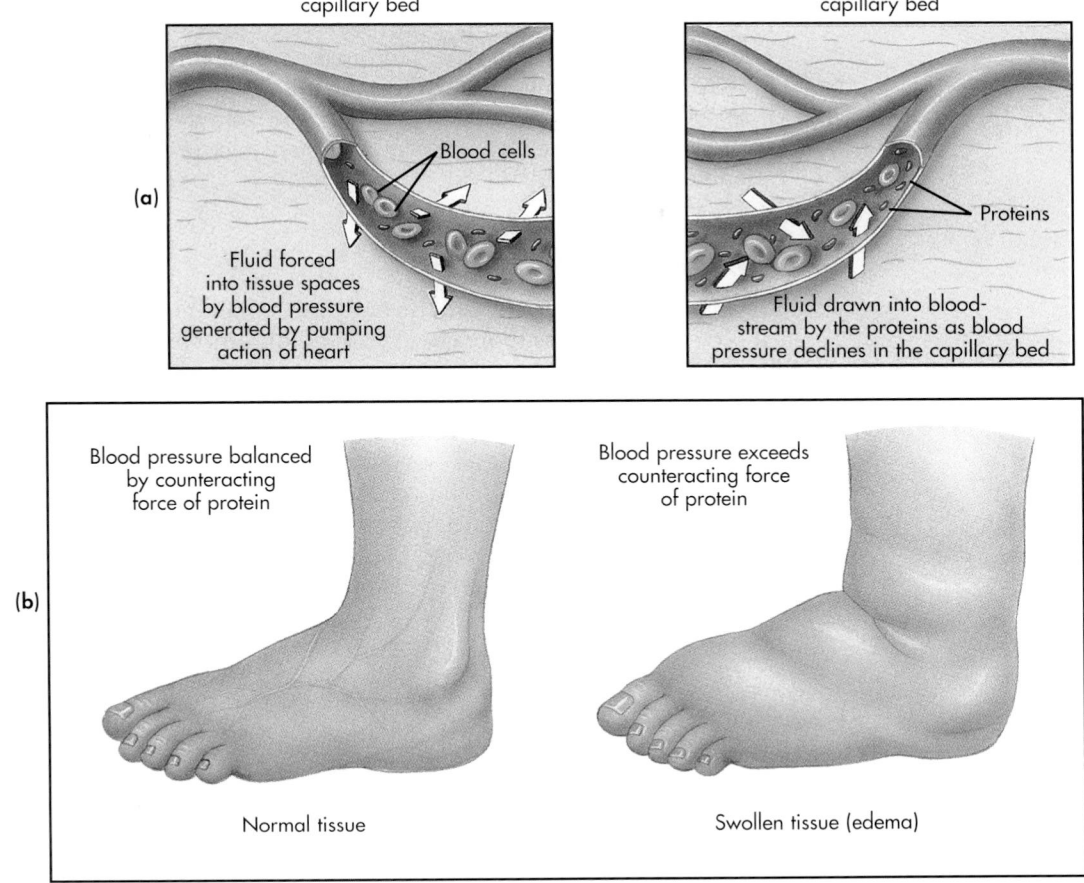

Figure 6.8 Blood proteins in relation to protein balance. (a) Blood proteins are important for maintaining the body's fluid balance. (b) Without sufficient protein in the bloodstream, edema develops.

factors, keeps the blood slightly alkaline. **Buffers**—compounds that maintain acid-base conditions within a narrow range—are another means of regulating acid-base balance in the blood. Some blood proteins are especially good buffers for the body.

buffers Compounds that cause a solution to resist changes in acid-base balance.

■ Forming Hormones and Enzymes

Amino acids are required for the synthesis of many hormones—our internal body messengers. Some hormones, such as the thyroid hormones, are made from only one amino acid, tyrosine. Insulin, on the other hand, is composed of 48 amino acids. These and other hormones classified as proteins perform important regulatory functions in the body, such as controlling the metabolic rate and the amount of glucose taken up from the bloodstream.

Almost all enzymes are proteins or have a protein component. Recall from Chapter 3 that enzymes are compounds that speed chemical reactions. Occasionally, a cell lacks the correct genetic information to make needed enzymes. For example, an infant who has the disease **galactosemia** can't make an enzyme needed to metabolize the single sugar galactose. If the infant is not started on a galactose-free diet soon after birth—which in practical terms means no cow's milk, human milk, liver, and certain other foods—its growth and mental development will be depressed. A special infant formula must be used. The galactose-free diet is then continued, ideally throughout life. This example underscores the crucial roles that enzymes and, thus, proteins, play in cell function.

Neurotransmitters, released by nerve endings, are often derivatives of amino acids. This is true for dopamine (synthesized from the amino acid tyrosine), norepinephrine (synthesized from the amino acid tyrosine), and serotonin (synthesized from the amino acid tryptophan). The way in which diet influences the synthesis of some of these neurotransmitters is currently under study. For example, high-carbohydrate meals can induce sleepiness as a result of increased serotonin synthesis in the brain.

■ Contributing to Immune Function

Proteins compose key parts of the cells used by the immune system. Also, the antibodies produced by one type of white blood cell are proteins. These antibodies can bind to foreign proteins in the body, an important step in removing invaders from the body. Without sufficient dietary protein, the immune system lacks the cells and other tools needed to function properly. This state can turn measles into a fatal disease for a malnourished child.

■ Forming Glucose

In Chapter 4 you learned that the body must maintain a fairly constant concentration of blood glucose to supply energy for red blood cells and nervous tissue. At rest, the brain uses about 19% of the body's energy requirements, and it gets most of that energy from glucose. If you don't consume enough carbohydrate to supply the glucose, your liver (and kidneys, to a lesser extent) will be forced to make glucose from amino acids present in body tissues (review Fig. 6.7).

Making some glucose from amino acids is normal. For example, when you skip breakfast and haven't eaten since 7 P.M. the preceding evening, glucose must be manufactured. Taken to an extreme, however, such as occurs in starvation, the conversion of amino acids into glucose wastes much muscle tissue and can produce edema.

■ Providing Energy

Proteins supply very little of the energy to the body, except during prolonged exercise (see Chapter 11 for information about the use of amino acids for energy during exercise). In this case, the amino group ($-NH_2$) from the amino acid is removed and the **carbon skeleton** is used for energy needs. Still, under most conditions, cells use primarily carbohydrates and fats for energy. Proteins and carbohydrates contain the same amount of usable energy—on average, 4 kcal per gram. However, proteins are a very costly source of energy, considering the amount of metabolism and processing the liver and kidneys must perform to use this energy source. The monetary cost of protein-rich foods is also a consideration.

> *The vitamin niacin can be made from the amino acid tryptophan, illustrating another role of proteins.*

carbon skeleton Amino acid structure that remains after the amino group has been removed.

Concept Check

Vital body constituents—such as muscle, connective tissue, transport proteins in the bloodstream, enzymes, hormones, buffers, and immune factors—are mainly proteins. Proteins can also provide fuel for the body and be used for glucose production.

Protein Needs

How much protein (actually, amino acids) do we need to eat each day? People who aren't growing need to eat only enough protein to match whatever they lose daily from protein breakdown. The amount of breakdown is determined by measuring the amount of urea and other nitrogen-containing compounds in the urine, as well as losses of protein as such from feces, skin, hair, nails, and so on. In short, people need to balance protein intake with losses. This maintains a state of protein equilibrium (Fig. 6.9).

When a body is growing or recovering from an illness, it needs a positive protein balance to supply the raw materials required to build new tissues. To achieve this, a person must eat more protein daily than he or she loses. In addition, the hormones insulin, growth hormone, and testosterone all stimulate positive protein balance. Resistance exercise (weight training) also enhances positive protein balance.

Positive protein balance	Protein equilibrium	Negative protein balance
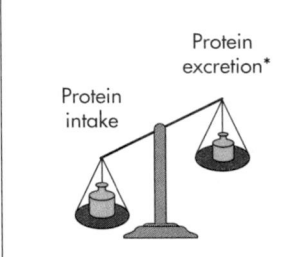	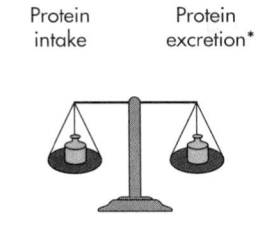	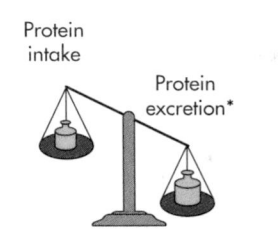

Situations in which protein balance is positive:

Growth
Pregnancy
Recovery stage after illness
Athletic training**
Increased secretion of hormones, such as insulin, growth hormone, and testosterone

Situations in which protein balance is negative:

Inadequate intake of protein (fasting, intestinal tract diseases)
Inadequate energy intake
Conditions such as fevers, burns, and infections
Bed rest (for several days)
Deficiency of essential amino acids (e.g., poor-quality protein consumed)
Increased protein loss (as in some forms of kidney disease)
Increased secretion of certain hormones, such as thyroid hormone and cortisol

---

*Based on losses of urea and other nitrogen-containing compounds in the urine, as well as protein itself lost from feces, skin, hair, nails, and other minor routes.

**Only when additional lean body mass is being gained. Nevertheless, the athlete is probably already eating enough protein to support this extra protein synthesis; protein supplements are not needed.

Figure 6.9   Protein balance in practical terms.

For healthy people, the amount of dietary protein needed to maintain protein equilibrium (wherein intake equals losses) can be determined by increasing protein intake until it just equals losses. Energy needs must be met so that amino acids are not diverted for energy use.

Today, the best estimate for the amount of protein required for nearly all adults to maintain protein equilibrium is 0.8 grams of protein per kilogram of healthy body weight. This is the RDA for protein. The amount approximately doubles during infancy. (Specific values for infants and children are discussed in Chapter 14 and the concept of healthy weight in Chapter 10.) Healthy weight is used as a baseline because excess fat storage doesn't contribute much to protein needs. This RDA works out to about 56 grams of protein daily for a typical 70-kilogram (154-pound) man and about 44 grams of protein daily for a typical 55-kilogram (120-pound) woman.

*T*he RDA for protein translates into about 8% to 10% of total calories. The National Cholesterol Education Program in the United States recommends up to 15% of total calories to provide more flexibility in diet planning, in turn allowing for the variety of protein-rich foods North Americans typically consume. This amount also generally provides enough protein for the active athlete.

Convert weight from pounds to kilograms:

$$\frac{154 \text{ pounds}}{2.2 \text{ pounds/kilogram}} = 70 \text{ kilograms}$$

$$\frac{120 \text{ pounds}}{2.2 \text{ pounds/kilogram}} = 55 \text{ kilograms}$$

Calculate RDA:

$$70 \text{ kilograms} \times \frac{0.8 \text{ grams protein}}{\text{kilogram body weight}} = 56 \text{ grams}$$

$$55 \text{ kilograms} \times \frac{0.8 \text{ grams protein}}{\text{kilogram body weight}} = 44 \text{ grams}$$

Table 6.3 The Protein Content of a 1200 kcal Diet and a 2400 kcal Diet*

1200 kcal Diet	Protein (grams)	2400 kcal Diet	Protein (grams)
Breakfast			
Nonfat milk, 1 cup	8	2% reduced-fat milk, 1 cup	8
Cheerios, 1 cup	2	Cheerios, 1 cup	2
Orange	1	Eggs, soft cooked, 2	12
		Orange	1
Lunch			
Whole-wheat bread, 2 slices	5	Whole-wheat bread, 2 slices	5
Chicken breast, 2 ounces	17	Chicken breast, 2 ounces	17
Mayonnaise, 1 teaspoon	—	Provolone cheese, 2 ounces	15
Tomato slices, 2	—	Tomato slices, 2	—
Carrot sticks, 1 cup	1	Mayonnaise, 1 teaspoon	—
Fig, 1 large	0.5	Oatmeal-raisin cookies, 2	2
Diet soda	—	Figs, 2	1
		Diet soda	—
Dinner			
Mixed green salad, ½ cup	—	Mixed green salad, ½ cup	—
Italian dressing, 2 teaspoons	—	Italian dressing, 2 teaspoons	—
Beef tenderloin, 2 ounces	14	Beef tenderloin, 4 ounces	28
Spinach pasta, 1 cup, with garlic butter, 1 teaspoon	7	Spinach pasta, 1 cup, with garlic butter, 1 teaspoon	7
Zucchini, ½ cup, sauteed in oil, 1 teaspoon	0.5	Zucchini, ½ cup, sauteed in oil, 1 teaspoon	0.5
Nonfat milk, 1 cup	8	Carrot sticks, ½ cup	0.5
Bagel, toasted, ½ of a 3½-inch bagel	4		
Jam, 2 teaspoons	—	**Snack**	
		2% reduced-fat milk, 1 cup	8
		Bagel, toasted, ½ of 3½-inch bagel	4
		Jam, 2 teaspoons	—
	—	Fruited yogurt, 1 cup	10
TOTAL	70		122

*This table illustrates how little energy need be consumed while still meeting the RDA for protein. It also shows how much protein we eat when we consume typical energy intakes. The amounts work out to be about 25% of total calories as protein, quite a generous amount.

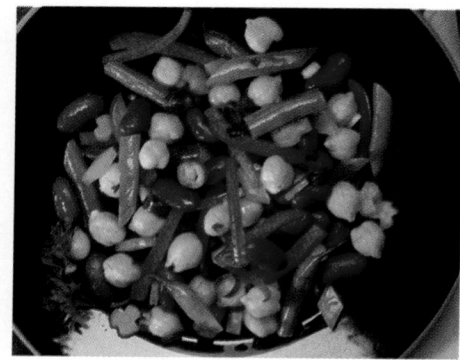

Keep in mind that amino acids in vegetables are best used when a combination of sources is consumed.

It is easy to consume the amount of protein currently suggested each day to meet body needs (Table 6.3). North American men typically consume about 95 grams of protein daily, whereas women typically consume 65 grams daily.

Thus, most of us consume much more protein than the RDA recommends because we like many high-protein foods and can afford to buy them. Excess protein eaten cannot be stored as such, so it is turned into glucose or fat and then either stored or metabolized for energy needs (review Fig. 6.7). Pregnancy raises protein needs by about 10 to 15 grams per day averaged over the 9 months and totaling 60 grams per day in all for the diet. However, mental stress, physical labor, and routine weekend sports activities do not require an increase in the protein RDA.

To support the training needs of endurance and highly trained athletes, the protein allowance can be increased to about 1.2–1.4 grams per kilogram (about 1.5 to 2 times the RDA, see Chapter 11 for details). There is no clear, demonstrated advantage however in exceeding 1.7–2 grams of protein per kilogram of healthy body weight per day (about 2½ times the RDA). In addition, athletes do not need individual amino-acid supplements. All of us, athletes included, can meet our protein needs using basic foods.

Surveys show that only older women as a group fail to eat enough protein to meet the RDA, and the deficiency is very slight. Older adults may also have slightly higher protein needs than those established by the RDA. Some researchers advocate an intake up to 1.2 grams of protein per kilogram of healthy body weight. To put this recommendation into practice, older adults should strive to include a rich protein source at every meal (and most snacks).

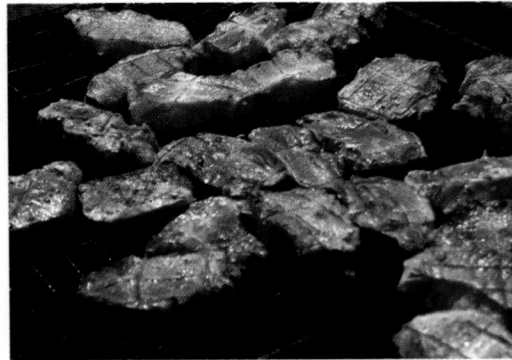

Animal protein foods are typically our favorite sources of amino acids.

Does Eating a High-Protein Diet Harm You?

People frequently ask whether the high protein intake of adults in North America is harmful. The extra vitamin B-6, iron, and zinc that accompany protein foods are often beneficial. However, high-protein diets typically are low in plant foods and, so, low in dietary fiber, some vitamins (e.g., folate), some minerals (e.g., magnesium), and phytochemicals. As well, these diets are typically rich in saturated fat. As a consequence, consumption of animal protein (if not well trimmed of fat) has been linked to cardiovascular disease in humans, likely due to this saturated fat content.

High-protein diets can increase calcium loss in urine. Certain types of amino acids—especially some of those rich in animal proteins—cause this effect. Based on the research to date, it is reasonable to assume that individuals who have inadequate calcium intakes are further compromising bone health by consuming excessive amounts of protein. People meeting their calcium needs should not be concerned about this effect of dietary protein. The increased calcium loss in the urine also may contribute to kidney stone formation in people who have this problem.

Excessive intake of red meat, especially processed meats like ham and salami, is linked to colon cancer in population studies. This link could be attributable to the protein or fat in the food products, to substances used in curing the meats, or to substances that form during cooking of red meat at high temperatures (heterocyclic amines; see the Nutrition Issue in Chapter 8). Excessive fat intake associated with diets rich in red meat, or low dietary fiber intake, may also be a contributing factor. Because of this concern with red meat, some nutrition experts suggest we focus more on poultry, fish, nuts, legumes (beans), and seeds to meet protein needs, and as well trim red and other forms of meat of visible fat before cooking.

Some researchers have also expressed the concern that a high protein intake may unduly burden the kidneys by forcing them to excrete the resulting excess nitrogen as urea. Low-protein diets marginally slow the decline in kidney function in humans if begun early in the course of developing kidney disease, and laboratory animal studies show that protein intakes that just meet nutritional needs preserve kidney function over time better than do high-protein diets. Preserving kidney function is especially important for people with diabetes, for people who show signs of kidney disease, and for people who have only one functioning kidney. High-protein diets are discouraged in these cases. For people without diabetes or kidney disease, the risk of suffering kidney failure is very low; thus, the risk of a high-protein diet's contributing to kidney disease (aside from kidney stones) in later life is also low.

Generally speaking, most experts recommend that not more than twice the RDA for protein be consumed on a regular basis (including any use of protein powders and related supplement forms). Reducing intake to approximate RDA amounts may benefit some of us, but the research is still too incomplete to permit a firm conclusion.

The amino acids most likely to cause toxicity when consumed in large amounts are methionine and tyrosine. Overall, the potential for amino acid imbalances and toxicities is too great to recommend that any be taken individually as supplements. As emphasized earlier, the body is designed to handle whole proteins as a dietary source of amino acids. When individual amino-acid supplements are taken, they can overwhelm the absorptive mechanism in the small intestine, triggering amino acid

*I*nfants' diets must be limited in protein because their kidneys have difficulty excreting large amounts of urea and minerals, which remain after protein metabolism. Thus, regular cow's milk must not be used for feeding young infants—it is too high in protein and other nutrients (see Chapter 14 for details).

imbalances in the body. These imbalances occur because groups of chemically similar amino acids compete for absorption sites in the absorptive cells. An excess of one can hamper other amino acids from being absorbed. We should stick to whole foods as sources for amino acids.

Concept Check

The Recommended Dietary Allowance (RDA) for adults is 0.8 grams of protein per kilogram of healthy body weight. This is approximately 56 grams of protein daily for a 70-kilogram (156-pound) person. The average North American man consumes about 95 grams of protein daily, and a woman consumes about 65 grams. Thus, typically we eat more than enough protein to meet our needs. Diets high in protein can increase calcium loss in the urine, compromise kidney health in people with diabetes and those with kidney disease or a history of kidney stones.

Protein-Energy Malnutrition

protein-energy malnutrition A condition resulting from regularly consuming insufficient amounts of energy and protein. The deficiency eventually results in body wasting, primarily of lean tissue, and an increased susceptibility to infections.

marasmus A disease that results from consuming a grossly insufficient amount of protein and energy; one of the diseases classed as protein-energy malnutrition. Victims have little or no fat stores, little muscle mass, and poor strength. Death from infections is common.

kwashiorkor A disease occurring primarily in young children who have an existing disease and consume a marginal amount of energy and considerably insufficient protein in relation to needs. The child generally suffers from infections and exhibits edema, poor growth, weakness, and an increased susceptibility to further illness.

Rarely an isolated condition, protein deficiency usually accompanies a deficiency of dietary energy and other nutrients resulting from insufficient food intake. In developing areas of the world, people often have diets low in energy and, as a result, protein. This state of undernutrition stunts the growth of children and makes them more susceptible to disease throughout life. (Note that undernutrition is a main focus of Chapter 17.) People who consume too little protein and food energy can go on to develop **protein-energy malnutrition (PEM),** also referred to as *protein-calorie malnutrition (PCM)*. In its milder form, it is difficult to tell if a person with PEM is consuming too little energy or protein, or both. But if the nutrient deficiency—especially for energy—is quite severe, a deficiency disease called **marasmus** can result. When an inadequate intake of nutrients, including protein, is combined with an already existing disease, a form of malnutrition called **kwashiorkor** can develop. Both are primarily seen in children, but can also develop in adults. These two conditions form the tip of the iceberg with respect to states of undernutrition, and symptoms of these two conditions even can be present in the same person (Fig. 6.10).

▌ Kwashiorkor

Kwashiorkor is a word from Ghana that means "the disease that the first child gets when the new child comes." From birth, an infant is usually breastfed. Typically, it is believed that by the time the child reaches 1 to 1.5 years of age, the mother is usually pregnant or has already given birth again, and breastfeeding is no longer possible for the first child. This child's diet abruptly changes from nutritious human milk to native starchy roots and gruels. These foods have low protein densities, compared with total energy. Additionally, the foods are usually full of plant fibers, which are often bulky, making it difficult for the child to consume enough to meet energy needs. The child may also have infections and parasites, which acutely raise energy and protein needs. For these reasons, energy needs of these children are met marginally, at best, and their protein needs are not met, especially when needs are greatly increased by infections and marginal energy intakes. Usually, many vitamin and mineral requirements are also far from being fulfilled. Famine victims face similar problems.

The major symptoms of kwashiorkor are apathy, listlessness, failure to grow and gain weight, and withdrawal from the environment. These symptoms complicate other diseases present. For example, a condition such as measles, a disease that normally makes a healthy child ill for only a week or so, can become severely debilitating and even fatal. Further symptoms of kwashiorkor are changes in hair color, potassium deficiency, flaky skin, fatty infiltration in the liver, reduced muscle mass, and massive edema in the abdomen and legs. The presence of edema in a child who has some

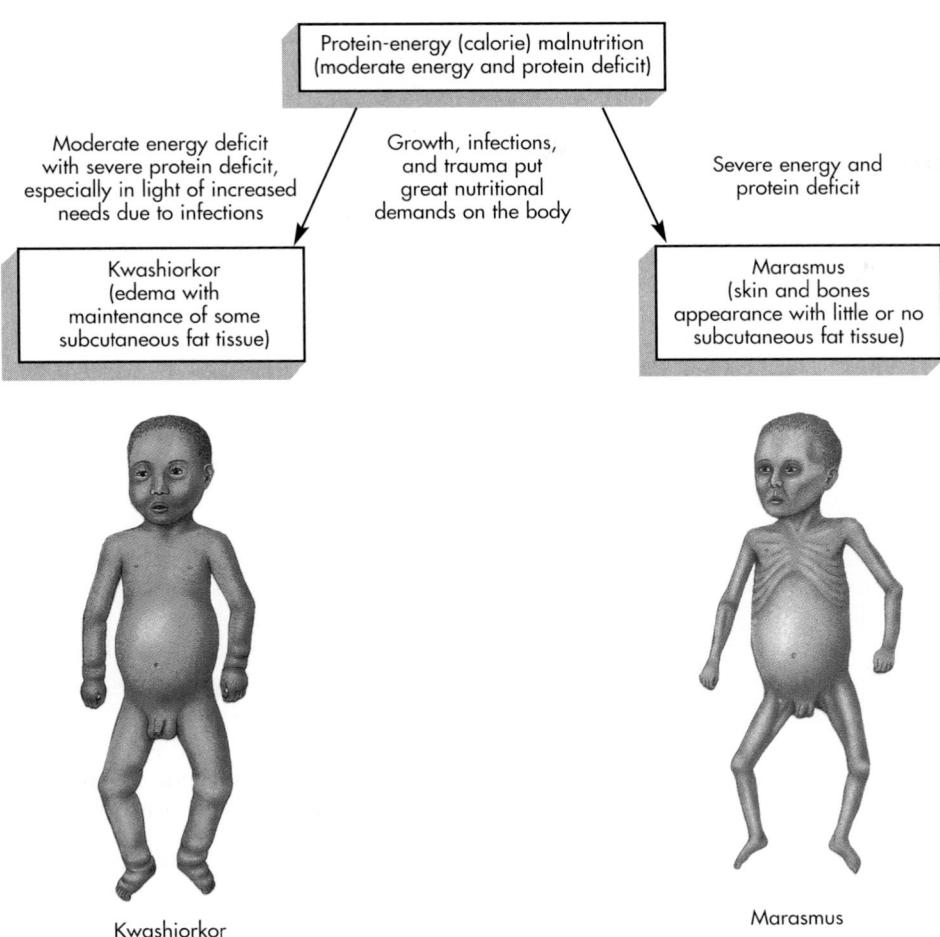

Protein-energy (calorie) malnutrition
(moderate energy and protein deficit)

Moderate energy deficit
with severe protein deficit,
especially in light of increased
needs due to infections

Growth, infections,
and trauma put
great nutritional
demands on the body

Severe energy and
protein deficit

Kwashiorkor
(edema with
maintenance of some
subcutaneous fat tissue)

Marasmus
(skin and bones
appearance with little or no
subcutaneous fat tissue)

Kwashiorkor

Marasmus

Figure 6.10 A schema for classifying undernutrition in children. The presence of subcutaneous fat (directly underneath the skin) is a diagnostic key for distinguishing kwashiorkor from marasmus.

subcutaneous fat (i.e., directly under the skin) still present is the hallmark of kwashiorkor (see Fig. 6.10). In addition, these children seldom move. If you pick them up, they don't cry. When you hold them, you feel the plumpness of edema, not muscle and fat tissue.

Many symptoms of kwashiorkor can be explained based on what we know about proteins. Proteins play important roles in fluid balance, lipoprotein transport, immune function, and production of tissues, such as skin, cells lining the GI tract, and hair. We should not expect children with an insufficient protein intake to grow and mature normally. And they don't.

If children with kwashiorkor are helped in time—if infections are treated and a diet ample in protein, energy, and other essential nutrients is provided—the disease process reverses. They begin to grow again and may even show no signs of their previous condition, except perhaps shortness of stature. Unfortunately, by the time many of these children reach a hospital or care center, they already have severe infections. In spite of the best care, they still die. Or, if they survive, they return home only to repeat the cycle.

■ Marasmus

Marasmus typically occurs as an infant slowly starves to death. It is caused by diets containing greatly insufficient amounts of protein, energy, and other nutrients.

As many as 2 million people worldwide die each year from tuberculosis, as this disease reemerges as the world's leading fatal infectious disease. In fact, up to one-third of the world population may be infected with the dreaded disease. A protein deficiency may lead to susceptibility to tuberculosis, and an improved diet may help delay fatalities. Unfortunately, as covered in Chapter 17, improving the diets for protein-malnourished people around the world remains an overwhelming task and will not likely be solved soon.

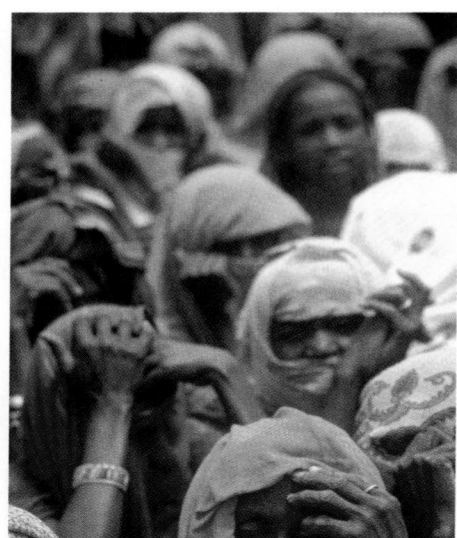

Famine conditions can provoke protein-energy malnutrition in adults as well as infants and children.

preterm An infant born before 37 weeks of gestation; also referred to as premature.

As previously noted, the condition is also commonly referred to as *protein-energy malnutrition*, especially when experienced by older children and adults. Typically, it occurs in infants who are slowly starving to death. The word *marasmus* means "to waste away," in Greek. Victims have a "skin-and-bones" appearance, with little or no subcutaneous fat (see Fig. 6.10).

Marasmus commonly develops in infants who either are not breastfed or have stopped breastfeeding in the early months. Often the weaning formula used is improperly prepared because of unsafe water and because the parents cannot afford sufficient infant formula for the child's needs. The latter problem may lead the parents to dilute the formula to provide more feedings, not realizing that this provides only more water for the infant.

Marasmus in infants commonly occurs in the large cities of poverty-stricken countries. In the cities, bottle-feeding is often necessary because the infant must be cared for by others when the mother is working or away from home. When people are poor and sanitation is lacking, bottle-feeding often leads to marasmus. An infant with marasmus requires large amounts of energy and protein—like a **preterm** infant—and, unless the child receives them, full recovery from the disease may never occur. The majority of brain growth occurs between conception and the child's first birthday. In fact, the brain is growing at its highest rate at birth. If the diet does not support brain growth during the first months of life, the brain may not grow to its full adult size. This reduced or retarded brain growth may lead to diminished intellectual function. Both kwashiorkor and marasmus wreak havoc on infants and children; mortality rates in developing countries are often 10 to 20 times higher than in North America.

Concept Check

Most undernutrition consists of mild deficits in energy, protein, and often other nutrients. If a person needs more nutrients because of disease and infection but does not consume enough energy and protein, a condition known as kwashiorkor can develop. The person suffers from edema and weakness. Children around age 2 are especially susceptible to kwashiorkor, particularly if they already have other diseases. Famine situations in which only starchy root products are available to eat contribute to this problem. Marasmus is a condition wherein people—infants, especially—starve to death. Symptoms include muscle wasting, absence of fat stores, and weakness. Both an adequate diet and the treatment of concurrent diseases must be promoted to maintain nutritional health.

Summary

1. Amino acids, the building blocks of proteins, contain a very usable form of nitrogen for humans. Of the 20 types of amino acids found in food, 9 must be consumed as food and the rest can be synthesized by the body.

2. High-quality, also called complete, protein foods contain ample amounts of all nine essential amino acids. Furthermore, foods derived from an animal source provide high biological value protein. Lower-quality, also called incomplete, protein foods lack sufficient amounts of one or more essential amino acids. This is typical of plant foods, especially cereal grains. Different types of plant foods eaten together often complement each other's amino-acid deficits, thereby providing high-quality protein in the diet.

3. Individual amino acids are bonded together to form proteins. The sequential order of amino acids determines the protein's ultimate shape and function. This order is directed by DNA in the cell nucleus. Diseases such as sickle cell anemia can occur if the amino acids are incorrect on a polypeptide chain. When the three-dimensional shape of a protein is unfolded—denatured—by treatment with heat, acid or alkaline solutions, or other processes, the protein also loses its biological activity.

4. Almost all animal products are nutrient-dense sources of protein. The high quality of these proteins means that they can be easily converted into body proteins.

5. Protein digestion begins in the stomach, dividing the proteins into breakdown products containing shorter chains of amino acids. In the small intestine, these polypeptide chains eventually separate into amino acids in the absorptive cells. These free amino acids then travel via the portal vein to the liver. Some then enter the bloodstream.

6. Important body components—such as muscles, connective tissue, transport proteins in the bloodstream, visual pigments, enzymes, some hormones, and immune bodies—are made of proteins. These proteins are in a state of constant turnover. Proteins also provide carbons which can be used to produce glucose when necessary.

7. The protein RDA for adults is 0.8 grams per kilogram of healthy body weight. For a typical 70-kilogram (156-pound) person, this corresponds to 56 grams of protein daily; for a 55-kilogram (120-pound) person, this corresponds to 44 grams per day. The North American diet generally supplies plenty of protein. Men typically consume about 95 grams of protein daily, and women consume closer to 65 grams. The combined protein intake is also of sufficient quality to support body functions.

8. Undernutrition can lead to protein-energy malnutrition in the form of kwashiorkor or marasmus. Kwashiorkor results primarily from an inadequate energy and protein intake in comparison with body needs, which often increase with concurrent disease and infection. Kwashiorkor often occurs when a child is weaned from human milk and fed mostly starchy gruels. Marasmus results primarily from extreme starvation—a negligible intake of both protein and energy. Marasmus commonly occurs during famine, especially in infants.

Study Questions

1. Discuss the relative importance of essential and nonessential amino acids in the diet. Why is it important for essential amino acids lost from the body to be replaced in the diet?
2. Describe the concept of complementary proteins.
3. What is a limiting amino acid? Explain why this concept is a concern in a vegetarian diet. How can a vegetarian compensate for limiting amino acids in specific foods?
4. Briefly describe the organization of proteins. How can this organization be altered or damaged? What might be a result of damaged protein organization?
5. Describe four functions of proteins. Provide an example of how the structure of a protein relates to its function.
6. How are DNA and protein synthesis related?
7. What would be one health benefit of reducing protein intake to RDA amounts for some people?
8. What characteristics of vegetable proteins could improve the North American diet? What foods would you include to provide a diet that has ample protein from both plant and animal sources but is moderate in fat?
9. Outline the major differences between kwashiorkor and marasmus.
10. What are the possible long-term effects of an inadequate intake of dietary protein among children between the ages of 6 months and 4 years?

Further Readings

1. Greaves KA, Thomson K: Soy protein comes to the aid of women. *Today's Dietitian*, p. 23, April 2001.
   There are multiple benefits from consumption of soy protein: heart health, bone health, and relief of menopausal symptoms. The benefits of a diet containing soy protein extend to people across the life cycle.
2. Henkel J: Soy: Health claims for soy proteins, questions about other components. *FDA Consumer*, p. 13, May–June 2000.
   In October 1999, FDA gave food manufacturers permission to put labels on products indicating that soy proteins in these foods may help lower cardiovascular disease risk. There is less evidence to support the consumption of other components of soy, especially when consumed as concentrated supplements.
3. How much protein is enough? *Consumer Reports on Health*, p. 8, February 2001.
   It is particularly important for pregnant women, breastfeeding women, young children, and older adults to meet protein needs. A daily intake of about 15% of total calorie intake is adequate to meet the protein needs of most people.
4. Is it time to stop eating meat? *Harvard Health Letter*, p. 6, September 2001.
   It is best to consume red meat on an occasional basis, rather than daily. Chicken, fish, legumes, and nuts are healthier, protein-rich alternatives.
5. Johnston TK: Nutritional implications of vegetarian diets. In Shils ME and others (eds.): *Modern nutrition in health and disease.* 9th ed. Baltimore: Williams & Wilkins, 1999.
   Vegetarian diets have a long history. There are many positive aspects of a primarily plant-based diet, including ample consumption of fruits and vegetables. Many typical diseases, such as cardiovascular disease and osteoporosis, are less common in vegetarians than in people consuming animal protein-rich diets. These findings are discussed in detail.
6. Kris-Etherton PM and others: The effects of nuts on coronary heart disease risk. *Nutrition Reviews* 59:103, 2001.
   Nuts have many nutritional attributes. They are rich in unsaturated fatty acids, dietary fiber, antioxidant vitamins, minerals, and numerous bioactive substances (i.e., flavonoids and plant sterols) that have many health benefits. A growing body of evidence demonstrates that nuts decrease cardiovascular disease risk.
7. Liebman B, Hurley J: Beans: No longer a bore. *Nutrition Action Health Letter*, p. 13, May 1999.
   If one hasn't consumed beans on a regular basis, it is best to start with small portions and increase this gradually over a few weeks, so one's GI tract has a chance to adjust. Use of the product Beano® can also help reduce intestinal gas-related discomfort.
8. Messina V, Mangels AR: Considerations in planning vegan diets: Children. *Journal of the American Dietetic Association* 101:661, 2001.
   Vegans must find good sources of vitamin B-12, riboflavin, zinc, calcium, and, if sun exposure is not adequate, vitamin D. This should not be problematic, due to the growing number and availability of fortified vegan foods that can help meet all nutrient needs. With appropriate food choices, vegan diets can be adequate, even for children. The article provides numerous examples of sources for the nutrients of concern in the vegan diet.
9. Norat T, Riboli E: Meat consumption and colorectal cancer: A review of epidemiologic evidence. *Nutrition Reviews* 59(2): 37, 2001.
   The risks of colorectal cancer are higher in people who consume diets rich in processed meat and red meat compared to individuals who consume small amounts. Total meat intake is not as much of a concern if one chooses a diet low in red meat and processed meats.
10. Smit E and others: Estimates of animal and plant protein intake in US adults: Results from the third National Health and Nutrition Examination Survey, 1988–1991. *Journal of the American Dietetic Association* 99:813, 1999.
    The main source of protein in the North American diet is animal protein (69%). Meat, fish, and poultry protein contributes most of the animal protein. Women tend to consume a lower percentage of red meat and a higher percentage of proteins from chicken, dairy, fruits, and vegetables.

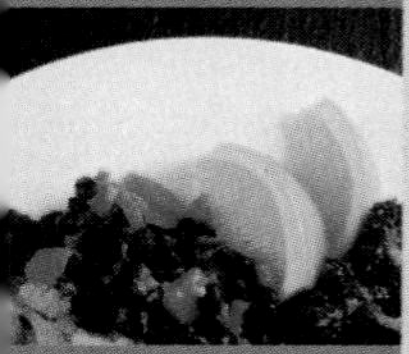

I. Is Your Protein Intake Sufficient to Meet Your Needs?

1. How much protein do you eat in a typical day? Look at the nutrition assessment you completed at the end of Chapter 2. Review it closely. Find the figure indicating the amount of protein you consumed on that day, and write it in the following space:

TOTAL PROTEIN _____

Compare your protein intake with your RDA for protein. Find your healthy weight for height in pounds using Figure 10.7 in Chapter 10. Choose a midrange value. Divide this number by 2.2 to reveal your healthy weight in kilograms. Next, multiply by 0.8 per kilogram of this weight or your current body weight if the numbers are close. This will indicate the RDA for protein for your weight and gender. Write it in the following space:

RDA FOR PROTEIN _____

How does your consumption compare with your RDA? _____

_____

If you consumed either more or less than the RDA, what foods could you add, delete, or eat more or less of? (Look at the foods you ate.)

_____

_____

Was most of your protein from animal or plant sources? _____

_____

If your protein intake was primarily from plants, did this come from a wide variety to encourage protein complementarity for the day?

_____

_____

II. Protein and the Vegetarian

Alana is excited about all the health benefits that might accompany a vegetarian diet. However, she is concerned that she will not consume enough protein to meet her needs. She is also concerned about possible vitamin and mineral deficiencies. Use your nutrition software to see if her concerns are valid.

Breakfast
Calcium fortified orange juice, 1 cup
Soybean milk, 1 cup
Fortified bran flakes, 1 cup
Banana, medium

Snack
Calcium-enriched granola bar

Lunch
Garden Burger, 4 ounces
Whole-wheat bun
Mustard, 1 tablespoon
Soy cheese, 1 ounce
Apple, medium
Green leaf lettuce, 1½ cups
Peanuts, 1 ounce
Sunflower seeds, ¼ cup
Tomato slices, 2
Mushrooms, 3
Vinaigrette salad dressing, 2 tablespoons
Iced tea

Dinner
Kidney beans, ½ cup
Brown rice, ¾ cup
Soft margarine, 2 tablespoons
Mixed vegetables, ¼ cup
Hot tea

Dessert
Strawberries, ½ cup
Angel food cake, 1 small slice
Soy milk, ½ cup

Alana's diet contained 2150 kcal, with _____ grams (you fill in) of protein (plenty for her), 360 grams of carbohydrate, 57 grams of total dietary fat (only 9 grams of which came from saturated fat), and 50 grams of fiber. Her vitamin and mineral intake with respect to those of concern in vegetarians—vitamin B-12, vitamin D, calcium, iron, and zinc—met her needs.

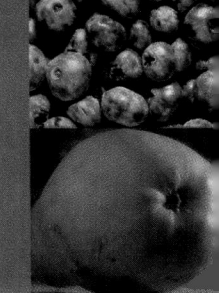

Vegetarianism has evolved over the centuries from a necessity into an option. Historically, vegetarianism was linked with specific philosophies and religions or with science. In the sixth century B.C., Pythagoras advocated a meatless diet for its physical health, ecological, religious, and philosophical benefits.

Today, there are about 12 million vegetarians in the United States alone, about double the number in 1985. Over the past two decades, vegetarian diets have gone from dull to delicious, with the inclusion of such new products as soy-based sloppy joes, chili, tacos, burgers, and more. In addition, cookbooks that feature the use of a variety of fruits, vegetables, and seasonings are enhancing food selection for vegetarians of all degrees.

Vegetarianism is popular among college students. Fifteen percent of college students in one survey said they select vegetarian options at lunch or dinner on any given day. In response, dining services offer vegetarian options at every meal, the most common being pastas with meatless sauce and pizza. Many teenagers are also turning to vegetarianism out of respect for animals. And a survey by the National Restaurant Association found that 20% of its customers want a vegetarian option when they eat out. Many customers cite health and taste as reasons for choosing vegetarian fare.

As nutrition science has grown, new information has enabled the design of adequate vegetarian diets. It is important for vegetarians to take advantage of this information because a diet of only plants can lead to various nutrient deficiencies and a substantial growth retardation in infants and children. People who choose a vegetarian diet can meet their nutritional needs by following a few basic rules and knowledgeably planning their diets (Table 6.4).

Table 6.4 Food-Group Plan for Lactovegetarians and Vegans[§]

	Servings		
Group[†]	Lactovegetarian[‡]	Vegan[§ll]	Key Nutrients Supplied
Grains[¶]	6–11	8–11	Protein, thiamin, niacin, folate, vitamin E, zinc, magnesium, iron, and dietary fiber
Legumes	1–2	2	Protein, vitamin B-6, zinc, magnesium, and dietary fiber
Nuts, seeds	1–2	2	Protein, vitamin E, and magnesium
Vegetables	3–5 (include one dark green or leafy variety daily)	4–6 (include one dark green or leafy variety daily)	Vitamin A, vitamin C, and folate
Fruits	2–4	4	Vitamin A, vitamin C, and folate
Milk	2–3	—	Protein, riboflavin, vitamin D, vitamin B-12, and calcium

[†]Base serving size on those listed for the Food Guide Pyramid (see Chapter 2). This plan yields about 1600 to 1800 kcal. Increase the number of servings, or add other foods to meet higher energy needs.

[‡]Contains about 75 grams of protein in 1650 kcal.

[§]A calcium-fortified food, such as orange juice or soy milk, is needed unless a calcium supplement is used. In addition, use of a supplemental source of vitamin B-12 or foods fortified with vitamin B-12 is a must. Overall, fortified soy milk makes a valuable contribution to a vegan diet.

[ll]Contains about 79 grams of protein in 1800 kcal.

[¶]One serving of vitamin- and mineral-enriched breakfast cereal is recommended. Alternately, a balanced multivitamin and mineral supplement can be used to help close possible nutrient gaps.

continued

Studies show that death rates from some chronic diseases, such as certain forms of cardiovascular disease, cancer, type 2 diabetes, and obesity, are lower for vegetarians than for nonvegetarians. Healthful lifestyles (not smoking, abstaining from alcohol and drugs, and increasing physical activity) and social class bias probably partially account for these findings.

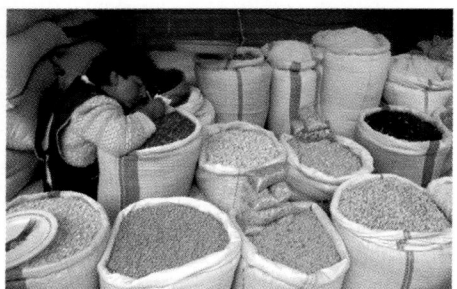

Primarily vegetarian diets are typical among rural peoples throughout the world.

Why Do People Become Vegetarian?

People choose vegetarianism for a variety of reasons. Some believe that killing animals for food is unethical. Hindus and Trappist monks eat vegetarian meals as a practice of their religion. In North America, many Seventh Day Adventists base their practice of vegetarianism on biblical texts and believe it is a more healthful way to live. Some people might pursue vegetarianism because meat is expensive.

People might choose vegetarianism after realizing that animals are not efficient protein factories. Animals actually use much of the protein they eat just to maintain themselves rather than to synthesize new muscle tissue. Note that 40% of the world's grain production is used to breed meat-producing animals. Animals that humans eat sometimes eat grasses that humans cannot digest. Many, however, also eat grains that humans can eat.

People might also practice vegetarianism because it encourages a high intake of carbohydrates; vitamins A, E, and C; carotenoids; magnesium; and dietary fiber while limiting saturated fat and cholesterol intake. This produces a diet closely resembling that suggested in the Dietary Guidelines for Americans, covered in Chapter 2.

Food Planning for Vegetarians

vegan A person who eats only plant foods.

fruitarian A person who primarily eats fruits, nuts, honey, and vegetable oils.

lactovegetarian A person who consumes plant products and dairy products.

lactoovovegetarian A person who consumes plant products, dairy products, and eggs.

There are a variety of vegetarian styles. **Vegans** eat only plant foods. **Fruitarians** primarily eat fruits, nuts, honey, and vegetable oils. This plan is not recommended because it can lead to nutrient deficiencies in people of all ages. **Lactovegetarians** modify vegetarianism a bit—they include dairy products and plant foods. **Lactoovovegetarians** modify the diet even further and eat dairy products and eggs, as well as plant foods. Including these animal products makes food planning easier because they are rich in some nutrients that are missing or present in low amounts in plants. The more variety in the diet, the easier it is to meet nutritional needs. Thus, the practice of eating no animal sources of food significantly separates the vegans and fruitarians from all other semivegetarian styles.

It has been suggested that "almost vegetarians" (those who allow some dairy and regular fish intake) are the healthiest group of all vegetarians. Perhaps this is due to the health benefits of a high fruit and vegetable diet, rather than the complete exclusion of all animal products.

Most people who call themselves vegetarians consume at least some dairy products, if not all dairy products and eggs. A food-group plan has been developed for lactovegetarians and vegans (review Table 6.4). This plan includes servings of nuts, grains, legumes, and seeds to help meet protein needs. There is also a vegetable group, a fruit group, and a milk group. Figure 6.11 shows a pyramid for vegetarians developed by Oldways Preservation & Exchange Trust. The base consists of fruits, vegetables, whole grains, and legumes (at every meal). The middle tier is nuts, seeds, egg whites, soy milks, dairy products, and plant oils (daily). Eggs and sweets form the tip (small quantities). Alcohol intake in moderation is optional and daily physical activity is recommended (see the Oldways Preservation & Exchange Trust website at www.oldwayspt.org for further information).

The Vegan

A vegan diet requires some creative planning. A real effort must be made to use grains and legumes to yield high-quality protein and other key nutrients in meals, especially when used with infants and children. Then, if energy needs are satisfied, protein needs should also be met. Including a wide variety of protein sources should provide all amino acids needed for a high-quality protein diet. The essential amino acids deficient from one food protein are supplied by

Table 6.2, earlier in this chapter, lists traditional dishes in which vegetable proteins combine to provide high-quality (complete) protein in the meal.

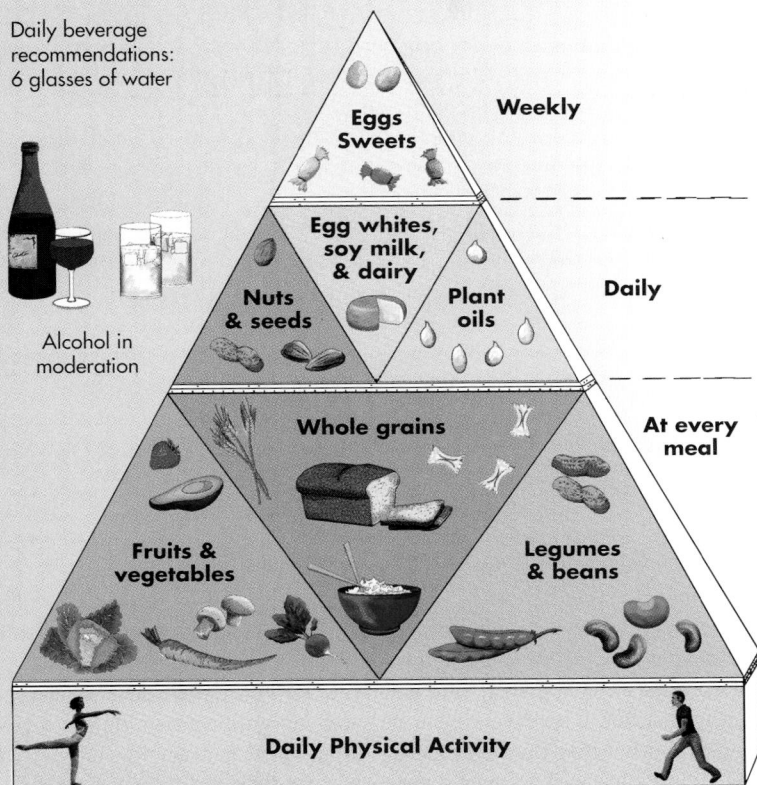

The Traditional Healthy
Vegetarian Diet Pyramid

Daily beverage
recommendations:
6 glasses of water

Alcohol in
moderation

Weekly

**Eggs
Sweets**

**Egg whites,
soy milk,
& dairy**

Daily

**Nuts
& seeds**

**Plant
oils**

At every
meal

Whole grains

**Fruits &
vegetables**

**Legumes
& beans**

Daily Physical Activity

Figure 6.11 The Oldways Preservation & Exchange Trust traditional vegetarian diet. Note that alcohol should only be used by adults of legal age. The organization emphasizes that such a diet has the advantage of being low in saturated fat, high in dietary fiber, and rich in antioxidants. However, it can pose a risk for an adequate iron, vitamin D, and vitamin B-12 intake. Inclusion of some fortified foods, such as a whole-grain, ready-to-eat breakfast cereal or a balanced vitamin and mineral supplement, is advised.

those of another protein in the same meal or in the next. For example, many legumes do not provide enough of the essential amino acid methionine, and cereals are limited in lysine. When a combination of these two foods is eaten, the body is supplied with adequate amounts of both amino acids, so cereals and legumes complement each other.

Purchasing some vegetarian cookbooks will simplify the task of menu planning. They provide numerous ideas for imaginative and nutritious ways to use plant foods.

The vegan diet must also include good sources of riboflavin, vitamins D and B-12, calcium, iron, and zinc. A typical ready-to-eat breakfast cereal provides a good start in meeting those needs. Riboflavin can be obtained from green leafy vegetables, whole grains, yeast, and legumes, part of most vegan diets. A major source of riboflavin in the typical North American diet is milk, which is omitted from the vegan diet. Vitamin D can be obtained through regular sun exposure and fortified margarine. Otherwise, a supplemental source of vitamin D should be considered (see Chapter 8).

The vegan should find a reliable source of vitamin B-12, such as fortified soybean milk or ready-to-eat breakfast cereals and special yeast grown on media rich in vitamin B-12. Use of a balanced vitamin and mineral supplement containing vitamin B-12 is another option. Vitamin B-12 occurs naturally only in animal foods, although plants can contain soil or microbial

hapter 5 noted that a vegan diet coupled with regular exercise and other lifestyle changes can lead to a reversal of atherosclerotic plaque in the coronary arteries.

continued

Fish oil supplements (about 900 milligrams per day of the omega-3 fatty acids) may be beneficial for the vegan to provide a concentrated source of long-chain omega-3 fatty acids (see Chapter 5 for details). In addition, regular use of canola oil, soybean oil, flax seeds, or walnuts is advised to obtain alpha-linolenic acid, another omega-3 fatty acid.

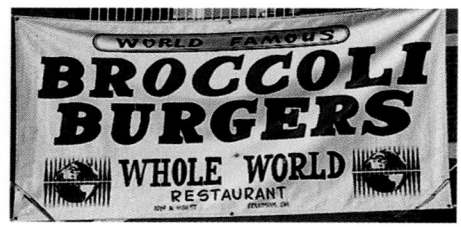

Vegetarian adaptations of traditional foods is a growing trend in our society.

contamination that provides at most a trace amount of vitamin B-12. Because the body can store enough vitamin B-12 for about 4 years, a deficiency can take a long time to develop after animal foods are removed from the diet. If a deficiency develops, nerves can be damaged irreversibly and brain function can decrease. Evidence of a vitamin B-12 deficiency has been noted in vegetarian mothers and their infants. The milk produced by the vegetarian mothers is low in vitamin B-12. The earliest sign of a vitamin B-12 deficiency is mental dysfunction; a prolonged deficiency can lead to irreversible nerve damage. Excess blood concentration of homocysteine has also been noted to vegans who underconsume vitamin B-12. This can lead to other health problems. Therefore, vegans need to be careful to prevent a vitamin B-12 deficiency.

To obtain calcium, the vegan can drink fortified soy milk or fortified orange juice and consume calcium-rich tofu (check the label) or other calcium-fortified foods, such as certain ready-to-eat breakfast cereals and snacks. Green leafy vegetables and nuts also contain calcium, but the calcium is either not well absorbed or not very plentiful. Calcium supplements are another option (see Chapter 9).

For iron, the vegan can consume whole grains, dried fruits and nuts, and legumes. The iron in these foods is not absorbed as well as that found in animal foods, but a good source of vitamin C taken with these foods modestly enhances iron absorption. Thus, a recommended strategy is to consume vitamin C with every meal that contains adequate iron-rich plant foods. Cooking in iron pots and skillets can also add iron to the diet (see Chapter 9).

The vegan can find zinc in whole grains, nuts, and legumes, but phytic acid and other substances in these foods limit zinc absorption. Grains are most nutritious when leavened, as in bread, because this process reduces the influence of phytic acid.

Of all these nutrients, calcium is the most difficult to consume in sufficient quantities. Special diet planning is required, as even a multivitamin and mineral supplement will not supply enough.

Veganism during childhood can pose problems. The most common nutritional concerns are deficiencies of iron, calcium, vitamin D, and vitamin B-12. Iron-deficiency anemia is a frequent occurrence during childhood; however, it can be avoided by supplementing the diet with iron-fortified cereals, and other iron-fortified foods. A supplement containing vitamin B-12 may be needed for children who exclude all animal products from their diets. A supplement containing vitamin D is recommended for children who do not get much sunlight exposure and who do not have any dietary source of vitamin D. Calcium can be obtained in the diet through dairy products or calcium-enriched products, such as tofu and orange juice. Finally, the fiber content of a child's diet may need to be decreased with high-fiber sources replaced with some refined grain products, fruit juices, and peeled fruit. Overall, vegan children need concentrated sources of energy to help avoid these problems. Examples include fortified soy milk, nuts, dried fruits, avocados, cookies made with vegetable oils or tub margarine, and fruit juices.

Soy milk, soy yogurt, and soy cheese are excellent choices for vegan children (and vegan adults). When fortified with calcium and vitamin B-12, these substitutes can provide many of the key nutrients found in milk.

Finding excellent iron and zinc sources is important in planning vegan diets, especially for infants and children. Overall, both infancy and childhood are life stages in which vegetarianism is appropriate, but it must be implemented with knowledge and, ideally, professional guidance. An especially informative website is www.ivu.org, supported by the International Vegetarian Union.

Scenario *Follow-Up*

Shannon is a vegan if she had no cheese on the sub sandwich, and a lactovegetarian if she did have cheese. Her diet plan is not healthy, as it does not come close to following the recommendations in this Nutrition Issue. Where are the whole grains, nuts, soy products, beans, two to four fruits, and three to five vegetables, that form the base of such diets? The diet is also low in the many phytochemicals under study. Overall, she is not benefiting as she had hoped to from her vegetarian diet, since so little care has gone into following a healthy pattern.

chapter 7

Alcohol

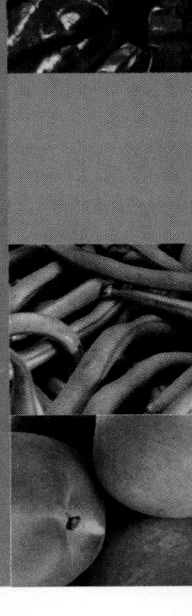

Chapter Outline

Alcohol use is an issue requiring careful attention by health professionals, law enforcement officials, the courts, elected officials, the entertainment industry, university professors, parents, students, and those engaged in the production and distribution of alcoholic beverages. Although not a nutrient per se, alcohol is a source of calories for about half of all adults, constituting about 5% of total calories in the North-American diet when averaged across the population. We also know that moderate consumption of alcohol by a person of legal age is an acceptable practice, and has some health benefits. But when it leads to excessive consumption, many unfortunate consequences are almost inevitable. By far the most commonly abused drug, alcohol can destroy families and friendships; spur deadly behaviors such as suicide, rape, and violence; and fill jails and prisons.

Over 8 million people in the United States alone are currently classified as having alcoholism, and another 31.9 million engage in binge drinking. Approximately 11 million of current drinkers are under the legal age of 21. From teenage through later years in life, excess alcohol intake has damaging effects on one's nutritional status and overall health. Alcohol abuse is also a major problem in Canada.

The American Medical Association defines alcoholism as an illness characterized by significant impairment directly related to persistent and excessive use of alcohol. Impairment can involve physiological and social dysfunction, and for psychological, social, and genetic reasons some people are more vulnerable to this disorder than others. Alcohol abuse touches many of our lives, so let's examine this substance in detail.

Check out the **Contemporary Nutrition: Issues and Insights Online Learning Center** www.mhhe.com/wardlawcont5 *for quizzes, flash cards, other activities, and web links designed to further help you learn about issues surrounding alcohol use and abuse.*

Chapter Objectives

Chapter 7 is designed to allow you to:

1. Describe the process of alcohol metabolism.

2. Describe some benefits of moderate alcohol consumption and define "moderate drinking."

3. List some nutrients that are most likely to be deficient in the diet of a person who abuses alcohol.

4. Explain how alcohol abuse damages body organs, such as the liver, heart, brain, and kidneys.

5. Identify body organs most likely to develop cancer because of alcohol abuse.

6. Outline the methods use to diagnose alcohol abuse.

7. List the typical strategies used in treating alcoholism, including the typical medications employed.

8. Describe the risks of binge drinking and the corresponding amount of alcohol this represents.

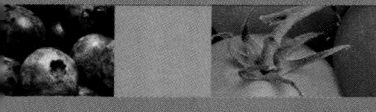

Refresh Your Memory

As you begin your study of alcohol in Chapter 7, you may want to review:

- The role of the GI tract, liver, and pancreas in digestion and absorption in Chapter 3

- The process of fermentation in Chapter 4

- Protein-energy malnutrition in Chapter 6

Real Life Scenario

Todd is a college junior. He was a very serious student in high school and achieved excellent grades, but as a college student he has begun binge drinking. As a result, his grades have fallen sharply and he is becoming socially isolated. He has been arrested once for drunk driving.

Last night, he had eight beers and three shots of whiskey at an off-campus party he attended with his girlfriend, Alyssa. Unfortunately, everyone who knows Todd says he tends to get angry and says things he doesn't mean when he drinks too much. He often becomes cruel and destructive to those he cares for and respects. He also has been involved in several fights.

As the party began to die down, Alyssa tried to get Todd to leave. He responded rudely and forcefully grabbed her arm. She became frightened with his aggressive behavior and left without him.

The next morning, Alyssa awoke early, still thinking about the hurtful events of the previous night. Having known of one student who died from an overdose of alcohol (he drank 23 shots of whiskey on his 21st birthday) Alyssa decided to email Todd, expressing her anxiety about his alcohol abuse. She did not want to see everything he had worked so hard for ruined by alcohol.

What should Alyssa say in the email about alcohol and how it affects various organs in the body? What long-term problems are associated with such alcohol abuse? Is Alyssa correct in taking the initiative in communicating to Todd her concerns about his drinking problem?

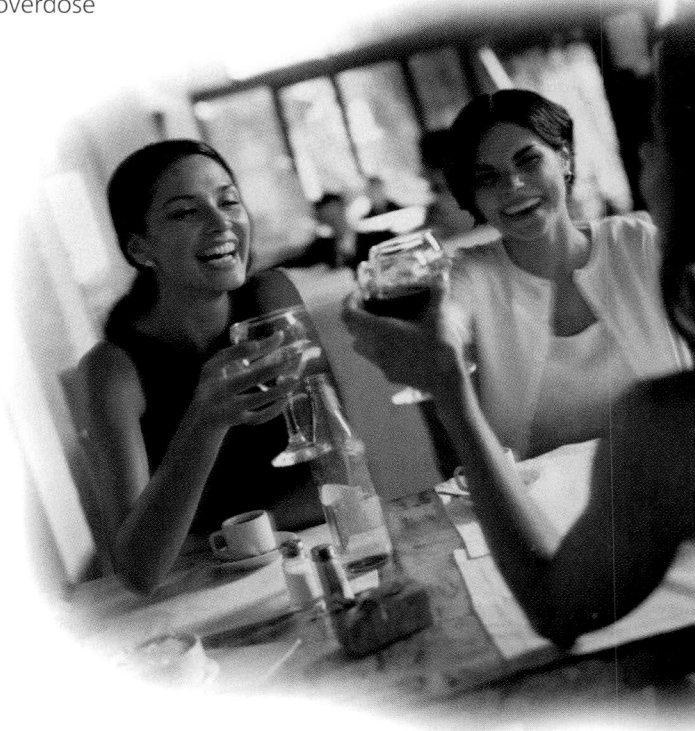

Nutrition Connection

FRANK & ERNEST

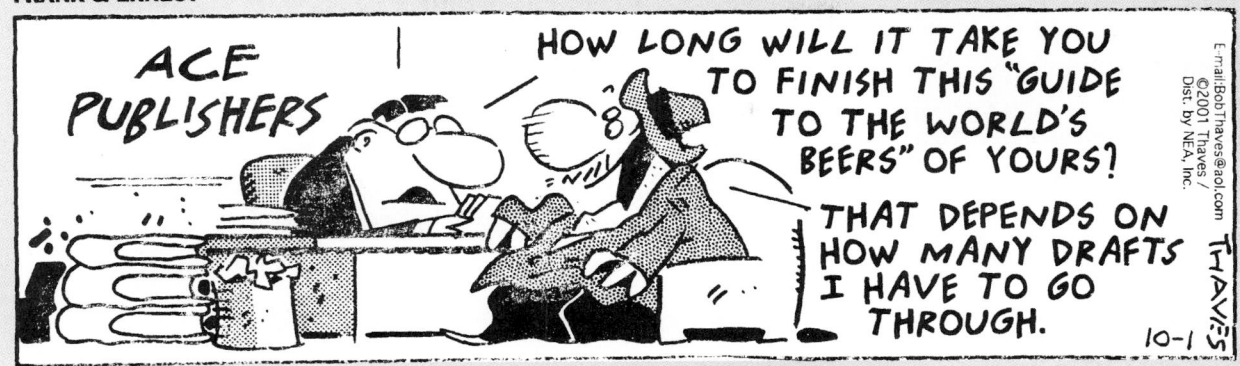

What are the pluses and minuses of alcohol use? And what constitutes alcoholism? Are some of us more susceptible to this chronic illness than others? How is it treated? Based on this relationship, should all adults of legal drinking age be abstainers? This chapter provides some answers.

FRANK & ERNEST © United Features Syndicate. Reprinted by Permission.

Alcohol—An Introduction

Given the wide spectrum of alcohol use and abuse—often starting in teenage and college years—knowledge of alcohol consumption and its relationship to overall health is essential to the study of nutrition. Alcohol, chemically known as ethanol, has played many roles throughout history (see the Nutrition Insight). Alcohol can be considered a food, primarily because it contributes energy to the diet (about 7 kcal per gram) (Table 7.1). It is also a social stimulant because it takes away inhibitions, it is a thirst quencher when used as a safe alternative to polluted water, and it is an analgesic to treat aches and pain.

Alcohol requires no digestion. It is absorbed rapidly from the GI tract by simple diffusion—no specific transport mechanisms are required for alcohol to enter a cell—so it is the most efficiently absorbed of all energy sources. Different parts of the GI tract absorb alcohol at different rates. The upper parts of the small intestine absorb alcohol fastest, depending on how quickly the stomach empties, which in turn depends on the kinds of foods consumed along with the alcohol. Alcohol then goes on to act on various organs as you will see, but has no cellular receptors per se, as do other compounds that affect the body, such as insulin and some fat-soluble vitamins.

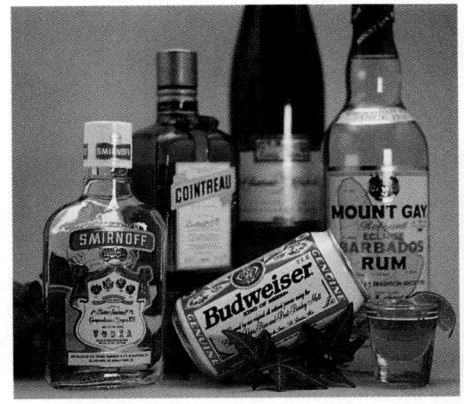

The following servings of each type of alcoholic beverage provide the same amount of alcohol (about 15 grams): wine—5 ounces, hard liquor—1.5 ounces, beer or wine cooler—12 ounces. In determining a safe level of intake, it is important to observe these serving sizes.

How Alcoholic Beverages Are Produced

Any number of natural foods can be fermented. Recall from Chapter 4 that this represents the breakdown of carbohydrates without the use of oxygen. Alcohol, carbon dioxide (CO_2), and various acids are byproducts. Production temperatures and composition of the food itself determine the characteristics of the final product. High-carbohydrate foods especially encourage the growth of yeast, the microbe responsible

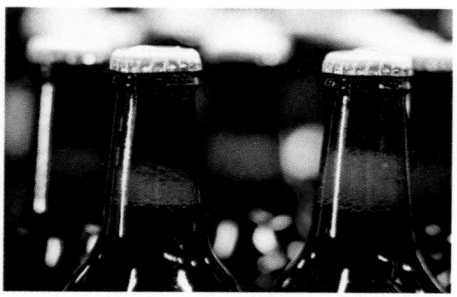

Beer is a source of alcohol and carbohydrates.

Table 7.1 Energy, Carbohydrate, and Alcohol Content of Alcoholic Beverages*

Beverage	Amount (fluid ounce)	Alcohol (grams)	Carbohydrates (grams)	Energy (kcal)
Beer				
Regular	12.0	13	13	146
Light	12.0	11	5	99
Distilled Spirits				
Gin, rum, vodka, bourbon, whiskey (80 proof)	1.5	14	—	105
Brandy, cognac	1.0	9	—	64
Wine				
Red	3.5	10	2	74
White	3.5	10	1	70
Dessert, sweet	3.5	16	12	158
Rosé	3.5	10	1	73
Mixed Drinks				
Manhattan	3.0	26	3	191
Martini	3.0	27	—	189
Bourbon and soda	3.0	11	—	78
Whiskey sour	3.0	15	5	122

*There is little to no fat or protein contribution to energy content.
Source: USDA.

for alcohol production. Brewer's yeast is one source of the enzyme that is necessary to make alcohol production possible.

The overall reaction for alcohol production is:

$$C_6H_{12}O_6 \rightarrow 2\ C_2H_5OH + 2\ CO_2 + 2\ H_2O$$

Glucose   Alcohol (ethanol)

The carbohydrate must be a simple sugar, such as maltose or glucose, in order for the yeast to use it as food. If the carbohydrate is a starch, such as that found in cereal grains, it must be broken down to these smaller forms, or "malted." During malting, the cereal grain seeds are allowed to sprout to produce the enzymes that break down the starches to simple sugars. The sprouting is then stopped by heating, and the yeast cells and water are added to the malt. The yeast grows using the sugars for energy. When the oxygen in the vat (the mixture of water, yeast, and malt) is used up, the yeast ferments the remaining sugar to produce alcohol and carbon dioxide. After fermentation has ceased, the product is finished in a variety of ways. In some cases, the alcohol itself is recovered from the product.

Beer is made from malted cereal grain, such as barley; it is flavored with hops and brewed by slow fermentation. The carbon dioxide released is collected and used to carbonate the beer, thus producing the desirable fizz associated with a quality beverage.

Wine is the fermented juice of grapes. Climate, geographic region, and variety of grape determine the quality of the wine. After fermentation, wines are aged in oak barrels to decrease the acidity and remove undesirable impurities.

Distilled spirits are made from the **distillation** of the alcohol after fermentation. Any number of fruits, vegetables, and grains can be fermented and the resulting mash distilled. The difference between the boiling point of water and the boiling point of alcohol allows these two liquids to be separated by distillation and the alcohol to be

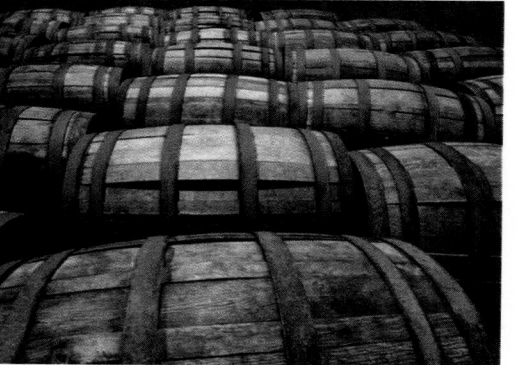

Wine is a historic beverage. It has been produced and consumed for more than 10,000 years.

distillation A physical method used to separate liquids based on their boiling points.

History of Alcohol

For thousands of years, alcoholic beverages have been produced from just about every plant material that can be fermented. Many important foods also have been produced by fermentation: Bread is leavened, milk is transformed into cheese, meat is aged, cabbage is made into sauerkraut, and soybeans become soy sauce.

Beer recipes, complete with illustrations, were discovered on Babylonian clay tablets dating more than 6000 years old. It is estimated that alcohol was probably known as early as the Stone Age, 10,000 years ago. The first encounter was most likely by accident. Sweet substances such as honey, dates, or sap were fermented into wines and related beverages after exposure to wild yeast. (Most wines from these times contained large amounts of acids as a result of such fermentation, much like vinegar today.) Beer had to wait for the later agriculture boom, as it depended upon the fermentation of starchy grains. From the river deltas of Egypt and Mesopotamia, crops of wheat and barley were harvested. This allowed beer production by the early Egyptians and Babylonians.

Overall, the process of production and consumption of alcohol has been a part of all but three or four modern-day cultures. It is only known to be absent from polar societies and Australian aborigines. In some early cultures, the production of alcohol fell under the domain of priests and clergy. The Catholic Church operated the biggest and finest vineyards for nearly 1300 years. The vineyards were inherited with the decline of the Roman Empire; the Catholic Church was the only group rich enough to be able to sustain wine production. Production of alcoholic beverages even occurs today in some European monasteries. Historically, some religions used alcohol to attain a divine state of drunkenness in religious rites and festivals. Today, many Christians consider alcohol a symbol of sacrificial blood. In contrast, some forms of religion, including Islam, devout Buddhism, Hinduism, Mormonism, and Quakerism, ban the use of alcohol mostly because of the abuse that often occurs.

Based on the earliest records, alcohol has provided a release from the drudgery of everyday life. Throughout history, alcohol also has been a valued beverage as an alternative to contaminated drinking water. As villages and cities began to expand, so did life in close quarters. Providing citizens with clean, pure water became a problem as the water supply rapidly became unfit to drink from pollution by waste products. Alcoholic beverages were free of pathogens and had antiseptic powers. Unclean water treated with the natural acidity of beer and wine was made safe to drink. In the Old and New Testaments, drinking water is seldom mentioned, whereas wine and beer are identified as thirst quenchers. Early founders of Christianity considered wine a gift from God. In sum, alcoholic beverages were a common hydration mechanism in former centuries, and remained so until the early nineteenth century, when microorganisms were discovered as causing disease. After that, water was made much safer as a beverage for the West by treating or filtering it for microorganisms before use.

Wine, beer, and mead were made for 9000 years with relatively low alcohol content. Users were focused more on taste issues, on quenching thirst, and on hunger satisfaction, than on intoxication. In A.D. 700, an Arab chemist, experimenting with alcohol, used the properties of boiling and condensation to distill beverages to their maximum alcohol content. This produced the known potent effect of hard liquor seen today. This distillation went on to give alcohol a confusing connotation in later centuries: nourishing food, numbing medication, and harmful drug. To our historical timeline, this concentrated form of alcohol is still new to human experience.

Early in the nineteenth century, the practice of medicine and known scientific principles gained common ground in diagnosing disease. Alcohol abuse was one of the first problems to be recognized as a chronic, life-threatening disease. Keep in mind that alcoholic beverage production was not intended for the destruction that it causes today. A majority of early cultures found alcoholic beverages to be an important source of fluid. Use of alcohol might be offensive to some today, but its original discovery was a true act of nature. Fermentation will continue, whether humans continue to abuse the process or not.

recovered. Some distilled spirits are marketed "unaged." Vodka and gin are examples of unaged beverages. Other spirits, such as whiskeys, rums, and brandies, are aged in oak barrels, some more than 20 years.

Government standards for each nation determine the kinds of alcoholic beverages allowed to be produced and sold. For instance, single malt scotch whiskey produced in Scotland for export to the United States must meet Bureau of Alcohol, Tobacco, and Firearms standards before it can be shipped from Scotland to the United States.

Alcohol proof represents ½% of the volume. 80 proof vodka is then 40% alcohol.

Alcohol Metabolism

After a person drinks an alcoholic beverage, his or her blood concentration of alcohol rises rapidly. Alcohol is readily absorbed into the blood from different segments of the GI tract by simple diffusion. You've probably been warned, with good reason, not to drink on an empty stomach. Alcohol absorption depends partly on the rate of stomach emptying. Food slows the stomach's emptying rate and stimulates secretions, such as gastric acid, which dilute the alcohol and slow its absorption into the bloodstream. Certain drugs also control stomach-emptying time and, thus, overall absorption. The type of beverage consumed also determines alcohol absorption. The alcohol in beer is absorbed more slowly than the alcohol in whiskey, which is slower than wine. Pure alcohol is absorbed fastest of all but, of course, such a beverage is not for sale, nor is it safe to consume (the risk of alcohol poisoning is significant; see the Nutrition Issue on binge drinking).

Alcohol is readily distributed in the fluid compartments within the body because alcohol is found wherever water is distributed in the body. Alcohol moves easily through the cell membranes; however, as it does, it damages proteins in the membranes. Most of alcohol's damaging effects are concentrated in the liver because this is the first organ that is exposed to alcohol after absorption, and the liver is the chief site for alcohol metabolism. Although it is true that cells of the GI tract are in contact with alcohol, they are constantly being replaced because of their naturally short life span. Thus, they are not subject to the same degree of damage as liver cells, which have a much longer life span.

alcohol dehydrogenase (ADH) An enzyme used in alcohol (ethanol) breakdown—metabolism; the major enzyme used in the liver when alcohol is in low concentration.

Metabolism of alcohol is dependent on numerous factors, such as gender, race, size, physical condition, what is eaten, the alcohol content of the beverage, and even how much sleep one has had. The ability to produce the enzyme **alcohol dehydrogenase (ADH)** is the key to alcohol metabolism, as it acts on about 90% of the dose consumed. Women absorb and metabolize alcohol differently than men do. A woman cannot metabolize much alcohol in the cells that line her stomach because of low activity of ADH. Women also have less body water in which to dilute the alcohol than do men. So, when a man and a woman of similar size drink equal amounts of alcohol, a larger proportion of the alcohol reaches and remains in the woman's bloodstream. Men metabolize about 30% of the alcohol ingested in this manner, but women metabolize only 10%. Overall, women develop alcohol-related ailments, such as **cirrhosis** of the liver, more rapidly than men do with the same alcohol-consumption habits. Also, certain drugs used to treat ulcers and heartburn inhibit ADH activity in the stomach, as does chronic alcohol abuse and aging.

cirrhosis A loss of functioning liver cells, which are replaced by nonfunctioning connective tissue. Any substance that poisons liver cells can lead to cirrhosis. The most common cause is a chronic, excessive alcohol intake.

Once acted on by ADH, alcohol turns into acetaldehyde. This goes on to eventually form carbon dioxide and water:

$$\text{Alcohol} \xrightarrow{\text{ADH}} \text{Acetaldehyde} \rightarrow \rightarrow \rightarrow CO_2 + H_2O$$

Most of the remaining alcohol consumed is then metabolized in the same way by alcohol dehydrogenase to carbon dioxide and water in the liver. Only a small percentage of alcohol intake is excreted as such through the lungs, urine, and sweat. (Since the alcohol content of expired air exhibits a constant relationship to the blood alcohol concentration in the lungs, it is used as the basis of the breathalyzer test.) As one continues to drink, one's blood alcohol concentration (BAC) continues to rise (Fig. 7.1). A social drinker who weighs 150 pounds and has normal liver function metabolizes about 5 to 7 grams of alcohol per hour. This is about one half of a beer or one fourth of an ordinary-sized drink. When the rate of alcohol consumption exceeds the liver's metabolic capacity, blood alcohol rises and symptoms of intoxication appear as the brain begins to be exposed to alcohol (Table 7.2). Because alcohol cannot be stored in the body, it has absolute priority in metabolism as a fuel source.

Two other enzyme systems in body cells also metabolize alcohol, especially when it is consumed in high amounts. Increased activity of one of these systems is the key reason for developing tolerance to the effects of alcohol—more rapid alcohol metabolism means that more alcohol is now needed to feel the effects.

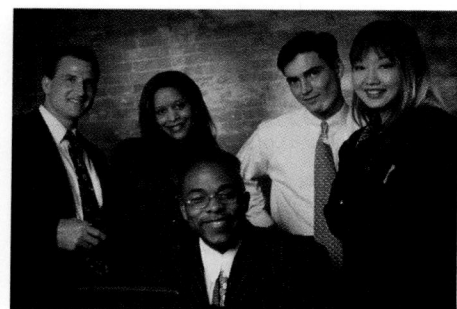

Compared with Caucasians, most Asians and Native Americans have a limited ability to metabolize alcohol.

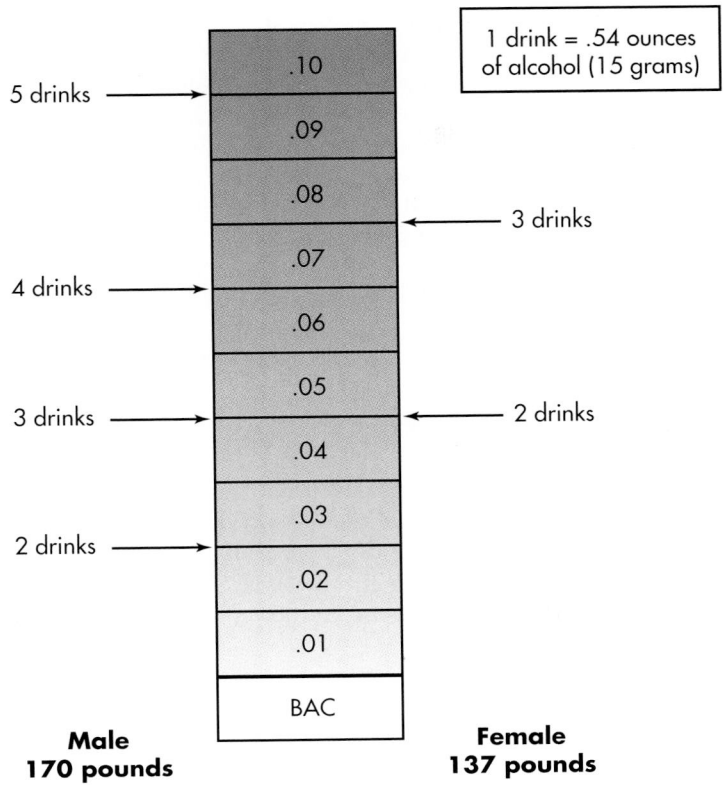

1 drink = .54 ounces
of alcohol (15 grams)

5 drinks → .10
.09
.08 ← 3 drinks
.07
4 drinks → .06
.05
3 drinks → .04 ← 2 drinks
.03
2 drinks → .02
.01
BAC

Male
170 pounds

Female
137 pounds

Figure 7.1 Approximate relationship between alcohol consumption and blood alcohol concentration (BAC). Note that effects can vary among people and whether food is also consumed. A BAC of 0.02 begins to impair driving. One is legally intoxicated at a BAC of 0.08 in most states in the United States and throughout Canada. In October 2003, 0.08 will be the U.S. standard; 0.1 will no longer be the limit.

Table 7.2 Blood Alcohol Concentration and Symptoms

Concentration*	Sporadic Drinker	Chronic Drinker	Hours for Alcohol to Be Metabolized
50 (party high) (0.05%)	Congenial euphoria; decreased tension; noticeable impairment in driving and coordination	No observable effect	2–3
75 (0.075%)	Gregarious	Often no effect	
100 (0.1%)	Uncoordinated; 0.1% is legally drunk (as in drunk driving) in most areas in the United States; note that 0.08% is legal drunkenness in Canada and in a growing number of areas in the United States	Minimal signs	4–6
125–150 (0.125–0.15%)	Unrestrained behavior; episodic uncontrolled behavior; legally drunk	Pleasurable euphoria or beginning of uncoordination	6–10
200–250 (0.2–0.25%)	Alertness lost; lethargic	Effort is required to maintain emotional and motor control.	10–24
300–350 (0.3–0.35%)	Stupor to coma	Drowsy and slow	
>500 (>0.5%)	Some will die	Coma	>24

*Milligrams of alcohol per 100 milliliters of blood.
Modified from Wyngaarder JB, Smith LH: *Cecil Textbook of Medicine*, fourth edition, Philadelphia, 1988, WB Saunders. Used with permission.

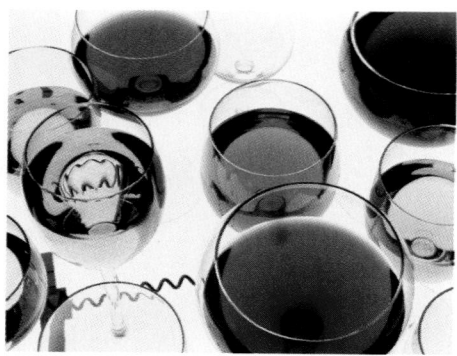

Of all the alcohol sources, red wine is often singled out as the best choice because of the added bonus of the many phytochemicals present. These were leached out from the grape skins as the red wine was fermented. Still, the American Heart Association recently stated that use of red wine does not substitute for controlling the other cardiovascular risk factors discussed in Chapter 5.

ischemic stroke A stroke caused by the absence of blood flow to a part of the brain.

Another Bite

Use of the primary alternate pathway for alcohol metabolism also increases the potential for a drug overdose. While this pathway is metabolizing alcohol in the liver, its capacity for metabolizing other drugs, such as many sedatives (barbiturates), is reduced, since both compounds are competing for the same enzymes. If large amounts of alcohol and sedatives are consumed simultaneously, the alcohol gets preferential treatment. This means the liver is not able to metabolize the sedatives fast enough, so the user may lapse into a coma and even die from the effects of the sedatives. This is due to a lack of enzymes to convert the sedatives to harmless substances. Alcohol itself is toxic in high quantities. Mixed with sedatives, it creates an extremely lethal combination.

Concept Check

Alcohol is not an essential nutrient, but does supply energy for the body. It requires no digestion, and alcohol metabolism takes precedence over metabolism of the other energy-yielding nutrients. Alcohol is metabolized in the liver and other tissues. Metabolism mostly depends on the enzyme alcohol dehydrogenase (ADH). A number of individual factors, such as gender, race, and body composition, determine how a person reacts to alcohol.

Benefits of Moderate Alcohol Use

The benefits of moderate alcohol use are linked to specific intakes of about one drink a day for men and slightly less than one for women. The benefits begin with the many pleasurable and social aspects of its use. People enjoy meeting a friend over a beer or settling down to a glass of wine with dinner in the evening. These behaviors are not considered excessive, as long as they are practiced by people of legal drinking age, remain under control, and cause no obvious harm. The risks of developing some forms of cardiovascular disease, such as coronary heart disease and **ischemic stroke,** are decreased in moderate drinkers as opposed to those who abstain from alcoholic beverages. These and other possible benefits of moderate alcohol use are discussed in Table 7.3.

Many of the benefits of moderate alcohol use are effective only in the short term. Previous consumers of alcohol no longer experience the benefits of alcohol when consumption ceases.

The benefits of alcohol use are realized with moderate consumption. Under the correct circumstances, alcohol can be pleasurable, adds to social occasions, decreases the risk of various forms of cardiovascular disease, in middle-aged and older adults at risk for the disease, and may lead to other health benefits. Mortality risk is somewhat greater in those who abstain from alcohol, and the risk appears to be decreased in those consuming up to one drink or so per day. The protective dose of alcohol is somewhat less in women.

Health Problems from Alcohol Abuse

Despite the few benefits of regular, moderate alcohol use, the risks of abuse are more numerous and harmful. Alcoholism, in and of itself, is one of the most preventable health problems in North America. Excessive consumption of alcohol contributes significantly to 5 of the 10 leading causes of death in North America—heart failure, certain forms of cancer, cirrhosis of the liver, motor vehicle and other accidents, and suicides (review Table 7.3). Tobacco, often used simultaneously, interacts with alcohol in a way that reinforces its effects and causes esophageal and oral cancer. In addition, excessive alcohol drinking increases the risk of heart rhythm disturbances, hypertension and hemorrhagic stroke, osteoporosis, brain damage, colorectal and

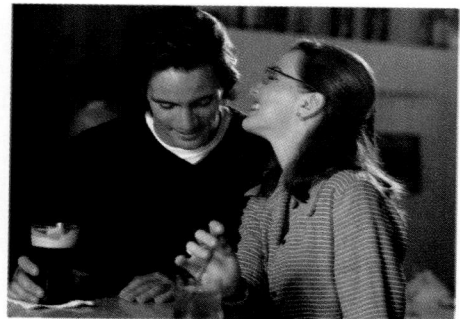

One attribute of alcohol use are the pleasurable and social aspects experienced.

Table 7.3 A Summary of Benefits and Risks of Alcohol Use

	Moderate Use	Alcohol Abuse
Coronary heart disease	Decreased risk of death in those at high risk for coronary heart disease-related death, primarily by increasing HDL-cholesterol and decreasing blood clotting	Heart rhythm disturbances, heart muscle damage, increased blood triglycerides
Hypertension and stroke	Mild decrease in blood pressure; less ischemic stroke	Increased blood pressure (hypertension); more hemmorhagic stroke
Blood glucose regulation and type 2 diabetes	Decreased risk of death from cardiovascular disease	Hypoglycemia and damage to pancreas (site of insulin production)
Bone and joint health	Some increase in bone mineral content in women, linked to increased estrogen output	Loss of active bone-forming cells and eventual osteoporosis (many nutrient deficiencies also contribute to the problem); increased risk of gout
Brain function	Enhanced brain function and decreased risk of dementia	Brain tissue damage and decreased memory
Skeletal muscle health	No benefit	Skeletal muscle damage
Cancer	No benefit	Increased risk of oral, esophageal, stomach, liver, lung, colorectal, and breast cancer, to name a few (especially if the person's diet is deficient in the vitamin folate)
Liver function	No benefit	Fat infiltration and eventual cirrhosis, especially if a person is also infected with hepatitis C
GI tract disease	Decreased risk of certain bacterial infections in the stomach	Inflammation of the stomach (and pancreas)
Immune system function	No benefit	Reduced function and increased infections
Nervous system function	No benefit	Loss of nerve sensation and nervous system control of muscles
Sleep disturbances	No benefit	Fragmented sleep patterns; worsens sleep apnea
Impotence and decreased libido	No benefit	Contributes to the problem in both men and women
Drug overdose	No benefit	Contributes to the problem, especially with sedatives
Obesity	No benefit	Increased abdominal fat distribution, contributes to positive energy balance
Nutrient intake	May supply some B vitamins and iron	Leads to numerous nutrient deficiencies: protein, vitamins, and minerals
Alcoholism	No benefit	Increases risk of developing alcoholism
Fetal health	No benefit	Variety of toxic effects on the fetus when alcohol is consumed by pregnant women (see Chapter 13)
Socialization and relaxation	Provides some benefit to socialization and leads to relaxation	Contributes to violent behavior and agitation
Traffic deaths and other violent deaths	No benefit (and likely even an increase in traffic accidents)	Contributes to both traffic death and violent death

The risks from alcohol abuse begin at intake of more than two to three drinks per day for men and one to two drinks per day for both women and adults over age 65. Binge drinking (more than four drinks in a row for women and more than five drinks for men can be especially harmful [see the Nutrition Issue]). The Swiss chemist Paracelsus (1493–1541) made the observation that "the dose determines the poison." This is especially true for alcohol.

breast cancer, inflammation of the stomach lining, suppression of the immune system (and, thus, an increased risk of infections), sleep disturbances, impotence, hypoglycemia, and high blood triglycerides. Figure 7.2 illustrates many of these risks. Alcohol ingestion also reduces use of fat by body cells and promotes a positive energy balance, thus contributing to risk for obesity, especially abdominal obesity. Finally, by reducing the action of antidiuretic hormone, alcohol increases urination. Death from alcohol abuse usually results from respiratory failure or inhalation of vomit (the latter if the blood alcohol concentration is lower).

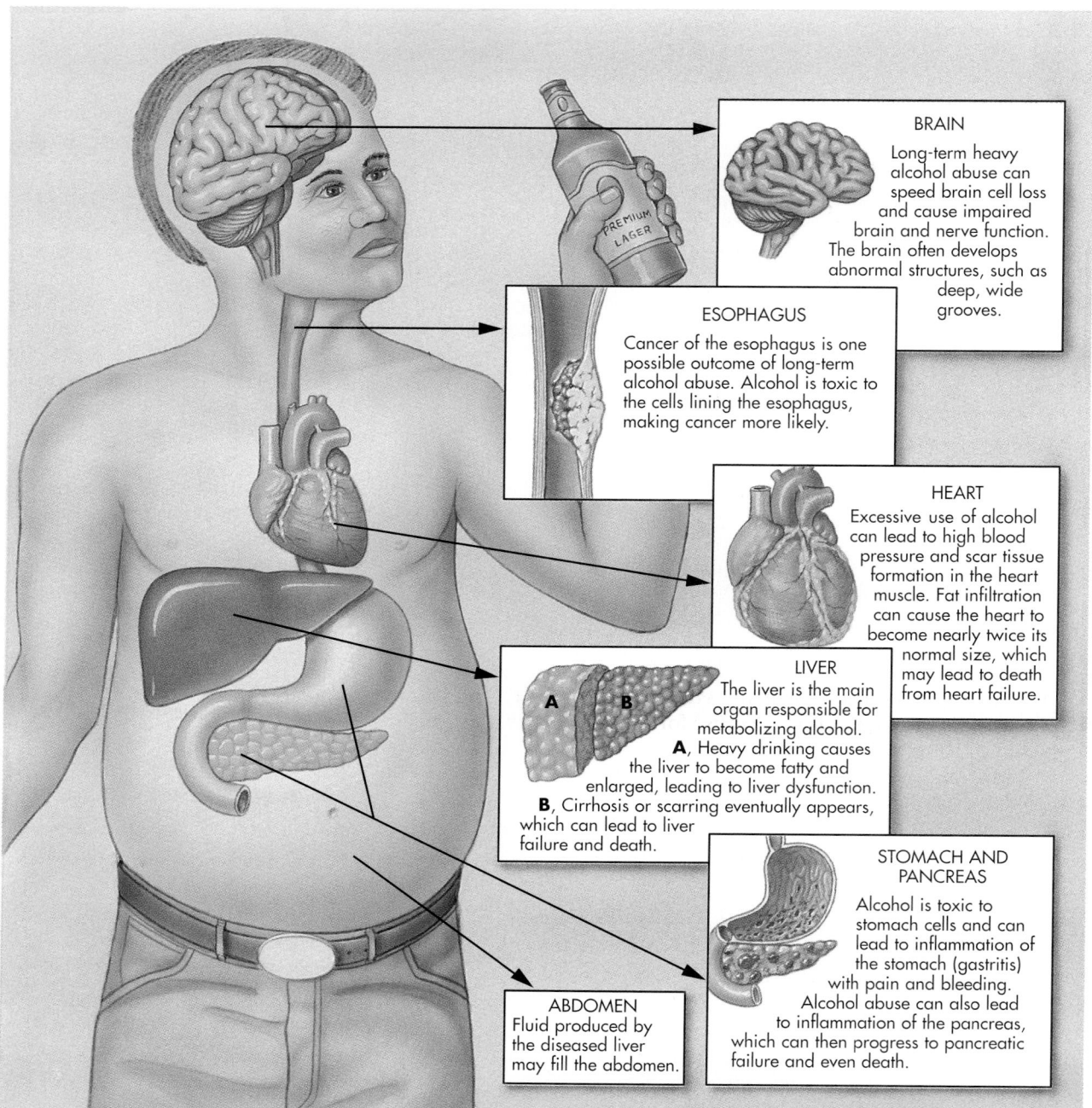

Figure 7.2 Some effects of alcohol abuse on the body. The mind-altering effects of alcohol begin soon after it enters the bloodstream. Virtually every organ system is affected by alcohol. Within minutes, alcohol inhibits nerve cells in the brain. The heart muscle strains to cope with alcohol's depressive action. If drinking continues, rising blood alcohol causes impaired speech, vision, balance, and judgment. With an extremely high blood alcohol content, respiratory failure is possible. Over time, alcohol abuse increases the risk of liver and pancreas failure and certain forms of heart damage and cancer, among other disorders. Table 7.3 summarizes all the negative effects of excessive alcohol use on physical health.
Illustration by William Ober.

As a nutrient source, alcohol has little nutritional value and, thus, nutrient deficiencies are also a common result of alcoholism. The protein and vitamin content is extremely low, except in beer, where it is marginal. Iron content varies from drink to drink, with red wine ranking especially high in iron. Excess use of some alcoholic beverages can even lead to iron toxicity, as well as that from lead or cobalt.

Another Bite

Typical deficiencies seen in alcoholism include the fat-soluble vitamins—vitamin A, vitamin D, vitamin E, and vitamin K—as well as the water-soluble vitamins— thiamin, niacin, vitamin B-6, folate, vitamin B-12, and vitamin C. Mineral deficiencies of calcium, phosphorus, potassium, magnesium, zinc, and iron are possible. These arise mostly due to poor nutrient intakes, but fat malabsorption linked to poor pancreatic function and increased urinary losses are also important in some cases. On the other hand, vitamin and mineral toxicity is also of concern, particularly with vitamin A and iron. In both cases, damage to the GI tract and liver enhance the potential for toxicity from these nutrients. The immediate aim in nutritional treatment of alcoholism is eliminating alcohol intake. Then attention turns to repleating nutrient stores, generally with nutrient supplements.

■ A Closer Look at Cirrhosis

Long-term alcohol use causes fatty liver, inflammation of the liver (alcoholic hepatitis), and eventually cirrhosis. Cirrhosis is a chronic and usually relentlessly progressive disease characterized by fatty infiltration of the liver. Fatty liver occurs in response to increased synthesis of fat and decreased utilization of energy by the liver. Eventually, the enlarged fat deposits choke off the blood supply, depriving the liver cells of oxygen and nutrients. Liver cells can accumulate so much fat that they burst and die and are replaced by connective (scar) tissue. This scarring process is called *cirrhosis.* When too many liver cells die, the liver dies, and the alcoholic patient dies. In North America, most cases of cirrhosis are caused by alcohol consumption. Cirrhosis develops in about 15% to 20% of cases of alcoholism and effects about 2 million people in the United States alone. It is the second leading cause for the need for liver transplant. In addition to the amount and duration of alcohol consumption, genetic factors and individual differences determine one's risk for the disease, such as obesity, exposure to hepatotoxins (e.g., acetaminophen [Tylenol]), and infections with hepatitis C. Note that about 4 million people in the United States are infected with the virus that causes hepatitis C. Once a person has cirrhosis, there is a 50% chance of death within 4 years, a far worse prognosis than many forms of cancer. Most of the deaths from alcoholic cirrhosis occur in people between the ages of 40 and 65 years. The actual death rate in the United States is 8.8 per 100,000 people.

A number of possible mechanisms underlie the liver damage from alcohol abuse. In chronic alcoholism, acetaldehyde concentration also increases in the liver, and is thought to be the underlying cause of the toxic effects of alcohol. Another cause of liver damage is the production of **free radicals** from alcohol metabolism. These highly reactive molecules destroy cell membranes and DNA. A by-product of free radical damage, inflammation, can destroy healthy liver tissue.

No specific amount of alcohol consumption guarantees cirrhosis. One perceptible pattern is that cirrhosis commonly results from a 10-year or longer consumption of approximately 80 grams of alcohol (the equivalent of seven beers) per day. Some evidence suggests that damage is caused by a dose as low as 40 grams per day for men and 20 grams per day for women. Early stages of alcoholic liver injury are reversible, but advanced stages usually are not. If a person is terminally ill, a liver transplant is necessary for survival.

A nutritious diet helps prevent some complications associated with alcoholism, but usually alcoholism brings about serious destruction of vital tissues regardless of the quality of the food consumed. Laboratory animal studies show clearly that, even when a nutritious diet is consumed, alcohol abuse can lead to cirrhosis. Still, deficient nutritional status compounds the problem of cirrhosis, as it makes the liver more vulnerable to toxic substances by depleting supplies of antioxidants, such as vitamins E and C. If present in adequate amounts, these two vitamins reduce free-radical

*I*f a person were to use beer as a nutrient source, he or she would need to consume daily:

- 40 to 55 bottles (12-ounce) to meet protein needs
- 65 bottles for thiamin needs
- 6 bottles for niacin needs

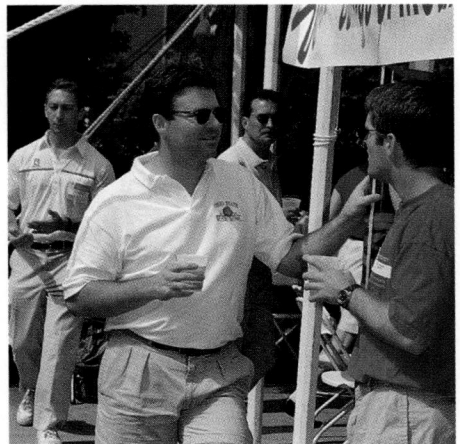

Excessive alcohol intake encourages fat deposition, especially in the abdominal region.

free radicals Short-lived forms of compounds that exist with an unpaired electron, causing it to seek an electron from another compound. Free radicals can be very destructive to electron-dense cell components, such as the DNA and cell membranes.

damage to the liver. A folate deficiency also compounds the damage. Because of this observation, daily use of a balanced multivitamin and mineral supplement is especially important for people who abuse alcohol.

*S*ome people even have food-related allergic and asthmatic reactions to alcohol.

Other Problems Associated with Alcohol Abuse

Many social problems accompany the medical problems associated with alcohol abuse.

▪ Problem Drinking in the Workplace

Problem drinking can result in decreased job performance, an increased number of sick days, interference with regular sleep at home, and increased sleeping on the job. Accidents, violence, suicide, and workplace problems are often caused in part by the misuse of alcohol. Rather than ignoring the issue, it is important that these alcohol-related problems be addressed. We all know people who dislike their jobs or a specific coworker. Because we spend about one-third of our lives working, the job environment can have a strong effect on quality of life. Workplace alienation can lead to drinking. Some workplace cultures accept and encourage alcohol consumption, whereas others forbid or discourage this behavior. Alcohol availability is strongly linked to consumption in the workplace. Sometimes it is very easy to bring alcohol onto the job site. Employer-sponsored health promotion programs may help reduce employee drinking and increase awareness of these issues.

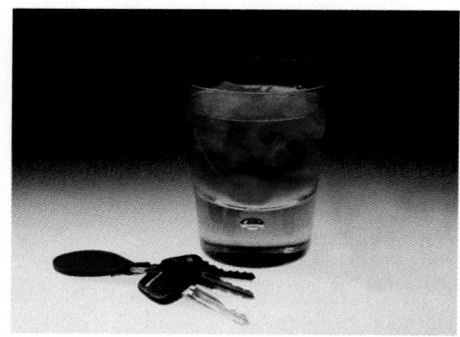

Drinking and driving should never be combined. The consequences are dangerous and possibly deadly.

▪ Operation of Motor Vehicles and Related Equipment

It is extremely dangerous to mix drinking with activities requiring sound judgment and responsibility. Driving, boating, athletics, and water sports are all activities in which alcohol does not belong. Consuming alcohol prior to or during these and many other activities increases the risk of injury to oneself and others because it reduces coordination and judgment. Note the warning label on alcoholic beverages.

▪ Sexually Transmitted Diseases

Due to the inhibition-reducing effect of alcohol, drinking increases the incidence of high-risk sexual activity and infection by a **sexually transmitted disease (STD).** Unplanned and unprotected sexual intercourse often results from overconsumption of alcohol. Multiple sex partners also increase the risk for contracting an STD, as well as hepatitis C and HIV/AIDS.

sexually transmitted disease (STD) A contagious disease usually acquired by sexual intercourse or genital contact. Common examples include AIDS, gonorrhea, and syphilis. Also called venereal disease.

fetal alcohol syndrome (FAS) A group of irreversible physical and mental abnormalities in the infant that result from the mother's consuming alcohol during pregnancy.

▪ Unplanned Pregnancy

Along with STDs, an unplanned pregnancy can be the result of unprotected sex while under the influence of alcohol. And, if the drinking continues during the first month of pregnancy, the chances of delivering an infant with **fetal alcohol syndrome** increase (see Chapter 13).

▪ Children of Alcoholics

Alcoholism affects the entire family. Children of alcoholics have a hard time developing in a normal way. Living with an alcoholic family member causes stress for everyone, and, for a child, this dysfunction reduces the chances of becoming intellectually, culturally, and socially independent. Almost 1 in 4 North American children grow up with an alcoholic in the family, and this environment influences children's perception of alcohol use, especially when it comes to their own decisions about this issue. Children of alcoholics often have long-lasting emotional problems, which carry over into adulthood.

Critical Thinking

When people consume alcohol, they often do things they would not normally do. Unplanned sexual activity, the damaging of property, and other harmful events can occur. For many people, drinking and smoking go hand-in-hand. What risks and diseases could correlate with the combination of these behaviors with excessive alcohol use?

*E*xcessive alcohol use can result in an array of medical problems. It increases the risk of developing hypertension, certain forms of strokes and heart damage, birth defects, inflammation of the pancreas, damage to the brain, and malnutrition, to name a few. Furthermore, alcoholism interferes with all aspects of family, professional, and social life.

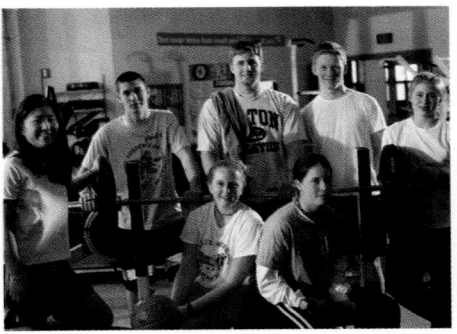

Young people benefit most from a healthy diet and exercise to decrease future risk of cardiovascular disease. There is no related benefit at this age for alcohol use.

Advice Regarding Alcohol Use

The U.S. surgeon general's office, the National Academy of Science, and the USDA/DHHS do not recommend drinking alcohol. The text of the *2000 Dietary Guidelines for Americans* (discussed in Chapter 2), contains this statement: "Drinking in moderation may lower risk for coronary heart disease, mainly among men over age 45 and women over age 55. However, there are other factors that reduce the risk of heart disease, including a healthy diet, physical activity, avoidance of smoking, and maintenance of a healthy weight. Moderate consumption provides little, if any, health benefit for younger people." All groups, however, caution that if adults do consume alcohol, they should (1) drink alcohol only in moderation with meals (no more than two drinks a day for men and one for women or anyone over age 65 years); (2) avoid drinking any alcohol before or while driving, operating machinery, taking medications, or engaging in any other activity requiring sound judgment; and (3) avoid drinking alcohol while pregnant.

There is no recommendation for a nondrinker to start consuming alcohol for the health benefits. Overall, people who have one drink or so a day and are not prone to abuse should know that there's nothing wrong with moderate drinking, as long as they are not putting themselves or others at risk.

The federal labels in the United States currently added to some wine bottles convey a noncommittal message. They state the positive and negative aspects of drinking wine, so that consumers are aware of both sides of the issue and can make up their own minds. These labels do not endorse drinking but refer consumers to other informative venues. It is unfortunate that the wine industry has become increasingly aggressive in promoting wine as a means of reducing the risk of heart disease. Producers and distributors have latched onto the *2000 Dietary Guidelines for Americans* as a means of marketing their product. Alcoholic beverages account for more than $50 billion in annual sales in the United States.

Currently, about 32% of all North American adults have three drinks or less each week, about 22% have two drinks or less a day, and only about 11% have more than two drinks a day.

*H*ealthy People 2010 *set an important goal regarding alcohol use: Reduce by 25% the proportion of adults who exceed the guidelines for appropriate alcohol use (currently, 73% of those who consume alcohol).*

Alcohol Dependency and Abuse

Many factors determine a person's chances of developing **alcohol dependence.** Studies have shown links tying gender, genetics, ethnicity, parental influence, nurture, and depression to alcohol dependency and abuse. For some people, alcohol can be addictive and dangerous, and can eventually lead to **alcohol abuse.** This is true for about 10% to 15% of men and 5% of women in Western countries who drink alcohol.

Some studies suggest that 40% to 60% of a person's risk for alcoholism comes from genetic factors, although the gene, or genes, have not been identified. The genetic influence on alcohol dependency and abuse has been indicated by a number of studies, including twin and adoption research. Twins and first-degree relatives share a tendency toward alcohol addiction. Children of alcoholics have a fourfold-increased risk of developing alcoholism, even when adopted by a family with no history of

alcohol dependence The person experiences repeated alcohol-related difficulties, such as inability to control use, spending a great deal of time associated with alcohol use, continued use of alcohol despite physical or psychological consequences, persistent desire or unsuccessful efforts to cut down or control alcohol use, and withdrawal symptoms. Tolerance is also seen.

alcohol abuse The person experiences severe alcohol-related problems, such as an inability to fulfill major obligations, use in hazardous situations (e.g., driving), related legal problems, or use despite social and interpersonal difficulties.

*A*bility to "hold one's liquor" is a strong indicator of genetic risk.

Critical Thinking

Jose is a well-liked 17-year-old. It always seems as if everything is going his way—an A on a test, a scholarship to his dream school, you name it. Lately, however, Jose has experienced some disappointments. His grandfather has just passed away, and he and his girlfriend of 6 months have broken up. When he arrived home late with the smell of alcohol on his breath, his parents started to worry. They talked to his school counselor, who suggested they look for certain signs that could indicate depression and/or alcohol dependence. What might those signs be?

alcoholism. This suggests that individuals with a family history of alcoholism need to be especially alert for evidence of the early signs of alcohol dependence.

It is suggested that children with a family history of alcoholism be warned of the dangers of drinking by the age of 10. At this age, they are old enough to understand the consequences of alcoholism but are not yet under the strong influence of their peers. Children as young as 10 may begin experimenting with alcohol to feel grown up, to fit in and belong to a group, to relax and feel good, to take risks and rebel against authority, or simply to satisfy curiosity. When there are alcoholic beverages available in the home, it is easy for a child to sample a variety of drinks and to share them with friends.

A low threshold of response to alcohol may be genetic. If this is the case, it requires greater amounts of alcohol to produce the desired effect. Other studies question the relative importance of the genetic component. Any one of us can become addicted if we drink long enough and consume ever-increasing quantities of alcohol.

Gender plays a key role in alcohol metabolism, dependency, and, surprisingly, treatment. The male:female ratio of alcohol dependency is 4:1, but there is evidence that women delay seeking treatment for alcohol abuse. As previously noted, the recommended limit for alcohol use is also different for men and women, as women's bodies have more fat and less muscle tissue than do men's. Alcohol can be diluted by water-holding muscle tissue, but not by adipose tissue. Therefore, alcohol is diluted more quickly in men than in women. As also mentioned before, women cannot metabolize alcohol as quickly as men and, so, it remains in their blood longer. Higher blood alcohol concentrations make women more susceptible to alcoholic liver disease, heart muscle damage, and brain injury.

Many ethnic distinctions play an important role in the probability of alcohol dependency and abuse. Compared with Caucasians, Asians and Native Americans are very susceptible to the damaging effects of alcohol for reasons discussed earlier. The major cause of death among Native Americans is unintentional injuries related to alcohol use, especially high rates of motor vehicle accidents. Other alcohol-related mortality statistics confronting Native Americans are suicide, homicide, domestic abuse, and fetal alcohol syndrome. African-American alcoholics are at greater risk than other racial groups for tuberculosis, hepatitis C, HIV/AIDS, and other infectious diseases. Hispanic Americans are at particular risk for cirrhosis-related death.

Depression and alcohol abuse often go hand-in-hand. Researchers have discovered that the risk for heavy drinking is higher among women with a history of depression than among women with no such history. This finding holds up even when other factors that increase the risk of heavy drinking, such as age, family history of drinking, and personality disorder, are accounted for. The more symptoms of depression women report, the more likely they are to drink heavily. There may be several reasons for this association. One reason is self-medication to relieve the symptoms of depression. Research has shown that, although alcohol may alleviate depression in the short term, it tends to increase it over time. A second reason is that women who are more depressed may not pay attention to their drinking and may not be concerned about the effects it can have on their health and behavior. More research is needed to determine if there is a genetic or environmental factor that links depression and heavy drinking.

The majority of suicides and interfamily homicides are alcohol-related. Clinicians need to be careful when dealing with depressed alcoholic patients to determine the psychological reasons for their drinking and how these behaviors might cause the death of the alcoholic or a family member. Alcohol consumption appears to be associated with youth suicide. The younger the drinker, the more likely he or she is to commit suicide.

Alcohol dependence is the most common psychiatric disorder, affecting 13% of the North American population. Overall, about $185 billion is spent annually in terms of lost productivity, premature deaths, direct treatment expenses, and legal fees associated with alcoholism in the United States alone. A liver transplant costs about

$150,000 and is needed in cases of excessive alcohol use. On the positive side, it costs only about $5000 to treat a person who is abusing alcohol. Identifying alcoholism early can be a way to control and decrease health-care costs.

■ Alcoholism Diagnosis

Alcoholism is often considered a two-phase problem. Initially, it begins as problem drinking. This includes the repetitive use of alcohol, often to alleviate anxiety or solve other emotional problems. Alcohol addiction, the second phase, is defined as a true addiction following the repeated use of alcohol.

Alcohol addiction is seen frequently among homeless individuals.

The diagnosis of alcoholism is based on a list of major criteria. These criteria do not fit every individual but are commonly seen in cases of alcoholism:

- Physiologic dependence on alcohol manifested by evidence of withdrawal symptoms when intake is interrupted
- Tolerance to the effects of alcohol, prompting greater alcohol intake to achieve the desired effect
- Evidence of alcohol-associated illnesses such as alcoholic liver disease or irreversible brain damage exhibited by memory loss, inability to concentrate, and decline in intellectual functions
- Continued drinking in defiance of strong medical and social contraindications and disruptions in normal life
- Depression and blackouts, as well as impairment in social and occupational functioning

Other signs of alcoholism include the basic alcohol stigmas: alcohol odor on the breath, flushed face and reddened skin (the latter due to breakage of small blood vessels, which allows blood to seep under the skin), and nervous system disorders, such as tremors. Unexplained work absences, frequent accidents, and falls or injuries of vague origin may all lead a clinician to consider the possibility of alcoholism. Laboratory tests are also helpful. These tests include measures of liver function, red blood cell synthesis, and triglyceride concentration in the blood.

■ Do You Have a Problem with Alcohol?

Asking a person about the quantity and frequency of alcohol consumption is an important means of detecting abuse and dependence. The questionnaire shown in Table 7-4 (CAGE) is commonly used in routine health care.

Other questions to ask along with the CAGE questionnaire are:

1. Have you had memory lapses or blackouts due to drinking?
2. Do you continue to drink even though you have health problems caused by alcohol?
3. Do you get withdrawal symptoms, such as headaches, chills, shakes, and a strong craving for alcohol, and, as a result, drink more to get rid of these symptoms?
4. Do you take part in high-risk behaviors, such as having unsafe sex in a non-monogamous relationship or driving a boat or car when under the influence of alcohol?
5. Has drinking caused trouble at home, at work, or in relationships with others?
6. Do you have to drink alcohol for any of the following reasons?
   a. To get through the day or unwind at the end of the day
   b. To cope with stressful life events
   c. To escape from ongoing problems

Answering yes to any of these questions should prompt the respondent to consult a family physician or a certified counselor for help.

Table 7.4 CAGE Questionnaire to Screen for Alcohol Abuse

C: Have you every felt you ought to *cut* down on drinking?

A: Have people *annoyed* you by criticizing your drinking?

G: Have you ever felt bad or *guilty* about your drinking?

E: Have you ever had a drink first thing in the morning to steady your nerves or get rid of a hangover (*eye-opener*)?

More than one positive response to the CAGE questionnaire suggests an alcohol problem. Another key point to probe is tolerance. Does it take more to make you inebriated than it did in the past?

Treatment of Alcoholism

Once a diagnosis of alcohol abuse or dependence is established, one should seek the guidance of a physician to arrange appropriate treatment and counseling for the person and family. An important goal of counseling is to identify ways to compensate for the loss of pleasure from drinking. This helps the drinker confront the immediate problem of how to stop drinking. Total abstinence must be the ultimate objective. For alcoholics, there is no such thing as controlled drinking. A problem drinker cannot return safely to social drinking.

The person should enter an Alcoholics Anonymous (AA) 12-step program (Al-Anon for the spouse), or another reputable therapy program for people with alcoholism. For more information, one can check with a local mental health treatment center for programs available in the community or call 800-245-4656. Substance Abuse and Mental Health Services can be reached at 800-729-6686 or www.health.org for alcohol and drug information. In addition, one may visit the Alcoholics Anonymous web page at www.alcoholics-anonymous.org or contact AA at:

AA World Services, Inc.
P.O. Box 459
New York, NY 10163
212-870-3400

According to AA's literature, "AA is a fellowship of men and women who share their experience, strength, and hope with each other that they may solve their common problem and help others recover from alcoholism." As an informal society chartered in 1935, Alcoholics Anonymous includes more than 2 million recovered alcoholics. The only requirement for membership is the desire to stop drinking. There are no rules, regulations, dues, or fees. In addition, the group is not a political or formal organization.

It is helpful for the spouse to join the treatment program as well. AA has two types of meetings—open and closed. Alcoholics and their families and friends are invited to the open meetings, whereas the closed meetings are reserved for alcoholics only.

Current research does not support the generally negative public opinion about the prognosis for alcoholism. In most job-related alcoholism treatment programs, wherein workers are socially stable and—because of the risk to jobs and pensions—well motivated, recovery rates reach 60% or more. This remarkably high cure rate is probably accounted for by early detection. Once a person moves from problem drinking to an advanced stage of alcoholism, success rates seldom exceed 50%. Early identification and intervention remain the most important steps in the treatment of alcoholism. Success is usually proportionate to participation in AA, other social agencies' programs, and religious counseling. About 2 years of treatment should be expected.

*T*o learn more about alcoholism, visit these websites:
www.niaaa.nih.gov
www.asam.org
www.mentalhelp.net/selfhelp.

Two medications are available to treat alcoholism. The medication naltrexone (Re-Via) blocks the craving for alcohol and the pleasure of intoxication. Disulfiram (Antabuse) causes physical reactions, such as vomiting, when drinking alcohol. It does so by blocking acetaldehyde metabolism. However, antabuse is rarely used today.

Concept Check

*T*reatment of alcoholism often includes the use of medicine, counseling, and social support. The clinicians involved must treat the entire person. Alcoholics Anonymous and other support groups are very helpful. Naltrexone can be prescribed to decrease alcohol cravings. Another option is disulfiram, which produces an ill feeling when the patient consumes both the medicine and alcohol. With all of the treatments for alcoholism, it is important to find the one that works best for the individual with alcoholism.

Scenario *Follow-Up*

Alcohol is a central nervous system depressant that affects both respiration and heart rate. In large quantities, alcohol can depress both systems to the point of terminating respiration and cardiac function. Obviously, this is fatal. Alcohol abuse is a common problem, and continued alcohol abuse can lead to dependence problems, although alcohol abuse and dependence are different.

As a close friend, Alyssa has a responsibility to hold Todd accountable for his actions. Sometimes it is difficult to realize that one has a drinking problem, although it may be obvious to others. Alyssa should talk privately to Todd when he is sober and calm about the most recent incident. It is important to deal with situations such as these very carefully, as the problem drinker will probably respond defensively. She could explain how his drinking is causing problems for both of them, she could tell him about the harmful consequences of his drinking, and she could refuse to go with him to any alcohol-related events, but she must be prepared to carry out the threat. Alyssa could talk with a counselor, who may help her learn ways to approach Todd effectively. Offering to go with Todd to a treatment program or an AA meeting and get help is one idea. There is strength in numbers, so other members of Todd's family or close friends also should be enlisted to help, under the guidance of a therapist trained in treating alcoholics.

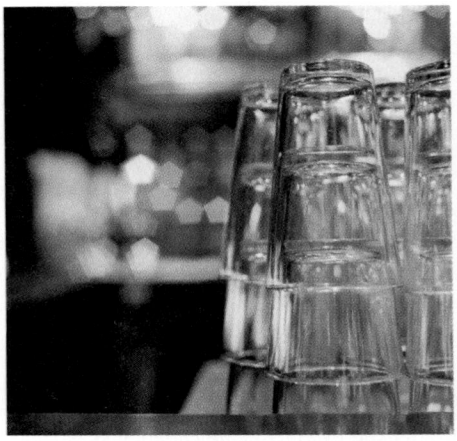

There is no such thing as controlled drinking once a person has alcoholism. Total abstinence is mandatory.

Summary

1. Alcohol use is a complex issue because it involves psychological, social, economic, health, legal, and family issues.
2. Since the Stone Age 10,000 years ago, alcohol has provided an alternative to unsafe drinking water and a pleasurable stimulant to social interaction.
3. Alcohol is metabolized in the liver and other tissues. Metabolism depends on the enzyme alcohol dehydrogenase. A number of factors, such as gender, race, and body composition, determine how a person reacts to alcohol.
4. The benefits of alcohol use are associated with low to moderate alcohol consumption. These benefits include the pleasurable and social aspects of alcohol use, a reduction in various forms of cardiovascular disease, increase in insulin action, and protection against some harmful stomach bacteria.
5. Alcohol use also creates many health risks. Excessive consumption of alcohol contributes significantly to 5 of the 10 leading causes of death in North America. Alcohol increases the risk of developing certain forms of heart damage, inflammation of the pancreas, GI tract damage, vitamin and mineral deficiencies, cirrhosis of the liver, certain forms of cancer, hypertension, and hemmorhagic stroke—to name a few.
6. If alcohol is consumed, it should be consumed in moderation with meals. Women are advised to drink no more than one drink per day, as are adults 65 years and older; men are advised to limit intake to two drinks a day.
7. Gender, genetics, ethnic background, and ongoing depression all determine a person's chances of becoming alcohol dependent.
8. Early detection of alcoholism is key to successful treatment and a reduction of health-care costs. The CAGE questionnaire can help a person determine whether or not he or she has an alcohol problem.
9. Many methods are available to treat alcoholism. Alcoholics Anonymous and the medication ReVia are among the typical approaches.

Study Questions

1. Where in the body does most of the metabolism of alcohol take place? What is a by-product of alcohol metabolism?
2. Why does it take a woman longer than a man to metabolize alcohol?
3. List two potential health benefits of alcohol use.
4. List four problems associated with alcohol abuse.
5. Which two nutrient deficiencies are common in alcoholism? Why?
6. Define the term *one drink*. How much alcohol use is considered to be moderate for men? for women?
7. Why can some ethnic groups hold their liquor better than others can?
8. Name four criteria that might indicate someone has a problem with alcohol. What is this group of criteria checklist called?
9. Describe a method used in treating alcoholism. List a pro and con.
10. After reading the Nutrition Issue, answer the following: What is binge drinking? Within which segment of the population is this increasing in popularity?

Further Readings

1. American Institute for Cancer Research: Alcohol: Healthy living and lower cancer risk. *Facts on Preventing Cancer* 1998.
   Alcoholic drinks increase the risk of cancers of the mouth, pharynx, larynx, and esophagus. Alcohol also increases risk of liver cancer and probably increases the risk for colon, rectal, and breast cancers.

2. Berger K and others: Light-to-moderate alcohol consumption and the risk of stroke among U.S. male physicians. *The New England Journal of Medicine* 341:1557, 1999.
   One to four drinks per week reduced the risks of total stroke and of ischemic stroke in a group of healthy, predominantly White physicians. The authors suggest, however, that any public health recommendation that emphasizes the positive aspects of alcohol would likely do more harm than good.

3. Health risks and benefits of alcohol consumption. *Alcohol Research & Health* 24 (1):5, 2000.
   The lowest observed risk for overall mortality is associated with an average of 10 grams of alcohol (<1 drink) per day for men, and slightly less for women. Still, in people at low risk for death from cardiovascular diseases, alcohol provides little or no reduction in overall mortality.

4. Klatsky AL: Should patients with heart disease drink alcohol? *Journal of the American Medical Association* 285:2004, 2001.
   From a health viewpoint, heavy drinkers would be better off to reduce drinking or abstain, and moderate drinkers and abstainers should be told to avoid heavy drinking. In light of current knowledge, a person with a history of cardiovascular disease and an established moderate drinking pattern should generally not be advised to abstain from alcohol. However, nondrinkers with these conditions should not be advised to start drinking for health reasons, especially because most have good reasons for abstinence.

5. Lieber CS: Alcohol: Metabolism and interaction with nutrients. *Annual Review of Nutrition* 20:325, 2000.
   Alcohol alters the metabolism of many vitamins and minerals.

6. National Institute on Alcohol Abuse and Alcoholism National Institutes of Health: What you don't know can harm you. *NIH Publication* 99-4324, 1999.
   The complications of alcohol abuse include drunk driving, interpersonal problems, alcohol-related birth defects, and long-term health problems. Also included in this pamphlet is a listing of support groups and the types and amounts of alcohol considered to be one serving.

7. Schuckit MA: New findings in the genetics of alcoholism. *Journal of the American Medical Association* 281:1875, 1999.
   A number of combined genetic factors appear to explain approximately half of the alcoholism risk, and the search for genes that have an effect on risk has important implications. The range of potential causes seen in genetic studies implies that there is not a single definitive treatment that will work for everyone.

8. Suter PM: Alcohol: Its role in health and nutrition in Bowman BA, RM Russell, eds Present Knowledge in Nutrition. *ILSI Press,* Washington, DC 2001.
   Alcohol contributes about 5% of calories to the U.S. diet, but in a heavy drinker, this would rise to 50%. A healthy person can metabolize abut 5–7 grams of alcohol per hour.

9. Vallee BL: Alcohol in the Western world. *Scientific American* 278 (June):80, 1998.
   The role of alcohol in Western civilization began 10 millennia ago. It is a popular and common daily beverage to dispense calories, fluid, and social stimulation in almost every culture. Early Hebrews, Greeks, and Romans cautioned about the dangers of drunkenness.

10. Valmadrid CT and others: Alcohol, heart disease, and type 2 diabetes. *Journal of the American Medical Association* 281:239, 1999.
    Cardiovascular disease is the leading cause of death in persons with type 2 diabetes. Moderate alcohol use reduces death from cardiovascular disease in type 2 diabetes.

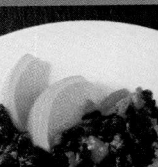

I. Could You or Someone You Know Have a Problem with Alcohol?

Problem drinking often has its seeds in the teen years. Significant health consequences of this typically arise in adulthood. A prominent contributor to 5 of the 10 leading causes of death in North America, misuse of alcohol is a common preventable health problem. The social consequences of alcohol dependency include divorce, unemployment, and poverty. The following questionnaire was developed by the National Council on Alcoholism. With this assessment, you can determine whether you or someone you know might need help. Answer the following questions by placing an "X" in the appropriate blank.

	Yes	No
1. Do you occasionally drink heavily after disappointment, after a quarrel, or when someone gives you a hard time?	___	___
2. When you have trouble or feel under pressure, do you drink more heavily than usual?	___	___
3. Have you ever noticed that you're able to handle liquor better than you did when you first started drinking?	___	___
4. Do you ever wake up the morning after you've been drinking and discover that you can't remember part of the evening before, even though your friends tell you that you didn't pass out?	___	___
5. When drinking with other people, do you try to have a few extra drinks when others won't know it?	___	___
6. Are there certain occasions when you feel uncomfortable if alcohol isn't available?	___	___
7. Have you recently noticed that when you begin drinking, you're in more of a hurry to get the first drink than you used to be?	___	___
8. Do you sometimes feel a little guilty about your drinking?	___	___
9. Are you secretly irritated when your family or friends discuss your drinking?	___	___
10. Have you recently noticed an increase in the frequency of memory blackouts?	___	___
11. Do you often find that you wish to continue drinking after your friends say they've had enough?	___	___
12. Do you usually have a reason for the occasions when you drink heavily?	___	___
13. When you're sober, do you often regret things you have done or said while drinking?	___	___
14. Have you tried switching brands or following different plans to control your drinking?	___	___
15. Have you often failed to keep promises you've made to yourself about controlling or stopping your drinking?	___	___
16. Have you ever tried to control your drinking by changing jobs or moving to a new location?	___	___
17. Do you try to avoid family or close friends while you're drinking?	___	___

continued

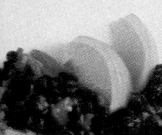

	Yes	No
18. Are you having an increasing number of financial and work problems?	_____	_____
19. Do more people seem to be treating you unfairly without good reason?	_____	_____
20. Do you eat very little or irregularly when you're drinking?	_____	_____
21. Do you sometimes have the "shakes" in the morning and find that it helps to have a little drink?	_____	_____
22. Have you recently noticed that you can't drink as much as you once did?	_____	_____
23. Do you sometimes stay drunk for several days at a time?	_____	_____
24. Do you sometimes feel very depressed and wonder whether life is worth living?	_____	_____
25. Sometimes after periods of drinking do you see or hear things that aren't there?	_____	_____
26. Do you get terribly frightened after you have been drinking heavily?	_____	_____

Interpretation

These are all symptoms that may indicate alcoholism. "Yes" answers to several of the questions indicate the following stages of alcoholism:

Questions 1–8:   Potential drinking problem
Questions 9–21:   Drinking problem likely
Questions 22–26:   Definite drinking problem

It is vital that people assess themselves honestly. If you or someone you know demonstrates some or a number of these symptoms, it is important that help be pursued. If there is even a question in your mind, go talk to a professional about it. Alcohol abuse is one of many problems adults, including older people, face.

II. Investigate Alcohol Use with the CAGE Questionnaire

Have a few of your friends complete the CAGE questionnaire in Table 7.4. What observations have you made? Alcoholism often has its seeds in young adulthood. Do you see evidence of that in you or your friends?

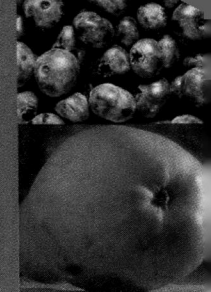

College students are drinking more heavily and more frequently than ever before. Excessive alcohol consumption is an even bigger problem than illicit drug use on college campuses today. Many college students consider drinking alcohol to be a "rite of passage" into adulthood. The heaviest drinking population in North America is young, Caucasian college students. Bars near campus typically promote heavy drinking. Alcohol producers frequently target college students with advertising and other marketing efforts. Adding to the overall problem is typically half of all college students are not of legal drinking age. In fact, the annual overall costs related to alcohol use by those under 21 is estimated at more than $58 billion dollars. This estimate includes costs associated with violent crime, traffic accidents, treatment, and alcohol poisonings, among other variables.

Binge drinking is also common among college students. Young athletes are more likely to abuse alcohol in such a way than their nonathlete peers. Drunken athletes are more likely to drive while drinking, fight, experience memory loss, and be in academic trouble. This binging is defined as four or more drinks in a row for women and five or more for men. **Acute alcohol intoxication** is a major cause of suicide and hazing deaths related to binge drinking. Regular binge drinking also often leads to academic failure. About 50% of college students practice binge drinking.

acute alcohol intoxication A temporary deterioration in mental function, accompanied by muscular incoordination and partial paralysis as a result of drinking alcoholic beverages too rapidly.

Another Bite

*I*n 2000, a student at the University of Michigan rapidly drank 20 shots to celebrate his 21st birthday and died shortly after with a blood alcohol concentration of 0.39 percent. A student at Old Dominion University choked to death on his own vomit during a pledge-week drinking binge. A student at Ohio State University on the diving team became so intoxicated he dove head-first while "mud-diving." He is lucky to be alive but is paralyzed from the neck down. Still other students have drowned while intoxicated, even though they knew how to swim.

*H*ealthy People 2010 *recommends an important goal regarding* binge drinking: Reduce by at least one-half the number of high school and college students engaging in binge drinking (currently estimated at 32% and 40%, respectively).

Binge drinking has a variety of contraindications. It can lead to unplanned sexual activity, damaged property, injury to oneself or others, and death. Death due to alcohol misuse can result, for example, from inhalation of vomit. In other cases, the body systems slowly shut down due to alcohol's overpowering depressant effect (Table 7.5). Other injuries can occur, resulting in paralysis or other lifelong medical problems.

Many problems associated with binge drinking can affect all aspects of life. Binge drinkers are more likely to miss class, damage property, and experience impaired academic performance than are students who are light drinkers or abstainers. Students that live around binge drinkers experience more unwanted sexual advances, assaults, and insults/humiliations. Bingers often do not think they have a problem because binge drinking has become so acceptable on college campuses.

According to U.S. law, one must be 21 years old to drink in all 50 states. In Canada, one must be age 18 or 19, depending on the province. However, alcohol use often begins in adolescence. For example, 31% of 12th-graders in the United States reported frequent drinking during 1999. Premature alcohol use is often seen in conjunction with athletics, as older, highly visible role models advertise products or are seen consuming alcohol. Peer pressure at school and on sports teams can cause many adolescents to drink. These habits become dangerous when young adults choose to drive drunk or ride with friends who are intoxicated. They are also creating habits that may continue and worsen throughout their lives. Education and prevention strategies should focus on behavioral and psychosocial consequences because athletic performance typically does not suffer yet.

continued

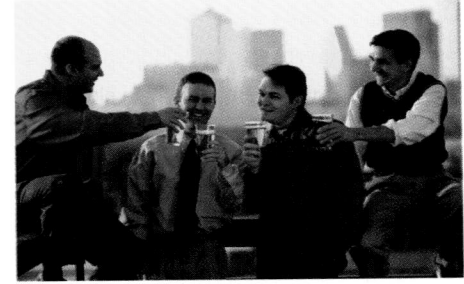

Alcohol use often begins in young adulthood and is carried into later years.

Table 8.1 Tips for Preserving the Vitamin Content of Foods

What to Do	Why
Keep fruits and vegetables cool.	Enzymes in food begin to degrade vitamins once the fruit or vegetable is picked. Chilling reduces this process. Refrigerate fresh produce (except for potatoes, onions, and bananas) until they are consumed.
Refrigerate foods in moisture-proof containers.	Nutrients keep best at temperatures near freezing, at high humidity, and away from exposure to air.
Avoid trimming and cutting fruits and vegetables into small pieces as much as possible.	The more surface exposed, the faster oxygen breaks down vitamins. Keep in mind the outer leaves of lettuce and other greens have higher values of vitamins and minerals than the inner, tender leaves or stems. Potato skins and apple skins are higher in vitamins and minerals than the inner parts.
To retain the maximum amounts of nutrients in vegetables, microwave cooking, steaming, or using a pan or wok with very small amounts of fat and a tight-fitting lid is best.	The less contact with water and the shorter the cooking time, the more nutrients are retained. Whenever possible, cook fruits or vegetables in their skins.
Minimize reheating food.	Prolonged reheating reduces vitamin content.
Do not add fats to vegetables during cooking if you plan to discard the liquid.	Discarding fat can lead to loss of fat-soluble vitamins in the liquid. Add fats to vegetables after they are fully cooked and drained.
Don't add baking soda to vegetables to enhance the green color.	Alkalinity destroys much vitamin D, thiamin, and other vitamins.
Store canned goods in a cool place.	To get maximal nutritive value from canned goods, serve any liquid packed with the food whenever possible. Canned foods vary in the amount of nutrients lost, largely because of differences in storage time and temperatures in the canning process.

consuming many vitamin pills, especially highly potent sources of vitamin A and vitamin D, can cause problems. In the 1930s, consumption of cod liver oil and other fish oils, which contain high concentrations of vitamin A and vitamin D, was quite common and often led to toxicity symptoms. Today, concentrated vitamin A and vitamin D supplements are widely available in grocery, drug, and health-food stores and still pose risks for toxicity when used inappropriately. See the Nutrition Insight in this chapter to find out whether you should take a vitamin and mineral supplement and, if so, how to do it safely.

▮ Preservation of Vitamins in Foods

Substantial amounts of vitamins in foods can be lost from the time a fruit or vegetable is picked until it is eaten. The water-soluble vitamins—particularly thiamin, vitamin C, and folate—can be destroyed with improper storage and excessive cooking. Heat, light, exposure to the air, cooking in water, and alkalinity are all factors that can destroy vitamins. The sooner a food is eaten after harvest, the less chance of nutrient loss.

In general, if the food is not eaten within a few days, freezing is the best method to retain nutrients. In fact, frozen vegetables and fruits are often as nutrient-rich as supermarket-fresh ones. Frozen foods are often processed immediately after harvesting. As part of the freezing process, vegetables are quickly blanched in boiling water. This destroys the enzymes that would otherwise degrade the vitamins. Table 8.1 provides some tips to aid in preserving the vitamins in food.

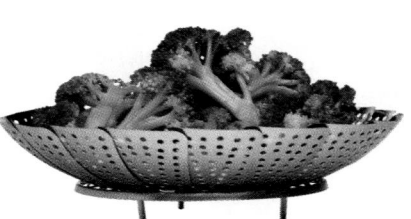

Rapid cooking of vegetables in minimal fluids aids in preserving vitamin content. Steaming is one effective method.

Concept Check

*I*n general, the fat-soluble vitamins—A, D, E, and K—are less readily excreted than are the water-soluble B-vitamins and vitamin C. When a person ingests a vitamin-free diet, the first deficiency signs will be due to a lack of thiamin and will appear after about 10 days. This shows that even water-soluble vitamins persist to some extent in the body, so an occasional inadequate daily consumption is of no health concern. It is important, however, to regularly consume foods rich in both water-soluble and

Table 8.2 Summary of the Fat-Soluble Vitamins, Their Functions, Deficiency Conditions, and Food Sources

Vitamin	Major Functions	Deficiency Symptoms	People Most at Risk	Dietary Sources	RDA or Adequate Intake	Toxicity Symptions
Vitamin A (retinoids) and Provitamin A (carotenoids)	Promote vision: light and color Promote growth Prevent drying of skin and eyes Promote resistance to bacterial infection and overall immune system function	Night blindness Xerophthalmia Poor growth Dry skin	People in poverty, especially preschool children (still very rare in North America) Alcoholics People with HIV/AIDS	Preformed: Vitamin A Liver Fortified milk Fortified breakfast cereals Provitamin A: Sweet potatoes Spinach Greens Carrots Cantaloupe Apricots Broccoli	Females: 700 micrograms RAE Males: 900 micrograms RAE (2300–3000 IU if as preformed vitamin A)	Fetal malformations, hair loss, skin changes, pain in bones, fractures Upper Level is 3000 micrograms of preformed vitamin A (10,000 IU)
Vitamin D (cholecalciferol and ergocalciferol)	Increase absorption of calcium and phosphorus Maintain optimal calcification of bone	Rickets in children Osteomalacia in adults	Some breastfed infants, older adults	Vitamin D-fortified milk Fortified breakfast cereals Fish oils Sardines Salmon	5–15 micrograms (200–600 IU)	Growth retardation, kidney damage, calcium deposits in soft tissue Upper Level is 25 micrograms (2000 IU)
Vitamin E (alpha-tocopherol)	Acts as an antioxidant: prevents breakdown of vitamin A and unsaturated fatty acids	Hemolysis of red blood cells Nerve degeneration	People with poor fat absorption Smokers	Plant oils Products made from plant oils Some greens Some fruits Nuts and seeds Fortified breakfast cereals	15 milligrams alpha-tocopherol (22 IU natural form, 33 IU synthetic form)	Muscle weakness, headaches, fatigue, nausea, inhibition of vitamin K metabolism Upper Level is 1000 milligrams (1100 IU synthetic form, 1500 IU natural form)
Vitamin K (phylloquinone and menaquinone)	Help form prothrombin and other factors for blood clotting and contribute to bone metabolism	Hemorrhage Fractures	People taking antibiotics for months at a time, possibly some older adults	Green vegetables Liver Some plant oils	90–120 micrograms	No Upper Level has been set (anemia and jaundice seen with medicinal forms)

Abbreviations: RAE = retinol activity equivalents, IU = international units.

fat-soluble vitamins. The fat-soluble vitamins A and D, when taken in supplement form, pose the greatest risk of toxicity. The water-soluble vitamins known to show toxic effects when taken in supplement form are niacin, vitamin B-6, and vitamin C. Vitamins obtained from food for the most part pose no health threat.

▮ The Fat-Soluble Vitamins—A, D, E, and K

First, let's look at what we know about the fat-soluble vitamins—vitamins A, D, E, and K (Table 8.2).

▮ Absorption of Fat-Soluble Vitamins

Vitamins A, D, E, and K are absorbed along with dietary fat. These vitamins travel with dietary fats through the bloodstream to reach body cells. Special carriers in the bloodstream help distribute some of these vitamins. Fat-soluble vitamins are stored mostly in the liver and fatty tissues.

When fat absorption is efficient, about 40% to 90% of the fat-soluble vitamins are absorbed. Anything that interferes with normal digestion and absorption of fats also interferes with fat-soluble vitamin absorption. For example, people with cystic fibrosis, or any other disease that hampers fat absorption, also absorb fat-soluble vitamins poorly. Some medications, such as the weight-loss drug orlistat (Xenical), also interfere with fat absorption. Unabsorbed fat carries these vitamins to the large intestine, where they are incorporated into the feces and excreted. People with such conditions are especially susceptible to vitamin K deficiency because body stores of vitamin K are lower than those of the other fat-soluble vitamins. Vitamin supplements, taken under a physician's guidance, are part of the treatment for preventing a vitamin deficiency associated with fat malabsorption (Chapter 10 discusses orlistat use in detail). Finally, people who use mineral oil as a laxative at mealtimes risk fat-soluble vitamin deficiencies because the intestine does not absorb mineral oil. Fat-soluble vitamins are simply eliminated with the mineral oil in the feces.

▌ Vitamin A

The amount of vitamin A you consume is very important. Either too much or too little vitamin A can cause severe problems. Vitamin A is found in foods in a variety of forms. Retinol is one example. As a family, the various forms are called *preformed vitamin A* or **retinoids** (and found naturally only in animal foods). Vitamin A activity in the diet also occurs in the form of common plant pigments—carotenoids—such as the yellow-orange, beta-carotene pigment in carrots. Thus, carotenoids can be termed provitamin A because parts can be turned into vitamin A as needed. Over 600 carotenoids are found in nature; three of them are known to serve as provitamin A in humans. The most potent form of provitamin A is beta-carotene. The other two are alpha-carotene and beta-cryptoxanthin. The preformed vitamin A and the provitamin A carotenoids both make up what is generically referred to as *vitamin A*.

retinoids Chemical forms of preformed vitamin A; one source is animal foods.

▪ Functions of Vitamin A and Carotenoids

Vitamin A performs many important functions in the body. Its importance to vision is perhaps its best-known role and the only role clearly understood. Body changes that occur when vitamin A is lacking provide clues to this and other functions.

Vision

The link between vitamin A and night vision has been known since ancient Egyptian times, when juice extracted from liver was used as a cure for night blindness. Vitamin A performs important functions in light-dark vision, and to a lesser extent, color vision. For a person to see in dim light, one form of vitamin A is required to start the chemical process that signals the brain that light is striking the eye. This allows the eye to adjust from bright to dim light (such as after seeing the headlights of an oncoming car). Without sufficient dietary vitamin A, eventually the eye cannot quickly readjust to dim light. The condition is known as **night blindness.**

If night blindness is not corrected and vitamin A deficiency progresses, the cells that line the cornea of the eye (the clear window of the eye) also lose their ability to produce mucus. The eye then becomes dry. Eventually, when dirt particles scratch the dry surface of the eye, bacteria infect it. The infection soon spreads to the entire surface of the eye and leads to blindness. This disease process is called **xerophthalmia,** which means *dry eye* (review Fig. 8.2).

Vitamin A deficiency is second only to accidents as a worldwide cause of blindness. North Americans are at little risk because of generally good diets. However, people—especially children—in less-developed nations are very susceptible to vitamin A deficiency. Poor dietary intakes, low fat intakes that do not allow for sufficient vitamin A

night blindness A vitamin deficiency condition in which the retina (in the eye) cannot adjust to low amounts of light.

xerophthalmia Literally "dry eye." This is a cause of blindness that results from a vitamin A deficiency. The specific cause is linked to a lack of mucus production by the eye, which then leaves it at a greater risk of damage from surface dirt and bacteria.

absorption, and low stores of vitamin A lessen the ability of the children to meet high needs during rapid childhood growth. Up to 500,000 children in developing nations, especially Asia, become blind each year because of vitamin A deficiency and die soon after from infections. As covered in more detail in Chapter 17, worldwide attempts to reduce this problem have included giving large doses of vitamin A twice yearly and supplementing sugar, margarine, and monosodium glutamate with vitamin A. These food vehicles are used because they are commonly consumed by the populations of less-developed nations. This effort has proven effective in some countries.

Age-related **macular degeneration** is a leading cause of legal blindness among North American adults over the age of 65. The disease is associated with changes in the macular area of the eye, which provides the most detailed vision. Age, smoking, and genetics seem to be risk factors. The macula contains the carotenoids lutein and zeaxanthin in high enough concentrations to impart a yellow color. In one study, the higher the total number of dietary carotenoids (beta-carotene, lutein, and zeaxanthin) consumed, the lower was the risk for age-related macular degeneration. These carotenoids may also decrease the risk of cataracts in the eyes. Although these are interesting hypotheses, it also may be that other factors, such as fruit and vegetable intake in general, may affect the risk for these eye disorders rather than the intake of these specific carotenoids. Note that Centrum Silver™ and other competing brands are marketing their supplements as a source of lutein.

Health of Other Cells

Vitamin A maintains the health of cells that line internal and external "skin" surfaces in the lungs, intestines, stomach, vagina, urinary tract, and bladder, as well as those of the eyes and skin. These cells (called **epithelial cells**) serve as important barriers to bacterial infection. As just noted for the eye, some epithelial cells secrete mucus, a needed lubricant. Without vitamin A, mucus-forming cells deteriorate and no longer synthesize mucus. Vitamin A deficiency also causes insufficient mucus production in the intestines and lung cells and poor health of cells in general. All of this increases the risk of body infections. Vitamin A deficiency also reduces the activity of certain immune system cells. Together, these effects leave the vitamin A–deficient person at great risk for infections. For many years, vitamin A has been dubbed the "anti-infection" vitamin.

Growth, Development, and Reproduction

Vitamin A is necessary for cell growth and development. Vitamin A binds to DNA and in turn causes a cell to increase its synthesis of proteins that stimulate proper growth and development. Supplementation with vitamin A has been shown to have an effect on the growth of children who have low amounts of vitamin A in their body.

One consequence of vitamin A deficiency in laboratory animals is that they cannot reproduce. Resorbing old bone, which must occur before new bone can be deposited, requires bone cells that also use vitamin A. In addition, producing some components of bone requires vitamin A.

Cardiovascular Disease Prevention

Carotenoids in general may play a role in preventing cardiovascular disease in persons at high risk, possibly linked to carotenoids' antioxidant capability. Until definitive studies are complete, many scientists recommend that we consume a total of at least 5 servings of a combination of fruits and vegetables per day as a part of an overall effort to reduce the risk of cardiovascular disease.

Cancer Prevention

Most forms of cancer arise from cells that are influenced by vitamin A. Coupled with its ability to aid immune system activity, vitamin A may be a valuable tool in the fight

*I*n North America the leading cause of blindness in adults is diabetes; in children, it is accidents.

mascular degeneration A painless condition leading to disruption of the central part of the retina and, in turn, blurred vision.

*C*hapter 9 discusses a recent study that showed the mineral zinc helps prevent macular degeneration in people who show evidence of the disease, as do vitamin C and vitamin E.

epithelial cells The cells that line the outside of the body and the inside of all external passages within it, such as the GI tract.

prostate gland A solid, chestnut-shaped organ surrounding the first part of the urinary tract in the male. The prostate gland secretes substances into the semen.

*R*ecently, derivatives of vitamin A have been put into creams (Renova) that reduce some effects of aging on the skin. Note that if the skin is already deeply wrinkled, these creams are ineffective.

analog A chemical compound that differs slightly from another, usually natural, compound. Analogs generally contain extra or altered chemical groups and may have similar or opposite metabolic effects compared with the native compound.

Food Sources of Vitamin A

Food item and amount	Vitamin A (RAE)
Fried liver beef, 1 ounce	3042
Sweet potato, ½ cup	958
Spinach, ⅔ cup	494
Mango, 1	402
Baby carrots, 5	375
Acorn squash, ⅔ cup	244
Cooked kale, ½ cup	206
Skim milk, 1 cup	150
Broccoli, 1 cup	138
Apricot, 3	137
Cheddar cheese, 1 ounce	78
Romaine lettuce, 1 cup	72
Margarine, 1 pat	50
Scallions, 1 tablespoon	32
Peach, 1	26

against cancer. This is especially true for skin, lung, bladder, and breast cancers. The results to date indicate that use of vitamin A supplements can lower the risk of breast cancer among women with very low intakes of dietary vitamin. Still, because of the potential for toxicity, unsupervised use of megadose vitamin A supplements to reduce cancer risk is not advised.

Carotenoids by themselves also may help prevent cancer, acting again as antioxidants. Population studies show that regular consumption of foods rich in carotenoids decreases the risk of lung and oral cancers. However, recall from Chapter 1 that recent studies from the United States and Finland failed to show a reduction in lung cancer in male smokers and nonsmokers who were given supplements of beta-carotene for 5 or more years. In fact, beta-carotene use increased the number of lung cancer cases compared with the control groups. No comparable studies have been done with women. Although further research continues, most researchers are now convinced that beta-carotene supplementation offers no protection against cancer. The overwhelming advice is to rely on food sources of this or any other carotenoids. Again, the best related advice is to eat a combination of at least five fruits and vegetables a day (and not smoke).

Prostate cancer is one of the most common cancers among North American men. The dietary carotenoid lycopene (the red pigment found in tomatoes, watermelon, and several other fruits) seems to protect against this type of cancer. The proposed biological role of lycopene again may be that of an antioxidant. Some food companies (e.g., Campbell Soup Company), are even marketing their products as important sources of lycopene.

Vitamin A Analogs for Acne

The acne medication tretinoin (Retin-A) is made of one **analog** form of vitamin A. It has been used as a topical treatment (applied to the skin) for acne for more than 10 years. It appears to work by altering cell activity in the skin. Another derivative of vitamin A, 13-*cis* retinoic acid (Accutane), is an oral drug used to treat serious acne. Note that taking high doses of vitamin A itself would not be safe. Even Accutane, a less potentially toxic form, can induce toxicity symptoms, as well as birth defects in the offspring of women using it during pregnancy.

■ Vitamin A in Foods and Needs

Preformed vitamin A is found in liver, fish, fish oils, fortified milk and yogurt, and eggs. Margarine is also fortified with vitamin A. The provitamin A carotenoids mentioned before are mainly found in dark green and yellow-orange vegetables and some fruits. Carrots, spinach and other greens, winter squash, sweet potatoes, broccoli, mangoes, cantaloupe, peaches, and apricots are examples of such sources. About 65% of the vitamin A in the typical North American diet comes from preformed vitamin A sources, whereas provitamin A dominates in the diet among poor people in other parts of the world (Fig. 8.3).

Among common foods, those having the highest nutrient density for vitamin A are carrots, liver, spinach and other greens, sweet potatoes, winter squash, romaine lettuce, broccoli, apricots, and nonfat and low-fat milk. Many of the vegetables listed are good sources of beta-carotene and the other two provitamin A carotenoids. Though rarely consumed in North America, the oils from the livers of saltwater fish and marine mammals are extremely rich sources of vitamin A. Consumption of large amounts of such foods can even lead to symptoms of vitamin A toxicity.

Beta-carotene accounts for some of the orange color of carrots. In vegetables such as broccoli, this yellow-orange color is masked by dark-green chlorophyll pigments. Still, green vegetables contain provitamin A. Green, leafy vegetables, such as spinach and kale, have a high concentration of lutein and zeaxanthin. Tomato juice and other tomato products, such as pizza sauce, contain significant amounts of lycopene.

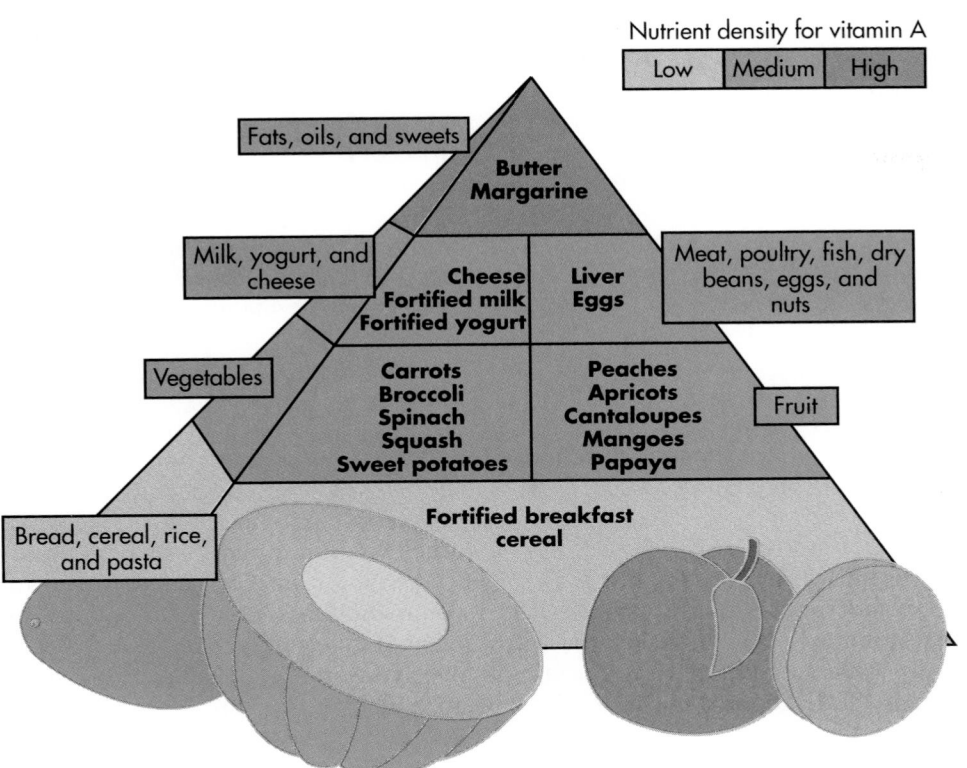

Nutrient density for vitamin A

| Low | Medium | High |

Figure 8.3 Food sources of vitamin A from the Food Guide Pyramid. The fruit and vegetable groups supply abundant carotenoids if they have an intense yellow-orange or green color. Three of these carotenoids are known to yield vitamin A in humans. Liver is the richest source of preformed vitamin A, because that is the major site of vitamin A storage in animals. Milk is often fortified with vitamin A. The background color of each food group indicates the average nutrient density (RAE per kcal) for vitamin A in that group.

The RDA for vitamin A is 700 to 900 micrograms of Retinol Activity Equivalents (RAEs). These Retinol Activity Equivalent units consider the activity of both preformed vitamin A and the three carotenoids that also yield vitamin A in humans. The total RAE value for a food is calculated by adding the actual weight of preformed vitamin A to the conversion equivalents for the provitamin A carotenoids in the food. The Daily Value used on food and supplement labels is 1000 milligrams (5000 IU).

Another Bite

Most nutrient amounts in foods, including vitamin A, were formerly expressed in less precise **International Units (IUs)**. Some food and supplement labels still show the IU value for vitamin A. To compare the older IU (or RE) standards to current RAE recommendations, assume that for any preformed vitamin A in a food or added to food, 3.3 IU (or 1 RE) = 1 RAE. The same is true for any beta-carotene added to foods.

There is no easy way to convert IU or RE units to RAE units for foods that naturally contain provitamin A carotenoids, such as carrots, spinach, and apricots. A general rule of thumb is to divide the older values for foods containing carotenoids by 2, and then do the conversion from IU to RAE as just discussed. There is also no easy way to do this calculation for food containing a mixture of preformed vitamin A and carotenoids. We will just have to wait for all of the food tables to be updated. Generally speaking, any values listed for such foods provide less vitamin A than the RE or IU values currently suggest. On a positive note, increasing intakes of provitamin A carotenoids poses no risk for toxicity (see later section on vitamin A toxicity). Thus, increasing provitamin A carotenoid intake to compensate for less efficient conversion to vitamin A is of no health concern, and likely produces some health benefits, as covered earlier in the section on Functions of Vitamin A and Carotenoids.

The retinal equivalent (RE) is an older unit for vitamin A. This RE assumed that there was a greater contribution to vitamin A needs from carotenoids than we assume today. Food composition tables and nutrient databases still contain this older RE standard, as is the case for Appendix A in this text. It will take some time to update these resources.

International Unit (IU) A crude measure of vitamin activity, often based on the growth rate of animals. Today these units have largely been replaced by more precise milligram and microgram measures.

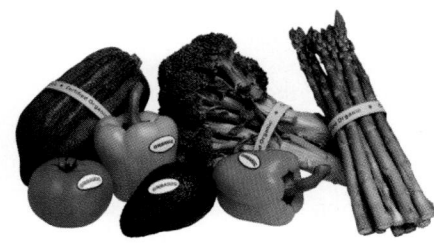

Many vegetables, such as asparagus and broccoli, are rich in provitamin A carotenoids.

fetus The developing human life form from 8 weeks after conception until birth.

Average intakes of vitamin A for North American adult men and women meet the RDA. Most adults in North America have liver reserves of vitamin A that are three to five times greater than needed to provide good health. Thus, the use of vitamin A supplements by most people is unnecessary. At present, there is no separate RDA for beta-carotene or any of the other provitamin A carotenoids.

Deficient vitamin A status in North America may be seen in preschool children who do not eat enough vegetables. The urban poor, older adults, and people with alcoholism or liver disease (which limits vitamin A storage) can also show diminished vitamin A status, especially with respect to stores. Finally, children and adults with severe fat-malabsorption or HIV/AIDS may also experience vitamin A deficiency.

▮ Toxicity of Vitamin A

The Upper Level for vitamin A intake is established at 3000 micrograms preformed vitamin A for adult men and women (10,000 IU). This amount is based on the risk of birth defects occurring during pregnancy and liver toxicity in general with intakes above this amount when consumed on a long-term basis. An increased risk of hip fracture is another possibility. A high preformed vitamin A intake is especially dangerous during the early months of pregnancy because it may cause **fetal** malformations and spontaneous abortions. FDA recommends that women in childbearing years limit their overall intake of preformed vitamin A to a total of about 100% of the Daily Value. In addition, it is also important to consume rich food sources, such as liver, in moderation. This also applies to women who may become pregnant. Because vitamin A is stored in the body for long periods, women who take large amounts during the months before pregnancy place their babies at risk.

The ingestion of large amounts of vitamin A–yielding carotenoids does not cause toxic effects. If someone consumes large amounts of carrots or takes pills containing beta-carotene (more than 30 milligrams daily), or if infants eat a great deal of squash, high carotenoid concentration in the blood can occur. This can turn the skin yellow-orange. The palms of the hand and soles of the feet in particular become colored. This condition does not appear to cause harm and disappears when the excess carotenoid intake decreases. Dietary carotenoids do not produce toxic effects because (1) their rate of conversion into vitamin A is relatively slow and regulated, and (2) the efficiency of carotenoid absorption from the small intestine decreases markedly as oral intake increases.

Vitamin D

Vitamin D is not just a vitamin. It is also considered a hormone because the cells in the skin can convert a cholesterol-like substance to vitamin D, using sunlight. Overall, sun exposure provides about 90% of our vitamin D needs. These skin cells are different from those cells that respond mostly to vitamin D, namely bone cells and kidney cells. This difference between the site of synthesis and action is characteristic of hormones.

The amount of sun exposure needed by individuals to produce vitamin D depends on their skin color, age, time of day, season, and location. Experts recommend that people should expose their hands, face, and arms two to three times a week to 25% of the amount of sun needed to cause a sunburn. In other words, for a person who would sunburn in just an hour, 15 minutes of exposure is recommended. Persons with dark skin would need additional exposure, but the amount is not known. This sun exposure is only effective for vitamin D synthesis if sunscreen over SPF 8 is not used during this time, and it is done between about 8:00 A.M. and 4:00 P.M. Still, this practice is not effective at all in the winter in northern climates. Some people also may be able to use vitamin D stored from summer months in their adipose cells, but most people in northern climates should find alternate vitamin D sources in the winter months. Overall, anyone who does not receive enough sunshine to synthesize an adequate amount of vitamin D must have a dietary source of the vitamin. About 80% of dietary vitamin D is absorbed.

■ Functions of Vitamin D

To become the active hormone, vitamin D must be acted on by the liver and then the kidneys. The main function of this vitamin D hormone (1,25 dihydroxyvitamin D) is to help regulate calcium and bone metabolism. In concert with other hormones, especially **parathyroid hormone (PTH)**, the vitamin D hormone closely regulates blood calcium to supply appropriate amounts of it to all cells. This task entails a variety of processes: the vitamin D hormone helps regulate absorption of calcium and phosphorus from the intestine, it reduces kidney excretion of calcium, and it helps regulate the deposition of calcium in the bones.

Even tissues in the brain, pancreas, and pituitary gland appear to be influenced by the vitamin D hormone. More interestingly, the vitamin D hormone is capable of influencing development in some cancer cells, such as skin, bone, and breast cancer cells. The vitamin D hormone also controls the growth of the parathyroid gland, aids in the function of the immune system, and contributes to skin cell development.

The most obvious result of the vitamin D hormone action is increased calcium and phosphorus deposition in bones. Without adequate calcium and phosphorus, bones weaken and bow under pressure. A child with these symptoms has the disease **rickets.** Symptoms also include enlarged head, joints, and rib cage and a deformed pelvis (review Fig. 8.2).

For the prevention of rickets, infants, especially those with dark skin and breastfed infants, should be provided supplemental vitamin D (under a physician's guidance) if sufficient exposure to sunlight is not possible. Recent studies have shown rickets to be a problem in breastfed infants with dark skin who receive little sun exposure. Keep in mind that supplements should be used very carefully to avoid vitamin D toxicity.

Vitamin D fortification of milk in North America has greatly reduced the risk of rickets in children. Today, rickets in children is most commonly associated with fat malabsorption, such as occurs in children with cystic fibrosis.

Osteomalacia, which means *soft bones,* is an adult disease comparable to rickets. It results when calcium is withdrawn from the bones to make up for inefficient absorption in the intestine or poor conservation by the kidneys. Both of these calcium-rated problems can be caused by vitamin D deficiency. Bones then lose their minerals and become porous and weak and break easily. This leads to fractures in the hip and other bones. One study showed that treatment with 10 to 20 micrograms per day (400 to 800 IU per day) of vitamin D (in conjunction with adequate dietary calcium) greatly decreased fracture risk in older people in nursing homes. Aging decreases production of vitamin D in the skin by about 75% when one reaches the age of 70.

Osteomalacia in adults occurs most commonly in people with kidney, stomach, gallbladder, or intestinal disease (especially when most of the intestine has been removed) and in people with cirrhosis of the liver. These diseases affect both vitamin D activation and calcium absorption. Adults with limited sun exposure may also develop the disease. Combinations of sun exposure, vitamin D intake, or both can prevent this problem. Older people are advised to get sun exposure during early morning and late afternoon when possible to receive the benefit of vitamin D synthesis without also increasing skin cancer risk.

■ Dietary Sources of Vitamin D and Needs

Few foods contain appreciable amounts of vitamin D. Rich sources are fatty fish (e.g., sardines and salmon), fortified milk and yogurt, and some ready-to-eat breakfast

Vitamin D
↓ Acted on by the liver
25-hydroxyvitamin D
↓ Acted on by the kidney
1,25 dihydroxyvitamin D
(active hormone form)

parathyroid hormone (PTH) A hormone made by the parathyroid glands that increases synthesis of the vitamin D hormone and aids calcium release from bone and calcium uptake by the kidneys, among other functions.

rickets A disease characterized by poor mineralization of bones because of low calcium content. This deficiency disease arises from insufficient amounts of the vitamin D hormone in the body.

osteomalacia Adult form of rickets. The weakening of the bones that is seen in this disease is caused by low calcium content. A reduction in the amount of the vitamin D hormone in the body is the cause.

B e careful not to confuse osteomalacia with osteoporosis, another type of bone disorder discussed in Chapter 9.

Food Sources of Vitamin D

Food item and amount	Vitamin D (micrograms)	Vitamin D (IU)
Baked herring, 3 ounces	44.4	1775
Smoked eel, 1 ounce	25.5	1020
Cod liver oil, 1 tablespoon	11.3	453
Baked salmon, 3 ounces	6.0	238
Sardines, 1 ounce	3.4	136
Canned tuna, 3 ounces	3.4	136
1% milk, 1 cup	2.5	99
Nonfat skim milk, 1 cup	2.5	98
Soft margarine, 1 teaspoon	1.5	60
Italian pork sausage, 3 ounces	1.1	44
Soy milk, 1 cup	1.0	40
Raisin Bran cereal, ¾ cup	1.0	38
Baked bluefish, 3 ounces	0.9	34
Special K cereal, ¾ cup	0.8	30
Cooked egg yolk, 1	0.6	25

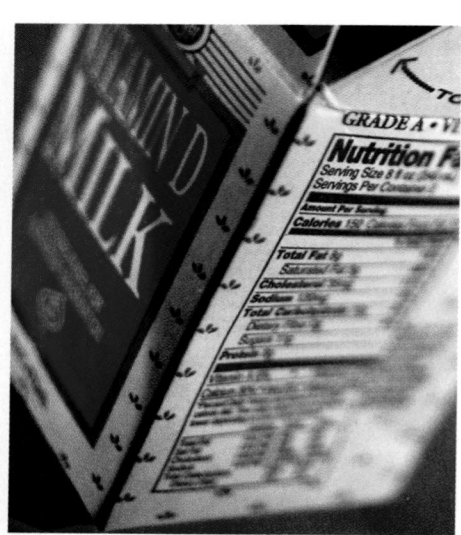

Milk is usually fortified with vitamin D, as well as vitamin A.

cereals. In the United States and Canada, milk usually is fortified with 10 micrograms (400 IU) per quart. Although eggs, butter, liver, and a few brands of margarine contain some vitamin D, large servings must be eaten to obtain an appreciable amount of the vitamin; thus these foods are not considered significant sources.

The Adequate Intake set for vitamin D is 5 micrograms per day (200 IU per day) for people under age 51 and increases two to three times for older adults. The Daily Value used on food and supplement labels is 10 micrograms (400 IU). As mentioned, young, light-skinned people can synthesize all the vitamin D needed from casual sun exposure on just the face and hands. A number of experts suggest older adults, especially those who experience limited sun exposure, receive about 15 to 20 micrograms (600 IU to 800 IU) from a combination of vitamin D-fortified foods and a multivitamin and mineral supplement, with an individual supplement of vitamin D added if needed.

■ Toxicity of Vitamin D

The Upper Level for vitamin D is 50 micrograms per day (2000 IU per day). Too much vitamin D taken regularly can create problems, especially in children. The Upper Level is based on the risk of overabsorption of calcium and eventual calcium deposits in the kidneys and other organs. The person also suffers the typical symptoms of high blood calcium: weakness, loss of appetite, diarrhea, vomiting, mental confusion, and increased urine output. Calcium deposits in organs cause metabolic disturbances and cell death. However, vitamin D toxicity does not result from tanning in the sun too long because the body regulates the amount made in the skin.

Concept Check

Vitamin A is found in foods as preformed vitamin A and as provitamin A carotenoids. The most fully understood function of vitamin A is its importance in vision. Blindness caused by vitamin A deficiency is a major problem in many parts of the world. Vitamin A is also needed to maintain the health of many types of cells, support the immune system, and promote proper growth and development. Vitamin A and some carotenoids may be important in preventing cancer. However, because taking supplements of preformed vitamin A can be toxic, especially in pregnancy, the best recommendation is to focus primarily on eating some vitamin A–rich foods and plenty of provitamin A–rich foods, such as fruits and vegetables.

Vitamin D is a true vitamin only for people who fail to produce enough from sunlight, such as some older people. Using a cholesterol-like substance, people synthesize vitamin D by the action of sunlight on their skin. The vitamin D is later acted on by the liver and kidneys to form the hormone 1,25 dihydroxyvitamin D. This hormone increases calcium absorption in the intestine and works with another hormone (PTH) to maintain calcium metabolism in bones and other organs in the body. Rich food sources of vitamin D are fish oils and fortified milk. Megadose vitamin D intake can be quite toxic, especially in childhood.

Vitamin E

Health-food literature attests to many benefits of vitamin E, including prevention of arthritis, cataracts, stroke, diabetes, cancer, and cardiovascular disease; increased immune function; delayed symptoms of Alzheimer's disease; relief of asthma; and protection of the skin from pollution. Though only some of these benefits are actually supported by reliable studies, North Americans are spending more than $1 billion on vitamin E supplements each year. The following section attempts to sort out fact from fiction in the debate over this high-profile vitamin.

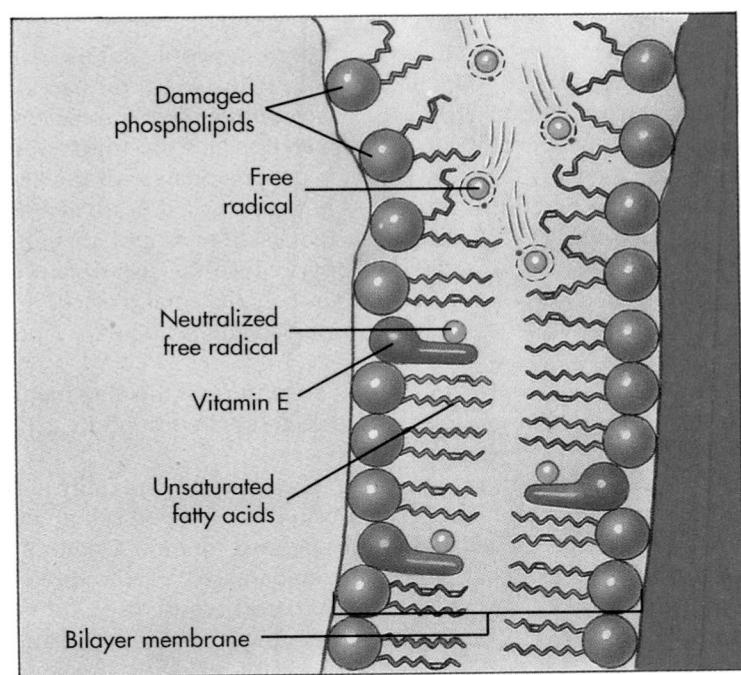

Figure 8.4 Fat-soluble vitamin E can insert itself into cell membranes, where it helps stop free-radical chain reactions. If not interrupted, these reactions cause extensive oxidative damage to cells and ultimately cell death.

■ Functions of Vitamin E

Acting as a fat-soluble antioxidant, vitamin E resides mostly in cell membranes. As discussed in Chapter 5, an antioxidant can form a barrier between a target molecule—an unsaturated fatty acid in a cell membrane, for example—and a compound seeking its electrons (Fig. 8.4). The antioxidant donates electrons or hydrogens to the electron-seeking compound. This protects other molecules or parts of a cell from having electrons nabbed. Note that vitamin C is a water-soluble antioxidant.

If vitamin E is not available to do its job, an electron-seeking compound, such as a free radical, can pull electrons from cell membranes, DNA, and other electron-dense cell components. This either alters the cell's DNA, which may increase the risk for cancer, or injures cell membranes, possibly causing the cell to die. Recall from Chapter 7 that free radicals are highly reactive compounds containing an unpaired electron. This free-radical production is a normal result of cell metabolism and immune system function. For example, white blood cells generate free radicals as part of their action to stop infection. Some exposure to free radicals, then, is part of life. Overall, however, the body needs to carefully regulate this exposure to avoid their undesirable effects. Once vitamin E acts on free radicals and related compounds, some of it is excreted and some of it is likely recycled by the addition of an electron from other antioxidants (e.g., vitamin C).

Many other antioxidant systems exist in cells as well, some of which utilize minerals such as copper, selenium, and manganese (see Chapter 9 for details). Overall, cells do not rely exclusively on vitamin E for protection from free radicals. Systems also exist in cells to repair molecules (such as DNA) that have been damaged by free radicals.

This discussion raises the question of the relative role of vitamin E in oxidant protection in the body. Experts do not know whether taking megadose vitamin E supplements by otherwise healthy people confers any additional protection against cardiovascular disease and cancer than that achieved by improving diet (especially fruit, vegetable, and whole-grain intake), performing regular physical activity, not smoking, and maintaining a healthy body weight. This advice has the widest scientific support in the battle against these diseases. Furthermore, the proven benefits of these lifestyle changes are far greater than the postulated benefits of supplemental antioxidants, including vitamin E. Thus, as reviewed in Chapter 5, even if antioxidant

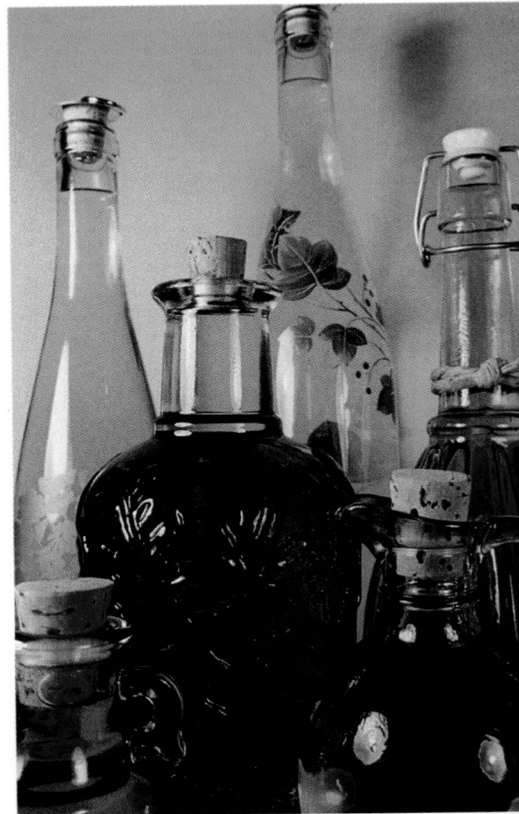

Plant oils are rich sources of vitamin E.

hemolysis Destruction of red blood cells. The red blood cell membrane breaks down, allowing cell contents to leak into the fluid portion of the blood.

tocopherols The chemical name for some forms of vitamin E. The alpha form is the most potent.

isomers Different chemical structures for compounds that share the same chemical formula.

Food Sources of Vitamin E

Food item and amount	Vitamin E (milligrams)	Vitamin E (IU)
Total Raisin Bran cereal, ¾ cup	22.5	33.5
Sunflower oil, 2 tablespoons	16.3	24.3
Dry-roasted sunflower seeds, 1 ounce	14.3	21.2
Dry-roasted almonds, 1 ounce	7.5	11.1
Safflower oil, 1 tablespoon	5.9	8.7
Canola oil, 2 tablespoons	5.7	8.5
Wheat germ, ¼ cup	5.2	7.7
Almonds, 1 ounce	4.5	6.8
Oil-roasted sunflower seeds, 1 tablespoon	3.4	5.0
Italian dressing, 2 tablespoons	3.1	4.5
Mayonnaise, 1 tablespoon	3.0	4.5
Avocado, 1	2.7	4.0
Chunky peanut butter, 2 tablespoons	2.4	3.6
Mango, 1	2.3	3.5
Peanuts, 1 ounce	2.1	3.1

supplements eventually are clearly determined to be effective in preventing cardiovascular disease (and cancer), they should be used (even in people at high risk) only as an adjunct—not as an alternative—to a healthful lifestyle. In fact, the American Heart Association recently stated that it is premature to recommend vitamin E supplements to the general populations, based on current knowledge, and the failure of most clinical trials to show any benefit. This conclusion is in agreement with the latest report on vitamin E by the Food and Nutrition Board of the National Academy of Sciences. In addition, as late as 2001, FDA has denied the request of the supplement industry to make a health claim that vitamin E supplements reduce the risk of cardiovascular disease and cancer. Still, some experts recommend a daily intake of 200 milligrams (13 times the RDA) while at the same time noting that that evidence supporting this recommendation is sketchy.

Finally, vitamin E can help improve vitamin A absorption if the dietary intake of vitamin A is low. In addition, vitamin E is used to metabolize iron in the cell and help maintain nervous tissue and immune function.

A deficiency of vitamin E causes cell membrane breakdown, especially in red blood cells of premature infants. Unsaturated fatty acids in the red blood cell membrane are very sensitive to attack by oxidizing compounds. Because vitamin E neutralizes these agents, it protects the red blood cell membrane from damage. Red blood cell breakage, called **hemolysis,** commonly occurs in preterm infants because they did not receive sufficient vitamin E from their mothers. The rapid growth of premature infants, coupled with the high oxygen concentration found in infant incubators, greatly increases the stress on red blood cells. This raises the risk of cell damage. Special formulas and supplements designed for preterm infants can help compensate for lack of vitamin E.

■ Vitamin E in Foods and Needs

Plant oils and foods rich in these, such as salad dressings and mayonnaise; ready-to-eat breakfast cereals; some fruits and vegetables, such as asparagus, tomatoes, and green leafy vegetables; eggs; and margarine are major sources of vitamin E. The vitamin E in plant oils is used to protect the unsaturated fats present in plant oils. Animal fats and fish oils, on the other hand, have practically no vitamin E (Fig. 8.5). Also, grain meals, such as oatmeal, nuts (e.g., almonds), and seeds (e.g., sunflower seeds) are good sources. The actual vitamin E content of a food depends on how it was harvested, processed, stored, and cooked because vitamin E is very susceptible to destruction by oxygen, metals, light, and especially repeated use of oils in deep-fat frying.

The RDA of vitamin E for adults is 15 milligrams per day of **alpha-tocopherol,** the active form of what is called vitamin E. This is about two-thirds of the amount we eat each day. Daily intake of nuts and seeds, or a ready-to-eat breakfast cereal containing vitamin E, or use of a multivitamin and mineral supplement would close this gap. To convert from the older IU system, 10 IU equals about 4.5 milligrams, based on the synthetic (dl **isomer**) form of vitamin E found in most supplements. If vitamin E is from a natural source (d isomer) 10 IU equals 6.7 milligrams, as the natural form of vitamin E is more potent than the synthetic form. Thus the 200 milligram recommendation above represents 300 IU (d isomer) to 450 IU (dl isomer). The Daily Value used on food and supplement labels is 30 IU.

The beneficial effects of vitamin E and other antioxidants in counteracting free-radical damage in biological systems is most apparent when viewed on a long-term basis because free-radical-related damage to cells occurs over time. Thus, current research can't rule out that some benefit for healthy adults may occur from intakes of vitamin E in excess of the RDA. Studies in otherwise healthy people are under way using megadoses from 45 IU to 800 IU per day.

Smokers are especially likely to develop a vitamin E deficiency. (Smoking readily destroys vitamin E in the lungs.) But one study showed that even using megadoses of vitamin E was ineffective in preventing this damage. Others at considerable risk of a vitamin E deficiency include adults on very low-fat diets or those with fat malabsorption.

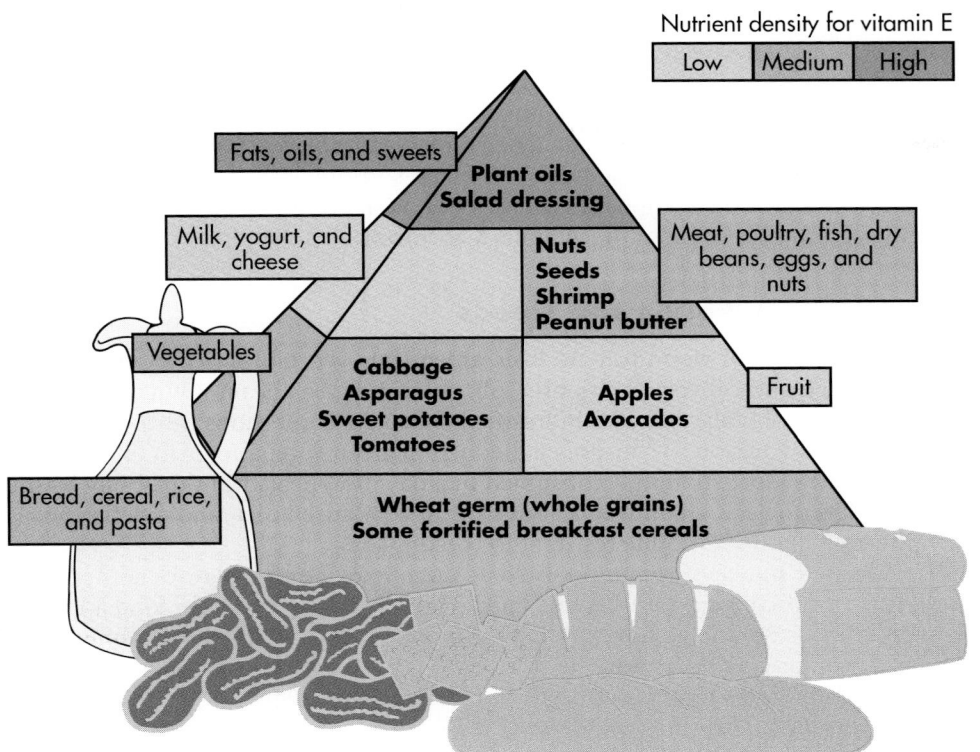

Nutrient density for vitamin E

| Low | Medium | High |

Figure 8.5 Food sources of vitamin E from the Food Guide Pyramid. Vitamin E is concentrated in plant oils, nuts, seeds, and some vegetables. The background color of each food group indicates the average nutrient density (milligram [or IU] per kcal) for vitamin E in that group.

■ Toxicity of Vitamin E

Excessive amounts of vitamin E can antagonize vitamin K's role in the clotting mechanism, leading to **hemorrhage.** The risk of insufficient blood clotting is especially high if vitamin E is taken in conjunction with anticoagulant medications. The Upper Level for vitamin E is based on reduced blood clotting in adults, and is 1000 milligrams per day of any form of supplemental alpha-tocopherol. Do not exceed this amount on a long-term basis if you decide to take vitamin E supplements. In International Units, the Upper Level is 1500 IU for vitamin E isolated from natural sources (d isomer) and 1100 IU for synthetic vitamin E (dl isomer). The lower IU value for the synthetic form reflects the greater number of forms present in the synthetic product, some of which do not contribute to vitamin E activity in cells but are still absorbed. This Upper Level also is confined to a healthy population. Again, individuals who are vitamin K-deficient or who are taking anticoagulants are especially at risk for hemorrhaging from megadose vitamin E use.

hemorrhage An escape of blood from blood vessels.

Vitamin K

A family of compounds known collectively as vitamin K is found in plants, plant oils, fish oils, and meats. One form is synthesized by bacteria in the human intestine. These bacteria supply us with about 10% of the vitamin K we need. The rest comes from diet.

Vitamin K is vital for blood clotting, working along with various proteins and calcium. The *K* stands for *koagulation,* as it is spelled in Denmark. This spelling is used because a Danish researcher first noted the relationship between vitamin K and blood clotting. Vitamin K contributes to the synthesis of several blood-clotting factors. Vitamin K also helps form proteins present in bone, muscle, and kidneys, thereby imparting calcium-binding potential to these organs. A poor intake has been linked to an increase in hip fractures because of its effect on various proteins in bone.

Inactive blood-clotting factors
↓ Action of vitamin K
Active blood-clotting factors

A newborn's intestinal tract lacks sufficient vitamin K–producing bacteria to allow for blood to clot effectively if the infant is injured. Therefore, vitamin K also is routinely given by injection shortly after birth to bridge the gap until enough bacteria are present to synthesize some of the vitamin K needed by the infant. In adults, deficiencies of vitamin K have occurred when a person takes antibiotics for a long period and in the presence of severe long-standing fat malabsorption. Long-term antibiotic use also can lead to this problem because it destroys many of the intestinal bacteria that normally account for some of the vitamin K absorbed.

■ Vitamin K in Foods and Needs

Major food sources of vitamin K are liver, green leafy vegetables (for example, kale, turnip greens, lettuce, and spinach), broccoli, peas, and green beans. Other sources are soybean and canola oils, and certain fortified chocolate confections (also contain extra calcium). One reason to consume a diet rich in green vegetables is to obtain sufficient vitamin K. Most vitamin K consumed in a day disappears from the body by the next day. Nevertheless, vitamin K is abundant in a balanced diet, and a deficiency is uncommon. Vitamin K is quite resistant to cooking losses.

The Adequate Intake for vitamin K is 90 to 120 micrograms per day for adults. Most North Americans consume at least this much. The Daily Value used on food and supplement labels is 80 micrograms. Older people may be at risk of a deficiency because of a scant green vegetable intake.

Oral vitamin K generally poses no risk of toxicity, so no Upper Level has been set. The main problem with megadose use is reduced effectiveness of oral medications used to reduce blood clotting. These medications are used by some people, especially those with blood-clotting disorders or those who have undergone recent cardiovascular surgery.

Food Sources of Vitamin K

Food item and amount	Vitamin K (micrograms)
Brussels sprouts, ½ cup	483
Raw kale, ½ cup	274
Cooked broccoli, ½ cup	211
Raw turnips, 1 cup	138
Raw spinach, 1 cup	120
Raw cauliflower, 3 florets	120
Looseleaf lettuce, 1 cup	118
Raw cabbage, 1 cup	101
Cooked green beans, ½ cup	49
Asparagus spears, 5	38
Boiled egg, 1	31
Sauerkraut, ½ cup	30
Green peas, ½ cup	26
Soybean oil, 1 tablespoon	25
Canola oil, 1 tablespoon	17

Concept Check

Vitamin E functions primarily as an antioxidant. It can donate electrons to electron-seeking free radical (oxidizing) compounds. By neutralizing these compounds, vitamin E helps prevent cell destruction, especially the destruction of red blood cell membranes. The richest sources of vitamin E are plant oils, foods rich in these oils, and nuts, but it occurs in a wide variety of foods. Studies using megadoses of vitamin E are under way. At present, it is not clear if such use provides health benefits.

Vitamin K plays a key role in efficient blood clotting; it contributes to the synthesis of certain blood-clotting proteins. In addition, vitamin K contributes to the synthesis of the calcium-binding proteins in some organs, such as bones. About 10% of the vitamin K we absorb every day is synthesized by intestinal bacteria; the rest comes from our diets. The amount in the diet alone generally meets our daily needs. Thus, except for newborns and possibly older adults, a deficiency of vitamin K is unlikely when one consumes green vegetables and certain plant oils on a regular basis.

Nutrient Supplements: Who Needs Them?

Today, supplements are marketed as good for anything that ails you. This cure-all approach is promoted by the supplement industry and countless health-food stores, pharmacies, and supermarkets.

Because recent research on a variety of nutrient supplements has revealed a lack of product quality, the USP (United States Pharmacopeia) designation is being extended to an increasing number of nutrient supplements. The USP standards designate strength, quality, purity, packaging, labeling, speed of dissolution, and acceptable length of storage of ingredients for drugs. The purpose of applying them to vitamin and mineral supplements is to establish professionally accepted standards for these products. Consumers who buy nutrient supplements should look for a USP label when comparing similar products, such as calcium supplements. If no USP label is present, the next best approach is to purchase nationally-advertised brands.

According to the Dietary Supplement Health and Education Act of 1994 (discussed in Chapter 1), a supplement in the United States is a product intended to supplement the diet that bears or contains one or more of the following dietary ingredients:

- A vitamin
- A mineral
- An herb or another botanical
- An amino acid
- A dietary substance to supplement the diet, which could be an extract or a combination of the first four ingredients in this list

The definition is very broad and covers a wide variety of nutritional substances. The use of supplements to the diet is a common practice among North Americans and generates about $14 billion annually for the industry in the United States alone. Recall also from the Nutrition Issue in Chapter 1 that unless FDA has evidence that a supplement is inherently dangerous or marketed with an illegal claim, it will not regulate such products closely. (The vitamin folate is an exception.) Currently, FDA has limited resources to police supplement manufacturers, and has to act against these manufacturers one at a time. Thus, we cannot rely on FDA to protect us from vitamin and mineral supplement overuse and misuse. We bear that responsibility ourselves, coupled with professional advice from a physician or registered dietitian.

Currently, the supplement makers can make broad claims about their products under the "structure or function" provision of the law, allowing the product onto the market without testing for safety or efficacy. The products, however, cannot claim to prevent, treat, or cure a disease. Since pregnancy, menopause, and aging are not diseases per se, products alleging to treat these conditions can be marketed without FDA approval. For example, a product that claims to treat morning sickness can be sold without any testing to prove that the product actually works, but a product that claims to decrease the risk of cardiovascular disease by reducing blood cholesterol must have scientific studies that justify the claim.

Why do people take supplements? Reasons that are frequently given include the following:

- To reduce susceptibility to health problems (e.g., colds)
- To prevent heart attacks
- To prevent cancer
- To reduce stress
- To increase "energy"

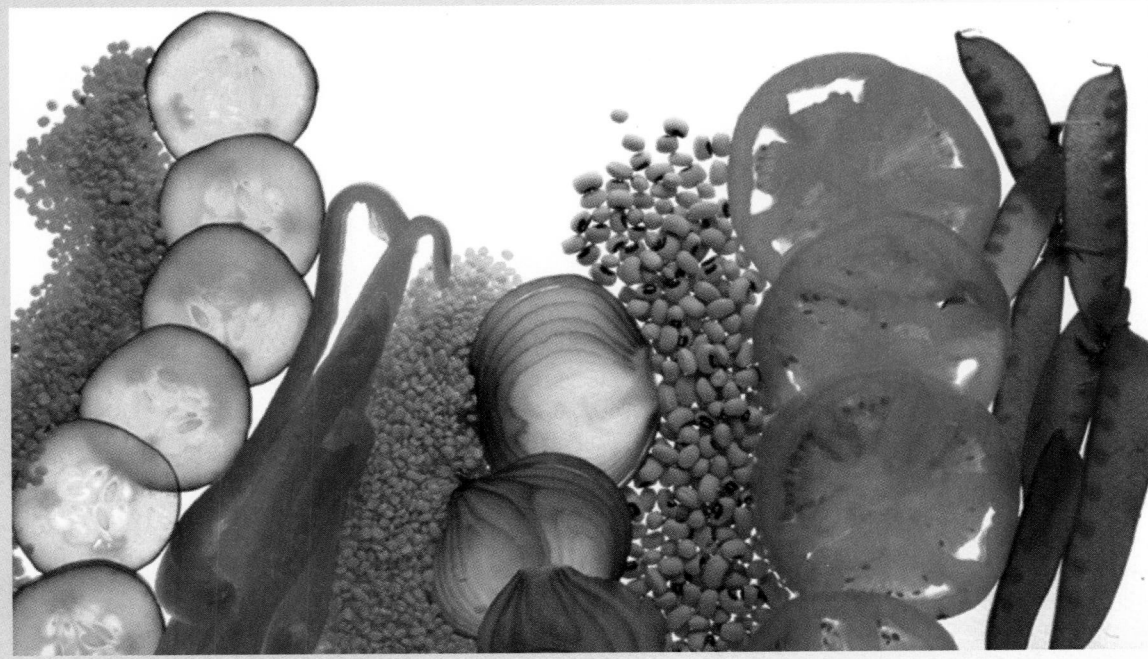

Focus first on foods that meet nutrient needs.

continued

Should you take a supplement? This is up to you. Currently, opinions vary about the wisdom and safety of supplement use even among knowledgeable scientists. Typically, nutrition scientists have recommended that supplement use is needed only by a few groups of our population at large. However, over the last few years many reputable nutrition scientists have recommended supplementation of specific nutrients for most adults.

This change in philosophy has arisen primarily because many North Americans have been unwilling to change their food habits, such as include ample fruits and vegetables. This gap can leave diets low in the vitamin folate. Adequate folate status when a woman becomes pregnant helps reduce the risk of certain birth defects in her offspring (400 micrograms per day of synthetic folic acid is recommended). Folate also limits homocysteine in the blood, a likely risk factor for cardiovascular disease that can affect all of us. In addition, the committee appointed by the Food and Nutrition Board that set current nutrient standards for vitamin B-12 suggested that adults over age 50 consume vitamin B-12 in a synthetic form, such as that added to ready-to-eat breakfast cereals or present in

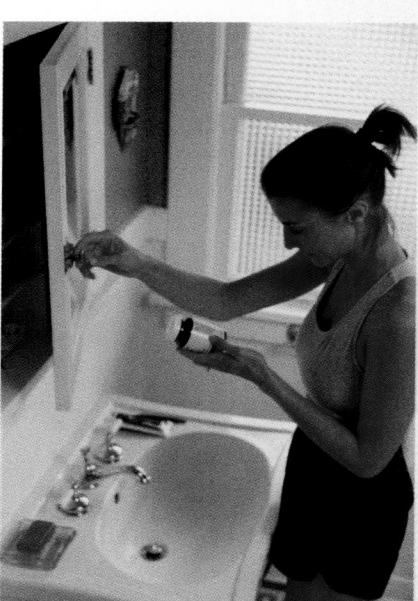

Long-term intake of just three or more times the Daily Value for some fat-soluble vitamins—particularly vitamins A and D—can cause toxic effects. Know what you are taking if you use supplements.

supplements. Synthetic vitamin B-12 is more easily absorbed than that found in food; this helps compensate for the fall in vitamin B-12 absorption typically seen as we age into our later years. This latter observation has caused nutrition experts at Tufts University to add a recommendation for vitamin B-12 supplements to the Food Guide Pyramid they developed for older persons. The Tufts scientists also include calcium and vitamin D supplements, as these nutrients can be deficient in the diets of older persons (see Chapter 15).

Nutrition expert Dr. Walter Willett also recommends in his book *Eat, Drink, and Be Healthy* (discussed in Chapter 2), that most people take a multivitamin and mineral supplement, citing that this is one inexpensive way to decrease the risk of developing a number of chronic diseases. A further example of this change in philosophy is a recent article in *The New England Journal of Medicine* entitled "What supplement should I be taking, doctor?" The authors recommended a multivitamin and mineral supplement and possibly some extra vitamin E. Still, they noted that all of the health-promoting effects of foods cannot be found in a bottle; recall the discussions of phytochemicals in Chapter 2 and the benefits of dietary fiber in Chapter 4. Few or no phytochemicals and no dietary fiber are present in supplements. Multivitamin and mineral supplements also contain little calcium in order to keep the pill size small.

Overall, supplement use cannot fix a poor diet in all respects. Uninformed megadose supplement use also can lead to harm. Currently, most nutrient toxicity is a result of supplement use. Thus, we are advised to first take a good look at our dietary habits and then improve them as possible, as outlined in Chapter 2. Finally, find out which nutrient gaps remain, and identify food sources that can help. Examples could be ready-to-eat breakfast cereals to increase vitamin E, folate, and vitamin B-6 intake and provide highly absorbable forms of vitamin B-12 (many currently contain RDA amounts or more per serving). One needs to be careful, however, as these products may provide the appropriate amount of nutrients in 1 serving, but the typical consumer may eat more than 1 serving. This can lead to an excessive intake of some nutrients, such as vitamin A, iron, and synthetic folic acid. Calcium-fortified orange juice could be

used to increase calcium intake, or milk and yogurt to increase vitamin D and calcium intake.

If supplement use is desired, one should discuss this practice with a physician, as some supplements can interfere with certain medicines. For example, vitamin B-6 can offset the action of L-dopa (used in treating Parkinson's disease), and high intakes of vitamin K or vitamin E alter the action of oral anticoagulants. Large doses of vitamin C can interfere with certain cancer therapy regimens. Excessive zinc intake can inhibit iron and copper absorption. Large amounts of folate can mask signs and symptoms of a vitamin B-12 deficiency (see the section on toxicity of folate in this chapter). Remember, you can get too much of a good thing.

V itamin and mineral supplements should generally be taken with or just after meals to maximize absorption.

People Most Likely to Need Supplements

Various medical and health-related organizations suggest that the following vitamin and mineral supplementation can be important for certain groups of healthy people:

- Women in their childbearing years may need extra synthetic folic acid if their dietary patterns do not supply enough (again, 400 micrograms).
- Women with excessive bleeding during menstruation may need extra iron.
- Women who are pregnant or breastfeeding may need extra iron, folate, and calcium.
- People with very low energy intakes (less than about 1200 kcal per day) may need a range of vitamins and minerals. This is true of some women and older people.
- Strict vegans may need extra calcium, iron, zinc, and vitamin B-12.
- Newborns, under the direction of a physician, need a single dose of vitamin K.
- Some infants may need fluoride supplements, as directed by a dentist.

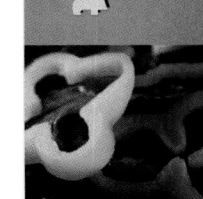

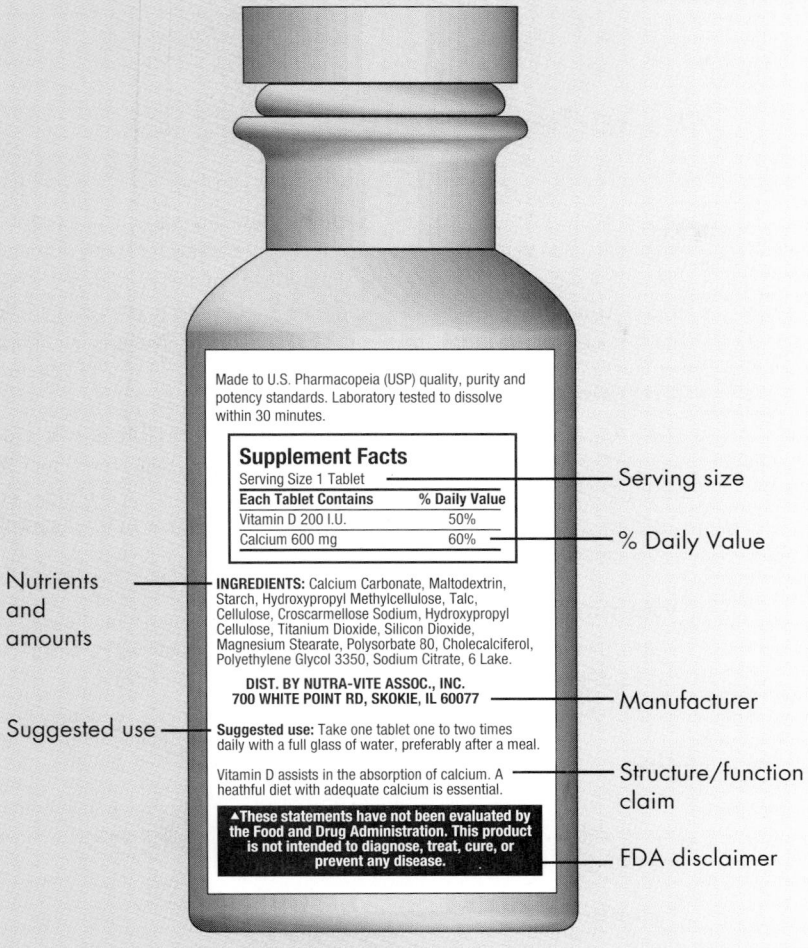

Serving size

% Daily Value

Nutrients and amounts

Suggested use

Manufacturer

Structure/function claim

FDA disclaimer

Made to U.S. Pharmacopeia (USP) quality, purity and potency standards. Laboratory tested to dissolve within 30 minutes.

Supplement Facts

Serving Size 1 Tablet

Each Tablet Contains	% Daily Value
Vitamin D 200 I.U.	50%
Calcium 600 mg	60%

INGREDIENTS: Calcium Carbonate, Maltodextrin, Starch, Hydroxypropyl Methylcellulose, Talc, Cellulose, Croscarmellose Sodium, Hydroxypropyl Cellulose, Titanium Dioxide, Silicon Dioxide, Magnesium Stearate, Polysorbate 80, Cholecalciferol, Polyethylene Glycol 3350, Sodium Citrate, 6 Lake.

DIST. BY NUTRA-VITE ASSOC., INC.
700 WHITE POINT RD, SKOKIE, IL 60077

Suggested use: Take one tablet one to two times daily with a full glass of water, preferably after a meal.

Vitamin D assists in the absorption of calcium. A healthful diet with adequate calcium is essential.

▲These statements have not been evaluated by the Food and Drug Administration. This product is not intended to diagnose, treat, cure, or prevent any disease.

Figure 8.6 Nutrient supplements display a nutrition label that is different from that of foods. This Supplement Facts label must list the ingredient(s), amount(s) per serving, serving size, suggested use, and % Daily Value if one has been established. Note that this label also includes structure/function claims. Thus, it also must include the FDA warning that these claims have not been evaluated by the agency.

- People with limited milk intake and sunlight exposure may need extra vitamin D. This includes many breastfed infants, especially those who are dark skinned (this reduces vitamin D synthesis by the skin), and many older people.
- People with lactose intolerance or allergies to dairy products may need extra calcium.
- Adults over age 50 need a synthetic source of vitamin B-12.
- People on very low-fat diets or diets low in plant oils and nuts may need some extra vitamin E.

Individuals with certain medical conditions (e.g., vitamin-resistance diseases or long-standing fat malabsorption) and those who use certain medications also may require supplementation with specific vitamins and minerals. Finally, smokers and alcohol abusers may benefit from supplementation, but cessation of these two activities is far more beneficial than any supplementation.

Which Supplement Should You Choose?

If you decide to take a multivitamin and mineral supplement, which one should you choose? As a start, choose a national brand (from a supermarket or pharmacy). Then intake from the total of this supplement, any other supplements used, and highly fortified foods such as ready-to-eat breakfast cereals should provide no more than the Upper Level for each vitamin and mineral. (See the inside cover of this textbook for Upper Levels.) Two exceptions are that men and older women should make sure any product used is low in iron or iron free to avoid possible iron overload (see Chapters 9 and 15 for details). One should read the labels carefully to be sure of what is being taken (Fig. 8.6).

Another consideration in choosing a supplement is avoiding superfluous ingredients, such as para-amino benzoic acid (PABA), hesperidin complex, inositol, bee pollen, and lecithins. These are not needed in our diets. They are especially common in expensive supplements sold in health-food stores and by mail. In addition, use of l-tryptophan and high doses of beta-carotene or fish oils are discouraged.

Five websites to help you evaluate ongoing claims and evaluate safety of supplements are:

www.acsh.org
www.quackwatch.com
www.ncahf.org
dietary-supplements.info.nih.gov
www.consumerlabs.com.

The sites are maintained by groups or individuals committed to providing reasoned and authoritative nutrition and health advice to consumers.

Scenario *Follow-Up*

Use of *Nutramega* poses some health risks for Kristen. Taking 2 to 3 tablets every 3 hours would mean taking at least 16 tablets per day. This alone would provide an intake of vitamin A, vitamin C, and zinc well in excess of the Upper Levels for these nutrients. Intake of preformed vitamin A would be 1.3 times the Upper Level, intake of vitamin C would be 3.4 times the Upper Level, and intake of zinc would be 3 times the Upper Level. Intake of selenium, however, falls well below the Upper Level set for that nutrient. This is how the math works out.

Vitamin A

33% (0.33) times the Daily Value of 1000 micrograms RAE equals 330 micrograms RAE per tablet. Sixteen tablets would yield 5280 micrograms RAE. The Upper Level is 3000 micrograms RAE for preformed vitamin A. Since 75% of the vitamin A is preformed vitamin A, this yields 3960 micrograms RAE of preformed vitamin A (5280 × 0.75 = 3960), or 1.3 times the Upper Level (3960/3000 = 1.3).

Vitamin C

700% (7) times the Daily Value of 60 milligrams equals 4200 milligrams per tablet. 16 tablets would yield 6720 milligrams. The Upper Level is 2000 milligrams. This would then yield 3.4 times the Upper Level (6720/2000 = 3.4).

Zinc

50% (0.5) times the Daily Value of 15 milligrams equals 7.5 milligrams per tablet. 16 tablets would yield 120 milligrams. The Upper Level is 40 milligrams. This would then yield 3 times the Upper Level (120/40 = 3).

Selenium

10% (0.1) times the Daily Value of 70 micrograms equals 7 micrograms per tablet. 16 tablets would yield 112 micrograms. This is less than the Upper Level of 400 micrograms.

The maintenance dose of two to three tablets per day poses no risk per se, but *Nutramega* is very expensive compared to the cost of the typical multivitamin and mineral supplement (a 1-month supply would cost about $2 compared to about $15 for *Nutramega*). Overall, Kristen is smart to be concerned about meeting her nutrient needs when under stress, but such stress does not increase nutrient needs. A balanced diet, as shown in Table 2.7 in Chapter 2, should be her primary focus. Taking a balanced multivitamin and mineral supplement is also a reasonable practice. Actually, however, it is most important for Kristen to get adequate sleep; this is the main health habit that will help her through her current schedule.

The Water-Soluble Vitamins and Choline

Most water-soluble vitamins are more readily excreted than are fat-soluble vitamins. Any excess generally ends up in the urine or stool, so consuming the water-soluble vitamins regularly is important. Because they dissolve in water, large amounts of these vitamins can be lost during food processing and preparation. Light cooking such as stir-frying, steaming, and microwaving best preserve vitamin content (review Table 8.1). A summary of much of what we know about water-soluble vitamins is presented in Table 8.3.

The B vitamins are thiamin, riboflavin, niacin, pantothenic acid, biotin, vitamin B-6, folate, and vitamin B-12. Choline is a related nutrient, but currently is not classified as a vitamin. Vitamin C rounds out the water-soluble vitamins.

Because they often occur in the same foods, a lack of one B vitamin may mean other B vitamins are also low. The B vitamins are all changed into coenzymes, small

*V*itamin status can be tested by measuring enzyme activities in red blood cells that require vitamins to function. Such biochemical tests for enzyme activity can be used to determine thiamin, riboflavin, and vitamin B-6 status.

Table 8.3 A Summary of the Water-Soluble Vitamins and Choline: Their Functions, Deficiency Conditions, and Food Sources

Name	Major Functions	Deficiency Symptoms	People Most at Risk	Dietary Sources*	RDA or Adequate Intake	Toxicity
Thiamin	Coenzyme involved in carbohydrate metabolism; nerve function	Beriberi: nervous tingling, poor coordination, edema, heart changes, weakness	People with alcoholism or in poverty	Sunflower seeds, pork, whole and enriched grains, dried beans, peas, brewer's yeast	1.1–1.2 milligrams	None
Riboflavin	Coenzyme involved in energy metabolism	Inflammation of mouth and tongue, cracks at corners of the mouth, eye disorders	Possibly people on certain medications if no dairy products consumed	Milk, mushrooms, spinach, liver, enriched grains	1.1–1.3 milligrams	None
Niacin	Coenzyme involved in energy metabolism, fat synthesis, fat breakdown	Pellagra: diarrhea, dermatitis, dementia (death)	People in areas of severe poverty where corn is the dominant food; alcoholism	Mushrooms, bran, tuna, salmon, chicken, beef, liver, peanuts, enriched grains	14–16 milligrams (Niacin Equivalents)	Upper Level is 35 milligrams from supplements based on flushing of skin
Pantothenic acid	Coenzyme involved in energy metabolism, fat synthesis, fat breakdown	No natural deficiency disease or symptoms	None	Mushrooms, liver, broccoli, eggs; most foods have some	5 milligrams	None
Biotin	Coenzyme involved in glucose production, fat synthesis	Dermatitis, tongue soreness, anemia, depression	People with alcoholism	Cheese, egg yolks, cauliflower, peanut butter, liver	30 micrograms	Unknown
Vitamin B-6,[†] pyridoxine, and other forms	Coenzyme involved in protein metabolism, neurotransmitter synthesis, hemoglobin synthesis, many other functions	Headache, anemia, convulsions, nausea, vomiting, flaky skin, sore tongue	Adolescent and adult women; people on certain medications; alcoholism	Animal protein foods, spinach, broccoli, bananas, salmon, sunflower seeds	1.3–1.7 milligrams	Upper Level is 100 milligrams based on nerve destruction
Folate[†] (folic acid)	Coenzyme involved in DNA synthesis, other functions	Megaloblastic anemia, inflammation of tongue, diarrhea, poor growth, depression	People with alcoholism, pregnancy, people on certain medications	Green leafy vegetables, orange juice, organ meats, sprouts, sunflower seeds	400 micrograms (Dietary Folate Equivalents)	None likely; nonprescription vitamin dosage is controlled by FDA; Upper Level for adults set at 1000 micrograms per day for synthetic folic acid, exclusive of food folate, based on masking vitamin B-12 deficiency
Vitamin B-12[†] (cobalamins)	Coenzyme involved in folate metabolism, nerve function, other functions	Macrocytic anemia, poor nerve function	Older adults because of poor absorption; vegans, people with HIV/AIDS	Animal foods, especially organ meats, oysters, clams (not natural in plants), fortified ready-to-eat breakfast cereals	2.4 micrograms (adults 51 and older: same, but use fortified foods or supplements)	None
Vitamin C (ascorbic acid)	Connective tissue synthesis, hormone synthesis, neurotransmitter synthesis	Scurvy: poor wound healing, pinpoint hemorrhages, bleeding gums	People with alcoholism, older men who eat poorly	Citrus fruits, strawberries, broccoli, greens	75–90 milligrams (smokers should add 35 milligrams)	Upper Level is 2 grams, based on development of diarrhea; can also alter some diagnostic tests
Choline[†]	Neurotransmitter and phospholipid synthesis	No natural deficiency	None	Widely distributed in foods, plus self-synthesis	425–550 milligrams	Upper Level is 3.5 grams per day based on development of fishy body odor and reduced blood pressure

*Fortified ready-to-eat breakfast cereals are good sources for most of these vitamins and a common source of B vitamins for many of us.

[†]These vitamins also participate in homocysteine metabolism, which in turn limits their ability to promote cardiovascular disease.

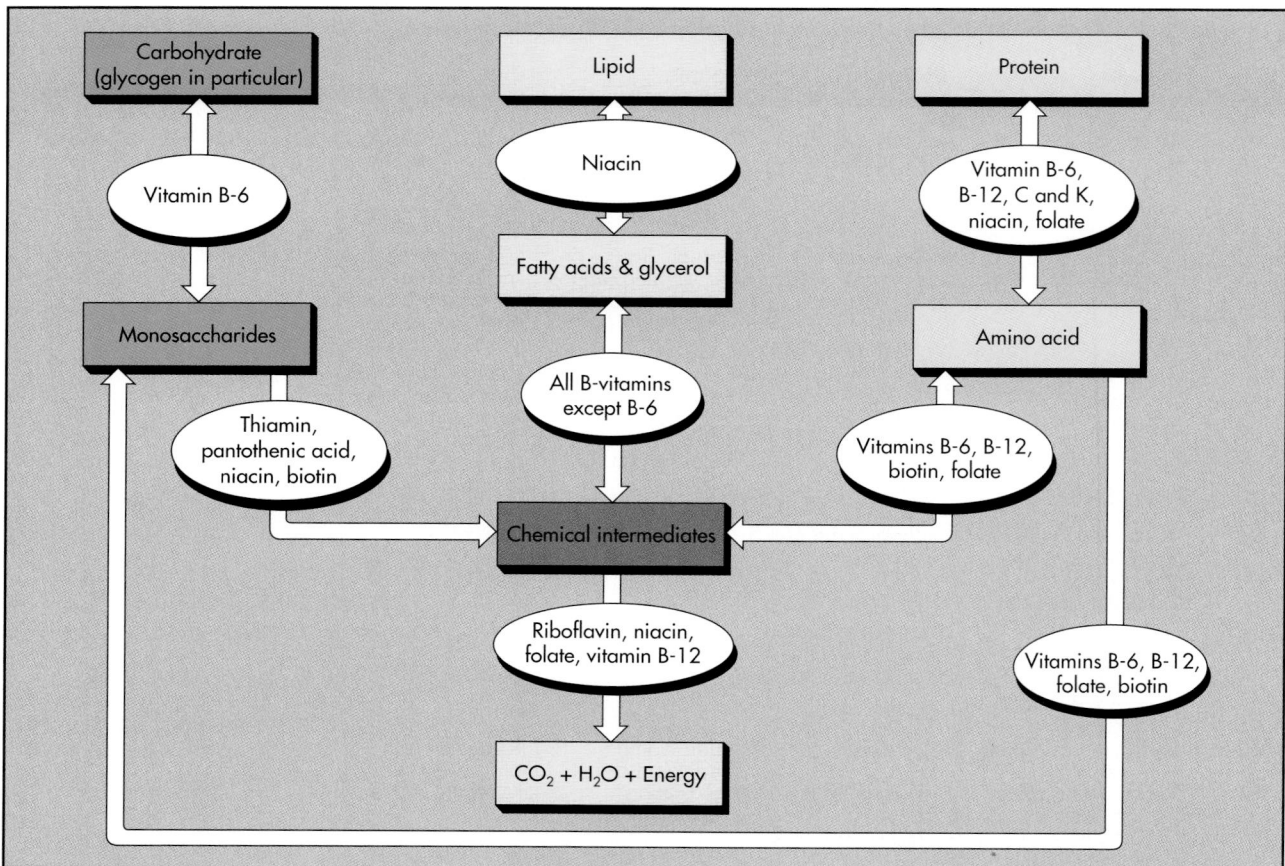

Figure 8.7 Examples of metabolic pathways for which vitamins are essential. The metabolism of energy-yielding nutrients requires vitamin input.

molecules that interact with enzymes to enable enzymes to function. In essence, the coenzymes contribute to enzyme activity (review Fig. 8.1).

As coenzymes, the B vitamins play many key roles in metabolism. The metabolic pathways used by carbohydrates, fats, and amino acids together require input from B vitamins. This makes many B vitamins interdependent because they participate in the same processes (Fig. 8.7).

After being ingested, the B vitamins are first broken down from their coenzyme forms into free vitamins in the stomach and small intestine. The vitamins are then absorbed, primarily in the small intestine. Typically, about 50% to 90% of the B vitamins in the diet are absorbed. Once inside cells, the coenzyme forms are resynthesized. Although certain forms are sold in health food stores, there is no need to consume the coenzyme forms themselves. We make them when needed.

■ B Vitamin Intakes of North Americans

The nutritional health of most North Americans with regard to the B vitamins is generally good. Typical diets contain plentiful and varied natural sources of these vitamins. In addition, many common foods, such as ready-to-eat breakfast cereals, are fortified with one or more of the water-soluble vitamins. In some developing countries, however, deficiencies of the water-soluble vitamins are more common, and the resulting deficiency diseases pose significant public-health problems. (A detailed discussion of nutritional deficiencies worldwide is presented in Chapter 17.)

Despite the generally good B vitamin status of North Americans, marginal deficiencies of the water-soluble vitamins may occur in some cases, especially in older people who eat little food, and in people who follow poor dietary patterns. The long-term effects of such marginal deficiencies are as yet unknown, but increased risk of cardiovascular disease, cancer, and cataracts of the eye is suspected. However, in the short run, such a marginal deficiency in most people likely leads only to fatigue or other bothersome and unspecific physical effects. With rare exceptions, healthy adults do not develop the more serious B vitamin deficiency diseases from diet alone. The main exceptions are people with alcoholism. The extremely unbalanced diets of some people with alcoholism, in combination with alcohol-induced alteration of vitamin absorption and metabolism, create significant risks for some serious nutrient deficiencies (review Chapter 7).

In the milling of grains, the seeds are crushed and the germ, bran, and husk layers are removed. This process leaves just the starch-containing endosperm, used to make flour, bread, and cereal products. Since the discarded fractions are rich in many nutrients, the time-honored milling process leads to loss of vitamins and minerals. To counteract this nutrient loss, bread and cereal products made from milled grains are enriched with four B vitamins—thiamin, riboflavin, niacin, and folic acid—and with the mineral iron. This fortification helps protect us from the common deficiency diseases associated with a dietary lack of the added nutrients, but still leaves the products with proportionately less vitamin B-6, vitamin E, magnesium, and zinc than in the whole grains. This is one reason why nutrition experts advocate regular consumption of whole-grain products, such as whole-wheat bread, rather than consuming mostly enriched grain products.

Thiamin

Thiamin (formerly called *vitamin B-1*) is used, among other purposes, to release energy from carbohydrate. Its coenzyme participates in reactions in which a carbon dioxide (CO_2) is lost from a larger molecule. This reaction is particularly important in metabolizing glucose, the primary nutrient yielded from carbohydrate digestion (review Fig. 8.7).

The thiamin deficiency disease is called **beriberi,** a word that means "I can't, I can't" in the Sri Lankan language of Sinhalese. The symptoms include weakness, loss of appetite, irritability, nervous tingling throughout the body, poor arm and leg coordination, and deep muscle pain in the calves. A person with beriberi often develops an enlarged heart and sometimes severe edema.

Beriberi is seen in areas where rice is a staple and the polished (white) form is consumed rather than the brown (whole-grain) form. In most parts of the world, brown rice has had its bran and germ layer removed to make white rice, a poor source of thiamin, unless later enriched.

Beriberi results when glucose, the primary fuel for brain and nerve cells, is poorly metabolized. Because the thiamin coenzyme participates in glucose metabolism, body functions associated with brain and nerve action quickly show signs of a thiamin deficiency. Symptoms of depression and weakness can be seen after only 10 days on a thiamin-free diet. Thiamin probably also contributes in other ways to nerve function.

Thiamin in Foods and Needs

Major sources of thiamin include pork products, whole grains (wheat germ), ready-to-eat breakfast cereals, enriched grains, green beans, milk, orange juice, organ meats, peanuts, dried beans, and seeds (Fig. 8.8).

The adult RDA for thiamin is 1.1 to 1.2 milligrams per day. The Daily Value used on food and supplement labels is 1.5 milligrams. Average daily intakes for men exceed this by 50% or more, and women generally meet the RDA. Some groups, such as low-income people and older people, may barely meet their needs for thiamin. A diet

beriberi The thiamin deficiency disorder characterized by muscle weakness, loss of appetite, nerve degeneration, and sometimes edema.

Food Sources of Thiamin

Food item and amount	Thiamin (milligrams)
Brewer's yeast, 2 tablespoons	2.4
Canned lean ham, 3 ounces	0.9
Pork chops, 4 ounces	0.6
Wheat germ, ¼ cup	0.5
Canadian bacon, 2 ounces	0.5
Acorn squash, 1 cup	0.4
Soy milk, 1 cup	0.4
Flour tortilla, 1	0.4
Ham lunch meat, 2 pieces	0.3
Watermelon, 1 slice	0.2
Fresh orange juice, 1 cup	0.2
Cooked green peas, ½ cup	0.2
Baked beans, ½ cup	0.2
Navy beans, ½ cup	0.2
Corn, ½ cup	0.2

Figure 8.8 Food sources of thiamin, riboflavin, and niacin from the Food Guide Pyramid. The meat, poultry, fish, dry beans, eggs, and nuts group and the bread, cereal, rice, and pasta group are especially nutrient-dense sources. Foods from the milk, yogurt, and cheese group are nutrient-dense sources of riboflavin. The background color of each food group indicates the average nutrient density (milligram per kcal) for the nutrients in that group as a whole. For this reason, individual foods are not listed.

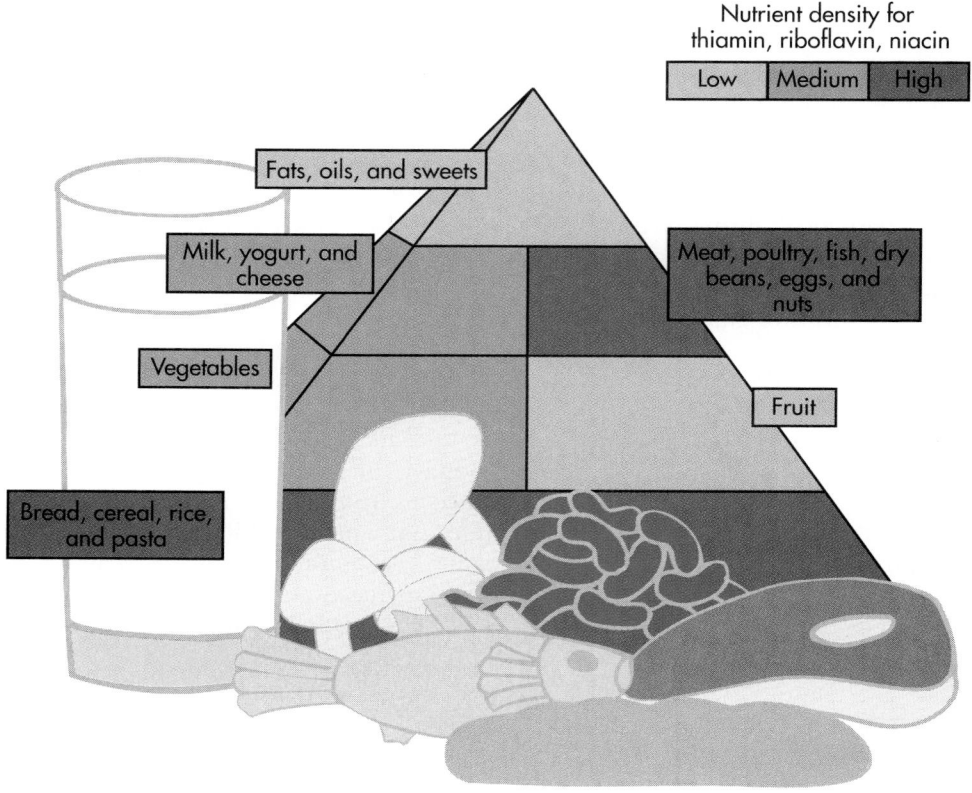

Nutrient density for thiamin, riboflavin, niacin

| Low | Medium | High |

Fats, oils, and sweets

Milk, yogurt, and cheese

Meat, poultry, fish, dry beans, eggs, and nuts

Vegetables

Fruit

Bread, cereal, rice, and pasta

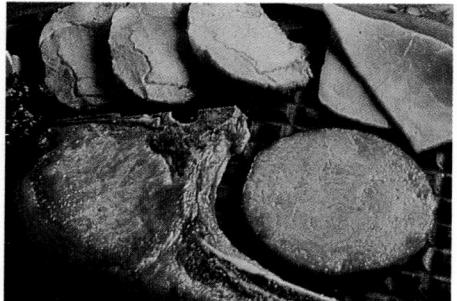

Pork is a nutrient-dense source of thiamin.

dominated by highly processed and unenriched foods, sugar, fat, and alcohol also creates a potential for thiamin deficiency. Oral thiamin supplements are essentially nontoxic since excess thiamin is rapidly lost in the urine. Thus, no Upper Level has been set for thiamin.

Another Bite

*P*eople with alcoholism are at the greatest risk for thiamin deficiency because absorption and use of thiamin are profoundly diminished and excretion is increased by alcohol consumption. Furthermore, the low-quality diet that often accompanies severe alcoholism makes matters worse. Since there is limited thiamin storage in the body, an alcoholic binge lasting 1 to 2 weeks may quickly deplete already diminished amounts of the vitamin and result in deficiency symptoms.

Riboflavin

The name *riboflavin* comes from its yellow color (*flavus* means yellow in Latin). Riboflavin was formerly referred to as *vitamin B-2*.

The coenzymes of riboflavin participate in many energy-yielding metabolic pathways. When cells form cellular energy using oxygen-requiring pathways, such as when fatty acids are broken down and burned for energy, the coenzymes of riboflavin are used (review Fig. 8.7). Some vitamin and mineral metabolism also requires riboflavin. In addition, because of its link to activity of certain enzymes, riboflavin has an antioxidant role in the body.

The symptoms associated with riboflavin deficiency include inflammation of the mouth and tongue, dermatitis, cracking of tissue around the corners of the mouth (called *cheilosis*), various eye disorders, sensitivity to the sun, and confusion (review

Fig. 8.2). The first symptoms of a deficiency are inflammation of the mouth and tongue. All symptoms associated with deficiency develop after approximately 2 months on a riboflavin-poor diet. In addition, riboflavin deficiencies probably do not exist by themselves. Instead, a riboflavin deficiency would occur with deficiencies of niacin, thiamin, and vitamin B-6 because these nutrients often occur in the same foods.

■ Riboflavin in Foods and Needs

Major sources of riboflavin are milk and milk products, enriched grains, ready-to-eat breakfast cereals, meat, and eggs (review Fig. 8.8). Vegetables such as asparagus, broccoli, and various greens (e.g., turnip and collard) are also good sources.

The adult RDA of riboflavin is 1.1 to 1.3 milligrams per day. The Daily Value used on food and supplement labels is 1.7 milligrams. On average, daily intakes of riboflavin are slightly above the RDA. People with alcoholism are those who primarily risk riboflavin deficiency because they generally eat nutrient-poor diets. No specific symptoms indicate that riboflavin taken in megadoses is toxic, so no Upper Level has been set.

Niacin

Niacin is actually composed of a pair of related compounds: nicotinic acid and nicotinamide. Both can function as niacin in the body. Niacin was formerly referred to as *vitamin B-3*.

The coenzyme forms of niacin function in many cellular metabolic pathways. In general, when cell energy is being utilized, a niacin coenzyme is used. Synthetic pathways in the cell—those that make new compounds—also often use a niacin coenzyme. This is especially true for fatty acid synthesis (review Fig. 8.7).

Because almost every cellular metabolic pathway uses a niacin coenzyme, a deficiency causes widespread changes in the body. The entire group of symptoms is known as *pellagra*, which means rough or painful skin. The symptoms of the disease are **dementia,** diarrhea, and dermatitis (especially on areas of skin exposed to the sun) (review Fig. 8.2). Later, death often results. Early symptoms include poor appetite, weight loss, and weakness.

Pellagra became epidemic in southern Europe in the early 1700s when corn, a poor source, became a staple food. It became a major problem in the southeastern United States in the late 1800s and persisted until the late 1930s when standards of living and diets improved. In fact, pellagra is the only dietary deficiency disease ever to reach epidemic proportions in the United States. Today, pellagra is rare in Western societies, but can be seen in the developing world.

> ### Another Bite
>
> Niacin in corn is bound by a protein that hampers its absorption. Soaking corn in an alkaline solution, such as lime water (water with calcium hydroxide), releases bound niacin and renders it more usable. Hispanic people traditionally soak corn in lime water before making tortillas. This treatment is one reason why Hispanic populations never suffered much pellagra.

■ Niacin in Foods and Needs

Major sources of niacin are poultry, ready-to-eat breakfast cereals, beef, wheat bran, tuna and other fish, asparagus, and peanuts (review Fig. 8.8). Coffee and tea also contribute some niacin to the diet. Niacin is very heat stable; little is lost in cooking.

Besides the preformed niacin found in protein foods, every 60 milligrams of the amino acid tryptophan in a food are metabolized into about 1 milligram of niacin. In this manner, we synthesize about 50% of the niacin we need.

Food Sources of Riboflavin

Food item and amount	Riboflavin (milligrams)
Multigrain Cheerios, ¾ cup	1.3
Fried beef liver, 1 ounce	1.2
Steamed oysters, 10	1.1
Plain yogurt, 1 cup	0.5
Brewer's yeast, 2 tablespoons	0.5
Raw mushrooms, 5	0.5
Braunschweiger sausage, 1	0.4
Cooked spinach, 1 cup	0.4
1% milk, 1 cup	0.4
Buttermilk, 1 cup	0.4
Boiled egg, 1	0.3
Sirloin steak, 3 ounces	0.3
Feta cheese, 1 ounce	0.2
Tortilla, 1	0.2
Lean ham, 3 ounces	0.2

dementia A general loss or decrease in mental function.

Food Sources of Niacin

Food item and amount	Niacin (milligrams)
Tuna, 3 ounces	11.3
Roasted chicken, 3 ounces	10.1
Peanuts, ½ cup	9.9
Baked salmon, 3 ounces	8.6
Turkey lunch meat, 3 ounces	5.4
Ground beef, 3 ounces	5.0
Raw mushrooms, 5	4.7
Lean steak, 4 ounces	4.5
Chunky peanut butter, 2 tablespoons	4.4
Fried beef liver, 1 ounce	4.1
Raisin Nut Bran cereal, ¾ cup	3.8
Tortilla, 1	2.6
Baked cod, 3 ounces	2.1
Potato, 1	2.1
Broiled halibut, 3 ounces	1.6

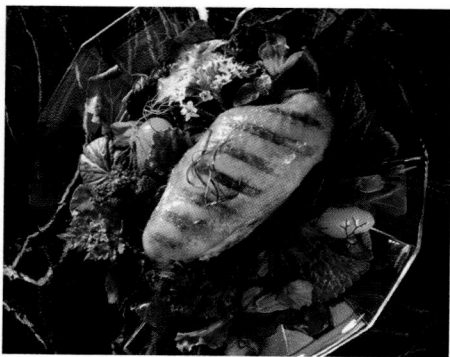

Chicken is a nutrient-dense source of niacin. The tryptophan present can also be metabolized to niacin.

Food Sources of Pantothenic Acid

Food item and amount	Pantothenic acid (milligrams)
Total corn flakes cereal, ¾ cup	11.8
Power bar, 1	10.0
Luna bar, 1	9.9
Sunflower seeds, ¼ cup	2.3
Fried beef liver, 1 ounce	1.7
Raw mushrooms, 5	1.7
Plain yogurt, 1 cup	1.5
Acorn squash, 1 cup	1.2
Peanuts, ½ cup	1.0
1% milk, 1 cup	0.9
Roasted chicken breast, 3 ounces	0.8
Broccoli, 1 cup	0.8
Baked potato, 1	0.7
Legumes, ½ cup	0.7
Cooked egg yolk, 1	0.6

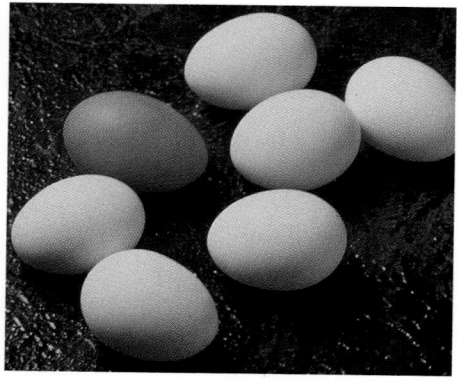

Egg yolks are one of the most nutrient-dense sources of biotin.

The adult RDA of niacin is 14 to 16 milligrams per day. The RDA is expressed as niacin equivalents (NE) to account for niacin received intact from the diet, as well as that made from tryptophan. The Daily Value used on food and supplement labels is 20 milligrams. Intakes of niacin by adults are about double the RDA for men and slightly greater than the RDA for women, without considering the contribution from tryptophan. Note that tables of food values also ignore this contribution. People with alcoholism and those with rare disorders of tryptophan metabolism are generally the only groups to show a niacin deficiency.

Niacin begins to become toxic at intakes of 35 milligrams of the nicotinic acid form. This is the Upper Level for niacin. Effects include headache, itching, and increased blood flow to the skin, causing a general blood vessel dilation or flushing in various parts of the body, especially when intakes are above 100 milligrams per day. In the long run, GI tract and liver damage is possible, so any use of megadoses, such as part of treatment for cardiovascular disease, requires close physician scrutiny (see Chapter 5).

Concept Check

The B vitamins thiamin, niacin, and riboflavin are all important in the metabolism of carbohydrates, proteins, and fats. Energy metabolism in particular requires adequate amounts of coenzymes of these three vitamins. Enriched grains are adequate sources of all three vitamins, as are ready-to-eat breakfast cereals. Otherwise, pork is an excellent source of thiamin, milk is an excellent source of riboflavin, and protein foods in general—such as chicken—are excellent sources of niacin. Deficiencies of all three vitamins can occur with alcoholism; a thiamin deficiency is the most likely.

Pantothenic Acid

Like the other B vitamins, pantothenic acid helps release energy from carbohydrates, fats, and protein. By forming its coenzyme, pantothenic acid allows many energy-yielding metabolic reactions to occur (review Fig. 8.7). This coenzyme makes other molecules much more reactive. In addition, this coenzyme must activate fatty acids before they can yield energy. It is also used in the beginning steps of fatty acid synthesis. Pantothenic acid is so widespread in foods that a nutritional deficiency among healthy people who eat varied diets is unlikely. *Pantothen* actually means "from every side" in Greek.

Pantothenic Acid in Foods and Needs

Rich sources of pantothenic acid are sunflower seeds, mushrooms, peanuts, and eggs. Other sources are meat, milk, and many vegetables.

The Adequate Intake set for pantothenic acid is 5 milligrams per day for adults, and we generally consume that amount or more. The Daily Value used on food and supplement labels is 10 milligrams. A deficiency of pantothenic acid might occur in alcoholism along with a very nutrient-deficient diet. However, the symptoms would probably be hidden among deficiencies of thiamin, riboflavin, vitamin B-6, and folate, so the pantothenic acid deficiency might be unrecognizable. No toxicity is known for pantothenic acid, so no Upper Level has been set.

Biotin

Biotin exists in two active forms in foods. In the ultimate coenzyme form, biotin acts in fat and carbohydrate metabolism.

Biotin assists the addition of carbon dioxide to other compounds. By doing so, it promotes the synthesis of glucose, fatty acids, and DNA, while helping to break down certain amino acids. Symptoms of biotin deficiency include a scaly inflammation of the skin, changes in the tongue and lips, decreased appetite, nausea, vomiting, a form of anemia, depression, muscle pain and weakness, and poor growth.

■ Biotin in Foods and Needs

Cauliflower, egg yolks, peanuts, and cheese are good sources of biotin. Intestinal bacteria synthesize and supply some biotin, making a biotin deficiency unlikely. However, scientists are not sure how much of the bacteria-synthesized biotin in our intestines is actually absorbed. If the intestinal bacteria are not sufficient, as in people who are missing a large part of the small intestine or who take antibiotics for many months, special attention should be paid to meeting biotin needs. A protein called *avidin* in raw egg whites binds biotin and inhibits its absorption. Consuming many raw egg whites eventually leads to the deficiency disease.

The Adequate Intake set for biotin is 30 micrograms per day for adults. Our food supply is thought to provide 40 to 60 micrograms per person per day. The Daily Value used on food and supplement labels is 300 micrograms, 10 times our current estimate of needs. Biotin is relatively nontoxic. Large doses have been given over an extended period without harmful side effects to children who exhibit defects in biotin metabolism. Thus, no Upper Level for biotin has been set.

Vitamin B-6

Vitamin B-6 is actually a family of three compounds. All can be changed to the active vitamin B-6 coenzyme. The general vitamin name is *pyridoxine*.

■ Functions of Vitamin B-6

The coenzymes of vitamin B-6 are needed for the activity of numerous enzymes involved in carbohydrate, protein, and fat metabolism. Because vitamin B-6 is needed in so many areas of metabolism, a deficiency results in widespread symptoms, such as depression, vomiting, skin disorders, irritation of the nerves, and impaired immune response.

A key function of vitamin B-6 concerns protein because metabolizing any amino acid requires the vitamin B-6 coenzyme (review Fig. 8.7). By helping to split the nitrogen group ($-NH_2$) from an amino acid, the coenzyme participates in reactions that allow a cell to synthesize nonessential (dispensable) amino acids.

Another important role of vitamin B-6 is the synthesis of many neurotransmitters. Recall from Chapter 3 that neurotransmitters allow nerve cells to communicate with each other and with other body cells. In the 1950s, infants fed oversterilized commercial formulas developed vitamin B-6 deficiency symptoms, particularly convulsions. Heat destroyed vitamin B-6 in the formulas. Today, manufacturers are more careful to maintain adequate vitamin B-6 content in formulas.

The vitamin B-6 coenzyme is important for the synthesis of hemoglobin and its later function as the oxygen-carrying part of the red blood cell. Vitamin B-6 is also necessary for the synthesis of white blood cells, which perform a major role in the immune system.

Vitamin B-6 participates in various aspects of carbohydrate, fat, and vitamin metabolism. Finally, vitamin B-6 plays a role in the recycling of homocysteine to the amino acid cysteine. This is important since elevated homocysteine in the blood likely increases the risk for cardiovascular disease. The B-vitamins folate and vitamin B-12 and the vitamin-like compound choline also participate in homocysteine metabolism.

■ Vitamin B-6 in Foods and Needs

Major sources of vitamin B-6 are animal products, ready-to-eat breakfast cereals, potatoes, and milk. Other sources are such fruits and vegetables as bananas, cantaloupe,

Food Sources of Biotin

Food item and amount	Biotin (micrograms)
Smooth peanut butter, 2 tablespoons	30.1
Cooked lamb liver, 1 ounce	11.6
Boiled egg, 1	9.3
Cooked egg yolk, 1	8.1
Low-fat yogurt, 1 cup	7.4
Wheat germ, ¼ cup	7.2
Roasted peanuts, 5	6.5
Wheat bran, ¼ cup	6.4
Skim milk, 1 cup	4.9
Salmon, 3 ounces	4.3
Egg noodles, 1 cup	4.0
Swiss cheese, 2 ounces	2.2
Cheddar cheese, 2 ounces	1.7
Raw cauliflower, 1 cup	1.5
American cheese, 2 ounces	1.4

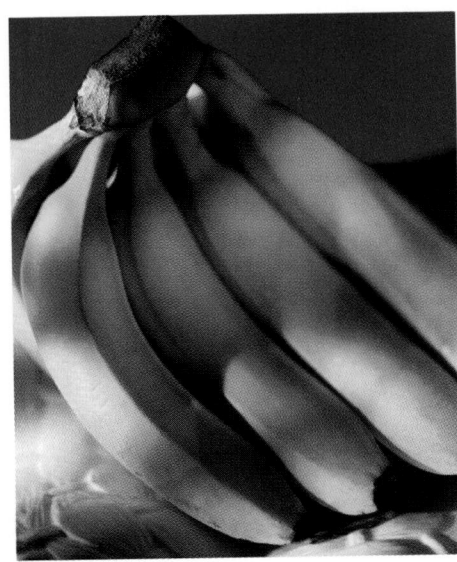

Bananas are a nutrient-dense plant source of vitamin B-6.

Figure 8.9 Food sources of vitamin B-6 from the Food Guide Pyramid. The meat, poultry, fish, dry beans, eggs, and nuts group is an especially nutrient-dense source. The background color of each food group indicates the average nutrient density (milligram per kcal) for vitamin B-6 in that group.

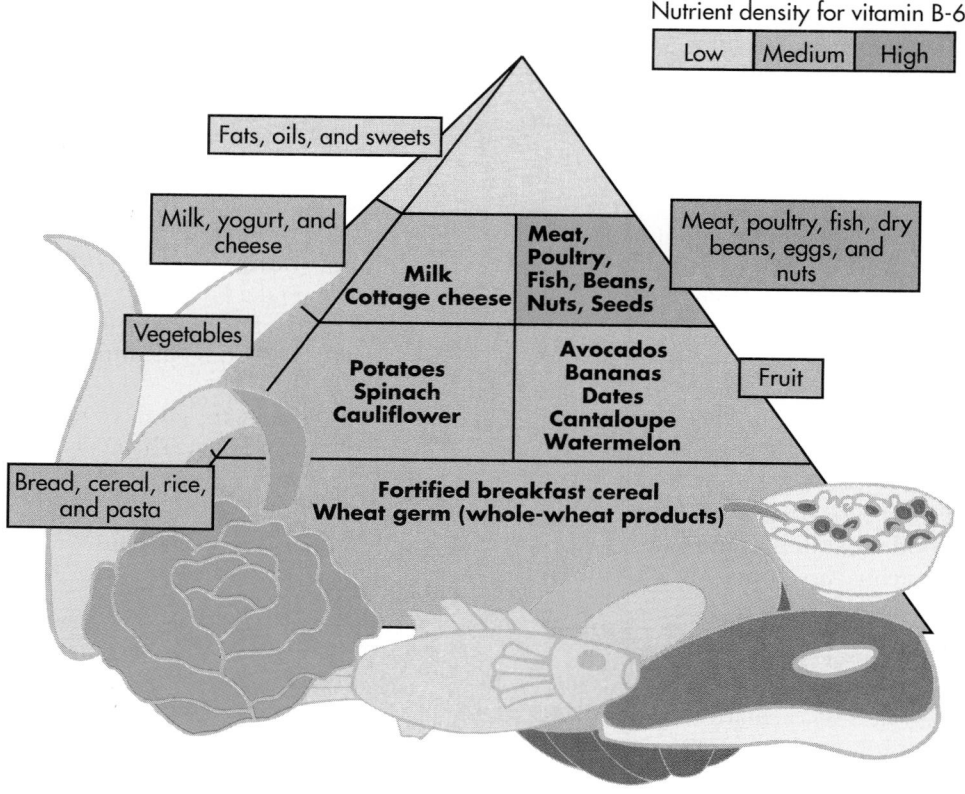

broccoli, and spinach (Fig. 8.9). Overall, animal sources and fortified products are the most reliable because the vitamin B-6 they contain is more absorbable than that in plant foods. Food tables listing vitamin B-6 are often incomplete because measuring this vitamin in foods is difficult.

The adult RDA of vitamin B-6 is 1.3 to 1.7 milligrams per day. The Daily Value used on food and supplement labels is 2 milligrams. Average daily consumption of vitamin B-6 for men and women is somewhat above the RDA.

Athletes may need slightly more vitamin B-6 because of their increased use of glycogen as a fuel (glycogen metabolism requires vitamin B-6), their increased use of amino acids for fuel, and their high protein intakes. Still, the protein foods in their diets should supply any extra vitamin B-6 needed.

People with alcoholism are susceptible to a vitamin B-6 deficiency because a metabolite formed in alcohol metabolism can displace the coenzyme form from enzymes, increasing its tendency to be destroyed. In addition, alcohol decreases the absorption of vitamin B-6 and decreases the synthesis of its coenzyme form. Cirrhosis and hepatitis (both of which may accompany alcoholism) also disable liver tissue from actively metabolizing vitamin B-6, which in turn decreases synthesis of its coenzyme form.

■ Toxicity of Vitamin B-6

The Upper Level for vitamin B-6 is 100 milligrams per day, based on the risk of developing nerve damage. Studies have shown that intakes of 2 to 6 grams of vitamin B-6 per day for 2 or more months especially can lead to irreversible nerve damage. Use, or more appropriately, misuse, of such megadoses of vitamin B-6 has occurred among body builders and in women attempting to treat themselves for **premenstrual syndrome.** Symptoms include walking difficulties and hand and foot numbness. Some nerve damage in individual sensory neurons is probably reversible, but damage to the ganglia (where many nerve fibers converge) is probably permanent. With 500 milligram tablets of vitamin B-6 available in health-food stores, taking a toxic dose is quite easy.

Food Sources of Vitamin B-6

Food item and amount	Vitamin B-6 (milligrams)
Baked salmon, 3 ounces	0.8
Baked potato, 1 medium	0.7
Banana, 1	0.7
Avocado, 1	0.6
Brewer's yeast, 2 tablespoons	0.5
Roasted chicken breast, 3 ounces	0.5
Acorn squash, 1 cup	0.5
Special K cereal, ¾ cup	0.5
Fried beef liver, 1 ounce	0.4
Roasted turkey lunch meat, 3 ounces	0.4
Sirloin steak, 3 ounces	0.4
Lean ham, 3 ounces	0.4
Watermelon, 1 slice	0.3
Sunflower seeds, ¼ cup	0.3
Cooked spinach, ½ cup	0.2

Pantothenic acid and biotin both participate in the metabolism of carbohydrate and fat. A deficiency of either vitamin is unlikely; pantothenic acid is found widely in foods, and our need for biotin is partially met by intestinal synthesis from bacteria. Vitamin B-6 is important for protein metabolism, neurotransmitter synthesis, homocysteine metabolism, and other key metabolic functions. Headache, a form of anemia, nausea, and vomiting can result from a vitamin B-6 deficiency. Increased risk of cardiovascular disease is also likely. Animal protein foods, ready-to-eat breakfast cereals, broccoli, spinach, and bananas are some food sources. Megadose supplements of vitamin B-6 can lead to nerve damage.

Folate

In the past, folate was referred to as *folic acid* and *folacin*. Today the term *folate* is preferred because it encompasses the variety of food forms of the vitamin. Folic acid, however, is the form added to foods and present in supplements.

Functions of Folate

A key role of the folate coenzymes is helping to form DNA. The active coenzymes help in this synthesis by supplying or accepting single carbon compounds. The coenzymes also help metabolize various amino acids and their derivatives, such as homocysteine.

One major result of a folate deficiency is that in the early phases of red blood cell synthesis, the immature cells cannot divide because they cannot form new DNA. The cells grow progressively larger because they can still synthesize enough protein and other cell parts to make new cells. When the time comes for the cells to divide, however, the amount of DNA is insufficient to form two nuclei. The cells then remain in a large immature form, known as a **megaloblast** (review Fig. 8.2).

Because the bone marrow of a folate-deficient person produces mostly immature megaloblast cells, few mature red blood cells (called **erythrocytes**) arrive in the bloodstream. When fewer mature red blood cells are present, the blood's capacity to carry oxygen decreases, causing a form of anemia. In short, a folate deficiency causes megaloblastic anemia (also called **macrocytic anemia**).

The changes in red blood cell formation occur after 7 to 16 weeks on a folate-free diet, depending on the person's folate stores. White blood cell formation is also affected, but to a lesser degree. In addition, cell division throughout the entire body is disrupted. Clinicians focus primarily on red blood cells because they are easy to examine. Other symptoms of folate deficiency are inflammation of the tongue, diarrhea, poor growth, mental confusion, depression, and problems in nerve function.

*F*olate differs from folic acid by containing extra units of the amino acid glutamic acid attached to the structure. These must be removed before absorption, yielding free folic acid. Thus folic acid is more reliably absorbed (1.7 times greater) than that shown for folate.

megaloblast A large, immature red blood cell that results from the particular cell's inability to divide when it normally should.

erythrocytes Mature red blood cells. These have no nucleus and a life span of about 120 days; they contain hemoglobin, which transports oxygen and carbon dioxide.

macrocytic anemia Anemia characterized by the presence of abnormally large red blood cells.

Some forms of cancer therapy provide a vivid example of the effects of a folate deficiency on DNA metabolism. A cancer drug, methotrexate, closely resembles a form of folate but cannot act in its place. Because of this resemblance, when methotrexate is taken in high doses, it hampers folate metabolism. In essence, methotrexate crowds out folate in the metabolic pathways. DNA synthesis and, consequently, cell division, then decreases. Because cancer cells are among the most rapidly dividing cells in the body, they are among those first affected. However, other rapidly dividing cells, such as intestinal cells and skin cells, are also affected. Not surprisingly, typical side effects of methotrexate therapy are diarrhea, vomiting, and hair loss. These are also typical symptoms of folate deficiency.

neural tube defect A defect in the formation of the neural tube occurring during early fetal development. This type of defect results in various nervous system disorders, such as spina bifida. Folate deficiency in the pregnant woman increases the risk that the fetus will develop this disorder.

Food Sources of Folate

Food item and amount	Folate (micrograms)
Asparagus, 1 cup	263
Cooked spinach, 1 cup	262
Cooked lentils, ½ cup	179
Black-eyed peas, ½ cup	179
Romaine lettuce, 1½ cups	114
Great Grains cereal, ¾ cup	114
Tortilla, 1	89
Cooked turnips, ½ cup	85
Cooked broccoli, 1 cup	78
Sunflower seeds, ¼ cup	76
Fresh orange juice, 1 cup	75
Cooked beets, ½ cup	68
Kidney beans, ½ cup	65
Fried beef liver, 1 ounce	62
Brewer's yeast, 1 tablespoon	60

Figure 8.10 Neural tube defects result from a developmental failure affecting the spinal cord or brain in the embryo. Very early in fetal development, a ridge of neural-like tissue forms along the back of the embryo. As the fetus develops, this material develops into both the spinal cord and body nerves at the lower end, and into the brain at the upper end. At the same time, the bones that make up the back gradually surround the spinal cord on all sides. If any part of this sequence goes awry, many defects can appear. The worst is total lack of a brain (anencephaly). Spina bifida, in which the back bones do not form a complete ring to protect the spinal cord, is much more common. Deficient folate status in the mother during the beginning of pregnancy greatly increases the risk of neural tube defects, as does a genetic predisposition.

A maternal deficiency of folate and a genetic predisposition have been linked to development of **neural tube defects** in the fetus (Fig. 8.10). These defects include spina bifida (spinal cord or spinal fluid bulge through the back) and anencephaly (absence of a brain). About 2000 infants are so affected annually in the United States alone. Victims of spina bifida exhibit paralysis, incontinence, learning disabilities, and other health problems. Children born with anencephaly die shortly after birth. Adequate folate nurture is crucial for all women of childbearing years since the neural tube closes within the first 28 days of pregnancy, a time when many women are not even aware that they are pregnant. Hence a recommendation is made that ample folate be consumed at least 6 weeks before conception, specifically 400 micrograms of synthetic folic acid per day. Note that almost all related research has been done with synthetic folic acid supplementation, and it appears that even women with varied diets may not consume adequate synthetic folic acid to prevent neural tube defects unless specific attention to rich sources is given. Perhaps as many as 50% of these defects could be avoided by adequate folate status before conception.

Consuming ready-to-eat breakfast cereals that contain 100% of the Daily Value for folate (this is the same as the RDA) is a good practice for meeting the goal for synthetic folic acid intake. A multivitamin and mineral supplement can also be used to supply adequate synthetic folic acid, but women should be careful to monitor the amount of any accompanying preformed vitamin A content.

Research is currently underway in the link between folate and cancer protection. Because folate aids in DNA synthesis, it is hypothesized that even mild folate deficiency contributes to abnormal DNA integrity, which in turn affects certain cancer-protecting genes. Meeting the RDA for folate is thought to be one way to reduce cancer risk.

A final function of folate is the formation of neurotransmitters in the brain. Meeting folate needs can improve the depressed state in some cases of mental illness.

■ Folate in Foods and Needs

Green, leafy vegetables (*folate* is derived from the Latin word *folium*, which means *foliage*), organ meats, sprouts, other vegetables, dried beans, and orange juice are the most rich sources of folate (Fig. 8.11). The vitamin C in orange juice also reduces folate destruction. Ready-to-eat breakfast cereals, milk, and bread also are important sources of folate for many adults.

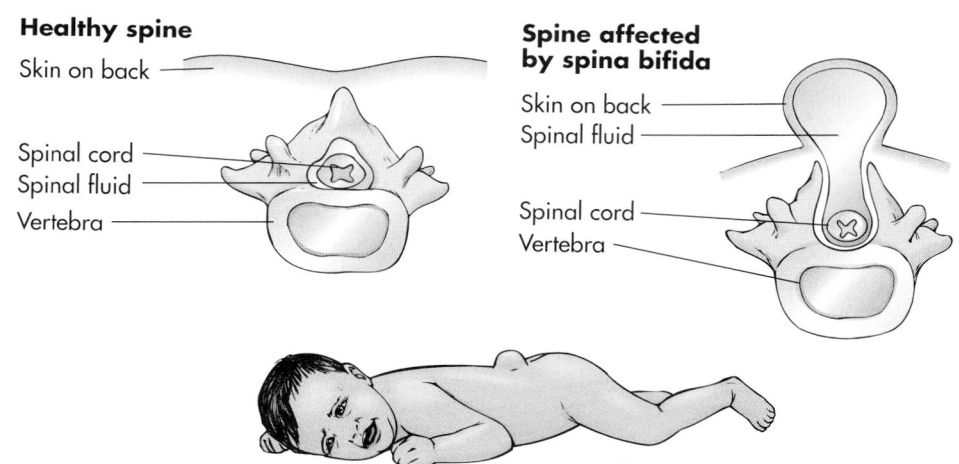

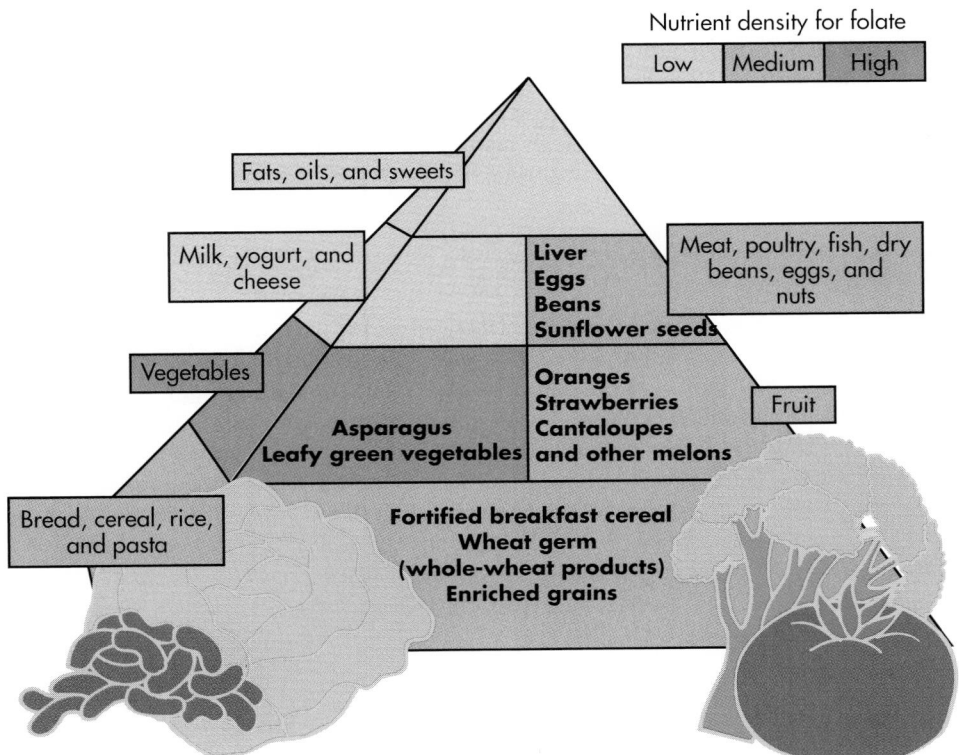

Nutrient density for folate

| Low | Medium | High |

Fats, oils, and sweets

Milk, yogurt, and cheese

Liver
Eggs
Beans
Sunflower seeds

Meat, poultry, fish, dry beans, eggs, and nuts

Vegetables

Oranges
Strawberries
Cantaloupes
and other melons

Asparagus
Leafy green vegetables

Fruit

Bread, cereal, rice, and pasta

Fortified breakfast cereal
Wheat germ
(whole-wheat products)
Enriched grains

Figure 8.11 Food sources of folate from the Food Guide Pyramid. The vegetable group is an especially nutrient-dense source. The background color of each food group indicates the average nutrient density (microgram per kcal) for folate in that group.

Food processing and preparation destroy 50% to 90% of the folate in food. Folate is very susceptible to destruction by heat. This underscores the importance of regularly eating fresh fruits and raw or lightly cooked vegetables. As mentioned before, vegetables retain their nutrients best when cooked quickly in minimal water—steaming, stir-frying, or microwaving (review Table 8.1).

The RDA of folate for adults is 400 micrograms per day, as is the Daily Value used on food and supplement labels. Folate recommendations for all but women of child-bearing years are based on dietary folate equivalents (DFE). (As just covered, those women should meet such recommendations with synthetic folic acid.) To compute folate intake in DFE units, one has to determine how much of a day's food intake comes from food folate and how much comes from synthetic folic acid added to foods. When in doubt, assume all folate in a diet is in the food form, except that coming from ready-to-eat breakfast cereals and refined grain products. Also include in this second category any folic acid consumed as part of supplements. To calculate the DFE, multiply total synthetic folic acid intake by 1.7, and add that value to the food folate consumed. For example, if a person consumed 300 micrograms as food folate and 200 micrograms from a ready-to-eat breakfast cereal, total folate DFE would be 640 micrograms ([200 × 1.7] + 300 = 600). Compared to the RDA of 400 micrograms, one's intake would be sufficient.

Average daily folate intake in the United States is approximately 320 micrograms for men and 220 micrograms for women. With the recent mandate for fortification of grain products with synthetic folic acid, these average intakes should increase by about 100 micrograms per day. Still, women in general should pay more attention to meeting folate needs. Recent studies have shown a decrease in neural tube defects in infants and blood homocysteine in adults in the United States since this fortification was enacted.

Folate deficiencies sometimes appear in pregnant women. They need extra folate (600 micrograms DFE per day) to meet an increased rate of cell division and, thus, of DNA synthesis in their own bodies and that of the developing fetus. Today, prenatal care often includes a multivitamin and mineral supplement enriched with synthetic

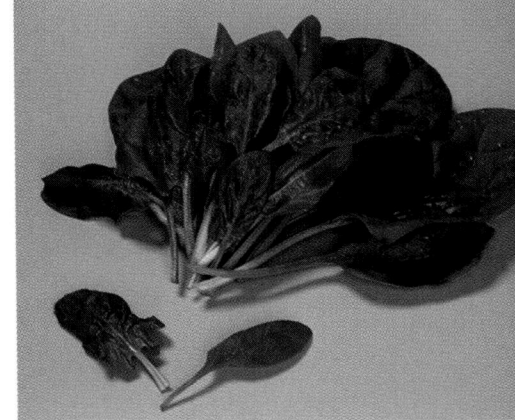

Spinach is a nutrient-dense source of folate.

Critical Thinking

Gary has alcoholism and pays no attention to his diet. In addition to the detrimental effects on the liver, excess alcohol consumption can cause deficiencies in certain B vitamins. Explain why this can occur.

folic acid to help compensate for the extra needs associated with pregnancy. Older people are also at risk for folate deficiency, probably because of inadequate folate intake and absorption. Perhaps these people failed to consume sufficient amounts of fruits and vegetables because of poverty or physical problems, such as poor dental health. In addition, folate deficiencies also often occur with alcoholism, due mostly to poor intake and absorption. Symptoms of a folate-related anemia can alert a physician to the possibility of alcoholism.

Another Bite

The use of dietary folate equivalents (DFEs) instead of the actual amount of folate in a food has some important implications. Typically, many foods will be richer in folate than the Nutrition Facts label suggests since folate content is due primarily to synthetic folic acid added to the foods, such as in enriched grains and ready-to-eat breakfast cereals. This contributes substantially to the DFE calculation. Another implication is that food composition tables (such as the one in the back of this book) and nutrition analysis software programs (such as that supplied with this book) also underestimate the true folate contribution of a diet compared to folate needs because these have not been updated to DFE units.

■ Toxicity of Folate

Large doses of folate complicate the diagnosis of vitamin B-12 deficiency. Regular consumption of large amounts of folate can prevent the appearance of the primary early warning sign of vitamin B-12 deficiency—enlarged red blood cell size. To prevent such masking of vitamin B-12 deficiency, it is the goal of FDA, through its recent enactment of folate fortification of grains, to increase the folate status of women of childbearing years without producing excessive intake by other groups (over 1 milligram of synthetic folic acid per day). This 1 milligram quantity is the Upper Level set for synthetic folic acid. Also, for this reason, FDA limits supplements for nonpregnant adults and food fortification to 400 microgram amounts. Note that the Upper Level does not apply to folate naturally present in foods since absorption is limited.

Vitamin B-12

Vitamin B-12 represents a family of compounds that contain the mineral cobalt. All vitamin B-12 compounds are synthesized by bacteria, fungi, and other lower organisms.

The body's complex means of absorbing vitamin B-12 is unique to this vitamin. Vitamin B-12 in food enters the stomach and is released from other materials by digestion, especially by stomach acid. The free vitamin B-12 binds with a substance produced by the salivary glands in the mouth and then later with **intrinsic factor** produced in the stomach. The resulting intrinsic factor/vitamin B-12 complex travels to the last portion of the small intestine for absorption. Utilizing this system, approximately 50% of dietary vitamin B-12 is absorbed, depending on the body's need for it. Any failure in this system results in only 1% to 2% absorption of dietary vitamin B-12.

intrinsic factor A protein-like compound produced by the stomach that enhances vitamin B-12 absorption.

If a defect in absorption develops, the person usually takes monthly injections of vitamin B-12 to bypass the need for absorption, uses vitamin B-12 nasal gels, or takes megadoses of a supplemental form (300 times the RDA). In this latter case, the vitamin B-12 absorption defect is overcome by providing enough of the vitamin via simple diffusion across the intestinal tract.

About 95% of all cases of vitamin B-12 deficiencies in healthy people result from defective vitamin B-12 absorption, rather than from inadequate intakes. This is especially true for older people. As we age, our stomachs lose their ability to synthesize the intrinsic factor needed for vitamin B-12 absorption.

■ Functions of Vitamin B-12

Vitamin B-12 participates in a variety of cellular processes. The most important function is in folate metabolism. Vitamin B-12 is required to convert folate coenzymes to the active forms needed for metabolic reactions, such as DNA synthesis. Without vitamin B-12, reactions that require certain active forms of folate do not take place in the cell. Thus, a vitamin B-12 deficiency contributes to a folate deficiency. Another vital function of vitamin B-12 is maintaining the myelin sheaths that insulate neurons from each other. People with vitamin B-12 deficiencies show patchy destruction of the myelin sheaths. This destruction eventually causes paralysis and, perhaps, death. Vitamin B-12 also participates in homocysteine metabolism and certain minor metabolic pathways.

In the past, the inability to absorb enough vitamin B-12 eventually led to death. Researchers in mid-nineteenth century England noted a form of anemia that caused death within 2 to 5 years of the initial illness, mainly because it destroyed the nerves. They called it **pernicious anemia** (*pernicious* literally means "leading to death"). Clinically the anemia looks much like a folate-deficiency anemia as many megaloblasts appear in the bloodstream. The vitamin B-12 anemia is typically called *macrocytic anemia*.

Besides the anemia, symptoms of pernicious anemia include weakness, sore tongue, back pain, apathy, and tingling in the extremities. Symptoms of nerve destruction generally develop after about 3 years from the onset of the disease. Unfortunately, significant nerve destruction often occurs before the anemia is seen, and this destruction is irreversible. Pernicious anemia and its accompanying nerve destruction generally start after middle age, affecting up to 10% to 20% of older adults. Both reduced liberation of vitamin B-12 from food due to a fall in stomach acid output and reduced absorption from a fall in intrinsic factor output with aging are to blame.

Infants who are breastfed by vegetarian or vegan mothers are at risk for vitamin B-12 deficiency accompanied by anemia and long-term nervous system problems, such as diminished brain growth, degeneration of the spinal cord, and poor intellectual development. The problems may have their origins during pregnancy, when the mother is deficient in vitamin B-12. Vegan diets supply little vitamin B-12 unless they include vitamin B-12–enriched food or supplements.

■ Vitamin B-12 in Foods and Needs

Major sources of vitamin B-12 include meat, milk, ready-to-eat breakfast cereals, poultry, seafood, and eggs. Organ meats (especially liver, kidneys, and heart) are especially rich sources of vitamin B-12. Adults over age 50 are encouraged to seek a synthetic vitamin B-12 source to aid absorption, which can be limited due to reduced intrinsic factor and stomach acid output seen in aging, as just mentioned. Synthetic vitamin B-12 is not food bound, so it doesn't need stomach acid to aid in liberation from foodstuffs. Thus, it will be more readily absorbed than the food form. Ready-to-eat breakfast cereals and multivitamin and mineral supplements are two possible synthetic sources.

The RDA of vitamin B-12 for adults is 2.4 micrograms per day. The Daily Value used on food and supplement labels is 6 micrograms. On average, men consume 3 times the RDA and women consume 2 times the RDA. This high intake provides the average meat-eating person with 2 to 3 years' storage of vitamin B-12 in the liver.

It takes approximately 20 years of consuming a diet essentially free of vitamin B-12 for a person to exhibit nerve destruction caused by a diet deficiency. Still, vegans, who eat no animal products, should find a reliable source of vitamin B-12. As noted earlier, older persons are at significant risk for developing pernicious anemia. This develops after a few years of the loss of vitamin B-12 absorption capacity. The quicker appearance is because of the reduced ability to reuse vitamin B-12 that is excreted into the GI tract during digestion, coupled with reduced absorption of dietary sources. Regular physical examinations should test for pernicious anemia. Vitamin B-12 supplements are essentially nontoxic, so no Upper Level has been set.

pernicious anemia The anemia that results from a lack of vitamin B-12 absorption; it is pernicious because of associated nerve degeneration that can result in eventual paralysis.

Food Sources of Vitamin B-12

Food item and amount	Vitamin B-12 (micrograms)
Fried beef liver, 1 ounce	31.7
Baked clams, 1 ounce	15.7
Boiled oysters, 2	14.4
Brewer's yeast, 2 tablespoons	3.0
Lobster, 3 ounces	2.7
Pot roast, 3 ounces	2.5
Plain yogurt, 1 cup	1.4
Corn Flakes cereal, ¾ cup	1.1
Shrimp, 3 ounces	1.0
1% milk, 1 cup	0.9
Soy milk, 1 cup	0.8
Boiled egg, 1	0.6
Lean ham, 3 ounces	0.6
Beef hot dog, 1	0.5
Ham lunch meat, 2 ounces	0.4

*P*eople with HIV/AIDS also are at risk of vitamin B-12 deficiency, linked to long-standing malabsorption that they often experience. Adequate vitamin B-12 status has been shown in a few studies to lessen the decline in health experienced by those with HIV/AIDS.

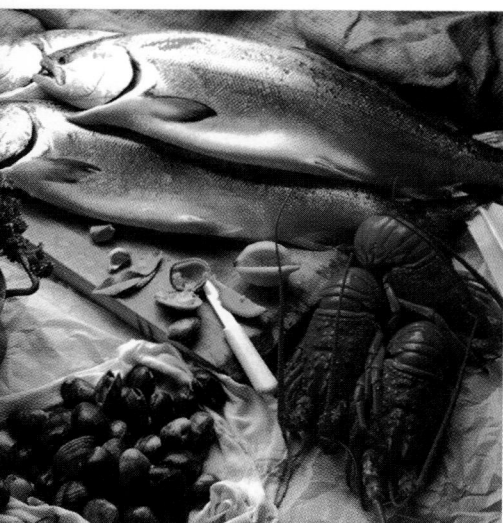

Fish, seafood, and related products are nutrient-dense sources of vitamin B-12.

Concept Check

*F*olate is needed for cell division because it influences DNA synthesis. A folate deficiency results in megaloblastic (macrocytic) anemia, as well as elevated blood homocysteine, inflammation of the tongue, diarrhea, and poor growth. Excess folate intake can mask a vitamin B-12 deficiency since these vitamins work together in metabolism. Folate is found in fruits and vegetables, beans, and organ meats. Emphasizing fresh and lightly cooked vegetables is important because much folate is lost during cooking. Women in their childbearing years should meet needs using a source of synthetic folic acid. Folate needs during pregnancy are especially high; deficiency may lead to neural tube defects in the fetus.

Vitamin B-12 is necessary for folate metabolism. Without dietary vitamin B-12, folate deficiency symptoms, such as macrocytic anemia, develop. In addition, vitamin B-12 is necessary for maintaining the nervous system. Paralysis can develop from a vitamin B-12 deficiency. The absorption of vitamin B-12 requires a number of specific factors. If absorption is inhibited, the resulting deficiency can lead to pernicious anemia and its associated nerve destruction. Concentrated amounts of vitamin B-12 are found only in animal foods; meat eaters generally have a 2- to 3-year supply stored in the liver. Vitamin B-12 absorption may decline as we age. Monthly injections, nasal gels, or megadoses can make up for this. Vitamin B-12 also participates with vitamin B-6 and folate in homocysteine metabolism.

Vitamin C

Scurvy, the vitamin C deficiency disease, was long ago a constant threat to the health of sailors. Its symptoms include weakness, opening of previously healed wounds, slower wound healing, bone pain, fractures, bleeding gums, diarrhea, and pinpoint hemorrhages around hair follicles on the back of the arms and legs. On long sea voyages, captains often lost half or more of their crews to scurvy. In 1740, the Englishman Dr. James Lind first showed that citrus fruits—two oranges and one lemon a day—could cure scurvy. Fifty years after Lind's discovery, rations for British sailors included limes to prevent scurvy.

Vitamin C (ascorbic acid) is a puzzling vitamin. It is found in all living tissues, and most animals synthesize their own from the simple sugar glucose. What is strange is that animals who synthesize vitamin C often make quite a lot of it. For instance, a pig produces 8 grams per day (though we do not benefit from it when we eat pork because it is lost in processing). This amount is over 80 times our human RDA of 75 to 90 milligrams. Why some animals make so much vitamin C, whereas other animals, including humans, appear to need so little has fueled much controversy.

Vitamin C is absorbed in the small intestine. About 70% to 90% of vitamin C is absorbed when a person eats between 30 and 180 milligrams of it per day. If someone ingests 1 gram (1000 milligrams) per day, absorption efficiency drops to about 50%. A common side effect of megadose vitamin C use is diarrhea. The unabsorbed vitamin C stays in the small intestine and attracts water, finally causing diarrhea (see the section on toxicity of vitamin C).

Functions of Vitamin C

The best understood function of vitamin C is its role in synthesizing the protein collagen. This protein is highly concentrated in connective tissue, bone, teeth, tendons, and blood vessels. It is very important for wound healing. Vitamin C increases the cross-connections between amino acids in collagen, greatly strengthening the tissues it helps form.

A vitamin C deficiency can cause widespread changes in tissue metabolism. Most symptoms of scurvy are linked to a decrease in collagen synthesis, such as in the skin. About 20 to 40 days with no vitamin C intake are required for the first symptoms of scurvy to appear (review Fig. 8.2).

Vitamin C is one of the cell's water-soluble antioxidants. Recall that vitamin E is a fat-soluble antioxidant for the cell membrane. The antioxidant capabilities of vitamin C can reduce the formation of cancer-causing nitrosamines in the stomach and also keep the folate coenzymes intact, preventing their destruction. Vitamin C and vitamin E work together as free-radical scavengers. Vitamin C also may aid in reactivating oxidized vitamin E so that it can be reused. Population studies suggest that vitamin C is effective in helping prevent certain cancers (such as esophageal, oral, and stomach cancers), cardiovascular disease, and cataracts in the eye, probably because of its antioxidant capabilities.

Vitamin C enhances iron absorption by keeping iron in its most absorbable form. The iron in the small intestine's alkaline environment is much more usable than other forms of iron. Thus, iron absorption is modestly enhanced, especially with an intake of 75 milligrams or more at a meal. Increasing intake of vitamin C–rich foods is beneficial for those people with poor iron stores.

Vitamin C is vital for the function of the immune system, especially for the activity of certain cells in the immune system. Thus, disease states can increase the need for vitamin C, although we don't know what amount above the RDA is needed (if any). Partly on the basis of this observation, Dr. Linus Pauling gained great notoriety by claiming that vitamin C could combat the common cold. He claimed that 1000 milligrams (1 gram) or more of vitamin C daily could reduce the number of colds for most people by nearly half. As a result of the popularity of his books and the respectability of his scientific credentials, millions of North Americans supplement their diets with vitamin C.

But does vitamin C reliably and effectively work against colds and other infections? Most medical and nutrition scientists disagree with Pauling's views of vitamin C. Numerous well-designed, double-blind studies have not shown megadoses of vitamin C to reliably prevent colds, though it seems to reduce duration of symptoms by a day or so.

Most vitamin C consumed in large doses ends up in the feces or the urine. Only a small fraction of such large doses can be used. The body is saturated at intakes of about 200 milligrams per day. This means that if more than 200 milligrams of vitamin C is ingested, it is quickly excreted. Finally, vitamin C is also necessary for the synthesis of a number of hormones, neurotransmitters, and other compounds, such as bile acids and DNA.

◾ Vitamin C in Foods and Needs

Major sources of vitamin C are green peppers, cauliflower, broccoli, cabbage, strawberries, papayas, and romaine lettuce. Citrus fruits, potatoes, ready-to-eat breakfast cereals, and fortified fruit drinks are also good sources of vitamin C (Fig. 8.12). The 5 to 9 servings of fruits and vegetables from the Food Guide Pyramid can easily provide enough vitamin C. Vitamin C is easily lost in processing and cooking as it is very unstable in contact with heat, iron, copper, or oxygen.

The adult RDA of vitamin C is 75 to 90 milligrams per day. The Daily Value used on food and supplement labels is 60 milligrams. Cigarette smokers need to add an extra 35 milligrams per day to the RDA because of the great stress on their lungs from oxygen and toxic by-products of cigarette smoke. Nearly all North Americans likely meet their daily needs for vitamin C. We consume an average 70 to 100 milligrams per day. Respected nutrition experts who advocate increased use of vitamin C often recommend intakes of about 200 milligrams per day. Still, this amount can be obtained by sufficient fruit and vegetable intake. Today, vitamin C deficiency appears mostly in alcoholic people who eat nutrient-poor diets and in some older persons who also eat poorly.

Critical Thinking

Carlos just returned from a local mall and is excited because he saw an advertisement claiming that vitamin C will cure just about everything, from colds to heart disease. How would you explain to him vitamin C's main functions in the human body?

Food Sources of Vitamin C

Food item and amount	Vitamin C (milligrams)
Orange, 1	98
Cooked brussels sprouts, 1 cup	97
Strawberries, 1 cup	94
Grapefruit juice, 1 cup	80
Red peppers, ¼ cup	71
Kiwi fruit, 1	57
Green pepper rings, 5	45
Tomato juice, 1 cup	45
Cooked broccoli, ½ cup	33
Kale, ½ cup	27
Raw cauliflower, ½ cup	23
Sweet potato, 1	17
Baked potato, 1 medium	16
Pineapple chunks, ½ cup	12
Cooked spinach, ½ cup	9

Figure 8.12 Food sources of vitamin C from the Food Guide Pyramid. The fruit group and the vegetable group are especially nutrient-dense sources. The background color of each food group indicates the average nutrient density (milligram per kcal) for vitamin C in that group.

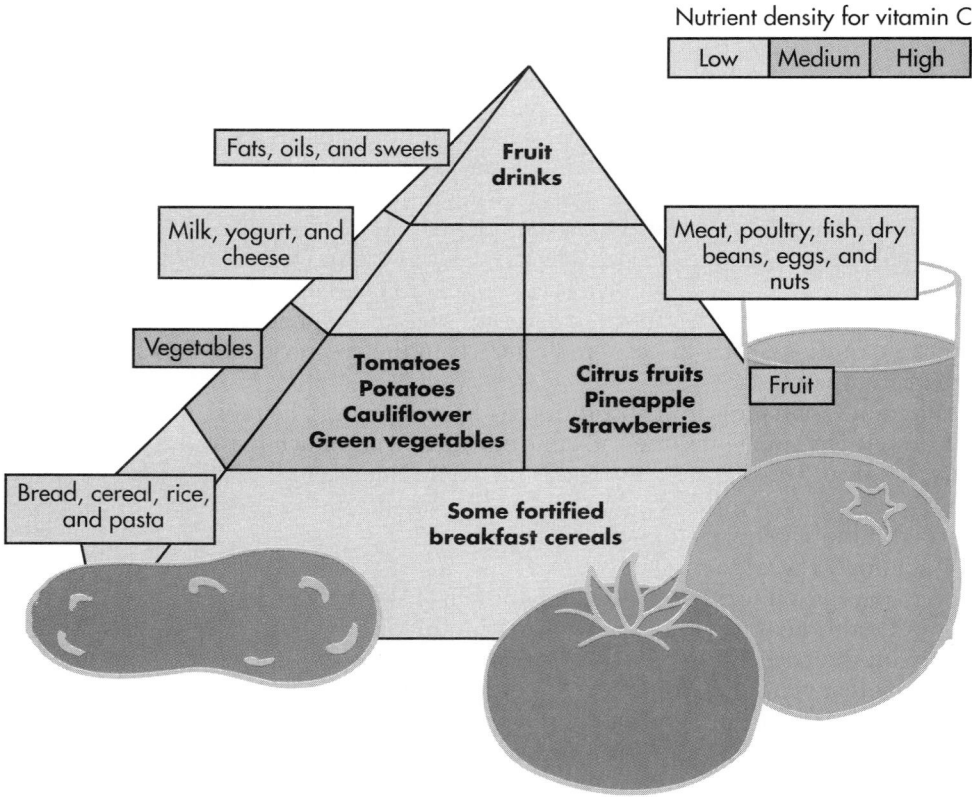

Nutrient density for vitamin C

| Low | Medium | High |

Fats, oils, and sweets

Fruit drinks

Milk, yogurt, and cheese

Meat, poultry, fish, dry beans, eggs, and nuts

Vegetables

Tomatoes Potatoes Cauliflower Green vegetables

Citrus fruits Pineapple Strawberries

Fruit

Bread, cereal, rice, and pasta

Some fortified breakfast cereals

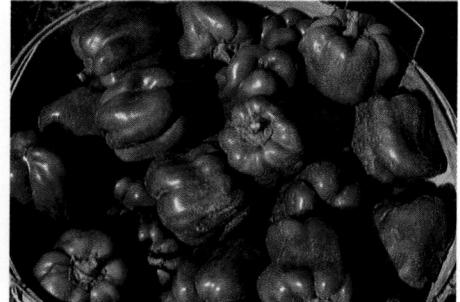

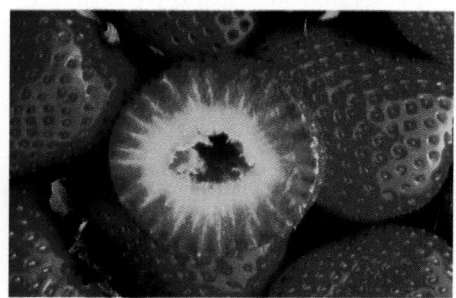

Vegetables such as green peppers are one nutrient-dense source of vitamin C, as are fruits such as strawberries.

■ Toxicity of Vitamin C

Vitamin C is probably not toxic when consumed in amounts less than about 2 grams per day. This is the Upper Level for vitamin C. Regularly consuming more than that may cause stomach inflammation and diarrhea.

Now that you have studied the vitamins, review the Food Guide Pyramid and note how each group makes an important vitamin contribution (Fig. 8.13).

Another Bite

*I*f people want to experiment with large doses of vitamin C, they should alert their physician, primarily because high doses of vitamin C can change reactions to medical tests for diabetes or blood in the feces. Physicians may misdiagnose conditions when large doses of vitamin C are consumed without their knowledge.

Concept Check

*V*itamin C is important in the synthesis of collagen, a major connective tissue protein. A vitamin C deficiency, known as scurvy, causes many changes in the skin and gums, such as small hemorrhages. This is mainly because of poor collagen synthesis. Vitamin C also modestly improves iron absorption, is involved in synthesizing certain hormones and neurotransmitters, and acts as a general body antioxidant. Citrus fruits, green peppers, cauliflower, broccoli, strawberries, and ready-to-eat breakfast cereals are good sources of vitamin C. As with folate, eating fresh or lightly cooked foods is important because vitamin C loses a lot of its potency in cooking. High doses of vitamin C can lead to diarrhea and foil various medical tests. These high doses do not prevent the common cold.

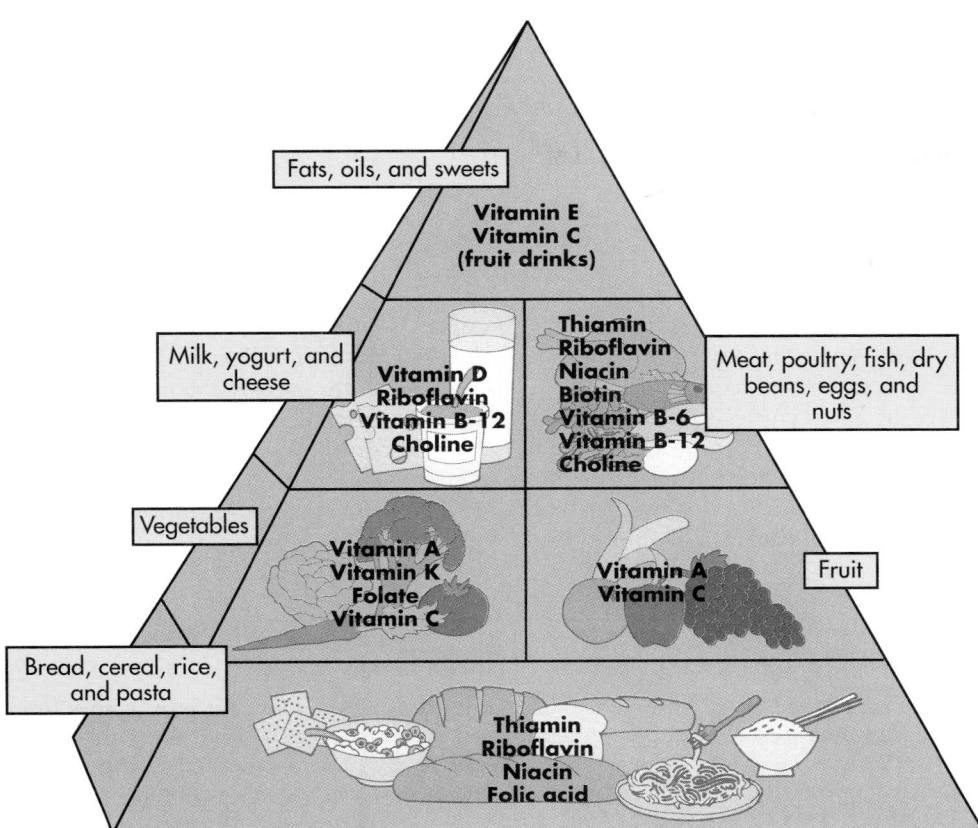

Figure 8.13 Certain groups of the Food Guide Pyramid are especially rich sources of various vitamins and choline. This is true for those listed. Each may be also found in other groups but in lower amounts. Pantothenic acid is also present in moderate amounts in many groups.

Choline

The dietary component choline is the latest addition to the list of essential nutrients. Choline is part of acetylcholine, a neurotransmitter associated with attention, learning and memory, muscle control, and many other functions. It is also part of phospholipids, such as lecithins, the major component of the cell membrane. Finally, choline participates in some aspects of homocysteine metabolism.

There has been only one published study examining the effect of inadequate dietary intake of choline in healthy humans. The study of male volunteers showed decreased choline stores and liver damage when humans were fed choline-deficient total parental nutrition solutions. Based on this one study, plus laboratory animal studies, choline has been deemed essential, but is not yet classified as a vitamin.

■ Choline in Foods and Needs

Choline is widely distributed in foods. Milk, liver, eggs, and peanuts are rich sources. Lecithins often are added to food during processing, so this is yet another source. There is so much choline available in ordinary foods that it is unlikely that a dietary deficiency exists. Choline also can be synthesized from the nonessential (dispensable) amino acid serine.

The Adequate Intake for choline for adults is 425 to 550 milligrams per day. Currently we don't know if a dietary supply is needed at all life stages. Although Adequate Intakes are set for choline, it may be that the choline requirement can be met by body synthesis at some or all stages of life. We consume ample choline from food, at least 700 to 1000 milligrams per day. The Upper Level for adults is 3.5 grams per day, based on development of a fishy body odor and low blood pressure.

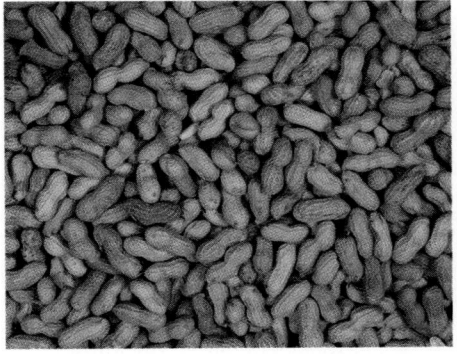

Nuts, such as peanuts, are a nutrient-dense source of choline. Body cells also produce choline.

A list of sources and amounts is not provided for choline, as current nutrient databases do not include these values.

Vitamin-Like Compounds

A variety of vitamin-like compounds are found in the body. These include the following:

- **Carnitine**
- Inositol
- Taurine
- Lipoic acid

All of these vitamin-like compounds are necessary to maintain proper metabolism in the body. They can be synthesized by cells using common building blocks, such as amino acids and glucose. Our diets are also a source. In disease states or periods of active growth, synthesis of vitamin-like compounds may not meet needs, so dietary intake can be crucial. The needs for vitamin-like compounds in certain groups of individuals, such as for premature infants, are being investigated. Although promoted and sold by health-food stores, these vitamin-like compounds need not be included in the diet of the average healthy adult.

Summary

1. Vitamins are carbon-containing compounds we generally need daily in small amounts from foods. They yield no energy directly, but many contribute to energy-yielding chemical reactions in the body and promote growth and development. Many vitamins act as coenzymes, which help enzymes function. Vitamins A, D, E, and K are fat soluble, whereas the B vitamins and vitamin C are water soluble.

2. Vitamin A consists of a family of compounds that includes several forms of preformed vitamin A. Some carotenoids function as antioxidants and three forms can also yield vitamin A. Vitamin A contributes to vision, immune function, and cell development. Vitamin A is found in liver and fish oils; carotenoids are especially plentiful in dark green and orange vegetables. Vitamin A can be quite toxic, even when taken at just 3 times the RDA for preformed vitamin A (the Upper Level). High vitamin A intakes are especially dangerous during pregnancy.

3. Vitamin D is both a hormone and a vitamin. Human skin synthesizes it using sunshine and a cholesterol-like substance. If we don't spend enough time in the sun, such foods as fish and fortified milk can supply the vitamin. The active hormone form of vitamin D helps regulate blood calcium in part by increasing calcium absorption from the intestine. Infants and children who don't get enough vitamin D may develop rickets, and adults with inadequate amounts in the body develop osteomalacia. Older people often need a supplemental source. Vitamin D is a very toxic substance. An intake just 5 times young adult needs (the Upper Level) can cause problems, especially in childhood.

4. Vitamin E functions primarily as an antioxidant and is found in plant oils. By donating electrons to electron-seeking, free-radical (oxidizing) compounds, it neutralizes them. This effect shields cell membranes and red blood cells from breakdown. Claims are made about the curative powers of vitamin E, but more information is needed before megadose vitamin E recommendations for healthy adults can be made with certainty. The Upper Level is set at about 50 times adult needs.

5. Vitamin K helps blood clot and increases the calcium-binding potential of some organs. Some vitamin K absorbed each day comes from bacterial synthesis in the intestine, but most comes from foods, primarily green, leafy vegetables. Vitamin K is poorly stored in the body, but our dietary intake alone is usually sufficient. People who can't absorb fat well or who are on antibiotics for long periods may need extra vitamin K. No Upper Level has been set.

6. Thiamin, riboflavin, and niacin play key roles as coenzymes in energy-yielding reactions. They help metabolize carbohydrates, fats, and proteins. Alcoholism and a poor diet can create deficiencies of these three nutrients. Enriched grain products are common sources of all three of these vitamins. Only niacin has an Upper Level (2.5 times adult needs).

7. Pantothenic acid, which participates in many aspects of cell metabolism, is widely distributed among foods. Biotin, which participates in glucose production, fatty acid synthesis, and DNA synthesis, can be synthesized by bacteria in the intestine. Biotin comes from foods such as eggs, peanuts, and cheese. No Upper Levels have been set for either vitamin.

8. Vitamin B-6 performs a vital role in protein metabolism, especially in synthesizing nonessential amino acids. It also helps synthesize neurotransmitters and performs other metabolic roles, such as metabolism of homocysteine. Headaches, a form of anemia, nausea, and vomiting result from a B-6 deficiency. Increased risk of cardiovascular disease is also possible, especially when coupled with inadequate folate or vitamin B-12 intake or both. Generally, women are more likely to have poor vitamin B-6 stores than men. Regular consumption of animal protein foods, and rich plant sources such as broccoli provides needed vitamin B-6. Taking high doses causes malfunction of the nervous system. The Upper Level is about 60 times adult needs.

9. Folate plays an important role in DNA synthesis and homocysteine metabolism. Symptoms of a deficiency include generally poor cell division in various areas of the body, megaloblastic anemia, tongue inflammation, diarrhea, and poor growth. Pregnancy puts high demands for folate on the body; deficiency can result in neural tube defects in offspring. A deficiency can also occur in people with alcoholism. Food sources are leafy vegetables, organ meats, and orange juice. Women in childbearing years need to

meet the RDA with synthetic folic acid. Great amounts of folate can be lost in prolonged cooking. Excess folate in the diet can mask a vitamin B-12 deficiency, so an Upper Level has been set at 2½ times adult needs (refers to synthetic folic acid only).

10. Vitamin B-12 is needed to metabolize folate (and, so, in addition homocysteine) and maintain the insulation surrounding nerves. A deficiency results in anemia (because of its relationship to folate) and nerve degeneration. Older people often absorb vitamin B-12 inefficiently. If so, they can benefit from monthly injections or megadoses of the vitamin. Generally a dietary deficiency is unlikely because vitamin B-12 is highly concentrated in animal foods, which constitute a major part of the North American diet. Vitamin B-12 does not occur naturally in plant foods. Vegans need a supplemental source, and adults over age 50 should consume a synthetic source, such as that in ready-to-eat breakfast cereals. No Upper Level has been set.

11. Vitamin C is mainly used to synthesize collagen, a major protein for building connective tissue. A vitamin C deficiency results in scurvy, which is evidenced by poor wound healing, pinpoint hemorrhages in the skin, and bleeding gums. Vitamin C also modestly enhances iron absorption, is a general antioxidant, and is needed for synthesizing some hormones and neurotransmitters. Fresh fruits and vegetables, especially citrus fruits, are generally good sources. Because a great amount of vitamin C is lost in cooking, a good diet should emphasize fresh or lightly cooked vegetables. Deficiencies can occur in people with alcoholism and those whose diets lack sufficient fruits and vegetables. Smoking makes matters worse for people already at risk. The Upper Level is set at about 20 times adult needs.

12. Choline is a dietary component that is available from a wide variety of foods and is synthesized in the body. It is used to form a neurotransmitter, among other functions. Nutritional needs have recently been set. No natural deficiency of choline has been reported. The Upper Level is set at about 8 times adult needs.

13. The vitamin-like compounds carnitine, inositol, taurine, and lipoic acid, while participating in many important chemical reactions in the body, are not true vitamins because they can be synthesized in the body from readily available building blocks; they are also obtained from the diet.

Study Questions

1. Why is the risk of toxicity greater with the fat-soluble vitamins A and D than with water-soluble vitamins in general?
2. How would you determine which fruits and vegetables displayed in the produce section of your supermarket are likely to provide plenty of carotenoids?
3. What is the primary function of the vitamin D hormone? Which groups of people likely need to supplement with vitamin D, and on what do you base your answer?
4. Describe how vitamin E functions as an antioxidant. Use the term *free radical*.
5. Describe how the RDA, Daily Value, and Upper Level for vitamin B-6 should be used in everyday life. How do the RDA and Daily Value differ?
6. The need for certain vitamins increases as energy expenditure increases. Name two such vitamins and explain why this is the case.
7. Take one of the B vitamins that might be low in the North American diet and explain why the lack might occur.
8. Which vitamins are lost from cereal grains as a result of the "refining" process? Which vitamins must be replaced by law in the subsequent enrichment process?
9. Why does FDA limit the amount of folate that may be included in supplements and fortified foods?
10. Is it necessary for North Americans to consume a great excess of vitamin C to avoid the possibility of a deficiency? Does the intake of vitamin C well above the RDA have any negative consequences?

Further Readings

1. ADA Reports: Position of the American Dietetic Association: Food fortification and dietary supplements. *Journal of the American Dietetic Association* 101:115, 2001.
   The best nutritional strategy for promoting optimal health and reducing the risk of chronic disease is to wisely choose a wide variety of foods. Additional vitamins and minerals from fortified foods and/or supplements can help some people meet their nutritional needs.

2. Feskanich D and others: Vitamin A intake and hip fractures among postmenopausal women. *Journal of the American Medical Association* 287:47, 2002.
   Intakes of preformed vitamin A at just two times the RDA may increase the risk of hip fracture in older women. Any supplement use should carefully consider preformed vitamin A intake and not exceed about two times the RDA.

3. Food and Nutrition Board, Institute of Medicine: *Dietary Reference Intakes for thiamin, riboflavin, niacin, vitamin B-6, folate, vitamin B-12, pantothenic acid, biotin, and choline.* Washington, DC: National Academy Press, 1998.
   Explanation as to how nutrient recommendations were established for the B-vitamins and choline, with specific reference to establishing RDA and related standards. The functions of each of the B-vitamins and choline are explained.

4. Food and Nutrition Board, Institute of Medicine: *Dietary Reference Intakes for vitamin C, vitamin E, selenium, and carotenoids.* Washington, DC: National Academy Press, 2000.
   The functions of antioxidant nutrients; how RDA and related standards were determined; and deficiency and toxicity symptoms are explained. This is the definitive report by the panel of experts on nutrient needs for dietary antioxidants.

5. Food and Nutrition Board, Institute of Medicine: *Dietary reference intakes for vitamin A, vitamin K, arsenic, boron chromium, copper, iodine, iron, manganese, molybdenum, nickel, silicon, vanadium, and zinc.* Washington, DC: National Academy Press, 2001.
   New nutrient recommendations have recently been set for vitamin A and vitamin K. The rationale used to set the RDA or Adequate Intake and Upper Level for these nutrients is discussed in detail.

6. Holick MF: Meeting vitamin D needs of the elderly. *Nutrition & the M.D.*, p. 1, May 2001.

   Older adults are likely to be deficient in vitamin D if they do not receive regular sun exposure or consume enough vitamin D-fortified foods, such as milk. Needs for vitamin D can usually be met by exposure to sunlight two to three times per week. Exposure time should be about 25% of that required to cause a sunburn. This may not provide vitamin D for older people, however, as aging decreases the ability of the skin to produce vitamin D. Thus, a yearly determination of vitamin-D status should be a part of the health evaluation by a physician for all older adults, and low status corrected with vitamin-D supplements.

7. Holt PR: Dairy foods and prevention of colon cancer: Human studies. *Journal of the American College of Nutrition*, 18:379S, 1999.

   Combined data from several studies suggest that daily consumption of 850 milligrams of calcium per day is accompanied by a reduced incidence of colon tumors. Low-fat dairy foods or supplemental calcium may reduce colon cancer incidence.

8. Lichtenstein P and others: Environmental and heritable factors in the causation of cancer—Analyses of cohorts of twins from Sweden, Denmark, and Finland. *The New England Journal of Medicine* 343:78, 2000.

   Inherited genetic factors make only a minor contribution to susceptibility to most types of cancers. Environmental factors, such as smoking, infections, and diet, play the principal role in causing cancer.

9. Mason JB: Folate in the prevention of cancer. *Nutrition & the M.D.*, p. 1, August 2001.

   Most experts in nutrition and the cancer prevention field feel that increasing folate intake to achieve a cancer-preventive effect is best accomplished by increasing consumption of foods that contain the vitamin, because these are likely to contain other cancer-preventive factors. However, as long as total intake does not exceed approximately 1000 micrograms per day, there is little risk associated with synthetic folic acid supplementation.

10. Multivitamins: Do you need one? Mayo Clinic Health letter, p. 4, April 2001.

    Multivitamins usually provide the RDA of most vitamins. Some contain the RDA of select minerals. Still, it is important to check the label to make sure one is not getting too much of any nutrient. In some cases an excess may be harmful.

11. Russell R: Vitamins and minerals: How much is too much? *Nutrition Action Healthletter*, p. 8, June 2001.

    People older than age 50 need at least 2.4 micrograms of vitamin B-12 from a supplement or fortified food like a ready-to-eat breakfast cereal. This should suffice to meet vitamin B-12 needs, even if the person has reduced stomach absorption of vitamin B-12. Most older people do not drink enough milk to meet the current RDA for vitamin D. For people over 70 years, vitamin D as part of supplement use is typically necessary, especially for older people living in northern climates. The article goes on to list the Upper Levels for vitamins and minerals, comparing these amounts to the RDAs or Adequate Intakes, as well as the Daily Values set by FDA.

12. Should you take a vitamin E supplement? *Harvard Health Letter* 26(11):1, September 2001.

    Meeting the RDA for vitamin E is an important goal for maintaining health. Whether consuming more vitamin E than the RDA provides further health benefits is under debate. Currently, experts suggest that it is safe to consume 200–400 IU of vitamin E each day in the form of a supplement, but solid evidence for the effectiveness of this practice in regard to health is lacking.

13. Willett WC: Diet, nutrition, and the prevention of cancer. In Shils ME and others (eds.): *Modern nutrition in health and disease.* 9th ed. Baltimore, MD: Williams & Wilkins, 1999.

    Excessive energy intake increases risk of cancer. The author recommends consuming more fruits and vegetables, avoiding excess intake of red meat and animal fat, and limiting alcohol intake.

14. Willet WC, Stampfer MJ: What vitamin should I be taking, doctor? *The New England Journal of Medicine* 345:1819, 2001.

    Use of a daily multivitamin and mineral supplement is a reasonable dietary practice, but it does not substitute for avoiding smoking, weight control, and regular physical activity. These supplement's also do not contain needed dietary fiber or essential fatty acids. Use of up to 400 IU of vitamin E may be considered, but evidence supporting specific health benefits is still a research question.

I. Measuring Your Vitamin Intake Against the RDAs

This activity requires you to reexamine the nutritional assessment you did for Chapters 1 and 2. You recorded all the foods and drinks you consumed for 1 day and their quantities. Then you assessed your intake by recording the total amounts of nutrients you consumed. You were then asked to compare your nutrient intake to the RDAs found on the inside front cover of this book. Take your completed assessment and look at your intakes of vitamins A, E, C, B-6, B-12, and thiamin, riboflavin, niacin, and folate. Record these numbers in the table. Next, record the RDAs for each of these nutrients from your assessment. Then, record the percentage of the RDA you consumed for each vitamin. Lastly, place a +, −, or = in the space provided, reflecting an intake higher than, lower than, or equal to the RDA.

Vitamin	Intake	RDA	% of RDA	+, −, =
A				
E				
C				
Thiamin				
Riboflavin				
Niacin				
B-6				
Folate				
B-12				

Analysis

1. Which of your vitamin intakes equaled or exceeded the RDA?

   _____

2. Which of your vitamin intakes were below the RDA?

   _____

3. What foods could you eat to improve your dietary intake of vitamins in low amounts in your diet? (Review sources of certain vitamins in this chapter.)

   _____

   _____

II. Spotting Fraudulent Claims on the Internet and in Popular Books for Sale at Health-Food Stores and Bookstores

Using the World Wide Web, search for vitamins and vitamin-like substances that are sold over the Internet. Are these websites really selling vitamins, or are they actually a cover for selling something else? Compare the price of the vitamins from these sites with the price you would pay at the local supermarket. Do any of these sites display any disclaimers or warnings about the products? Then visit a health-food store to examine the books that are for sale. How many books represent sound nutrition, and how many are mostly filled with nutrition quackery? Also, consult last Sunday's edition of *The New York Times* best-seller list. How many books represent sound nutrition, and how many are nutrition quackery? Write a report comparing the various sources of nutrition information available to the public.

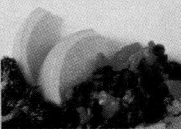

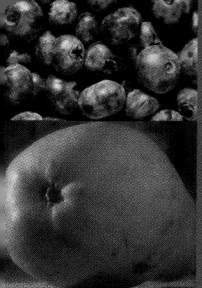

Nutrition and Cancer

Cancer is currently the second leading cause of death for North American adults. It is further estimated that more than 1500 people die each day of cancer in the United States alone, yielding a cost of about $100 billion from all cancer-related expenses. The top four cancers, causing more than 50% of cancer deaths, are lung, colorectal, breast, and prostate cancers. Of those, lung cancer in female smokers is the only form that is increasing on a yearly basis.

Cancer is actually many diseases; these differ in the types of cells affected and, in some cases, in the factors contributing to cancer development (Fig. 8.14). For example, the factors leading to skin cancer differ from those leading to breast cancer. Similarly, the treatments for the different types of cancer often differ.

Cancer essentially represents abnormal and uncontrollable division of cells; if untreated or not treatable, it leads to death. Most cancers take the form of tumors, although not all tumors are cancers. A tumor is simply spontaneous new tissue growth that serves no physiological purpose. It can be **benign,** like a wart, or **malignant,** like most lung cancers. The terms *malignant tumor* and *malignant neoplasm* are synonymous with cancer.

Benign tumors are made up of cells similar to the surrounding normal cells and are enclosed in a membrane that prevents them from penetrating other tissues. They are dangerous only if their physical presence interferes with normal functions. A benign brain tumor, for example, can cause illness or death if it blocks blood flow in the brain. In contrast, a malignant tumor, or cancer, is capable of invading surrounding structures, including blood vessels, the lymph system, and nervous tissue. It can also spread, or **metastasize,** to distant sites via the blood and lymphatic circulation, thereby producing invasive tumors in almost any part of the body (Fig. 8.15). A few cancers, such as leukemia, a form of cancer found in white blood cells, don't produce a mass and so aren't properly classified as tumors. But since leukemic cells exhibit the fundamental property of rapid and inappropriate growth, they are still malignant and therefore represent a form of cancer.

benign Noncancerous; tumors that do not spread.

malignant Essentially to do anything malicious. In reference to a tumor, the property of spreading locally and to distant sites.

metastisis The spreading of disease from one part of the body to another, even to parts of the body that are remote from the site of the original tumor. Cancer cells can spread via blood vessels, the lymphatic system, or direct growth of the tumor.

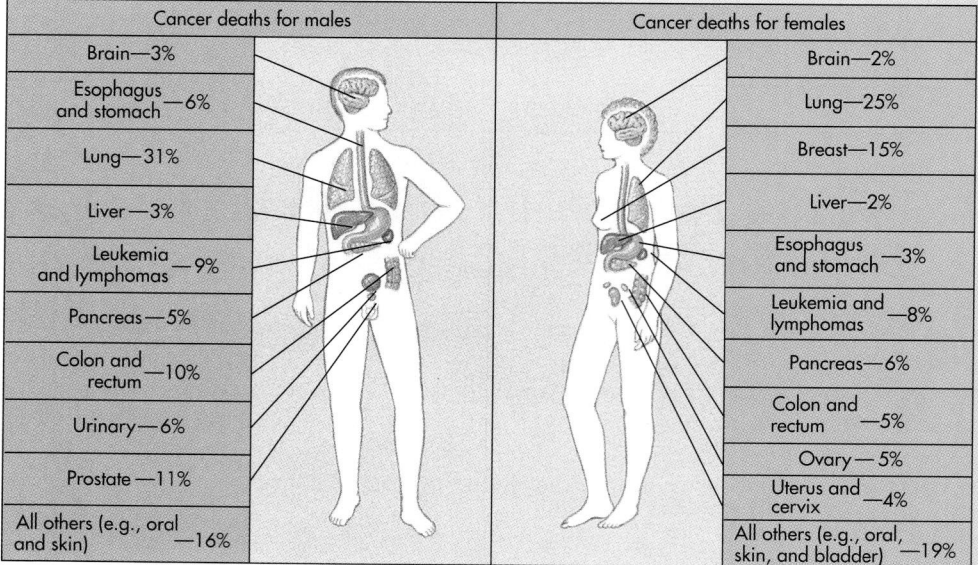

Cancer deaths for males	Cancer deaths for females
Brain—3%	Brain—2%
Esophagus and stomach—6%	Lung—25%
Lung—31%	Breast—15%
Liver—3%	Liver—2%
Leukemia and lymphomas—9%	Esophagus and stomach—3%
Pancreas—5%	Leukemia and lymphomas—8%
Colon and rectum—10%	Pancreas—6%
Urinary—6%	Colon and rectum—5%
Prostate—11%	Ovary—5%
All others (e.g., oral and skin)—16%	Uterus and cervix—4%
	All others (e.g., oral, skin, and bladder)—19%

Figure 8.14 Cancer is actually many diseases. Numerous types of cells and organs are its target. Note that about one-third of all cancers arise from smoking.
Illustration by William Ober.

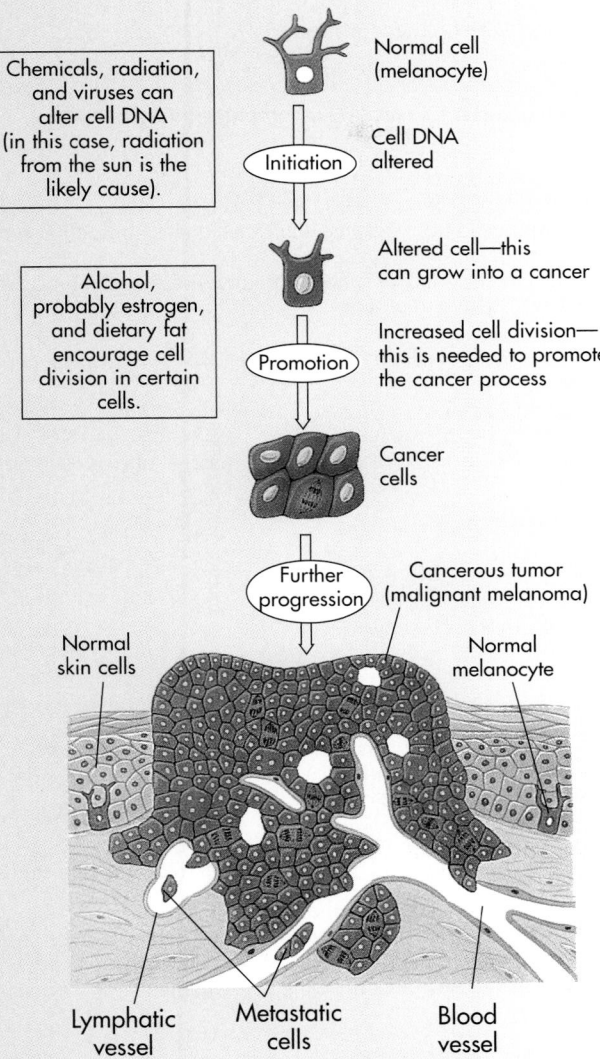

Chemicals, radiation, and viruses can alter cell DNA (in this case, radiation from the sun is the likely cause).

Normal cell (melanocyte)

Initiation

Cell DNA altered

Altered cell—this can grow into a cancer

Alcohol, probably estrogen, and dietary fat encourage cell division in certain cells.

Promotion

Increased cell division— this is needed to promote the cancer process

Cancer cells

Further progression

Cancerous tumor (malignant melanoma)

Normal skin cells

Normal melanocyte

Lymphatic vessel

Metastatic cells

Blood vessel

Figure 8.15 Progression from a normal skin cell to skin cancer through the initiation, promotion, and progression stages. The ball of cells is a developing tumor. As the mass of cells grows, it can invade surrounding tissues, eventually penetrating into both lymph and blood vessels. These vessels carry spreading (metastatic) cancer cells throughout the body, where they can form new cancer sites.

Both genetics and lifestyle are potent forces that influence the risk for developing cancer. Certain cancers tend to occur in some families more than in others. Thus persons within high-risk families are said to be genetically predisposed, or at risk for developing specific types of cancer. A genetic predisposition is especially important in development of colon cancer, some types of breast cancer, and prostate cancer (35%, 27%, and 42%, respectively). About 30 cancer-susceptibility genes have been isolated. However, experts estimate that only 1% to 5% of most cancers can be explained by inheriting a cancer gene. Overall, lifestyle is also a critical factor in most forms of cancer, as evidenced by the variation in cancer rates from country to country. In fact, diet likely accounts for more than 30% to 40% of all cancers.

Although we have little control over our genetic risks for cancer, we do have a great deal of choice in deciding which risks to take with respect to lifestyle, especially with regard to smoking, alcohol abuse, physical activity, and nutrient intake (food choice). It is well established that one-third of all cancers in North America are due directly to tobacco use. About half of the cancers of the mouth, pharynx, and larynx are associated with heavy use of alcohol. A combination of alcohol use and smoking increases cancer risks even higher. In addition, it has become increasingly apparent that certain dietary factors and degree of physical activity either promote or inhibit cancer. With diet, as with tobacco and alcohol use, imprudent choices today likely cause medical problems tomorrow.

continued

Researchers are attempting to attack cancer from all sides. For example, cancer cells contain an enzyme called **telomerase** *that allows cancer tumors to indefinitely divide by continually lengthening the cap on the ends of DNA strands. This cap shortens as a cell multiplies, eventually preventing further cell division. Studies are ongoing to discover a way to attack telomerase. In addition, angiostatin and endostatin are two natural proteins that are being studied for their ability to inhibit the growth of blood vessels that facilitate cancer metastasis.*

Table 8.4 The Cancer Development Process

Cancer Initiation

Process: DNA alteration occurs in this relatively short phase (minutes to days).

Causes:
Radiation: e.g., sun overexposure
  Cross-links double strands of DNA or breaks them into fragments.
Chemicals: e.g., aflatoxin (mold from peanuts and cereal grains), benzo(a)pyrene (smoke from charbroiled meat fat)
  Transformed by body to highly reactive cancer initiators. These compounds are then able to cause mutations in DNA, RNA, and proteins.
Biological agents: e.g., viruses
  Promote uncontrolled growth of cells by inserting viral DNA or RNA into normal cells, which alters the cell's genes.

Cancer Promotion

Process: DNA alterations are "locked" into the genetic material of cells over a period of months to more than 10 years.

Causes:
Excess estrogen exposure
Excess alcohol
Excess dietary fat (controversial)
Bacterial infections: e.g., *Helicobacter pylori*

Cancer Progression

Process: Cells that can grow autonomously appear. These cells spread to surrounding tissue and other sites.

Causes:
Excess energy intake
Lack of early detection
Development of blood supply to the tumor
  The tumor uses newly formed capillaries to grow and spread cancer cells to remote sites in the body.

Anything that increases the rate of cell division decreases the chance that the repair enzymes will find the altered part of the DNA in time to do their work. Once a cell multiplies and incorporates its newly altered DNA into its genetic instructions, the repair enzymes can no longer detect the changes in DNA.

Mechanisms of Carcinogenesis

To understand how cancer can be prevented, let's first examine how cancer develops in the body. This process involves multiple steps, starting with exposure of a cell to a carcinogen (Table 8.4).

Cancer Initiation

mutation A permanent change in a cell's DNA; includes changes in sequence, alteration of gene position, gene loss or duplication, and insertion of foreign gene sequences.

cancer initiation The stage in the process of cancer development that begins with alterations in DNA, the genetic material in a cell. This may cause the cell to no longer respond to normal physiological controls.

Cancer begins with a **mutation** of DNA, the genetic material in a cell. As a result, the cell no longer responds to normal physiological controls on cell division. **Cancer initiation** can develop spontaneously, or it can be induced by specific agents. The affected cell now can dictate its own rate of division and is not inhibited from doing so at the expense of surrounding cells. Alteration of DNA can occur within a few minutes to days. Among the factors that can initiate cancer development are radiant energy, certain chemical agents, and biological agents. In addition, some metabolism that occurs in the body can contribute harmful substances. For example, certain products of liver metabolism cause cancer.

Potentially thwarting this process of cancer development are other human genes, called *tumor suppressors.* These may step in to prevent the abnormal growth, slowing cell turnover. However if mutations cause the tumor suppressor to fail, this block against cancer development also fails. Mutations of this and other tumor-suppressor genes are often linked to cancer. Generally speaking, one or more mutations of various genes may be required for a tumor to develop.

Cancer Promotion

The initiation stage of carcinogenesis, during which DNA is altered, is relatively short (minutes to days). In contrast, the **cancer promotion** stage may last for months or more than 10 years before the final stage, progression, appears. During the promotion stage the DNA alterations are "locked" into the genetic material of cells.

Anything that increases the rate of cell division decreases the chance that the repair enzymes will find the altered part of the DNA in time to do their work. Once a cell multiplies and incorporates its newly altered DNA into its genetic instructions, the repair enzymes can no longer detect the changes in DNA.

Compounds that increase cell division are estrogen, alcohol (especially if one's diet is also low in folate), and probably high intakes of dietary fat. Bacterial infections in the stomach are also suspected agents, such as with *Helicobacter pylori*.

Studies with experimental animals have revealed that some substances can inhibit this promotion stage. Compounds present in cruciferous vegetables, onions, garlic, and citrus fruits—as well as vitamin A, vitamin D, and calcium—are thought to do so. Phytochemicals in general were discussed in Chapter 2. Cancer experts agree that a diet rich in fruits and vegetables is a key cancer-preventive measure. Relying on supplementation with individual nutrients, such as vitamin A and vitamin C, does not enjoy as much support, partly because this practice doesn't contribute phytochemicals, as food choices supplying these nutrients do.

Cancer Progression

The final stage in carcinogenesis begins with the appearance of cells that can grow autonomously (i.e., without normal controls on growth). During the **cancer progression** stage these malignant, or cancer, cells proliferate, invade the surrounding tissue, and spread (metastasize) to other sites. Early in this stage, the immune system may find the altered cells and destroy them. Or the cancer cells may be so defective that their own DNA limits their ability to grow, and they die. If nothing impedes growth of cancer cells, one or more tumors eventually develop that are large enough to affect body functions, and signs and symptoms of cancer appear (review Table 8.4).

Diet and Cancer

Cancer quackery aside, a nutritious diet, as well as other factors related to lifestyle, can reduce the risk of cancer initiation and promotion. Some food constituents may contribute to cancer development, whereas others have a protective effect (Table 8.5). First the association between fat/energy intake and cancer is discussed, and then some of the food constituents that may reduce the risk for cancer are covered.

▌ Contribution of Fat and Energy Intakes to Cancer Risk

Excess energy intake, leading eventually to obesity, is related to all major forms of cancer with the exception of lung cancer. This is the main diet-cancer risk factor. This includes cancer of the breast (especially in postmenopausal women), pancreas, kidney, gallbladder, colon, **endometrium,** and prostate gland. The link probably occurs between adipose tissue and the synthesis of estrogen from other hormones in the blood. High concentrations of circulating estrogen in the blood are thought to promote cancer. Excess insulin output resulting from an obese, insulin-resistant state is also implicated.

A long-standing excess energy intake also may promote cancer. In one study, people with the highest calorie intakes had a 70% higher risk of getting colon cancer than the control group. When laboratory animals are fed diets high in fat or total energy, they tend to experience more cancers, especially in the colon and breast. The effect is most apparent when an agent is used to

continued

cancer promotion The stage in the cancer process when cell division increases, in turn decreasing the time available for repair enzymes to act on altered DNA and encouraging cells with altered DNA to develop and grow.

cancer progression The final stage in the cancer process, during which the cancer cells proliferate, forming a mass large enough to significantly affect body functions.

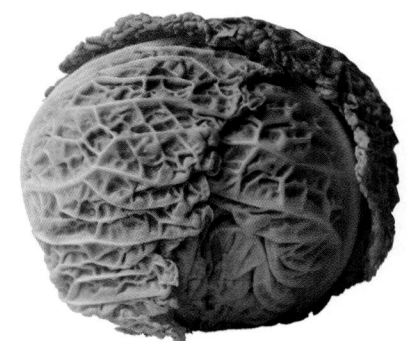
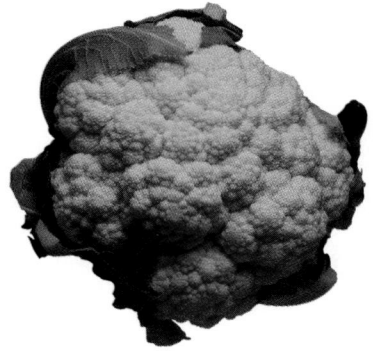

Cruciferous vegetables such as cabbage and cauliflower are rich in cancer-preventing phytochemicals.

endometrium The membrane that lines the inside of the uterus. It increases in thickness during the menstrual cycle until ovulation occurs. The surface layers are shed during menstruation if conception does not take place.

Table 8.5 Some Food Constituents Suspected of Having a Role in Cancer

Constituent	Dietary Sources	Action
Possibly Protective*		
Vitamin A	Liver, fortified milk, fruits, vegetables	Encourages normal cell development and differentiation
Vitamin D	Fortified milk	Increases production of a protein which suppresses cell growth, such as in the colon
Vitamin E	Whole grains, vegetable oil, green, leafy vegetables	Antioxidant; prevents formation of nitrosamines
Vitamin C	Fruits, vegetables	Antioxidant; can block conversion of nitrites and nitrates to potent carcinogens
Folate	Fruits, vegetables, whole grains	Encourages normal cell development. Especially reduces the risk of colon cancer
Selenium	Meats, whole grains	Part of antioxidant system that inhibits tumor growth and kills early cancer cells in the promotion stage
Carotenoids, such as lycopene	Fruits, vegetables	Likely act as antioxidants; some of these possibly influence cell metabolism. Lycopene in particular may reduce the risk of prostate cancer
Indoles, phenols, and other plant substances	Vegetables,[†] especially cabbage, cauliflower, broccoli, brussels sprouts, garlic, onions, tea	May reduce carcinogen activation in the liver and other cells
Calcium	Milk products, green vegetables	Slows cell division in the colon, binds bile acids and free fatty acids, thus reducing colon cancer risk
Omega-3 fatty acids	Cold-water fish, such as salmon and tuna	May inhibit tumor growth
Soy products		Phytic acid present possibly binds carcinogens in the intestinal tract; the genistein component possibly reduces growth and metastasis of malignant cells
Conjugated linoleic acid	Milk products, meats, fish	May inhibit tumor development and act as an antioxidant
Possibly Carcinogenic		
Excessive energy intake	All macronutrients can contribute	Excess fat mass; linked to increased synthesis of estrogen and other sex hormones, which in excess may themselves increase the risk for cancer; resulting excess insulin output from creation of an insulin-resistant state is also implicated
Total fat	Meats (especially in red meat), high-fat milk and milk products, vegetable oils	The strongest evidence is for excessive saturated and polyunsaturated fat intake. Saturated fat is linked to an increased risk of prostate cancer
Alcohol	Beer, wine, liquor	Contributes to cancers of the throat, liver, bladder, breast, and colon (especially if the person does not consume enough folate); increased cell turnover and liver metabolism of carcinogens are the main mechanism
Nitrites, nitrates	Cured meats, especially ham, bacon, and sausages	Under very high temperatures will bind to amino acid derivatives to form nitrosamines, potent carcinogens
Multi-ring compounds: Aflatoxin	Formed when mold is present on peanuts and other grains	May alter DNA structure and inhibit its ability to properly respond to physiologic controls; aflatoxin linked to liver cancer
Benzo(a)pyrene	Charcoal-broiled foods, especially meats	Benzo(a)pyrene linked to stomach and colon cancer. To limit this risk, trim fat from meat before cooking, cut barbecuing time by partially cooking meat (such as in a microwave oven), and don't consume blackened parts

*Many of the actions listed for these possibly protective agents are speculative and have been verified only by experimental animal studies.
[†]Some are part of the family of cruciferous vegetables, which includes cabbage, brussels sprouts, and broccoli.

deliberately initiate the cancer process, and the laboratory animals then are fed a high-fat or energy-rich diet. Fat and food energy are not considered initiators of cancer, but rather promoters.

The National Cancer Institute (NCI) believes there is a sufficient link between dietary fat and cancer to encourage North Americans to reduce fat intake. It recommends initially decreasing dietary fat to about 30% of total energy intake and eventually to 20% or less of total energy if the person is at high risk and can follow such a dietary pattern.

Some scientists, however, believe that the NCI has overreacted to the fat and cancer issue. Although epidemiological evidence does link fat and certain forms of cancer, the evidence is not strong. A stronger link actually exists between cancer and total energy in the diet. If rats or mice are treated with a carcinogen to promote either breast or colon cancer and then one group consumes a typical energy intake while a second group consumes a reduced energy intake, the group with the low energy intake will exhibit about a 40% reduction in tumor development. The amount of fat in the diet is not important, as long as energy intake is about 70% of the usual intake of the laboratory animals. Energy restriction is currently the most effective technique for preventing cancer in laboratory animals.

The mechanism behind this effect of total energy intake is probably mostly hormonal in nature. Unfortunately, it is very difficult for humans to reduce dietary energy to 70% of usual intake. So while the data obtained from laboratory animal studies are interesting, nutritionists do not see any practical way to make recommendations on the basis of these studies. In addition, once cancer is present, energy restriction is no longer helpful.

▌ Cancer-Inhibiting Food Constituents

Many single nutrients may have cancer-inhibiting properties. These anticarcinogens include antioxidants and certain phytochemicals (review Table 8.5).

The antioxidant activity of vitamin C and vitamin E helps to prevent formation of **nitrosamines** in the gastrointestinal tract, thus preventing formation of a potent carcinogen. Vitamin E also helps protect unsaturated fatty acids from damage by free radicals. Overall, carotenoids, vitamin E, vitamin C, and selenium function as or contribute to antioxidant systems in the body. These antioxidant systems help prevent the alteration of DNA by electron-seeking compounds.

In addition, phytochemicals from fruits and vegetables, and even tea, block cancer development in some cases. Numerous studies suggest that fruit and vegetable intake reduces the risk of nearly all types of cancer. These foods are normally rich in carotenoids, vitamin C, and vitamin E. Adequate vitamin D intake is suspected of reducing breast, colon, and prostate cancer. Calcium is also linked to a decreased risk for developing colon cancer. In sum, a diet that follows the Food Guide Pyramid (or related pyramid), so that fruits, vegetables, whole grains, low-fat and nonfat dairy products, and some plant oils are eaten daily, is a rich source of anticarcinogens. It is likely that all of these foods have a "cocktail" effect, in that no one food is likely to prevent cancer alone.

▌ The Bottom Line

A variety of dietary changes will reduce your risk for cancer. Start by making sure that your diet is moderate in energy and fat content and that you consume many fruits and vegetables, whole grains, beans, some fish, and low-fat or nonfat milk products (Table 8.6). In addition, remain physically active, avoid obesity, and moderate alcohol intake if used, and limit intake of animal fat and salt-cured, smoked, and nitrate-cured foods.

Remember also that if a cancer is left untreated, it can spread quickly throughout the body. When this happens, it is much more likely to lead to death. Thus early detection is critical. Aids to early detection include the following warning signs (acronym is CAUTION):

- A **c**hange in bowel or bladder habits
- **A** sore that does not heal
- **U**nusual bleeding or discharge
- A **t**hickening or lump in the breast or elsewhere
- **I**ndigestion or difficulty in swallowing
- An **o**bvious change in a wart or mole
- A **n**agging cough or hoarseness

A large-scale study called the Women's Health Initiative is testing the hypothesis that a diet with 20% or less energy from fat reduces cancer occurrence in the breast and other sites in adult women (ages 59–70 years). The study is due for completion in 2005. Currently, the research community is divided on whether this will be an effective therapy for reducing breast cancer.

nitrosamine A carcinogen formed from nitrates and breakdown products of amino acids; can lead to stomach cancer.

continued

Unexplained weight loss is an additional warning sign.

There are still other ways to detect cancer early. Colonoscopy examinations for middle-age and older adults, PSA (prostate-specific antigen) tests for middle-age and older men, and Papanicolaou tests (Pap smears) and regular breast examinations (and mammograms starting about age 40) for women are recommended by the American Cancer Society. Finally, to learn still more about cancer, review these sources of credible cancer information on the Internet:

American Cancer Society
www.cancer.org
CancerNet
www.icic.nci.nih.gov
Oncolink
cancer.med.upenn.edu.

Table 8.6 Example of a Diet Intended to Limit the Risk for Cancer—Low in Fat and High in Fruits and Vegetables and Provides Plenty of Calcium

Breakfast	Dinner
6 ounces orange juice ¾ cup ready-to-eat breakfast cereal 1 cup 1% fat milk 1 banana 1 slice whole-wheat toast, jelly, soft margarine Hot tea	3 ounces baked fish (e.g., cod, white fish, salmon) Baked potato topped with shredded mozzarella cheese (⅓ cup) Roasted corn on the cob, soft margarine Fresh garden salad with "lite" Italian dressing 1 whole-wheat dinner roll 1 scoop lemon ice or orange sherbet Hot tea
Lunch	**Snack**
Sandwich: ½ cup chicken salad served on ½ bagel or 1 slice of whole-wheat bread Assorted raw vegetables: carrots, celery, broccoli, chopped lettuce 1 cup 1% fat milk Fresh fruit in season: strawberries, melon, grapes, apple (1½ cups) 2 fig cookies	12-ounce can diet cola 2 cups popcorn ¼ cup mixed nuts

Nutrient breakdown:
kcal: 2300 kcal
% calories from fat: 25%

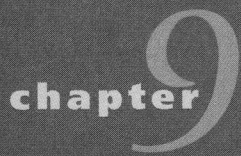
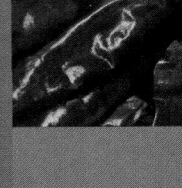
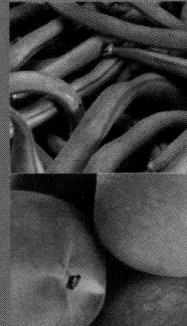

chapter 9

Water and Minerals

Chapter Outline

W ater—the most versatile medium for a variety of chemical reactions—constitutes the major portion of the human body. Without water, biological processes necessary to life would cease in a matter of days. We operate on about 2 quarts (2 liters) of water daily and must replenish it regularly because the body does not store water per se. We experience this constant demand for water as thirst. Many nutrients, including minerals, exist in the body dissolved in water. Because the functioning of minerals is related to the characteristics of water, water and its roles in the body are explored first in this chapter.

Many minerals, like water, are vital to health. They are considered inorganic because they are typically not bonded to carbon atoms. Minerals are key participants in body metabolism, muscle movement, body growth, and water balance, among other wide-ranging processes. Some of the minerals found in our bodies—for example, vanadium and arsenic—may not be necessary to sustain human life. Nevertheless, we know that some mineral deficiencies can cause severe health problems. For this reason, the study of minerals is critical to understanding human nutrition.

Based on the amount we need each day, minerals are categorized as major (requiring over 100 milligrams per day) or trace (requiring 100 milligrams or less per day). These categories do not reflect the importance of those minerals to the body; deficiencies of some trace minerals can cause severe health problems. In this chapter, you will see why the study of water and minerals is critical for understanding human nutrition, and that misuse of supplement forms of many of the minerals easily can lead to toxicity.

Check out the **Contemporary Nutrition: Issues and Insights Online Learning Center** www.mhhe.com/wardlawcont5 *for quizzes, flash cards, other activities, and web links designed to further help you learn about issues surrounding water and minerals.*

Chapter Objectives

Chapter 9 is designed to allow you to:

1. Classify the minerals as major or trace minerals.

2. List conditions of the body, dietary factors, and other pertinent relationships that influence the absorption, retention, and availability of specific minerals.

3. List and briefly explain the functions of water in the body.

4. List key functions of the major and trace minerals.

5. Identify possible deficiency and toxicity symptoms associated with the major and trace minerals.

6. List at least two food sources for each of the major and trace minerals.

7. Describe the processes involving minerals that aid in maintaining bone health as well as those that aid in control of blood pressure.

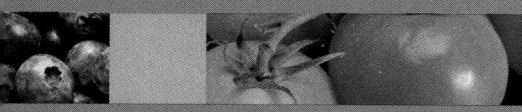

Refresh Your Memory

As you begin your study of water and minerals in Chapter 9, you may want to review:

- Cell structure and function, digestion and absorption of nutrients, cardiovascular transport, immunity, and endocrine function in Chapter 3

- The health risks of high-protein diets in Chapter 6

- The functions of vitamin D and vitamin K related to calcium and bone health in Chapter 8

- The role of vitamin C in collagen synthesis in Chapter 8

Real Life Scenario

*J*ana, a sophomore in high school, recently became a vegan. Her mother is concerned about her diet, because she is not a vegan herself, and worries about Jana's health. One of her primary concerns is osteoporosis, particularly because she knows that 95% of bone growth occurs by ages 16–17. Jana needs an adequate source of calcium in her diet to aid with her rapid bone development. Jana also recently started smoking, and her only physical activity is choir practice.

Jana's diet on a recent day consisted of the following items. For breakfast, she had oatmeal made with water, a banana, and a cup of fruit juice. At midmorning, she bought a snack cake from the vending machine. At lunch, she had vegetable pasta, bread with olive oil, a side salad, 1 ounce of mixed nuts, and a soft drink. For dinner, she had a soy burger along with mixed vegetables and rice. As an evening snack, she had some cookies and another soft drink.

What factors place Jana at risk for osteoporosis in the future? Suggest any necessary changes to her current diet.

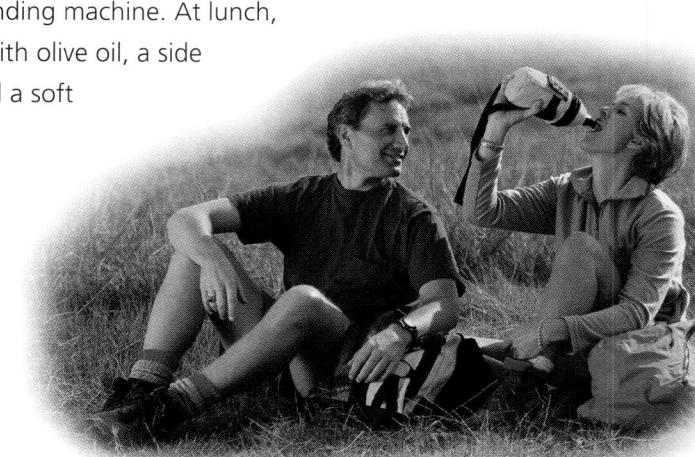

Nutrition Connection

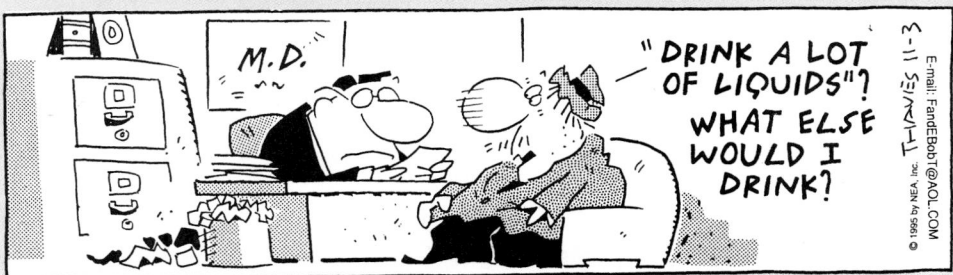

FRANK & ERNEST by Bob Thaves

Replacing fluids—water as part of foods, beverages, and water itself—is an important daily task. Why is this so critical for maintaining health? And why are infants, athletes, and older adults particularly at risk for dehydration? In addition, how does water interact with some of the minerals used by the body? This chapter provides some answers.

FRANK & ERNEST © Reprinted by permission of Newspaper Enterprise Association, Inc.

Water

To appreciate how minerals operate in the body, it helps to understand the nature and general chemical properties of water, as well as specific nutrient-related functions.

Life as we know it could not exist without water. Water is the perfect medium for body processes because it enables chemical reactions to occur. Water even participates directly in many of these reactions. It forms the greatest component of the human body, making up 50% to 70% of the body's weight (about 10 gallons or 40 liters). Lean muscle tissue contains about 73% water. Adipose tissue is about 20% water. Thus, as fat content increases (and the percentage of lean tissue decreases) in the body, total body water content drifts toward 50%.

Depending on the amount of fat stores present, an adult can survive for about 8 weeks without eating food but only a few days without drinking water. This occurs not because water is more important than carbohydrate, fat, protein, vitamins, or minerals, but rather because we can not conserve water as well as we can the other components of our diet.

Water in the Body—Intracellular and Extracellular Fluid

Water flows in and out of body cells through cell membranes. Water inside cells forms part of the **intracellular fluid**—the fluid within the cells. When water is outside cells or in the bloodstream, it is part of the **extracellular fluid**—that outside cells (Fig. 9.1). Because cell membranes are permeable to water, water shifts freely in and out of cells. For example, if blood volume decreases, water can move from the areas inside and around cells to the bloodstream to increase blood volume. On the other hand, if blood volume increases, water can shift out of the bloodstream into cells and the surrounding areas, leading to edema (see Chapter 6).

The body controls the amount of water in the intracellular and extracellular compartments mainly by controlling *ion* concentrations. Ions have electrical charges, and so are called *electrolytes*. Water is attracted to ions, such as sodium, potassium,

intracellular fluid Fluid contained within a cell; it represents about two-thirds of all body fluid.

extracellular fluid Fluid present outside the cells; represents about one-third of all body fluid.

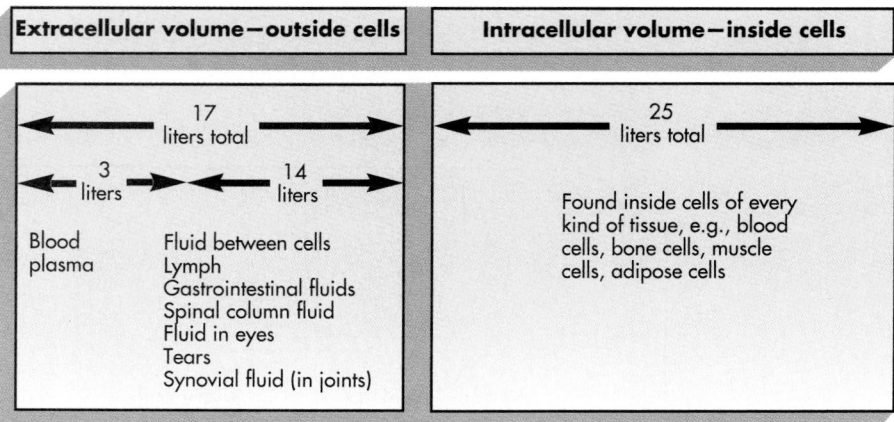

Extracellular volume—outside cells	Intracellular volume—inside cells

Figure 9.1 The fluid compartments in the body.

chloride, phosphate, magnesium, and calcium. By controlling the movements of ions in and out of the cellular compartments, the body maintains the appropriate amount of water in each compartment. Where ions go, water follows.

Positive ions, such as sodium and potassium, end up pairing with negative ions, such as chloride and phosphate. Intracellular water volume depends primarily on intracellular potassium and phosphate concentrations. Extracellular water volume depends primarily on the extracellular sodium and chloride concentrations.

■ Water Contributes to Temperature Regulation

Water changes temperature slowly because it has a great ability to hold heat. It takes much more energy to heat water than it does to heat fat. Water molecules are attracted to each other, and it takes much energy to separate them. Foods with high water content heat up and cool down slowly. Because water requires so much energy to change states—for example, from a liquid to a gas—it forms an ideal medium for removing heat from the body.

The body then secretes fluids in the form of perspiration, which evaporates through skin pores. To evaporate water, heat energy is required. So, as perspiration evaporates, heat energy is taken from the skin, cooling it in the process. Each quart (liter) of perspiration evaporated represents approximately 600 kcal of energy lost from the skin and surrounding tissues. For this reason, fever increases one's need for energy.

About 60% of the chemical energy in food is turned directly into body heat; the other 40% is converted to forms of energy cells can use, and almost all of that energy eventually leaves the body in the form of heat. If this heat could not be dissipated, the body temperature would rise enough to prevent enzyme systems from functioning efficiently. Perspiration is the primary way to prevent this rise in body temperature.

Another Bite

*T*o cool efficiently, perspiration must be allowed to evaporate. If it simply rolls off the skin or soaks into clothing, perspiration doesn't cool us much. Evaporation of perspiration occurs readily when humidity is low. This is why humans often tolerate hot, dry climates far better than they do hot, humid climates.

■ Water Helps Remove Waste Products

Water is an important vehicle for ridding the body of waste products. Most unusable substances in the body can dissolve in water and exit the body through the urine.

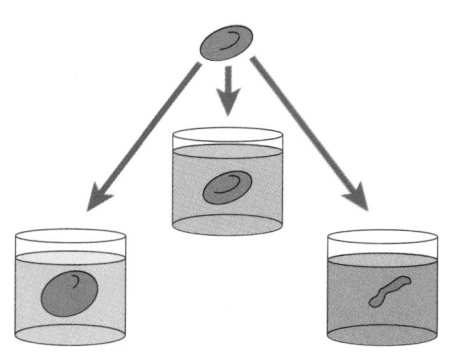

The effects of ion and water balance are easily demonstrated with red blood cells. Water can easily pass through its semipermeable membrane, but ions cannot. When water is added to the fluid surrounding the cells, thereby diluting the fluid, water moves into the cells, causing them to expand. Conversely, when particles (e.g., sodium and chloride ions as table salt) are added to the fluid, thereby concentrating it, water moves out of the cells, causing them to shrink. Sugar added to strawberries acts in the same way to draw water out of the fruit. The process of water crossing a semimembrane from a lower to a higher concentration is called **osmosis.**

osmosis The passage of a solvent such as water through a semipermeable membrane from a less concentrated compartment to a more concentrated compartment.

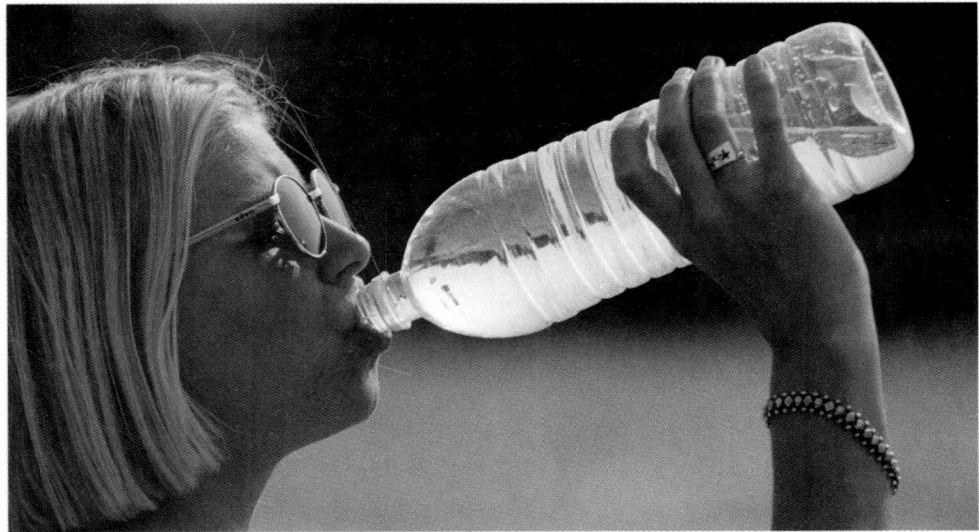

Regular intake of water and water-rich fluids are essential to replace daily fluid losses. A recent trend in North America is to carry this water with us.

Urea is a major body waste product. This by-product of protein metabolism contains nitrogen. The more protein we eat in excess of needs, the more nitrogen we excrete—in the form of urea—in the urine. Likewise, the more sodium we consume, the more sodium we excrete in the urine. Overall, the amount of urine a person needs to produce is determined primarily by excess protein and sodium chloride (salt) intake. By limiting excess protein and salt intakes, it is possible to limit urine output—a useful practice, for example, in space flights. This type of diet is also used to treat some kidney diseases wherein the ability to produce urine output is hampered.

A typical urine volume is about 1 to 2 liters (1 to 2 quarts) per day, depending mostly on the amount of fluid, protein, and sodium intake. Somewhat more urine output than that is fine, but less—especially less than 600 milliliters (2½ cups)—forces the kidneys to form a very concentrated urine. This is noticeable as a very dark yellow urine. The heavy ion concentration in turn increases the risk of kidney stone formation in susceptible people, generally men. Kidney stones are simply minerals and other substances that have precipitated out of the urine and accumulated in kidney tissues.

▪ Other Functions of Water

Water helps form the lubricants found in knees and other joints of the body. It is the basis for saliva, bile, and **amniotic fluid.** Amniotic fluid acts as a shock absorber surrounding the growing fetus in the mother's womb. Ion concentrations vary in each fluid compartment to accommodate specific needs, such as the ability to transfer nerve impulses.

▪ How Much Water Do We Need?

Adults need roughly 1 milliliter of water per kcal expended. We consume about 1 liter (1 quart) of water a day in various liquids, such as fruit juice, coffee, tea, soft drinks, and water itself (see margin). Foods supply another liter of fluid; many fruits, vegetables, and beverages are more than 80% water. Water as a by-product of metabolism provides approximately 350 milliliters (1½ cups) of additional water. This yields a total of about 2.4 liters (10 cups) of water for a 2400 kcal diet, or about 1 milliliter per kcal expended. One way to determine if water intake is adequate is to observe the color of one's urine: it should be clear to pale yellow.

Of the 2.4 liters of water needed, about 1.4 liters is used to produce urine. The rest, about 1 liter, compensates for typical water losses through the lungs (400 milliliters),

amniotic fluid Fluid contained in a sac within the uterus. This fluid surrounds and protects the fetus during development.

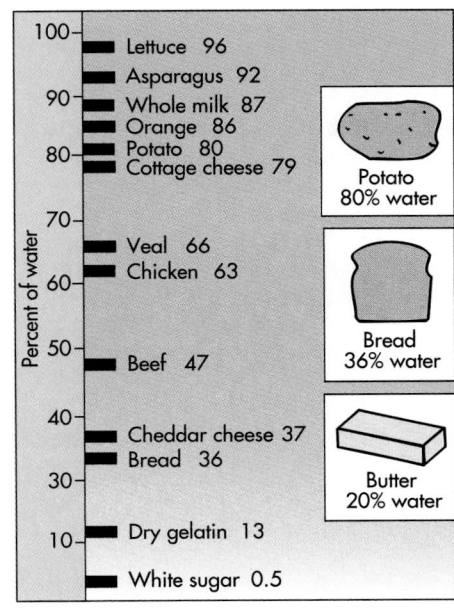

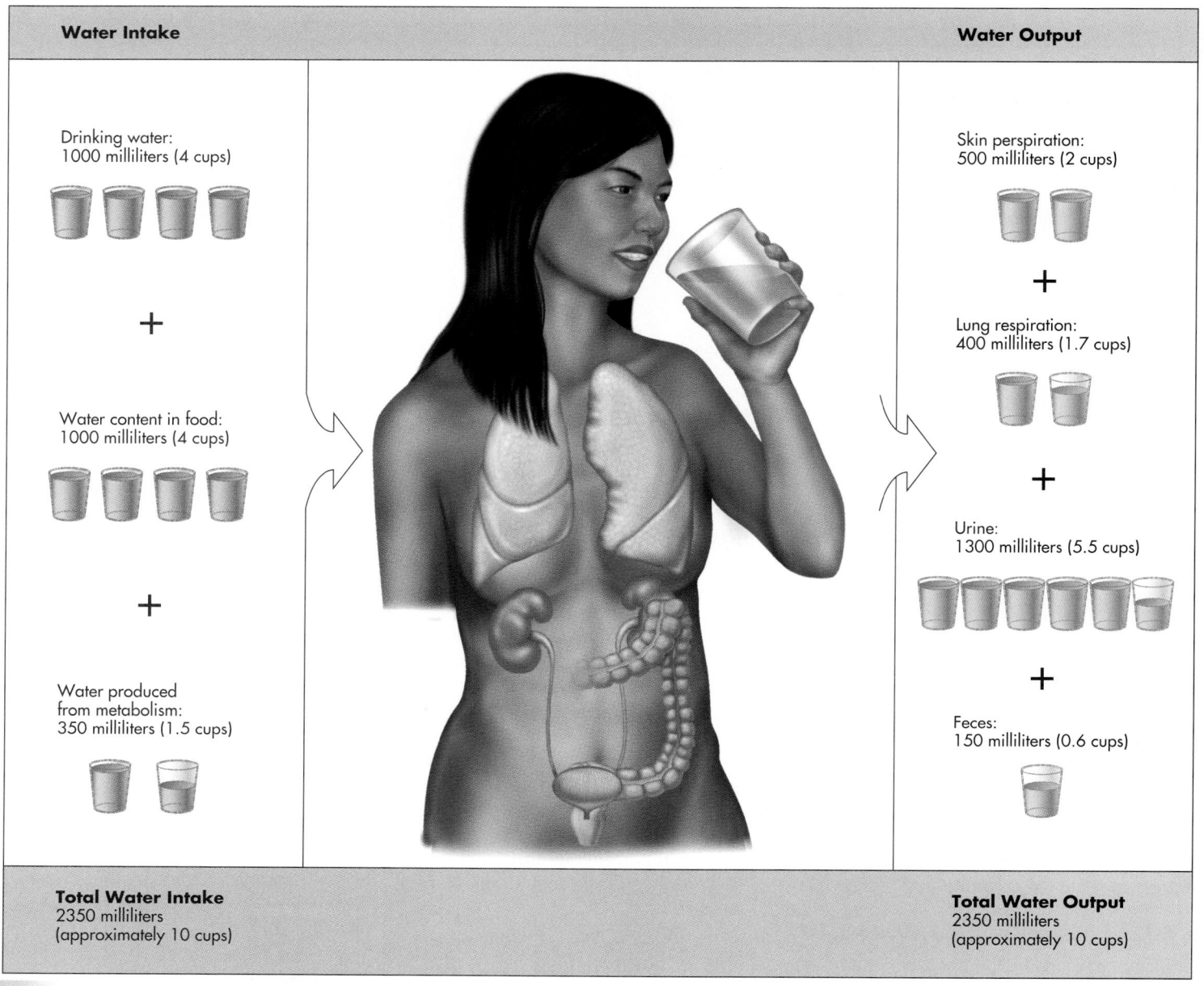

Figure 9.2 Water balance—intake versus output. We maintain body fluids at an optimum amount of adjusting water intake and output. Most water comes from the liquids we consume. Some comes from the moisture in more solid foods, and the remainder is manufactured during metabolism. Water output includes that lost via lungs, kidneys, skin, and feces.

Water can be classified by whether it is hard or soft. Hard water generally comes from underground wells and usually contains calcium, magnesium, and iron. The more minerals the water contains, the harder it is. Soft water has a low content of these minerals and is often produced by replacing other minerals with sodium.

feces (150 milliliters), and skin (500 milliliters) (Fig. 9.2). Note also that when we consider the large amount of water used to lubricate the gastrointestinal (GI) tract, the loss of only 150 milliliters of water a day through the feces is remarkable. About 8000 milliliters of water enter the GI tract daily via secretions from the mouth, stomach, intestine, pancreas, and other organs, while the diet supplies an additional 2000 milliliters or more. The kidneys also greatly conserve water. They reabsorb about 97% of the water filtered from waste products.

■ Thirst

If you don't drink enough water your body often lets you know by signaling thirst. Your brain is communicating the need to drink. This thirst mechanism is not always reliable, however, especially during infancy, illness, in one's older years, and during vigorous exercise. For this reason, athletes especially should monitor fluid status—they should weigh themselves before and after training sessions to determine their rate of water loss and, thus, their water needs. The current goal for athletes is to consume 3 cups of fluid for every pound lost. Two of the cups replace fluid losses, while the third cup compensates for extra urine output that results from the fluid replacement, as well as any extra sweating that occurs in the exercise recovery period. Note that two cups (½ liter) of water weigh about a pound (about half a kilogram) (see Chapter 11 for more details on fluid use in athletics). Ailing youngsters—especially those with fever, vomiting, diarrhea, and increased perspiration—and older persons often need to be reminded to drink plenty of fluids (see Chapters 14 and 15 for details). As Chapter 14 discusses in further detail, infants easily become dehydrated.

What If the Thirst Message Is Ignored?

Once the body registers a shortage of available water, it increases fluid conservation. Two hormones that participate in this process are **antidiuretic hormone (ADH)** and **aldosterone.** The pituitary gland releases ADH to force the kidneys to conserve water. The kidneys respond by reducing urine flow. At the same time, as fluid volume decreases in the bloodstream, blood pressure falls. This eventually triggers the release of the hormone aldosterone, which signals the kidneys to retain more sodium and, in turn, more water.

However, despite mechanisms that work to conserve water, fluid is constantly lost via the insensible routes—feces, skin, and lungs. Those losses must be replaced. In addition, there is a limit to how concentrated urine can become. Eventually, if fluid is not consumed, the body becomes dehydrated and suffers ill effects.

By the time a person loses 1% to 2% of body weight in fluids, he or she will be thirsty. And this small water deficit can cause one to feel tired. At a 4% loss of body weight, muscles lose significant strength and endurance. By the time body weight is reduced by 10% to 12%, heat tolerance is decreased and weakness results. At a 20% reduction, coma and death may soon follow.

■ Water Safety: How Safe Is the Water We Consume?

These days, it is common to see 5-gallon bottles of water being delivered to homes. Grocery store shelves are now stocked with many kinds of bottled waters—ranging from simple plastic jugs containing "pure spring water" to fancier, imported varieties of mineral water in glass bottles. In Europe, bottled water is an institution, as popular as soft drinks are in North America.

Currently, it is quite fashionable to order a bottle of Evian at a restaurant or bar. Not only are people looking for alternatives to alcoholic beverages and soft drinks, but they are also attracted to the perceived health value or taste of bottled water. Is this practice of bottled water use worth the effort and expense?

Most people in the United States enjoy very safe tap water. The Environmental Protection Agency (EPA) in the United States and local municipalities pay careful attention to possible contaminants that can appear in tap water, and 90% of public water facilities have been found to be in compliance with current regulations. Local municipalities in the United States also are required by law to inform customers of any dangerous amounts of contaminants and indicate specific actions to take, such as the need to boil water. These agencies also have to provide a yearly report of ongoing water quality evaluations.

Currently, it is estimated that 10 million people in the United States are at risk for consuming tap water that does not meet EPA guidelines. These individuals are primarily in rural communities, where agricultural runoff from farmlands can pollute both ground water used for wells and streams and rivers used as a water source. These individuals may have their water tested to see if a water purifier or bottled water is indicated. Testing is available through the local health department or county extension agencies. The cost for this testing is minimal.

antidiuretic hormone (ADH) A hormone that is secreted by the pituitary gland and that acts on the kidneys to cause a decrease in water excretion.

aldosterone A hormone produced by the adrenal glands that acts on the kidneys to cause sodium, and so water, conservation.

Alcohol inhibits the action of ADH. One reason people feel so weak the day after heavy drinking is that they are very dehydrated. Even though they may have consumed a lot of liquid in their drinks, they have lost even more liquid because alcohol has inhibited ADH. Caffeine also produces a diuretic effect on the body.

Too much water—whatever amount the kidneys are unable to excrete—can also lead to ill health. However, an excessive amount would have to approach many quarts (liters) each day. When excessive water overwhelms the kidneys' capacity to excrete, blurred vision is one resulting symptom.

cryptosporidiosis An intestinal disease, characterized by diarrhea, that originates from a protozoan parasite of the genus *Cryptosporidium*.

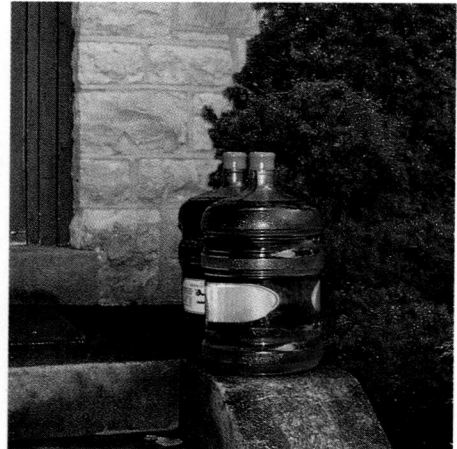

Concern over tap water quality has led some North Americans to purchase bottled water. This concern has merit, especially in rural communities.

*A*s bottled water becomes more and more popular, the industry now generates more than $3 billion per year. In 1996, FDA instituted definitions for the various types of bottled water on the market; FDA also tests products for microbial and chemical content. For a list of manufacturers that meet federal guidelines, contact the International Bottled Water Association at 1-800-928-3711 or www.nsf.org. Some experts recommend that children not be given bottled water exclusively, as it does not contain an adequate fluoride supply to protect against dental caries. For adults, bottled water is typically an unnecessary expense, as it is often very similar to tap water.

Another threat to water safety comes from a parasite called *Cryptosporidium*. **Cryptosporidiosis** is an intestinal disease that can spread from hand to mouth by having direct contact with infected human or animal feces, by swallowing the parasite via tap water or swimming pool water, or by consuming undercooked contaminated food.

In 1993, 400,000 people in Milwaukee, Wisconsin, became ill and 100 died from water contaminated with *Cryptosporidium*. Another recent attack happened in Sydney, Australia. This parasite poses little risk to healthy people—other than a case of diarrhea—but this is not true for people who have HIV/AIDS or other diseases that compromise function of the immune system (such as some forms of cancer therapy or organ transplant therapy). Recently, these high-risk patients have been advised to boil for 1 minute tap water they use for cooking or drinking to ensure the parasite is destroyed. Alternatively, one can purchase a water filter that screens out *Cryptosporidium* (the National Sanitation Foundation at 800-673-8010 can provide a list of manufacturers) or use bottled water that is certified to be free of this parasite (contact the supplier if in doubt). Generally, distilled water or that which has undergone reverse osmosis is free of *Cryptosporidium*.

As a safeguard against microbial contamination, chlorine and ammonia are added to water to kill bacteria (although such chlorination does not kill *Cryptosporidium*). The addition of such chemicals has raised concern that drinking water may increase rectal and bladder cancer risk, although there is currently no conclusive proof of such risk. If chlorine in tap water does increase cancer risk, the risk is extremely small (perhaps two cases of cancer per 1 million people).

If you find the taste of chlorinated tap water unpleasant or are concerned about the slight cancer risk, you can remove the chlorine from tap water by boiling it or by letting a large container filled with water stand uncovered overnight. In both cases, the chlorine will evaporate, taking its characteristic flavor with it. Alternatively, you can install a filter on the household spigot from which you obtain your water. It should be designed to remove trihalomethanes, common chlorine by-products.

Overall, if you are concerned about the safety of your tap water, you can ask the municipal water department for the most current test results, or, if you have well water (or are just interested), you can have the water tested yourself. Compared with the cost of bottled water or water filters, the testing fee is insignificant. As noted in Chapter 16, letting cold water run for a minute or so before taking a drink or before using it in meal preparation is a good way to limit possible lead exposure, especially if the water has been off for more than an hour. In addition, for the same reason, avoid using hot tap water for food preparation. If you want further information on water safety, call the EPA's Safe Drinking Water Hotline at 800-426-4791 or visit the web page www.epa.gov/safewater.

Concept Check

*B*ecause the body can neither readily store nor conserve water, we can survive only a few days without it. Water dissolves substances, serves as a medium for chemical reactions and as a lubricant, and aids in temperature regulation. Water accounts for 50% to 70% of body weight and distributes itself all over the body: among lean and other tissues (in both intracellular and extracellular fluids) and in urine and other body fluids. Adults need about 1 milliliter of water or other fluids for each kcal expended. Thirst is the body's first sign of dehydration. If this thirst mechanism is faulty, as it may be during illness or vigorous exercise, hormonal mechanisms also help conserve water by reducing urine output. Overall, the U.S. water supply is generally safe; thus, bottled water and home water purification are unnecessary in most communities. Excess fluid intake can be hazardous to a person's health.

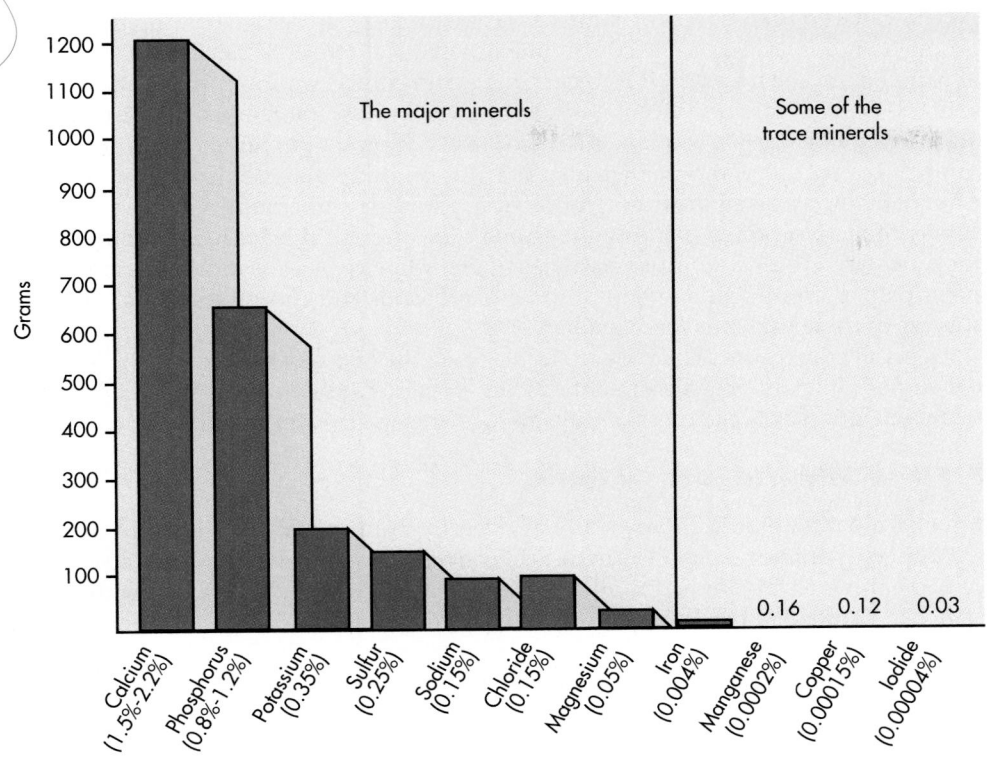

Figure 9.3 Approximate amounts of various minerals present in the average human body. The percent values in parentheses indicate the amounts as percentages of body weight. Other trace minerals of nutritional importance not listed include chromium, fluoride, molybdenum, selenium, and zinc.

Minerals—An Overview

The metabolic roles of minerals and the amounts of them in the body vary considerably (Fig. 9.3). Some minerals, such as copper and selenium, work as **cofactors,** enabling enzymes to function. Minerals also contribute to many body compounds. For example, iron is a component of hemoglobin in red blood cells. Sodium, potassium, and calcium aid in the transfer of nerve impulses throughout the body. Body growth and development also depend on certain minerals, such as calcium and phosphorus. Water balance requires sodium, potassium, calcium, and phosphorus. At all levels—cellular, tissue, organ, and whole body—minerals clearly play important roles in maintaining body functions.

Minerals are categorized based on the amount we need per day. Recall from Chapter 1 that if we require greater than 100 milligrams (1/50 of a teaspoon) of a mineral, it is considered a major mineral; otherwise, it is considered a trace mineral. Using these criteria, calcium and phosphorus are major minerals and iron and zinc are trace minerals.

The roles and nutritional significance of both the major and the trace minerals are discussed in this chapter. But before examining the properties of the individual minerals, let's consider some topics relevant to all these nutrients.

Mineral Bioavailability

Foods contain and supply us with many minerals, but our bodies vary in their capabilities to absorb and use available minerals. Although minerals may be present in foods, they are not **bioavailable** unless the body can absorb them. The ability to absorb minerals from a diet depends on many factors. The number listed in a food composition table for the amount of a mineral in a food is just a starting point for estimating the actual contribution the food will make to our mineral needs. Spinach, for example, contains plenty of calcium, but only about 5% of it can be absorbed because of the vegetable's high concentration of **oxalic acid,** a calcium-binder. Usually, about 25% of

cofactor A mineral or other substance that binds to a specific region on an enzyme and is necessary for the enzyme's activity.

bioavailability The degree to which the amount of an ingested nutrient is absorbed and is available to the body.

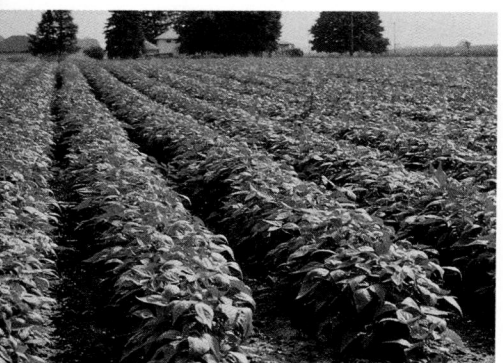

The trace mineral content of plant foods reflects the trace mineral concentration in the soil in which they were grown.

dietary calcium is absorbed by adults, with the higher percentage coming from dairy products, and in those people consuming moderate amounts of calcium.

Minerals in the average North American's diet come from both plant and animal sources. Overall, minerals from animal products are absorbed better, because binders and dietary fiber (as will soon be discussed) are not present to hinder absorption. The mineral content of plants also greatly depends on mineral concentration in the soil. Animals, however, may consume foods from multiple soil conditions and may eat a variety of plant products, because the animals are often shipped across country during their growth, so soil conditions have less of an influence. Vegans must be aware of the potentially poor mineral content of some plant foods and choose some concentrated sources of these minerals (see Chapter 6).

Generally the more refined a plant food—as in the case of white flour—the lower its content of minerals. The enrichment process for grains adds only the mineral iron. The selenium, zinc, copper, and other minerals lost when grains are refined are not replaced.

■ Fiber-Mineral Interactions

Mineral bioavailability can be greatly affected by nonmineral substances in the diet. Components of fiber, especially **phytic acid** (phytate) in grain fiber, can limit absorption of some minerals by binding to them. Oxalic acid, mentioned before, is another substance in plants that binds minerals and makes them less available to the body. High-fiber diets can decrease the absorption of iron, zinc, magnesium, and probably other minerals. An intake above the recommendation of 20 to 30 grams of dietary fiber per day can cause problems with mineral status of the body, as noted in Chapter 4.

If grains are leavened with yeast, as they are in bread, enzymes produced by the yeast can break some of the bonds between phytic acid and minerals. This increases mineral absorption. The zinc deficiencies found among some Middle Eastern populations are attributed partly to their consumption of unleavened breads, resulting in low bioavailability of dietary zinc. This is discussed more in a later section on zinc.

■ Mineral-Mineral Interactions

Many minerals are of similar sizes and chemical charges, such as magnesium, calcium, iron, and copper. Having similar sizes and the same chemical charge causes these minerals to compete with each other for absorption, and so they affect each other's bioavailability. Because of this, people should avoid taking individual mineral supplements, unless a medical condition specifically warrants it. This is because an excess of one mineral influences the absorption and metabolism of other minerals. For example, the presence of a large amount of zinc in the diet decreases copper absorption. Food sources pose little risk for mineral interactions.

■ Vitamin-Mineral Interactions

When consumed in conjunction with vitamin C, absorption of certain forms of iron improves. The active vitamin D hormone improves calcium absorption. Many vitamins require specific minerals to act as components in their structure and function. For example, the thiamin coenzyme requires magnesium or manganese to function efficiently.

■ Mineral Toxicities

Excess mineral intake can lead to toxic results, especially with the trace minerals, such as iron and copper. Again, supplement use poses the biggest risk; foods are unlikely causes. This potential for toxicity is yet another reason to carefully consider the use of mineral supplements. Every year, people poison themselves using mineral supplements, even though their intent is to improve health. Many trace minerals are quite toxic at doses not much above typical needs. Mineral supplements exceeding 100% of the Daily Values on the supplement label should be taken only under a physician's supervision, because toxicity and nutrient interactions are possible. An intake above this amount should especially not exceed any Upper Level set if consumed on a long-term basis. In addition, contamination in mineral supplements such as with lead is a possibility. Use of United States Pharmacopeia (USP)-approved brands lessens this risk.

Concept Check

Minerals are vital to the functioning of many body processes. Their bioavailability depends on many factors, including a mineral's interaction with dietary fiber, vitamins, and other minerals. Animal products often yield better mineral absorption than do plants. Still, both animal and plant sources help us meet our mineral needs. Taking megadoses of an individual mineral supplement can greatly diminish the absorption and metabolism of other minerals. In addition, some minerals are potentially toxic in amounts not much in excess of body needs. These are two good reasons to consider carefully any use of mineral supplements, especially in excess of any Upper Level set if consumed on a long-term basis.

Major Minerals

Up to now some general characteristics of minerals and how some of them interact with water in the body have been covered. Now let us review the individual properties of the major minerals in the context of the North American diet (Table 9.1).

Sodium (Na)

We both crave and hear concerns about sodium and its primary dietary source, table salt. Some of this concern is warranted, but it is an essential part of a diet.

The human body absorbs almost all sodium that gets eaten. This sodium then becomes the major positive ion in extracellular fluid and a key factor for retaining body water. Fluid balance throughout the body depends partly on varied sodium and other ion concentrations among the water-containing compartments in the body. Sodium ions also function in nerve impulse conduction and absorption of some nutrients (e.g., glucose).

A low-sodium diet—coupled with excessive perspiration, persistent vomiting, or diarrhea—has the ability to deplete the body of sodium. This state can lead to muscle cramps, nausea, vomiting, dizziness, and later shock and coma. The likelihood of this happening, however, is low because early kidney responses to low sodium status eventually trigger the body to conserve sodium. In addition, people generally eat a lot of sodium. Body conservation of sodium demonstrates how important small amounts are to body functions.

Only when weight loss from perspiration exceeds 2% to 3% of total body weight (or about 5 to 6 pounds) should sodium losses raise concern. Even then, merely salting foods is sufficient to restore body sodium for most people. Endurance athletes, however, may need to consume sports drinks during competition to avoid depletion of sodium (see Chapter 11). Note also that although perspiration tastes salty on the skin, sodium is not highly concentrated in perspiration. Rather, water evaporating from the skin leaves concentrated sodium behind. Perspiration contains about two-thirds the sodium concentration found in blood.

Sodium in Foods and Needs

About one-third to one-half the sodium we consume is added during cooking or at the table. Most of the rest is added during food manufacturing. Many health authorities are calling for manufacturers to use less sodium so that our total sodium intakes

Chapter 8 noted that if men, in general, and older women take a multivitamin and mineral supplement, it should be low in iron or iron-free because of their increased risk for iron toxicity.

For your information, the chemical symbols for the minerals discussed are given next to each mineral heading.

The importance of salt to human health has been recognized since antiquity. Salt was a commodity in the classical world. Indeed, the Latin word salary reflects the way a soldier's wages were paid.

Table 9.1 A Summary of the Major Minerals: Their Functions, Deficiency Conditions, and Food Sources

Name	Major Functions	Deficiency Symptoms	People Most at Risk	RDA, Adequate Intake, or Minimum Requirement	Nutrient-Dense Dietary Sources	Results of Toxicity
Sodium	Functions as a major positive ion of the extracellular fluid; aids nerve impulse transmission; water balance	Muscle cramps	People who severely restrict sodium to lower blood pressure (250–500 milligrams per day); excessive sweating	500 milligrams	Table salt, processed foods, condiments, sauces, soups, chips	Contributes to hypertension in susceptible individuals; leads to increased calcium loss in urine
Potassium	Functions as a major positive ion of intracellular fluid; aids nerve impulse transmission; water balance	Irregular heart beat, loss of appetite, muscle cramps	People who use potassium-wasting diuretics or have poor diets, as seen in poverty and alcoholism	2000 milligrams	Spinach, squash, bananas, orange juice, other vegetables and fruits, milk, meat, legumes, whole grains	Slowing of the heartbeat, as seen in kidney failure
Chloride	Functions as a major negative ion of the extracellular fluid; participates in acid production in stomach; aids nerve transmission; water balance	Convulsions in infants	No one	750 milligrams	Table salt, some vegetables, processed foods	Linked to hypertension in susceptible people when combined with sodium
Calcium	Provides bone and tooth structure, blood clotting; aids nerve impulse transmission; required for muscle contractions; contributes to other cell functions	Increased risk of osteoporosis	Women, especially those who consume few dairy products	1000–1200 milligrams (age > 18 years) 1300 milligrams (age 9–18 years)	Dairy products, canned fish, leafy vegetables, tofu, fortified orange juice (and other fortified foods)	Intakes > 2.5 grams/day (Upper Level) may cause kidney stones and other problems in susceptible people; poor mineral absorption in general
Phosphorus	Required for bone and tooth strength; serves as part of various metabolic compounds; functions as major ion of intracellular fluid; acid-base balance	Possibility of poor bone maintenance DEFICIENCIES ARE UNLIKELY	Older people consuming very nutrient-poor diets; possibly vegans and people with alcoholism	700 milligrams (age > 18 years) 1250 milligrams (age 9–18 years)	Dairy products, processed foods, fish, soft drinks, bakery products, meats	Impairs bone health in people with kidney failure; results in poor bone mineralization if calcium intakes are low; Upper Level is 3–4 grams/day
Magnesium	Provides bone strength; aids enzyme function; aids nerve and heart function	Weakness, muscle pain, poor heart function	Women and patients on certain forms of diuretics	Men: 400–420 milligrams Women: 310–320 milligrams	Wheat bran, green vegetables, nuts, chocolate, legumes	Causes diarrhea, as well as weakness in people with kidney failure; Upper Level of 350 milligrams per day refers to nonfood sources (e.g., supplements) only
Sulfur	Comprises part of vitamins and amino acids; aids drug detoxification; participates in acid-base balance	None have been described	No one, as long as protein needs are met	None	Protein foods	None are likely

fall. To some extent this is taking place (for example, low sodium soups and crackers). Almost all foods naturally contain a little sodium; the higher amount found in milk (about 120 milligrams per cup) is one exception. The more processed food one consumes, generally the higher sodium intake. Conversely, the more home cooking one does, the more sodium control that person has. Major contributors of sodium in the adult diet are white bread and rolls, hot dogs and lunch meats, cheese, soups, and foods with tomato sauce, partly because these foods are eaten so often. Other foods that generally are especially high in sodium include salted snack foods, French fries and potato chips, and sauces and gravies.

If we ate only unprocessed foods and add no salt, we would consume about 500 milligrams of sodium per day. This is also the recommended minimum sodium requirement for adults (see the inside cover for references to mineral needs for other age groups). Even this is a generous amount, considering that we really need only about 100 to 200 milligrams a day.

If we compare 500 milligrams of sodium from unprocessed food with the 4000 to 7000 milligrams or more typically eaten by adults, it is clear that food processing and cooking contribute most of our dietary sodium. As discussed in Chapter 2, nutrition labels list a food's sodium content. When dietary sodium must be severely restricted, these labels become very helpful. Under FDA food and supplement labeling rules, the Daily Value for sodium is 2400 milligrams. FDA established this value because it is consistent with U.S. government reports that encourage reduced sodium intakes.

Most humans can adapt to various dietary salt intakes, though very high intakes can be toxic. For most people who eat a typical diet, today's sodium intake is simply tomorrow's urine output. However, approximately 10% to 15% of adults are sodium sensitive, especially people who are overweight. For these people, high sodium intakes increase blood pressure, and lower-sodium diets (about 2 to 3 grams daily) often help correct the problem (see the Nutrition Insight on minerals and hypertension). Still, keep in mind that other lifestyle factors also contribute to hypertension, and even more so than does sodium intake. Scientific groups typically suggest that all adults reduce intake to 2.4 grams, mostly to limit the risk of later developing hypertension. Following this advice also helps maintain healthy calcium status, as sodium intake greater than about 2 grams per day increases urinary calcium loss as the sodium is excreted.

You can evaluate your sodium habits by completing the questionnaire in Table 9.2. The more checks in the "often" or "regularly" columns, the higher your dietary sodium intake. However, not all the habits in the table contribute the same amount of sodium. For example, many natural cheeses are relatively moderate in sodium, whereas processed cheeses and cottage cheese are much higher. You can choose to reduce your sodium intake by cutting back on those items for which you checked "often" or "regularly." You needn't suddenly eliminate foods from your diet. Rather, to moderate sodium intake, choose lower-sodium foods from each food group more often and balance high-sodium food choices with low-sodium ones. It is also important to pay attention to the sodium values listed on food labels, and taste foods before adding salt. In addition, when eating out, avoid foods commonly prepared with lots of sodium. Ask to have sauces served on the side and then use only small amounts.

It is also a good idea to have your blood pressure checked regularly. If you have hypertension, you should try to reduce your sodium intake as you follow a comprehensive plan to treat this disease.

It is actually not that hard to eventually adapt to a low-sodium diet. At first, foods will taste quite bland, but eventually you will perceive more flavor as the tongue becomes more sensitive to the salt content of foods. By slowly reducing dietary sodium and substituting oregano, lemon juice, and other herbs and spices, you can eventually become accustomed to a diet that contains only 2.4 grams of sodium daily but does not result in much of a flavor trade-off. Many new cookbooks offer excellent recipes for flavorful low-sodium foods.

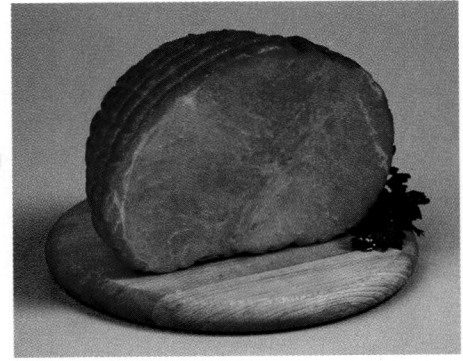

Cured meats, such as ham, are very high in sodium (salt).

*T*able salt is 40% sodium and 60% chloride. The range of sodium intakes seen in adults of 4 to 7 grams per day translates to 10 to 17.5 grams of salt. A teaspoon of salt contains about 2 grams of sodium (2000 milligrams).

Table 9.2 Questionnaire for Evaluating Your Sodium Habits with Respect to Typically Rich Sources

HOW OFTEN DO YOU:	Rarely	Occasionally	Often	Regularly (daily)
1. Eat cured or processed meats, such as ham, bacon, sausage, frankfurters, and other luncheon meats?	☐	☐	☐	☐
2. Choose canned or frozen vegetables with sauce?	☐	☐	☐	☐
3. Use commercially prepared meats, main dishes, or canned or dehydrated soups?	☐	☐	☐	☐
4. Eat cheese, especially processed cheese?	☐	☐	☐	☐
5. Eat salted nuts, popcorn, pretzels, corn chips, or potato chips?	☐	☐	☐	☐
6. Add salt to cooking water for vegetables, rice, or pasta?	☐	☐	☐	☐
7. Add salt, seasoning mixes, salad dressings, or condiments—such as soy sauce, steak sauce, catsup, and mustard—to foods during preparation or at the table?	☐	☐	☐	☐
8. Salt your food before tasting it?	☐	☐	☐	☐
9. Ignore labels for sodium content when buying foods?	☐	☐	☐	☐
10. When dining out, choose foods at restaurants with sauces, or foods that are obviously salty?	☐	☐	☐	☐

The more checks you have in the last two columns, the higher your dietary sodium intake.

Adapted from USDA *Home and Garden Bulletin* No. 232–6, April 1986.

Critical Thinking

Mrs. Massa has recently seen and heard a lot about the amount of salt (sodium) in foods. She has been surprised by the number of articles that advise the public to decrease the amount of salt in their food. If sodium is such a bad thing, Mrs. Massa wonders, why do you need to have any at all? How would you explain this need for some sodium to her?

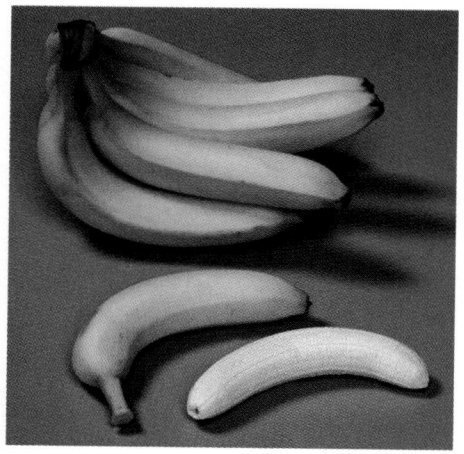

Bananas are a rich source of potassium.

Concept Check

Sodium is the major positive ion in the extracellular fluid. It is important for maintaining fluid balance and conducting nerve impulses. Sodium depletion is unlikely, since the typical North American's diet has abundant sources of sodium and most of it gets absorbed. The more foods prepared at home, the more control we have over our sodium intake. The minimum sodium requirement for adults is 500 milligrams per day. The average adult consumes 4000 to 7000 milligrams or more daily. About 10% to 15% of the population is sensitive to sodium, especially overweight individuals. In these people, hypertension can develop as a result of high-sodium diets, but many other lifestyle habits are also important. Many scientific groups suggest that for all adults, sodium intake should be limited to about 2.4 grams (2400 milligrams). Sodium in the North American diet is provided predominantly through processed foods and salt added in cooking and at the table.

Potassium (K)

Potassium performs many of the same functions as sodium, such as fluid balance and nerve impulse transmission. However, it operates inside, rather than outside cells. Intracellular fluids—those inside cells—contain 95% of the potassium in the body. Also, unlike sodium, potassium is associated with lower rather than higher blood pressure values. We absorb about 90% of the potassium we eat.

Low blood potassium is a life-threatening problem. Symptoms often include a loss of appetite, muscle cramps, confusion, and constipation. Eventually, the heart beats irregularly, decreasing its capacity to pump blood.

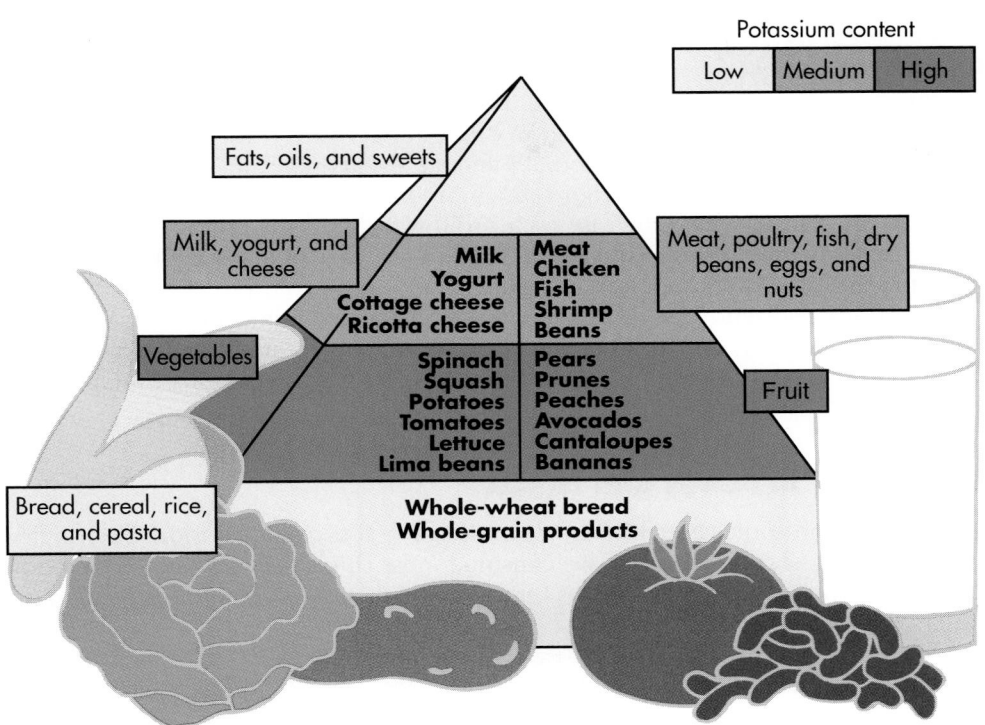

Figure 9.4 Food sources of potassium from the Food Guide Pyramid. The fruit group and the vegetable group are the most nutrient-dense sources of potassium, but it is widely distributed in foods. The background color of each food group indicates the amount of potassium in that group.

■ Potassium in Foods and Needs

Generally, unprocessed foods are rich sources of potassium. This includes fruits, vegetables, milk, whole grains, dried beans, and meats. Major contributors of potassium to the adult diet include milk, potatoes, beef, coffee, tomatoes, and orange juice (Fig. 9.4).

The adult minimum potassium requirement for health is 2000 milligrams (2 grams) per day. The Daily Value used on food and supplement labels is 3500 milligrams. Typically, an adult gets enough potassium by eating a wide variety of foods. North Americans average 2 to 3 grams per day

Diets are more likely to be low in potassium than sodium because we generally do not add potassium to foods. Some **diuretics** used to treat high blood pressure also deplete the body's potassium. Thus, people who take potassium-wasting diuretics need to monitor their potassium intakes carefully. For these people, high-potassium foods—such as fruits, fruit juices, and vegetables—are good additions to the diet, and if recommended by a physician, so are potassium chloride supplements.

A continually deficient food intake, as may be the case in alcoholism, can also result in potassium deficiency. People with certain eating disorders, whose diets are poor and whose bodies can be depleted of nutrients because of vomiting, are also at risk for potassium deficiency (see Chapter 12). People on very low-calorie diets are also at risk and so are athletes who exercise heavily. As covered in Chapters 10 and 11, all of these people should compensate for potentially low body potassium by consuming potassium-rich foods.

If the kidneys function normally, typical intakes of dietary potassium are not toxic. When the kidneys function poorly, potassium builds up in the blood. This inhibits heart function, causing slowed heartbeat. If untreated, this can be fatal, as the heart eventually stops beating. Consequently, in cases of reduced kidney function, close control of potassium intake becomes critical.

diuretic A substance that increases the flow of urine.

Food Sources of Potassium

Food item and amount	Potassium (milligrams)
Kidney beans, 1 cup	715
Winter squash, ¾ cup	670
Plain yogurt, 1 cup	570
Orange juice, 1 cup	495
Cantaloupe, 1 cup	495
Lima beans, ½ cup	480
Banana, 1 medium	470
Zucchini, 1 cup	450
Soybeans, ½ cup	440
Artichoke, 1 medium	425
Tomato juice, ¾ cup	400
Pinto beans, ½ cup	400
Baked potato, 1 small	385
Buttermilk, 1 cup	370
Sirloin steak, 3 ounces	345

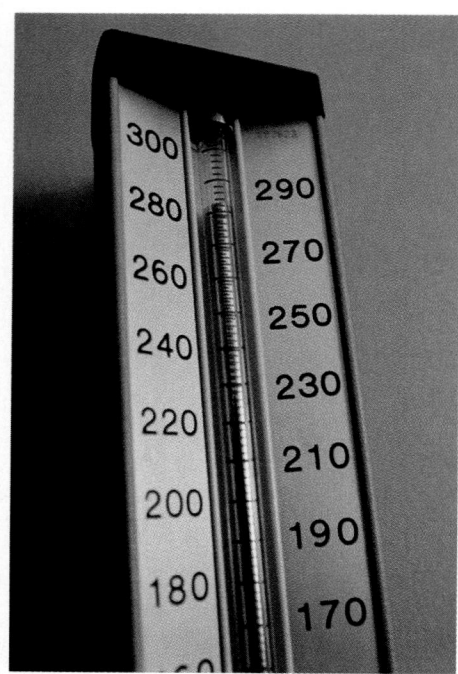

High blood pressure is harmful to many organs in the body. Chloride is likely part of the blood pressure-raising property of sodium chloride (salt).

Chloride (Cl)

Chlorine is a very poisonous gas. In our bodies, chloride—an ion form of chlorine—forms an important negative ion for the extracellular fluid. These ions are a component of the acid produced in the stomach and are also used during immune responses as white blood cells attack foreign cells. In addition, nerve function relies on the presence of chloride. As is the case with sodium, most of the body's chloride is excreted by the kidneys; some is lost in perspiration. It is also implicated in the blood pressure-raising ability of sodium chloride.

A chloride deficiency is unlikely because our dietary sodium chloride (salt) intake is so high. Frequent and lengthy bouts of vomiting—if coupled with a nutrient-poor diet—can contribute to a deficiency because stomach secretions contain much chloride.

■ Chloride in Foods and Needs

A few fruits and some vegetables are naturally good sources of chloride. Chlorinated water is also a source. However, we consume most chloride as salt added to foods. Knowing a food's salt content allows for a close prediction of its chloride content; recall salt is 60% chloride.

The minimum chloride requirement for health in adults is 750 milligrams per day. The Daily Value used on food and supplement labels is 3400 milligrams. Assuming that the average adult consumes at least 7.5 grams of salt daily, that yields 4.5 grams (4500 milligrams) of chloride, an abundance of this ion.

Concept Check

*P*otassium performs functions similar to those of sodium, except that it is the main positive ion found inside, not outside, cells. Potassium is vital to fluid balance and nerve transmission. A potassium deficiency—caused by an inadequate intake of potassium, persistent vomiting, or use of some diuretics—can lead to loss of appetite, muscle cramps, confusion, and heartbeat irregularities. Fruits and vegetables are generally rich sources of potassium. Potassium intake can be toxic if a person's kidneys do not function properly. Chloride is the major negative ion of extracellular fluid. Chloride also functions in digestion as part of stomach acid and in immune and nervous system responses. Deficiencies of chloride are highly unlikely because we eat so much sodium chloride (salt), the major source. Chloride is implicated in the blood pressure-raising ability of sodium chloride.

Minerals and Hypertension

An estimated 1 in 4 North American adults have hypertension, as does one out of two of those over age 65. Blood pressure is expressed by two numbers. The higher number represents systolic blood pressure, which is the pressure in the arteries when the heart actively pumps blood. The second value is for diastolic blood pressure, which is the artery pressure when the heart is relaxed. Optimal systolic blood pressure is less than 120 mm of mercury (mm Hg). Optimal diastolic blood pressure is less than 80 mm Hg. A high diastolic pressure shows a strong relationship to various diseases (especially strokes), as does a high systolic pressure.

Hypertension is defined as sustained systolic pressure exceeding 140 mm Hg or diastolic blood pressure exceeding 90 mm Hg. Most cases of hypertension (about 95% of cases) have no clear-cut cause. It is described as primary, or essential, in nature (e.g., essential hypertension). Kidney disease, sleep-disordered breathing (sleep apnea), and other causes often lead to the other 5% of cases, known as secondary hypertension. African-Americans are more likely than Caucasians to develop hypertension and to do so earlier in life. As a result, they also experience more from hypertension-related diseases and, so, are particularly advised to have their blood pressure checked regularly and to have any evidence of hypertension treated aggressively.

Unless blood pressure is measured periodically, the development of hypertension is easily overlooked. Thus, it's described as a silent disorder, because it usually does not cause symptoms.

Why Control Blood Pressure?

Blood pressure needs to be controlled mainly to prevent cardiovascular disease, kidney disease, strokes and related declines in brain function, poor blood circulation in the legs, problems with vision, and sudden death. All of these conditions are much more likely to be found in individuals with hypertension than in people with normal blood pressure. Smoking and elevated blood lipoproteins make these diseases even more likely. Individuals with hypertension need to be diagnosed and treated as soon as possible, as the condition generally progresses to a more serious stage over time and even resists therapy if it persists for years.

Causes of Hypertension

A family history of hypertension is a risk factor, especially if both parents have (or had) the problem. Blood pressure also usually increases as a person ages. Some increase is caused by atherosclerosis. As plaque builds up in the arteries, the arteries become less flexible and cannot expand. When vessels remain rigid, blood pressure remains high. Eventually, the plaque begins to choke off the blood supply to the kidneys, decreasing their ability to control blood volume and, in turn, blood pressure.

An enzyme secreted by the kidneys and some hormonelike compounds affect blood pressure. Medications are available to reduce their effect.

Obesity is often associated with hypertension, especially in women. In fact, overweight people have six times greater risk of having hypertension than lean people. Overall, obesity is considered the number 1 lifestyle factor related to hypertension. The increase in fat mass increases the need for blood circulation. The extra miles of associated blood vessels increases work by the heart and increases blood pressure. Elevated blood insulin concentration associated with insulin-resistant adipose cells is another reason for this link to obesity. Insulin increases sodium retention in the body and accelerates atherosclerosis. Additionally, an estimated 65% of people with diabetes also have hypertension.

A weight loss of as little as 10 to 15 pounds often can help treat hypertension. This, then, can decrease the need for hypertension drugs, which, by themselves may cause headache, impotence, reduced exercise tolerance, persistent cough, and other side effects. The sleep apnea linked to hypertension also typically improves with weight loss.

Inactivity also is associated with hypertension. It is considered the number 2 lifestyle factor related to hypertension. If an obese person can engage in regular physical activity (at least 5 days per week for 30 to 45 minutes per session) and lose weight, blood pressure often returns to normal.

Excess alcohol intake is responsible for about 10% of all cases of hypertension, especially in middle-aged males and among African-Americans in general. It is considered the number 3 lifestyle factor related to hypertension. When hypertension is caused by excessive alcohol intake, it is usually reversible. A sensible intake for people with hypertension is two or fewer drinks per day for men and one or no drinks per day for women, the same recommendation given to healthy adults. As discussed in Chapter 7, some studies suggest that such a minimal alcohol intake may reduce the risk of ischemic stroke. These data, however, should not be used to encourage alcohol use in nonconsumers.

Preliminary studies show a link between bone lead concentrations and increased risk of hypertension. More information is needed, but it is suspected that even small amounts of lead stored

continued

Another Bite

*I*ndividuals experiencing any of the following symptoms of stroke should seek immediate treatment. This is because physicians can administer drugs that can reduce the extent of the damage caused by most strokes (i.e., ischemic strokes).

- Sudden disturbances in sight, speech, and steadiness
- Sudden sleepiness or severe headache
- Sudden temporary blindness in one eye or other visual effects
- Sudden numbness, weakness, or paralysis of an arm, a leg, or an entire side of the body
- Sudden difficulty with speech or the ability to swallow
- Coma or convulsions

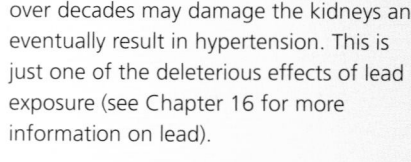

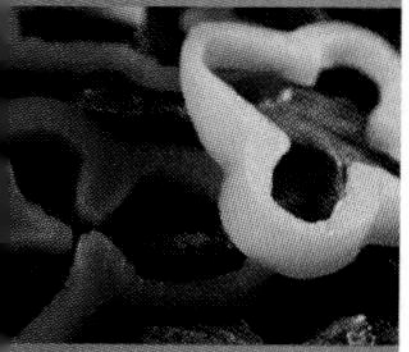

Nutrition Insight

Salt and Blood Pressure

Excess salt intake tends to increase blood pressure, particularly in African-Americans, older overweight persons, and people in general who are susceptible to developing a problem regulating sodium concentration in the body. It is not clear whether the sodium ion or the chloride ion is most responsible for the effect. Still, as reviewed in this chapter, if one reduces sodium intake, chloride intake naturally falls; the opposite is also true. For the most part, when nutrition recommendations suggest consuming less sodium, that is equivalent to saying consume less salt. Since only some North Americans are very susceptible to increases in blood pressure from salt intake, it is likely only the number 4 lifestyle factor related to hypertension. Thus, it is unfortunate that salt intake receives the major portion of public attention with regard to hypertension; obesity, inactivity, and alcohol abuse should be given much more attention.

The latest dietary advice from the Dietary Guidelines for Americans and the American Heart Association suggests that adults consume no more than the Daily Value for sodium (2400 milligrams). Currently, North Americans consume daily, on average, almost double that amount (4–7 grams). Both sets of recommendations note that there is no risk in reducing sodium intake to that amount.

over decades may damage the kidneys and eventually result in hypertension. This is just one of the deleterious effects of lead exposure (see Chapter 16 for more information on lead).

The exact mechanism whereby sodium increases blood pressure is not clear. Studies suggest that there is a genetically influenced ability that determines the ease at which the body can excrete sodium. In salt-sensitive individuals, the kidneys require a higher blood pressure in order to excrete sodium from the body, compared with salt-resistant people. This causes salt-sensitive individuals to retain more sodium. This sodium retention in the body then leads to fluid retention. Ultimately, the fluid retention leads to increased blood volume and, in turn, the increased blood pressure needed to maintain sodium excretion.

Physicians usually resort to a combination of antihypertensive medications, such as diuretics (to increase urine output) and moderate sodium restriction (3–4 grams per day) as an initial form of therapy. This reduces blood volume and, therefore, is often effective in controlling blood pressure.

Other Minerals and Blood Pressure

Minerals such as calcium, potassium, and magnesium also deserve attention when it comes to prevention and treatment of hypertension. People often register slightly lower blood pressures—especially the systolic component—when they consume at least the 1000 milligrams of calcium per day, as compared with one-third to one-half that amount. It is reasonable for a person with hypertension to experiment, in consultation with a physician, with increasing calcium intake to see if that produces the desired effect.

Adequate potassium intake also has been shown to moderately decrease blood pressure compared to people consuming far below this amount. FDA recently approved the following health claim for potassium and a reduction in blood pressure: "Diets containing foods that are good sources of potassium and low in sodium may reduce the risk of high blood pressure and stroke." This health claim will be allowed on foods that contain at least 350 milligrams of potassium (10% of the Daily Value) and 140 milligrams or less of sodium. In addition, qualifying foods must have less than 3 grams of fat, 1 gram or less of saturated fat, and 20 milligrams or less of cholesterol. Some studies indicate that magnesium also is capable of lowering blood pressure at intakes of about twice the RDA.

Recent studies show that a diet rich in calcium, potassium, and magnesium and low in sodium can lead to a decrease in blood pressure within days of beginning a specific diet, especially among African-Americans. The response is even similar to that seen with commonly used medications. The diet, called the DASH diet, closely follows the Food Guide Pyramid, with a few modifications (Table 9.3). The DASH diet is seen as a total dietary approach to treating hypertension. It is not clear which of the many factors contributed by this diet are responsible for the fall in blood pressure. An additional attribute of the DASH diet is that the participants in the study also experienced a fall in blood homocysteine, which should contribute to a lower risk of cardiovascular disease and stroke. Other studies also show a reduction in stroke risk among

Table 9.3 The DASH Diet—A Sample Menu (Provides Approximately 2000 Calories)

Breakfast		**Snack**	
Shredded Wheat, 1 cup		Mixed nuts, ¾ ounce	1 nut
1% low-fat milk, 8 ounces	1 milk	Grape juice, 4 ounces	1 fruit
Sugar, 1 teaspoon		**Dinner**	
Banana, 1 medium	1 fruit	Baked orange roughy, 3 ounces	1 meat
Grapefruit juice, 4 ounces	1 fruit	Rice, 1 cup	2 grains
Snack		Steamed broccoli, 1 cup	2 vegetables
Bread sticks, ¾ ounce	1 grain	Mixed greens salad, 2 cups	1 vegetable
Diet soft drink, 12 ounces		(made with vegetables)	
Lunch		Light Italian dressing, 1 tablespoon	½ fat
Chicken salad, ¾ cup	1 meat	Whole-wheat roll, 1 small	1 grain
(made with reduced-fat	1 fat	Margarine, 1 teaspoon	1 fat
mayonnaise)		1% low-fat milk, 8 ounces	1 milk
Whole-wheat bread, 2 slices	2 grains	**Snack**	
Carrots, 5 baby	1 vegetable	Watermelon, 1¼ cup	1 fruit
Low-fat yogurt, 1 cup	1 milk		
(with artificial sweetener)			
Applesauce, ½ cup	1 fruit		

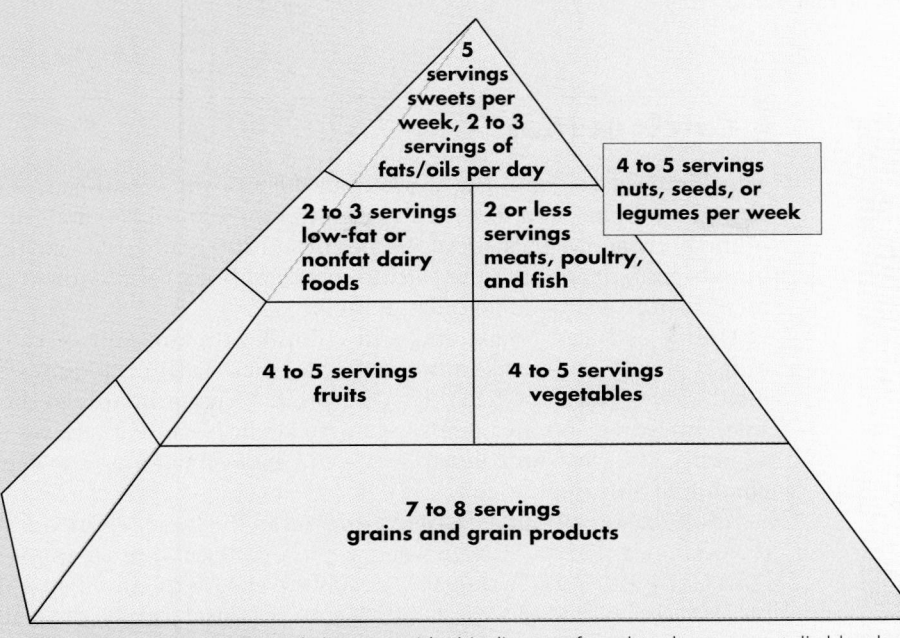

The Dietary Approaches to Stop Hypertension (DASH) diet pyramid. This diet was found to decrease systolic blood pressure by 5.5 mm Hg and diastolic blood pressure by 3.0 mm Hg more than the control diet. Overall, this diet provides approximately 18% of energy as protein, 55% as carbohydrate, and 27% as fat, with 6% from saturated fat. The diet contains more fruit and vegetable servings than the Food Guide Pyramid, contains less fat, and includes a serving of nuts. All DASH participants consumed no more than 3 grams of sodium and one to two alcoholic drinks per week. Researchers estimate that if North Americans were to follow the DASH diet, there would be a 15% decrease in cardiovascular disease and 27% fewer strokes.

A DASH 2 diet trial tested three daily sodium intakes (3300 milligrams, 2400 milligrams, and 1500 milligrams). People showed a steady decline in blood pressure on the DASH diet as sodium intake declined (see Sacks FM and others: Effects on blood pressure of reduced dietary sodium and the dietary approaches to stop hypertension (DASH) diet. *The New England Journal of Medicine* 344:3, 2001).

people who consume a diet rich in fruits, vegetables, and vitamin C (recall that fruits and vegetables are rich vitamin C sources). Overall, a diet rich in low-fat and nonfat dairy products, fruits, vegetables, whole grains, and some nuts can substantially reduce blood pressure and stroke risk in many people. The current challenge is to find a way to convince North Americans to follow such a diet.

Prevention of Hypertension

Many of these and other risk factors for hypertension and stroke are controllable, and appropriate lifestyle changes can reduce a person's risk (Table 9.4). Experts typically recommend that those with hypertension lower blood pressure through diet and lifestyle changes before resorting to blood pressure medications. Such a focus on diet and lifestyle is important because many people discontinue their blood pressure medications because of expense and side effects. Currently, physicians have a long way to go in establishing good blood pressure control among people with hypertension.

Medications to Treat Hypertension

Diuretic medications are one class of agents used to treat hypertension. These work to reduce blood volume by increasing fluid output in the urine. The resulting fall in blood volume then reduces blood pressure. Other medications act by slowing heart rate or by causing relaxation of blood vessels. A combination of two or more medications is commonly required to treat hypertension that does not respond to diet and lifestyle therapy.

Table 9.4 A Nutritional Plan to Minimize Hypertension and Stroke Risk*

1. Follow the Food Guide Pyramid (or related pyramid). Also consider going beyond this to include more fruit, vegetables, and some nuts (e.g., DASH diet), especially if one has hypertension.
2. Make sure to meet nutrient recommendations for calcium, potassium, and magnesium listed in this chapter.
3. Attain and maintain a healthy body weight.
4. Incorporate regular physical activity (at least five times per week for 30 to 45 minutes per session).
5. Consume alcoholic beverages in moderation, if at all (two drinks per day maximum for men and one drink per day maximum for women).
6. Consume moderate amounts of sodium (salt) and see if this helps. The Daily Value is a reasonable limit (2400 milligrams sodium or 6 grams salt [1¼ tsp]). One might even try to lower intake to 1500 milligrams of sodium. This was shown to lower blood pressure even more than the DASH diet alone did.
7. Don't smoke.
8. Maintain blood lipoproteins in the normal range (see Chapter 5).

*In addition, make sure to have blood pressure measured on a regular basis (i.e., yearly physician checkups).

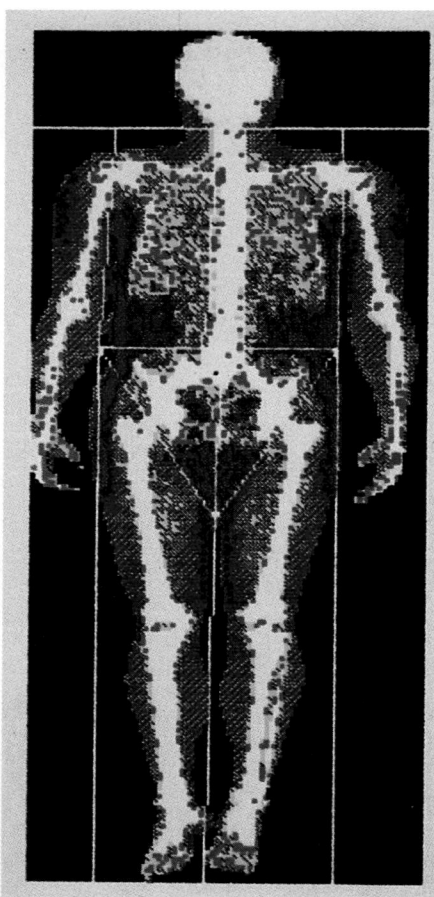

Ninety-nine percent of calcium in the body is in bones.

tetany A body condition marked by sharp contraction of muscles and failure to relax afterward; usually caused by abnormal calcium metabolism.

*D*iets that are low in natural sources of calcium tend also to be low in other essential nutrients found in dairy products such as riboflavin, vitamin A, and potassium. Thus, a low calcium intake generally reflects poor dietary patterns. Individuals who increase their calcium intake through foods, rather than supplements, increase their intake of many other nutrients as well.

Calcium (Ca)

All cells need calcium, but more than 99% of the calcium in the body is used to strengthen bones and teeth. This calcium represents 40% of all the minerals present in the body and equals about 2.5 pounds (1200 grams). As calcium circulates in the bloodstream, it supplies the calcium needs of body cells. Growth and bone development require an adequate calcium intake.

Unlike sodium, potassium, and chloride, the amount of calcium in the body hinges greatly on its absorption from the diet. Calcium requires an acidic environment to be absorbed efficiently. Absorption occurs primarily in the upper part of the small intestine. This area tends to remain acidic because it receives the acidic stomach contents. Much calcium absorption in the upper small intestine depends on the active vitamin D hormone.

Adults absorb about 25% of the calcium in the foods eaten, but during times when the body needs extra calcium—such as in infancy and pregnancy—absorption might reach as high as 60%. Young people tend to absorb calcium better than do older people, especially those older than 70. Postmenopausal women generally absorb the least calcium, unless they receive supplements of the hormone estrogen. Estrogen therapy is associated with an increased synthesis of the active vitamin D hormone, which aids calcium absorption.

Many other factors end up enhancing calcium absorption: parathyroid hormone, dietary glucose, and lactose; and normal intestinal motility (flow). Factors limiting calcium absorption include large amounts of phytic acid in dietary fiber from grains; great excess of phosphorus in the diet; polyphenols (tannins) in tea; a vitamin D deficiency; menopause; diarrhea; and old age.

Because we have excellent hormonal systems to control blood calcium, a normal value can be maintained despite an inadequate calcium intake. The bones, however, pay the price. Bone loss caused by insufficient calcium intake proceeds slowly. Only after many years are clinical symptoms apparent. By not meeting calcium needs, some people—especially women—are most likely setting the stage for future bone fractures. However, because we don't know how efficiently each individual absorbs calcium, we often cannot predict who is at the highest risk.

■ Functions of Calcium

Forming and maintaining bones are calcium's major roles in the body. This is discussed in detail in the Nutrition Issue on osteoporosis. However, calcium is important in many other processes as well. Calcium is essential for blood clotting and for muscle contraction. If blood calcium falls below a critical point, muscles cannot relax after contraction; the body stiffens and shows signs of **tetany**. In nerve transmission, calcium works to release neurotransmitters and permits the flow of ions in and out of nerve cells. Without sufficient calcium, nerve function fails, opening another path to tetany. Finally, calcium helps regulate cellular metabolism by influencing the activities of various enzymes and hormonal responses. It is the hormonal regulation of blood calcium that keeps all of these processes going, even if you fail to consume enough calcium on a daily basis.

Other Possible Health Benefits of Dietary Calcium

Adequate dietary calcium can reduce the risk of colon cancer, especially in people who consume a high-fat diet. A decreased risk of some forms of kidney stones and reduced lead absorption are other possible benefits. Calcium intakes of 800 to 1200 milligrams per day also can decrease blood pressure, compared with intakes of 400 milligrams per day or less (see the Nutrition Insight). In addition, as covered in

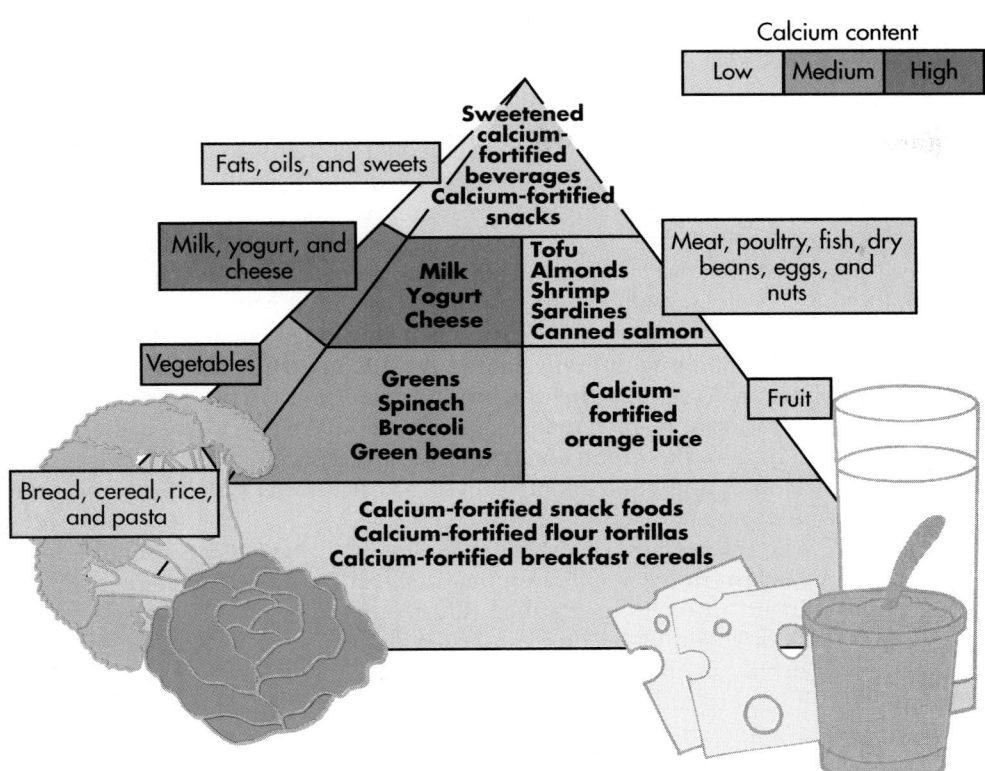

Calcium content

| Low | Medium | High |

Figure 9.5 Food sources of calcium from the Food Guide Pyramid. The milk, yogurt, and cheese group includes the most nutrient-dense sources of calcium. The background color of each food group indicates the average amount of calcium in that group. Additional calcium-fortified foods appear in stores each year and thus will add to the food sources currently listed for various groups.

Chapter 5, when people with elevated LDL-cholesterol consume a low-fat, low-cholesterol diet, intakes of calcium at 1200 milligrams per day further reduces LDL-cholesterol. An adequate calcium intake might also reduce the risk of premenstrual syndrome in women. Practical dietary recommendations stemming from all of this research indicate that meeting the Adequate Intake for calcium or exceeding it somewhat may be beneficial for a variety of conditions, not just bone health.

■ Calcium in Foods and Needs

Dairy products, such as milk and cheese, provide about 75% of the calcium in North American diets. The exception is cottage cheese, because most calcium is lost during production. Bread, rolls, crackers, and other foods made with milk products are secondary contributors. Other calcium sources are leafy greens (such as spinach), broccoli, sardines, and canned salmon. However, much of the calcium in some leafy green vegetables, notably spinach, is not absorbed because of the presence of oxalic acid. This effect is not as strong, however, in kale, collard, turnip, and mustard greens. Overall, nonfat milk is the most nutrient-dense (milligrams per kcal) source of calcium because of its high bioavailability and low energy value, with some of the vegetables just noted following close behind (Fig. 9.5). The new calcium-fortified versions of orange juice and other beverages, as well as calcium-fortified cottage cheese, breakfast cereals, breakfast bars, snacks, and certain chewable chocolate candies, also follow as close competitors. Another source of calcium is soybean curd (tofu) if it is made with calcium carbonate (check the label). Note that it is the bones in canned fish, such as salmon and sardines, that supply the calcium.

One reason why the Food Guide Pyramid contains a milk, yogurt, and cheese group is to supply calcium to the diet. People who do not like milk can use products

Food Sources of Calcium

Food item and amount	Calcium (milligrams)
Parmesan cheese, 2 ounces	780
Romano cheese, 2 ounces	605
Swiss cheese, 2 ounces	545
Plain yogurt, 1 cup	450
Fortified orange juice, 1 cup	350
Cheddar cheese, 1.5 ounces	305
1% milk, 1 cup	300
Buttermilk, 1 cup	285
Spinach, 1 cup	250
Salmon, 3 ounces	210
Total Raisin Bran cereal, ¾ cup	180
Sardines, 2 ounces	170
Chocolate pudding, ½ cup	160
Tofu, ½ cup	140

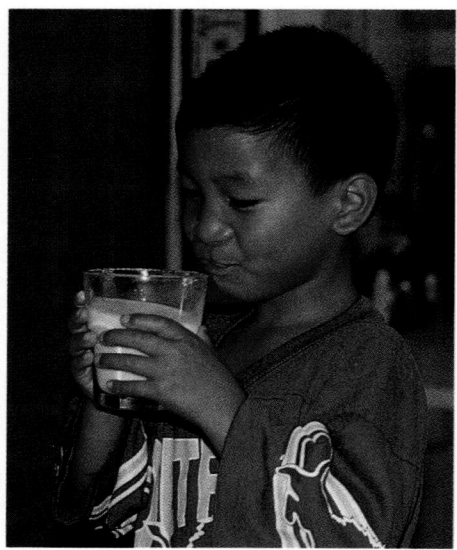

Milk products, and milk itself, are common sources of calcium in the North American diet.

made with milk, such as chocolate milk, yogurt, cheese, and ice cream. All forms of milk, yogurt, and cheese allow about the same degree of calcium absorption. Moderation in use of either cheese or ice cream as a calcium source is advised, because they are usually high in saturated fat. However, some low-fat cheeses and frozen desserts are good calcium sources and have a low saturated fat content.

Information about calcium is mandatory on food labels. The Daily Value for calcium used for food and supplement labels is 1000 milligrams.

The Adequate Intake for calcium for adults ranges from 1000 to 1200 milligrams per day. In the United States, average calcium intakes range from only approximately 600 to 800 for women and 800 to 1000 for men. Thus, dietary intakes of calcium by many women, especially young women, are well below the Adequate Intake, whereas intakes by most men are roughly equivalent to the Adequate Intake. The greater food consumption by men, to support their higher energy outputs, accounts for part of the difference. An easy way for women to increase calcium intake is to increase their physical activity and, in turn, their food consumption. It is especially important for vegetarians to focus on eating good plant sources of calcium as well as on the total amount of calcium ingested.

To estimate your calcium intake, use the rule of 300s. Give yourself 300 milligrams to account for calcium in the small amounts provided by a moderate energy intake from foods scattered throughout the diet. Add to that another 300 milligrams for every cup of milk or yogurt or 1.5 ounces of cheese. If you eat a lot of tofu, almonds, or sardines, or drink calcium-fortified beverages, use Table 9.5 or your diet analysis software to get a more accurate account of your calcium intake.

■ Calcium Supplements

Calcium supplements can be used by people who don't like milk or who can't incorporate enough milk products, foods made with milk, or calcium-fortified foods into their diet. Calcium carbonate, the form commonly found in calcium-based antacid tablets, is the most common supplement used. People with ample output of stomach acid should take this supplement at bedtime or between meals in doses of about 500 milligrams. This practice enhances absorption and limits its negative impact on absorption of other minerals. People with low acid production, such as older adults, should take the calcium carbonate supplement with meals, so that what little acid is produced during digestion can aid absorption. People with low acid production also can use a supplement containing calcium citrate, which is acidic itself, between meals.

Overall, taking 1000 milligrams of calcium daily in divided doses of about 500 milligrams in the form of calcium carbonate or calcium citrate is probably safe, but people using a supplement should notify their physician of the practice. Still, many people have difficulty adhering to a supplement regimen. In contrast, regular food habits can likely be integrated easily into a routine. In addition, it is difficult to consume an excess amount of calcium using foods. All of this points to focusing first on improving diet when addressing calcium needs.

Some calcium supplements pose a risk for lead toxicity. Chapter 16 points out that lead produces an array of deleterious effects on the body. Currently, FDA has no standards for lead in food supplements. However, FDA does plan to regulate the lead content of supplements, including calcium, in the future. Until then, it is important to avoid bonemeal, the worst offender when it comes to lead. Tablet or liquid calcium supplements with the USP seal of approval are less likely than others to contain high concentrations of lead or other contaminants.

An intake of more than 2000 milligrams of calcium per day in some people can cause high blood and urinary calcium concentrations, irritability, headache, kidney failure, soft tissue calcification, kidney stones, decreased absorption of other minerals, and possibly prostate cancer. Note that the Upper Level for calcium intake is 2500 milligrams per day, based on the observation that greater intakes increase the risk for some forms of kidney stones.

*S*ome calcium supplements are poorly digested because they do not readily dissolve. To test for this, put a supplement in ¾ cup of cider vinegar. Stir every 5 minutes. It should dissolve within 30 minutes.

Table 9.5 A Tool for Estimating Current Calcium Intake

For all of the following foods, write the number of servings eaten in a day. Total the number of servings in each category and then multiply the totals by the milligrams of calcium for each category. Finally, add the total milligrams to estimate calcium intake for that day.

Food	Serving Size	Number of Servings	Calcium (milligrams)	Total Calcium (milligrams)
Plain low-fat yogurt	1 cup	_____		
Nonfat dry milk powder	½ cup	_____		
	Total servings	_____	× 400	= _____ milligrams
Canned sardines (with bones)	3 ounces	_____		
Fruit-flavored yogurt	1 cup	_____		
Skim or low-fat milk, buttermilk	1 cup	_____		
Whole milk, chocolate milk	1 cup	_____		
Parmesan cheese (grated)	¼ cup	_____		
Swiss cheese	1 ounce	_____		
	Total servings	_____	× 300	= _____ milligrams
Cheese (all other hard cheese)	1 ounce	_____		
Pancakes	3	_____		
	Total servings	_____	× 200	= _____ milligrams
Canned pink salmon	3 ounces	_____		
Tofu (processed with calcium)	4 ounces	_____		
	Total servings	_____	× 150	= _____ milligrams
Collards or turnip greens, cooked	½ cup	_____		
Ice cream or ice milk	½ cup	_____		
Almonds	1 ounce	_____		
	Total servings	_____	× 75	= _____ milligrams
Chard, cooked	½ cup	_____		
Cottage cheese	½ cup	_____		
Corn tortilla	1 medium	_____		
Orange	1 medium	_____		
	Total servings	_____	× 50	= _____ milligrams
Kidney, lima, or navy beans, cooked	½ cup	_____		
Broccoli	½ cup	_____		
Carrot, raw	1 medium	_____		
Dates or raisins	¼ cup	_____		
Egg	1 large	_____		
Whole-wheat bread	1 slice	_____		
Peanut butter	2 tablespoons	_____		
	Total servings	_____	× 25	= _____ milligrams
Calcium-fortified orange juice	6 ounces	_____		
Calcium-fortified snack bars	1 each	_____		
Calcium-fortified breakfast bars	½ bar	_____		
	Total servings	_____	× 200	= _____ milligrams
Calcium supplements	1 each	_____	× 500	= _____ milligrams
			Total calcium intake	= _____ milligrams

Other calcium sources to consider include many breakfast cereals (100 to 250 milligrams per cup), calcium-fortified chewable chocolate candies (500 milligrams per serving), and some vitamins/mineral supplements (up to 500 milligrams per tablet).

Reprinted with permission from *Topics in Clinical Nutrition,* "Putting Calcium into Perspective for Your Clients," G. Wardlaw and N. Weese; 11:1, p. 29. © 1995 Aspen Publishers, Inc.

Scenario Follow-Up

Jana is increasing her chances of developing osteoporosis later in life because of her current high-risk lifestyle. Many factors contributing to her potential risk include physical inactivity, smoking, and poor dietary intake of calcium and other important minerals. If Jana remains a vegan, she especially needs to find some reliable sources of calcium. These could include calcium-fortified juices, calcium-fortified bread and snack bars, and calcium-fortified chewable chocolate candies. Tofu (made with calcium) is another potential source, as well as calcium-fortified soy milk. Meeting the Adequate Intake of 1300 milligrams per day for her age would not be that hard if she were to make a conscious effort to use these calcium-rich foods and/or find other rich sources.

Concept Check

About 99% of calcium in the body is found in the bones. Aside from its critical role in bone, calcium also functions in blood clotting, muscle contraction, nerve- impulse transmission, and cell metabolism. Calcium requires a slightly acid pH and the vitamin D hormone for efficient absorption. Factors that reduce calcium absorption include a vitamin D deficiency, large amounts of dietary fiber (especially excess wheat bran), decreased estrogen in the bloodstream, and old age in general. Blood calcium is regulated primarily by hormones and does not closely reflect daily intake.

Dairy products are rich food sources of calcium. Other foods, such as calcium-fortified beverages, are rich sources as well. Supplemental forms, such as calcium carbonate, are well-absorbed by most people. However, overzealous supplementation can also result in the development of kidney stones and other health problems.

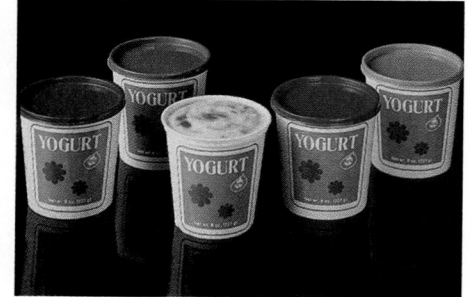

Milk products provide much of the phosphorus we consume, as do meat and grain products.

Food Sources of Phosphorus

Food item and amount	Phosphorus (milligrams)
Plain yogurt, 1 cup	350
Swiss cheese, 2 ounces	345
Almonds, ½ cup	340
Sunflower seeds, 1 ounce	330
1% milk, 1 cup	235
Cheddar cheese, 1.5 ounces	220
Salmon, 3 ounces	220
Sirloin steak, 3 ounces	210
Raisin Bran cereal, 1 cup	215
Egg, 2 hard-boiled	200
Chicken breast, 3 ounces	180
Roasted turkey, 3 ounces	180
Pot roast, 3 ounces	170
Lean ham, 3 ounces	165
American cheese, 1 slice	155

Phosphorus (P)

Although no disease is currently associated with an inadequate phosphorus intake, a deficiency may contribute to bone loss in older women. The body absorbs phosphorus quite efficiently, about 70% of dietary intake. This high absorption, plus the wide availability of phosphorus in foods, makes this mineral less important than is calcium in diet planning. The active vitamin D hormone enhances phosphorus absorption, as it does for calcium. Kidney excretion primarily regulates blood phosphorus. This regulating mechanism differs from that of calcium, wherein changes in the degree of absorption are a more significant factor.

Phosphorus is a component of enzymes, other key metabolic compounds (many of which are involved in energy metabolism), DNA (genetic material), cell membranes, and bone. About 85% of the body's phosphorus is inside bone. The remaining phosphorus circulates freely in the bloodstream and functions inside cells.

■ Phosphorus in Foods and Needs

Milk, cheese, meat, and bread provide most of the phosphorus in the adult diet. Breakfast cereals, bran, eggs, nuts, and fish are also good sources. About 20% to 30% of dietary phosphorus comes from food additives, especially in baked goods, cheeses, processed meats, and many soft drinks (about 75 milligrams per 12-ounce—⅓-liter—serving of soft drinks). Next time you have a soft drink, look for a listing of phosphoric acid on the label.

The RDA for phosphorus for adults over age 18 is 700 milligrams daily. The Daily Value used on food and supplement labels is 1000 milligrams. Adults consume from about 1000 to 1600 milligrams of phosphorus per day. Thus, deficiencies of phosphorus are unlikely in healthy adults, especially because it is so efficiently absorbed.

Marginal phosphorus status can be found in premature infants, vegans, people with alcoholism, older people on nutrient-poor diets, and people with long-term bouts of diarrhea.

Typical phosphorus intakes in and of themselves do not appear to be toxic for healthy adults, but high amounts can lead to problems in people with certain kidney diseases. In addition, chronic imbalance in the calcium-to-phosphorus ratio in the diet, resulting from a high phosphorus intake coupled with a low calcium intake, also can contribute to bone loss. This situation most likely arises when the Adequate Intake for calcium is not met, as can occur in adolescents and adults who regularly substitute soft drinks for milk or otherwise underconsume calcium. The Upper Level for phosphorus intake is 3 to 4 grams per day. Intakes greater than this impair kidney function.

Magnesium (Mg)

Magnesium is important for nerve and heart function and aids many enzyme reactions. It is found mostly in the plant pigment chlorophyll, where it functions in respiration. We normally absorb about 40% to 60% of the magnesium in our diets, but absorption efficiency can increase up to about 80% if intakes are low.

Bone contains 60% of the body's magnesium. The rest circulates in the blood and operates inside cells. Over 300 enzymes use magnesium, and many energy-yielding compounds in cells require magnesium to function properly, as does the hormone insulin.

Animals deficient in magnesium become very irritable and, with severe deficiency, eventually suffer convulsions and often die. In humans, a magnesium deficiency causes an irregular heartbeat, sometimes accompanied by weakness, muscle pain, disorientation, and seizures. Other possible benefits of magnesium in relation to heart disease include decreasing blood pressure by dilating arteries, preventing heart rhythm abnormalities, and inhibiting blood clotting. People with cardiovascular disease should closely monitor intake, especially because they are often on medications such as some diuretics that reduce magnesium status. Keep in mind that a magnesium deficiency develops very slowly, because our bodies store it readily.

■ Magnesium in Foods and Needs

Rich sources for magnesium are plant products, such as whole grains (like wheat bran), broccoli, potatoes, squash, beans, nuts, and seeds. Animal products, such as milk and meats, and even chocolate supply some magnesium, although less than the foods in the previous list (Fig. 9.6). Two other sources of magnesium are hard tap water, which contains a high mineral content, and coffee.

The adult RDA for magnesium is about 420 milligrams per day for men and about 320 milligrams per day for women. The Daily Value used on food and supplement labels is 400 milligrams. Adult men consume an average of 325 milligrams daily, whereas women consume closer to 225 milligrams daily. Women especially should find some good sources of magnesium that they like and eat them regularly. In addition, a balanced multivitamin and mineral supplement generally yields 100 milligrams, and so closes this gap if one is taken on a regular basis.

Poor magnesium status is especially found among users of certain diuretics, as noted earlier. In addition, heavy perspiration for weeks in hot climates and bouts of long-standing diarrhea or vomiting all cause significant magnesium loss. Alcoholism also increases the risk of a deficiency because dietary intake may be poor and because alcohol increases magnesium excretion in the urine. The disorientation and weakness associated with alcoholism closely resemble the behavior of people with low blood magnesium.

Food Sources of Magnesium

Food item and amount	Magnesium (milligrams)
Spinach, 1 cup	157
Squash, 1 cup	105
Wheat germ, ¼ cup	90
Raisin Bran cereal, 1 cup	90
Navy beans, ½ cup	54
Peanut butter, 2 tablespoons	51
Black-eyed peas, ½ cup	46
Plain yogurt, 1 cup	43
Kidney beans, ½ cup	43
Sunflower seeds, ¼ cup	41
Broccoli, 1 cup	37
Banana, 1 medium	34
1% milk, 1 cup	34
Watermelon, 1 slice	32
Oatmeal, ½ cup	28
Whole-wheat bread, 1 slice	25

Figure 9.6 Food sources of magnesium from the Food Guide Pyramid. The vegetable group and whole-grain choices in the bread, cereal, rice, and pasta group are the most nutrient-dense sources of magnesium. The background color of each food group indicates the average amount of magnesium in that group.

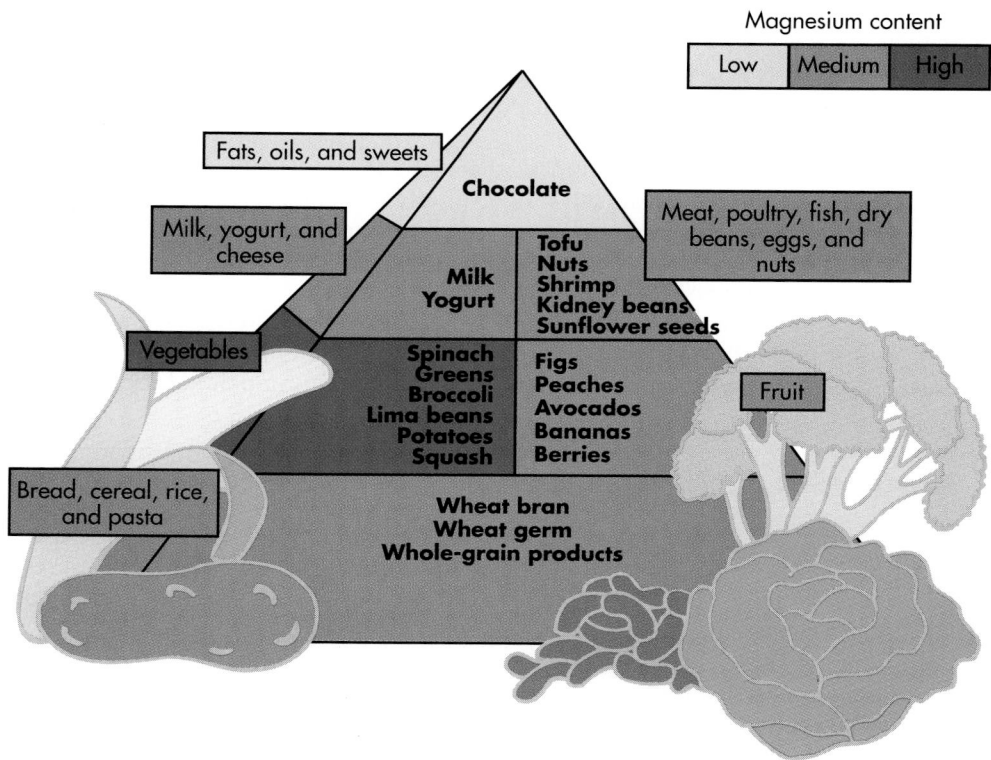

Magnesium content

| Low | Medium | High |

Fats, oils, and sweets
Chocolate

Milk, yogurt, and cheese

Tofu
Nuts
Shrimp
Kidney beans
Sunflower seeds

Meat, poultry, fish, dry beans, eggs, and nuts

Milk
Yogurt

Vegetables

Spinach
Greens
Broccoli
Lima beans
Potatoes
Squash

Figs
Peaches
Avocados
Bananas
Berries

Fruit

Bread, cereal, rice, and pasta

Wheat bran
Wheat germ
Whole-grain products

Magnesium toxicity typically occurs only in people who have kidney failure or who overuse over-the-counter medications that contain magnesium, such as certain antacids and laxatives. Older people are at particular risk, as kidney function may be compromised. The Upper Level for magnesium intake is 350 milligrams per day, based on the risk of developing diarrhea. Note, however, that this guideline refers only to nonfood sources such as the medications listed previously or supplements.

Sulfur (S)

Sulfur is found in many important compounds in the body, such as some amino acids (like methionine) and the vitamins biotin and thiamin. Sulfur helps in the balance of acids and bases in the body and is an important part of the liver's drug-detoxifying pathways. Because proteins supply the sulfur we need, sulfur is naturally a part of a healthy diet. Sulfur compounds are also used to preserve foods (see Chapter 16).

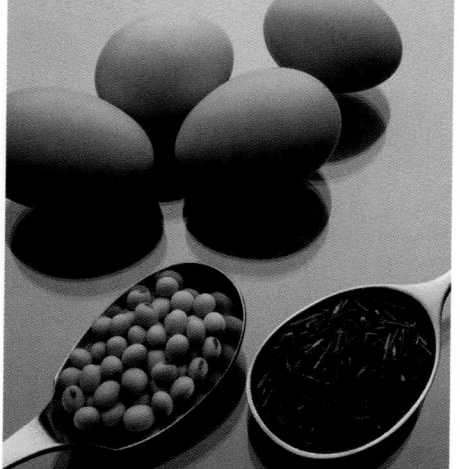

Protein-rich foods supply sulfur in the diet.

Concept Check

Phosphorus absorption is quite efficient and is enhanced by the active vitamin D hormone. Urinary excretion mainly controls body content. Phosphorus aids enzyme function and is part of key metabolic compounds and cell membranes. No distinct deficiency symptoms caused by an inadequate phosphorus intake have been reported. Food sources for phosphorus include dairy products, baked goods, and meat. The RDA is met by most North Americans. An excess intake of phosphorus can compromise bone health if sufficient calcium is not otherwise consumed, and can impair kidney function. Magnesium is required for nerve and heart function; it also aids activity for many enzymes. Food sources of magnesium are whole grains (wheat bran), broccoli, squash, beef, coffee, beans, nuts, and seeds. People using certain diuretics and people with alcoholism are at greatest risk of developing a deficiency. Magnesium toxicity is most likely in people with kidney failure or people using certain forms of laxatives and antacids. Sulfur is a component of certain vitamins and amino acids. The protein we consume supplies sufficient sulfur for the body's needs.

Trace Minerals—An Overview

Information about trace minerals is perhaps the most rapidly expanding area of knowledge in nutrition. With the exceptions of iron and iodine, the importance of trace minerals to humans has been recognized only within the last 30 years. Although we need only about 20 milligrams—or less—of each trace mineral daily, they are just as essential to good health as are major minerals.

In some cases, discovering the importance of a trace mineral reads like a detective story, and the evidence is still unfolding. In 1961, researchers linked dwarfism in Middle Eastern villagers to a zinc deficiency. Other scientists recognized that a rare form of heart disease in an isolated area of China was linked to a selenium deficiency. In North America, some trace mineral deficiencies were first observed in the late 1960s and early 1970s when the minerals were not added to synthetic formulas used for intravenous feeding.

It is difficult to define precisely our trace mineral needs because we need only minute amounts. Highly sophisticated technology is required to measure such small amounts in both food and body tissues.

See Table 9.6 to see what we know about the trace minerals.

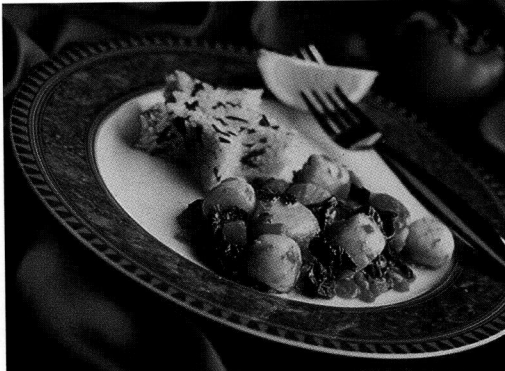

Seafood, like scallops, is a rich source of many trace minerals.

Iron (Fe)

The importance of dietary iron has been recognized for centuries. In 4000 B.C., the Persian physician Melampus gave iron supplements to sailors to make up for iron lost from bleeding wounds during battles. Today, iron deficiency is one of the most common nutrient deficiencies worldwide. Iron is the only nutrient for which adult women have a greater RDA than do adult men. Iron is found in every living cell, adding up to about 5 grams (1 teaspoon) for the entire body.

■ Absorption and Distribution of Iron

The body uses several mechanisms to regulate iron absorption. Controlling absorption is important because our bodies cannot easily eliminate excess iron once it is absorbed. Iron absorption from foods is about 15% of that present for healthy people, and up to 20% in people with iron deficiency. Overall, iron absorption depends on its form in the food, the body's need for it, and a variety of other factors.

The form of iron in foods especially influences how much is absorbed. About 40% of the total iron in animal flesh is in the form of **hemoglobin** (the same form as in red blood cells) and **myoglobin** (pigment found in muscle cells). This **heme iron** is absorbed more than twice as efficiently as the simple elemental iron, called **nonheme iron.** Nonheme iron is also present in animal flesh, as well as in eggs, milk, vegetables, grains, and other plant foods.

hemoglobin The iron-containing part of the red blood cell that carries oxygen to the cells and some carbon dioxide away from the cells. It is also responsible for the red color of blood.

myoglobin Iron-containing compound that binds oxygen in muscle tissue.

heme iron Iron provided from animal tissues in the form of hemoglobin and myoglobin. Approximately 40% of the iron in meat is heme iron; it is readily absorbed.

nonheme iron Iron provided from plant sources and animal tissues other than in the forms of hemoglobin and myoglobin. Nonheme iron is less efficiently absorbed than heme iron.

Table 9.6 A Summary of Key Trace Minerals: Their Functions, Deficiency Conditions, and Food Sources

Mineral	Major Functions	Deficiency Symptoms	People Most at Risk	RDA or Adequate Intake	Nutrient-Dense Dietary Sources	Results of Toxicity
Iron	Functional component of hemoglobin and other key compounds used in respiration; immune function; cognitive development	Fatigue; small, pale red blood cells; low blood hemoglobin values	Infants, preschool children, adolescents, women in childbearing years	Men: 8 milligrams Women: 18 milligrams	Meats, seafood, broccoli, peas, bran, enriched breads	Gastrointestinal upset; toxicity especially seen when children consume many iron pills; toxicity also seen in people with hemochromatosis; Upper Level is 45 milligrams per day
Zinc	Required for nearly 100 enzymes, including enzymes involved in growth, immunity, alcohol metabolism, sexual development, reproduction	Skin rash, diarrhea, decreased appetite and sense of taste, hair loss, poor growth and development, poor wound healing	Vegetarians, elderly people, people with alcoholism	Men: 11 milligrams Women: 8 milligrams	Seafoods, meats, greens, whole grains	Supplement use can reduce copper absorption; can cause diarrhea, cramps, depressed immune function; Upper Level is 40 milligrams per day
Copper	Aids in iron metabolism; works with many antioxidant enzymes, and those involved in protein metabolism and hormone synthesis	Anemia, low white blood cell count, poor growth	Infants recovering from semistarvation, overzealous supplementation of zinc	900 micrograms	Liver, cocoa, beans, nuts, whole grains, dried fruits	Supplement use can cause vomiting; nervous system disorders; Upper Level is 8–10 milligrams per day
Selenium	Part of an antioxidant system	Muscle pain, muscle weakness, form of heart disease	Unknown	55 micrograms	Meats, eggs, fish, seafoods, whole grains	Supplement use can cause nausea, vomiting, hair loss, weakness, liver disease; Upper Level is 400 micrograms per day
Iodide	Component of thyroid hormones	Goiter; mental retardation, poor growth in infancy when mother is iodide deficient during pregnancy	Few people in North America, because salt is usually fortified	150 micrograms	Iodized salt, white bread, saltwater fish, dairy products	Inhibition of function of the thyroid gland; Upper Level is 1.1 milligrams per day
Fluoride	Increases resistance of tooth enamel to dental caries	Increased risk of dental caries	Areas where water is not fluoridated and dental treatments do not make up for a lack of fluoride	Men: 3.8 milligrams Women: 3.1 milligrams	Fluoridated water, toothpaste, dental treatments, tea, seaweed	Stomach upset; mottling (staining) of teeth during development; bone pain; Upper Level is 10 milligrams per day
Chromium	Enhances insulin action	High blood glucose after eating	People on intravenous total parenteral nutrition, perhaps older adults with type 2 diabetes	25–35 micrograms	Egg yolks, whole grains, pork, nuts, mushrooms, beer	Caused by industrial contamination, not dietary excess; no Upper Level set
Manganese	Cofactor of some enzymes, such as those involved in carbohydrate metabolism	None in humans	Unknown	1.8–2.3 milligrams	Nuts, oats, beans, tea	Nervous system disorders; Upper Level is 11 milligrams per day
Molybdenum	Aids action of some enzymes	None in healthy humans	Unsupplemented total parenteral nutrition support	45 micrograms	Beans, grains, nuts	Poor growth in laboratory animals; Upper Level is 2 milligrams per day

Consuming heme iron and nonheme iron together increases nonheme iron absorption. A protein factor in meats may also aid nonheme absorption. Overall, eating meat with vegetables and grain products enhances the absorption of all nonheme iron present.

Vitamin C in amounts of about 75 milligrams can increase nonheme iron absorption. So when taking an iron supplement, one should consider drinking a glass of orange juice with it. Consuming more foods rich in vitamin C is particularly desirable if dietary iron is inadequate or if blood iron is low. Iron use in the body is also aided by copper, as explained in the later section on copper.

Several dietary factors interfere with our ability to absorb iron. Phytic acid and other factors in grain fibers and oxalic acid in vegetables can all bind iron and reduce its absorption. Polyphenols (tannins) found in tea also reduce iron absorption. It is a good idea to moderate intake of tannins if one has iron deficiency and keep dietary-fiber intake within 30 grams a day. Zinc also interferes with iron by competing with it for absorption. Finally, high-dose calcium supplements can also bind with iron when both are in the same meal—an important consideration when taking more than 500 milligrams in supplement form per occasion. In fact, experts suggest that adolescents, and menstruating and pregnant women take any calcium supplements at bedtime or between meals to avoid this interference, as noted earlier.

Overall, the most important factor influencing iron absorption is the body's need for it. In a deficiency state, iron absorption can increase. When iron stores are inadequate, the main blood protein that carries iron readily binds more iron, shifting it from intestinal cells into the bloodstream. If iron stores are adequate and the iron-binding protein in the blood is fully saturated with iron, little will be absorbed from the intestinal cells. It stays bound in the intestinal cells.

By this mechanism, in normal circumstances, iron is absorbed for the most part as needed. If not needed, when intestinal cells are shed at the end of their 2- to 5-day cycle, the iron returns to the lumen of the intestinal tract. This whole process is referred to as a "mucosal block" against excess iron absorption. High doses of iron can still be toxic, but absorption is carefully regulated under typical dietary conditions in most people.

Most iron in the body is contained in the hemoglobin molecules of the red blood cells. Some iron is stored in the bone marrow, and a small portion goes to other body cells, such as the liver, for storage. As iron is needed, it can be mobilized from body stores. If dietary intake is inadequate, these iron stores become depleted. Only then do signs of an iron deficiency appear.

■ Functions of Iron

Iron forms part of the hemoglobin in red blood cells and myoglobin in muscle cells. Hemoglobin molecules in red blood cells transport oxygen (O_2) from the lungs to cells and assist in the return of some carbon dioxide (CO_2) from cells to the lungs for excretion. In addition, iron is used as part of many enzymes, some proteins, and compounds that cells use in energy production. Iron is also needed for brain and immune function, and contributes to drug detoxification in the liver.

If neither the diet nor body stores can supply the iron needed for hemoglobin synthesis, the number of red blood cells decreases in the bloodstream. The blood hemoglobin concentration also falls. When both the percentage of red blood cells (called the **hematocrit**) and the hemoglobin concentration fall, a physician suspects iron deficiency. Physicians also use these two measures to assess iron status, along with the amount of iron and iron-containing proteins in the bloodstream. In severe deficiency, hemoglobin and hematocrit fall so low that the amount of oxygen carried in the bloodstream is decreased. Such a person has anemia, defined as a decreased oxygen-carrying capacity of the blood.

While there are many types of anemia, iron-deficiency anemia is the major type worldwide. About 30% of the world's population is anemic, and about half of those

hematocrit The percentage of blood that is made up of red blood cells.

cases are caused by an iron deficiency. Probably about 10% of North Americans in high-risk categories have iron-deficiency anemia. This appears most often in infancy, the preschool years, and at puberty for both males and females. Growth, with accompanying expansion of blood volume and muscle mass, increases iron needs, making it difficult to consume enough iron. Women are also very vulnerable during childbearing years when menstruation occurs. In addition, anemia is often found in pregnant women, as discussed in Chapter 13. Iron-deficiency anemia in adult men is usually caused by blood loss from ulcers, colon cancer, or hemorrhoids. Finally, athletes can develop anemia, as discussed in Chapter 11.

Clinical symptoms of iron-deficiency anemia primarily include pale skin, fatigue upon exertion, poor temperature regulation, loss of appetite, and apathy. Insufficient iron for the synthesis of red blood cells and key cell compounds may cause the fatigue. Poor iron stores may also decrease learning ability, attention span, work performance, and immune status even before a person is actually anemic.

More North Americans have an iron deficiency than iron-deficiency anemia. Their blood hemoglobin values are still normal, but they have no stores to draw from in times of pregnancy or illness, and basic functioning may not be up to par. That could mean anything from too little energy to perform everyday tasks in an efficient manner to difficulties staying alert in school or on the job.

To speed the cure of iron-deficiency anemia, a person needs to take iron supplements. A physician should also find the cause—an inadequate diet or a bleeding ulcer, for example—so that the anemia does not recur. Changes in diet may prevent iron-deficiency anemia, but supplemental iron is the only reliable cure.

◼ Iron in Foods and Needs

Animal sources contain some heme iron, the most bioavailable form. These then end up our best iron sources. Iron present in supplements is also absorbed well. The major iron sources in the adult diet are ready-to-eat breakfast cereals, animal products, and bakery items, such as bread (Fig. 9.7). Most of the iron in these bakery items has been added to refined flour in the enrichment process. Other iron sources are spinach, peas, and legumes, but the iron is less available in these foods than in animal products.

The use of iron-fortified formulas and cereals in the Special Supplemental Nutrition Program for Women, Infant, and Children (WIC) in the United States has been a major contributor to decreasing rates of iron-deficiency anemia in infants and preschool children (see Chapter 14).

Milk is a very poor source of iron. A common cause of iron-deficiency anemia in children is an overreliance on milk, coupled with an insufficient meat intake. Total vegetarians (vegans) are particularly susceptible to iron-deficiency anemia because of their lack of dietary heme iron.

The daily adult RDA for iron is 8 milligrams for men, as well as for women over 50 years, and 18 milligrams for women ages 19 to 50 years. The Daily Value used on food and supplement labels is 18 milligrams. The RDA value assumes that on average 18% of dietary iron is absorbed. If iron absorption exceeds that, less dietary iron is needed.

The higher RDA for young and middle-aged women is primarily because of menstrual blood loss. Women who menstruate more heavily and longer than average may need even more dietary iron, and those who have lighter and shorter flows may need less iron. The variation in menstrual blood loss, and hence, loss of iron, makes it difficult to set an RDA for iron for women.

By recording dietary intakes from a variety of young and middle-aged women, researchers find that most women do not consume 18 milligrams of iron daily. The average daily value is closer to 12 milligrams, while in men it is about 17 milligrams per day. Women can easily close this gap between average daily intakes and needs by

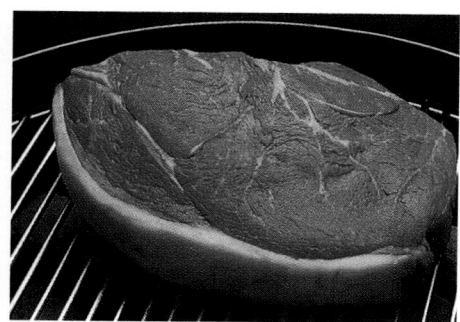

Red meat is a major source of iron in the North American diet. Currently, many experts suggest we limit red meat intake to two to three times per week because it is linked to an increase in colon cancer risk and instead seek other iron-rich sources.

Food Sources of Iron

Food item and amount	Iron (milligrams)
Oat bran cereal, 1 cup	15.0
Baked clams, 3 ounces	14.0
Spinach, 1 cup	6.4
Kidney beans, 1 cup	5.3
Pot roast, 4 ounces	3.9
Sirloin steak, 4 ounces	3.8
Parsley, 1 cup	3.7
Fried beef liver, 2 ounces	3.6
Shrimp, 3 ounces	2.7
Braunschweiger sausage, 1 piece	2.7
Flour tortilla, 1	2.4
Garbanzo beans, ½ cup	2.4
Navy beans, ½ cup	2.3
Baked potato, 1	1.7
Artichoke, 1	1.6

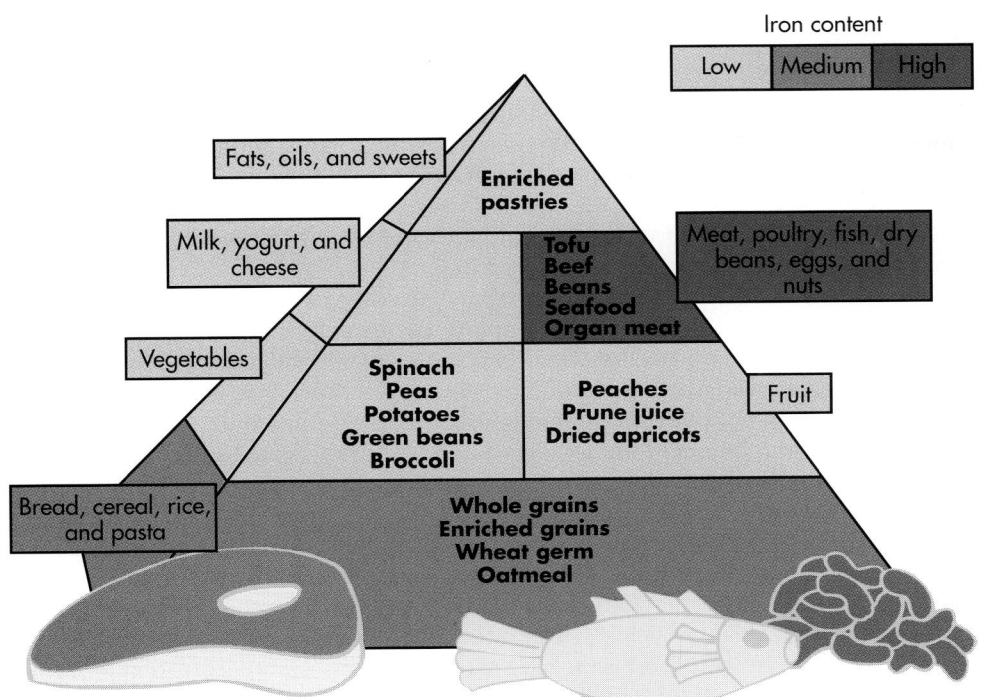

Iron content

| Low | Medium | High |

Fats, oils, and sweets

Enriched pastries

Milk, yogurt, and cheese

**Tofu
Beef
Beans
Seafood
Organ meat**

Meat, poultry, fish, dry beans, eggs, and nuts

Vegetables

**Spinach
Peas
Potatoes
Green beans
Broccoli**

**Peaches
Prune juice
Dried apricots**

Fruit

Bread, cereal, rice, and pasta

**Whole grains
Enriched grains
Wheat germ
Oatmeal**

Figure 9.7 Food sources of iron from the Food Guide Pyramid. The meat, poultry, fish, dry beans, eggs, and nuts group and the bread, cereal, rice, and pasta group are the most nutrient-dense sources of iron. The heme iron in the meat, poultry, fish, dry beans, eggs, and nuts group is especially well absorbed. The iron content of a food containing mostly nonheme iron is only an approximate measure of the amount delivered to body cells, as body need greatly influences the absorption of nonheme iron. The background color of each food group indicates the average amount of iron in that group.

seeking out iron-fortified foods, such as ready-to-eat breakfast cereals that contain at least 50% of the Daily Value. Use of a balanced multivitamin and mineral supplement containing up to 100% of the Daily Value for iron is another option. Consuming more than that much iron is not advised unless a physician suggests otherwise, such as to compensate for heavy monthly menstrual losses.

Another Bite

*T*he adult human body contains about 21 cups (5 liters) of blood. Blood donations are generally 2 cups (500 milliliters). Thus, a blood donor gives about a tenth of his or her total supply. Healthy people generally can donate blood two to four times a year without harmful consequences. As a precaution, blood banks first screen potential donors' blood for the presence of anemia.

■ Toxicity of Iron

The Upper Level for iron is 45 milligrams per day. Higher amounts can lead to stomach irritation. Although iron overload is not as common as iron deficiency, it can be a serious result of misuse because it can easily build up in the body and lead to toxic symptoms. Even a large single dose of iron of 60 milligrams can be life-threatening to a 1-year-old. Children are frequently victims of iron poisoning because iron pills and nutrient supplements containing iron are tempting targets on kitchen tables and in cabinets. FDA has recently ruled that all iron supplements must carry a warning about toxicity, and those with 30 milligrams of iron or more per tablet must be individually wrapped.

Smaller does of iron (but still greater than what is needed) over a long period can also cause problems. A form of iron toxicity, for example, has been observed in an African tribe that brews beer in iron pots. Some people of Mediterranean descent have

hemochromatosis A disorder of iron metabolism characterized by increased iron absorption and deposition in the liver and heart tissue. This eventually poisons the cells in those organs.

a type of anemia caused by increased destruction of red blood cells; low-dose iron therapy used to treat this disease can lead to toxicity symptoms. Repeated blood transfusions can also lead to iron toxicity.

In addition, iron toxicity accompanies the genetic disease called hereditary **hemochromatosis.** The disease is associated with a substantial increase in iron absorption. For people with this disease, iron in the body eventually builds up to dangerous amounts, especially in the blood and liver. Some iron is deposited in the muscles, pancreas, and heart. If not treated, the excess iron deposits contribute to severe organ damage, especially in the liver and heart.

Hereditary hemochromatosis requires that a person carry two defective copies of a particular gene to develop the disease. People with one defective gene and one normal gene, called carriers, may also absorb too much dietary iron but not to the same extent as those with two defective genes. About 5% to 10% of North Americans of Northern European extraction are carriers of hemochromatosis. Approximately 1 in 250 North Americans has both hemochromatosis genes. These numbers are high considering the fact that many physicians regard hemochromatosis as a rare disease and thus do not routinely test for it.

Carriers of one hemochromatosis gene may be prime candidates for cardiovascular disease, especially men. As noted in Chapter 5, excess iron in the blood may accelerate atherosclerosis in people with elevated LDL-cholesterol by contributing to oxidation of lipids in the LDL particles. This in turn allows LDL to be taken up more readily by scavenger cells in the blood vessels. However, the importance of iron in stimulating atherosclerosis is still hotly debated. Because of its relatively efficient absorption, dietary heme iron, such as that found in red meats, poses the greatest risk in this regard. To put this relatively new research area into perspective, a reasonable approach is for you to ask to be screened for iron overload at your next visit to a physician (ask for a transferrin saturation test). Because hemochromatosis can go undetected until a person is in their fifties or sixties, some experts recommend screening for anyone over the age of 20. If the disease goes untreated, many organs will have literally rusted away by one's fifties or sixties. If you show evidence of hemochromatosis, it would be wise to undergo therapy. This includes regular blood donations and avoidance of both iron-rich foods and iron supplements (see the website www.americanhs.org).

Ideally, consent of a physician should precede any intake of iron from supplements, especially by men. When iron supplements are advised, there should be adequate follow-up so that supplementation does not exceed what is necessary. Probably the only factor keeping many people with hemochromatosis and carriers of one gene from experiencing serious effects of the disease is that they consume only a moderate amount of iron.

Concept Check

Iron is absorbed depending mostly on its form and the body's need for it. Absorption is affected by a "mucosal block," but excess iron intake can override the system, leading to toxicity. Iron absorption increases somewhat in the presence of vitamin C and meat protein and decreases in the presence of large amounts of calcium and some components of grain fiber, such as phytic acid. Iron is used in synthesizing hemoglobin and myoglobin, in supporting immune function, and in energy metabolism. An iron deficiency can cause decreased red blood cell synthesis, which can lead to anemia. It is particularly important for women of childbearing age to consume adequate iron, primarily to replace that lost in menstrual blood. Sources include red meat, pork, liver, enriched grains and cereals, and oysters. Iron toxicity usually results from a genetic disorder called hemochromatosis. This disease causes overabsorption and accumulation of iron, which can result in severe liver and heart damage. Because of the risk of toxicity, any use of iron supplements should be supervised by a physician.

Zinc (Zn)

Although zinc has been recognized as an essential nutrient in farm animals since the early 1900s, zinc deficiency was first recognized in humans in the early 1960s in Egypt and Iran. Zinc deficiencies were determined to cause growth retardation and poor sexual development in some groups of people, even though the zinc content of their diets was fairly high. However, the customary diet contained unleavened bread almost exclusively and little animal protein. Unleavened bread is very high in phytic acid and other factors that decrease zinc bioavailability. Parasite infestation and the practice of eating clay and other parts of soil also probably contributed to the severe zinc deficiency.

In North America, zinc deficiencies were first observed in the early 1970s in hospitalized patients who were fed only intravenously via total parenteral nutrition. Zinc was not added to those solutions at that time, but the protein source in the solutions was based on milk protein or a blood protein, which are both naturally rich in zinc. When the solutions were changed in the early 1970s to include mostly individual amino acids as the protein source, deficiency symptoms quickly developed because amino-acid formulas are low in zinc.

Symptoms of adult zinc deficiency include an acnelike rash, diarrhea, lack of appetite, reduced sense of taste and smell, and hair loss. In children and adolescents with zinc deficiency, growth, sexual development, and learning ability may also be hampered.

Like iron, zinc absorption is influenced by the foods a person ingests. About 40% of dietary zinc is absorbed, especially when animal protein sources are used and when the body needs more zinc. Most people worldwide rely on cereal grains (low in zinc) for their source of protein, energy, and zinc. This makes consuming adequate zinc a problem. In addition, high-dose calcium supplementation with meals causes up to a 50% decrease in zinc absorption. For this reason, groups of people with high calcium needs may need to increase zinc intake, as well as not take calcium supplements with meals that are rich in zinc. Finally, zinc competes with copper and iron absorption.

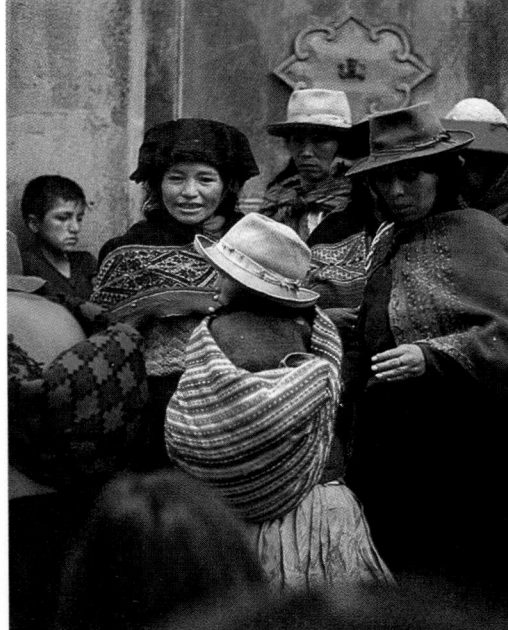

Minimal intakes of protein and zinc limit the growth of people worldwide.

Functions of Zinc

Nearly 100 enzymes require zinc as a cofactor for optimal activity, such as alcohol dehydrogenase. Adequate zinc intake is necessary to support many bodily functions, such as:

- DNA synthesis and function
- Protein metabolism, wound healing, and growth
- Immune function (intakes in excess of the RDA do not provide any extra benefit to immune function)
- Development of sexual organs and bone
- Storage, release, and function of insulin
- Cell membrane structure and function
- Component of superoxide dismutase, an enzyme that aids in the prevention of oxidative damage to cells

Other possible functions of zinc are slowing the progression of macular degeneration of the eye and reducing the risk for developing certain forms of cancer.

A recent study showed that megadose zinc supplements (80 milligrams per day) reduced progression of macular degeneration in people who showed evidence of the disease. The zinc supplements worked even better when provided in combination with 400 IU of vitamin E, 500 milligrams of vitamin C, and 15 milligrams of beta-carotene. Experts suggest that adults who have evidence of macular degeneration talk to their physicians about possibly following such a protocol.

Zinc in Foods and Needs

In general, protein-rich diets are also rich in zinc. Animal foods supply almost half our zinc intake. Major sources of zinc are beef, fortified breakfast cereals, milk, poultry, and bread. As with iron, bioavailability is also important to consider for zinc.

Figure 9.8 Food sources of zinc from the Food Guide Pyramid. The meat, poultry, fish, dry beans, eggs, and nuts group includes the most nutrient-dense sources of zinc. Some zinc is supplied by whole grains and fortified breakfast cereals from the bread, cereal, rice, and pasta group. The background color of each food group indicates the average amount of zinc in that group.

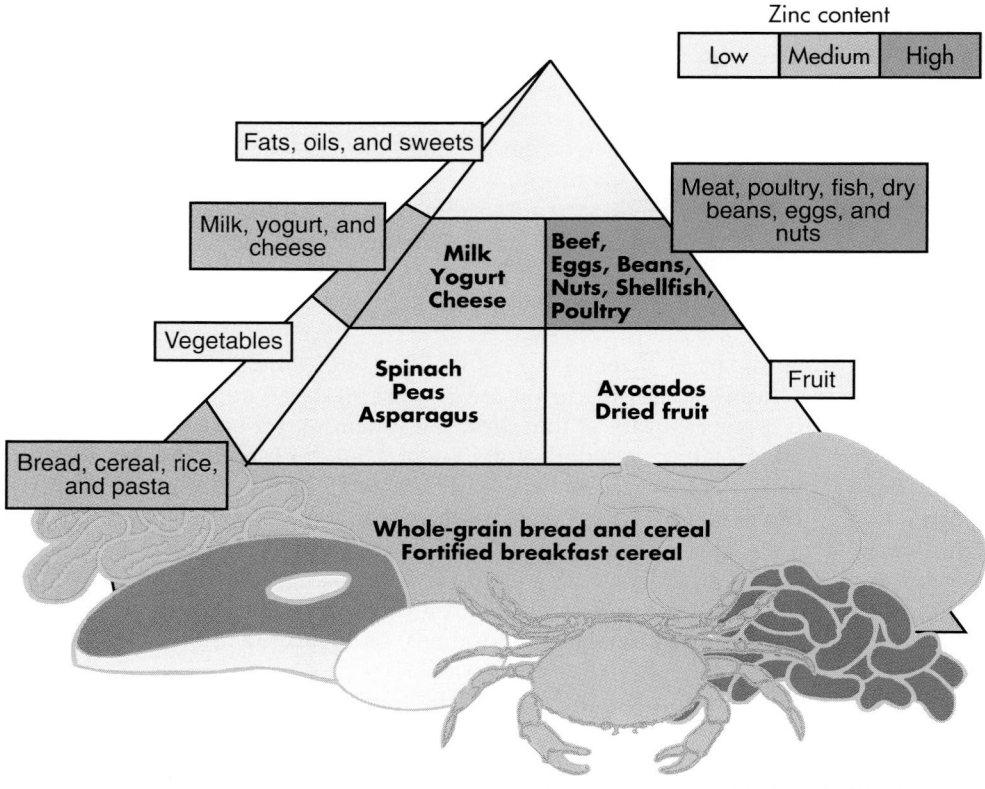

Zinc content

| Low | Medium | High |

Fats, oils, and sweets

Milk, yogurt, and cheese

Meat, poultry, fish, dry beans, eggs, and nuts

Milk Yogurt Cheese

Beef, Eggs, Beans, Nuts, Shellfish, Poultry

Vegetables

Fruit

Spinach Peas Asparagus

Avocados Dried fruit

Bread, cereal, rice, and pasta

Whole-grain bread and cereal Fortified breakfast cereal

Food Sources of Zinc

Food item and amount	Zinc (milligrams)
Steamed oysters, 6	49.9
Sirloin steak, 4 ounces	7.4
Peanuts, 1 cup	4.8
Pot roast, 3 ounces	4.6
Special K cereal, 1 cup	3.8
Wheat germ, ¼ cup	3.5
Lamb chops, 3 ounces	2.7
Black-eyed peas, 1 cup	2.2
Plain yogurt, 1 cup	2.2
Lean ham, 3 ounces	1.9
Swiss cheese, 1.5 ounces	1.7
Ricotta cheese, ½ cup	1.7
Sunflower seeds, 1 ounce	1.5
Cheddar cheese, 1.5 ounces	1.3
Enriched white rice, ½ cup	1.1

Animal foods are again our prime sources because zinc from animal sources is not bound by phytic acid. However, good plant sources of zinc—such as whole grains, peanuts, and beans—should not be discounted. They can deliver substantial amounts of zinc to body cells (Fig. 9.8).

The adult RDA for zinc is 11 milligrams for men and 8 milligrams for women. The Daily Value used on food and supplement labels is 15 milligrams. The average North American takes in 9 to 13 milligrams of zinc a day, with men showing the higher values. There are no indications of moderate or severe zinc deficiencies in an otherwise healthy adult population. It is likely, however, that some North Americans—especially some women, poor children, vegans, older people, and people with alcoholism—have a marginal zinc status. However, because we lack a sensitive marker for zinc status, a body must be very zinc-depleted for clinical tests to register a deficiency. Furthermore, absorption and excretion can maintain an adequate zinc status even when intakes are somewhat lower than those furnished by typical diets of North Americans. However, the long-term effects of marginal zinc intakes are not known. People who show deterioration in taste sensation, recurring infections, poor growth, or depressed wound healing should have zinc status checked.

Excessive zinc intakes, greater than about 3 to 4 times the RDA, over time can also lead to problems, as just mentioned. One study has shown that zinc supplements at approximately 5 to 20 times the RDA can reduce HDL-cholesterol by about 15%, perhaps by interfering with copper metabolism. That is disturbing for two reasons. First, low HDL-cholesterol is associated with an increased risk of developing cardiovascular disease. Second, many people who take zinc supplements do in fact consume an excessive amount. The interference with copper metabolism is the basis for setting the Upper Level for zinc at 40 milligrams per day. Overall, if a person uses megadose zinc supplements, such as to try to slow macular degeneration, he or she should be under close medical supervision and also take a supplement containing copper (2 milligrams per day). Zinc intakes over 100 milligrams per day also result in diarrhea, cramps, nausea, vomiting, and depressed immune system function, especially if intake exceeds 2 grams per day.

Another Bite

Many companies are singing the praises of zinc as a cold remedy. Products such as Cold Eeze are lozenges that contain zinc, and their claims are based largely on one study done with 100 participants. The 50 individuals in the experimental group took 13 milligrams of zinc via the lozenges every 2 hours for the duration of their symptoms. Cold symptoms subsided after 4 days in the experimental group and 7 days in the control group. Nausea was a common side effect of the zinc lozenges. Of 10 other follow-up studies, however, only half have shown beneficial results from zinc. This may be due to different bioavailability of various forms of zinc, or simply due to the more bitter flavor of the lozenges used in some studies (placebo effect). Adults can determine if the benefits outweigh the taste. Zinc expert Dr. Ananda Prasad recommends discontinuing use of zinc lozenges after 3 to 4 days unless they are showing evidence of effectiveness. Use in children is not helpful. Any use of such amounts beyond a week or so also is potentially dangerous.

Selenium (Se)

Selenium exists in many forms that are readily absorbed. Selenium's best understood role is aiding the activity of an enzyme that participates in reducing the damage that electron-seeking, free-radical (oxidizing) compounds can do to cell membranes. It also contributes to thyroid hormone metabolism.

In Chapter 8 you saw that vitamin E helps prevent attacks on cell membranes by electron-seeking compounds. Thus, vitamin E and selenium work together toward the same goal. Chapter 8 also discussed how free-radical compounds can cause cancer. Although selenium could prove to have a role in cancer prevention, such as prostate cancer, it is premature to recommend megadose selenium supplementation for this purpose. Animal studies in this area are conflicting; current studies with humans are under way to help clarify what role, if any, selenium plays in cancer prevention (supplemental intake of 200 micrograms per day).

Selenium deficiency symptoms in farm animals and humans include muscle pain and wasting and a certain form of heart damage. Farm animals in areas with low selenium soil concentration, such as New Zealand, and humans in some areas of China develop characteristic muscle and heart disorders associated with inadequate selenium intake. Other factors probably also contribute.

■ Selenium in Foods and Needs

Fish, meats (especially organ meats), eggs, and shellfish are good animal sources of selenium. Grains and seeds grown in soils containing selenium are good plant sources. Major selenium contributors to the adult diet are animal and grain products. Because we eat a varied diet of foods supplied from many geographic areas, it is unlikely that low soil selenium in a few locations will mean inadequate selenium in our diets.

The RDA for selenium is 55 micrograms per day for adults. The Daily Value used on food and supplement labels is 70 micrograms. In general, adults meet the RDA, consuming on average 105 micrograms of selenium each day. The Upper Level is 400 micrograms per day for adults, based on overt signs of selenium toxicity, such as hair loss.

Critical Thinking

Tammy read an article about antioxidants and their role in preventing free-radical damage to cells. When Tammy went to the drugstore to take a closer look at such supplements, she saw that selenium was one of the antioxidants in the supplements. Why does selenium deserve consideration as an antioxidant?

Food Sources of Selenium

Food item and amount	Selenium (micrograms)
Tuna, 3 ounces	68
Sirloin steak, 5 ounces	47
Lean ham, 3 ounces	42
Clams, 3 ounces	41
Salmon, 3 ounces	40
Egg noodles, 1 cup	35
Chicken breast, 3 ounces	20
Special K cereal, 1 cup	17
Oat bran cereal, 1 cup	14
Whole-wheat bread, 1 slice	10
Cooked oatmeal, ½ cup	10
White bread, 1 slice	9
Raisin Bran cereal, 1 cup	4

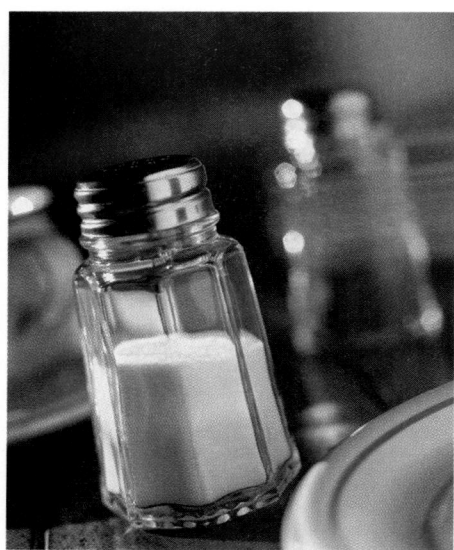

Iodized salt is the predominant source of dietary iodine in North American diets.

goiter An enlargement of the thyroid gland; this is often caused by insufficient iodide in the diet.

Food Sources of Iodide

Food item and amount	Iodide (micrograms)
Table salt, ½ teaspoon	195
Plain yogurt, 1 cup	87
Buttermilk, 1 cup	60
1% fat milk, 1 cup	59
Luna bar, 1	38
Soy protein bar, 1	38
Egg, 1 large	35
1% cottage cheese, ½ cup	28
Mozzarella cheese, 1 ounce	10

Concept Check

Zinc functions as a cofactor for many enzymes and is important for growth, immune function, and sense of taste. Beef, seafood, and whole grains are good food sources. As in the case of iron, zinc absorption is regulated according to the body's needs for the mineral. If taken in excess amounts, zinc competes with copper for absorption. Selenium activates an enzyme that helps change electron-seeking, free-radical (oxidizing) compounds into less toxic compounds so these do not attack and break down cell membranes. By helping to dismantle the free-radical compounds, selenium works toward the same goal as vitamin E. A selenium deficiency results in muscle and heart disorders. Animal products and grains are good selenium sources; however, the selenium content in plants depends on the selenium concentration in the soil. The misuse of both selenium and zinc supplements can readily lead to toxic results.

Iodine (I)

Iodine in foods is actually found in an ion form, called iodide. During World War I, a link was discovered between a deficiency of iodide and the production of a **goiter,** an enlarged thyroid gland (review Fig. 8.2). Men drafted from the Pacific Northwest and the Great Lakes Region of the United States had a much higher rate of goiter than did men from other areas of the country. The soils in these areas have very low iodide contents. In the 1920s, researchers in Ohio found that low doses of iodide given to children over a 4-year period could prevent goiter. That finding led to the addition of iodide to salt beginning in the 1920s.

Today, many nations such as Canada require iodide fortification of salt. In the United States, salt can be purchased either iodized or plain. Check for this on the label of a package of salt next time you are in a grocery store. Some areas of Europe, such as northern Italy, have very low soil levels of iodide, but have yet to adopt the practice of fortifying salt with iodide. People in these areas, especially women, still suffer from goiter, as do people in areas of Central America, South America, and Africa. The World Health Organization estimates that 250 million people in the world are at risk of iodide deficiency; 20% of these people have goiter. Eradication of iodide deficiency is a goal of many health-related organizations worldwide.

■ Function of Iodide

The thyroid gland actively accumulates and traps iodide from the bloodstream to support its hormone synthesis. Thyroid hormones are synthesized using iodide. These hormones help regulate metabolic rate and promote growth and development throughout the body, including the brain.

If a person's iodide intake is insufficient, the thyroid gland enlarges as it attempts to take up more iodide from the bloodstream. This eventually leads to goiter. Simple goiter is a painless condition, but if uncorrected can lead to pressure on the trachea (windpipe), which may cause difficulty in breathing. Although iodide can prevent goiter formation, it does not significantly shrink a goiter once it has formed. Surgical removal may be required in severe cases.

If a woman has an iodide-deficient diet during the early months of her pregnancy, the fetus suffers iodide deficiency because the mother's body uses up the available iodide. The infant then may be born with short stature and develop mental retardation. This stunted growth that results is part of what is known as *cretinism*. Cretinism appeared in North America before iodide fortification of table salt began. Today, cretinism still appears in Europe, Africa, Latin America, and Asia.

■ Iodide in Foods and Needs

Saltwater fish, seafood, iodized salt, dairy products, and grain products contain various forms of iodide. Sea salt found in health-food stores, however, is not a good source because the iodide is lost during processing.

The RDA for iodide for adults is 150 micrograms. This is the same as the Daily Value used on food and supplement labels. A half teaspoon of iodide-fortified salt (about 2 grams) supplies that amount. Most adults consume more iodide than the RDA—an estimated 190 to 300 micrograms daily, not including that from use of iodized salt at the table. This extra amount adds up because dairies and quick-service restaurants use it as a sterilizing agent, bakeries use it as a dough conditioner, food producers use it as part of food colorants, and it is added to salt.

When very high amounts of iodide are consumed, thyroid hormone synthesis is inhibited, as in a deficiency. The Upper Level of 1.1 milligram per day is based on such an effect. This can appear in people who eat a lot of seaweed, since some seaweeds contain as much as 1% iodide by weight. Total iodide intake then can add up to 60 to 130 times the RDA.

Copper (Cu)

Copper contributes to the metabolism of iron; it operates in processes that form hemoglobin and transport iron. A copper-containing enzyme aids in the release of iron from storage. Copper is needed by enzymes that create cross-connections in connective tissue proteins. Copper is also needed by other enzymes, such as those that defend the body against free-radical (oxidizing) compounds and those that act in the brain and nervous system. Finally, copper performs in immune system function, blood clotting, and blood lipoprotein metabolism. About 12% to 75% of dietary copper is absorbed, with higher intakes associated with lower absorption. This absorption takes place primarily in the stomach and upper small intestine, with copper excretion via the gallbladder. Phytates, certain amino acids, vitamin C, dietary fiber, zinc, and iron may all interfere with copper absorption. Symptoms of copper deficiency include a form of anemia, low white blood cell count, bone loss, poor growth, and some forms of cardiovascular disease.

■ Copper in Foods and Needs

Copper is found primarily in liver, seafood, cocoa, legumes, nuts, seeds, and whole-grain breads and cereals.

The RDA for copper is 900 micrograms daily for adults. The Daily Value used on food and supplement labels is 2 milligrams. The average adult intake is about 1 to 1.6 milligrams per day. Women generally consume the smaller amount. The copper status of adults appears to be good, though we lack sensitive measures to determine copper status. It is wise, however, to regularly eat good sources of copper.

The groups most likely to develop copper deficiencies are premature infants, infants recovering from semistarvation on a milk-dominated diet (which is a poor source of copper), and people recovering from intestinal surgery (during which time copper absorption decreases). Recall that a copper deficiency can also result from overzealous supplementation of zinc, because zinc and copper compete with each other for absorption. Copper can cause toxicity, including vomiting, at single doses of greater than 10 milligrams. Other forms of toxicity are also possible with megadose uses, such as liver toxicity. This risk is the basis for setting the Upper Limit at 10 milligrams per day.

Food Sources of Copper

Food item and amount	Copper (micrograms)
Fried beef liver, 3 ounces	3800
Power bar, 1	700
Walnuts, ½ cup	600
Sunflower seeds, ¼ cup	600
Kidney beans, 1 cup	500
Lobster, 3 ounces	400
Molasses, 3 tablespoons	300
Sunflower seeds, 2 tablespoons	300
Shrimp, 3 ounces	300
Raisin Bran cereal, 1 cup	300
Great Grains cereal, 1 cup	300
Black-eyed peas, ½ cup cooked	200
Wheat germ, ¼ cup	200
Milk chocolate, 1 ounce	110
Whole-wheat bread, 1 slice	80

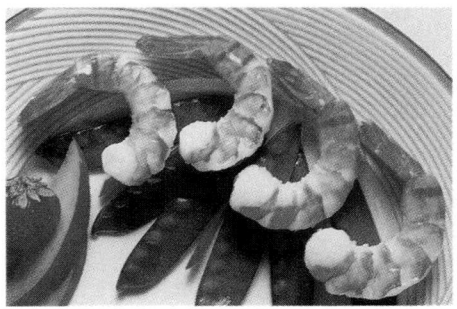

Seafood is one source of copper for a diet.

Fluoride (F)

Like chlorine, fluorine (F_2) is a poisonous gas. The fluoride ion (F^-) is the form of this trace mineral essential for human health. This link was found as dentists in the early 1900s noticed a lower rate of dental caries (cavities) in the southwestern United States. These areas contained high amounts of fluoride in the water. The amounts were sometimes so high that small spots on the teeth, called *mottling,* appeared. Even though mottled teeth were quite discolored, they contained very few dental caries. After experiments showed that fluoride in the water did indeed decrease the rate of dental caries, controlled fluoridation of water in parts of the United States began in 1945.

Those of us who grew up drinking fluoridated water generally have 40% to 60% fewer dental caries than people who did not drink fluoridated water as children. Dentists can provide fluoride treatments, and schools can provide fluoride tablets, but it is much less expensive and more reliable to simply add fluoride to a community's drinking water. State and private water sources do not always contain enough fluoride, however. When in doubt, contact your local water plant or have the water in your home analyzed for fluoride content. If it is less than 1 part fluoride per million parts of water (1 ppm), talk to your dentist about the best means to obtain the fluoride.

■ Functions of Fluoride

Dietary fluoride consumed during childhood, when bones and teeth are developing, aids the synthesis of tooth crystals that strongly resist acid. Therefore, teeth become very resistant to dental caries. Fluoride also inhibits metabolism and growth of the bacterium that causes dental caries, and fluoride present in saliva directly inhibits tooth demineralization and enhances tooth remineralization.

Fluoride applied to the surface of the teeth by dentists or from toothpaste adds additional protection against dental caries. Thus, people of all ages benefit from the topical effects of fluoride, whether or not they consumed fluoridated water or fluoride supplements as children.

High doses of fluoride (20 or more milligrams per day) are being used experimentally in adults to treat severe osteoporosis, especially that seen in the spine. Such high fluoride dosages can cause significant side effects, such as stomach upset and bone pain. Ongoing research is attempting to establish a dose, form, and duration of treatment that aid in increasing bone mass and contribute to reduced fracture risk.

■ Fluoride in Foods and Needs

Tea, seafood, seaweed, and some natural water sources are the only good food sources of fluoride. Most of our fluoride intake comes from fluoride added to drinking water and toothpaste and from fluoride treatments performed by dentists.

The Adequate Intake for fluoride for adults is 3.1 to 3.8 milligrams per day. This range of intake provides the benefits of resistance to dental caries without causing ill effects. Typical fluoridated water contains about 0.2 milligrams per cup.

Children may consume large amounts of fluoridated toothpaste as part of daily tooth care. Not swallowing toothpaste and limiting the amount used to "pea" size are the best ways to prevent this problem. In addition, children under 6 years should have toothbrushing supervised by an adult. When fluoride intakes reach 20 milligrams per day during tooth development, the tooth structure is weakened, and skeletal bones can deteriorate. With all of these problems in mind, the Upper Level for fluoride is set at 1.3 to 2.2 milligrams per day for young children, and 10 milligrams per day for children over 9 years of age and adults. Note however, that high fluoride intake in adults does not cause mottling.

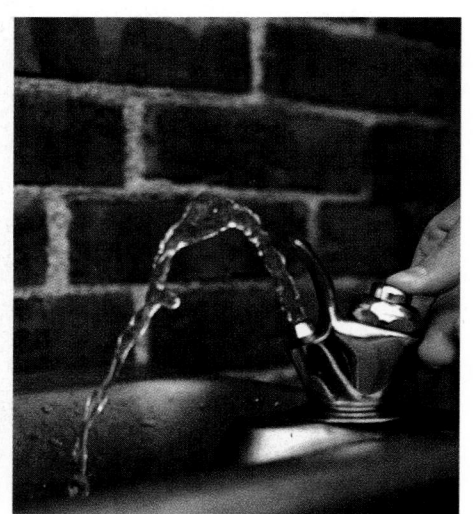

Fluoridated water is responsible for much of the decrease in dental caries throughout North America in recent years.

Concept Check

*I*odide is vital for the synthesis of thyroid hormones. A prolonged insufficient intake causes the thyroid gland to enlarge, resulting in a goiter. The use of iodized salt in America has virtually eliminated this condition. Copper functions mainly in iron metabolism and in the cross-bonding of connective tissue. A deficiency can result in a type of anemia. Good food sources of copper are seafoods, legumes, nuts, dried fruits, and whole grains. Fluoride aids in tooth development. When incorporated into the teeth during development and present in saliva, fluoride makes them resistant to acid and bacterial growth, in turn reducing development of dental caries. Fluoride also aids in remineralization of teeth once decay begins. Most of us receive adequate amounts of fluoride from that added to drinking water and toothpaste. A high fluoride intake during tooth development can lead to spotted, or mottled, teeth and possibly weakened tooth structure.

Chromium (Cr)

The importance of chromium in human diets has been recognized only in the past 40 years. There is much we do not understand about this mineral, but chromium deficiency may be related to type 2 diabetes in some individuals.

The most-studied function of chromium is the maintenance of glucose uptake into cells. Our current understanding is that chromium enters the cell and acts to enhance the transport of glucose across the cell membrane by interacting with insulin function.

A chromium deficiency is characterized by impaired blood glucose control and elevated blood cholesterol and triglycerides. The mechanism by which chromium influences cholesterol metabolism is not known but may involve enzymes that control cholesterol synthesis. Chromium deficiency appears in people maintained on total parenteral nutrition solutions not supplemented with chromium and in children with malnutrition. Because sensitive measures of chromium status are not available, marginal chromium deficiencies may go undetected.

■ Chromium in Foods and Needs

Specific data regarding the chromium content of various foods are scant, and most food composition tables do not include values for this trace mineral. Egg yolks, whole grains (bran), organ meats, other meats, mushrooms, nuts, and beer are good sources. Yeast is also a source. The amount of chromium in foods is closely tied to the local soil content of chromium. To provide yourself with a good chromium intake, regularly choose whole grains in preference to mostly refined grains.

The Adequate Intake for chromium is 25 to 35 micrograms per day. The Daily Value used on food and supplement labels is 120 micrograms, about 4 times greater. Average adult intakes in North America are estimated at about 30 micrograms per day, but could be somewhat higher. Marginal to low chromium intakes (about 20 micrograms, per day) may contribute to an increased risk for developing type 2 diabetes.

Some research also shows that an intake of 200 micrograms per day may improve blood glucose regulation in type 2 diabetes and may raise HDL-cholesterol. More studies are needed on these effects. Chromium toxicity has been reported in people exposed to industrial waste and in painters who use art supplies with a very high chromium content. Liver damage and lung cancer can result. Because of the risk of toxicity, any supplement use should normally not exceed the Daily Value set unless supervised by a physician. No Upper Level for chromium has been set since toxicity for that present in foods has not been observed.

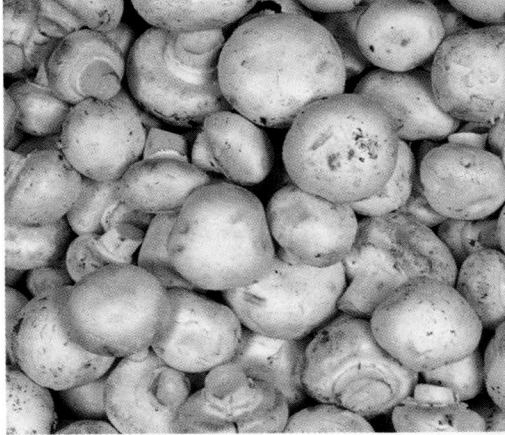

Mushrooms are a good source of chromium.

Nuts are rich in manganese.

Manganese (Mn)

The mineral manganese is easily confused with magnesium. Not only are their names similar, but they also often substitute for each other in metabolic processes. Manganese is needed by some enzymes, such as those used in carbohydrate metabolism. Manganese is also important in bone formation.

No human deficiency symptom is associated with a low manganese intake. Animals on manganese-deficient diets suffer alterations in brain function, bone formation, and reproduction. If human diets were low in manganese, these symptoms would probably appear as well. As it happens, our need for manganese is very low, and our diets tend to be adequate in manganese.

Good food sources of manganese are nuts, rice, oats and other whole grains, beans, and leafy vegetables. The Adequate Intake for manganese is 1.8 to 2.3 milligrams. Average intakes generally fall within this range. The Daily Value used on food and supplement labels is 2 milligrams. Manganese is toxic at high doses. The Upper Level is 11 milligrams per day, based on the development of nerve damage.

Molybdenum (Mo)

Several human enzymes use molybdenum. No molybdenum deficiency has been noted in people who consume normal diets, though deficiency symptoms have appeared in people maintained on intravenous total parenteral nutrition feedings. These symptoms include increased heart and respiration rates, night blindness, mental confusion, edema, and weakness.

Good food sources of molybdenum include milk and milk products, beans, whole grains, and nuts. The RDA for molybdenum is 45 micrograms. The Daily Value used on food and supplement labels is 75 micrograms. Our daily intakes average 75 to 110 micrograms. When consumed in high doses, molybdenum causes toxicity in laboratory animals, with weight loss and decreased growth. This is the basis of setting the Upper Level at 2 milligrams per day. Figure 9.9 summarizes the various contributions of groups in the Food Guide Pyramid to mineral needs.

Other Trace Minerals

Although a variety of other trace minerals is found in humans, many of them have not yet been shown to be required. The list of minerals in this category includes boron, nickel, vanadium, arsenic, and silicon (Table 9.7). Widespread deficiency symptoms in humans have never been noted, probably because typical diets provide adequate amounts and they are needed by very few enzymes and metabolic systems. Their potential for toxicity should make one question any supplementation not supervised by a physician. These trace minerals may achieve more importance as more research is reported.

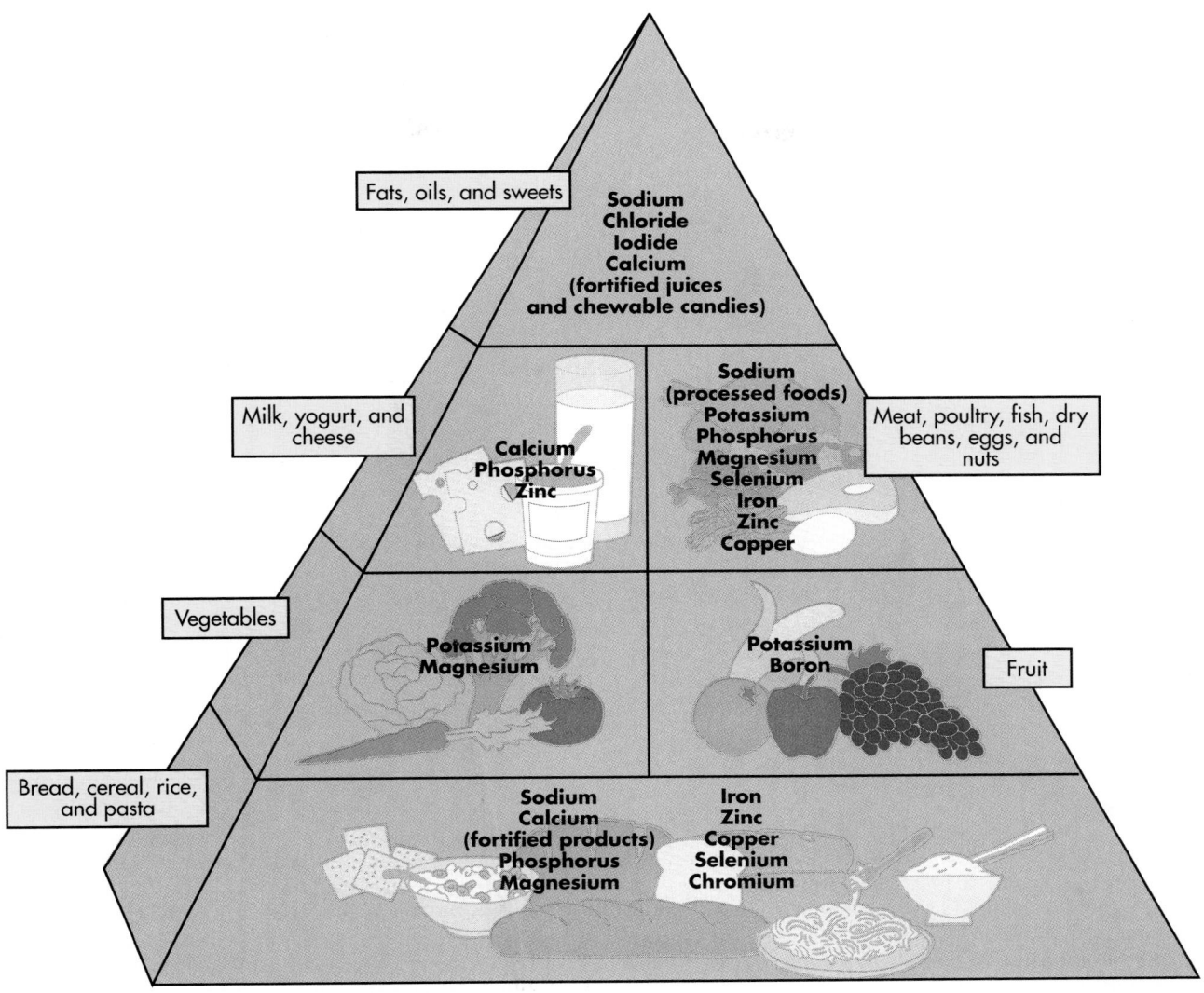

Figure 9.9 Certain groups of the Food Guide Pyramid are especially rich sources of various minerals. This is true for the minerals listed. Each mineral may also be found in other groups but in lower amounts. Other trace minerals are also present in moderate amounts in many groups. With regard to the bread, cereal, rice, and pasta group, whole-grain varieties are the richest sources of most trace minerals listed.

Concept Check

Chromium acts to increase the action of the hormone insulin. The amount of chromium found in food depends on soil content. Meats, whole grains, and egg yolks are some good sources. Manganese is a component of bone and used by many enzymes, including those involved in glucose production. Because our need for manganese is low, deficiencies are rare. Nuts, rice, oats, and beans are good food sources. Molybdenum is another trace mineral required by a few enzymes. Good sources include milk, beans, whole grains, and nuts. Deficiencies have appeared only in unsupplemented total parenteral nutrition. The needs for some other trace minerals—such as boron, nickel, arsenic, and vanadium—have not been fully established in humans. If required, these minerals are needed in such small amounts that our current diets are probably adequate sources of them.

Table 9.7 A Summary of Trace Minerals for Which Human Needs Have Not Been Established

Mineral	Proposed Function	Estimates of Daily Human Needs	Dietary Sources
Arsenic	Amino acid and fatty acid metabolism; DNA function	12–25 micrograms	Fish, grains, cereal products
Boron	Cell membrane function (ion transport); hormone metabolism in some cases	1–13 milligrams	Fruits, leafy vegetables, nuts, beans
Nickel	Amino acid and fatty acid metabolism	25–35 micrograms	Chocolate, nuts, beans, whole grains
Silicon	Bone formation	25–30 milligrams	Root vegetables, whole grains
Vanadium	Mimics action of insulin	10 micrograms*	Shellfish, mushrooms, black pepper

Human needs have not been established in any case; deficiency symptoms have been produced in experimental animals. All of these trace minerals pose a high risk for toxicity. Any supplement use should not exceed the estimates of daily human needs listed above.

*Upper Level is 1.8 milligrams per day (180 times estimated human needs)

Summary

1. Water constitutes 50% to 70% of the human body. Its unique chemical properties enable it to dissolve substances as well as serve as a medium for chemical reactions, temperature regulation, and lubrication. Water also helps regulate the acid-base balance in the body. For adults, daily water needs are estimated at 1 milliliter per kcal expended.

2. Overall, North Americans enjoy a very safe water supply. However, those with poor immune status should boil water used for drinking and cooking in order to avoid water-borne illness. Bottled water can also be used if desired.

3. Many minerals are vital for sustaining life. For humans, animal products are the most bioavailable sources of most minerals. Supplements of minerals exceeding 100% of the Daily Values listed on the label should be taken only under a physician's supervision. Toxicity and nutrient interactions are especially likely if the Upper Level (when set) is exceeded on a long-term basis.

4. Sodium, the major positive ion found outside cells, is vital in fluid balance and nerve impulse transmission. The North American diet provides abundant sodium through processed foods and table salt. About 10% to 15% of the adult population is sodium-sensitive and is at risk for developing hypertension from consuming excessive sodium, especially people who are overweight. One out of four North Americans suffers from high blood pressure. Controlling weight and alcohol intake, exercising, decreasing sodium intake, and ensuring adequate potassium, magnesium, and calcium in the diet all can play a part in controlling high blood pressure.

5. Potassium, the major positive ion found inside cells, has a similar function to sodium. Milk, fruits, and vegetables are good sources.

Chloride is the major negative ion found outside cells. It is important in digestion as part of stomach acid and in immune and nerve functions. Table salt supplies most of the chloride in our diets.

6. Calcium forms a part of bone structure and plays a role in blood clotting, muscle contraction, nerve transmission, and cell metabolism. Calcium absorption is enhanced by stomach acid and the active vitamin D hormone. Dairy products are important calcium sources. Women are particularly at risk for not meeting calcium needs.

7. Phosphorus aids enzyme function and forms part of key metabolic compounds, cell membranes, and bone. It is efficiently absorbed, and deficiencies are rare, although there is concern about possibly poor intake by some elderly women. Good food sources are dairy products, bakery products, and meats. Sulfur is incorporated into certain vitamins and amino acids. Magnesium is a mineral found mostly in plant food sources. It is important for nerve and heart function and as an activator for many enzymes. Whole grains (bran portion), vegetables, nuts, seeds, milk, and meats are good food sources.

8. Iron absorption depends mainly on the form of iron present and the body's need for it. Heme iron from animal sources is better absorbed than the nonheme iron obtained primarily from plant sources. Consuming vitamin C or meat simultaneously with iron increases nonheme absorption. Iron operates mainly in synthesizing hemoglobin and myoglobin and in the action of the immune system. Women are at great risk for developing iron deficiency, which decreases blood hemoglobin and red blood cell number. When this condition is severe enough to decrease the amount of oxygen carried in the blood, iron-deficiency anemia

develops. Iron toxicity usually results from a genetic disorder called hemochromatosis. This disease causes overabsorption and accumulation of iron, which can result in severe liver and heart damage.

9. Zinc aids in the action of nearly 100 enzymes that are important for growth, development, immune function, wound healing, and taste. A zinc deficiency results in poor growth, loss of appetite, reduced sense of taste and smell, hair loss, and a persistent rash. Zinc is best absorbed from animal sources. The richest sources of zinc are oysters, shrimp, crab, and beef. Good plant sources are whole grains, peanuts, and beans.

10. An important role of selenium is decreasing the action of free-radical (oxidizing) compounds. In this way, selenium acts along with vitamin E. Muscle pain, muscle wasting, and a form of heart damage may result from a selenium deficiency. Meats, eggs, fish, and shellfish are good animal sources of selenium. Good plant sources include grains and seeds.

11. Iodide forms part of the thyroid hormones. A lack of dietary iodide results in the development of an enlarged thyroid gland or goiter. Iodized salt is a major food source.

12. Copper is important for iron metabolism, cross-linking of connective tissue, and other functions. A copper deficiency can result in a form of anemia. Copper is found mainly in liver, seafood, cocoa, legumes, and whole grains.

13. Fluoride as part of regular dietary intake or toothpaste use makes teeth resistant to dental caries. Most North Americans receive the bulk of their fluoride from fluoridated water and toothpaste.

14. Chromium aids in the action of the hormone insulin. Egg yolks, meats, and whole grains are good sources of chromium. Manganese and molybdenum are used by various enzymes. Clear deficiencies in otherwise healthy people are rarely seen for any of these three nutrients. Human needs for other trace minerals are so low that deficiencies are uncommon.

Study Questions

1. Approximately how much water do you need each day to stay healthy? Identify at least two situations that increase the need for water. Then list three sources of water in the average person's diet.

2. What is the relationship between sodium and water balance, and how is that relationship monitored as well as maintained in the body?

3. Identify four factors that influence the bioavailability of minerals from food.

4. What are two similarities and differences between sodium and potassium? Sodium and chloride?

5. In terms of total amounts in the body, calcium and phosphorus are the first and second most abundant minerals, respectively. What function do these minerals have in common?

6. What are the best food sources for zinc and copper?

7. Describe the symptoms of iron-deficiency anemia and explain possible reasons why they occur.

8. Which trace minerals are lost from cereal grains when they are refined? Are any of these nutrients replaced by enrichment?

9. Describe the chief function of fluoride, copper, and chromium in the body.

10. What are the practical consequences of the Daily Values on food and supplement labels exceeding the RDA or Adequate Intake for many trace minerals?

Further Readings

1. ADA Reports: Position of the American Dietetic Association: The impact of fluoride on health. *Journal of the American Dietetic Association* 101:126, 2001.
   The American Dietetic Association reaffirms that fluoride is an important element for all mineralized tissues in the body. Appropriate fluoride intake is beneficial to bone and tooth health.

2. Anderson JJB: The important role of physical activity in skeletal development: How exercise may counter low calcium intake. *American Journal of Clinical Nutrition* 71:1384, 2000.
   A greater bone mass gained early in life is now considered a critical factor in protecting against osteoporotic fractures later in life. The critical years for skeletal growth and accumulation of bone mass are in the prepubertal and pubertal decades. These years are a particularly good time for regular physical activity, as it, along with adequate diet, increases bone mass.

3. Andrews NC: Disorders of iron metabolism. *The New England Journal of Medicine* 341:1986, 1999.
   Iron is able to accept and donate electrons, so it is capable of binding oxygen and participating in many enzyme systems. However, iron can damage tissues by causing the conversion of hydrogen peroxide to free radicals. Iron can't be readily excreted from the body; the cells that line the gastrointestinal tract act as a barrier to overabsorption.

4. Dawson-Hughes B: Osteoporosis. In Bowman BA, RM Russell (eds.): *Present Knowledge in Nutrition.* ILSI Press, Washington, DC 2001.
   Heredity has a pronounced effect on the amount of bone one builds in youth. Also important are adequate calcium, vitamin D, and protein. Weight-bearing physical activity also contributes to a healthy skeleton.

5. Food and Nutrition Board, Institute of Medicine: *Dietary Reference Intakes for calcium, phosphorus, magnesium, vitamin D, and fluoride.* Washington, DC: Standing Committee on the Scientific Evaluation of Dietary Reference Intakes National Academy Press, 1997.
   Dietary standards have recently been set for many major minerals. The rationale used to set RDA or Adequate Intakes and Upper Levels for these nutrients is discussed in detail.

6. Food and Nutrition Board, Institute of Medicine: *Dietary Reference Intakes for vitamin A, vitamin K, arsenic, boron, chromium, copper, iodine, iron, manganese, molybdenum, nickel, silicon, vanadium, and zinc.*

Washington, DC: Standing Committee on the Scientific Evaluation of Dietary Reference Intakes National Academy Press, 2001.

Dietary standards have recently been set for many trace minerals. The rationale used to set RDA or Adequate Intakes and Upper Levels for these nutrients is discussed in detail.

7. Heaney RP: Calcium, dairy products and osteoporosis. *Journal of the American College of Nutrition* 19(2):83S, 2000.

The results of several studies have shown that there is no single intervention, whether nutritional, hormonal, or pharmacologic, that can solve the problem of osteoporosis. Instead, what is needed is a combination of approaches, such as adequate calcium intake for women on medical therapy for osteoporosis.

8. Jackson JL and others: Zinc and the common cold: A meta-analysis revisited. *Journal of Nutrition* 130:1512S, 2000.

An analysis of current studies using zinc supplements to treat the common cold failed to find evidence of a significant reduction in cold duration. Studies reporting a benefit from zinc therapy have been criticized for poor blinding of the study subjects.

9. Kleiner SM: Water: An essential but overlooked nutrient. *Journal of the American Dietetic Association* 99:200, 1999.

Dehydration of as little as a 2% loss of body weight results in decreased physiological responses. New research indicates that fluid consumption in general and water consumption in particular can reduce the risk of kidney stones, certain cancers, obesity, and mitral valve prolapse. Adequate fluid intake is especially important for the overall health of older adults.

10. Liebman B: High blood pressure: The end of an epidemic? *Nutrition Action Health Letter*, p. 1, December 2000.

The DASH-Sodium trial included intakes of 3300 milligrams per day, 2400 milligrams per day, or 1500 milligrams per day of sodium in addition to the standard DASH diet plan. Each reduction in sodium intake resulted in a further fall in both systolic and diastolic blood pressure. Thus, people with hypertension should consider following the basic DASH diet and lowering sodium intake as much as possible.

11. Loria CM and others: Choose and prepare foods with less salt: Dietary advice for all Americans. *Journal of Nutrition* 131:536S, 2001.

Most North American adolescents and adults consume much more sodium than is recommended. Dietary advice to prepare foods with less salt is critical to reducing the number of cases of hypertension and its associated disease risks.

12. Miller GD and others: The importance of meeting calcium needs with foods. *Journal of the American College of Nutrition* 20(2):168S, 2001.

Milk and other dairy foods are the major sources of calcium in the North American diet. In addition to calcium, these foods provide substantial amounts of other essential nutrients. Consequently, a regular intake of dairy foods improves the overall nutrition quality of a diet. Currently, many North Americans are missing out on the attributes of this food group.

13. NIH Consensus Development Panel on Osteoporosis Prevention, Diagnosis, and Treatment; (Osteoporosis prevention, diagnosis, and treatment). *Journal of the American Medical Association* 285:785, 2001.

Osteoporosis is a major health threat. In the United States alone, 10 million persons already have osteoporosis, and 18 million more have low bone mass, placing them at increased risk for this disorder. Assessment of bone mass, identification of fracture risk, and determination of who should be treated are the optimal goals when evaluating patients for osteoporosis.

14. Schardt D: Water, water, everywhere. *Nutrition Action Health Letter*, 41, June 2000.

On the whole, people in the United States can feel confident about the quality of their drinking water. Almost 90% of public water systems in the United States report no violations of EPA limits for drinking water contaminants. The main individuals at risk from contaminated drinking water are those with compromised immune systems and possibly people in rural communities. The former persons should take the extra precaution to boil tap water for at least 1 minute, whereas the latter may consider having their tap water tested to see if it meets current EPA standards.

15. Vincent J: The biochemistry of chromium. *Journal of Nutrition* 130:715, 2000.

Chromium has been known to be an essential micronutrient for mammals for four decades. However, the most popular form of chromium in dietary supplements, chromium picolinate, appears to be absorbed in a different fashion than from dietary chromium and can lead to the production of harmful free radicals.

16. What's best for your bones? *Consumer Reports on Health* 3(7):1, 2001 (July).

Many factors contribute to optimal bone health, including meeting calcium and vitamin D needs, regular strength training and aerobic physical activities that put stress on bones, not smoking, and drinking alcohol moderately if one drinks. Bisphosphonates currently are becoming the first choice of drug therapy for preventing or treating osteoporosis; newer versions need be taken only once per week.

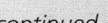

I. How Does Your Mineral Intake Measure Up?

To complete this activity, reexamine your nutritional assessment from Chapter 2. Compare your intake of selective minerals with the RDA, AI, or other established standard. Use your completed nutritional assessment to complete the table. For each mineral, record your intake, the intake recommended, the percentage of that intake you consumed, and a +, −, or = to indicate an intake higher, lower, or equal to that intake. Note that for sodium and potassium, minimum requirements for health are designated and already recorded in the table (these can also be found on the inside front cover of the book).

Mineral	Intake	RDA/Adequate Intake	% of Needs	+/−/=
Calcium				
Phosphorus				
Sodium		500 milligrams		
Potassium		2000 milligrams		
Iron				
Zinc				

Analysis

1. Which of your mineral intakes equaled or exceeded the RDA (or other standard set)? Do the nutrients for which you exceeded the desired amounts pose a likely risk for toxicity, based on the total amount consumed?

   _____

2. Which of your intakes were below the RDA (or other standard)?

   _____

3. What foods and cooking practices could be emphasized or de-emphasized to modify your weaknesses? Indicate for each food the specific amount of the missing nutrient(s) supplied.

   _____

   _____

   _____

   _____

   _____

continued

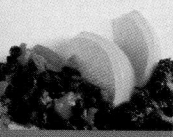

II. *Working for Denser Bones*

In the Nutrition Issue, you will learn important information about the disease osteoporosis, which is characterized by thinning and brittle bones.

Osteoporosis affects more than 28 million people in the United States. One-third of all women experience fractures because of this disease, amounting to about 1.3 million bone fractures per year. Given the rise in the number of older people in North America, osteoporosis-related illness and death are anticipated to increase dramatically in coming years.

This is a disease you can do something about. Some risk factors can't be changed, but others can. To what degree are you doing the things that can help prevent this debilitating disease? Answer yes or no to the following questions by placing an X in the appropriate blank.

	Yes	No
1. Do you average at least 20 minutes of sun exposure per day to at least your hands and face to get vitamin D, or do you drink vitamin D-fortified milk regularly?	_____	_____
2. Do you engage in weight-bearing physical activity (jogging, brisk walking, etc.) for at least 30 minutes on most or all days of the week?	_____	_____
3. If you are a woman, do you experience regular menstruation?		
4. Do you avoid smoking cigarettes?	_____	_____
5. Do you avoid regular consumption of large amounts (greater than one to two drinks per day) of alcohol?	_____	_____
6. Do you consume milk and other dairy products regularly, or substitute other sources to meet at least the Adequate Intake for calcium?	_____	_____
7. Do you moderate intake of phosphorus, sodium, protein, and caffeine?	_____	_____

The more *yes* answers you have, the more you are actively preserving your bone density for the future. Also, remember that this is not just a consideration for women, because if men plan to live well into their eighties and nineties, they are at risk for osteoporosis. In fact, about 14% of all spine fractures and 25% of all hip fractures linked to osteoporosis occur in men.

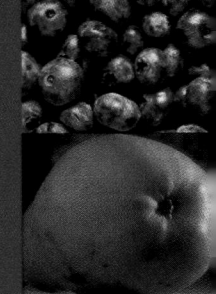

Widespread advertising has made it almost impossible for women to ignore osteoporosis. The crippling effect this disease has on older persons is now recognized as a major medical problem. The disease affects more than 28 million people in the United States and 200 million worldwide, most of them women. Osteoporosis leads to approximately 1.3 million bone fractures per year in the United States, usually in the hip, spine, or wrist, leading to about $14 billion per year in health-care costs. About one-half of Caucasian women (and one-third of all women) in North America experience osteoporosis-related fractures in their lifetimes.

The slender, inactive woman who smokes is most susceptible to osteoporosis, but any person who lives long enough can suffer from the disease, including men. About 25% of women older than age 50 develop osteoporosis. Among people older than age 80, osteoporosis becomes the rule—not the exception. The spine fractures commonly found in women with osteoporosis cause considerable pain and deformity and decrease physical ability (Fig. 9.10); hip fractures are seen in both men and women with osteoporosis. Not only is this disease debilitating, it also can be fatal. Up to one-fifth of all older persons who suffer hip fractures eventually die from fracture-related complications.

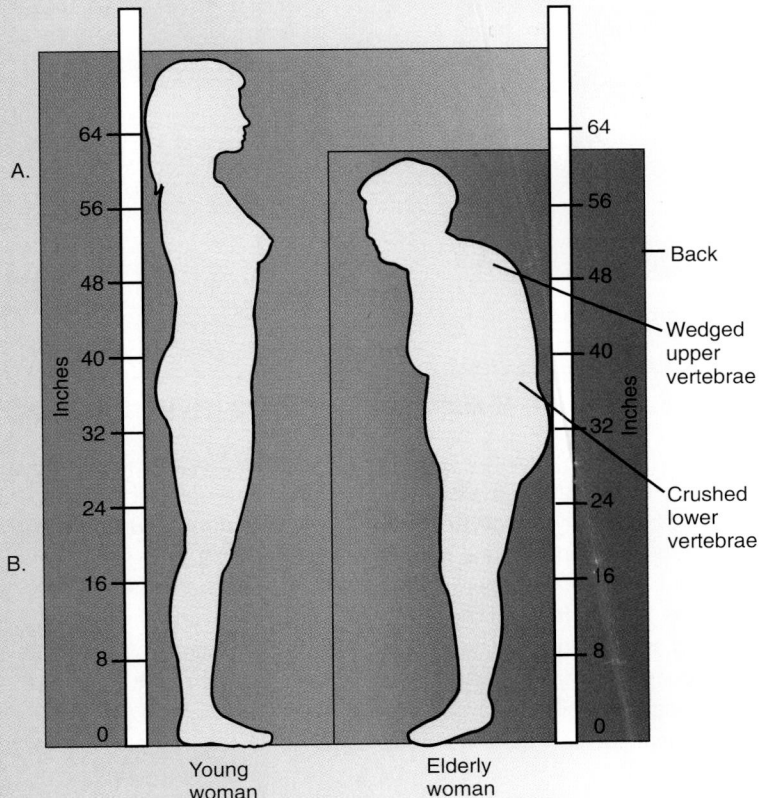

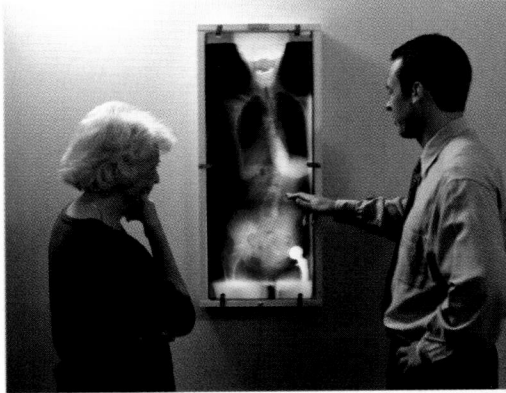

Fractures of the vertebrae in the spine are a typical result of osteoporosis in older women.

Figure 9.10 A loss of height and a distorted body shape are commonly seen in osteoporosis. Monitoring changes in adult height is one way to detect early evidence of osteoporosis.

continued

Figure 9.11 Cortical and trabecular bone. Cortical bone forms the shafts of bones and the outer mineral covering. Trabecular bone supports the outer shell of cortical bone in various bones of the body, as in the upper bone pictured. Note how in the lower picture there is much less trabecular bone. This leads to a more fragile bone and is not reversible to any major extent with current therapies.

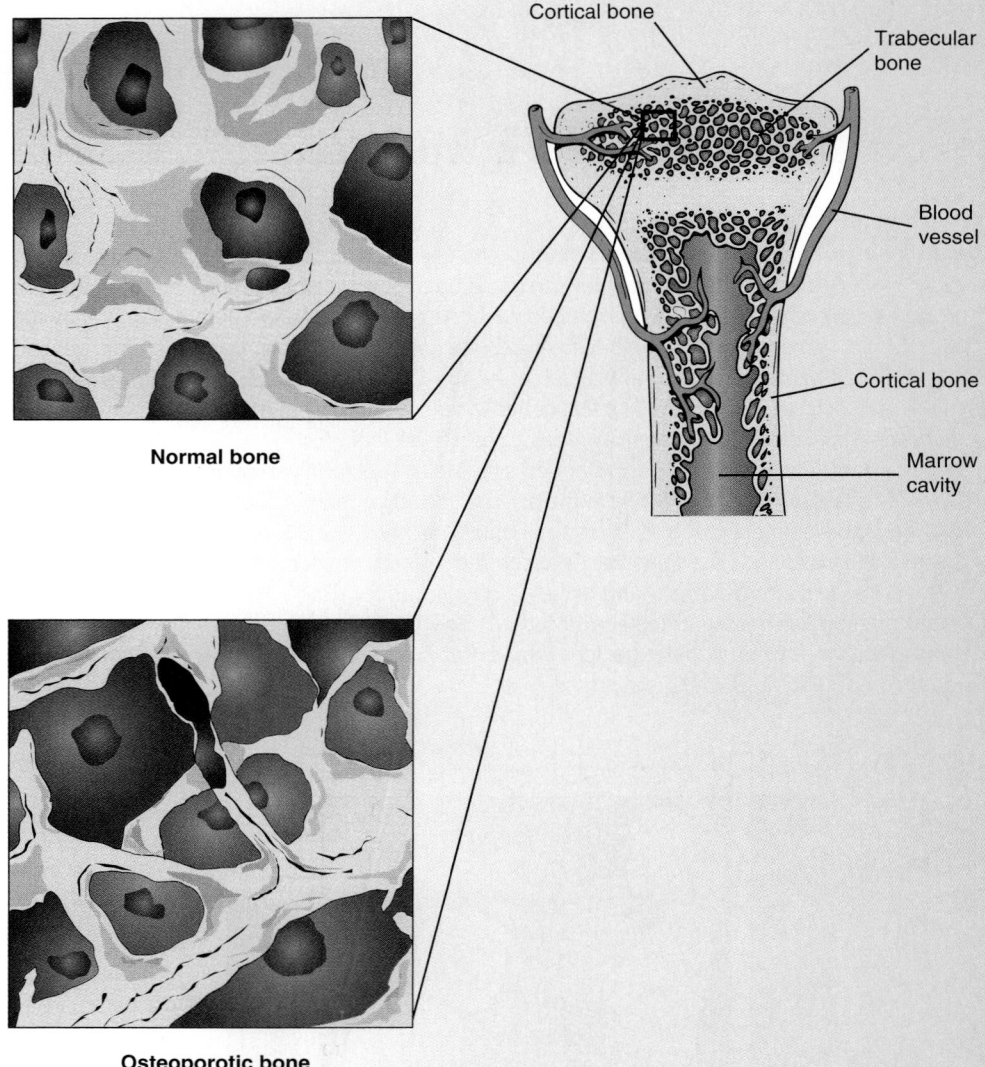

Normal bone

Osteoporotic bone

Cortical bone

Trabecular bone

Blood vessel

Cortical bone

Marrow cavity

cortical bone Dense, compact bone that comprises the outer surface and shafts of bone; also called compact bone.

trabecular bone The spongy, inner matrix of bone, found primarily in the spine, pelvis, and ends of bones; also called spony or cancellous bone.

bone mass Total mineral substance (such as calcium or phosphorus) in a cross section of bone, generally expressed as grams per centimeter of length.

bone mineral density Total mineral content of bone at a specific bone site divided by the width of the bone at that site, generally expressed as grams per cubic centimeter.

A Quick Look at Bone Structure and Strength

To better understand the role calcium plays in bone health and osteoporosis, it is important to understand how bone is constructed. Visual observation of the cross-sections of a bone reveals two primary bone structural types: **cortical bone** and **trabecular bone.** These interact within each bone to form quite an engineering marvel of strength (Fig. 9.11).

The entire outer surface of all bones is composed of cortical bone, which is very dense. The shafts of long bones, such as those of the arm, are almost entirely cortical bone. Trabecular bone is found in the ends of the long bones, inside the spinal vertebrae, and inside the flat bones of the pelvis. Trabecular bone forms an internal scaffolding network for a bone. It supports the outer cortical shell of the bone, especially in heavily stressed areas, such as joints.

Bone strength depends on a person's **bone mass** and **bone mineral density.** The more bone there is, and especially the more densely packed bone crystals are in the bone, the stronger the bone structure. Another important element of bone strength is the trabecular bone support network inside a bone. It is especially critical for the horizontal trabeculae to extend continuously—without breaks—between the areas of vertical trabeculae. Any break in either the horizontal or more vertical trabecular beams weakens the support system of a bone and increases the risk for bone fracture. And once these beams are broken, there is no way to rebuild them. This is why it is so important to limit bone loss as people age.

Table 9.8 Diet and Lifestyle Factors Associated with Bone Status and Related Action Plans to Implement

Positive Diet and Lifestyle Factors	Action Plans to Implement
Adequate diet containing a sufficient amount of protein, calcium, phosphorus, magnesium, potassium, vitamin A, vitamin C, vitamin D, vitamin K, zinc, copper, fluoride, and manganese (and boron?)	Follow a diet plan such as the Food Guide Pyramid with special emphasis on adequate amounts of fruits and vegetables. Consider use of fortified foods (or supplements) to make up for specific nutrient shortfalls, such as vitamin D and calcium.
Healthy body weight	Be aware that low body weight (slender figure) increases the risk for low bone mass.
Normal menses	During childbearing years, seek medical advice if menses cease (such as in cases of anorexia nervosa or extreme athletic training). Women at menopause and beyond should consider use of current medical therapies to reduce bone loss linked to the fall in estrogen output.
Weight-bearing physical activity	Perform weight-bearing activity as this contributes to bone maintenance, whereas bed rest and a sedentary lifestyle lead to bone loss. Strength training is especially helpful to bone maintenance.
Negative Diet and Lifestyle Factors	**Action Plans to Implement**
Excessive intake of protein, phosphorus, sodium, caffeine, wheat bran, and alcohol	Moderate intake of these dietary constituents is recommended. Problems primarily arise if adequate calcium is not consumed. Excessive soft drink consumption is especially discouraged.
Smoking	Since smoking lowers estrogen output in women, smoking cessation is advised.

Bone Mass Is Related to Age and Gender

Rapid and continual bone growth and calcification occur throughout the adolescent years, ultimately resulting in what is called *peak bone mass*. In the adolescent growth spurt, bone mass is increasing at the rate of about 8.5% per year. Small increases in bone mass then continue between 20 and 30 years of age.

The ultimate amount of bone built by a person is clearly dependent on gender, race, familial patterns seen in the mother and father, and probably other genetically determined factors, such as the degree of calcium absorption. In addition, men have higher bone mass value than women, and African-Americans have heavier skeletons than Caucasians. As a direct consequence, men and African-Americans in general have a somewhat lower risk of fractures than do other populations. Slender, small-framed Caucasian and Asian women show the lowest bone mass values. Peak bone mass is also related to dietary intake of calcium and other nutrients, such as protein, phosphorus, vitamin A, vitamin D, vitamin K, magnesium, zinc, and copper (Table 9.8).

Bone mass varies among young adults, some have much denser bone than others, perhaps because they built more bone when they were young. Some people also may more easily adapt to lower-calcium diets, as has been recently shown in Chinese women in one study. People who have developed more bone by early adulthood can sustain greater age-related bone loss with less fracture risk compared with those who have less bone. Thus, osteoporosis is considered to be a "pediatric disease" with geriatic (old age) consequences.

For women, bone loss begins about age 30 and proceeds slowly and continuously to menopause (approximately age 50). It often speeds up at menopause and continues at a high rate for the next 10 years. By age 65 to 70, the rate of bone loss falls to about the same rate as before menopause. In men, bone loss is slow and steady from around age 30. Overall, this bone loss in both males and females progresses without noticeable symptoms.

Osteoporosis

Failure to maintain enough bone mass in the body can be caused by the vitamin D deficiency disease osteomalacia, the use of certain medications (such as cortisol, antiseizure drugs, and thyroid hormones), and cancer. If these or similar causes are not present, the diagnosis is osteoporosis.

continued

R esearchers in New Zealand have uncovered what they think is one reason why hip fractures are more common in Western countries than in the developing world. Because children in Western countries have higher average nutrient intakes than those in developing countries, they grow faster and to a greater extent. As a result, the part of the thigh bone that fits into the pelvis becomes quite long, increasing the risk for hip fracture, especially as bone mass decreases with advanced age. This suggests that people in Western countries especially must pursue strategies to avert hip fracture, notably in later years.

DEXA bone scan Method to measure bone density that uses small amounts of x-ray radiation. The ability of a bone to block the path of the radiation is used as a measure of bone density at that bone site. DEXA stands for dual energy, x-ray absorptiometry.

Research is also ongoing in the area of phytoestrogens, plant compounds that have hormonelike effects in the body. Phytoestrogens can come in the form of isoflavones from soy products or lignans from grains (flaxseed), fruits, and vegetables. It is hoped that these phytoestrogens will act like estrogen in the body, such as on bone. If soy is used to help reduce bone loss, intakes of about 40 grams per day of soy protein are needed. Experts currently do not recommend the use of soy isoflavone supplements. More information is needed to discover the full potential of these foodborne substances.

bisphosphonates Compounds primarily composed of carbon and phosphorus that bind to bone mineral and in turn reduce bone breakdown.

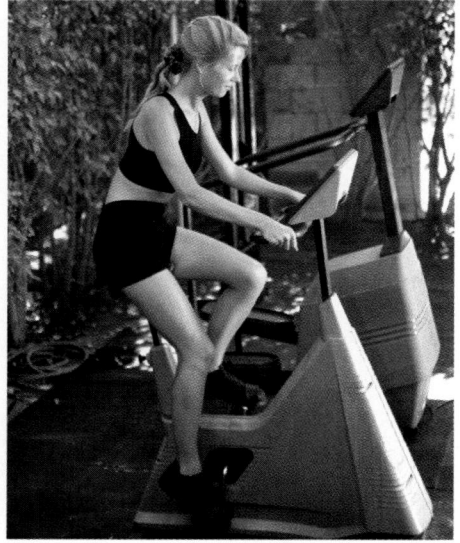

Regular, moderate physical activity contributes to bone health.

All women 65 years and older should be screened for this disease. Medicare covers the cost of the needed **DEXA bone scan.** Younger women are advised to do the same at menopause if they have associated risk factors, or if the results of the screening would help them decide what treatment plan is appropriate.

Bone composition in osteoporosis is essentially normal; basically there is just less bone throughout the body. Because these bones have less substance, osteoporosis generally leads to fractures in old age, loss of height, distorted body shape, and loss of teeth.

Preventing Osteoporosis

As women mature, different strategies for preventing osteoporosis are needed, based on the risk factors present. Young women should meet calcium, vitamin D, and other nutrient needs, as well as see a physician with any sign of irregular menstruation. In young women, regular menstruation is a main contributor to bone maintenance, as evidenced by low bone mass in some non-menstruating female athletes and other women with irregular menstruation (e.g., anorexia nervosa). An active lifestyle that includes weight-bearing physical activity is also important (to build and maintain muscle mass). Greater muscle mass linked to physical activity is associated with greater bone mass, as muscle keeps tension on bone. Still, physical activity cannot prevent the bone loss associated with irregular menstruation. Thus, female athletes with irregular menstruation should be closely monitored by a physician.

Smoking and excessive alcohol intake decrease bone mass at any age. Smoking lowers the estrogen concentration in the blood in women, increasing bone loss. Alcohol is toxic to bone cells, and alcoholism is probably a major undiagnosed and unrecognized cause of osteoporosis. Moderation in phosphorus, caffeine, sodium, and protein intake is also advised. These are especially problematic when insufficient calcium is consumed.

At menopause, women should discuss estrogen replacement and other related therapies with a physician. They also need to accurately track their height. A decrease of more than 1½ inches from premenopausal values is a sign that significant bone loss is taking place. Currently, there are four medical therapies that can be used to slow bone loss at menopause in women. Some can even be used in men who develop low bone mass. The approved drugs are estrogen (various forms are available; some contain added progestins); **bisphosphonates** (alendronate [Fosamax] and risedronate [Actonel]), selective estrogen receptor modulators (SERMs) (raloxifene [Evista]); and calcitonin (nasal form is Miacalcin). Estrogen and SERMs blunt bone turnover by binding to receptors on bone; bisphosphonates blunt bone resorption by binding to bone mineral; and calcitonon inhibits the bone cells that participate in bone resorption. All of these medications have side effects, so use needs to be tailored to a person's current health status. The latest thinking is that estrogen replacement is most useful for treating menopausal symptoms such as hot flashes. The bisphosphonates are most useful for preventing bone loss. The recent trend to use bisphosphonates as the major form of medical therapy for osteoporosis rather than estrogen replacement stems from the observation that greater than 5 to 10 years of estrogen use increases the risk for breast and some other forms of cancer. If a woman at menopause begins estrogen therapy to relieve related symptoms, experts suggest she should consider switching to another form of osteoporosis therapy after 5 to 10 years of such use. Any use of these medications also benefits from meeting calcium and vitamin D needs.

Older men and women need to stay physically active—including some weight-bearing and resistance activities—and they should meet the Adequate Intake for calcium set for their particular age. This physical activity and calcium intake are most likely to limit bone loss in some areas of the body, such as the hip. Older people also need to minimize the risk for falls, especially by limiting their use of medications and alcohol, which might disturb coordination, and they should take corrective measures if visual function is impaired. Hip protective garments are also available to reduce hip fracture risk. Regular sun exposure and the consumption of food sources of vitamin D are very important. Supplements containing up to 20 micrograms (800 IU) are also appropriate (see Chapter 8). To find out more about osteoporosis, check out the website of the National Osteoporosis Foundation (www.nof.org) or call (800) 464-6700. Another helpful website is that of the National Dairy Council (www.nationaldairycouncil.org).

Chapter Outline

O f people you see on the street, one-fourth of the men and nearly half the women are struggling to control their weight. Still, despite all their efforts, the ranks of the obese in America and worldwide are growing. Recall from Chapter 1 that it is estimated that 1.1 billion people in the world are overweight. This problem is increasing not only in the United States but also in affluent peoples in Brazil, China, India, Russia, the United Kingdom, and Germany. This excess weight increases the likelihood of many health problems, such as cardiovascular disease, cancer, hypertension and strokes, certain bone and joint disorders, and type 2 diabetes.

Currently, most weight-reduction efforts fizzle before bodies fall into a healthy weight range. Monotonous, ineffective, and confusing, typical fad diets even endanger some populations, such as children, teenagers, pregnant women, and people with various health disorders. Yet a more logical approach to weight loss is actually very straightforward: (1) Eat less; (2) increase physical activity; and (3) change problematic eating behaviors.

Experts are calling for a national commitment to address the growing weight problem in North America. They suspect that, without a national commitments to weight maintenance and effective new approaches to making the environment more favorable to maintaining healthy weight, the current trends will not be reversed. This chapter discusses these recommendations to help you understand obesity's effects, causes, and potential treatments.

Check out the **Contemporary Nutrition: Issues and Insights Online Learning Center** *www.mhhe.com/wardlawcont5 for quizzes, flash cards, other activities, and web links designed to further help you learn about weight control.*

Chapter Objectives

Chapter 10 is designed to allow you to:

1. Describe the uses of energy by the body and what constitutes energy balance.

2. Describe various ways to diagnose overweight and obesity.

3. Outline the risks to health posed by overweight and obesity.

4. List and discuss factors affecting energy balance in overweight and obesity with respect to nature and nurture, and describe the concept of set point with regard to body weight.

5. Describe why and how reduced energy intake, behavior modification, and increased physical activity fit into a weight-loss plan.

6. Outline the benefits and hazards of various weight-loss methods for severe obesity.

7. Describe possible reasons and treatments for underweight status.

8. Evaluate fad weight-reduction diets and determine which are unsafe, doomed to fail, or both.

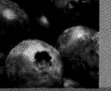 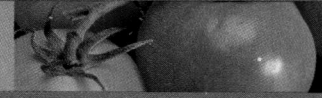

Refresh Your Memory

As you begin your study of weight control in Chapter 10, you may want to review:

- Biological and social dimensions of food intake in Chapter 1

- The concept of energy density and appropriate single serving sizes for foods in Chapter 2

- The causes and consequences of ketosis in Chapter 4

- The fat content of various foods in Chapter 5

- The long-term risks of high protein diets in Chapter 6

Real Life Scenario

Crystal has a hectic schedule. She works during the day for a "temp" agency, primarily performing secretarial duties. Three times a week she attends night classes at the local community college in pursuit of computer certification. She has little time to think about what she eats—convenience rules. Unfortunately, over the past few years Crystal's weight has been climbing. Watching television a few night ago, she saw an infomercial for a product that promises she can eat large portions of tasty foods but not gain weight. Famous celebrities support the claim that this product allows one to eat at will and not gain weight. She doesn't have a lot of spare money, but the claim that by taking this product you can eat whatever you want and never gain weight is tempting. What do you think she should do?

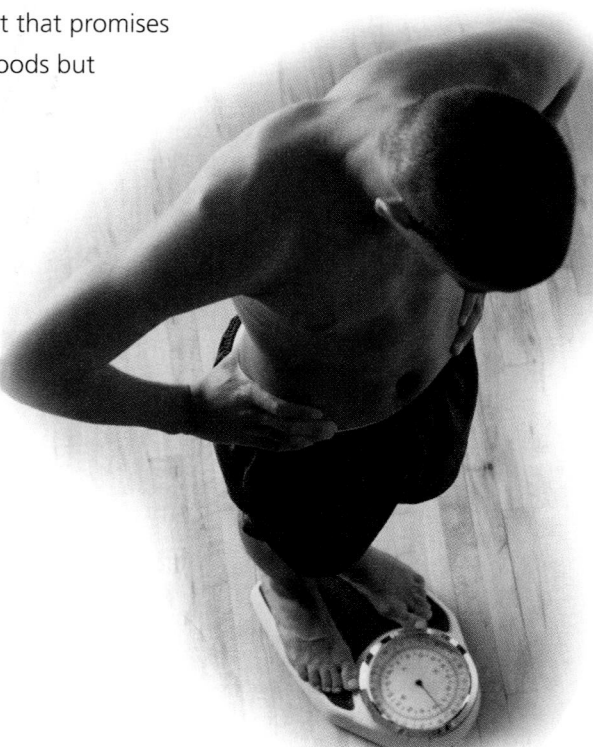

Nutrition Connection

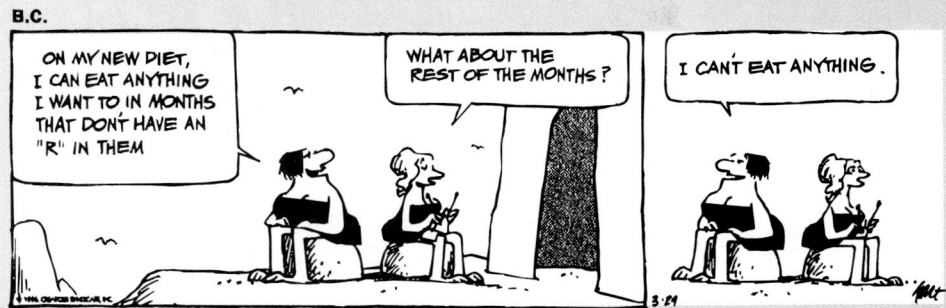

B.C.

What components make up a successful diet plan? What typically characterizes fad diets? Why is overweight and obesity a growing problem worldwide? What might be the future consequences of this trend? This chapter provides some answers.

B.C. ©*United Features Syndicate. Reprinted by Permission.*

Energy Balance

This chapter on weight control starts with some good news and some bad news. The good news is that, as a college student, you are probably at a healthy body weight. An important life goal is to stay within the recommended range for healthy body weight. The bad news is that over 60% of all North American adults are overweight (about 40% of these people are obese). As well, there is a good chance that any of us can join those ranks if we don't pay attention to the prevention of significant adult weight gain. Gaining more than 10 pounds or 2 inches in waist circumference should be a red flag that diet and physical activity re-evaluation is in order. This preventive strategy is currently considered the most potent form of therapy for the problem of overweight in our society. Other strategies do exist; however, as you will see, they have not shown to be as successful as prevention.

■ Positive and Negative Energy Balance

Bathroom scales keep many of us emotionally off balance. We would all benefit by paying more attention to another scale—that of **energy balance**. This balance depends on energy input and energy output. These in turn influence energy stores, primarily, the amount of triglyceride in adipose tissue (Fig. 10.1). Energy balance can be thought of as an equation: energy consumed minus energy expended. You are in positive energy balance when energy consumed is greater than energy expended. The result of **positive energy balance** is the storage of the excess energy.

Pregnancy is an example of when positive energy balance is necessary because the surplus of energy supports the developing fetus. Infants and children also need to be in positive energy balance to grow. In adults, however, positive energy balance causes creeping weight gain.

Negative energy balance results from an energy deficit. Energy consumed is less than energy expended. Weight loss occurs when a person is in a state of negative energy balance. In adulthood, however, the weight that is lost consists of a combination of lean and adipose tissue.

energy balance The state in which energy intake, in the form of food and/or alcohol, matches the energy expended, primarily through basal metabolism and physical activity.

positive energy balance The state in which energy intake is greater than energy expended, generally resulting in weight gain.

negative energy balance The state in which energy intake is less than energy expended, resulting in weight loss.

Figure 10.1 A model for energy balance (a). The model of a laboratory scale incorporates the major variables that influence energy balance. Note that alcohol is an additional source of energy for some of us (b). The different states of energy balance are shown.

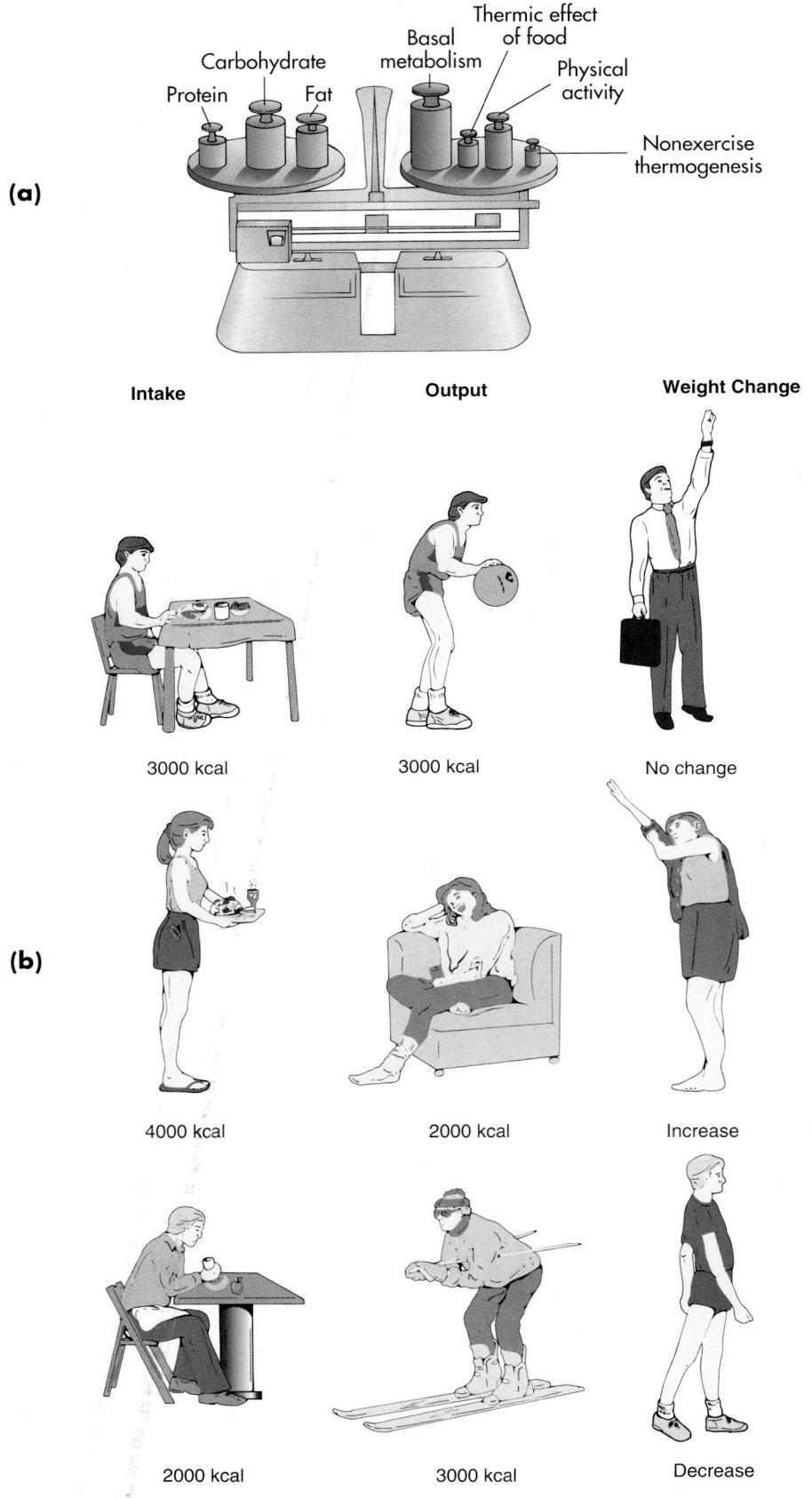

Critical Thinking

A 26-year-old classmate of yours has been thinking about the process of aging. One of the things she fears most as she gets older is gaining weight. How would you explain energy balance to her?

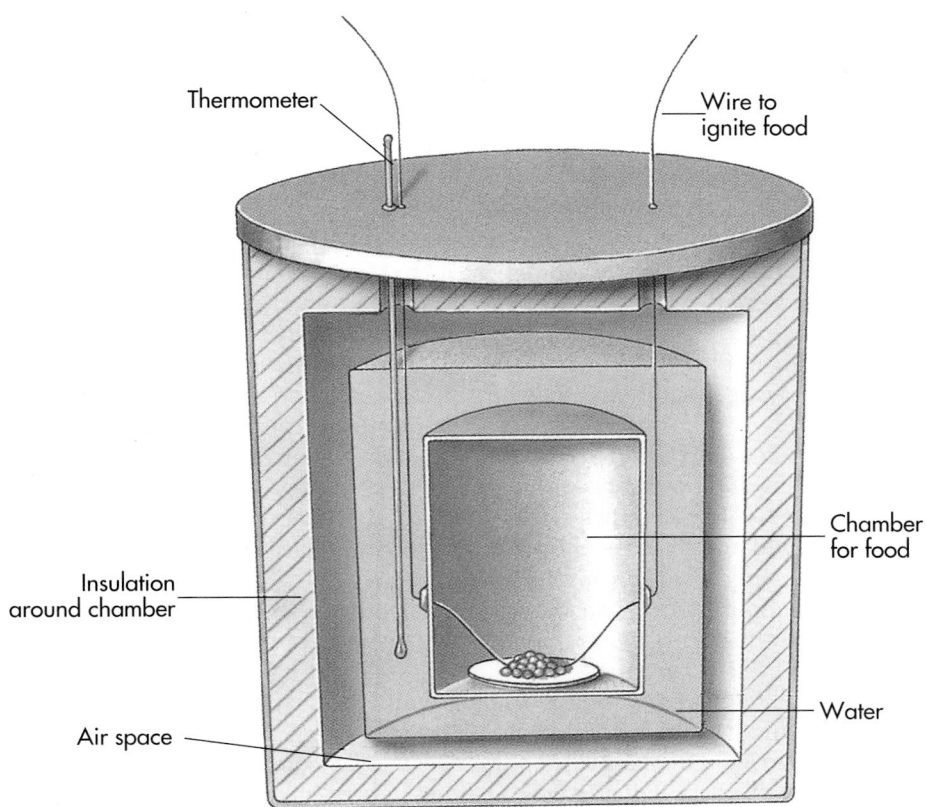

Figure 10.2 Cross-section of a bomb calorimeter. A dried portion of food is burned inside a chamber charged with oxygen and surrounded by water to determine energy content. As the food is burned, it gives off heat, which raises the temperature of the water surrounding the chamber. The amount of increase in water temperature indicates the number of kcal contained in the food, because 1 kcal equals the amount of heat needed to raise the temperature of 1 kilogram of water 1 degree Celsius.
Illustration by William Ober

As noted in the overview, the maintenance of energy balance—energy intake matching energy output over the long run—substantially contributes to health and well-being in adults by minimizing the risk of developing many common health problems. As well, adulthood is often a time of creeping weight gain, which eventually turns into obesity if not checked. However, increasing age is not the primary reason for this weight gain; it is caused primarily by the pattern of excess food intake and limited physical activity. Let's look in detail at the factors that affect the relationship between positive and negative energy balance.

▮ Energy Intake

Energy needs are met by food intake, represented by the number of kcal eaten each day. Determining the appropriate amount and type of food to match energy needs over the long run is a challenge for many of us. Our ability to consume food and use it efficiently is an evolutionary survival mechanism. We are by nature food-seeking and fat-storing organisms. However, given modern North American food supplies, many of us are now too successful in obtaining food energy. Given the wide availability of food in vending machines, drive-up windows, social gatherings, and fast-food (quick-service) restaurants—combined with the all too common *super-sized* portions—it is no wonder that the average adult is 8 pounds heavier than just 10 years ago. You might say "food hunts man" today, rather than man hunting food as in earlier times.

How much food energy actually is contained in a meal? A **bomb calorimeter** is used to determine the amount of energy in a food (Fig. 10.2). The process involves burning a portion of food inside a chamber of the calorimeter that is surrounded by water. As the food burns, it gives off heat, which raises the temperature of the water surrounding the chamber. The increase in water temperature measured after the food has burned indicates the amount of energy in the food. Recall from Chapter 1 that 1 kcal is the amount of energy required to increase the temperature of 1 kilogram (about 2.2 pounds) of water 1° Celsius.

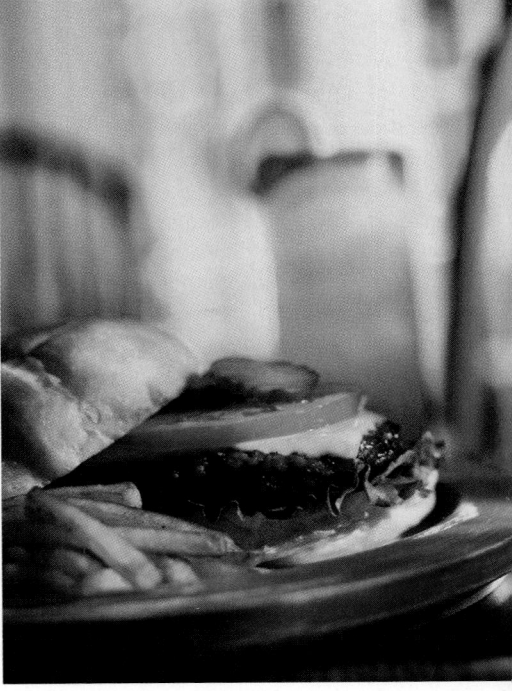

Today we demand food that is immediately available, tastes great, requires little or no preparation, and is served in generous quantities. Of all these characteristics, the generous quantities are the most troublesome for many of us.

The bomb calorimeter provides values for the amount of energy that can be derived from carbohydrate, fat, protein, and alcohol. Recall also from Chapter 1 that carbohydrates yield about 4 kcal per gram, proteins yield about 4 kcal per gram, fats yield about 9 kcal per gram, and alcohol yields about 7 kcal per gram. These energy figures have been adjusted for (1) digestibility and (2) substances in food, such as fibrous plant parts, that burn in the bomb calorimeter but are unusable by the human body for energy needs. The figures are then rounded to whole numbers.

In bomb calorimeter studies, fats produce close to 9 kcal per gram. This value alone should warn us about the overconsumption of fat. However, most absorbed fats are not immediately burned in the body for energy needs. Instead, much fat goes directly into storage in adipose tissue. We have an essentially unlimited ability to do this.

In contrast, most of the carbohydrate eaten is used at the time of consumption for energy needs or glycogen synthesis; generally little is converted to fat for storage in the body. This is not to say, however, that infinite amounts of carbohydrate can be consumed: Excessive amounts lead to decreased use of fat for energy needs and possibly increased fat synthesis—both changes contribute to fat storage.

Protein is used for tissue synthesis, but adults generally eat more than enough protein for this. Beyond body needs, excess amounts of amino acids are generally metabolized for energy; only some are metabolized as fat.

Carbohydrate and protein intake also stimulate body use of these fuels. This is not true for fat. Finally, the body must expend much energy if carbohydrate or protein is turned into fat—if this occurs at all.

Based on these observations, experts suggest that, ideally, fat intake should not exceed the amount of fat burned by the body. Active people can achieve this more easily than can those who are sedentary, since physical activity encourages burning of dietary fat. For a person who is sedentary and consumes a large amount of dietary fat, it is thought that any obesity that results actually represents an adaptation to this high-fat diet. This is because it is thought that only by reaching a certain point of body fatness will this sedentary person be able to balance the amount of fat burned by the body with fat intake: The greater fat mass present now allows for more release of body fat as fatty acids into circulation, so more fat is available for use. In other words, one needs enough fat mass to be able to burn the great amount of fat consumed over a long-term basis.

As noted in Chapters 2 and 5, it is also easier to overeat high-fat foods because they are energy dense and highly palatable. We can more easily eat a few extra cookies than a few extra apples, even though both may contain about the same amount of food energy. Laboratory animals become more obese when provided with high-fat foods than with their typical leaner fare. All of these findings suggest that, to reduce or control body fatness, monitor fat intake, substituting instead moderate amounts of carbohydrate foods rich in dietary fiber (i.e., low energy density).

Recall from Chapter 5 that some experts suggest adults should follow a relatively high-fat diet, up to 40% of calories. Such a diet requires careful monitoring of total energy intake, as weight gain is likely on this dietary pattern.

basal metabolism The minimal energy the body requires to support itself in a fasting state when resting and awake in a warm, quiet environment. It amounts to roughly 1 kcal per kilogram per hour for men and 0.9 kcal per kilogram per hour for women; these values are often referred to as basal metabolic rate (BMR).

While a person is resting, the percentage of total energy use by various organs is about as follows:

Liver	27%
Brain	19%
Skeletal muscle	18%
Kidneys	10%
Heart	7%
Other	19%

■ Energy Output

So far, some factors concerning energy intake have been discussed. Now let's look at the other side of the relationship—energy output.

The body uses energy for three general purposes: basal metabolism, physical activity, and the thermic effect of food. Fidgeting demonstrates another minor form of energy turned into heat production, and is part of what is called *nonexercise activity thermogenesis* (NEAT) (review Fig. 10.1).

Basal Metabolism

Basal metabolism represents the minimum energy expended in a fasting state (12 hours) to keep a resting, awake body alive in a warm, quiet environment. This requires about 60% to 70% of total energy use by the body. The processes involved include maintaining a heartbeat, respiration, temperature, and other functions. It does not include energy used for physical activity or food digestion. For an example of how basal metabolism contributes to energy needs, consider a 130 pound woman. Convert her weight, in pounds, into kilograms (130 ÷ 2.2 = 59 kilograms). Then, multiply 59 kilograms × 0.9 kcal per kilograms per hour × 24 hours = 1274 kcal needed for basal metabolism. Note that basal metabolism varies 25% to 30% among individuals.

The amount of **energy** used for basal metabolism depends primarily on **lean body mass.** That is, basal metabolism is generally higher in people with greater amounts of lean body mass than in those with large proportions of fat mass. The participating tissues in basal metabolism—such as muscle, liver, brain, and kidney—show high metabolic activity at rest and have high energy needs. Other influences that determine basal metabolism include the following:

- The amount of body surface (the greater the area, the greater the heat loss)
- Gender (males average higher energy use because of greater lean body mass)
- Body temperature (fever and cold conditions both increase basal metabolism)
- Thyroid hormones (increase basal metabolism)
- Aspects of nervous system activity, such as norepinephrine release (increases basal metabolism)
- Age (basal metabolism rate falls as we age through adulthood)
- Nutritional state (eating less slows basal metabolism rate in the short term)
- Pregnancy (increases basal metabolism)
- Caffeine and tobacco use (increase basal metabolism)

A low energy intake decreases the basal metabolism by about 10% to 20%, or about 150 to 300 kcal per day. This makes losing weight difficult. In addition, the effects of aging make weight maintenance hard. Basal metabolism declines about 2% each decade past age 30 as activity-metabolizing cells slowly and steadily decrease. However, because physical activity helps maintain lean body mass, remaining active as one ages helps maintain a high basal metabolism and, in turn, aids in weight control.

Energy for Physical Activity

Physical activity increases energy expenditure above and beyond basal energy needs by as much as 25% to 40%. In choosing to be active or inactive, we determine much of our total energy expenditure for a day. Unlike basal metabolism, energy expenditure from physical activity varies widely among people.

Climbing stairs rather than riding the elevator, walking rather than driving, riding a bicycle to class, and standing in a bus rather than sitting increase physical activity and, hence, energy use.

The alarming rate of and recent increase in obesity in North America are caused in part by our inactivity. We eat little more than people did at the turn of the twentieth century, but we are less active. Jobs demand less physical activity, and leisure time is usually spent slouched before a television or computer.

Thermic Effect of Food (TEF)

In addition to basal metabolism and physical activity, the body uses energy to digest, absorb, and further process food nutrients. Energy used for these tasks accounts for the **thermic effect of food (TEF).** The energy cost of this thermic effect is analogous to a sales tax. It is like being taxed about 5% to 10% for the total energy you eat. The charge covers the cost of processing that energy. To supply the body with 100 kcal for basal metabolism and physical activity, you must eat between 105 and 110 kcal. The processes of digestion, absorption, and metabolism use the extra 5 to 10 kcal to modify the energy-yielding nutrients for use. Given a daily energy intake of 3000 kcal, the thermic effect of food uses 150 to 300 kcal (3000 × 0.05 = 150; 3000 × 0.1 = 300). However, the total amount can vary somewhat among individuals.

The TEF value for a carbohydrate-rich or a protein-rich meal is higher than for a fat-rich meal. This is because it takes less energy to transfer absorbed fat into adipose stores than to convert glucose into glycogen or to metabolize excess amino acids into

lean body mass Body weight minus fat storage weight equals lean body mass. This includes organs such as the brain, muscles, and liver, as well as blood and other body fluids.

*W*hen planning a smoking cessation program, a plan to limit weight gain should also be implemented. Smoking cessation is linked to an increased risk of weight gain and obesity. Any form of regular physical activity can be extremely beneficial in an attempt to keep weight in check. Various risk factors associated with smoking, however, make it essential that this population obtain approval from a physician before beginning an intensive exercise regimen.

thermic effect of food (TEF) The increase in metabolism occurring during the digestion, absorption, and metabolism of energy-yielding nutrients. This represents 5% to 10% of energy consumed.

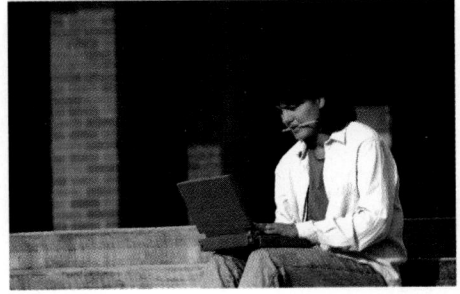

Classwork leads to mental stress but puts little physical stress on the body. Hence, energy needs are only about 1.5 kcal per minute.

*O*ther names for the thermic effect of food include specific dynamic action and diet-induced thermogenesis.

nonexercise activity thermogenesis (NEAT) Adaptive energy expended in heat production, such as fidgeting when one is subjected to overfeeding.

brown adipose tissue A specialized form of adipose tissue that produces large amounts of heat by metabolizing energy-yielding nutrients without synthesizing much useful energy for the body. The unused energy is released as heat.

fat. In addition, large meals show higher values for TEF than the same amount of food eaten over many hours. Some possible mechanisms for this phenomenon include changes in central nervous system activity, greater production and release of hormones (such as insulin) and enzymes, and the rate of absorption and storage of macronutrients.

Nonexercise Activity Thermogenesis (NEAT)

Nonexercise activity thermogenesis (NEAT) represents the increase in nonvoluntary physical activity triggered by overeating. This activity includes fidgeting, maintenance of muscle tone, and maintenance of body posture when not lying down. Studies have shown that some people resist weight gain from overfeeding by inducing NEAT, whereas other people are not able to do so to as great an extent.

Another Bite

*B*rown adipose tissue is a specialized form of adipose tissue found in small amounts in infants. The brown appearance results from its rich blood flow. Brown adipose tissue contributes to nonexercise activity thermogenesis by disconnecting the use of energy-yielding nutrients and the production of energy for cell use (see Chapter 11 for details on energy use by cells). In brown adipose tissue, compared to other types of cells, more of the energy released from metabolism is simply lost as heat. The role of brown adipose tissue in adults in unknown; it appears that adults have little brown adipose tissue. One interesting finding regarding brown adipose tissue is that hibernating animals contain much of it. This allows them to create the heat needed to withstand a long winter.

Overall, a sedentary person uses 70% to 80% of energy for a combination of basal metabolism and the thermic effect of food. The remainder is used for physical activity and nonexercise activity thermogenesis.

Concept Check

*E*nergy balance compares energy intake with energy output. Energy content of food is expressed in kcal and is determined using a bomb calorimeter. This analysis yields the 4-9-4-7 estimates for the energy content of carbohydrate, fat, protein, and alcohol, respectively.

The body uses this energy for four main purposes:

1. Basal metabolism represents the minimal amount of energy needed to maintain a body in a resting state. The rate of a person's basal metabolism depends greatly on the amount of lean body mass, the amount of body surface, and thyroid hormone concentrations in the bloodstream.
2. Physical activity expenditure represents energy use for total body cell metabolism above what is needed during rest (that is, basal metabolism).
3. The thermic effect of food represents the energy needed to digest, absorb, and process absorbed nutrients. This corresponds to 5% to 10% of energy used for basal metabolism and physical activity.
4. Nonexercise activity thermogenesis (NEAT) is heat production in response to overfeeding and other stimuli. Increased fidgeting is generally seen.

In a sedentary person, 70% to 80% of energy is used for basal metabolism and the thermic effect of food; the remainder is used for physical activity and nonexercise adaptive thermogenesis.

Determination of Energy Use by the Body

The amount of energy a body uses can be measured by both direct and indirect calorimetry or can be simply estimated based on height, weight, degree of physical activity, and age.

■ Direct and Indirect Calorimetry

Direct calorimetry measures the amount of body heat released by a person. The subject is put into an insulated chamber, often the size of a small bedroom, and body heat released raises the temperature of a layer of water surrounding the chamber. A kcal, as you recall, is related to the amount of heat available to raise the temperature of the water. By measuring the water temperature in the direct calorimeter before and after the body releases heat, scientists can determine the energy expended. This method resembles the bomb calorimeter method for measuring the energy content in food.

Direct calorimetry works because almost all the energy used by the body eventually leaves as heat. However, few studies use direct calorimetry, mostly because of its expense and complexity.

For **indirect calorimetry,** instead of measuring heat output, the most commonly used method measures the amount of oxygen a person uses (Fig. 10.3). A predictable relationship exists between the body's use of energy and oxygen. For example, when metabolizing a mixed diet of carbohydrate, fat, and protein—a typical blend of nutrients—the human body needs 1 liter of oxygen to metabolize about 4.85 kcal.

Instruments used to measure oxygen consumption for indirect calorimetry have great versatility. They can be mounted on carts and rolled up to a hospital bed or carried in backpacks while a person plays tennis or jogs. Tables showing energy demands of exercises rely on information gained from indirect calorimetry studies. There are also other methods of determining energy use by indirect calorimetry, but these will not be covered.

direct calorimetry A method of determining a body's energy use by measuring heat that emanates from the body, usually using an insulated chamber.

indirect calorimetry A method to measure the energy use by the body by measuring oxygen uptake. Formulas are then used to convert this gas exchange value into energy use.

■ Estimates of Energy Needs

A rough estimate for energy needs uses a person's weight and degree of physical activity. Total energy needs for a sedentary person are set at 25 to 30 kcal per kilogram. The value may then decrease by 100 kcal for every 10 years of age over age 30. People performing moderate activity, such as routine walking, start with 35 kcal per kilogram; those regularly performing heavy activity, as required in some sports play, start at 40 kcal per kilogram. These values can then be adjusted for age, as mentioned previously. For example, a 66 kilogram (145 pound), 40-year-old woman performing moderate activity needs to eat about 2200 kcal ([66 kilogram × 35 kcal per kilogram] − 100) to meet total energy needs.

Rough guidelines for energy needs found in the Food Guide Pyramid publication are as follows:

- Sedentary women and some older adults — 1600 kcal
- Children, teenage girls, active women, most men — 2200 kcal
- Teenage boys, active men, very active women — 2800 kcal
- Young children, pregnant and breastfeeding women — Check with a registered dietitian

These values then need to be fine-tuned based on personal characteristics and experiences, such as amount of physical activity performed.

A simple method of tracking your energy expenditure, and thus your energy needs, is to use the forms in Appendix E. Begin by taking an entire 24-hour period and listing all activities performed, including sleep. Record the number of minutes spent in

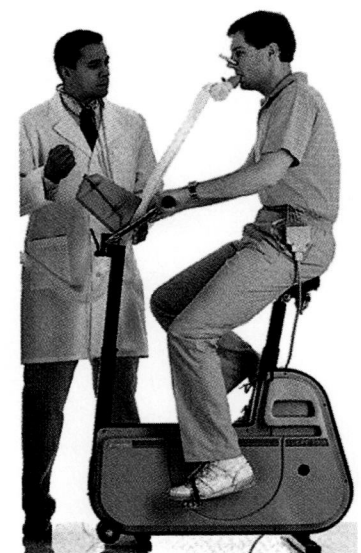

Figure 10.3 Indirect calorimetry. The method of measuring oxygen use and carbon dioxide output can determine energy output during daily activities.

each activity; the total should equal 1440 minutes (24 hours). Next record the energy cost for each activity in kcal per minute following the directions in Appendix E; these values are based on your weight in kilograms (pounds ÷ 2.2). Multiply the energy cost by the minutes. This gives the energy expended for each activity. Total all the kcal values. This gives your estimated energy expenditure for the day.

Concept Check

*E*nergy use by the body can be measured by direct calorimetry as heat given off and by indirect calorimetry as oxygen used. Total energy needs can be estimated based on a person's characteristics: weight, age, and amount of physical activity. In addition, the Food Guide Pyramid publication provides rough guidelines for energy intake.

*H*ealthy weight is currently the preferred term to use for weight recommendations. Older terms, such as ideal weight and desirable weight, are no longer used in the medical literature.

Estimation of a Healthy Weight

Numerous methods are used to set what body weight should be, typically called *healthy body weight*. Several tables exist, generally based on weight-for-height. These tables arise from studies of large population groups. When applied to a population, they provide good estimates of weight associated with health and longevity. These tables, however, do not necessarily refer directly to an individual's weight and health status.

Ideally, family history of weight-related disease and current health parameters should be considered when establishing a healthy weight for an individual, in addition to weight-for-height. Evidence of the following weight-related conditions is important:

- Hypertension
- Elevated LDL-cholesterol
- Family history of obesity, cardiovascular disease, or certain forms of cancer (e.g., breast, colon)
- Pattern of fat distribution in the body
- Elevated blood glucose

On a more practical note, other questions can be pertinent: What is the least one has weighed as an adult for at least a year? What is the largest size clothing one would be happy with? What weight has one been able to maintain during previous diets without feeling constantly hungry? Overall, the individual, under a physician's guidance, should establish a "personal" healthy weight (or need for weight reduction) based on weight history, fat distribution patterns, family history of weight-related disease, and current health status. This assessment points out how well the person is tolerating any existing excess weight. Thus, current height/weight standards are only a rough guide. Furthermore, a healthy lifestyle may make a more important contribution to a person's health status than the number on the scale. Fit and overweight are, for the most part, not mutually exclusive. And neither is thin synonymous with healthy if the person is also not physically active. This topic is discussed at greater length later in the chapter with regard to the appropriateness of a recommendation for weight loss.

■ Using Body Mass Index (BMI) to Set Healthy Weight

Body mass index (BMI) is the current method for calculating healthy body weight. It is based on the study of a wide variety of people from many countries. The older method, using the Metropolitan Life Insurance tables, is a less accurate way of establishing healthy body weight. The Metropolitan Life Insurance tables do not represent the North American population as a whole because these tables were based on people who had life insurance policies (see Appendix G for the Metropolitan Life Insurance

Women Men

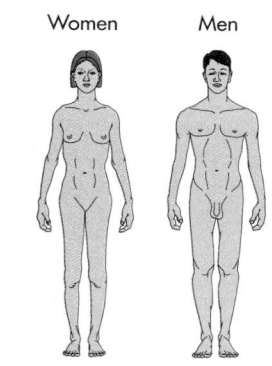

BMI 20

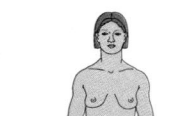
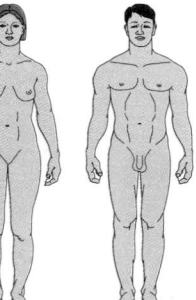

BMI 25

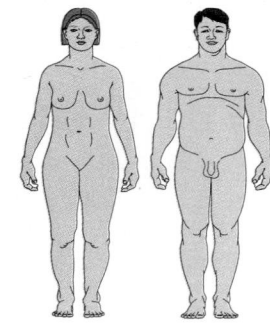

BMI 30

Estimates of body shapes at different BMI values.

Table 10.1 Body Weight in Pounds According to Height and Body Mass Index (BMI)

	BMI (kilogram per meter^2)													
	19	20	21	22	23	24	25	26	27	28	29	30	35	40
Height (Inches)	Body Weight (Pounds)													
58	91	96	100	105	110	115	119	124	129	134	138	143	167	191
59	94	99	104	109	114	119	124	128	133	138	143	148	173	198
60	97	102	107	112	118	123	128	133	138	143	148	153	179	204
61	100	106	111	116	122	127	132	137	143	148	153	158	185	211
62	104	109	115	120	126	131	136	142	124	153	158	164	191	218
63	107	113	118	124	130	135	141	146	152	158	163	169	197	225
64	110	116	122	128	134	140	145	151	157	163	169	174	204	232
65	114	120	126	132	138	144	150	156	162	168	174	180	210	240
66	118	124	130	136	142	148	155	161	167	173	179	186	216	247
67	121	127	134	140	146	153	159	166	172	178	185	191	223	255
68	125	131	138	144	151	158	164	171	177	184	190	197	230	262
69	128	135	142	149	155	162	169	176	182	189	196	203	236	270
70	132	139	146	153	160	167	174	181	188	195	202	207	243	278
71	136	143	150	157	165	172	179	186	193	200	208	215	250	286
72	140	147	154	162	169	177	184	191	199	206	213	221	258	294
73	144	151	159	166	174	182	189	197	204	212	219	227	265	302
74	148	155	163	171	179	186	194	202	210	218	225	233	272	311
75	152	160	168	176	184	192	200	208	216	224	232	240	279	319
76	156	164	172	180	189	197	205	213	221	230	238	246	287	328

Each entry gives the body weight in pounds for a person of a given height and BMI. The values apply to both men and women. Pounds have been rounded off. To use the table, find the appropriate height in the far left column. Move across the row to a weight. The number at the top of the column is the BMI for the height and weight. As a rough estimate, 1 BMI unit equals 6–7 pounds.

tables). Also, body mass index is the weight-for-height standard that is most closely related to body fat content.

Body mass index is calculated as

$$\frac{\text{body weight (in kilograms)}}{\text{height}^2\text{ (in meters)}}$$

An alternate method for calculating BMI is

$$\frac{\text{weight (pounds)} \times 703.1}{\text{height}^2\text{ (inches)}}$$

Table 10.1 lists BMI for various heights and weights. Health risks from excess weight begin when the body mass index reaches 25. A healthy weight-for-height is a BMI of 18.5 to 24.9. What is your BMI? How much would your weight need to change to yield a BMI of 25? 30? These are general cut-off values for the presence of overweight and obesity, respectively.

The concept of body mass index is convenient to use because the values apply to both men and women. However, any body weight-for-height standard is actually a crude measure because we are concerned about overfat, not simply overweight, individuals when setting guidelines for healthy weight. The husky athlete is a notable exception; he or she may be overweight but not overfat because the excess weight is from muscle mass, not fat mass. For this reason, any weight-for-height measurement such as BMI should be used only as a screening test for obesity.

BMI is not a standard for everyone. Adult BMI should not be applied to children, adolescents who are still growing, frail elderly people, pregnant and lactating women, and highly muscular individuals. Children and pregnant women have unique BMI standards (see Chapters 13 and 14).

*F*ormer Surgeon General Dr. C. Everett
Koop is currently spearheading a
campaign called "Shape Up America," to
convince overweight people to lose weight
and increase physical activity. According to Dr.
Koop, obesity is the number two killer in the
United States. What many North Americans
don't understand, he explains, is how serious
the problem of excess pounds is. Although
many North Americans are aware that
smoking is responsible for many deaths each
year, they are not aware that obesity is
responsible for nearly as many—300,000—
deaths annually in the United States alone.
Before long, obesity will surpass cigarette
smoking as a leading cause of death in
North America.

Still, overfat and overweight conditions generally appear together. The focus is on
body weight-for-height standards in clinical settings mainly because these are easier to
measure than total body fat.

■ Putting Healthy Weight into Perspective

One current school of thought is to let nature take its course with regard to body
weight. According to this proposal, by trying to lose weight in order to fall within a
specific (often unrealistic) height/weight range, people often regain their original
weight plus more. In contrast, listening to the body for hunger cues, eating a healthy
diet, and remaining physically active eventually help one maintain an appropriate
height/weight value. This concept will be further addressed in the upcoming discussion
on treatment for obesity. It is a cornerstone of the current "size acceptance"
movement. The clearest idea regarding a healthy weight is that it is personal. Weight
has to be considered in terms of health, not simply fashion.

Concept Check

*T*oday healthy body weight is generally determined using body mass index. The
presence of existing weight-related disease should be considered in determining
healthy body weight. Total health and a healthy lifestyle, not simply fashion, should be
the major considerations when determining healthy weight.

Energy Imbalance

If energy intake exceeds expenditure over time, obesity is likely to result. Often, health
problems eventually follow (Table 10.2). In this context, medical experts recommend
that an individual's cutoff value for obesity should not be based primarily on body
weight but, rather, on the total amount of fat in the body, the location of body fat, and
the presence or absence of weight-related medical problems.

■ Estimating Body Fat Content and Diagnosing Obesity

Body fat can range from 2% to 70% of body weight. In this regard, men with over
25% body fat and women with over about 35% body fat are considered obese. Desirable
amounts are about 8% to 25% body fat for men and 20% to 35% for women.
Women need more body fat because some "sex-specific" fat is associated with reproductive
functions. This fat is normal and factored into calculations.

Various methods are used to estimate body fat content. **Underwater weighing**
(most accurate) works because fat tissue is less dense than lean tissue; because fat
floats, the more fat tissue present, the less a person weighs when submerged. This procedure
requires a trained technician and submersion (Fig. 10.4).

Although there are some limits to its accuracy, skinfold thickness is the method
most widely used to estimate total body fat. Clinicians use calipers to measure the fat
layer directly under the skin at multiple sites (Fig. 10.5).

Clinicians have begun measuring total body fat using **bioelectrical impedance.**
This technique sends a painless, low-energy electrical current to and from the body via
wires and electrode patches. Researchers surmise that fat resists electrical flow, so more
fat proportionately means greater electrical resistance. Within a few minutes, bioelectrical
impedance analyzers convert body electrical resistance into an approximate estimate
of total body fat, as long as body hydration status is normal (Fig. 10.6).

Another method for estimating total body fat exposes the biceps to infrared light,
assessing the interactions with the fat and protein in arm muscle. After only 2 seconds,
this flashlight-size device can give an estimate.

underwater weighing A method of
estimating total body fat by weighing the
individual on a standard scale and then
weighing him or her again submerged in
water. The difference between the two
weights is used to estimate total body fat.

bioelectrical impedance The method to
estimate total body fat that uses a low-energy
electrical current. The more fat storage a
person has, the more impedance (resistance)
to electrical flow will be exhibited.

Table 10.2 Health Problems Associated with Excess Body Fat

Health Problem	Partially Attributable To
Surgical risk	Increased anesthesia needs and greater risk of wound infections
Pulmonary disease and sleep disorders	Excess weight over lungs and pharynx
Type 2 diabetes	Enlarged adipose cells, which poorly bind insulin and poorly respond to the message insulin sends to the cell
Hypertension	Increased miles of blood vessels found in the adipose tissue, increased blood volume, and increased resistance to blood flow
Cardiovascular disease	Increases in LDL-cholesterol and triglyceride values, low HDL-cholesterol, and decreased physical activity
Bone and joint disorders (including **gout**)	Excess pressure put on knee, ankle, and hip joints
Gallstones	Increased cholesterol content of bile
Skin disorders	Trapping of moisture and microbes in tissue folds
Various cancers (e.g., breast, colon, pancreas, gallbladder)	Estrogen production by adipose cells; animal studies suggest excess energy intake encourages tumor development
Shorter stature (in some forms of obesity)	Earlier onset of puberty
Pregnancy risks	More difficult delivery, increased number of birth defects, and increased needs for anesthesia
Reduced physical agility and increased risk of accidents and falls	Excess weight that impairs movement
Menstrual irregularities and infertility	Hormones produced by adipose cells, such as estrogen
Premature death	A variety of risk factors for disease, listed in this table

The greater the degree of obesity, the more likely and the more serious these health problems generally become. They are much more likely to appear in people who show an upper-body fat distribution pattern and/or greater than twice healthy body weight. Overall, obese people typically have numerous chronic health problems and poor physical health.

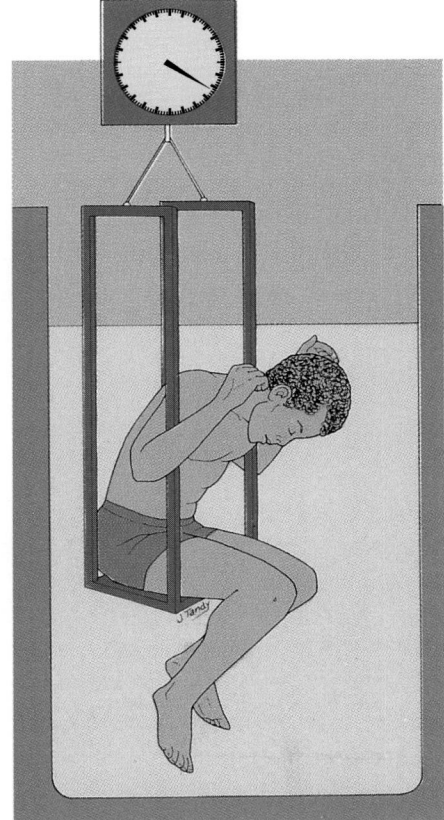

Figure 10.4 Underwater weighing. To get an accurate estimate of body fat, the subject exhales as much air as possible and then holds his or her breath and bends over at the waist. Once the subject is totally submerged, the underwater weight is recorded. For example, the loss of weight when submerged might yield a body density of 1.06 grams per centimeter^3. This would be put into the formula: % body fat = (495 ÷ body density) − 450. The subject is 17% body fat based on use of this formula.

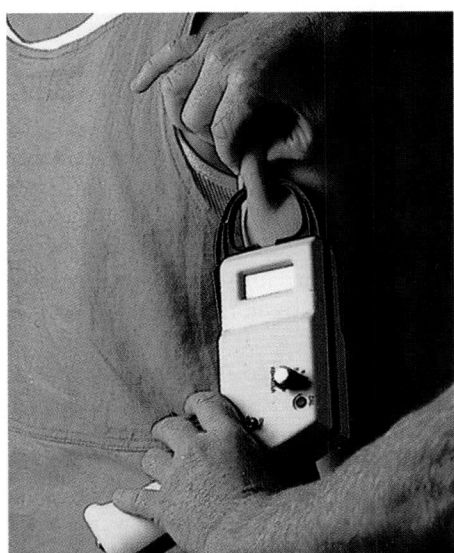

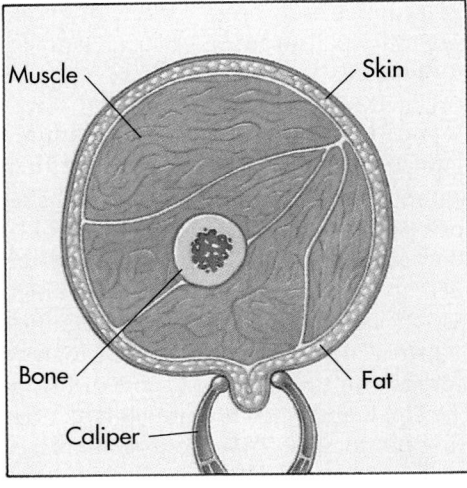

Muscle Skin

Bone Fat

Caliper

Figure 10.5 Skinfold measurements. Use of proper technique, calibrated equipment, and some practice skinfold measurements can predict body fat content.

Figure 10.6 Bioelectrical impedance. This method can estimate total body fat in less than 5 minutes and is based on the principle that fat in the body resists the flow of applied low-energy electricity. The degree of resistance to the flow of electricity per increment of body height is used to estimate body fatness.

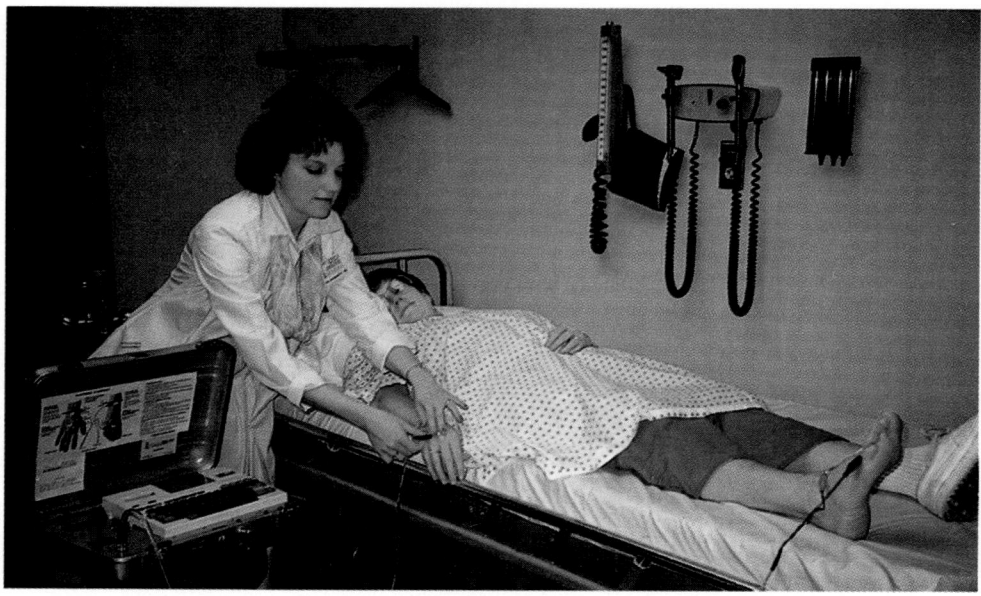

Still other methods to estimate body fat include using instruments to measure air displacement by the body (Bod Pod is one instrument used) and total-body electrical conductance when placed in an electromagnetic field (TOBEC).

A further advance in determining body fat is use of dual x-ray photon absorptiometry (DEXA). This x-ray system allows the clinician to separate body weight into three components—fat, fat-free soft tissue, and bone mineral. The usual whole-body scan requires about 5 to 20 minutes and delivers a minimal radiation dose. Obesity, osteoporosis, and other aspects of nutritional health can be investigated using this method.

BMI offers an alternative way to define overweight and obesity (Fig. 10.7):

25–29.9	Overweight	At risk for obesity and related health problems
30–39.9	Obese	Increases health risk
>40	Severely obese	Major health risk

A planned treatment program should be implemented after BMI reaches 30.

▌ Using Body Fat Distribution to Establish Obesity

Where we store fat, as well as how much, can predict health risks. Some people store fat in upper-body areas. Others hold fat lower on the body. Excess fat in either place generally spells trouble, but each storage space also has its unique risks. Fat deposited in the lower body often resists being shed. However, **upper-body (android) obesity** is related to more cardiovascular disease, hypertension, and type 2 diabetes.

High blood testosterone (a primarily male hormone) levels apparently encourage upper-body obesity, as does alcohol intake. This characteristic male pattern of fat storage appears in the "apple-on-a-stick" shape (large abdomen[pot belly] and small buttocks and thighs). This type of android-related risk is assessed by simply measuring the waist at the widest point (relaxed). A waist circumference more than 40 inches in men and more than 35 inches in women indicates such a shape (Fig. 10.8). If BMI is also 25 or more, health risks are significantly increased.

Estrogen and progesterone (primarily female hormones) encourage lower-body fat storage and **lower-body (gynecoid or gynoid) obesity**—the typical female pattern. The small abdomen and much larger buttocks and thighs give a pearlike appearance. After menopause, blood estrogen falls, encouraging upper-body fat distribution.

Overall, researchers suggest that women with lower-body fat distribution must be about 20 pounds more obese than men with a "pot belly" shape before they show the same health risks from an overfat state. Only some women have upper-body obesity. Note also that the cutoff values are based on studies of Caucasians. More study of minorities is needed to verify use in those populations.

upper-body (android) obesity The type of obesity in which fat is stored primarily in the abdominal area; defined as a waist circumference >40 inches (102 centimeters) in men and >35 inches (89 centimeters) in women; closely associated with a high risk for cardiovascular disease, and type 2 diabetes.

lower-body (gynecoid, gynoid) obesity The type of obesity in which fat storage is primarily located in the buttocks and thigh area.

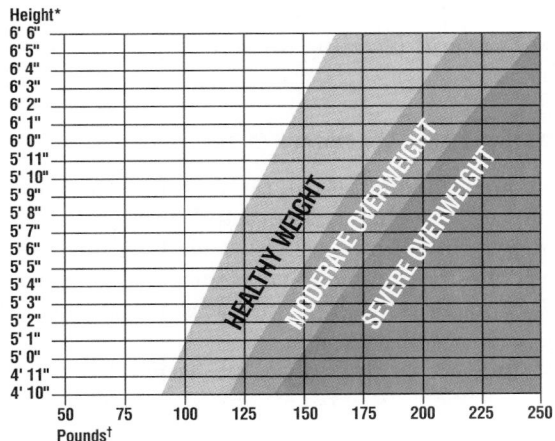

Figure 10.7 Height/weight table included as part of the latest Dietary Guidelines publication. The upper ends of the healthy weight ranges correspond to a body mass index of 25.

* Without shoes.
† Without clothes. The higher weights apply to people with more muscle and bone, such as many men.

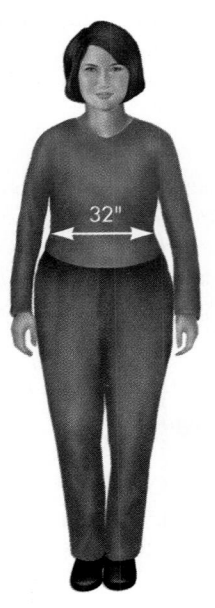
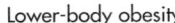
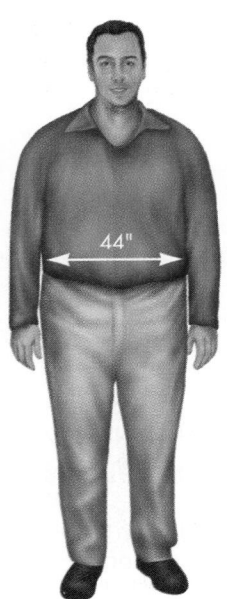

Lower-body obesity   Upper-body obesity

Figure 10.8 Body fat distribution, showing upper-body and lower-body obesity. The upper-body (android) form brings higher risks for ill health associated with obesity. The woman has a waist circumference of 32 inches. The man has a waist circumference of 44 inches. Thus, the man has upper-body obesity, but the woman does not, based on a cutoff of greater than 40 inches for men and greater than 35 inches for women.

■ Using Age of Onset in the Evaluation of Obesity

Obesity can be classified as juvenile-onset or adult-onset. When obesity develops in infancy or childhood, numerous adipose cells develop, each with the ability to grow larger. (This is discussed further in Chapter 14, particularly in reference to weight control in childhood.) In adult obesity, fewer adipose cells are usually present, but these contain an excess amount of fat. Still, as obesity progresses in adulthood, adipose cells can increase in number again.

Juvenile-onset obesity presents a special concern because the greater number of adipose cells may increase the body's resistance to cutting down fat stores. Adipose cells have a long life span and apparently need to store some fat. If more adipose cells

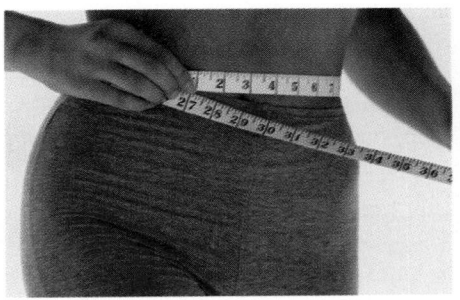

Waist circumference is an important measure of weight-related health risk.

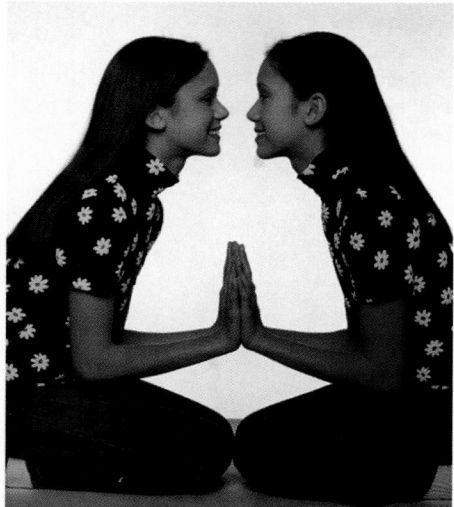

Figure 10.9 Nature or nurture: What causes these twins to have similar body weights?

automatically require more fat storage, reducing total body fat becomes a tough task. Although the reasons are still puzzling, long-term obesity appears to make losing weight more difficult.

■ Putting Obesity into Perspective

Obesity is a very personal disorder. It can be measured in many ways, but statistics aside, each person has unique characteristics and problems. Treatment needs to account for current energy expenditure, weight range in adulthood, fasting blood glucose, family history of obesity, number of years the person has been obese, and extent of erroneous nutrition practices. Each person faces possible complications requiring individual treatment plans.

On a positive note, however, only about a 10% weight loss is often needed for people to lower the risk for developing most weight-related diseases. Researchers are calling this a healthier weight. Although a person might not achieve a BMI of 25, he or she might still be healthier after a small weight loss.

Concept Check

Obesity is a state of excessive body fat storage. The risk of health problems related to obesity increases under the following conditions:

- A man's percentage of body fat exceeds 25%; a woman's exceeds about 35%.
- Body mass index (BMI) reaches 30 or more (calculated as weight in kilograms divided by height squared in meters).

However, if a healthy lifestyle is being followed and no current health problems exist, these guidelines need to be re-evaluated.

Body fat storage can be estimated clinically using skinfold thickness or bioelectrical impedance. Fat storage distribution further specifies an obese state as either upper body or lower body. Obesity leads to an increased risk for cardiovascular disease, some types of cancer, hypertension, type 2 diabetes, certain bone and joint disorders, and some digestive disorders. The risks for some of these diseases are greater with upper-body fat storage.

Why Some People Are Obese— Nature Versus Nurture

Both genetic traits and psychological factors can increase the risk for obesity. These diverse influences spark controversies concerning which factor yields the greater influence.

■ How Does Nature Contribute to Obesity?

Identical twins raised apart tend to show similar weight gain patterns, whether lean or obese (Fig. 10.9). It appears that nurture—what we learn about eating habits and nutrition, which varies between twins who are raised apart—has less to do with obesity than genes do. In fact, research using twins suggests that genetic background accounts for up to 70% of weight differences between people. Twins even tend to accumulate fat in the same body sites. Our genes help determine rates of metabolism, fuel use, and differences in brain neurotransmitter activity. All affect weight.

We also inherit specific body types, such as pencil-thin or muscular. The specific body types—known as **endomorph, mesomorph,** and **ectomorph**—greatly determine human size and shape. Endomorphs, with their stocky builds, have short, stubby bones; short trunks; round heads; wide chest and hips; and very short fingers. Ectomorphs, such as Abraham Lincoln, are tall and slender with long, thin bones and narrow chests, hips, heads, and fingers. Mesomorphs exhibit a medium, muscular build.

identical twins Two offspring who develop from a single ovum and sperm and consequently have the same genetic makeup.

endomorph A body type characterized by short, stubby bones, a short trunk, and short fingers.

mesomorph A body type associated with average bone size, trunk size, and finger length.

ectomorph A body type associated with very long, thin bones and very long, thin fingers.

A Set Point for Body Weight

The **set-point theory** of weight maintenance espouses the notion that weight is closely regulated by the body. It proposes that humans have a genetically predetermined body weight or body fat content, which the body attempts to defend. Some research suggests that the hypothalamus monitors the amount of body fat in humans and tries to keep that amount constant over time. This regulation of body fat content is referred to as a "set point." You have already seen in Chapter 1 that the hormone *leptin* produced by adipose cells forms one communication link between adipose cells and the brain that allows for some weight regulation.

Analogies to the tight regulation of blood pressure and body temperature are used to support this concept of set point. You could view the set point as a coiled spring: The further you stray from your usual weight, the harder the force acts to pull you back to that weight.

In the major studies of humans cited to support the set-point theory, volunteers who lost weight through starvation later ate in a way to regain their original weight or a little more. In addition, studies in the 1960s using prisoners with no history of obesity found it was hard for some men to gain weight. This was supported by later studies in the 1990s (see the section on nonexercise adaptive thermogenesis). Also, after an illness is resolved, a person generally gains lost weight.

Sound physiological evidence also suggests that body weight tends to be regulated. If energy intake is reduced, the blood concentration of the thyroid hormones fall, and the metabolic rate slows. In addition, lower body weight decreases the energy cost of each future weight-bearing activity, and the total energy used by lean tissue falls because some of these tissues are also lost. Furthermore, the enzyme used by adipose and muscle cells to take up fat from the bloodstream (lipoprotein lipase) often increases its activity. Through these changes, the body resists further weight loss.

If a person overeats, in the short run the metabolic rate tends to increase, in part because the thermic effect of food and total body mass increases. This causes some resistance to further weight gain. People often recognize the body's resistance to weight loss when dieting but do not think much about the resistance to weight gain after a holiday weekend. However, in the long run, resistance to weight gain is much less than resistance to weight loss. When a person gains weight and stays at that weight for a while, the body tends to defend the new weight.

Arguments against the set-point theory cite the fact that, during pregnancy, women slowly increase body weight and fat. Also, an average person's weight does not remain constant throughout adulthood; it usually increases slowly, at least until old age. This means that a person must be able to shift his or her set point. It is also argued that, if an individual is placed in a different social, emotional, or physical environment, weight can become markedly higher or lower and is maintained. These arguments suggest that humans, rather than having a set point determined by genetics or number of adipose cells, actually settle into a particular stable weight based on an interaction between nature and nurture influences.

In the final analysis, we must bear much of the responsibility for weight maintenance ourselves since set point is weaker in preventing weight gain than in preventing weight loss. The odds are against the likelihood that, even with a set point helping us, we can avoid creeping weight gain in adulthood without great attention to this tendency—and serious, consistent effort to achieve weight maintenance.

Ectomorphs appear to have an inherently easier time maintaining healthy body weight. Basal metabolism increases as body surface increases. Tall people have more body surface (based on body weight comparisons) than do short, stocky people. Therefore, taller people use more energy than do shorter ones, even when resting.

Some rats and mice have a genetic predisposition to obesity. They inherit a **thrifty metabolism,** one that uses energy frugally. This enables them to store fat more readily than the typical animal. Some people probably inherit a thrifty metabolism as well. Farmers once bred cows and hogs based on their ability to acquire fat. Today, because we know that eating too much animal fat can increase the risk of cardiovascular disease, farmers breed leaner animals.

A thrifty human metabolism requires less energy to get through the day. In earlier times, when food supplies were scarce, a thrifty metabolism helped protect people against starvation. With today's general abundance of food, people operating in this low gear require a high-energy output and wise food choices to prevent obesity.

If you think your metabolism promotes weight gain, you may have inherited a thrifty metabolism. It is likely that this is true for many of us. As a consequence, a child with no obese parent has only a 10% chance of becoming obese. A child with one obese parent (common in North American society) has a 40% risk, and one with two obese parents has an 80% risk. It can be argued that these probabilities are related, in part, to the eating behaviors a child learns.

Fraternal twins vary less in weight than do two unrelated people. This pattern supports the theory that environment, or nurture, affects obesity. Still, the close

thrifty metabolism A metabolism that characteristically conserves more energy than normal, so that it increases the risk of weight gain and obesity.

fraternal twins Offspring that develop from two separate ova and sperm and therefore have separate genetic identities, although they develop simultaneously in the mother.

The importance of environment in the development of obesity is exhibited in the treatment of Prader-Willi syndrome. Children with this inherited disorder have an extreme appetite and become very obese if food availability is not carefully controlled. If such a child has become obese, however, further careful control of food availability (e.g., locking all kitchen cabinets and not allowing the child access to money) can lead to significant weight loss, often 100 pounds or more. This environmental therapy is effective, despite the fact that the children maintain their extreme appetite.

Little relationship exists between how an infant was fed or how much weight was gained in the first year of life and the presence or absence of obesity in later childhood. The exception could be the infant who gains weight very rapidly in the first 6 weeks of life. Most overweight or obese infants become normal-weight schoolchildren. However, if a child has become obese by 5 years of age, immediate attention is necessary. Obesity in childhood is strongly related to obesity in adulthood.

association of body weights between identical twins strongly supports a genetic linkage. This varied evidence shows how complicated it is to separate nature from nurture when searching for the causes of obesity.

■ Does Nurture Have a Role?

Genetic factors determine some differences in energy metabolism and explain certain weight-gain variations among people. However, environmental factors, such as high-fat diets and inactivity, can literally shape us as well. Consider that human genetic makeup hasn't changed much in the past 50 years, but the ranks of obese people in North America have grown, and dramatically so in just the last 10 years.

Family members often have similar eating habits and choose similar foods. Even husbands and wives—who have no genetic link—may behave similarly toward food and eventually assume similar degrees of leanness or chunkiness. Therefore, family members who bond at the local quick-service (fast food) restaurant can influence each other's eating habits and, ultimately, fatness.

Is poverty associated with obesity? Ironically, the answer is often yes. Americans of lower socioeconomic status, especially females, are more likely to be obese than those in upper socioeconomic groups. Are cultural expectations or socioeconomic stress the cause of this?

Adult obesity in women is often rooted in childhood obesity. In addition, relative inactivity, periods of stress and boredom, as well as excess weight gain in pregnancy, contribute to female obesity. (Chapter 13 notes that breastfeeding one's infant contributes to loss of some of this excess fat associated with pregnancy.) These patterns suggest both social and genetic links. Male obesity, however, is not strongly linked to childhood obesity and, instead, tends to appear after age 30. In part, marriage and a working life encourage a sedentary state for many men. This powerful and prevalent pattern suggests a primary role of nurture in obesity, with less genetic influence.

■ Nature and Nurture Together

Overall, both nature and nurture influence the tendency toward obesity (Table 10.3). Consider the possibility that obesity is nurture allowing nature to express itself, like an accident waiting to happen. Some people begin life with a slower metabolism. Put these people in an inactive environment, feed them lots of energy dense foods, and praise them for eating. Like any of us, they can be nurtured into gaining weight, which may then allow their natural tendency for obesity to blossom. The eventual location of fat storage is strongly influenced by genetics.

If your parents are obese, you're likely to be at risk for obesity all your life. To avoid it will require eternal vigilance. Eat the right foods at the right times for the right reasons. And, whatever the answer to the nature versus nurture question is, it is likely that all obese people or those at risk for obesity will face this lifelong struggle as well. Still, genes do not control this destiny. With increased physical activity and decreased food consumption, even those with a genetic tendency toward obesity can maintain a healthy or "healthier" body weight.

Concept Check

Genetic background plays a role in obesity, influencing body shape, sites of fat deposition, and rate of basal metabolism. The role of nurture is evident in families, who tend to have similar eating habits, activity patterns, and degrees of fatness. Men tend to develop obesity after age 30, and women tend to have both childhood and adult roots for obesity; this suggests an especially important influence of nurture in men. Because both factors have an impact, it makes sense to assume that nurture serves as a catalyst for expressing or denying a genetic tendency toward obesity.

Table 10.3 What Encourages Excess Body Fat Stores and Obesity?

Factor	How Fat Storage Is Affected
Age	Excess body fat is more common in young and middle-aged adults, brought on to a great extent by sedentary lifestyle patterns.
Menopause	Increase in abdominal fat deposition is favored.
Gender	Females have more fat.
Insulin resistance	This often develops as obesity develops.
Positive energy balance	This is especially important if over a relatively long period.
Composition of diet	High fat intake, excess alcohol intake, and preference for sugary, fat-rich foods are likely to contribute to obesity.
Physical activity	Low or decreasing amount of physical activity ("couch potato") affects energy balance and body fat stores.
Basal metabolism	A low value with respect to lean body mass is linked to weight gain.
Thermic effect of food	This is low for some obesity cases.
Use of fat for energy	There is limited fat release into the bloodstream.
Total fat mass	Leptin, produced by adipose cells, affects food intake. Greater adipose cell mass then eventually leads to greater leptin production.
Ratio of fat to lean tissue	A high ratio of fat mass to lean body mass is correlated with weight gain.
Fat uptake by adipose tissue	This is high in some obese individuals and remains high (perhaps even increases) with weight loss.
Variety of social and behavioral factors	Obesity is associated with socioeconomic status; familial conditions; network of friends; busy lifestyles that discourage balanced meals; binge eating; easy availability of inexpensive, "super-sized" high-fat food (such as in quick-service restaurants); pattern of leisure activities; television time; smoking cessation; excessive alcohol intake; and number of meals eaten away from home. These meals are often served in large portions and are high in fat and energy content. Today, "food hunts man" to a great extent in Western societies.
Undetermined genetic characteristics	These affect energy balance, particularly via the energy expenditure components, the deposition of the energy surplus as adipose or lean tissue, and the relative proportion of fat and carbohydrate use by the body.
Race	In some ethnic groups, higher body weight may be more socially acceptable.
Certain medications	Food intake increases.
Childbearing	Women may not lose all weight gained in pregnancy, leading to creeping weight gain.
National region	Regional differences, such as high-fat diets and sedentary lifestyles in the Midwest and areas of the South, cause different rates of obesity in different places.

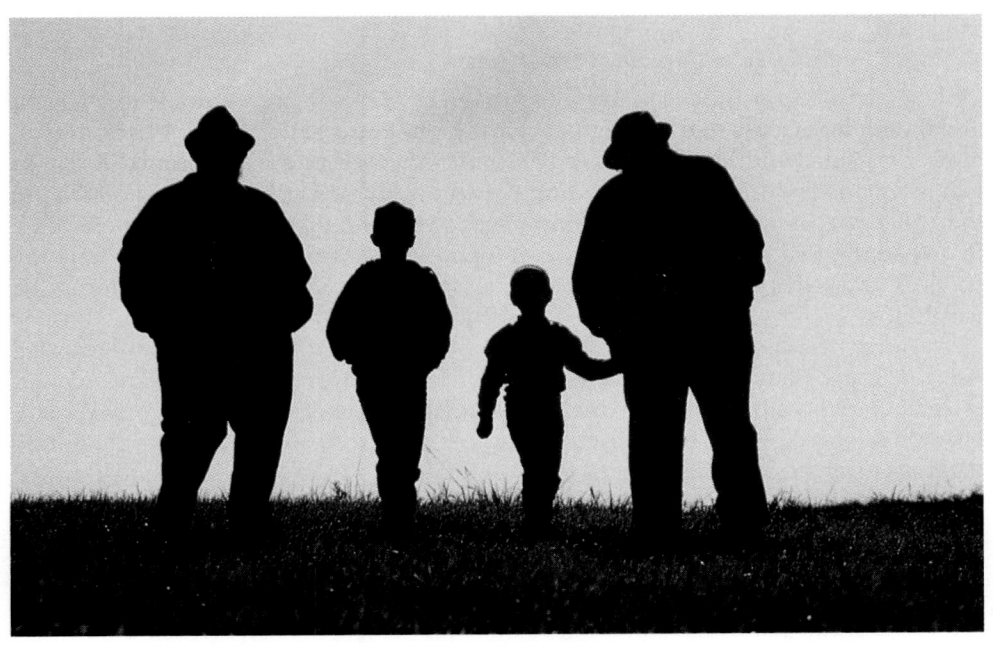

Does the difference in body fat between the grandfathers and the grandsons arise from nature or nurture, or both?

The total costs attributable to weight-related disease currently approaches $100 billion annually in the United States.

Here are some practices that can stimulate metabolism while one is dieting:

- Perform physical activity regularly throughout the day. Find opportunities for increasing activity, such as quick walks, stair climbing, or calisthenics (crunches, push-ups, etc.).
- Fidget when sitting and standing.
- Eat breakfast, so that food intake is spread throughout the day. Each time food is consumed, metabolism increases.
- Follow a carbohydrate-rich diet; much of this is further processed by the liver, which uses energy.
- Avoid "crash" dieting. Slow weight loss is a better idea because it leads to a smaller decline in basal metabolism during a diet.

Critical Thinking

Hal has been dieting to lose weight for 2½ months. However, like many dieters, he has reached a plateau. Although he continues to restrict his kcal intake, he's no longer losing weight. How would you explain to Hal the physical factors that fight weight loss?

Treatment of Obesity

Obesity should be considered similar to any chronic disease. Treatment requires long-term lifestyle changes, rather than simply taking medicine for 2 weeks, as for a sore throat, or following a quick fix promoted by a fad diet book. We often, however, view a "diet" as something one goes on temporarily, only to resume prior (typically poor) habits once satisfactory results have been achieved. It is for this reason that so many people regain lost weight. In place of this, healthy, active living with dietary modifications one can live with should be the emphasis for both obese and thin people. Let's explore why obesity must be regarded and treated in this way.

■ Some Basic Premises of Weight Loss

As you begin to consider current treatment options for obesity, first focus on five important, general principles concerning weight loss for adults. (Chapter 14 provides weight-loss strategies for children.)

Much of the Current Mania Surrounding Dieting Is Misdirected

People on diets often fall within a BMI of 18.5 to 24.9. Rather than worrying about weight loss, these individuals should be focusing on a healthy lifestyle that allows for weight maintenance. Incorporating necessary lifestyle changes and learning to accept one's particular body characteristics—such as an endormorphic shape—should be the overriding goal.

Actually, this dieting mania can be viewed as mostly a social problem, stemming from unrealistic weight expectations (especially for women) and lack of appreciation for the natural variety in body shape and weight. Not every woman can look like a Hollywood actress, nor can every man look like a Greek god, but all of us can strive for good health and, if physically possible, an active lifestyle.

The Body Defends Itself Against Weight Change

As noted in the Nutrition Insight on set point, the body makes numerous physiological adjustments during times of underfeeding or overfeeding that resist weight change. The compensation is most pronounced during times of underfeeding.

Weight Cycling Is a Common Phenomenon

Only about 5% of people who follow commercial diet programs actually lose weight and then remain close to that weight. Typically, one-third of the weight lost during dieting is regained within 1 year of the end of dietary restriction, and almost all weight lost is regained within 3 to 5 years. Some programs have slightly higher success rates than 5%, as do some people who simply lose weight on their own without enrolling in any supervised plan. Overall, however, the statistics are grim. Currently, only the surgical approaches to obesity treatment show routine success in maintaining the weight loss in most people.

Negative health consequences associated with this weight cycling are an increased risk for upper-body-fat deposition, profound discouragement and erosion of self-esteem, and possibly a fall in blood HDL-cholesterol. Nevertheless, experts still encourage obese people to attempt weight loss, with a strong focus on maintaining that lower weight. Still, dieters need to be aware of the trap of today's crash diet, which too often leads to the next month's weight gain. Weight-loss programs that claim you can lose weight and keep it off without changing food intake or increasing physical activity are selling a fantasy and are potentially dangerous. A weight-loss program should be considered successful only when the subjects involved in the process remain at or close to their lower weights.

Weight Gain in Adulthood Is All Too Common

In adulthood, weight gain is common, especially in those aged 25–44 years. Particular care should be practiced in these decades, although childhood and the adolescent years also deserve attention. Adults should generate a goal of not gaining greater than about 10 to 16 pounds more than their weight was on reaching age 21. People who gain weight rapidly should closely monitor food intake and activity patterns to discover the causes and then moderate the increases or reverse the trend in appropriate ways.

Changes in Body Composition Deserve a Primary Focus in Weight Loss

Weight should be lost mostly from adipose stores, not from muscle and other lean tissues. Rapid weight loss at the start of a diet program often represents water lost as a result of decreased salt intake and loss of glycogen from the liver and muscle. Substantial muscle tissue may be lost as well, and this is mostly (about 73%) water. People are fooled when they weigh themselves after starting a fad diet. They lose weight, but very little of it represents fat loss. Any loss of lean tissue means a decrease in basal metabolism and thus a decrease in overall energy expenditure.

Weight Loss in Perspective

All of this shows the importance of preventing obesity. This concept has wide support because curing the disorder is very difficult. Public health and political strategies to address the current obesity epidemic in North America must begin with weight maintenance for the adult population and increased physical activity. There is a particular need to focus on children and adolescents, in which excess weight and sedentary lifestyle may form the basis for a lifetime of weight-related illness and increased mortality.

Only the very motivated person should try to lose weight. Ideally, this attempt should also be preceded by a period of weight maintenance for about 6 months in order to begin the process of balancing energy intake with a degree of energy output that can be maintained.

■ Wishful Shrinking—Why Can't Quick Weight Loss Be Mostly Fat?

Rapid weight loss cannot consist mostly of fat loss because such a high energy deficit is needed to lose a large amount of adipose tissue. The body fat present in adipose tissue contains about 3500 kcal per pound. Fat storage, which includes body fat tissue plus supporting lean tissues, contains approximately 2700 kcal per pound. To lose ½ to 1 pound of adipose stores per week, energy intake must be decreased by approximately 300 to 500 kcal per day, with the addition of participating in at least 30 minutes of physical activity on most days of the week. A goal of 2 pounds per week would require a 1000 kcal deficit. Behavioral strategies to reinforce lifestyle changes are also effective for weight loss and later weight maintenance. Diets that promise 10 to 15 pounds of weight loss per week can't ensure that the weight loss is from adipose stores alone. Producing an energy deficit sufficient to lose that amount of fat mass simply isn't practical. Lean tissue, rather than fat, accounts for the major part of the weight lost.

■ What to Look for in a Sound Weight-Loss Diet

A dieter can try to devise a plan of action by seeking advice from health professionals or consulting current books. Either way, a sound weight-loss program should include three components: control of energy intake; increased energy expenditure through physical activity; and acknowledgment that a lifelong change in habits is required, not simply a short-term weight-loss period. Focusing on just consuming less energy represents a difficult path to success. As just noted, adding regular physical activity and an appropriate psychological component contributes to success and later maintenance of the weight loss (Table 10.4).

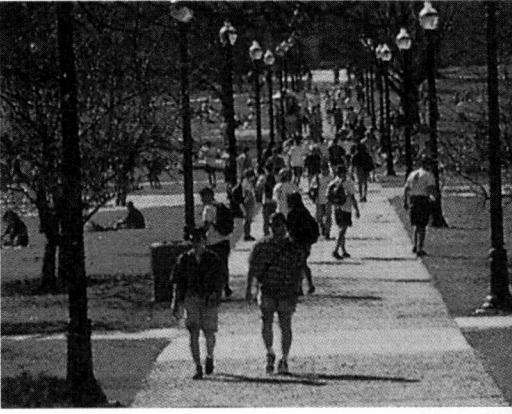

Student life is often full of physical activity. This is not necessarily true for a person's later working life; hence, weight gain is a strong possibility.

A typical fast-food hamburger in 1957 contained little more than 1 ounce of cooked meat, compared with up to 6 ounces or more today. A theater serving of popcorn was 3 cups in 1957, compared with 16 cups (medium-size popcorn) today.

When you read brochures or research reports about specific diet plans, ask not only whether the people lost weight but also whether they maintained much of that weight loss. If this did not happen, the entire dieting program was in vain.

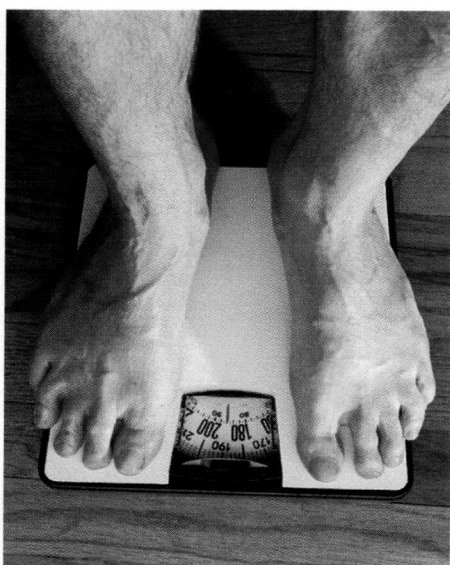

Slow, steady weight loss is one of the characteristics of a sound weight-loss program.

Table 10.4 Characteristics of a Sound Weight-Loss Diet

Rate of Loss

1. Slow and steady weight loss, rather than rapid weight loss, is encouraged.
2. Goal is 1 pound or so of loss of fat storage per week.
3. A period of weight maintenance for a few months following a loss of 10% of body weight.
4. Evaluation of need for further dieting before more weight loss begins.

Flexibility

1. Ability to participate in normal activities (e.g., parties, restaurants).
2. Adaptations to individual habits and tastes.

Intake

1. Nutritional needs are met (except for energy).
2. Hunger and fatigue are minimized by providing at least 1200 to 1500 kcal per day. (1000 kcal per day may be enough for a very sedentary person but is generally not recommended. Increasing energy output in order to consume more calories is a better strategy.)
3. Common foods are included, with no certain foods being promoted as magical.
4. Use of a fortified, ready-to-eat breakfast cereal or balanced multivitamin/mineral supplement is recommended, especially when consuming less than 1600 kcal per day.
5. Use the Food Guide Pyramid (or other related pyramid) as a pattern for food choices.

Behavior Modification

1. Maintenance of healthy lifestyle (and weight) is a key concern; there is a lifetime focus.
2. Changes are reasonable and can be maintained.
3. Social support is encouraged.
4. Plans for relapse so one does not quit after a setback.

Overall Health

1. Screening by a physician is required for persons with existing health problems, those over 40 (men) to 50 (women) years of age who plan to substantially increase physical activity, and those who plan to lose weight rapidly.
2. Regular physical activity, proper rest, stress reduction, and other healthy changes in lifestyle are encouraged.
3. Underlying psychological weight issues are addressed, such as depression or marital stress.

Weight-Control Objectives from

Healthy People 2010

Increase by 40% the proportion of adults who are at a healthy weight (body mass index between 18.5 and 25).

Reduce by 50% the proportion of adults who are obese (body mass index of 30 or more).

Reduce by 50% the proportion of children and adolescents who are overweight or obese.

Concept Check

Obesity is a chronic disease that necessitates lifelong treatment. Key points to consider when attempting to treat obesity include the following: (1) The primary focus should be on a healthy lifestyle that can be maintained; (2) the body resists weight loss; (3) typical weight-loss attempts often are followed by weight regain; (4) emphasis should be placed on preventing obesity, since curing this disorder is very difficult; (5) weight should be lost from adipose stores, not mostly from lean tissues. Appropriate weight-loss programs have the following characteristics in common: (1) They meet nutritional needs—this can be evaluated by checking for mostly low energy density choices from the Food Guide Pyramid (or related pyramid); (2) they can adjust to accommodate habits and tastes; (3) they emphasize readily obtainable foods; (4) they promote changing habits that discourage overeating; (5) they encourage regular physical activity; and (6) they help change obesity-promoting beliefs and rally healthy social support.

Control of Energy Intake—The First Key to Weight Loss

A goal of losing ½ to 1 pound of stored fat per week may require limiting energy intake to 1200 kcal per day for women and 1500 kcal for men, with 30% or less of energy intake coming from fat. For a very sedentary obese person energy intake may need to be as low as 1000 calories per day to allow for weight loss. Each calorie allowance could also be higher for very active people. Keep in mind that, in a very sedentary society, decreasing fat (and calories) is important because it is difficult to use much of either without ample physical activity.

Traditionally, dieters have counted calories. Some experts recommend counting fat grams, assuming that control of energy intake follows. Chapter 5 contains a tool to convert energy intake into an appropriate fat gram allowance. Food labels simplify the task of counting fat grams. Note that not all food choices need to be low fat. Total fat intake for the day is the focus. A low-fat diet is easy to follow indefinitely if it allows the consumption of enough food—especially low energy density foods such as fruits, vegetables, and whole grains—to satisfy hunger. However, this method will work only if high-calorie, fat-free foods—such as fat-free cakes and cookies—are not overeaten.

Another Bite

As discussed in Chapter 5, many of the fat-reduced products flooding the market substitute sugar for fat to maintain flavor. Consequently, they tend to be slightly lower in energy content. This makes it easy to gain weight, even on a low-fat diet, without careful portion control of fat-reduced foods. In addition, some experts think that certain fat-reduced foods, such as nonfat sour cream, merely remind dieters of what they are missing, driving them back to the high-fat food choice. In addition, some studies have shown that people eat more when told a food is fat reduced, even if it is not. This suggests it may be better to avoid high-fat foods and their fat-reduced counterparts, instead replacing them with a food choice naturally low in fat, such as nonfat yogurt for sour cream or a plain warm, whole-wheat bagel for a doughnut.

In any case, dieters should ideally consume at least 1200 kcal daily; fewer than that causes so much hunger that they will probably not be able to stick to the plan. A better idea is to first increase physical activity, allowing closer to 1600 kcal to be eaten each day.

One way for a dieter to monitor energy intake at the start of a weight-loss program is to read labels. Label reading is important because many foods are more energy dense than people suppose and the serving size may be smaller than suspected (Fig. 10.10). Another method is to write down food intake for 24 hours and then calculate energy intake from the food table in Appendix A or your diet analysis software, adjusting future food choices as needed. Because people often underestimate portion size when recording food intake, measuring utensils can help.

Whatever the method chosen, it is unreasonable to think that measuring food and keeping records will continue for a lifetime. These methods are suggested as a temporary practice for people who need to get a handle on their portion size. Once the eyes and stomach are trained to know what constitutes a specific portion size, it will be possible to then "eyeball" appropriate meals.

Decreasing fat in the diet from 40% to 30% does not result in much compensation. That is, people do not often feel the need to eat large volumes of food to make up for the missing fat. On the other hand, reducing dietary fat to 20% of calories frequently leaves people feeling hungry and leads to the overeating of fat-free foods, many of which are high in calories. It is only when the dietary fat is replaced by carbohydrate foods rich in dietary fiber that this compensation can be minimized.

Liquids are getting more attention, since liquid calories do not stimulate satiety mechanisms to the same extent as solid foods. The advice from experts is to use beverages that have few or no calories and limit calorie-containing beverages.

Compared with the eating habits in the late 1970s, the average North American now eats about 160 calories more each day.

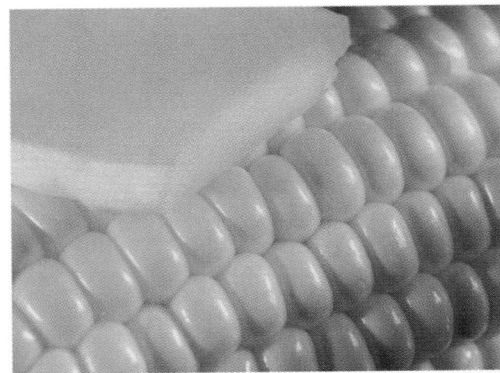

It is important to watch the amount of added fats when controlling energy intake.

Figure 10.10 Reading labels helps you choose foods with less fat and calories. Which frozen dessert is the best choice, per ½ cup serving, for a person on a weight-loss diet? The % Daily Values are based on a 2000 kcal diet.

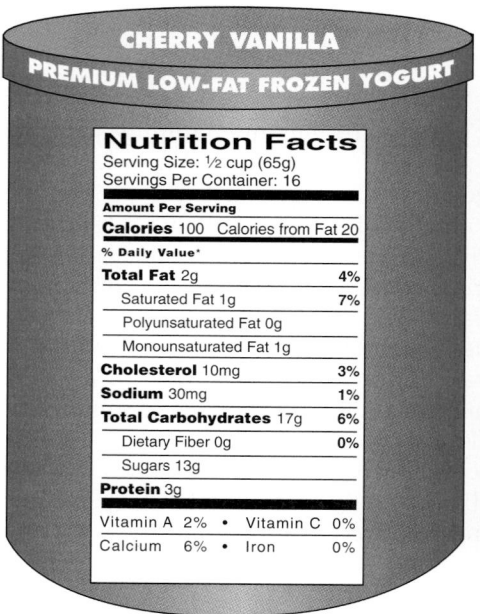

Table 10.5 shows how to start reducing energy intake. As you should realize by now, it is best to consider healthy eating a lifestyle change, rather than simply a weight-loss plan.

Regular Physical Activity—A Second Key to Weight Loss and Especially Important for Later Weight Maintenance

Regular physical activity is very important for everyone, especially those who are trying to lose weight or maintain a lower body weight. Fat use is enhanced. Therefore, it greatly complements a reduction in energy intake for weight loss, but does not substitute for it. Many of us rarely do more than sit, stand, and sleep. Obviously, much more energy is used during physical activity than at rest. In addition, expending only 200 to 300 extra kcal per day above and beyond normal daily activity, while controlling energy intake, can lead to about a half pound of fat loss per week, or about 25 pounds of fat loss per year. Furthermore, physical activity often boosts overall self-esteem.

Adding any of the activities listed in Table 10.6 to one's lifestyle leads to more energy expenditure. Duration and regular performance, rather than intensity, are the keys to success with this approach to weight loss. One should search for activities than can be continued over time. In this regard, walking vigorously 2 to 3 miles per day can be as helpful as aerobic dancing or jogging if it is maintained. Moreover, walking is less likely to lead to injuries. Some resistance exercises (weight training) should also be added to increase lean body mass and, in turn, fat use (see Chapter 11). Exercise also helps maintain bone health during weight loss. Keep in mind that bone health suffers most in those involved in weight-reduction programs that do not include a weight-bearing exercise component.

Daily opportunities to expend energy have diminished. Technology is systematically eliminating almost every reason to move our muscles. The easiest way to increase physical activity is to make it part of a daily routine. To start, one could consider walking every day and then incorporating some regular stair climbing. A simple trick is to park the car farther from campus, work, and the shopping mall, so that one must walk farther. Overall, physical activity is a key to weight loss and weight maintenance—30

*H*ealthy People 2010 *aims for 30% of adults to exercise 30 minutes at least 5 days a week. Currently, only about 15% of adults do this.*

*D*igiwalker is a device that monitors activity. It costs about $35.00. An often-stated goal for activity is to take at least 10,000 steps per day—typically we take half that many or less. Digiwalker tracks this activity.*

Table 10.5 Saving Kcal: Ideas to Help Get Started

Instead of	Try	Number of kcal Saved
3 oz well-marbled meat (prime rib)	3 oz lean meat (eye of round)	140
½ chicken breast, batter-fried	½ skinless chicken breast, broiled with lemon	175
½ cup beef stroganoff	3 oz lean roast beef (or use a fat-reduced recipe)	210
½ cup home-fried potatoes	1 medium baked potato	65
½ cup green bean-mushroom casserole	½ cup cooked green beans	50
½ cup potato salad	1 cup raw vegetable salad	140
½ cup pineapple chunks in heavy syrup	½ cup pineapple chunks canned in juice	25
2 tbsp bottled French dressing	2 tbsp low-calorie French dressing	150
⅙ 9-inch apple pie	1 baked apple	185
3 oatmeal-raisin cookies	1 oatmeal-raisin cookie	125
½ cup ice cream	½ cup low-fat ice cream	45
1 danish pastry	½ English muffin	150
1 cup sugar-coated corn flakes	1 cup plain corn flakes	60
1 cup whole milk	1 cup 1% low-fat milk	45
7-fluid-oz gin and tonic	6-fluid-oz wine cooler made with sparkling water	150
1-oz bag potato chips	1 cup plain popcorn	120
¹⁄₁₂ 8-inch white layer cake with chocolate frosting	¹⁄₁₂ angel food cake, 10-inch tube	185
Regular beer	Light beer	40

minutes per day is a minimum, while 60 minutes per day greatly increases the likelihood of such success.

The physical activity and reduced calorie intake then must be maintained after achieving the weight loss (goal weight) to prevent weight regain. This is a lifestyle change that must be maintained. The goal is to attain and maintain a healthy weight, body, and mind.

Behavior Modification—The Third Strategy for Weight Loss

Controlling energy intake, so important to weight loss, also means modifying *problem* behaviors. Only the dieter can decide what behaviors keep him or her from reaching for the wrong foods at the wrong times for the wrong reasons.

What events start (or stop) eating? What factors influence food choices? Psychologists often use terms such as **chain-breaking, stimulus control, cognitive restructuring, contingency management,** and **self-monitoring** when discussing behavior modification (Table 10.7). This terminology helps place the problem in perspective and organizes the intervention strategy into manageable steps.

Chain-breaking separates behaviors that tend to occur together—for example, snacking on chips while watching television. Although these activities do not have to occur together, they often do. Dieters may need to break the chain reaction (see the Rate Your Plate at the end of this chapter for more details).

Stimulus control puts us in charge of temptations. Options include pushing tempting food to the back of the refrigerator, removing fat-laden snacks from the kitchen counter, and avoiding the path by the vending machines. Provide a positive stimulus by keeping low energy density snacks ready to satisfy hunger/appetite. Note that alcohol and foods offer quick, easy stress relief. We need to plan healthful alternatives.

chain-breaking Breaking the link between two or more behaviors that encourage overeating, such as snacking while watching television.

stimulus control Altering the environment to minimize the stimuli for eating—for example, removing foods from sight and storing them in kitchen cabinets.

cognitive restructuring Changing one's frame of mind regarding eating—for example, instead of using a difficult day as an excuse to overeat, substituting other pleasures for rewards, such as a relaxing walk with a friend.

contingency management Forming a plan of action to respond to a situation in which overeating is likely, such as when snacks are within arm's reach at a party.

self-monitoring Tracking foods eaten and conditions affecting eating; actions are usually recorded in a diary, along with location, time, and state of mind. This is a tool to help people understand more about their eating habits.

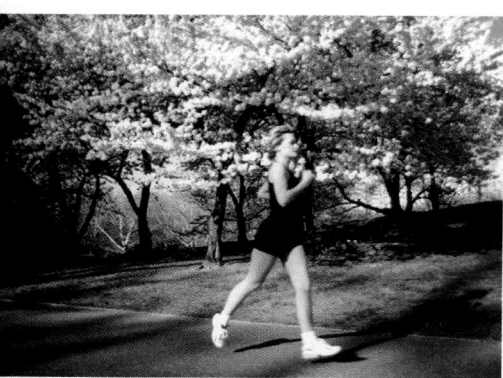

Physical activity complements any diet plan.

Table 10.6 Approximate Energy Costs of Various Activities for a 150 pound (68 kilogram) Person

Activity	Kcal per Kilogram per Hour	Number of kcal per Hour
Aerobics—heavy	8.0	544
Aerobics—light	3.0	204
Aerobics—medium	5.0	340
Backpacking	9.0	612
Basketball—vigorous	10.0	680
Bicycling (5.5 mph)	3.0	204
Bowling	3.9	265
Calisthenics—heavy	8.0	544
Calisthenics—light	4.0	272
Canoeing (2.5 mph)	3.3	224
Cleaning (female)	3.7	253
Cleaning (male)	3.5	236
Cooking	2.8	190
Cycling (13 mph)	9.7	659
Dressing/showering	1.6	106
Driving	1.7	117
Eating (sitting)	1.4	93
Food shopping	3.6	245
Football—touch	7.0	476
Golf	3.6	244
Horseback trotting	5.1	346
Ice skating (10 mph)	5.8	394
Jogging—medium	9.0	612
Jogging—slow	7.0	476
Lying—at ease	1.3	89
Racquetball—social	8.0	544
Roller-skating	5.1	346
Running or jogging (10 mph)	13.2	897
Skiing (10 mph)	8.8	598
Sleeping	1.2	80
Swimming (.25 mph)	4.4	299
Tennis	6.1	414
Volleyball	5.1	346
Walking (2.5 mph)	3.0	204
Walking (3.75 mph)	4.4	299
Water skiing	7.0	476
Weightlifting—heavy	9.0	612
Weightlifting—light	4.0	272
Window cleaning	3.5	240
Writing (sitting)	1.7	148

The values in the table refer to total energy expenditure, including that needed to perform the physical activity, plus that needed for basal metabolism, the thermic effect of food, and nonexercise activity thermogenesis. Use your diet analysis software for your personal estimate.

Table 10.7 Behavior Modification Principles for Weight Loss

Stimulus Control

Shopping

1. Shop for food after eating—buy nutritious foods.
2. Shop from a list; limit purchases of irresistible "problem" foods.
3. Avoid ready-to-eat foods.
4. Shop for one or more weeks at a time rather than more often. Also avoid shopping when hungry.

Plans

1. Plan to limit food intake as needed.
2. Substitute periods of physical activity for snacking.
3. Eat meals and snacks at scheduled times; don't skip meals.

Activities

1. Store food out of sight, preferably in the freezer, to discourage impulsive eating.
2. Eat all food in the same place.
3. Keep serving dishes off the table, especially dishes of sauces and gravies.
4. Use smaller dishes and utensils.

Holidays and Parties

1. Drink fewer alcoholic beverages.
2. Plan eating behavior before parties.
3. Eat a low-calorie snack before parties.
4. Practice polite ways to decline food.
5. Don't get discouraged by an occasional setback.

Eating Behavior

1. Put fork down between mouthfuls.
2. Chew thoroughly before taking the next bite.
3. Leave some food on the plate.
4. Pause in the middle of the meal.
5. Do nothing else while eating (for example, reading, watching television).

Reward

1. Plan specific rewards for specific behavior (behavioral contracts).
2. Solicit help from family and friends and suggest how they can help you. Encourage family and friends to provide this help in the form of praise and material rewards.
3. Use self-monitoring records as basis for rewards.

Self-Monitoring

1. Note the time and place of eating.
2. List the type and amount of food eaten.
3. Record who is present and how you feel.
4. Use the diet diary to identify problem areas.

Cognitive Restructuring

1. Avoid setting unreasonable goals.
2. Think about progress, not shortcomings.
3. Avoid imperatives such as *always* and *never*.
4. Counter negative thoughts with positive restatements.

Portion Control

1. Make substitutions, such as a regular hamburger instead of a "quarter pounder" or cucumbers instead of croutons in salads.
2. Think small. Order half, and save the other half. Order half of an entrée and share it with another person. Order a cup of soup instead of a bowl or an appetizer in place of an entrée.
3. Use a doggie bag. Ask your server to put half the entrée in a doggie bag before bringing it to the table.

In sum, become a "defensive eater." Know when to refuse food after satiety registers and reduce portion sizes.

*S*uccessful weight losers and maintainers from the National Weight Control Registry:

- Eat a low-fat, high-carbohydrate diet (on average 24% of calories as fat).
- Eat breakfast almost every day.
- Self-monitor by weighing themselves regularly and keeping a food journal.
- Exercise for a total of about 1 hour per day.
- Eat at restaurants only once or twice per week.

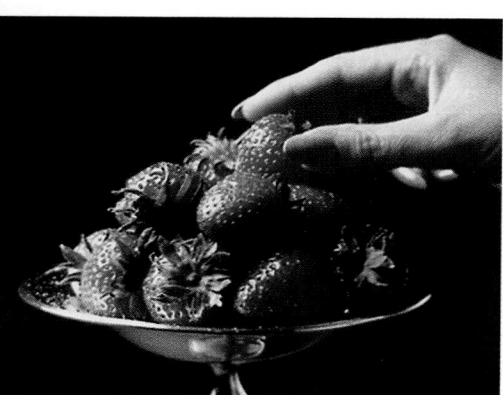

Fruit is a great low-cal snack—high nutrient density and low energy density.

relapse prevention A series of strategies used to help prevent and cope with weight-control lapses, such as recognizing high-risk situations and deciding beforehand on appropriate responses.

*T*he motivation to lose weight and keep it off generally comes with a proverbial "flip of the switch," in which the desire to lose weight finally becomes more important than the desire to overeat.

Cognitive restructuring changes our frame of mind. For example, after a hard day, respond with a walk or satisfying talk with a friend instead of a binge. Replace eating reactions to stress with healthful, relaxing alternatives.

Decreeing some food off limits sets up an internal struggle to resist the urge to eat that food. This hopeless battle can keep us feeling deprived. We lose the fight. Managing food choices with the principle of moderation is best. If a favorite food becomes troublesome, place it off limits only temporarily, until it can be enjoyed in moderation.

Contingency management prepares us for potential pitfalls and high-risk situations. We might rehearse in advance some appropriate responses to pressure—such as food being passed at a party.

Did you keep a record of what you ate and what catalysts urged you to pick up the fork or put it down as suggested in Rate Your Plate in Chapter 1? If so, you already know one key tool in modifying behavior—self-monitoring. A self-monitoring record can reveal patterns—such as unconscious overeating—that may explain problem eating habits. This record can encourage new habits to counteract unwanted behaviors. Obesity experts note that this is the key behavioral tool to use in any weight-loss program.

Overall, it's important to *address specific* problems, such as snacking, compulsive eating, and mealtime overeating. Behavior modification principles end up as critical components of weight reduction and maintenance. To succeed with behavior modification, one must emphasize the desirable changes in eating behavior, have rewards for objectives that have been met, and, more importantly, incorporate strategies that sustain physical activity. Without behavior modification, it is difficult to make lifelong lifestyle changes needed to meet weight-control goals.

■ Relapse Prevention Is Important

A dieter can tolerate an occasional lapse but needs to plan for lapses, encouraging not overreacting, but taking charge immediately. Change responses such as "I ate that cookie; I'm a failure" to "I ate that cookie, but I did well to stop after only one!" An occasional cookie is fine; a pound of cookies in an afternoon deserves reconsideration. When dieters lapse from their diet plan, newly learned food habits should steer them back toward the plan. This should enable dieters to avoid the lapse-relapse-collapse trap. Without a strong behavioral program for **relapse protection** in place, a lapse frequently turns into a relapse. Once a pattern of poor food choices begins, dieters may feel that they have failed and stray further from the plan. As the relapse lengthens, the diet plan collapses, and dieters fall short of their weight-loss goal. Even with a good behavioral plan, one may fail at a diet. Losing weight is difficult. Overall, maintenance of weight loss is fostered by the "3 Ms": motivation, movement, and monitoring.

■ Social Support Aids Behavioral Change

Healthy social support is helpful in weight control. Helping others understand how they can be supportive can make weight control easier. Family and friends can provide praise and encouragement. A weight-control professional can keep dieters accountable and help them learn from difficult situations. Long-term contact with a professional can be quite helpful for later weight maintenance. Groups of individuals attempting to lose weight or maintain losses can provide empathetic support.

■ A Recap

Sometimes, dieters emphasize the need for immediate results through unreasonable restrictions, willpower, and perfection. A healthier emphasis is on a well-balanced diet containing whole grains, fruits, and vegetables; regular physical activity; and behavior modification (Fig. 10.11). These components should be a part of an overall lifestyle change that is permanent. No foods should be forbidden, and occasional overindulgence should be expected. Managing weight can be described as practicing healthy eating and maintaining a physically active lifestyle. In turn, this lifestyle can be continued for a lifetime and will result in improved health for the mind and the body.

Would-be dieters should choose and follow weight-control plans that are appropriate for them. They have a smorgasbord of options: lowered energy and fat intakes, behavior modification, increased physical activity, and group or individual counseling. Many tools are effective, but some are more useful than others, depending on the individual's lifestyle, personality, and motivation. Generally the more tools used, the greater the success.

Figure 10.11 The weight-loss triad. The key to weight loss and maintenance can be thought of as a triangle in which the three corners consist of (1) controlling energy intake, (2) performing regular physical activity, and (3) making needed lifestyle changes. The three corners of the triangle support each other in that without one corner the triangle becomes incomplete. In the same way, without one of the three keys to weight loss, weight loss and later maintenance become unlikely.

Concept Check

*I*ncreasing physical activity in daily life should be part of any weight-loss plan. Daily activity, such as walking and stair climbing, is recommended. Behavior modification can improve conditions for losing weight. One behavioral area that requires change is habit chains that encourage overeating, such as snacking while watching television. Another tactic is to modify the environment to reduce temptation; for example, put foods into cupboards to keep them out of sight. In addition, rethinking attitudes about eating—for example, substituting pleasures other than food as a reward for coping with a stressful day—can be important for altering undesirable behavior. Advanced planning to prevent and deal with lapses is vital, as is rallying healthy social support. Finally, the careful observation and recording of eating habits can reveal subtle cues that lead to overeating. Overall, weight loss and maintenance are fostered by controlling energy intake, performing regular physical activity, and modifying problem behaviors.

Professional Help for Weight Loss

The first professional to see for advice about a weight-loss program is the family physician. Doctors are best equipped to assess overall health and the appropriateness of weight loss. The physician may then recommend a registered dietitian for a specific weight-loss plan and answers to diet-related questions. Registered dietitians are uniquely qualified to help design a weight-loss plan because they understand both food composition and the psychological importance of food. Exercise physiologists can provide advice about programs to increase physical activity.

Many communities have a variety of weight-loss organizations. These include self-help groups, such as Take Off Pounds Sensibly and Weight Watchers. Other programs, such as Jenny Craig and Nutri/System, are less desirable for the average dieter. Often, the employees are not dietitians or other appropriately trained health professionals. These programs also tend to be expensive because of their requirements for intense counseling or mandatory diet foods and supplements. In addition, the U.S. Federal Trade Commission has charged some commercial diet-program companies with misleading consumers through unsubstantiated weight-loss claims and deceptive testimonials.

*A*t a time when quick fixes for weight are not only expected but are, in fact, demanded, many of us are willing to try almost anything to shed unwanted pounds. Operation Waistline is a program designed by the U.S. Federal Trade Commission to terminate fraudulent claims being made by the weight-loss and health-store industry with regard to diet products. The program hopes to put an end to the $6 billion spent in the United States each year on counterfeit products.

■ Medications for Weight Loss

People who are candidates for medications for obesity treatment include those with a BMI of 30 or more or a BMI of 27 or more with weight-related conditions, such as type 2 diabetes, cardiovascular disease, hypertension, or excess waist circumference; those with no contraindications to use of the medication; and those ready to undertake lifestyle change. Success with such medications has been shown only in those who modify their behavior and energy intake and increase their physical activity. Medications alone have not been found to be successful. In addition, if a person has not lost at least 4.4 pounds (2 kilogram) after 4 weeks, it is not likely that the person will benefit from further use of the medication.

amphetamine A group of medications that stimulate the central nervous system, among other effects. Abuse is linked to physical and psychological dependence.

*T*he only two medications approved by FDA for long-term use are sibutramine (Meridia) and orlistat (Xenical).

*C*hapter 8 discussed the risks of self-diagnosis and self-treatment of disease with megadose vitamin and mineral supplements. An even bigger danger exists using herbal substances to foster weight loss. Chapter 15 will discuss herbal remedies in detail. For now, know that, despite widespread advertising, ephedrine (also known as ephedra or ma huang) and St. John's wort are not safe treatments for weight loss. Ephedrine has been linked to numerous health problems and even deaths in recent years. FDA warns any use should not exceed 24 milligrams per day. St. John's wort should not be taken with any other antidepressants. Many experts advise staying away from any over-the-counter diet pills, and especially these herbal combinations.

very-low-calorie diet (VLCD) Known also as *protein-sparing modified fast* (PSMF), this diet allows a person 400 to 800 kcal per day, often in liquid form. Of this, 120 to 480 kcal is carbohydrate, where the rest is mostly high-quality protein.

With regard to the agents used, an **amphetamine**-like medication (phenteramine [Fastin or Ionamin]) is available. It prolongs the activity of epinephrine and norepinephrine in the brain. This therapy is effective for some people in the short run but has not yet been proved effective in the long run. Most state medical boards currently limit use to 12 weeks unless the person is participating in a medical study using the product. The drug should not be used in pregnant or nursing women or those under 18 years of age.

Sibutramine (Meridia) has been approved by FDA for weight loss. It enhances both norepinephrine and serotonin activity in the brain by reducing reuptake of these neurotransmitters by the secreting neurons. The neurotransmitters then remain active in the brain for a longer period of time, and so prolong a sense of reduced hunger. The most common side effects are constipation, dry mouth, insomnia, and a mild increase in blood pressure. Thus, sibutramine should be used with caution in people with a history of hypertension (or cardiovascular disease). Studies have shown that it is effective in helping some people who already eat healthy diets but just eat too much. The main effect is to moderately reduce appetite to allow people to eat less. Sibutramine is safe and effective only when combined with a comprehensive weight-control program and when supervised by a physician.

Orlistat (Xenical) is another medication approved by FDA for weight loss. This medication inhibits lipase action in the small intestine, reducing fat digestion and the subsequent absorption of dietary fat by one-third for about 2 hours when taken along with a meal containing fat. This malabsorbed fat simply is deposited in the feces. *Fat intake has to be controlled,* however, because large amounts of fat in the feces cause numerous side effects, such as gas, bloating, and oil discharge. Interestingly, orlistat use can actually remind the person to follow a fat-controlled diet, as the symptoms resulting from consuming a high-fat meal quickly develop. Orlistat is taken with each meal. One way to reduce the cost of orlistat use is to eat a very-low-fat breakfast (e.g., cereal, juice, and skim milk) and use the medication to inhibit fat absorption at lunch and dinner.

Since the malabsorbed fat carries fat-soluble vitamins into the feces, the person taking orlistat must take a multivitamin and mineral supplement at bedtime. In this way, any micronutrients not absorbed during the day can be replaced; fat malabsorption from the dinner meal will not greatly influence micronutrient absorption in the late evening.

Overall, in skilled hands, prescription medications can aid weight loss in some instances. However, they do not replace the need for reducing energy and fat intake, modifying problem behavior, and increasing physical activity, both during and after therapy. And, more times than not, any weight loss during drug treatment can be attributed mostly to the individual's hard work.

▪ Treatment of Severe Obesity

Severe (morbid) obesity—weighing at least 100 pounds over healthy body weight (or twice one's healthy body weight)—requires professional treatment. Because of the serious health problems related to severe obesity, drastic measures may be necessary. Such treatments are recommended only when traditional diets fail. Drastic weight-loss procedures are not without side effects, both physical and psychological, making careful physician monitoring a necessity.

Very-Low-Calorie Diets

If more traditional diet changes have failed, treating severe obesity with a **very-low-calorie diet (VLCD)** is possible. Optifast is one such commercial program. Some researchers believe that people with body weight greater than 30% above their healthy weight are also appropriate candidates. The diet allows a person to consume 400 to 800 kcal per day, often in liquid form. (These diets were known earlier as protein-sparing modified fasts.) Of this amount, about 30 to 120 grams (120 to 480 kcal) is carbohydrate. The rest is high-quality protein, which supplies about 70 to 100 grams per day (280 to 400 kcal). This low carbohydrate intake often causes ketosis, which may decrease hunger. However, the main reasons for weight loss are the minimal energy allowed and the absence of food choice. About 3 to 4 pounds can be lost per week; men tend to lose at a faster rate than women. When physical activity and resistance training augment this diet, a greater loss of adipose tissue occurs. Careful physician monitoring is crucial throughout this very restrictive form of diet therapy during weight loss, refeeding, and later maintenance. Major health risks include heart problems and gallstones.

Weight regain remains a nagging problem with this type of therapy. If behavioral therapy and physical activity supplement a long-term support program, maintenance of the weight loss is more likely but still difficult. Any program under consideration should include a maintenance plan. Today, antiobesity medications also may be included in this phase of the program.

Gastroplasty

Gastroplasty, or stomach stapling, is the most common surgical procedure for treating severe obesity. The most common procedure works by reducing stomach volume to about 30 milliliters (size of a golf ball). Another method uses a band placed around the entire stomach. It is then tightened to reduce upper stomach volume. In either case overeating of solid foods is consequently less likely, because rapid vomiting would result. The smaller stomach volume also promotes more rapid satiety. With the enforced food reduction, about 75% of people with severe obesity eventually lose 50% or more of excess body weight. When gastroplasty leads to success at long-term maintenance of this weight loss, it also often leads to dramatic health improvements, such as reduced blood pressure and elimination of type 2 diabetes. Risk of death from the surgery itself is about 1%.

Gastroplasty has disadvantages. The surgery is costly and may not be covered by medical insurance. In addition, follow-up surgery is often needed after weight loss to correct stretched skin, which used to be filled with fat. Furthermore, months of difficult adjustments regarding reduced food intake face the dieter who has chosen this drastic approach to weight loss. Nutrient deficiencies are also possible if an appropriate diet and nutrient supplement plan is not followed.

This surgery is not reversed, even after the desired weight loss is attained. Thus, however successful for weight loss, gastroplasty still requires major, lifelong lifestyle changes, such as control of energy intake and regular physical activity.

Concept Check

Severly obese people who have failed to lose weight with conservative weight-loss strategies may consider other options. Their doctors may recommend undergoing surgery to reduce the volume of the stomach to approximately 30 milliliters or following a very-low-calorie diet plan containing 400 to 800 kcal per day. Careful physician monitoring is crucial in both cases.

Treatment of Underweight

Underweight can be caused by a variety of factors, such as anorexia nervosa (see Chapter 12 for details), cancer, infectious disease, digestive tract disorders, and excessive physical activity. Genetic background may also lead to a higher resting metabolic rate, a slight body frame, or both. Significant underweight is also associated with increased death rates, especially when combined with cigarette smoking. Health problems associated with underweight include the loss of menstrual function, complications with pregnancy and surgery, and slow recovery after illness. We frequently hear

Spot-reducing using diet and physical activity is not possible. "Problem" local fat deposits can be reduced in size, however, using suction lipectomy (also called liposuction). Lipectomy means surgical removal of fat. A pencil-thin tube is inserted into an incision in the skin, and the fat tissue, such as that in the buttocks and thigh area, is suctioned. This procedures carries some risks, such as infection, lasting depressions in the skin, and blood clots, which can lead to kidney failure and sometimes death. The procedure is designed to help a person lose about 4 pounds per treatment. Cost is about $1600 per site; total costs range as high as $2600–$9000.

gastroplasty Surgery performed on the stomach to limit its volume to approximately 30 milliliters.

underweight A body mass index below 18.5. The cutoff is less precise than that for obesity because this condition has been less studied.

about the risks of obesity, but seldom of underweight. In our culture, being underweight is much more socially acceptable than being obese.

Sometimes being underweight requires medical intervention. A physician should be consulted first to rule out hormonal imbalances, depression, cancer, infectious disease such as tuberculosis, certain digestive tract disorders, excessive physical activity, and other hidden disease, such as the eating disorder anorexia nervosa (see Chapter 12 for a detailed discussion of eating disorders).

The causes of underweight are not altogether different from the causes of obesity. Internal and external satiety-signal irregularities, the rate of metabolism, hereditary tendencies, and psychological traits can all contribute to underweight.

In growing children, the demand for energy to support physical activity and growth can cause underweight. During growth spurts in adolescence, active children may not take the time to consume enough energy to support their energy needs. Moreover, gaining weight can be a formidable task for an underweight person. More than 500 extra kcal per day may be required to gain weight, even at a slow pace, in part because of the increased expenditure of energy in nonexercise activity thermogenesis. In contrast to the weight loser, the weight gainer may need to increase portion size.

When underweight requires a specific intervention, one approach for treating adults is to gradually increase their consumption of energy-dense foods (foods that provide a great deal of energy in a small volume), especially those high in vegetable fat. Italian cheeses, nuts, and granola can be good energy sources with low saturated-fat content. Dried fruit and bananas are energy-dense fruit choices. If eaten at the end of a meal, they don't cause early satiety. Underweight people should replace such foods as diet soft drinks with good energy sources, such as fruit juices.

Encouraging a regular meal and snack schedule aids in weight gain and maintenance. Sometimes people who are underweight have experienced stress at work or have been too busy to eat. Making regular meals a priority may not only help them attain an appropriate weight, but also help with digestive disorders such as constipation, which are sometimes associated with irregular eating times.

Excessively physically active people can reduce activity. If their weight remains low, they can add muscle mass through a resistance training (weightlifting) program, but they must increase their energy intake to support that physical activity. Otherwise, weight gain will be hindered.

If these efforts fail to achieve the desired weight, they should at least prevent the health problems associated with being underweight. After achieving that, they may have to accept their lean frames.

*F*or more information on weight control obesity, and nutrition, visit the Weight-Control Information Network (WIN) at *www.niddk.nih.gov/NutritionDocs.html* or call 800-WIN-8098. Other websites include *www.caloriecontrol.org*, *www.weight.com, www.obesity.org, and www.cyberdiet.com.*

▮ Summary

1. Energy balance is energy intake minus energy output. Negative energy balance occurs when energy output surpasses energy intake, resulting in weight loss. Positive energy balance occurs when energy intake is greater than energy output. The result is weight gain.

2. Basal metabolism, the thermic effect of food, physical activity, and nonexercise activity thermogenesis account for total energy use by the body. Basal metabolism, which represents the minimum energy expenditure needed to keep the resting, awake body alive, is primarily affected by lean body mass, surface area, and thyroid hormone concentrations. Physical activity represents energy use above that expended at rest. The thermic effect of food represents the increase in metabolism to facilitate the digesting, absorbing, and processing of nutrients recently consumed. Nonexercise activity thermogenesis is heat production caused by overfeeding and

other stimuli. About 70% to 80% of energy use is accounted for by basal metabolism and the thermic effect of food in a primarily sedentary person.

3. Energy use by the body can be measured directly from heat output or indirectly from oxygen uptake, carbon dioxide output, or both. Energy use by the body can be estimated using formulas based on various combinations of body height and weight with degree of physical activity and age.

4. A person of healthy weight shows good health and performs daily activities without weight-related problems. A body mass index (weight [in kilograms] ÷ height^2 [in meters]) of 18.5 to 24.9 is one measure of healthy weight, although weight in excess of this value may not lead to ill health. This suggests that healthy weight is best determined in conjunction with a thorough health evaluation by a physician.

5. Obesity is usually defined as total body fat percentage over 25% in men and about 35% in women. A body mass index of 30 or more also represents obesity.

6. Fat distribution partially determines health risks from obesity. Upper-body fat-storage distribution (waist circumference greater than 40 inches in men and greater than 35 inches in women) suggests higher risks of hypertension, cardiovascular disease, and type 2 diabetes associated with obesity than does lower-body fat distribution.

7. Genetic factors influence the tendency toward obesity. Basal metabolism and body fat distribution both have genetic links. How a person is raised (or nurtured) also influences the tendency toward obesity because family members often develop similar eating habits and activity patterns. Obesity can be viewed as nurture allowing nature to be expressed.

8. Those in search of a treatment for obesity should remember these five points: (1) A focus on healthy lifestyle rather than weight loss per se is more appropriate for many potential and current dieters; (2) the body resists weight loss; (3) the emphasis should be on preventing obesity because curing the disorder is very difficult; (4) weight loss should represent mostly a loss of fat storage and not primarily the loss of muscle and other lean tissues; and (5) rapid weight loss and quick regain can be especially harmful to emotional health.

9. A sound weight-loss program meets the dieter's nutritional needs by emphasizing a wide variety of low energy density food choices from the Food Guide Pyramid (or related pyramid), it adapts to the dieter's habits, consists of readily obtainable foods, strives to change poor eating habits, stresses regular physical activity, and stipulates the participation of a physician if weight is to be lost rapidly or if the person is over 40 (men) or 50 (women) years of age and plans to perform substantially greater physical activity than usual.

10. A pound of fat contains about 3500 kcal. A pound of adipose tissue—the fat itself plus lean support tissue—lost or gained represents approximately 2700 kcal. Thus, if energy output exceeds energy intake by about 500 kcal per day, a pound of adipose tissue can be lost per week. Decreasing the intake of high-fat foods is one way to obtain this energy deficit, along with increasing physical activity.

11. Physical activity as part of a weight-loss program should be focused on duration rather than intensity. Ideally, vigorous activity for 30 to 60 minutes should be part of each day; both during weight loss and then indefinitely.

12. Behavior modification is a vital part of a weight-loss program because the dieter may have many habits that encourage overeating and thus discourage weight maintenance. Specific behavior-modification techniques, such as stimulus control and self-monitoring, can be used to help change problem behavior.

13. Medications to blunt appetite, such as phenteramine (Fastin) and sibutramine (Meridia), can aid weight-reduction strategies. Orlistat (Xenical) reduces fat absorption in a meal when taken with the meal. Use is reserved for those who are obese or have or weight-related problems, and they must be administered under strict physician supervision. These medications may promote weight loss but they are not meant for long-term usage. In addition, individuals must learn a new lifestyle and eating habits.

14. The treatment of severe obesity may include surgery to reduce stomach volume to approximately 30 milliliters or very-low-calorie diets containing 400 to 800 kcal per day. Both of these measures should be reserved for people who have failed at more conservative approaches to weight loss. They require close medical supervision and lifelong adjustments in eating habits.

15. Underweight can be caused by a variety of factors, such as excessive physical activity and genetic background. Sometimes being underweight requires medical intervention. A physician should be consulted first to rule out ongoing disease. The underweight person may need to increase portion sizes and learn to like energy-dense foods. In addition, encouraging a regular meal and snack schedule aids in weight gain and maintenance. A physically active person can reduce excessive activity and substitute some resistance exercise (weight training).

Study Questions

1. How is the energy content of a food determined? How is this similar to one method of determining total energy use by the body?

2. Knowing the four contributors to human energy expenditure, propose two hypotheses for the development of obesity, based on the classes of energy expenditure.

3. Define a healthy weight in a way that makes the most sense to you.

4. Describe a practical method to define obesity in a clinical setting.

5. What are the two most convincing pieces of evidence that both genetic and environmental factors play significant roles in the development of obesity?

6. What three health problems do obese people typically face? Describe a possible reason that each problem arises.

7. When searching for a sound weight-loss program, what three key characteristics would you look for?

8. Why is the claim for quick, effortless weight loss by any method necessarily misleading?

9. Define the term *behavior modification*. Relate it to the terms *stimulus control*, *self-monitoring*, *chain-breaking*, *relapse prevention*, and *cognitive restructuring*. Give examples of each.

10. Why should the treatment of obesity be viewed as a lifelong commitment rather than just a short episode of weight loss?

Further Readings

1. Allara L: The return of the high-protein, low-carbohydrate diet: Weighing the risks. *Nutrition in Clinical Practice* 15:26, 2000.
The weight problem in this country is not seen as being due to one particular nutrient ingested—for example, too much carbohydrate or too little protein—but, instead, to an increase in total calorie intake without some compensation, such as increased physical activity.

2. Atkinson RL: A 33-year-old woman with morbid obesity. *Journal of the American Medical Association* 283:3236, 2000.
The history of an African-American woman who has struggled with weight control since her teenage years is presented. Dr. Atkinson reviews much of what is known about obesity treatment as he presents the options suggested to the patient, such as the use of diet control, exercise, behavior modification, medications, and possible gastroplasty.

3. Bren L: Losing weight: More than counting calories. *FDA Consumer*, p. 16, January–February 2002.
Losing weight requires great commitment. Important lifestyle changes are eating less, regular physical activity, and behavior modification, but it is worth the effort as it can improve one's health.

4. Dickerson LM, Carek PJ: Drug therapy for obesity. *American Family Physician* 61:2131, 2000.
If drug therapy is recommended in the management of obesity, it should be used in combination with a structured diet and exercise program to achieve the greatest and longest-lasting results. The use of phenteramine (Ionamin), sibutramine (Meridia), and orlistat (Xenical) is reviewed.

5. Expert panel on the identification, evaluation, and treatment of overweight in adults: Clinical guidelines on the identification, evaluation, and treatment of overweight and obesity in adults: Executive summary. *American Journal of Clinical Nutrition* 68:899, 1998.
Step-by-step plans are provided for the evaluation and treatment of weight and obesity. After successful weight loss, the likelihood of weight-loss maintenance is enhanced by a program consisting of diet therapy, physical activity, and behavior therapy—this should be continued indefinitely.

6. Kennedy ET and others: Popular diets: Correlation of health, nutrition, and obesity. *Journal of the American Dietetic Association* 101:411, 2001.
For the most part, individuals successful at weight loss and later weight control restrict intake of certain types or classes of foods, eat all types of foods but in limited quantity, count calories, limit percentage of daily energy intake from fat, and participate in regular physical activity.

7. Liebman B: Defensive eating: Staying lean in a fattening world. *Nutrition Action Health Letter*, p. 1, December 2001.
Food in North America is widely available and generally inexpensive, and the number of opportunities to eat has risen dramatically—drugstores, gas stations, and shopping malls to name a few. In response, one strategy for weight control is to fill your plate with salad greens and vegetables and use calorie-dense foods as condiments. Also watch portion size—the bigger the portion, the more people eat.

8. Lyznicki JM and others: Obesity: Assessment and management in primary care. *American Family Physician* 63:2185, 2001.
Basic treatment of overweight and obese patients requires a comprehensive approach involving diet and nutrition, regular physical activity, and behavioral change, with an emphasis on long-term weight management rather than short-term extreme weight reduction. The article discusses these interventions in detail.

9. Kushner R: Medical management of the bariatric surgery patient. *Nutrition and the M.D.*, p. 1, July 2001.
Gastroplasty is now considered a well-established treatment for patients with severe obesity. Patients can expect to lose approximately one-third of their initial body weight with resolution of existing medical conditions and improvement in quality of life. Ongoing nutritional and medical management is required to prevent nutritional deficiencies and optimize post-operative care.

10. Marcus J: Dietitians come in all sizes. *Today's Dietitian*, p. 26, October 1999.
People who weigh more than current healthy BMI standards undergo unfair social hardships that erode self-esteem. Some health professionals are calling for size acceptance—less emphasis on body size and more emphasis on healthy eating and personal fitness.

11. Mokdad AH and others: The continuing epidemics of obesity and diabetes in the United States. *Journal of the American Medical Association* 286:1195, 2001.
The percentage of the U.S. population that has obesity and/or type 2 diabetes has increased in recent years. This is likely to be even a bigger problem in the future if more attention to preventive measures, such as healthy eating and regular physical activity, are not implemented on a widespread basis. Restoring physical activity to daily routines is especially important.

12. Peter JC and others: Control of energy balance in Stipanuk MH, *Physiological Aspects of Human Nutrition*, Philadelphia, PA: W.B. Saunders, 2000.
Set point with respect to body weight is more effective in preventing weight loss than weight gain. Throughout adult life a person may settle at a variety of "set-point" weights, rather a single weight. For a person who is sedentary and consumes a large amount of dietary fat, it is thought that any increase in body weight actually represents an adaptation to this high-fat diet. This is because it is thought that only by reaching a certain point of body fatness will this sedentary person be able to balance the amount of fat consumed with the amount released from adipose tissue and burned by the body.

13. St. Jeor ST and others: Dietary protein and weight reduction. *Circulation* 104:1869, 2001.
High-protein diets are not recommended for weight loss because they restrict healthful foods that provide essential nutrients and do not provide the variety of foods needed to adequately meet nutritional needs. Individuals who follow these diets are therefore at risk for compromised vitamin and mineral intake, as well as potential decline in heart, kidney, bone, and liver health.

I. A Close Look at Your Weight Status

Determine the following two indices of your body status: body mass index and waist circumference.

Body Mass Index (BMI)

Record your weight in pounds: _155_ pounds
Divide your weight in pounds by 2.2 to determine your weight in kilograms: _70.5_ kilograms
Record you height in inches: _72_ inches
Divide your height in inches by 39.3 to determine your height in meters: _1.8_ meters
Calculate your BMI using the following formula:
BMI = weight (kilograms)/height^2 (meters)
BMI = _70.5_ kilograms/ _1.8_ meters^2 = _21.8_

Waist Circumference

Use a tape measure to measure the circumference of your waist (at the umbilicus with stomach muscles relaxed): Circumference of waist (umbilicus) = _30_ inches

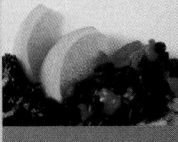

Interpretation

1. When BMI is 25 or greater, health risks from obesity often begin. It is especially advisable to consider weight loss if your BMI is 30 or more. Does your BMI reach 25 or more?

    Yes _____   No _X_

2. When a person has a BMI of 25 or more and a waist circumference of more than 40 inches in men or 35 inches in women, there is an increased risk of cardiovascular disease, hypertension, and type 2 diabetes. Does your circumference exceed the standard for your gender?

    Yes _____   No _X_

3. Do you feel you need to pursue a program of weight loss?

    Yes _____   No _X_

Application

From what you've learned in this chapter, what habits can you change in patterns of eating and physical activity to lose weight and help ensure maintenance of any loss:

_____NONE_____

_____

_____

II. An Action Plan to Change Weight Status

Now that you have assessed your current weight status, do you feel that you would like to make some changes? Following is a step-by-step guide to behavioral change. This process can be useful even for those who are satisfied with their current weight, as it can be applied to changing exercise habits, self-esteem, and a variety of other behaviors (Fig. 10.12).

Becoming Aware of the Problem

By calculating your current weight status, you have already become aware of the problem, if one exists. From here, it is important to find out more information about the cause of the problem and whether it is worth working toward a change.

continued

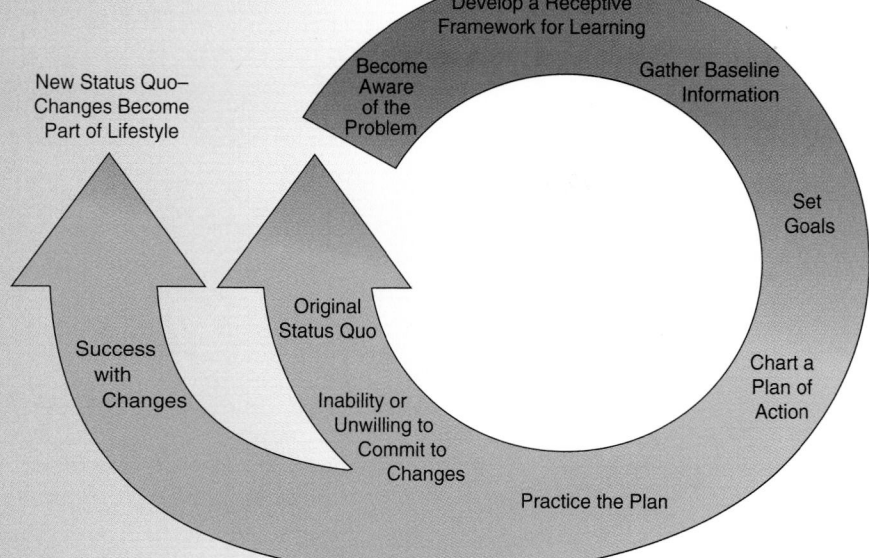

Figure 10.12 A model for behavior change. It starts with awareness of the problem and ends with the incorporation of new behaviors intended to address the problem.

1. Looking back at the food diary you completed in Chapter 1, what are some of the factors that most influence your eating habits? Do you eat due to stress, boredom, or depression? Is volume of food your problem, or do you eat mainly the wrong foods for you? Take some time to assess the root causes of your eating habits.

2. Once you have more information about your specific eating practices, you must decide if it is worth changing these practices. A benefits-and-costs analysis can be a useful tool in evaluating whether or not it is worth your effort to make life changes. Use the following examples as a guide for listing benefits and costs pertinent to your own situation (Fig. 10.13).

Setting Goals

What can we accomplish, and how long will it take? Setting a realistic, achievable goal and allowing a reasonable amount of time to pursue it increases the likelihood of success.

1. Begin by determining the final outcome you would like to achieve. If you are trying to change your eating behaviors to be more healthy, list your reasons for doing so (e.g., overall health, weight loss, self-esteem).

   Overall goal:

   _____

   _____

   _____

   Reasons to pursue goal:

   _____

   _____

   _____

   _____

2. Now list several steps that will be necessary to achieve your goal. Keep in mind, however, that it is generally best to change only a few specific behaviors at first—walking briskly for 30 minutes five times a week, reducing fat intake, using more whole-grain products, and not eating after 7 P.M. Many experts suggest that attempting small and perhaps easier dietary changes first reduces the scope of the problem and so can increase the likelihood of success.

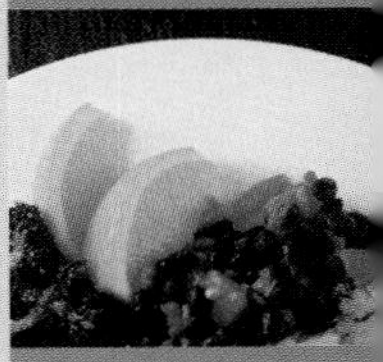

BENEFITS AND COSTS ANALYSIS

1 Benefits of changing eating habits?

What do you expect to get, now or later, that you want? What do you get to avoid that would be unpleasant?

— *feel better physically and psychologically*
— *look better*
—
—
—
—

3 Costs involved in changing eating habits?

What do you have to do that you don't want to do? What do you have to stop doing that you would rather continue doing?

— *take time to plan meals and shop*
— *must give up some food volume*
—
—

2 Benefits of not changing eating habits?

What do you get to do that you enjoy doing? What do you avoid having to do?

— *no need for planning*
— *can eat without feeling guilty*
—
—
—

4 Costs of not changing eating habits?

What unpleasant or undesirable effects are you likely to experience now or in the future? What are you likely to lose?

— *creeping weight gain*
— *low self-esteem and poor health*
—
—
—

Figure 10.13 Benefits and costs analysis applied to increasing physical activity. This process helps put behavior change into the context of total lifestyle.

Steps toward achieving goal:

1. _____

2. _____

3. _____

Note that, if you are having trouble deciphering the steps needed to achieve your goal, health professionals are an excellent resource for aid in planning.

Measuring Commitment

Now that you have collected information and know what is required to reach your goal, you must ask yourself, "Can I do this?" Commitment is an essential component in the success of behavioral change. Be honest with yourself. Permanent change is not quick or easy. Once you have decided that you have the commitment required to see this through, continue on to the following sections.

Making It Official with a Contract

Drawing up a behavioral contract often adds incentive to follow through with a plan. The contract could list goal behaviors and objectives, milestones for measuring progress, and regular rewards for meeting the terms of the contract. After finishing a contract, you should sign it in the presence of some friends. This encourages commitment.

Initially, plans should reward positive behaviors, and then they should focus on positive results. Positive behaviors, such as regular physical activity, eventually lead to positive outcomes, such as increased stamina.

Figure 10.14 is a sample contract for increasing physical activity. Keep in mind that this sample contract is only a suggestion; you can add your own ideas as well.

continued

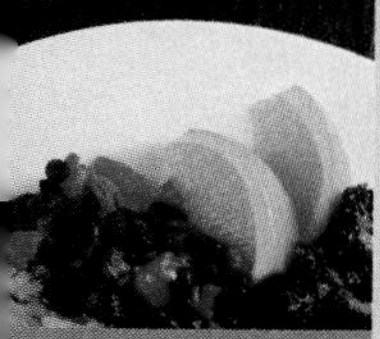

Name _Alan Young_

Goal

I agree to _ride my exercise bike_
                                    (specify behavior)

under the following circumstances _for 30 minutes, 4 times per week_
in the evening
                                    (specify where, when, how much, etc.)

Substitute behavior and/or reinforcement schedule _I will reinforce myself_
if I've achieved my goal after a month with a weekend off
campus with my roommate.

Environmental planning

In order to help me do this, I am going to (1) arrange my physical and social environment
by _buying a new jogging suit at the local sporting goods_
store

and (2) control my internal environment (thoughts, images) by _coordinating riding_
the bike with the first T.V. watching I do in the evening

Reinforcements

Reinforcements provided by me daily or weekly (if contract is kept):
I will buy myself a new piece of clothing for off campus
trip

Reinforcements provided by others daily or weekly (if contract is kept):
at the end of a month if I've completed my goal my parents will
buy me a fitness club membership for winter.

Social support

Behavior change is more likely to take place when other people support you. During the
quarter/semester please meet with the other person at least three times to discuss your
progress.

The name of my "significant helper" is: _Mr. and Mrs. Young_

This contract should include:

1. Baseline data (one week)
2. Well-defined goal
3. Simple method for charting progress (diary, counter, charts, etc.)
4. Reinforcements (immediate and long-term)
5. Evaluation method (summary of experiences, success, and/or new learnings about self).

Figure 10.14 Alan's behavior contract. Completing such a contract can help generate commitment to behavior change. What would your contract look like? You'll have a chance to develop one in the Rate Your Plate section later in the chapter.

Psyching Yourself Up

Once your contract is in place, you need to psych yourself up. Discouragement from peers and your own temptations to stray from your plan need to be anticipated. Psyching yourself up can enable you to progress toward your goals in spite of others' attitudes and opinions. Almost everyone benefits from some assertiveness training when it comes to changing behaviors. The following are a few suggestions. Can you think of any others?

- No one's feelings should be hurt if you say, "No, thank you," firmly and repeatedly when others try to dissuade you from a plan. Rather, ask them—and yourself—why they want you to eat their way. Your needs are as important as anyone else's.

- You don't have to eat a lot to accommodate anyone—your mother, business clients, or the chef. For example, at a party with friends, you may feel you have to eat a lot to participate, but you don't. Another trap is ordering a lot just because someone else is paying for the meal.

- Learn ways to handle put-downs—inadvertent or conscious. An effective response can be to communicate feelings honestly, without hostility. Tell criticizers that they have annoyed or offended you, that you are working to change your habits and would really like understanding and support from them.

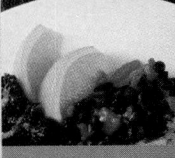

Practicing the Plan

Once you've set up a plan, the next step is to implement it. Start with a trial of at least 6 to 8 weeks. Thinking of a lifetime commitment can be overwhelming. Aim for a total duration of 6 months of new activities before giving up. We may have to persuade ourselves more than once of the value of continuing the program. The following are some suggestions to help keep a plan on track:

- *Focus on reducing, but not necessarily extinguishing, undesirable behaviors.* For example, it's usually unrealistic to say, "I'll never eat a certain food again." It's better to say, "I won't eat that problem food as regularly as before."

- *Monitor progress.* Note your progress in a diary and reward yourself according to your contract. While conquering some habits and seeing improvement, you may find yourself quite encouraged, even enthusiastic, about your plan of action. That can give you the impetus to move ahead with the program.

- *Control environments.* In the early phases of behavioral change, try to avoid problem situations, such as parties, coffee breaks, and favorite restaurants. Once new habits are firmly established, you can probably more successfully resist the temptations in these environments.

Re-evaluating and Preventing Relapse

After practicing a program for several weeks to months, it is important to reassess the original plan. In addition, you may now be able to pinpoint other problem areas for which you need to plan appropriately.

1. Begin by taking a close and critical look at your original plan. Does it actually lead to the goals you set? Are there any new steps toward your goal that you feel capable of adding to your contract? Do you need reinforcements? It may even be necessary to make a new contract. For permanent change, it is worth this time of reassessment.

2. In practicing your plan over the past weeks or months, you have likely experienced relapses. What triggered these relapses? To prevent a total retreat to your old habits, it is important to set up a plan for such relapses. You can do this by identifying high-risk situations, rehearsing a response, and remembering your goals.

You may have noticed a behavior chain in some of your relapses. That is, the relapse may stem from a series of interconnected habitual activities. The way to break the chain is to first identify the activities, pinpoint the weak links, break those links, and substitute other behaviors. Figure 10.15 is a sample behavior chain and a substitute activities list. Consider compiling your own list based on your behavior chains.

Epilogue

If you have used the activities in this section, you are well on your way to permanent behavioral change. Recall that this exercise can be used for a variety of desired changes, including quitting smoking, increasing physical activity, and improving study habits. It is by no means an easy process, but the results can be well worth the effort. Overall, the keys to success are motivation (keeping the problem in the forefront of your mind), having a plan of action, securing the resources and skills needed for success, and looking for help from family, friends, or a group.

continued

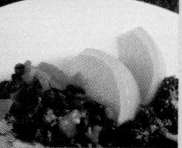
ALTERNATIVE ACTIVITY SHEET

SUBSTITUTE ACTIVITIES

Pleasant activities
1. _Singing / washing hair_
2. _Reading comics / biking_
3. _Sewing / calling a friend_

Necessary activities
1. _Ironing_
2. _Vacuuming_
3. _Straightening apartment_

Situations when used
1. _Wanted ice cream – delayed with bath_
2. _Wanted wheat thins – cleaned up apt._
3. _Wanted snack – went for walk_
4. _Wanted cookies – did dishes first_
5. _Saw leftovers – went for bike ride_
6. _Tempted by cookies – set timer_
7. _Wanted snack – read comics_

BEHAVIOR CHAIN

Identify the links in your eating response chain on the following diagram. Draw a line through the chain where it was interrupted. Add the link you substituted and the new chain of behavior this substitution started.

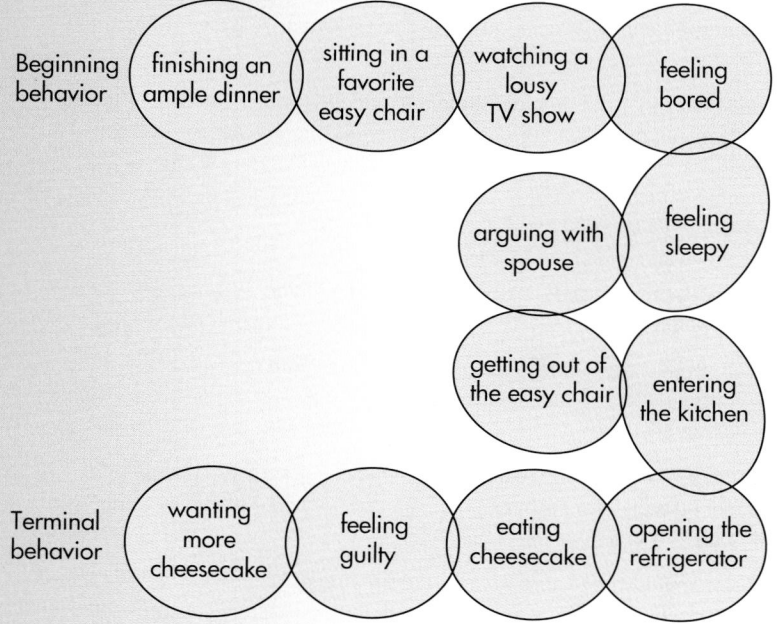

Figure 10.15 Identifying behavior chains. This is a good tool for understanding more about your habits and pinpointing ways to change unwanted habits. The earlier in the chain you substitute a nonfood link, the easier it is to intervene. Four types of behaviors can be substituted in an ongoing behavior chain.

1. Fun activities (taking a walk, reading a book)
2. Necessary activities (cleaning a room, balancing your checkbook)
3. Incompatible activities (taking a shower)
4. Urge-delaying activities (setting a kitchen timer for 20 minutes before allowing yourself to eat)

Using activities to interrupt behavior patterns that lead to inappropriate eating (or inactivity) can be a powerful means of changing eating habits.

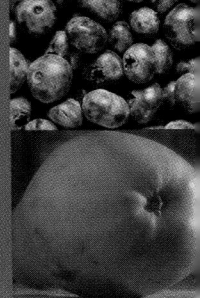

Many overweight people try to help themselves by using the latest fad diet book. But, as you will see, most of these diets do not help, and some can actually harm those who follow them (Table 10.8).

Recently, weight-loss experts came together at the request of the USDA to evaluate weight-loss diets. They came to this conclusion: Forget fads when it comes to dieting. Most of the popular fad diets are nutritionally inadequate and include certain foods that people would not normally choose to consume in such amounts. The experts stated that eating less of one's favorite foods and becoming more physically active can be much more effective when trying to implement a weight-loss diet. People need a plan that they can live with in the long run so that weight control becomes permanent. The goal should be weight control over a lifetime, not immediate weight loss. Every fad diet leads to some immediate weight loss because daily intake is monitored—not necessarily because of certain imposed practices—and because monotonous food choices are typically part of the plan. Overall, a traditional reduced calorie, moderate-fat diet coupled with regular physical activity is adequate for weight loss.

You may wonder why fad diet books exist at all. Why doesn't the government put a stop to them? Many contain blatant misinformation. However, FDA concerns itself only when products are suspected of doing serious harm, as in the case of earlier forms of liquid protein diets. FDA is too busy and too underfunded to pursue every new fad diet plan. Ancient advise is still valid: "Let the buyer beware." Responsibility rests with the authors and publishers, who want to sell books and earn money and know there is little risk involved. Making outrageous claims sells more books than writing "eat less fat and walk more."

I t is illegal in the United States to falsely represent worthless or dangerous cures and medical devices. Thus, U.S. citizens can use their rights under federal law to have FDA pursue a seller of a dangerous fad diet book in an attempt to have it removed from the market.

How to Recognize a Fad Diet

The criteria for evaluating weight-loss programs with regard to their safety and effectiveness were discussed previously. In contrast, fad diets typically share some different common characteristics:

1. They promote quick weight loss. As mentioned before, this loss primarily results from glycogen, sodium, and lean muscle mass depletion. All lead to a loss of body water.
2. They limit food selections and dictate specific rituals, such as eating only fruit for breakfast or cabbage soup every day.
3. They use testimonials from famous people and tie the diet to well-known cities, such as Beverly Hills and New York.
4. They bill themselves as cure-alls. These diets claim to work for everyone, whatever the type of obesity or the person's specific strengths and weaknesses.
5. They often recommend expensive supplements.
6. No attempts are made to change eating habits permanently. Dieters follow the diet until the desired weight is reached and then revert to old eating habits—they are told, for example, to eat rice for a month, lose weight, and then return to old habits.
7. They are generally critical of and skeptical about the scientific community. They suggest that physicians and registered dietitians do not really want people to lose weight. They encourage people to look outside the medical establishment for correct advice.

Probably the cruelest characteristic of fad diets is that they essentially guarantee failure for the dieter. These diets are not designed for permanent weight loss. Habits are not changed, and the food selection is so limited that the person cannot follow the diet in the long run. Although dieters assume they have lost fat, they have actually lost mostly muscle and other lean tissue mass. As soon as they begin eating normally again, the lost tissue is replaced. In a matter of weeks,

A practical example of the effectiveness of monotony in contributing to weight loss is the experience of Jerad Fogle. He primarily ate Subway® sandwiches for 11 months and lost 245 pounds. He notes, however, that this is not a miracle diet—it takes a lot of hard work to lead to the success he experienced. There are also many other examples where diet monotony has led to weight loss.

continued

Table 10.8 Summary of Popular Diet Approaches to Weight Control

Approach and Examples*		Characteristics and Possible Negative Health and Other Consequences
Moderate Calorie Restriction		
The Setpoint Diet	Living Without Dieting	Usually 1000–1800 kcal per day, with moderate fat intake
Slim Chance in a Fat World	Volumetrics	Reasonable balance of macronutrients
Weight Watcher's Diet	Lose the Last 10 Pounds	Encourage exercise
Mary Ellen's Help Yourself Diet Plan	Dieting with the Dutchess	May use behavioral approach
The Beyond Diet	Dieting for Dummies	
Staying Thin	The Wedding Dress Diet	Acceptable if a multivitamin and mineral supplement is used and
The Callaway Diet	Dr. Shapiro's Picture Perfect Diet	permission of family physician is granted
Macronutrient Restriction		
Low or Restricted Carbohydrate		
Dr. Atkins' Diet Revolution	Endocrine Control Diet	Generally less than 100 grams of carbohydrate per day
Calories Don't Count	Enter the Zone	
Miracle Diet for Fast Weight Loss	Protein Power	Ketosis if carbohydrate is greatly restricted; reduced exercise capacity due to
Woman Doctor's Diet for Women	The Five-Day Miracle Diet	poor glycogen stores in the muscles; excessive animal fat intake
The Doctor's Quick Weight Loss Diet	Healthy for Life	
The Complete Scarsdale Medical Diet	Carbohydrate Addicts Diet	
Four Day Wonder Diet	Sugar Busters	
Low Fat		
The Rice Diet Report	The Maximum Metabolism Diet	Less than 20% of energy from fat
The Macrobiotic Diet (some versions)	The Pasta Diet	Limited (or elimination of) animal protein sources; also limited fats, nuts,
The Pritikin Diet	The McDougall Plan	seeds
Eat More, Weigh Less	Ultrafit Diet	Little satiety; flatulence; possibly poor mineral absorption from excess
The 35+ Diet	Stop the Insanity	dietary fiber; limited food choices sometimes leads to deprivation
20/30 Fat and Fiber	G-Index Diet	
Fat to Muscle Diet	Outsmarting the Female Fat Cell	Not necessarily to be avoided, but certain aspects of many of the plans
T-Factor Diet	Foods That Cause You to Lose	possibly unacceptable
Fit or Fat	Weight	
Two Day Diet	Lean Bodies	
Complete Hip and Thigh Diet	Turn Off the Fat Genes	
Novelty Diets		
Dr. Abravenel's Body Type and	Eat to Succeed	Promotes certain nutrients, foods, or combinations of foods as having
Lifetime Nutrition Plan (or his	The Underburner's Diet	unique, magical, or previously undiscovered qualities
other books)	Eat to Win	
Dr. Berger's Immune Power Diet	Two Day Diet	Malnutrition; no change in habits leads to relapse; unrealistic food choices
Fit for Life	Paris Diet	lead to possible bingeing
The Hilton Head Metabolism Diet	Cabbage-Soup Diet	
The Beverly Hills Diet	Eat Great, Lose Weight	
Dr. Debetz Champagne Diet	Eat Smart Think Smart	
Sun Sign Diet	*Scent*sational Weight Loss	
F-Plan Diet	Eat Right 4 Your Type	
Fat Attack Plan	The Greenwich Diet	
Autohypnosis Diet	3 Season Diet	
The Ultrafit Diet	Metabolize	
The Princeton Diet	God's Diet	
The Diet Bible	The Weigh Down Diet	
Very-Low-Calorie Diets (VLCDs)		
Optifast	Ultrafast	Less than 800 kcal per day
Cambridge Diet	Thin So Fast	Also known as protein-sparing modified fasts
HMR		Must be under close physician scrutiny
		Organ tissue loss—especially from the heart; low blood potassium leads to
		heart failure; expense; kidney stones; gout
Formula Diets		
Optifast	Cambridge Diet	Can help people who find it easier not to eat whole foods while dieting to
Genesis	Slimfast	lose weight
		Based on formulated or packaged products
		Tend to be very-low-calorie regimens; no change in habits, possibly leading
		to increased chance of relapse; expense; constipation
Premeasured Diets		
Jenny Craig		Most food supplied in premeasured servings to take much of the decision
Nutri/System		making out of the process of eating
		Expense; may not allow for easy, sound eating later

*Diets may be listed in more than one category if multiple characteristics apply.

most of the lost weight is back. The dieter appears to have failed, when actually the diet has failed. This whole scenario can add more blame and guilt, challenging the self-worth of the dieter. If someone needs help losing weight, professional help is advised. It is unfortunate that current trends suggest people are spending more time and money on "quick fixes" rather than on such professional help.

Types of Fad Diets

Low- or Restricted-Carbohydrate Approaches

This is the most common form of fad diet. As discussed in Chapter 4, a very low-carbohydrate intake forces the liver to produce needed glucose. The source of carbons for this glucose is mostly tissue proteins. Thus, a low-carbohydrate diet results in protein tissue loss, as well as urinary loss of essential ions, such as potassium. Since protein tissue is mostly water, the dieter loses weight very rapidly. When a normal diet is resumed, the protein tissue is rebuilt and the weight is regained.

Low carbohydrates primarily work in the short run because they limit total food intake. Consider a visit to a fast-food restaurant. You plan to order a hamburger, French fries, and a soft drink and pay a bit more for the *super-size* option. This will yield about 1500 kcal. If you were on a low-carbohydrate diet plan, you can't have the French fries or the soft drink, as they contain too much carbohydrate. You can have the hamburger, but you will have to discard the bun. This leaves a lunch containing about 240 kcal of mostly fat and protein. You will also soon tire of the limited food choices, and this will cause you to eat less.

In the short run, this low-carbohydrate gimmick can lead to weight loss. But this plan does not include the fruits, vegetables, and whole grains that nutrition experts point out are important components of a healthy diet. Thus, the low-carbohydrate diet is not intended for long-term use (no more than 4 to 6 weeks). The American Heart Association recently warned against following such a diet.

Diet plans that use a low-carbohydrate approach are the Dr. Atkins' Diet Revolution, Dr. Stillman's Calories Don't Count Diet, the Scarsdale Diet, and the Four Day Wonder Diet. More moderate approaches are found in the various Zone diets (40% of energy intake as carbohydrate) and Sugar Busters diet. When you see a new fad diet advertisement, look first to see how much carbohydrate it contains. If breads, cereals, fruits, and vegetables are extremely limited, you are probably looking at a low- or restricted-carbohydrate diet.

Low-Fat Approaches

The very-low-fat diet turns out to be a very-high-carbohydrate diet. These diets contain approximately 5% to 10% of energy intake as fat. The most notable is the Pritikin Diet and the Dr. Dean Ornish diet plans. This approach is not harmful for healthy adults, but it is extremely difficult to follow. People get bored with this type of diet very quickly because they can't eat many of their favorite foods. These dieters eat primarily grains, fruits, and vegetables, which most people cannot do for very long. Eventually, the person wants some foods higher in fat or protein. Thus, the dieter suffers a lapse, then a relapse, and probably a collapse. These diets are just too different from the typical North American diet for many adults to follow consistently, but may be acceptable for some people.

Novelty Diets

A variety of fad diets are built on gimmicks. Some novelty diets emphasize one food or food group and exclude almost all others. A rice diet was designed in the 1940s to lower blood pressure; now it has resurfaced as a weight-loss diet. The first phase consists of eating only rice and fruit until you can't stand them any longer. Another novelty diet is the egg diet, on which you eat all the eggs you want. On the Beverly Hills Diet, you eat mostly fruit.

The rationale behind these diets is that you can eat only eggs, fruit, or rice for just so long before becoming bored and, in theory, reducing your energy intake. However, chances are that you will abandon the diet entirely before losing much weight.

continued

Since the 1960s, grapefruit has been touted for supposed unique ability to cause weight loss. No studies back up this claim. To add appeal to a grapefruit diet, proponents even suggest adding several "diet aids": lecithin to help release fat from the tissues, vitamin B-6 to act as a diuretic, vinegar to provide potassium, and kelp to stimulate the thyroid gland.

The most bizarre of the novelty diets proposes that "food gets stuck in your body." Fit for Life, the Beverly Hills Diet, and Eat Great, Lose Weight are examples. The supposition is that food gets stuck in the intestine, putrefies, and creates toxins, which invade the blood and cause disease. This is utter nonsense. Nevertheless, the same idea has been promoted in health-food books since the 1800s. Today, Fit for Life suggests that meat eaten with potatoes is not digested and that fresh fruit should be consumed only before noon. These recommendations are absurd. They are gimmicks that appear controversial but are really designed to sell books.

Finally, some commercial schemes are used to sell diet books. Books describing the allergy approach to dieting, for instance, suggest that diseases, including obesity, are due to food allergies. Supposedly, once your food allergies are found and treated, you will no longer have the disease. However, no research supports the claim. In addition, see the Sun Sign Diet if you believe in astrology, the Champagne Diet if you need a drink, the Cabbage Soup Diet if you want to eat it every day, or the Body Type and Lifetime Nutrition Diet if you have a "dominant" gland.

Quackery Is Characteristic of Fad Diets

Fad diets fall under the category of quackery—people taking advantage of others. They usually involve a product or service that costs a considerable amount of money. Often, those offering the product or service don't realize that they are promoting quackery, because they were victims themselves. For example, they tried the product and by pure coincidence it worked for them, so they wish to sell it to all their friends and relatives.

Recent examples of dubious recommendations in the field of weight loss are herbal laxative teas and chromium picolinate. These laxative teas, many of which have oriental-type labels, contain senna, which induces diarrhea. However, this diarrhea does not sufficiently reduce the absorption of calories from the diet. FDA is concerned that these teas may also result in serious injury or death linked to the diarrhea and related intestinal damage that is inducted. To date, these teas are linked to deaths of four young women.

Chromium picolinate, a nutritional supplement, has been touted as an aid for reducing body fat, increasing lean body mass, suppressing hunger, and increasing metabolic rate. However, chromium picolinate has not been approved for weight loss by FDA, nor has the agency seen any convincing data on the claims being made (see Chapter 9).

Numerous other gimmicks for weight loss have come and gone and are likely to resurface. If in the future an important aid for weight loss is discovered, you can feel confident that major journals, such as the *Journal of the American Dietetic Association,* the *Journal of the American Medical Association,* or *The New England Journal of Medicine,* will report it. You don't need to rely on paperback books or newspaper advertisements for information about weight loss.

Usually, quackery reduces only the bank account. Currently, $6 billion dollars per year are spent on such false hope in the United States alone. However, it can lead to life-threatening results. The rule of thumb on seeing a new diet aid on the market is that, if it sounds too good to be true, it is.

*F*DA recently announced that a weight-loss product sold over the Internet has been linked to six cases of liver failure. The product, called Lipokinetix, contains a form of thyroid hormone and other unsafe substances. This is another reason to avoid any weight-loss medicine or supplement that is not prescribed by a physician.

Scenario Follow-Up

As you have probably surmised, Crystal will just be wasting her money if she buys the product seen in the infomercial. Unfortunately, regulation of the supplement industry currently is woefully lacking. In the future, if there is such a breakthrough in weight loss and weight control, authorities such as the Surgeon General's Office or the National Institutes of Health will make North Americans aware of that fact. At this time, Crystal would be better off simply paying more attention to what she is eating and trying to find time for daily physical activity.

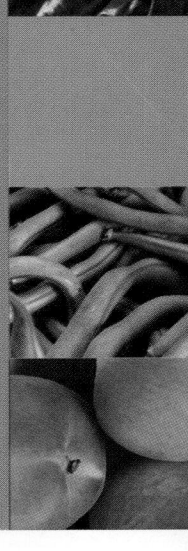

chapter 11

Nutrition: *Fitness and Sports*

A thletes invest a lot of time and effort in training. Because they are often seeking ways to modify their diets to improve their performances, athletes make easy targets for purveyors of nutrition misinformation. Still, most athletes don't want to miss out on any advantage, whether real or perceived, that might give them the winning edge.

Although good eating habits can't substitute for physical training and genetic endowment, proper diet choices are crucial to top-notch performance, contributing to endurance and helping speed the repair of injured tissues.

In this chapter, you will discover how physical fitness benefits the entire body; it is an essential ingredient in achieving maximal health. Experts might disagree on how much carbohydrate, protein, and fat we should consume, but there is no argument over the health benefits of regular physical activity. It is even beneficial for overweight people who remain at that excess weight.

Some people are active simply because they enjoy it, whether they're swimming, playing basketball, walking briskly, or engaging in any of innumerable other activities. Let's now look further at nutrition as it relates to fitness.

Check out the **Contemporary Nutrition: Issues and Insights Online Learning Center** www.mhhe.com/wardlawcont5 *for quizzes, flash cards, other activities, and web links designed to further help you learn about nutrition as it relates to fitness and sports.*

Chapter Objectives

Chapter 11 is designed to allow you to:

1. Design a fitness regimen that begins with no physical activity, moves to a first goal of at least 30 minutes of such activity on most (or all) days of the week, and then advances to more vigorous activity for a total of about 1 hour per day.

2. Describe when and how glycogen, blood glucose, fat, and protein are used to meet energy needs during different types of physical activity.

3. Differentiate between anaerobic and aerobic use of glucose and identify advantages and disadvantages of each.

4. Show how muscles and related organs adapt to an increase in physical activity.

5. Outline how to estimate an athlete's energy needs and discuss the general principles for meeting overall nutrient requirements in the training diet, focusing specifically on carbohydrate intake.

6. Examine the problems associated with rapid weight loss by dehydration and outline the importance of use of water and/or sports drinks during exercise.

7. Show an understanding of the importance of maintaining a healthy status of various vitamins and minerals during training.

8. List several ergogenic aids and describe their effects on an athlete's performance.

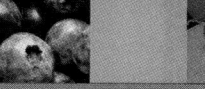 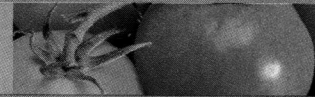

Refresh Your Memory

As you begin your study of nutrition for fitness and sports in Chapter 11, you may want to review:

- The current trend of consuming "energy bars" in Chapter 1
- The components of the cell in Chapter 3
- The concept of glycemic index in Chapter 4
- The various food sources of carbohydrates, proteins, and lipids in Chapters 4–6
- Food sources of calcium and iron in Chapter 9

Real Life Scenario

Marcella has become hooked on fitness in the past year and is training for a 10K run coming up in 3 weeks. She has read a lot about sports nutrition, and especially about the importance of eating a high-carbohydrate diet while in training. She also has been struggling to keep her weight in a range that she feels contributes to better speed and endurance. Consequently, she is also trying to eat as little fat as possible. Unfortunately, over the past week her workouts in the afternoon have not met her expectations. Her run times are slower, and she shows signs of fatigue after just 20 minutes into her training program.

Her breakfast yesterday was a large bagel, a small amount of cream cheese, and orange juice. For lunch, she had a small salad with fat-free dressing, a large plate of pasta with tomato marinara sauce and broccoli, and a diet soft drink. For dinner, she had a small broiled chicken breast, a cup of rice, some carrots, and iced tea. Later, she snacked on fat-free pretzels.

What advice would you provide Marcella regarding her training diet? Note current strengths and weaknesses. Is her diet likely contributing to her recent fatigue during workouts?

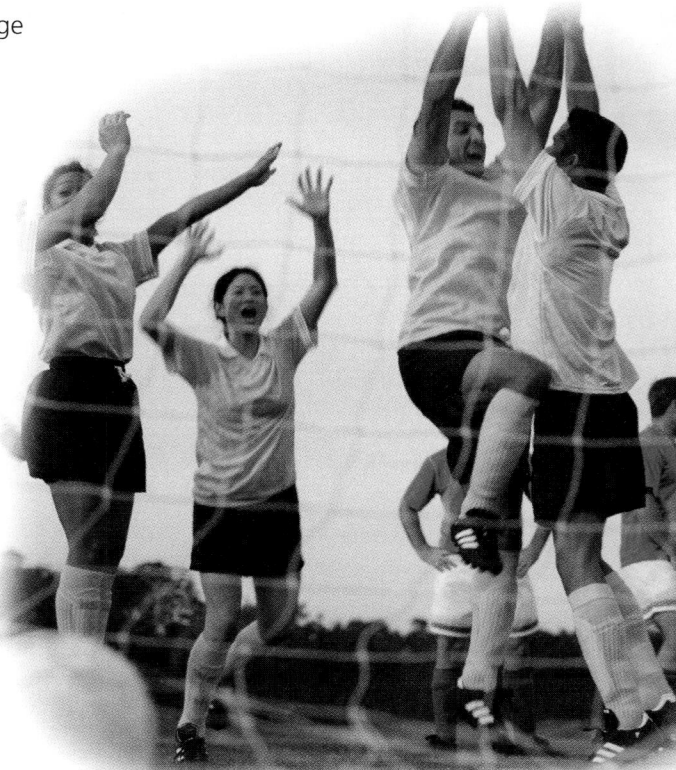

Nutrition Connection

FRANK & ERNEST

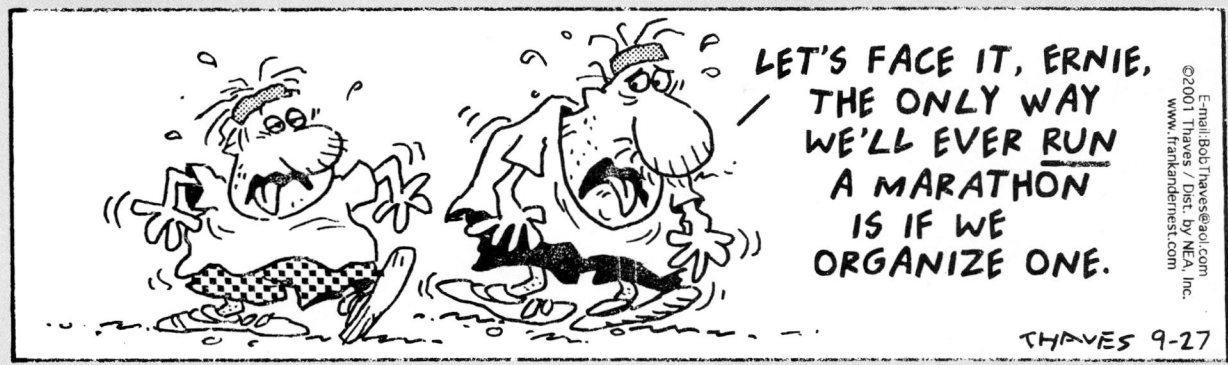

E-mail:BobThaves@aol.com
©2001 Thaves / Dist. by NEA, Inc.
www.frankandernest.com

THAVES 9-27

Why is daily physical activity generally advocated for all of us? What benefits accrue from this practice? How do athletes need to tailor their diets to support the vigorous physical activity typically performed? This chapter provides some answers.

FRANK & ERNEST Reprinted by permission of Newspaper Enterprise Association, Inc.

The Close Relationship Between Nutrition and Fitness

The ability to engage routinely in vigorous physical activity requires good health. The ability to perform also depends on a nutritious diet that supplies all the needed nutrients.

Once muscles have nutrients available to them, what determines the type of fuel muscles will use? Athletes do to an extent, depending on how physically fit the athletes are and how hard each one performs. This physical fitness—defined as the ability to do moderate to vigorous activity without undue fatigue—especially affects fat use by the body. The greater one's fitness, the more fat used to supply energy needed for activity, and even more so if the activity lasts for 20 minutes or more.

Beyond affecting fuel use, the benefits of regular physical activity include improvement in several aspects of heart function, less injury, better sleep habits, and improvement in body composition (less body fat, more muscle mass). Physical activity also can reduce stress and positively affect blood pressure, blood cholesterol, and blood glucose regulation. In addition, it aids in weight control, both by raising resting energy expenditure for a short period of time after exercise and by increasing overall energy expenditure. See Table 11.1 for a further look at the benefits of a physically active lifestyle.

Unfortunately, as noted in Chapter 10, many North American adults lead sedentary lives. Only about 15% of adults practice moderate to vigorous physical activity on a regular basis, and about half of all adults quit their exercise program within 3 months of onset. Does this discussion motivate you to assess your activity patterns and improve them as needed? The Nutrition Insight in this chapter will help you plan your exercise program.

Healthy People 2010 has set a number of specific objectives for adults related to physical activity:

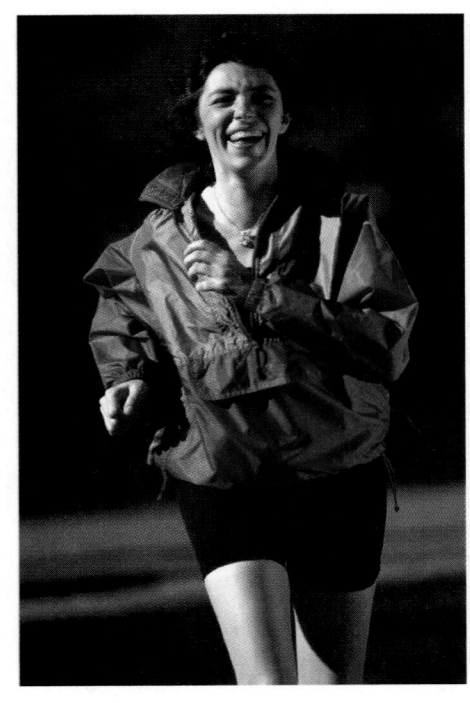

What is the best exercise? One you enjoy.

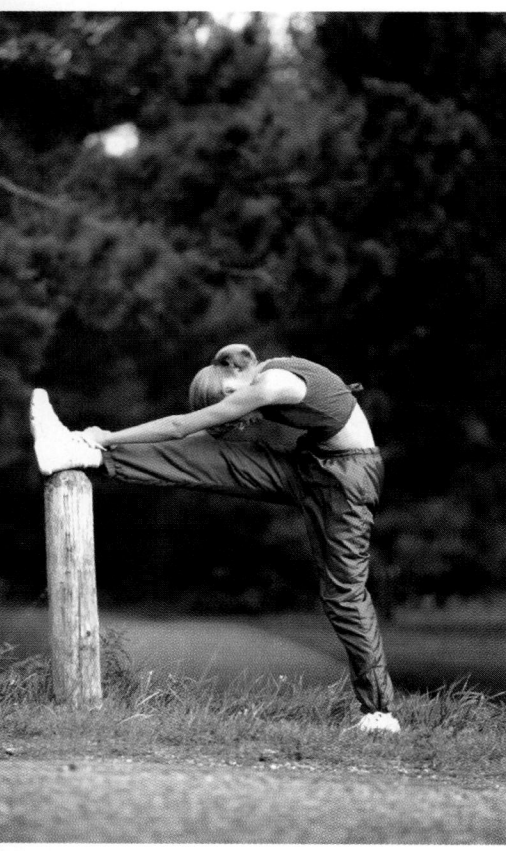

Stretching should be part of warm-up and cooldown activities.

Table 11.1 Exercise Is Medicine—the Benefits of Regular, Moderate Physical Activity

Cardiovascular health	Increases heart strength and overall cardiovascular function, which decreases chance of developing the many forms of cardiovascular disease, such as heart attacks and strokes Helps maintain healthy blood pressure Can increase HDL-cholesterol and lower LDL-cholesterol and triglycerides in the blood Aids in smoking-cessation programs
Obesity	Helps maintain lean tissue and promotes loss of fat tissue Assists in better control of appetite and increases energy expenditure Helps prevent or reverse development of diseases associated with obesity, including type 2 diabetes and various forms of cardiovascular disease, even if one can't attain a more healthy weight
Muscular health	Contributes to building and maintaining muscle mass and muscle tone
Diabetes	Increases glucose uptake by muscle tissue cells independent of insulin action Contributes to energy balance, which decreases risk of type 2 diabetes and related complications
Osteoporosis	Helps strengthen bones and contributes to joint health
Infections	Reduces susceptibility to respiratory and other infections by enhancing various functions of the immune system
Cancer	Reduces risk of colon cancer, and likely breast cancer
Gastrointestinal health	Improves peristaltic function in the small intestine and colon mass movements Lessens risk for gallstones and related gallbladder disease
Fewer injuries (e.g., from falls)	Contributes to balance and agility, especially in older adulthood
Psychological health	Reduces depression, anxiety, and mental stress while enhancing a sense of well-being and self-image and improving sleep patterns May also help treat chronic fatigue syndrome

Can you pass the U.S. military minimum fitness standards?

25-year-old males: 40 push-ups, 50 sit-ups, and 2 miles in 16:36

25-year-old females: 17 push-ups, 50 sit-ups, and 2 miles in 19:36

35-year-old males: 34 push-ups, 38 sit-ups, and 2 miles in 18:18

35-year-old females: 13 push-ups, 38 sit-ups, and 2 miles in 22:42

- Reduce by 50% the proportion of adults engaging in no leisure-time physical activity (currently 40% of adults)
- Double the proportion of adults engaging regularly, preferably daily, in moderate physical activity for at least 30 minutes per day (currently 15% of adults)
- Increase by 30% the proportion of adults engaging in vigorous physical activity that promotes the development and maintenance of cardiovascular and respiratory fitness 3 or more days per week for 20 or more minutes per occasion (currently 23% of adults)
- Increase by 50% the proportion of adults who perform physical activities that enhance and maintain muscular strength and endurance (currently 19% of adults)

To help yourself stay with an exercise program, experts recommend the following:

- Start slowly
- Vary your workouts; make it fun
- Work out with friends and others
- Set specific attainable goals and monitor progress
- Set aside a specific time each day for exercise; build it into your routine, but make it convenient
- Reward yourself for being successful in keeping up with your goals
- Don't worry about occasional setbacks; focus on the long-term benefits to your health

Designing a Fitness Program

For healthy people, a gradual increase to a goal of regular physical activity is recommended. Men 40 years of age or older and women 50 years of age or older who have been inactive for many years, or who have an existing health problem, should talk to a physician before increasing activity. Health problems that require medical evaluation before beginning an exercise program are obesity, cardiovascular disease (or family history of it), hypertension, diabetes (or family history), shortness of breath after mild exertion, and arthritis.

Phase 1: Getting Started Means Getting Going

During the first phase of a fitness program to promote health, you should begin to incorporate short periods of physical activity into the daily routine. This includes walking, some stair climbing, house cleaning, gardening, and other activities that cause you to "huff and puff" a bit. The goal is a total of 30 minutes of this moderate type of physical activity on most (and preferably all) days. If necessary, this can be broken up into increments lasting at least 10 minutes. Experts suggest starting small, building up to a total of 30 minutes of activity incorporated into each day's tasks. If there is not much time for activity, you can even go for more intensity in the activities over shorter periods to get the same benefits (Fig. 11.1).

The easiest way to increase physical activity is to make it part of a daily routine, similar to other regular activities, such as eating. You do not need to join a gym or attend aerobic classes. Daily activities can meet the Phase 1 goal. Many people find that the best time to exercise is when they need an energy pick-me-up or a break from work. Rather than abandoning an exercise program entirely when obstacles impede you, strive to use any small periods of available time, such as breaks between classes or "coffee breaks" at work. Once you reap the benefits of exercise, you will tend to spend more time at it.

Clearly, many of the activities recommended for Phase 1 are not very vigorous. By recommending Phase 1 for those starting an exercise program, fitness experts have not given up on the value of more vigorous physical activity. They're just making concessions to human nature. Still, most of the possible benefits from physical activity are seen if this Phase 1 goal is met.

Phase 2: Guidelines for Achieving and Maintaining Even Greater Physical Fitness

Once you can perform physical activity for 30 minutes per day, turn your attention to more specific activities, such as increasing muscle mass and strength, to reap even more benefits.

Warm-up

Stretch the whole torso for 5–10 minutes. Start with smaller muscle groups (arms) and work toward larger muscle groups (legs and abdomen).

Do 5–10 more minutes of low-intensity exercises, such as walking, slow jogging, or any slow version of anticipated activity. This warms up your muscles so that muscle filaments slide more easily over one another to increase range of motion and decrease the risk of injury.

Workout

Both daily aerobic activity and strength training two to three times per week are recommended.

Aerobic Activity

An aerobic workout prescription considers mode, duration, frequency, intensity, and progression.

Mode

The mode of exercise is the type of exercise prescribed. It must be one that uses large muscle groups in a rhythmic fashion, such as brisk walking, running, and cycling.

Duration

Duration is the amount of time spent in an exercise session. It should generally last at least 20–30 minutes, depending on intensity, not counting time for warm-up and cooldown. Ideally, this should be continuous (without stopping) exercise, but multiple 10-minute bouts with rest periods in between are also acceptable.

Frequency

The frequency of the exercise describes the number of times that the activity is performed. The frequency of exercise should be at least five times per week. Daily exercising will lead to even further benefits related to physical fitness.

Intensity

Intensity is defined as the level of exertion that indicates the degree of energy expenditure required to sustain the activity. In other words, intensity is used to describe how hard you are working and to what extent you can maintain that intensity over time. Health benefits are especially seen when you can achieve a moderate level of intensity of exercise.

There are a few ways to establish the intensity of exercise. One of the most popular, and simplest, methods is using a percentage of your age-predicted maximum heart rate. Subtract your age from 220 (this is considered your maximal heart rate), and then multiply by 70% and 85%. The heart rate range that results is sometimes called the *target zone*. When beginning, you should stay closer to the lower end of this range to achieve the appropriate duration—then work up from there. Taking a pulse reading during exercise is easy (stop and count your pulse for 10 seconds and then multiply that number by 6 to determine your heart rate for 1 minute). There are also watches available that contain heart rate monitors.

Another way of determining the intensity of exercise is the Rating of Perceived Exertion Scale (RPE). One version includes a range of 1–10, with each number corresponding to a subjective feeling of exertion. For example, the number 0 is "nothing at all" (sitting at a table) and the number 10 is considered close to maximal effort or very, very strong (all-out sprint).

continued

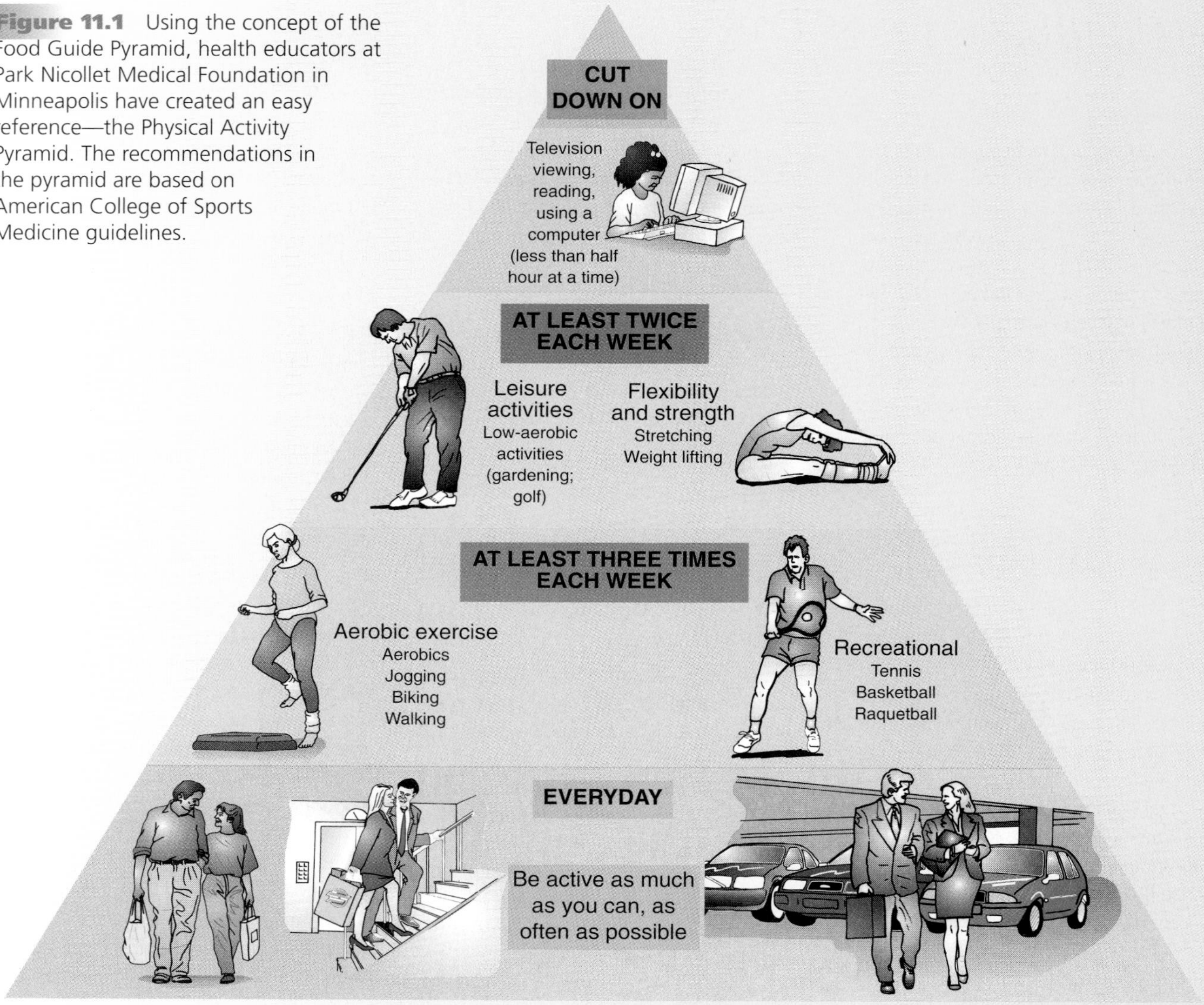

Figure 11.1 Using the concept of the Food Guide Pyramid, health educators at Park Nicollet Medical Foundation in Minneapolis have created an easy reference—the Physical Activity Pyramid. The recommendations in the pyramid are based on American College of Sports Medicine guidelines.

CUT DOWN ON

Television viewing, reading, using a computer (less than half hour at a time)

AT LEAST TWICE EACH WEEK

Leisure activities
Low-aerobic activities (gardening; golf)

Flexibility and strength
Stretching
Weight lifting

AT LEAST THREE TIMES EACH WEEK

Aerobic exercise
Aerobics
Jogging
Biking
Walking

Recreational
Tennis
Basketball
Raquetball

EVERYDAY

Be active as much as you can, as often as possible

When using the RPE scale, the goal is to aim for the number 4 to 6, which corresponds to "Somewhat strong." This is the point at which you begin to see significant fitness results. You should be working hard, but still be able to talk to an exercise partner (sometimes called the "talk test").

Progression

Progression, the final component, describes how the frequency, intensity, and duration of exercise have increased over a period of time. The first 3–6 weeks of your new exercise program are the initiation, or "getting started," phase. This phase corresponds to the time it takes for your body to adapt to the exercise program. The next 5 or 6 months of training are the improvement stage, in which the intensity and duration are increased to a point of tapering off. In other words, you notice no further appreciable gains in fitness. This plateau marks the beginning of your maintenance stage, when you evaluate your goals, but need make no changes to your exercise program in order to maintain the gains already achieved.

Strength Training

Strength training should be done at least 2, and preferably 3, days per week. It is recommended that a group of 8–10 exercises be performed in a circuit (all in

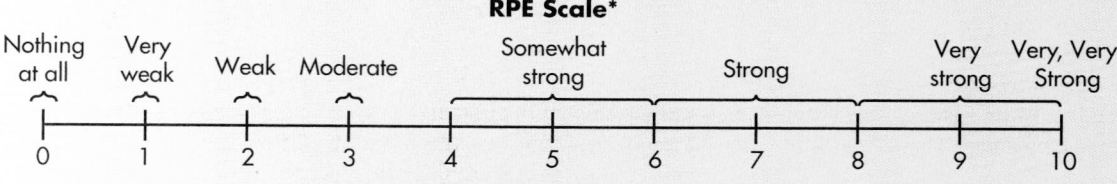

RPE Scale*

Nothing at all	Very weak	Weak	Moderate		Somewhat strong		Strong		Very strong	Very, Very Strong
0	1	2	3	4	5	6	7	8	9	10

* Perceived exertion beyond 10 is considered maximal

one exercise session) to condition major muscle groups of the upper body and lower body. When selecting the proper weight to use, make sure that the weight allows you to perform one (or more) set(s) of at least 8 repetitions, but no more than 12. (However, 10 to 15 repetitions is fine for older adults using lighter weights.) Proper form when doing these exercises is also important. Generally, if more than 12 repetitions can be performed with relative ease, the weight can then be increased in moderate increments.

Cooldown

Follow a reverse pattern of warm-up: 5–10 minutes of low-intensity activity and 5–10 minutes of stretching. The same exercises performed during warm-up are appropriate. The cooldown is essential to the prevention of injury and soreness.

Following these Phase 2 guidelines will aid in the development of an individualized exercise prescription that will safely optimize your efforts in achieving health, fitness, and wellness goals and improve your overall quality of life.

Including several types of enjoyable physical activities in a fitness program may also be helpful. For example, jogging one day might be followed by swimming the next day. Adding variety to a program not only keeps you mentally fresh but also strengthens different muscle groups and reduces risk of injury. This also keeps the program interesting. An exercise partner may offer additional motivation.

Vigorous programs for overweight people should be non-weight-bearing activities, such as swimming, water aerobics, and bicycling. Note also that even if weight loss is not possible, overweight people still benefit from regular physical activity.

Whatever physical activities you choose to include in your fitness program, they should be enjoyable and done regularly and willingly. This way they can become routine. Consider convenience, cost, and options for bad weather so that when motivation wanes, you are not adding further obstacles. Overall, do what you enjoy, but start out small, committing to keep on track and maintaining reasonable expectations. Positive results may take a month or so to be noticeable.

Realize also that harmful side effects may accompany excessive physical activity. The list of complications includes an increased risk of muscular-skeletal injuries, heat illness, sudden (heart-related) death, respiratory infections, GI tract problems, and disturbances in mood and sleeping habits, not to mention impaired performance. These complications are most common in competitive runners, swimmers, and cyclists. Still, although prolonged vigorous exercise poses some health risks, far greater risks exist for those who are and remain primarily sedentary.

Another Bite

*C*onsider applying the dietary principles of variety, balance, and moderation to your exercise plan:

- Variety: Enjoy many different activities to exercise different muscles.
- Balance: Different activities have different benefits, so balance your exercise pattern. For overall fitness, you need exercises that build cardiovascular endurance, muscular strength, and flexibility.
- Moderation: Exercise to keep fit without overdoing it. You don't need a heavy workout every day to achieve fitness.

Concept Check

*R*egular physical activity is a vital part of a healthy lifestyle, ideally constituting a total of at least 30 minutes of aerobic activity on most (or all) days. Including some strength training and daily stretching activities adds further benefits. People over age 40 years (men) to 50 years (women) should first discuss plans with a physician. Physically active people show lower risks of cardiovascular disease, type 2 diabetes, obesity, and other common chronic diseases.

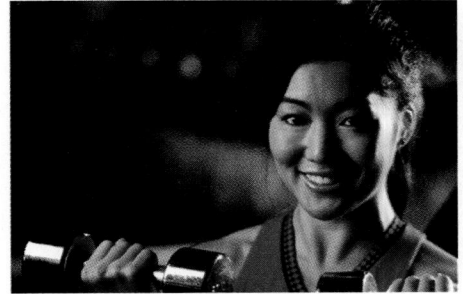

Resistance activities complement aerobic activities and regular stretching exercises, rounding out a total fitness plan.

Energy Sources for Muscle Use

To allow for the many benefits of locomotion, muscle cells need a specific form of energy for contraction. These and other cells can't directly use the energy released from breaking down glucose or triglycerides. Rather, to utilize the energy in foods, body cells must first convert the energy to a specific form called **adenosine triphosphate (ATP)**.

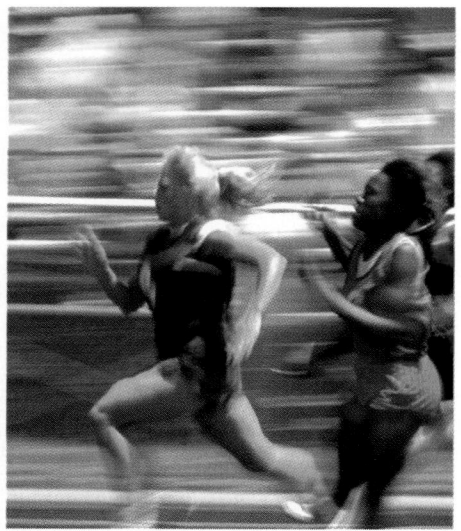

Bursts of muscle activity use a variety of energy sources, including PCr and ATP.

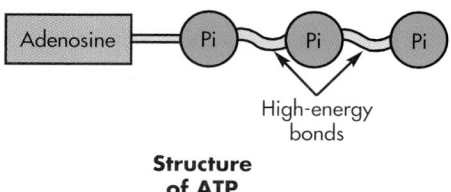

High-energy bonds

Structure of ATP

adenosine triphosphate (ATP) The main energy currency for cells. ATP energy is used to promote ion pumping, enzyme activity, and muscular contraction.

adenosine diphosphate (ADP) A breakdown product of ATP. ADP is synthesized into ATP using energy from foodstuffs and a phosphate group (abbreviated Pi).

phosphocreatine (PCr) A high-energy compound that can be used to re-form ATP. It is used primarily during bursts of activity, such as lifting and jumping.

*S*trength-training athletes have begun to use creatine supplements (see the Nutrition Issue at the end of this chapter for details).

Table 11.2 Energy Sources Used by Resting and Working Muscle Cells

Source/System*	When in Use	Examples of an Exercise
ATP	At all times	All types
Phosphocreatine (PCr)	All exercise initially; extreme exercise thereafter	Shotput, high jump
Carbohydrate (anaerobic)	High-intensity exercise, especially lasting 30 seconds to 2 minutes	200-yard (about 200 meters) sprint
Carbohydrate (aerobic)	Exercise lasting 2 minutes to 3 hours or more; the higher the intensity (for example, running a 6-minute mile), the greater the use	Basketball, swimming, jogging
Fat (aerobic)	Exercise lasting more than a few minutes; greater amounts are used at lower exercise intensities	Long-distance running, long-distance cycling; much of the fuel used in a 30-minute brisk walk is fat
Protein (aerobic)	Low amount during all exercise; slightly more in endurance exercise, especially when carbohydrate fuel is lacking	Long-distance running

*Note that at any given time, more than one system is operating.

Cells make ATP from its breakdown product **adenosine diphosphate (ADP)** and a phosphate group (abbreviated Pi). Again, the cells are using the energy obtained from foodstuffs. Conversely, to release energy from APT, cells partially break down ATP to ADP and Pi. This releases usable energy for cell functions.

$$\text{ADP} + \text{Energy from food} + \text{Pi} \rightarrow \text{ATP}$$
$$\text{ATP} \rightarrow \text{Energy to do work} + \text{ADP} + \text{Pi}$$

Essentially, ATP is the immediate source of energy for body functions (Table 11.2). The primary goal in the use of any fuel, whether carbohydrate, fat, or protein, is to make ATP. A resting muscle cell contains only a small amount of ATP that can be used. If no resupply of ATP were possible, this amount of ATP could keep the muscle working maximally for only about 2 to 4 seconds. Fortunately, another type of high-energy compound—**phosphocreatine (PCr)**—can be broken down to release enough energy to make more ATP. This helps resupply ATP until use of carbohydrate and fat fuels begins in earnest. Overall, cells must constantly and repeatedly use and then re-form ATP, using a variety of energy sources.

■ Phosphocreatine Is the First Line of Defense for Resupplying ATP in Muscles

As soon as the muscle ATP begins to be used, another source of ATP begins to be produced in the muscle. This ATP comes from PCr. An enzyme in the muscle cell is activated to split PCr. This releases energy that can be used to re-form ATP from its breakdown products. If no other source of energy for ATP re-supply were available, PCr could probably maintain maximal muscle contractions for about 10 seconds. Because other ATP resupply sources kick in, however, PCr ends up a source of energy for all events lasting about 1 minute or less.

$$\text{PCr} + \text{ADP} \rightarrow \text{ATP} + \text{Cr}$$

The main advantage of PCr is that it can be activated instantly and can replenish ATP at rates fast enough to meet the energy demands of the fastest and most powerful actions, including jumping, lifting, throwing, and sprinting. The disadvantage of PCr is that not much of it is made and stored in the muscles.

■ Carbohydrate Fuel for Muscles

Carbohydrates are an important fuel for muscles. The most useful form of carbohydrate fuel is the simple sugar glucose, available to all cells from the bloodstream. The breakdown of liver glycogen (a storage form of glucose) helps maintain blood glucose. Breakdown of glycogen stored in a specific muscle also helps meet the carbohydrate demand of that muscle, but the actual amount of glycogen stored is limited (more on this in a later section on aerobic glucose breakdown).

When glucose is used to make ATP, two metabolic processes can be used depending on the availability of oxygen. When oxygen supply in the muscle is limited (anaerobic conditions), such as when the exercise is intense (for example, running 400 meters or swimming 100 meters), a three-carbon compound called **pyruvic acid** accumulates in the muscle and is converted to **lactic acid.** About 5% of the energy capable of forming ATP has been extracted at this point.

If plenty of oxygen is available in the muscle (aerobic condition), such as when the exercise is of moderate to low intensity (for example, jogging or distance swimming), the bulk of the three-carbon pyruvic acid is shuttled to the mitochondria of the cell, where it is further metabolized into carbon dioxide (CO_2) and water (H_2O) (Fig. 11.2). This aerobic stage of glucose breakdown yields approximately 95% of the ATP made from complete glucose metabolism to carbon dioxide and water.

pyruvic acid A three-carbon compound formed during glucose metabolism; also called pyruvate.

lactic acid A three-carbon acid formed during anaerobic cell metabolism; a partial breakdown product of glucose; also called lactate.

glucose (6 carbons)

2 ATP for cell use

2 three-carbon compounds (pyruvic acid)

anaerobic

aerobic

about 28 to 30 ATP for cell use

lactic acid

$CO_2 + H_2O$

Anaerobic Glucose Breakdown Yields Energy Fast

The advantage of anaerobic glucose breakdown is that it is the fastest way to resupply ATP, other than PCr breakdown. This provides most of the energy for events ranging from about 30 seconds to 2 minutes. The two major disadvantages of the anaerobic process are that (1) the high rate of ATP production cannot be sustained for long events and (2) the rapid accumulation of lactic acid greatly increases the acidity of the muscle. This acid inhibits the activities of key enzymes in the muscle cells, slowing anaerobic ATP production and causing short-term fatigue. We learn by trial-and-error a pace for these events that controls muscle lactate concentrations.

For the most part, lactic acid accumulates in active muscle cells until it is released into the bloodstream. The liver picks up the lactic acid and resynthesizes it into glucose. Glucose can then reenter the bloodstream, where it is available for cell uptake and breakdown. The heart can also use the lactic acid directly for its energy needs, as can less active muscle cells situated near active ones.

Aerobic Glucose Breakdown Yields Energy More Slowly But Does Not Produce Lactic Acid

Aerobic glucose breakdown supplies ATP more slowly than does the anaerobic process, but it releases more energy. Furthermore, the slower rate of aerobic energy supply can be sustained for hours. Moreover, the end products are carbon dioxide and

As people start exercising regularly four or five times a week, they experience a "training effect." Initially these people might be able to exercise for 20 minutes before tiring. Months later, exercise can be extended to an hour before they feel tired. During the months of training, muscle cells have produced more mitochondria and can burn more fat. Training also increases the number of capillaries in muscles. This increases oxygen supply to muscles. As a result, lactic acid production from glucose metabolism decreases. Because it contributes to short-term muscle fatigue, the less lactic acid produced, the longer the exercise can continue. Part of the training effect derives also from the increased aerobic efficiency of heart and muscle action and increased muscle triglyceride content, as well as increased use of that fuel for energy needs.

Figure 11.2 Simplified view of ATP formation from carbohydrate, fat, and protein in muscles. All three nutrients may be used to form ATP, but glucose and fatty acids are the major sources for oxygen-requiring (aerobic) metabolism. Glucose may be used to produce small amounts of ATP under oxygen-free (anaerobic) conditions, thus providing us with the ability to produce energy rapidly without oxygen for relatively short periods. Lactic acid is a by-product. Note that blood glucose is not an important source of energy during exercise for muscles, but it is important for the brain and certain other body cells. [Any lactic acid produced in a muscle cell is eventually transported out of the muscle cell. The lactic acid can then be used for energy by nearby muscle cells.] In addition, heart tissue can use the lactic acid once it is transported to the bloodstream. The lactic acid can also be transformed back to glucose by the liver once it is transported to the bloodstream.

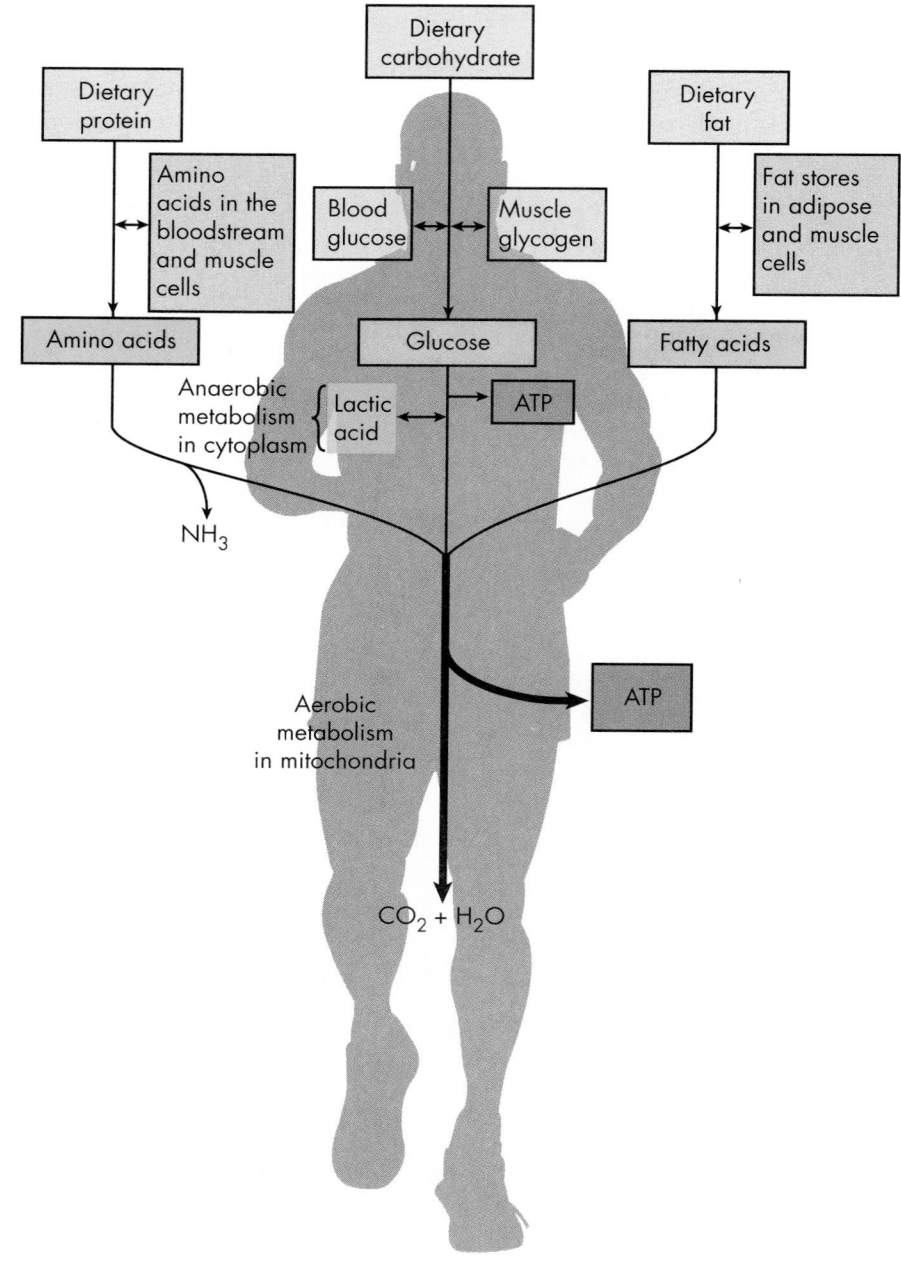

Critical Thinking

Marty started going to the gym about 8 weeks ago. At first, he noticed that he began "huffing and puffing" about 7 minutes into his aerobic workout. Now, however, he can work out for about 25 minutes without tiring. What is a possible explanation for this ability to work out longer?

water, not lactic acid. Aerobic glucose breakdown makes a major energy contribution to activities that last anywhere from 2 minutes to 3 hours or more (review Table 11.2).

Many researchers have studied various types of carbohydrate feedings to maximize glucose supply to muscles during prolonged exercise. Overall, the techniques have succeeded. Carbohydrate feedings of about 30 to 60 grams per hour during strenuous endurance exercise that lasts 1 hour or more, such as cycling, can aid in maintaining adequate blood glucose, resulting in delay of fatigue by 30 to 60 minutes. A later section on sports drinks discusses this in more detail. This attention to carbohydrate intake also helps one tolerate vigorous training on a daily basis.

Without the maintenance of blood glucose in such endurance activities, there is a decline in mental function associated with low blood glucose (cyclists call this mental decline "bonking"). Note that the fall in blood glucose is related to depletion of liver glycogen, not muscle glycogen.

Carbohydrate intake during exercise is not as important for the muscles in shorter events (e.g., one-half hour or so) because the muscles do not take up much blood glucose during short-term exercise, relying instead primarily on their glycogen stores for carbohydrate fuel. This is because the action of the hormone insulin to increase glucose uptake by muscles is blunted by other hormones, such as epinephrine and glucagon, that increase initially during exercise.

■ Fat: The Main Fuel for Prolonged Low-Intensity Activity

When fat stores in body tissues are broken down for energy, one triglyceride first yields three fatty acids and a glycerol. The majority of the stored energy is found in the fatty acids. During physical activity, the fatty acids are released from various adipose tissue depots into the bloodstream and travel to the muscles, where they are taken into each cell and broken down aerobically to carbon dioxide and water. Some of the fat stored in muscles also is used.

The rate at which muscles ultimately use fatty acids partly depends on the concentration of fatty acids in the bloodstream. In other words, the more fatty acids that are released from adipose tissue stores into the bloodstream, the more fat will be used by the muscles. Recently, some cyclists and other endurance athletes have attempted to raise their blood concentrations of fatty acids by consuming caffeinated beverages. This practice can actually increase fatty acid release from the adipose tissue depots and is therefore helpful to certain athletes, but it is illegal under International Olympic rules if the amount of caffeine in the body exceeds the equivalent of 6 to 8 cups of coffee (see the Nutrition Issue at the end of the chapter).

Fat, as a general muscle fuel, is ultimately not a very useful fuel for intense, brief exercise, but it becomes a progressively more important energy source as duration increases, especially when exercise remains at a low or moderate (aerobic) rate for more than 20 minutes (Fig. 11.3). The reason for this is that some of the steps involved in fat breakdown simply cannot occur fast enough to meet the ATP demands of short-duration, high-intensity exercise. If fat were the only available fuel, we would be unable to exercise beyond a fast walk or jog.

The advantage of fat fuel is that it provides tremendous stores of energy in a relatively concentrated form, and we generally have a lot stored. For a given weight of fuel, fat supplies more than twice as much energy as supplied by carbohydrate. For very lengthy activities at a moderate pace (for example, hiking) or even sitting at a desk for 8 hours a day, fat supplies about 70% to 90% of the energy required. Carbohydrate use is much less. As intensity increases, such as in a 3-hour marathon run at a competitive pace, muscles use about a 50:50 ratio of fat to carbohydrate. In comparison, for short events, such as a 100-meter sprint or even a 1500-meter race, the contribution of fat used to resupply ATP is minimal. Keep in mind that the only fast-paced (anaerobic) fuel we eat is carbohydrate; slow and steady (aerobic) activity uses much fat in addition to carbohydrate.

■ Protein: A Minor Fuel Source, Primarily for Endurance Exercise

Although amino acids derived from protein are used to fuel muscles, their contribution is relatively small, compared with that of carbohydrate and fat. As a rough guide, only about 5% of the body's general energy needs, as well as the typical energy needs of exercising muscles, is supplied by the metabolism of amino acids.

However, proteins can contribute significantly to energy needs in endurance exercise, perhaps as much as 10% to 15%, especially as glycogen stores in the muscle are exhausted. Most of the energy supplied from protein comes from metabolism of the branched-chain amino acids—leucine, isoleucine, and valine. Because a normal diet provides enough protein to supply this amount of fuel, protein supplements or amino acid supplements are not needed. Contrary to what many athletes believe, protein is used for fuel less in resistance types of exercise (e.g., weightlifting) compared

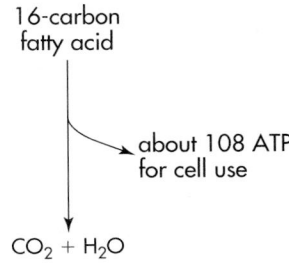

16-carbon fatty acid

about 108 ATP for cell use

$CO_2 + H_2O$

The fatty acids can come from all over the body, not necessarily from depots near the active muscles. This is why spot reducing does not work. Exercise can tone the muscles underlying adipose tissue but does not preferentially use those stores. If this was not the case, we would all have lean cheeks and necks, because muscles in that vicinity are regularly used!

Figure 11.3 Rough estimates of fuel use during various forms of physical activity. With regard to the weightlifting session, carbohydrate use could be somewhat greater if the session is intense and fast-paced.

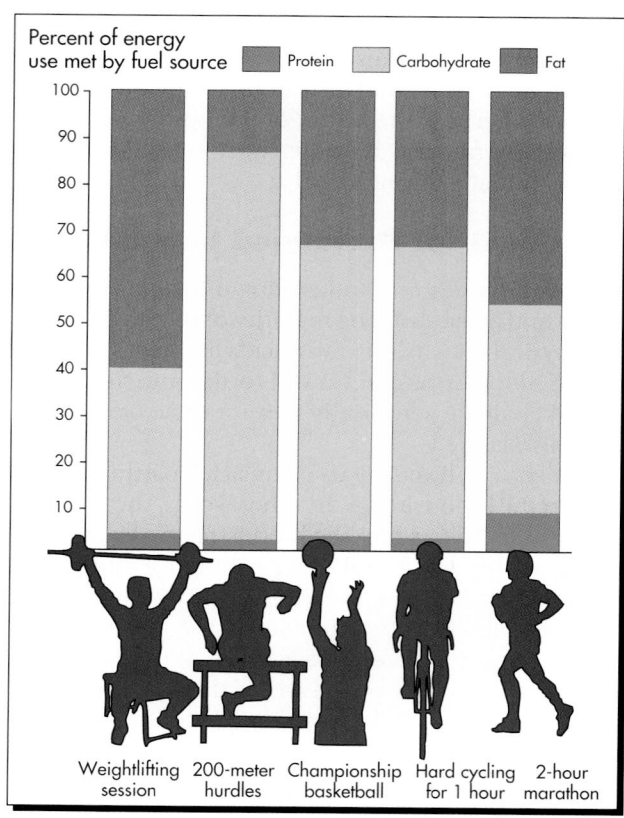

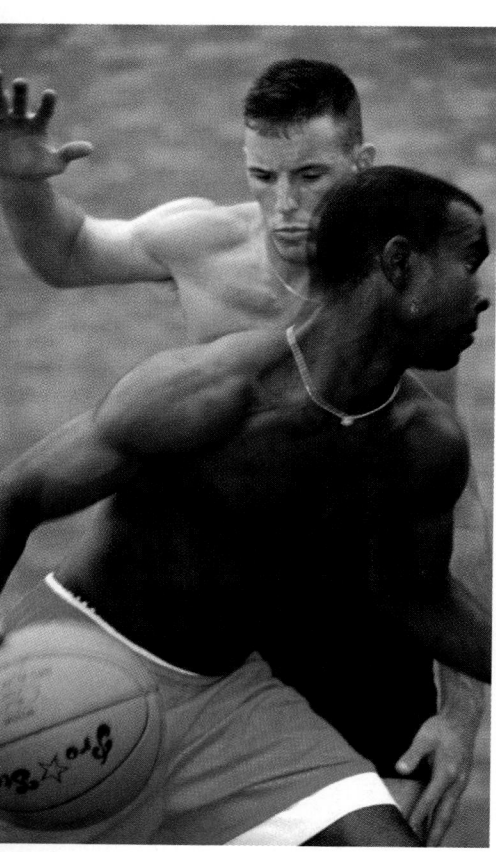

The energy to perform comes from carbohydrate, fat, and protein. The relative mix depends on the pace.

to endurance exercise (e.g., running) (review Fig. 11.3). The primary muscle fuels for weightlifting are phosphocreatine (PCr) and carbohydrate, with fat providing comparably less energy and little use of protein. Despite this fact, high-protein products such as Pro-Complex, Amino Fuel 2000, High Voltage Protein Drink, and Instant Egg Protein are marketed in nearly every health-food and fitness store, specifically for weightlifters and bodybuilders. Note also that consuming high-carbohydrate, moderate-protein foods immediately after a weight-training workout enhances the anabolic effect of the activity, most likely by increasing the concentrations of insulin and growth hormone released into the blood and contributing to protein synthesis.

Concept Check

Adenosine triphosphate (ATP) is the main form of energy used by cells. Cells use food energy to form ATP. Phosphocreatine (PCr) can rapidly re-form ATP from its breakdown product adenosine diphosphate (ADP), but PCr supplies are limited. Carbohydrate metabolism to form ATP begins as glucose becomes available from the bloodstream or glycogen breakdown. In a muscle cell, each glucose molecule is broken down through a series of steps to yield either lactic acid or carbon dioxide (CO_2) plus water (H_2O). The process that occurs when glucose is broken down into carbon dioxide and water is called *aerobic* because oxygen is used. The conversion of glucose to lactic acid is called *anaerobic* because no oxygen is used. This latter process allows the cell to quickly re-form ATP and supports the demand for energy during intense exercise. Fat is a key aerobic fuel for muscle cells, especially at low exercise outputs. At rest and light activity, muscles burn primarily fat for energy needs. In comparison, little protein generally is used to fuel muscles. Protein supplies at most 10% to 15% of energy needs during endurance activities, especially when glycogen stores are depleted.

Still, it is impossible to increase muscle mass by simply eating protein. Putting physical strain on muscle through strength training or other physical activity is needed.

Power Food: Dietary Advice for Athletes

Athletic training and genetic makeup are two very important determinants of athletic performance. A good diet won't substitute for either factor, but diet can further enhance and maximize an athlete's potential. More important, a poor diet can certainly harm performance.

■ Energy Needs

Athletes need varying amounts of food energy, depending on each athlete's body size and current body composition and on the type of training or competition being considered. A small person may need only 1700 kcal daily to sustain normal daily activities without losing body weight; a large, muscular man may need 4000 kcal. These rough estimates can be viewed as starting points that need to be individualized by trial and error for each athlete.

The energy required for sports training or competition has to be added to the energy needed just to carry on normal activities. Energy use averages 5 to 8 kcal per minute for moderate activity; again, this is just an estimate. For example, an hour of bowling requires little energy in addition to that required to sustain normal daily living. At the other extreme, a 12-hour endurance bicycle race over mountains can require an additional 4000 kcal per day. Therefore, some athletes may need as much as 7000 kcal or more daily just to maintain body weight while training, whereas others may need 1700 kcal or less. If an athlete experiences daily fatigue, the first consideration should be if he or she is consuming enough food. Up to six meals per day may be needed, including one before each workout.

How can we know if an athlete is getting enough energy from food? Estimating daily intake from a food diary by the athlete is one way. Another step is to estimate the athlete's body fat percentage by measuring skinfold thicknesses, by using bioelectrical impedance, or by using the underwater weighing technique (see Chapter 10). Body fat should be the typical amount found for athletes in the specific sport practiced. This corresponds to 5% to 18% for most male athletes and 16% to 28% for most female athletes. Then one goes on to monitor body weight changes on a daily or weekly basis. If body weight starts to fall, food energy should be increased; if weight rises and it is because of increases in body fat, the athlete should eat less.

If the body composition test shows that an athlete has too much body fat, the athlete should lower food intake by about 200 to 500 kcal per day, while maintaining a regular exercise program, until the desirable fat percentage is achieved. Reducing fat intake is the best nutrient-related approach. On the other hand, if an athlete needs to gain weight, increasing food intake by 500 to 700 kcal per day will eventually lead to the needed weight gain. A mix of carbohydrate, fat, and protein is advised, coupled with exercise to make sure this gain is mostly from lean tissue, and not mostly added fat stores.

Wrestlers, boxers, judoists, jockeys, and oarsmen often try to lose weight, so that they can be certified to compete in a lower weight class. This helps them gain a mechanical advantage over an opponent of smaller stature. They usually lose this weight before stepping on the scale for weight certification. Athletes can lose up to 22 pounds (10 kilograms) of body water in 1 day by sitting in a sauna, exercising in a plastic sweat suit, or taking diuretic drugs, which speed water loss from the kidneys. Losing as little as 2% to 3% of body weight by dehydration can adversely affect endurance performance. A pattern of repeated weight loss or gain of more than 5% of body weight by dehydration carries some risk of kidney malfunction and heat-related illness. Death is also a possibility, as was seen in three collegiate wrestlers in late 1997.

As noted in Chapter 1, "energy" bars are becoming popular, especially with athletes. A wide variety of bars is on the market, some with a mixture of protein, carbohydrate, and fat, whereas others are mostly protein. Choosing a bar with about 40 grams of carbohydrate and no more than 10 grams of protein, 4 grams of fat, and 5 grams of fiber is recommended. The bars are typically fortified with vitamins and minerals, often to 100% of the Daily Values. Overall these can be seen as a convenient, although somewhat expensive, source of nutrients. The need for a high-protein bar is especially questionable (see the Nutrition Issue at the end of this chapter).

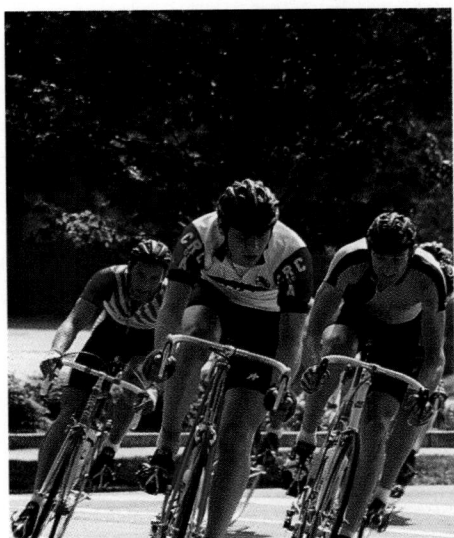

Athletes often expend much energy. In such cases, their resulting food intake should easily provide ample protein and other nutrients to support activity.

To prevent such deaths in the future, the National Collegiate Athletic Association has begun requiring that a minimum safe weight be set by a physician or an athletic trainer for each wrestler at the start of the season. Several states also have adopted this practice. If athletes, such as wrestlers, wish to compete in a lower-body-weight class and have enough extra fat stores, they should begin a gradual, sustained reduction in food-energy intake long before the competitive season starts. In so doing, the athlete attains a healthier body composition (less fat) while avoiding the potentially harmful and certainly misery-creating effects of severe dehydration. Athletes who have no extra body fat should not attempt to compete at a lower-body-weight class. Coaches and trainers should be aware of the decreased performance and serious side effects of severe dehydration to wrestlers.

■ Carbohydrate Needs

Anyone who exercises vigorously, especially for more than 1 hour per day on a regular basis, needs to consume a diet that includes moderate to high amounts of carbohydrates. The diet should include a variety of foods, such as those recommended by the Food Guide Pyramid. Numerous servings of grains, starchy vegetables, and fruits provide enough carbohydrate to maintain adequate liver and muscle glycogen stores, especially for replacing glycogen losses from workouts on the previous day. Relatively low carbohydrate/high-protein diets, such as *The Zone Diet*, are not recommended (recall that Chapter 10 discussed the Zone Diet. The carbohydrate content of this diet is only 40% of calories, rather than 50% or more that is typically recommended for athletes).

Carbohydrate intake should be at least 5 grams per kilogram body weight. People engaged in aerobic training and endurance athletes (duration >60 minutes per day) may need as much as 6 to 10 grams per kilogram body weight. In other words, triathletes and marathoners should consider eating close to 500 to 600 grams of carbohydrates daily, and even more if necessary, to (1) prevent chronic fatigue and (2) load the muscles and liver with glycogen. This is especially important when performing multiple training bouts in a day, such as swim practices, or heavy training on successive days, as in cross-country running. Depletion of carbohydrate ranks just behind depletion of fluid and electrolytes as a major cause of fatigue. Table 11.3 shows sample menus, based on the Food Guide Pyramid, for diets providing food energy ranging from 1500 to 5000 kcal per day. In addition, the Exchange System described in Appendix C is a very useful tool for planning all types of diets, including high-carbohydrate diets for athletes.

Note that one does not have to give up any specific food when planning a high-carbohydrate diet. The focus is to include more high-carbohydrate foods and moderation with concentrated fat sources. Sports nutritionists emphasize the difference between a high-carbohydrate meal and a high-carbohydrate/high-fat meal. Before endurance events, such as marathons or triathlons, some athletes seek to increase their carbohydrate reserves by eating potato chips, French fries, banana cream pie, and pastries. Although such foods contain carbohydrate, they also contain a lot of fat. Better high-carbohydrate food choices include pasta, rice, potatoes, bread, fruit and fruit juices, and many breakfast cereals (check the label for carbohydrate content) (Fig. 11.4). Sport drinks appropriate for carbohydrate loading, such as GatorLode and UltraFuel, can also help. Consuming a moderate amount of dietary fiber during the final day of training is a good precaution to reduce the chances of bloating and intestinal gas during the next day's event.

As a general rule, athletes should obtain at least 60% of their total energy needs from carbohydrate, rather than the 50% typical of most North American diets, especially if exercise duration is expected to exceed 2 hours and total caloric intake is about 3000 kcal per day or less. Diets containing 4000 to 5000 kcal per day can be as low as 50% carbohydrate, as these will still provide sufficient carbohydrate (500–600 grams per day).

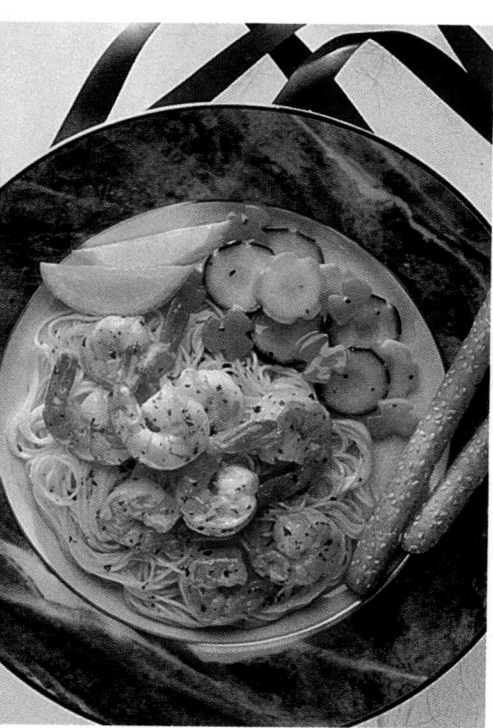

The athlete's plate should be about two-thirds grains and vegetables to provide ample carbohydrates.

Table 11.3 Sample Daily Menus Based on the Food Guide Pyramid That Provide Various Total Energy Intakes

1500 kcal Diet
Breakfast
Skim milk, 1 cup
Cheerios, ½ cup
Bagel, ½
Cherry jam, 2 tsp
Margarine, 1 tsp

Lunch
Chicken breast (roasted), 2 oz
Figs, 1
Skim milk, ½ cup
Banana, 1

Snack
Oatmeal-raisin cookie, 1
Low-fat fruit yogurt, 1 cup

Dinner
Spaghetti w/meatballs, 1 cup
Romaine lettuce, 1 cup
Italian dressing, 2 tsp
Green beans, ½ cup
Cranberry juice, 1½ cups

18% protein (68 grams)
64% carbohydrate (240 grams)
19% fat (32 grams)

2000 kcal Diet
Breakfast
Skim milk, 1 cup
Cheerios, 1 cup
Bagel, ½
Cherry jam, 1 tbsp
Margarine, 1 tsp

Lunch
Chicken breast (roasted), 2 oz
Wheat bread, 2 slices
Mayonnaise, 1 tsp
Raisins, ¼ cup
Cranberry juice, ½ cup
Banana, 1

Snack
Oatmeal-raisin cookies, 3
Low-fat fruit yogurt, 1 cup

Dinner
Broiled beef sirloin, 3 oz
Romaine lettuce, 1 cup
Italian dressing, 2 tsp
Green beans, 1 cup
Skim milk, ½ cups

17% protein (85 grams)
63% carbohydrate (315 grams)
20% fat (44 grams)

3000 kcal Diet
Breakfast
Skim milk, 1 cup
Cheerios, 2 cups
Bagel, 1
Cherry jam, 2 tbsp
Margarine, 1 tsp
Oat bran muffins, 2

Lunch
Chicken breast (roasted), 2 oz
Wheat bread, 2 slices
Provolone cheese, 1 oz
Mayonnaise, 1 tsp
Raisins, ½ cup
Cranberry juice, 1½ cups
Low-fat fruit yogurt, 1 cup

Snack
Banana, 1
Oatmeal-raisin cookies, 3

Dinner
Broiled beef sirloin, 3 oz
Romaine lettuce, 1 cup
Garbanzo beans, 1 cup
Italian dressing, 2 tsp
Spinach pasta noodles, 1½ cups
Margarine, 1 tsp
Green beans, 1 cup

Skim milk, ½ cups

17% protein (128 grams)
62% carbohydrate (465 grams)
21% fat (70 grams)

4000 kcal Diet
Breakfast
Orange, 1
Cheerios, 2 cups
Skim milk, 1 cup
Bran muffins, 2

Snack
Chopped dates, ¾ cup

Lunch
Romaine lettuce, 1 cup
Garbanzo beans, 1 cup
Grated carrots, ½ cup
French dressing, 2 tbsp
Macaroni and cheese, 3 cups
Apple juice, 1 cup

Snack
Wheat bread, 2 slices
Margarine, 1 tsp
Jam, 2 tbsp

Dinner
Skinless turkey breast, 2 oz
Mashed potatoes, 2 cups
Peas and onions, 1 cup
Banana, 1
Skim milk, 1 cup

Snack
Pasta, 1 cup cooked
Margarine, 2 tsp
Parmesan cheese, 2 tbsp
Cranberry juice, 1 cup

14% protein (140 grams)
61% carbohydrate (610 grams)
26% fat (116 grams)

5000 kcal Diet
Breakfast
Cheerios, 2 cups
Bran muffins, 2
Orange, 1
2% milk, 1 cup

Snack
Low-fat yogurt, 1 cup
Chopped dates, 1 cup

Lunch
Apple juice, 1 cup
Chicken enchilada, 1 cup
Romaine lettuce, 1 cup
Garbanzo beans, 1 cup
Shredded carrots, ¾ cup
Chopped celery, ½ cup
Seasoned croutons, 1 oz
French dressing, 2 tbsp
Wheat bread, 2 slices
Margarine, 1 tbsp

Snack
Banana, 1
Bagel, 1
Cream cheese, 1 tbsp

Dinner
2% milk, 1 cup
Beef sirloin, 5 oz
Mashed potatoes, 2 cups
Spinach pasta noodles, 1½ cups
Grated parmesan cheese, 2 tbsp
Green beans, 1 cup
Oatmeal-raisin cookies, 3

Snack
Cranbery juice, 1 cup
Air-popped popcorn, 4 cups
Raisins, ⅓ cup

14% protein (175 grams)
63% carbohydrate (813 grams)
24% fat (136 grams)

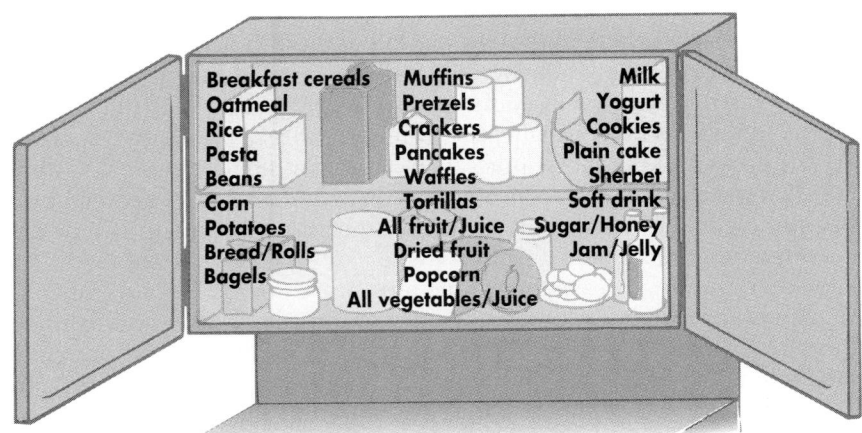

Breakfast cereals
Oatmeal
Rice
Pasta
Beans
Corn
Potatoes
Bread/Rolls
Bagels

Muffins
Pretzels
Crackers
Pancakes
Waffles
Tortillas
All fruit/Juice
Dried fruit
Popcorn
All vegetables/Juice

Milk
Yogurt
Cookies
Plain cake
Sherbet
Soft drink
Sugar/Honey
Jam/Jelly

Figure 11.4 Foods rich in carbohydrate are a key part of a training diet. Many typical foods are carbohydrate-rich. For the specific amount of carbohydrate in each food choice, see Appendix A.

When carbohydrate fuel (glycogen) in muscles is eventually used up, maintaining the high initial workload is difficult unless normal blood glucose concentrations are maintained by carbohydrate feedings. Athletes call this point of glycogen depletion "hitting the wall," because further exertion is hampered.

Appropriate Activities for Carbohydrate Loading

Marathons
Long-distance swimming
Cross-country skiing
30-kilometer runs
Triathlons
Tournament-play basketball
Soccer
Cycling time trials
Long-distance canoe racing

Inappropriate Activities for Carbohydrate Loading

American football games
10-kilometer or shorter runs
Walking and hiking
Most swimming events
Single basketball games
Weightlifting
Most track and field events

For athletes who compete in continuous, intense aerobic events lasting more than 60 to 90 minutes (or in shorter events repeated over a 24-hour period), undertaking a **carbohydrate-loading** regimen is often advantageous to maximizing muscle glycogen fuel. (Note, however, that this duration applies to few athletes.) One possible regimen includes a gradual reduction, or "tapering," of exercise intensity and duration, coupled with a gradual increase in dietary carbohydrate as a percentage of energy intake. The procedure can begin 6 days before competition, with the athlete completing a hard workout lasting about 60 minutes. Workouts for the next 4 days then last about 40, 40, 20, and 20 minutes, respectively, with exercise intensities being progressively reduced each day. On the final day before the competition, the athlete rests.

The dietary carbohydrate on the first 3 days of this regimen (about 450 grams per day) contributes 45% to 50% of energy intake. The carbohydrate contribution rises to 70% to 80% (about 400 to 700 grams per day depending on body weight) for the last 3 days before competition. This carbohydrate-loading technique usually increases muscle glycogen stores by 50% to 85% over typical conditions (that is, when dietary carbohydrate constitutes about 50% of the total energy intake). A typical carbohydrate-loading schedule looks like this:

Days Before Competition	6	5	4	3	2	1
Exercise time (minutes)	60	40	40	20	20	Rest
Carbohydrate (grams)	450	450	450	600	600	600

Total energy intake should also decrease as exercise time decreases.

A potential disadvantage of carbohydrate loading is that some water is incorporated in the muscles with the extra glycogen. Although it aids in maintaining hydration, in some individuals this additional water weight and related muscle stiffness are sufficient to detract from their sports performance, making carbohydrate loading inappropriate. Athletes considering carbohydrate loading should try it during training (and well before an important competition) to experience its effects on performance. They can then determine whether it is worth the effort. Note also that carbohydrate feeding during exercise provides about the same advantage as carbohydrate loading. In fact, the trend is currently toward this second method coupled with a daily diet high in carbohydrate.

▪ Fat Needs

A diet containing up to 30% of calories from fat is recommended for athletes. Rich sources of monounsaturated fat, such as canola oil, should be emphasized, and saturated fat and trans fat intake should be limited.

▪ Protein Needs

Looking at protein intake more specifically, typical recommendations for athletes range from 1.2 to 1.4 grams of protein per kilogram of body weight, considerably higher than the RDA of 0.8 grams per kilogram body weight for nonathletes (Table 11.4). Again, athletes engaged in endurance sports should aim for the higher value (1.4 gram per kilogram body weight), as protein supplies a greater percentage of the energy used (up to 15%) in these sports than in other athletic endeavors. Overall, the vast majority of athletes can meet protein needs without having to exceed twice the RDA. In addition, energy needs must be met or much of this protein will be diverted to fuel use instead of maintaining muscle tissue.

For athletes beginning a strength-training program, some experts recommend up to 1.7 to 2 grams of protein per kilogram of body weight. That is up to approximately 2½ times the RDA for protein. To date, the importance of such an excessive protein intake during the initial phases of strength training has not been supported by sufficient research. In addition, protein intakes above this amount simply result in an increased use of amino acids for energy needs; no further increase in muscle protein synthesis is

Table 11.4 Grams of Protein That Meet Recommendations for Individuals of Different Weights

Pounds	Kilograms	RDA (0.8 g/kg)	1.5 × RDA (1.2 g/kg)	2 × RDA (1.6 g/kg)
110	50	40	60	80
130	60	48	72	96
155	70	56	84	112
175	80	64	96	128
200	90	72	108	144
220	100	80	120	160

Compare these quantities with protein intake from the diets listed in Table 11.3. Note that diets supplying enough total energy for athletes yield plenty of protein, even for those who make no special attempt to consume high-protein foods.

seen. Note also that energy needs for strength training itself are not the reason for the high protein recommendation, as the fuel used in this activity is primarily fat and carbohydrate. The extra protein, theoretically, is required for the synthesis of new tissue brought on by the loading effect of strength training. Once the desired muscle mass is achieved, protein intake need not exceed twice the RDA.

Any athlete not specifically on a low-calorie regimen can easily have a protein intake twice or more of the RDA simply by eating a variety of foods (review Table 11.3). For example, a 123 pound (53-kilogram) woman can consume 82 grams of her upper range of 85 grams of protein (twice the RDA) by eating 4 ounces of chicken (one chicken breast), 3 ounces of beef (a small lean hamburger), and ½ cup of cooked beans and by drinking two glasses of milk during a single day. A 180-pound (77-kilogram) man needs to consume only 6 ounces of chicken (a large chicken breast), ½ cup of cooked beans, a 6-ounce can of tuna, and two glasses of milk a day to consume 122 grams of his upper range of 123 grams of protein (twice the RDA). And, for both athletes this does not even include the protein in the grains or vegetables they will also eat. In meeting their energy needs, many athletes consume even more protein. Thus, protein supplements are not needed despite marketing claims.

Athletes who either feel they must significantly limit their energy intake or are vegetarians should specifically determine how much protein they eat. They should make sure to follow a diet that provides at least 1.2 grams of protein per kilogram of body weight per day.

▪ Vitamin and Mineral Needs

Vitamin and mineral needs are the same or slightly higher for athletes, compared with those of sedentary adults. Still, because athletes usually have such high food-energy intakes, they tend to consume plenty of vitamins and minerals. An exception is athletes consuming low-calorie diets (about 1200 kcal or less), such as seen with some female athletes participating in events in which maintaining a low body weight is crucial. They may not be meeting B-vitamin and other micronutrient needs. Vegetarian athletes are also a concern. In these cases, consuming fortified foods, such as ready-to-eat breakfast cereals, or a balanced multivitamin and mineral supplement is recommended. Athletes' needs for vitamin E and vitamin C may be somewhat greater because of the antioxidant protection these nutrients provide; this effect could be especially important in the face of high oxygen use by muscles. Still, the use of megadoses of vitamin E and vitamin C requires more study and is not currently an accepted part of the dietary guidance for athletes. Experts first suggest following a diet containing foods rich in antioxidants, such as fruits, vegetables, whole grains, and vegetable oils. This diet is rich in vitamin C (200 milligrams per day is a reasonable target for athletes), but still does not supply the amount of vitamin E currently used in studies

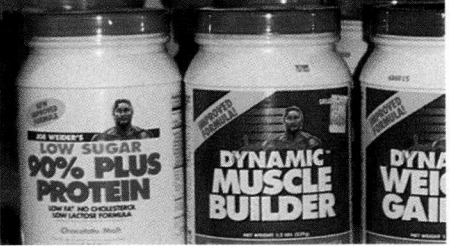

High-protein products, which are often marketed to athletes, are unnecessary. The same holds true for high-protein bars, a current trend in marketing products to athletes.

*C*onsuming excessive amounts of protein is not without its drawbacks. As noted in Chapter 6, it increases calcium loss in the urine. It also leads to increased urine production, possibly compromising body hydration. It also may lead to kidney stones in people with a history of such stones or other kidney problems.

of athletes (200 milligrams per day; about 400 IU per day). Adding this amount of vitamin E to a diet is generally safe; it provides no benefit to exercise performance but may offer some protection from exercise-induced muscle damage, especially for endurance athletes competing at high altitudes. Currently, however, the evidence regarding the importance of this practice is sketchy. For other nutrients, if supplements are used, intakes below the Upper Level set for each is a safe guide. (Still, iron may be one exception; see the Nutrition Insight in Chapter 8).

Iron Deficiency Impairs Performance

Athletes, especially female and adolescent athletes (if they experience heavy monthly menstrual flows or follow a low-calorie diet), vegetarians, and distance runners in general, should pay special attention to their iron intake. They are at risk of what is called *sports anemia*. Much of the anemia results because plasma volume in the blood expands to a greater extent than the red blood cells in response to training. Although an athlete has increased synthesis of red blood cells, this increase is diluted by an even larger plasma volume and, so, the red blood cell concentration falls. Iron deficiency may also be a cause. Iron status may be compromised by the loss of iron in sweat, urine, and gastrointestinal blood and by the increased use of iron required for the elevated production of red blood cells associated with physical fitness.

If iron status is low and not replenished, iron-deficiency anemia and markedly impaired endurance performance can eventually result. Although true anemia (noted as a depressed blood hemoglobin) is not that common among athletes, it is a good idea, especially for adult women athletes, to have their iron status checked about once a year and to monitor dietary iron intake.

Because iron deficiency can be caused by blood loss, it is important that physicians also investigate the cause of the deficiency. If caught early, some serious medical conditions can be treated or prevented. And, if blood iron is consistently low, the use of iron supplements by an athlete may be advisable. However, indiscriminate use of iron supplements is not advised because toxic effects are possible.

Some studies have suggested that iron deficiency without anemia may still have a negative effect on physical activity and performance. For this reason, athletes must be especially careful not to deplete iron stores.

Calcium Intake Deserves Attention, Especially in Women

Athletes, especially women trying to lose weight by restricting their intake of dairy products, can have marginal or low dietary intakes of calcium. This practice compromises optimal bone health. Of still greater concern are women athletes who have stopped menstruating because their arduous exercise training interferes with the normal secretion of the reproductive hormones. Disturbing reports show that female athletes who do not menstruate regularly have far less dense spinal bones than both nonathletes and female athletes who menstruate regularly. This places them at increased risk for osteoporosis in later life, a risk that outweighs the benefits of weight-bearing exercise on bone density. This is discussed further in Chapter 12, with respect to the Female Athlete Triad, and in Chapter 9, where osteoporosis was reviewed in detail.

Research has clearly documented the importance of regular menstruation to maintain bone mineral density. Current studies imply that a woman runner who does not menstruate regularly may also have a higher risk for the development of a **stress fracture.** Thus, female athletes whose menstrual cycles become irregular should consult a physician to ascertain the cause. Decreasing the amount of training or increasing energy intake and body weight often restores regular menstrual cycles. If irregular menstrual cycles persist, severe bone loss and osteoporosis can result. Extra calcium in the diet does not necessarily compensate for the effects of menstrual loss, but inadequate dietary calcium can make matters worse.

*A*t one time in his career, long-distance runner Alberto Salazar experienced problems sleeping and performed poorly because of low iron intake and related iron-deficiency anemia.

stress fracture A fracture that occurs from repeated jarring of a bone. Common sites include bones of the foot.

■ Fluid Needs

Water (fluid) needs for an average adult are about 1 milliliter per kcal expended, or about 8 cups per day. Athletes need this and generally even more water intake to maintain the body's ability to regulate internal temperature and to keep cool. Most energy released during metabolism appears immediately as heat. Furthermore, heat production in contracting muscles can rise 15 to 20 times above that of resting muscles. Unless this heat is quickly dissipated, heat exhaustion, heat cramps, and deadly heatstroke may ensue. In fact, typically three to five athletes die each year of heatstroke. In 2001, both college football players and a professional football player died in such a way.

Heat exhaustion occurs when heat stress causes loss of body fluid and then depletion of blood volume. As environmental temperature rises about 95°F (35°C), virtually all body heat is lost through the evaporation of sweat from the skin. Sweat rates during prolonged exercise range from 3 to 8 cups (750 to 2000 milliliters) per hour. However, as the humidity rises, especially when it rises about 75%, evaporation slows and sweating becomes inefficient. The result is rapid fatigue, increased work for the heart, and difficulty with prolonged exertion. Clearly, the combination of high heat and humidity (e.g., 95°F and 90% humidity) can be as dangerous for athletes as extreme cold.

Increased body temperature associated with dehydration is most evident when the amount of water loss exceeds 3% of body weight. This dehydration then leads to a decline in endurance, strength, and overall performance. Wearing football equipment in hot weather can lead to a loss of 2% of body weight in 30 minutes. Marathon runners have been shown to lose 6% to 10% of body weight during a race.

Common symptoms of heat exhaustion include profuse sweating, headache, dizziness, nausea, vomiting, muscle weakness, visual disturbances, and flushing of the skin. A person with heat exhaustion should be taken to a cool environment immediately, and excess clothing should be removed. The body should be sponged with tap water. Fluid replacement, as tolerated, then should suffice.

Heat cramps are a frequent complication of heat exhaustion, but they may appear alone, without other symptoms of dehydration. They usually occur in individuals exercising for several hours in a hot climate who have large sweat losses and have consumed a large volume of water. It is important not to confuse heat cramps with other forms of muscle cramps, such as those caused by gastrointestinal upset. Heat cramps occur in skeletal muscles, including those of the abdomen and the extremities. They consist of a contraction for 1 to 3 minutes at a time. The cramp moves down the muscle and is associated with excruciating pain. The best way to prevent heat cramps is to exercise moderately at first in the heat, and have an adequate salt intake, before engaging in long, strenuous exercise.

Heatstroke can occur when internal body temperature reaches 105°F or more. Related symptoms include nausea, confusion, irritability, poor coordination, seizures, and coma (in severe cases). Exertional heatstroke results from high blood flow to exercising muscles, which overloads the body's cooling capacity. Sweating generally ceases, and the body temperature may become dangerously high. If left untreated, circulatory collapse, nervous system damage, and death are likely. Death rate is high, approximately 10%.

Many individuals who suffer heatstroke faint, and their skin becomes hot and dry. Cooling the skin with ice packs or cold water is the usual recommended immediate treatment until medical help can be summoned. To decrease the risk of developing heatstroke, athletes should replace lost fluids, watch for rapid body-weight changes (2% to 3% or more of body weight), and avoid exercise under extremely hot, humid conditions.

Since dehydration during exercise sets the stage for heat exhaustion, heat cramps, and potentially fatal heatstroke, athletes must avoid becoming dehydrated. Fluid intake during exercise, when possible, should be adequate to minimize body-weight loss; this practice is a good idea even when sweating can go unnoticed, such as swimming or during the winter.

heat exhaustion The first stage of heat-related illness that occurs because of depletion of blood volume from fluid loss by the body. This increases body temperature and can lead to headache, dizziness, muscle weakness, and visual disturbances, among other effects.

heat cramps A frequent complication of heat exhaustion. They usually occur in people who have experienced large sweat losses from exercising for several hours in a hot climate and have consumed a large volume of water. The cramps occur in skeletal muscles and consist of contractions for 1 to 3 minutes at a time.

heatstroke Heatstroke can occur when internal body temperature reaches 105°F. Sweating generally ceases if left untreated, and blood circulation is greatly reduced. Nervous system damage may ensue, and death is likely. Often the skin of individuals who suffer heatstroke is hot and dry.

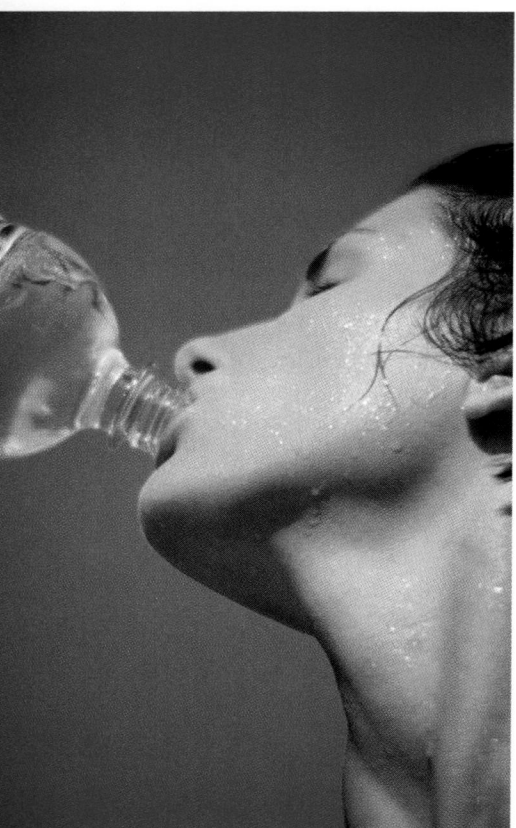

Fluid intake during physical activity is important.

*S*ports drinks containing glucose polymers (several glucose molecules chemically linked) or simple sugars (e.g., glucose, sucrose) have similar benefits for exercise if the carbohydrate concentration is between 6% and 10%. In addition, both types of sports drinks empty the stomach at similar times. Fructose is the exception, in that it takes longer to empty the stomach and may cause bloating or diarrhea when it is the primary sweetener in a product.

The recommended goal is a loss of no more than 3% of body weight during exercise. Athletes should first calculate 2% to 3% of their body weight and then by trial and error determine how much fluid they must take in to avoid losing more than this amount of weight during exercise. This determination will be most accurate if an athlete is weighed before and after a typical workout. For every 1 pound (½ kilogram) lost, 3 cups (0.75 liters) of water should be consumed during exercise or immediately afterward. Experts now recommend a total of 3 cups (0.75 liters) of water per pound lost, rather than the previous recommendation of 2 cups per pound, as some of the fluid replacement will quickly be lost via increased sweating after exercise and increased urine output. Much of this fluid replacement will have to take place after exercise since it is difficult to consume enough fluid during exercise to prevent weight loss. If weight change can't be monitored, urine color is another measure of hydration status. Urine color should be no more yellow than that of lemonade.

Thirst is not a reliable indicator of an athlete's need to replace fluid during exercise. An athlete who drinks only when thirsty is likely to take 48 hours to replenish fluid loss. After several days of training, an athlete relying on thirst as an indicator can build up a large enough fluid debt to impair performance. The following fluid replacement approach can meet athletes' fluid needs in most cases:

- Freely drink beverages (e.g., water, diluted fruit juice, sports drinks) during the 24-hour period before an event, even if not particularly thirsty.
- Drink 1½ to 2½ cups of fluid (400 to 600 milliliters) 2 to 3 hours before exercise. This allows time for both adequate hydration and excretion of excess fluid.
- During events lasting more than 30 minutes, consume about ½ to 1½ cup (150 to 350 milliliters) of fluid every 15 to 20 minutes beginning at the start of the exercise. Consuming more than 1 quart (1 liter) per hour can cause discomfort. On hot days, cold drinks are preferable to help cool the body. Again, the athlete should not wait until he or she feels thirsty. In many cases, athletes, especially children and teenagers, need to be reminded to do this.
- After exercise, about 3 cups of fluid should be consumed for every pound lost, as just mentioned. It is also important that weight be restored before the next exercise period. Skipping fluids before or during events will almost certainly cause problems.

A question that often arises is whether to drink water or a sports-type carbohydrate-electrolyte drink (e.g., All Sport, Exceed Energy Drink, Gatorade, PowerAde, and Amino Force) during competition (Fig. 11.5). For sports that require less than 60 minutes of exertion or when total weight loss is less than 5 to 6 pounds, the primary concern is replacing the water lost in sweat, because losses of carbohydrate stores and electrolytes (sodium, chloride, potassium, and other minerals) are not usually too great. Although electrolytes are lost in sweat, the quantities lost in exercise of brief to moderate duration can be easily replaced later by consuming normal foods, such as orange juice, potatoes, and tomato juice. Keep in mind that sweat is about 99% water and only 1% electrolytes and other substances.

Beyond 60 minutes of exertion, electrolyte (especially sodium) and carbohydrate replacement becomes increasingly important, and more so in hot weather. Use of a sports drink then is important to provide water for hydration, electrolytes both to enhance water and glucose absorption from the intestine and to help maintain blood volume, as well as carbohydrate to provide energy.

An advantage of sports drinks over water is that sports drinks taste better than water. This may help the athlete drink more often. In addition, the carbohydrate in these drinks quickly replaces carbohydrate used during practice or competition, and the sodium present aids in glucose uptake in the small intestine. Finally, the sodium content stimulates thirst, so athletes drink more. Thus, some experts prefer sport drinks over water for all athletes.

As mentioned before, optimum performance in endurance activities can be enhanced when carbohydrate is replaced throughout exercise as opposed to replacement only near the end of exercise. For this reason, it may be beneficial for endurance athletes to begin carbohydrate replacement using sports drinks or another convenient source early (see below for some ideas).

Overall, the decision to use a sports drink hinges primarily on the duration of the activity. As the projected duration of continuous activity approaches 60 minutes or longer, the advantages of the use of a sports drink over plain water clearly emerge. However, athletes should first experiment with the suggested protocol during practice, instead of trying it for the first time during competition.

As an alternative to the use of sports drinks for providing a source of carbohydrate during prolonged physical activity, some athletes have begun to use carbohydrate gels (e.g., PowerGel, GU, and ClifShot) and so-called energy bars (e.g., PowerBar). The amount to use can be calculated as follows. If one was to use 6 ounces of a sports drink every 15 minutes, this would provide 13 grams of carbohydrate, or a total of 52 grams after 1 hour. One can use gels or energy bars in order to provide the same amount of carbohydrate (check the label for carbohydrate content. Gels contain about 25 grams per serving.). Interestingly, one fig cookie also provides the 13 gram carbohydrate dose (Gummy Bears and jellybeans work as well). Note that any use of these alternate carbohydrate sources must be accompanied by water consumption. In this way, the goal of fluid *and* carbohydrate replacement from the sports drink will be realized. Another thing to consider when using gels and energy bars is that they are relatively expensive.

It is also possible to drink too much water. Ultra-endurance athletes compete at relatively low exercise intensities for prolonged periods of time and therefore may not sweat as much as one might predict. Thus, water losses are not very high. In addition, some of these athletes have used one-half strength Coca-Cola as their fluid-replacement beverage, which is relatively low in sodium, and they drink this at every rest stop. This combination leads to an eventual fall in blood sodium and chloride, which is not desirable. Drinking less fluid and choosing a sports drink containing sodium and chloride can help prevent this problem.

■ Meals Before Endurance Events Should Emphasize Carbohydrate

A light meal supplying up to about 1000 kcal should be eaten about 2 to 4 hours before an endurance event to top off muscle and liver glycogen stores, prevent hunger during the event, and provide extra fluid. The longer the period before an event, the larger the meal can be, as there will be more time available for digestion. A pre-event meal should consist primarily of carbohydrate (about 200 grams), have little fat or dietary fiber, and include a moderate amount of protein (Table 11.5). A pre-event meal eaten 1 to 2 hours before an event should be blended or liquid to promote rapid stomach emptying.

Good food choices for a pre-event meal include spaghetti, bagels, muffins, bread, bananas, apples, oranges, and breakfast cereals with low-fat or nonfat milk. Liquid meal-replacement formulas, such as Carnation Instant Breakfast, also can be used. Foods rich in dietary fiber should be eaten the previous day to help empty the colon

Figure 11.5 Sports drinks for fluid and electrolyte replacement typically contain a form of simple carbohydrate plus sodium and potassium. The various sugars in this product total 14 grams per 1 cup (240 milliliters) serving. In percentage terms based on weight, the sugar content is about 6% ([14 grams sugar per serving ÷ 240 grams per serving] × 100 = 5.8%). Sports drinks typically contain about 6% to 8% sugar. This provides ample glucose and other monosaccharides to aid in fueling working muscles, and it is well tolerated. Drinks with a sugar content above 10%, such as soft drinks or fruit juices, may cause stomach distress.

Alcohol and caffeine both have a dehydrating effect on the body, so fluids containing them should not be part of any hydration plan for exercise.

Table 11.5 Convenient Pre-event Meals

Breakfast

Cheerios, ¾ cup 2% milk, 1 cup Blueberry muffin, 1 Orange juice, 4 oz	450 kcal 82% carbohydrate (92 grams)
Low-fat fruit yogurt, 1 cup Plain bagel, ½ Apple juice, 4 oz Peanut butter (for bagel), 1 tbsp	482 kcal 68% carbohydrate (84 grams)
Whole-wheat toast, 1 slice Apple, 1 large 2% milk, 1 cup Oatmeal, ½ cup 2% milk, ½ cup	491 kcal 73% carbohydrate (94 grams)

Lunch or Dinner

Chili; with beans, 8 oz Baked potato with sour cream and chives Chocolate Frosty	900 kcal 65% carbohydrate (150 grams)
Spaghetti noodles, 2 cups Spaghetti sauce, 1 cup 2% milk, 1½ cups Green beans, 1 cup	761 kcal 66% carbohydrate (129 grams)
Orange, 1 large 2% milk, 1½ cups Chicken noodle soup, 1 cup Saltine crackers, 12 Buttered beans, 1 cup Corn, 1 cup Angel food cake, 1 slice	829 kcal 70% carbohydrate (160 grams)

With regard to the timing of preactivity meals, the rule of thumb is to allow 4 hours for a big meal (about 1200 kcal), 3 hours for a moderate meal (about 800–900 kcal), 2 hours for a light meal (about 400–600 kcal), and an hour or less for a snack (about 300 kcal).

Rule of Thumb for Approximate Pre-event Carbohydrate Intake (grams)

Hours Before	Grams per Kilogram Body Weight (70 kilogram person)
1	1 (70)
2	2 (140)
3	3 (210)
4	4 (280)

before an event, but they should not be eaten the night before or in the morning before the event. Foods to avoid are those that are fatty or fried, such as sausage, bacon, sauces, and gravies. A meal high in carbodydrate is quickly digested, promotes maintenance of blood glucose, and avoids the need to dip right away into glycogen stores.

The selection of carbohydrates for the pre-event meal (and postevent meal) based on their glycemic index is becoming increasingly popular among athletes (see Chapter 4 for a review of glycemic index and a table of values for specific foods). The rationale behind this practice is that the glycemic index of a carbohydrate is a major influence on the insulin response to that carbohydrate: high-glycemic-index carbohydrates generally cause high insulin responses, and low-glycemic-index carbohydrates result in lower insulin responses. You know, of course, from Chapter 4 that insulin is one of the hormones that regulates blood glucose.

An endurance athlete may wish to choose a low-glycemic-index food before an event in the attempt to achieve a moderate and sustained increase in blood glucose, which will lessen the insulin response (review Table 4.7). This decreased insulin response, in turn, may allow for greater access to the fatty acids from the adipose tissue as a fuel source, preserving glycogen stores for when they are needed late in the race.

In such a pre-event situation, a number of studies have examined the impact of the feeding of low-glycemic-index foods and high-glycemic-index foods 45 minutes to 1 hour prior to exercise. In general, these studies have shown a more favorable metabolic profile for endurance performance—lower blood insulin, higher blood free fatty acids, and more stable blood glucose—with low- versus high-glycemic-index pre-event meals. However, not all of these studies have shown improved endurance exercise performance with low-glycemic-index foods. Still, no detrimental effects have been observed, compared with higher-glycemic-index foods. If an athlete feels a pre-event meal harms performance, eating a high-carbohydrate diet the day and night before can help meet the same goal. The pre-event meal could then be moderate to low in carbohydrate content.

Another Bite

*I*t cannot be emphasized enough that any nutrition strategies should be tested during practice and trial runs before being used in a meet or key event. An athlete should never try a new food or beverage on the day of competition. Some food items and beverages may not be well tolerated, and the day of competition is not the time to find this out.

■ Carbohydrate Intake During Recovery from Prolonged Exercise

Carbohydrate-rich foods providing about 1 to 1.5 grams of carbohydrate per kilogram body weight should be consumed within 2 hours after extended (endurance) exercise, and the sooner the better. This is when glycogen synthesis is greatest, as the muscles are very insulin-sensitive at this point. This process should then be repeated over the next 2-hour interval. Athletes who are training hard can consume a simple sugar candy, sugared soft drink, fruit or fruit juice, or a sports-type carbohydrate supplement right after training as they attempt to reload their muscles with glycogen. Later, bread, mashed potatoes, and rice can contribute further carbohydrate. All of these high-glycemic-index carbohydrates especially contribute to glycogen synthesis. Adding some rich protein sources is also recommended, with carbohydrate to protein in a 3:1 ratio. For a 154-pound (70-kilogram) athlete, this corresponds to about 70 grams carbohydrate and 25 grams protein in each 2-hour interval (see Table 11.6 for sample meals of this composition). In summary, the following are key factors for achieving the most rapid replenishment of muscle glycogen after exercise: (1) availability of adequate carbohydrate, (2) ingestion of carbohydrate as soon as possible after completion of exercise, (3) selection of high-glycemic-index carbohydrates, (4) combination of carbohydrate and protein foods, rather than either carbohydrate or protein alone.

*F*or more information on sports nutrition, visit the Gatorade Sport Science Institute web page (www.gssiweb.com). For more information on sports medicine, visit www.physsportsmed.com. *This home page of* The Physician and Sportsmedicine *journal details current issues in sports medicine, including injury prevention, nutrition, and exercise. Also helpful are the web pages of the American College of Sports Medicine (www.acsm.org), Centers for Disease Control (www.cdc.gov/nccdphp/dnpa), and the American Council on Exercise (www.acefitness.org). A recent book that provides much practical information on sports nutrition is* Eat Smart, Play Hard *by Dr. Liz Applegate (Rodale, 2001).*

Table 11.6 Sample Postexercise Meals for Rapid Muscle Glycogen Replacement

Option 1

1 regular bagel
2 tbsp peanut butter, smooth
8 fl oz skim milk
1 medium banana
562 kcal, 77 grams carbohydrate, 23 grams protein, 18 grams fat

Option 2

1 packet Carnation Instant Breakfast
8 oz skim milk
1 medium banana
1 tbsp peanut butter
Blend until smooth
438 kcal, 70 grams carbohydrate, 17 grams protein, 10 grams fat

Option 3

1.5 cans GatorPro (11 fl oz per can)
559 kcal, 89 grams carbohydrate, 26 grams protein, 11 grams fat

Fluid and electrolyte (i.e., sodium and potassium) intake is also an essential component of an athlete's recovery diet. This helps replenish body fluids as quickly as possible. This is especially important if two workouts a day are followed and if the environment is hot and humid. If food and fluid intake is sufficient to restore weight loss, it generally will also supply enough electrolytes to meet needs during recovery from endurance activities.

Concept Check

All athletes would do well to plan a diet following the Food Guide Pyramid. High-carbohydrate foods should be emphasized, and these should dominate in pre-event meals. Protein intake above twice the RDA is not needed in most cases. Most athletes easily consume enough protein from typical food choices. If nutrient supplements are used, dosages generally should not exceed the Upper Level set for each nutrient. Fluid should be consumed as liberally as possible before, during, and after an event. Carbohydrate and electrolytes in the fluid are especially helpful when exercise duration is expected to exceed 60 minutes to help delay fatigue and maintain electrolyte balance.

Scenario *Follow-Up*

Marcella is correct in following a high-carbohydrate diet. However, in her effort to minimize her fat intake, she is probably not consuming enough calories to support her training routine. Her diet is also low in protein. She has fallen into the bagel, pasta, and pretzel routine that sports nutritionists warn is not conducive to peak performance. Marcella would be smart to have a high-protein source at each meal. She could include milk with breakfast and possibly some low-fat yogurt or low-fat cheese at lunch. She should have a carbohydrate/protein snack before her workout, such as a half a sandwich and fruit and some water. The sandwich and fruit will help provide her with fuel to support her vigorous training. During her workouts, she could consume a sports drink to meet fluid needs and supply some carbohydrate, or she could consume water, along with a few fig cookies or other high-carbohydrate food. In the evenings, she could substitute oil and vinegar dressing for the fat-free dressing on her salad and cheese and crackers for the pretzels to improve protein intake. Overall, it is important for Marcella to fuel her body before, during, and after workouts.

Summary

1. A gradual increase in regular physical activity is recommended for all healthy persons. A minimum plan includes at least a total of 30 minutes of physical activity on most (or all) days. A more intense program lasting about 60 minutes should begin with warm-up exercises to increase blood flow and warm the muscles, and end with cooldown exercises. Regular resistance activities and stretching add further benefits.

2. Human metabolic pathways extract chemical energy from food and transform it into ATP, the compound that provides energy for body functions.

3. In carbohydrate fuel use, glucose is broken down into the three-carbon compound pyruvic acid, yielding some ATP. This is metabolized further via the aerobic pathway to form carbon dioxide (CO_2) and water (H_2O) or via the anaerobic pathway to form lactic acid.

4. At rest, muscle cells mainly use fat for fuel. For intense exercise of short duration, muscles mostly use phosphocreatine (PCr) for energy. During more sustained intense activity, muscle glycogen breaks down to lactic acid, providing a small amount of ATP. For endurance exercise, both fat and carbohydrate are used as fuels; carbohydrate is used increasingly as activity intensifies. Little protein is used to fuel muscles.

5. Anyone who exercises regularly should consume a diet that meets energy needs and is moderate to high in carbohydrates and fluid, and adequate in other nutrients such as iron and calcium.

6. Athletes should consume enough fluid to both minimize loss or body weight and ultimately restore preexercise weight. Sports drinks aid fluid, electrolyte, and carbohydrate replacement. Their use especially should be considered when continuous activity lasts beyond 60 minutes.

7. High-glycemic-index carbohydrates should be consumed by an athlete within 2 hours after a workout to begin restoration of muscle glycogen stores. Some protein in the meal is also helpful. The use of low-glycemic-index carbohydrates in the pre-event meal may help some endurance athletes.

Study Questions

1. How does greater physical fitness contribute to greater overall health? Explain the process.
2. The store of ATP in muscle is rapidly depleted once contraction begins. For physical activity to continue, ATP must be resupplied immediately. Describe how this occurs after initiation of exercise and at various times thereafter.
3. What is the difference between anaerobic and aerobic exercise? Explain why aerobic metabolism is increased by a regular exercise routine.
4. What is glycogen? How is it used during exercise?
5. Is fat from adipose tissue stores used as an energy source during exercise? If so, when?
6. What are some typical measures used to assess whether an athlete's energy intake is adequate?
7. List five specific nutrients that athletes need and appropriate food sources from which these nutrients can be obtained.
8. What conditions might contribute to the inability to get all required nutrients from food, thus requiring use of a multivitamin and mineral supplement?
9. What advice would you give your neighbor, who is planning to run a 50-kilometer (km) race, concerning fluid intake before and during the event?
10. One of your friends, a competitive athlete, asks your opinion about a nutritional supplement sold in a local sporting-goods store. She has read that such supplements, which contain amino acids, can help improve athletic performance. What would you tell her about the general effectiveness of such products?

Further Readings

1. Ahrendt DM: Ergogenic aids: Counseling the athlete. *American Family Physician* 63:913, 2001.
   New products with ergogenic claims appear on the market almost daily. Most are classified as supplements, which means the contents of the product and the claims on the label have not been evaluated by FDA and therefore may not have any scientific basis. Supplying adequate fluid and energy intake, and carbohydrate and protein in the diet, and timing these to be used efficiently by the body will provide the most effective and safe results.

2. American College of Sports Medicine and others: Nutrition and Athletic Performance, *Medicine & Science in Sports & Exercise* 32:2130, 2000.
   The athlete who wants to optimize exercise performance needs to follow good nutrition and hydration practices, use supplements and ergogenic aids carefully, minimize severe weight loss practices, and eat a variety of foods in adequate amounts. The various recommendations for carbohydrate, protein, fat, vitamins, minerals, and fluids in this chapter were taken from this article.

3. Beard J, Tobin B: Iron status and exercise. *American Journal of Clinical Nutrition* 72 (Suppl): 594S, 2000.
   Athletes most likely to develop iron deficiency anemia are female athletes in general, distance runners, and vegetarian athletes. These groups are advised to pay particular attention in maintaining adequate amounts of iron in their diets. They also may want to consider using low-dose iron supplements under medical supervision.

4. Clarkson PM, Thompson HS: Antioxidants: What role do they play in physical activity and health? *American Journal of Clinical Nutrition* 92 (Suppl): 637S, 2000.
   There is general agreement that following a diet rich in antioxidants for all those who exercise regularly is beneficial. At present, data are insufficient to recommend antioxidant supplements for athletes or other persons who exercise regularly. With respect to vitamin E, such supplements do not appear to enhance exercise performance but may offer protection from exercise-induced muscle damage, although study results are equivocal.

5. Coyle E: Physical activity as a metabolic stressor. *American Journal of Clinical Nutrition* 72 (Suppl): 512S, 2000.
   Blood glucose is a minor source of fuel during exercise lasting less than 30 minutes. As exercise duration increases to an hour or more, blood glucose becomes increasingly important, especially after 2 hours. Consuming carbohydrate during endurance exercise can help maintain blood glucose and reduce fatigue.

6. Kesaniemi YA and others: Dose-response issues concerning physical activity and health: An evidence-based symposium. *Medicine & Science in Sports & Exercise* 33 (Suppl): S351, 2001.
   There is a clear relationship between physical activity and reduced risk of all-cause mortality, cardiovascular disease, and type 2 diabetes. Other health benefits may also accrue, but the relationship for these health outcomes is more difficult to determine given our current knowledge.

7. Ling N: Performance foods for active individuals: Sports drinks, energy bars and energy gels. *Today's Dietitian*, p. 26, March 2000.
   Sports drinks, energy bars, and energy gels are unnecessary for short workouts. If a pre-exercise meal or snack has been consumed, use need not begin until an hour into a workout. Bars and gels should be consumed with at least 8 ounces of water, but not with sports drinks. For high-intensity workouts, such as track running or swimming, an energy gel may be a better choice than an energy bar.

8. Manore MM: Effect of physical activity on thiamine, riboflavin, and vitamin B-6 requirements. *American Journal of Clinical Nutrition* 72 (Suppl): 598S, 2000.
   Active individuals who restrict their energy intake or make poor dietary choices are at risk for poor B-vitamin status. However, the amount of these nutrients needed to cover losses or increased needs resulting from physical activity is small and can be met easily through wise food choices.

9. Sarubin A: *The health professionals' guide to popular dietary supplements*, The American Dietetic Association, Chicago Ill, 2000.
   The author provides a detailed look at individual dietary supplements, including those used by athletes. One example is creatine, which can increase strength/power during short bouts of exercise.

10. Williams MH: *Nutrition for health, fitness, & sport.* 6th ed. Boston: McGraw-Hill, 2002.
    Excellent textbook for reviewing nutrient needs of athletes, as well as learning more about ergogenic aids; also provides a detailed look at metabolism in exercise.

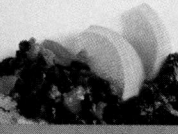
I. Is Your Diet Measuring Up to the Numbers?

In this chapter, several key nutrients were discussed in relation to exercise performance. The following guidelines were mentioned, not only for athletes but for everyone maintaining generally good fitness.

- Eat a moderate to high amount of carbohydrates (generally 60% or more of total energy intake).

- Athletes should eat a minimum of 1.2 grams of protein per kilogram of body weight.

- Consume the recommended standards of vitamins and minerals, making sure iron and calcium intakes are adequate (especially for women).

- Consume enough fluid, especially to approximately maintain weight during prolonged exercise or in hot conditions.

Review the results of the dietary assessment you completed in Chapter 2. Remember that you analyzed a 1-day food intake. Now answer the following questions, whether or not you consider yourself an athlete.

1. What percentage of your energy intake came from carbohydrate? Was your carbohydrate intake 60% or more of your total energy intake?

   _____

2. Did you eat at least 0.8 grams of protein per kilogram of body weight? If you are an athlete, did you consume at least 1.2 grams per kilogram of body weight? Did intake exceed 2 grams per kilogram of body weight?

   _____

   _____

3. Did you consume your estimated needs of all vitamins and minerals, especially iron and calcium? Which ones were below the current nutrient standards?

   _____

   _____

4. For nutrients low in your diet, list one rich food source (see Chapters 8 through 9).

   _____

   _____

5. Did you consume sufficient fluid—about 8 cups for a good starting point?

   _____

   _____

6. What can you do to improve your dietary intake to aid general fitness and, if you are an athlete, to promote maximal performance in your chosen event(s)?

   _____

   _____

   _____

   _____

   _____

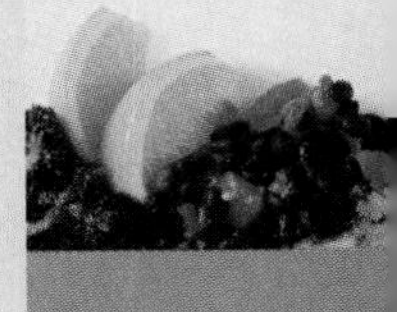

II. *Evaluating Protein Intake—A Case Study*

Marcus is a college student who has been lifting weights at the student recreation center. The trainer at the center recommended a protein drink to help Marcus build muscle mass. Evaluate Marcus's current food intake and determine whether a protein drink is needed to supplement Marcus's diet.

1. The following is a tally of yesterday's intake.

Breakfast	Frosted Mini-Wheats cereal, 2 oz
	1% milk, 1½ cups
	Orange juice, chilled, 6 oz
	Glazed yeast doughnut, 1
	Brewed coffee, 1 cup
Lunch	Double hamburger with condiments, 1
	French fries, 30
	Cola, 12 oz
	Medium apple, 1
Dinner	Frozen lasagna w/meat, 2 pieces
	1% milk, 1 cup
	Looseleaf lettuce, chopped, 1 cup
	Creamy Italian salad dressing, 2 tsp
	Medium tomato, ½
	Whole carrot, raw, 1
Evening snack	Vanilla ice milk, 1 cup
	Hot fudge chocolate topping, 2 tsp
	Soft chocolate chip cookies, 2

   Evaluate Marcus's diet—is he meeting the minimum recommendations of the Food Guide Pyramid? _____

2. Marcus's weight has been stable at 70 kilograms (154 pounds). Determine his protein needs based on the RDA (0.8 grams per kilogram).

   a. Marcus's estimated protein RDA: _____

   b. What are the maximum recommendations for protein intake for strength-training athletes (see p. 398)? _____

   c. Apply the maximum recommendations to Marcus. _____

   _____

3. An analysis of the total kcal and protein content of Marcus's current diet is 3470 kcal, 125 grams of protein (14% of total calories supplied by protein). This diet is representative of the food choices and amounts of food that Marcus chooses on a regular basis.

   a. What is the difference between Marcus's estimated protein needs as an athlete (from Exercise 2) and the amount of protein that his current diet provides? _____

   b. Is his current protein intake inadequate, adequate, or excessive? _____

4. Marcus takes his trainer's advice and goes to the supermarket to purchase a protein drink to add to his diet. Four products are available; they contain the following label information.

	Amino Fuel	Joe Weider's Sugar-Free 90% Plus Protein	Joe Weider's Dynamic Muscle Builder	Victory Super Mega Mass 2000
Serving size	3 tbsp	3 tbsp	3 tbsp	¼ scoop
Kcal	104	110	103	104
Protein (grams)	15	24	10	5

   continued

The trainer recommends adding the supplement to Marcus's diet two times a day. Marcus chooses Joe Weider's Dynamic Muscle Builder.

a. How much protein would be added to Marcus's diet daily from two servings of the supplement alone (prior to mixing it with a beverage)?

b. Marcus mixes the powder with the milk he already consumes at breakfast and dinner. How much protein total would Marcus now consume in 1 day? (Add the protein amount from the nutrition analysis to the value from the previous question.)

c. What is the difference between Marcus's estimated protein needs as an athlete and this total value?

5. What is your conclusion—does Marcus need the protein supplement?

Answers to Calculations

2a. Marcus's estimated protein RDA: 70 kilograms × 0.8 grams per kilogram = 56 grams

2b. Maximum recommendation for protein intake for athletes = 1.7–2 grams/kilogram (use the approximate midpoint of 1.8 for the calculation)

2c. Applied to Marcus: 1.8 × 70 = 126 grams

3a. Difference between Marcus's estimated maximum protein needs if an athlete and the amount of protein provided by his current diet: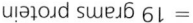
126 − 125 = 1 gram protein

3b. Marcus's current diet is adequate

4a. Two servings of protein supplement alone = 20 grams of protein

4b. Marcus's total protein consumption: 125 grams + 20 grams = 145 grams protein

4c. Difference between Marcus's estimated maximum protein needs as an athlete and total value (from above): 145 grams − 126 grams = 19 grams protein

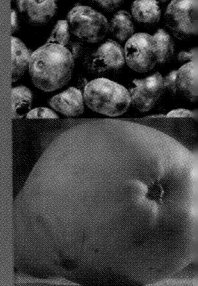

Evaluating Ergogenic Aids to Enhance Athletic Performance

Diet manipulation to improve athletic performance is not a recent innovation. As long as 30 years ago, American football players were encouraged on hot practice days to "toughen up" for competition by liberally consuming salt tablets before and during practice and by not drinking water. Now it is widely recognized that this practice can be fatal. Today's athletes are as likely as their predecessors to experiment with artichoke hearts, bee pollen, dried adrenal glands from cattle, seaweed, freeze-dried liver flakes, gelatin, and ginseng. These are just some of the ineffective substances used by athletes in hopes of gaining an **ergogenic** (work-producing) edge.

Ergogenic aids are classified into five categories:

1. *Mechanical aids* are designed to increase energy efficiency—to provide a mechanical edge. Runners may use lightweight racing shoes in place of heavier ones to increase the economy of running.
2. *Psychological aids* are designed to enhance psychological processes during sport performance—to increase mental strength. Hypnosis, through posthypnotic suggestion, may help remove psychological barriers that can limit physiological performance.
3. *Physiological aids* are designed to augment natural physiological processes to increase physiological power. Some athletes use creatine supplements to increase creatine phosphate in muscles. One intent is to provide more energy for activities that use primarily creatine phosphate, such as weightlifting and sprinting.
4. *Pharmacological aids* are drugs designed to influence physiological or psychological processes to increase physical power or mental strength. Some athletes use androstenedione to boost testosterone levels with the intent of increasing muscle mass. (This practice, however, can lead to many side effects, as discussed later in this Nutrition Issue.)
5. *Nutritional aids* are nutrients designed to influence physiological or psychological processes to increase physical power or mental strength. Sports drinks have been used to supply fluid, electrolytes, and glucose to offset that used (or lost) during prolonged physical activity.

Of these five classes of ergogenic aids, the final three will be discussed. Based on what is known at this time, today's athletes can benefit from recent scientific evidence documenting the ergogenic properties of a few dietary substances. These ergogenic aids include sufficient water and electrolytes, lots of carbohydrates, and a balanced and varied diet consistent with the Food Guide Pyramid or related pyramid. Protein and amino acid supplements are not among those aids because athletes can easily meet protein needs from foods, as Table 11.3 demonstrated. The use of nutrient supplements should be designed to meet a specific dietary shortcoming, such as an inadequate iron intake. These and other aids, which often have dubious benefits and may pose health risks, must be given close scrutiny before use. The risk-benefit ratio of any ergogenic aids especially needs to be examined.

As summarized in Table 11.7, no scientific evidence supports the effectiveness of many substances touted as performance-enhancing aids. Many are useless; some are dangerous. Athletes should be skeptical of any substance until its ergogenic effect is scientifically verified. FDA has a limited ability to regulate these dietary supplements (see the Nutrition Issue in Chapter 1). As well, the manufacturing processes for dietary supplements are not as tightly regulated by FDA as they are for prescription drugs. Some may contain substances that will cause athletes to "test positive" for various banned substances. Recent studies also have called into question the quality control associated with the manufacturing of dietary supplements. For example, a study looked at 16 brands of dehydroepiandrosterone (DHEA) purchased from health-food stores. As noted in Table 11.7, DHEA is a supplement that is claimed to increase muscle mass, decrease body fat, and increase blood testosterone. The study showed that only 7 of the 16 brands had a DHEA content within 90% to 110% of the stated label claim; 3 products had essentially no DHEA at all.

continued

ergogenic Work-producing. An ergogenic acid is a mechanical, nutritional, psychological, pharmacological, or physiological substance or treatment that is intended to directly improve exercise performance.

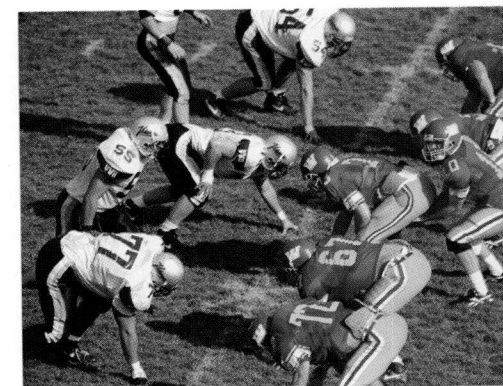

Attention to carbohydrate and fluid needs—along with meeting overall nutrient needs—is the most important ergogenic aid.

Table 11.7 An Evaluation of Ergogenic Aids Currently in the Limelight

Substance/Practice	Rationale	Reality
Useful in Some Circumstances		
Creatine	Increase phosphocreatine (PCr) in muscles to keep ATP concentration high	Use of 20 grams per day for 5 to 6 days and then a maintenance dose of 2 grams per day may improve performance in those who undertake repeated bursts of activity, such as in sprinting and weightlifting. Some of the muscle weight gain noted with use results from water retention. Endurance athletes do not benefit from use. Little is known about the safety of long-term creatine use. Continual use of high doses has led to kidney damage in a few cases. Cost: $25–$65 per month.
Sodium Bicarbonate	Counter lactic acid buildup	Partially effective in some circumstances, such as wrestling, but induces nausea and diarrhea. The dose used is 300 milligrams/kilogram, given 1–3 hours before exercise. Cost: nil.
Caffeine	Increase use of fatty acids to fuel muscles, promote psychological effects	Drinking two to three 5-ounce cups of coffee (equivalent to 3–9 milligrams of caffeine per kilogram of body weight) about 1 hour before events lasting about 5 minutes or longer is useful for some athletes; benefits are less apparent in those who have ample stores of glycogen, are highly trained, or habitually consume caffeine; intake of more than about 600 milligrams (six to eight cups of coffee) elicits a urine concentration illegal under Olympic rules (12 micrograms per milliliter). NCAA rules allow 15 micrograms per milliliter. A possible side effect is reduced body hydration. Cost: $0.08 per 300 milligrams.
Possibly Useful, Still Under Study		
Beta-hydroxy-beta methylbutyric acid (HMB)	Decrease protein catabolism, causing a net growth-promoting effect	Research in livestock and humans suggests that supplementation with this may increase muscle mass. Still, safety and effectiveness of long-term HMB use in humans is unknown. Cost: $100 per month.
Glutamine (an amino acid)	Enhance immune function, preserve lean body mass	Glutamine is the most abundant amino acid in plasma, and preservation of lean body mass levels fall in glycogen-depleted athletes. Overtrained athletes also have lower glutamine levels. Glutamine may be needed during metabolic stress and critical illness, and it is important for immunity. Some preliminary studies show decreased occurrence of upper respiratory tract infections in athletes with use. It also may promote muscle growth, but long-term studies are lacking. Protein foods are a rich source of glutamine. Cost: $10–$20 per month for 1–2 grams per day.
Branched-chain amino acids (BCAA) (leucine, isoleucine, valine)	Important energy source, especially when carbohydrate stores are depleted. A high ratio of free tryptophan:BCAA in the brain increases serotonin in the brain, which depresses the central nervous system and causes fatigue	Supplementation of BCAA during exercise can increase BCAA in the blood when it has been lowered due to exercise, but there is no consistent evidence of improved performance. Carbohydrate feeding, by delaying use of BCAA as fuel, may negate the need for BCAA supplementation. Preliminary studies show that BCAA use increases muscle mass more than does carbohydrate supplementation alone in swimmers, but there are no studies regarding resistance training. Protein-rich foods are also rich in BCAA. Cost: $20 per month.
Useful in Some Circumstances, But Dangerous or Illegal		
Anabolic steroids	Increase muscle mass and strength	Although effective for increasing protein synthesis, are illegal in the United States; have numerous potential side effects, such as premature closure of growth plates in bones (thus possibly limiting the adult height of a teenage athlete), bloody cysts in the liver, increased risk of cardiovascular disease, increased blood pressure, and reproductive dysfunction. Possible psychological consequences include increased aggressiveness, drug dependence (addiction), withdrawal symptoms (such as depression), sleep disturbances, and mood swings (known as "roid rage"). Use of needles for injectable forms adds further health risk. Banned by the International Olympic Committee.
Growth hormone	Increase muscle mass	At critical ages may increase height; may also cause uncontrolled growth of the heart and other internal organs and even death; potentially dangerous; requires careful monitoring by a physician. Use of needles for injections adds further health risk. Banned by the International Olympic Committee.
Insulin-like growth factor (IGF-1)	Increase muscle mass, enhance fat metabolism	Use can lead to enlargement of organs (as with growth hormone, as they have related functions in the body), back pain, headache, and difficulty breathing. Use of needles for injections adds further health risk. Cost: $30 per month. Bovine colostrum is a new and expensive source of IGF-1.
Blood doping	Red blood cells harvested previously from the athlete and then injected into the bloodstream, or alternately the athlete may use the hormone erythropoietin (Epogen) to increase red blood cell number in order to try to enhance aerobic capacity	May offer aerobic benefit; very serious health consequences are possible, including thickening of the blood, which puts extra strain on the heart; is an illegal practice under Olympic guidelines.

Table 11.7 continued

Substance/Practice	Rationale	Reality
Gamma hydroxybutyric acid (GHB)	Promoted as a steroid alternative for bodybuilding	FDA has never approved it for sale as a medical product; is illegal to produce or sell GHB in the United States. GHB-related symptoms include vomiting, dizziness, tremors, and seizures. Many victims have required hospitalization, and some have died. Clandestine laboratories produced virtually all of the chemical accounting for GHB abuse. FDA is working with the U.S. Attorney's office to arrest, indict, and convict individuals responsible for the illegal operations.
Androstenedione	Increase muscle mass	Possibly converted to testosterone and estrogen but does not increase muscle mass. Its use is banned by the NFL, NCAA, and International Olympic Committee. Side effects are acne, fits of rage, baldness, development of breasts in men, stunted growth, lower HDL-cholesterol in the blood, and sterility. Cost: $30 per month.
Insulin	Promote muscle development and inhibit muscle breakdown	Use can lead to seizures, hypoglycemia, and resulting brain damage. The need for injection can lead to increased risk of hepatitis and other viral diseases. Overall, unsupervised use of this powerful hormone is fraught with danger to one's health.
Ephedrine	Increase stamina and exercise performance. When combined with caffeine, thought to decrease appetite and increase fat use	No evidence that it enhances performance. Ephedrine (ephedra or ma juang in the herbal form) is currently under scrutiny by FDA due to more than 1000 reports of detrimental effects and at least 100 deaths. FDA is currently reviewing rules that would dictate amount of ephedrine allowed in each pill and taken within a 24-hour period, as well as a warning system on labels. Provisional advice is to consume no more than 25 milligrams per day for a total of 7 days, if at all. Ephedrine has caused heart attack, stroke, anxiety, seizure, and death. People who have hypertension, cardiovascular disease, diabetes, thyroid gland disorders, prostate gland enlargement, or nerve disease should not take ephedrine. Use is especially risky when combined with large quantities of caffeine (this is common). Cost: $0.08 per 25 milligrams.

Effectiveness Not Clearly Demonstrated (or No Benefit)

Substance/Practice	Rationale	Reality
Alcohol	Reduce fatigue, provide energy	Not a muscle fuel; actually impairs performance; abuse can lead to hypoglycemia and dehydration.
Medium chain triglyceride (MCT oil)	Excellent fuel for muscles; transfers directly from GI tract into bloodstream	Can provide a source of energy for muscles but provides no advantage over carbohydrate intake alone, as is very expensive. Doses over 25–30 grams at one time lead to nausea and diarrhea, also it is not tolerated well by athletes. Cost: $50 per month.
Phosphate loading	Improve oxygen delivery to muscles	Not effective. A current trend is to combine phosphates with creatine when using the latter. Cost: $2 per month for phosphate supplement.
Inosine	Increase protein and ATP synthesis	Not effective. Cost: $18 per month.
Coenzyme Q-10	Increase energy metabolism	Sufficient amount is produced by the body for energy metabolism. May also lead to increased free radical damage in cells during exercise. Cost: $16 per month.
Carnitine	Shuttle fatty acids into mitochondria of cells	Body cells produce enough; therefore, use is ineffective. Cost: $14 per month.
Chromium	Enhance insulin function	No benefit in performance. American College of Sports Medicine states that supplementation is unnecessary. Generally, we consume enough chromium to meet needs. Large doses can lead to kidney failure and possible damage to DNA in cells. Cost: $2 per month.
Conjugated linoleic acid (CLA)	Reduce body fat and increase lean mass	May be effective at doses of 3–7 grams per day. Many supplements on the market are of poor quality. Cost: $30-$70 per month.
Ornithine, arginine (human growth hormone releasers)	Used to increase human growth hormone output for muscle growth	Studies with unrealistically high doses of these amino acids (over 10 grams per day) given intravenously have been shown to increase human growth hormone. However, recent studies with more reasonable doses (2–4 grams per day) as commercial dietary supplements have shown no effects on human growth hormone. In addition, the increase in human growth hormone (even if the amino acids were effective) would be of questionable value and may even be harmful (see the section in this table on growth hormone). Cost: $15 per month.
Amino acids not already mentioned	Increase bioavailability to promote protein synthesis and lessen the muscle loss that occurs during both strength and endurance exercise	Of no value; dietary protein intake is sufficient to meet amino acid needs.
Deyhdroepiandrosterone (DHEA)	Increase production of testosterone and provide an anabolic steroid effect	Studies to date are inconclusive. Side effects are masculine traits in women, including hair loss and voice deepening. Men may develop irreversible breast development and prostate gland enlargement, possibly leading to prostate cancer. Recently banned by International Olympic Committee. Use is not recommended. Cost: $14–$52 per month.

continued

Table 11.7 continued

Substance/Practice	Rationale	Reality
Albuterol and Clembuterol	Train harder as to increase muscle strength and mass	No immediate ergogenic effect on either power or endurance in humans.
Pyruvic acid (Pyruvate)	Increase energy available to muscles	No benefit with use in trained athletes. Cost: $125 per month.
Vanadyl sulfate (vanadium)	Has insulin-like effects on carbohydrate and amino acid metabolism; used to promote muscle growth and decrease body fat	Doses of 0.5 milligrams per kilogram/day for 12 weeks did not alter body composition in weight trainers (normal diet contains about 0.1–0.3 milligrams per day). Exceeding the Upper Level (1.8 milligrams per day) can lead to kidney toxicity (see inside cover). Cost: $20 per month.
Hydroxycitrate (HCA) (*Garcinia cambogia*)	HCA is a competitive inhibitor of an enzyme involved in the synthesis of fat from carbohydrate; used as a fat-burner	Some poorly designed studies found body fat loss with HCA; however, the HCA was often given in combination with other herbs, vitamins, or minerals. A recent study with a more appropriate experimental design showed no impact of HCA (1500 milligrams per day), along with a 1200-kcal diet, on weight loss or body fat loss, compared to the diet alone. Cost: $30 per month.
Glycerol	Increase fluid retention in the body mass, enhancing body hydration	Limited research and small numbers of subjects used in studies provide conflicting evidence regarding the usefulness of glycerol in enhancing physical performance. Until more studies are completed, the claim that glycerol enhances sports performance is unsupported. Use of glycerol may produce headache and blurred vision, which could interfere with athletic performance. Cost: $30 per month.
Aspartates	May help reduce ammonia accumulation in muscles	Magnesium and/or potassium salts of aspartic acid have been used as potential aids to endurance performance. The small number of subjects used in current studies makes interpretation of the results difficult. To date, aspartate salts do not appear to reduce accumulation of ammonia in the blood. Until additional controlled trials with larger numbers of subjects are conducted, supplementation is not warranted. There appears to be no toxicity with the doses used in reported studies. Cost: $11 per month.
Ribose	Increase ATP synthesis	Although the monosaccharide ribose is part of the ATP molecule, no studies support the concept that increasing ribose intake increase ATP availability during physical activity, but studies are underway with the product. Cost: $50 per month.

These results add yet another worry for the athlete. Not only must the athlete determine whether there is evidence that a dietary supplement is safe and effective (FDA does not regulate dietary supplements), but now must also question if the dietary supplement contains what it is supposed to contain. To obtain information on independent laboratory tests on the quality of dietary supplements, the following website is helpful: www.consumerlab.com.

Even substances whose ergogenic effects have been supported by systematic scientific studies should be used with caution, as the testing conditions may not match those of the intended use.

Finally, rather than waiting for a magic bullet to enhance performance, athletes are advised to concentrate their efforts on improving their training routines and sport technique and consuming well-balanced diets, as described in this chapter.

Another Bite

The NCAA's Committee on Competitive Safeguards and Medical Aspects of Sports has developed lists of supplements that are permissible and nonpermissible for athletic departments to dispense. Following are key examples:

Permissible

Vitamins and minerals
"Energy" bars (if no more than 30% protein)
Sports drinks
Meal replacement drinks such as Ensure Plus or Boost

Nonpermissible

Amino acids
Creatine
Glycerol
HMB
L-carnitine
Protein powders

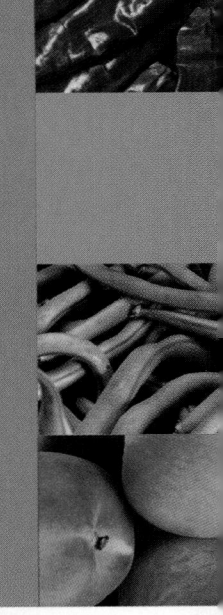

chapter *12*

Eating Disorders: *Anorexia Nervosa, Bulimia Nervosa, and Other Conditions*

*M*any of us occasionally eat until we're stuffed and uncomfortable, such as at Thanksgiving dinner. Faced with savory and tempting foods, we find that we can't easily stop eating. Usually we forgive ourselves, vowing not to overeat the next time. Nevertheless, many of us have problems controlling our weight. Although creeping weight gain can eventually lead to medical problems, it is usually associated with simple overeating, coupled with too little physical activity.

Although obesity is the most common eating disorder in our society, the eating disorders explored in this chapter involve much more severe distortions of the eating process. The eating disorders discussed here are serious and can develop into life-threatening conditions if left untreated. What's most alarming about these disorders—anorexia nervosa, bulimia nervosa, female athlete triad, binge-eating disorder, baryophobia and related disorders—is the increasing number of cases for many of these disorders reported each year.

Some people are more receptive and vulnerable to these disorders than other people are—for genetic, psychological, and physical reasons. And keep in mind that eating disorders are not restricted to any socioeconomic class or ethnicity. They can also strike at any age in both females and males. Let's examine the causes and treatments of these conditions in detail, because these eating disorders touch many of our lives.

Check out the **Contemporary Nutrition: Issues and Insights Online Learning Center** *www.mhhe.com/wardlawcont5* *for quizzes, flash cards, other activities, and web links designed to further help you learn about eating disorders.*

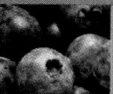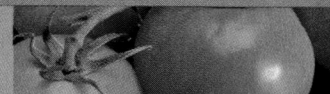

Real Life Scenario

At age 16, Sarah suddenly became self-conscious about her weight when the neighborhood children teased her about being overweight. She began exercising to an aerobics video for an hour each day and found that she had success in losing weight; this was just the beginning of her obsession to be thin. Next, Sarah turned to eating less food to lose even more weight and began eliminating certain foods from her diet, such as candy and meat. She increased her water and vegetable intake and chewed sugarless gum to curb her appetite. Once she began dieting, it was impossible for her to stop. She really enjoyed having a high degree of self-control over her body. She was literally obsessed with food and stared at others while they were eating a meal. She cooked large meals and then refused to eat all but a few bites. By the time Sarah was 19 years old and 5'6" tall, her weight had dropped from 150 pounds to 85 pounds in 20 months. Her family was concerned about her weight status, demanding that she go to a physician for an evaluation. Sarah was not happy about this idea but believed that her family would stop pestering her if she just did this. Sarah did not think she had a problem; she truly thought she was still grotesquely overweight. She did notice, however, that she was intolerant of cold temperatures and had not menstruated in a year.

Does Sarah have an eating disorder? What types of therapy do you think the physician will suggest for Sarah? Where could she go for such therapy? What is the likelihood that she will fully recover from her condition?

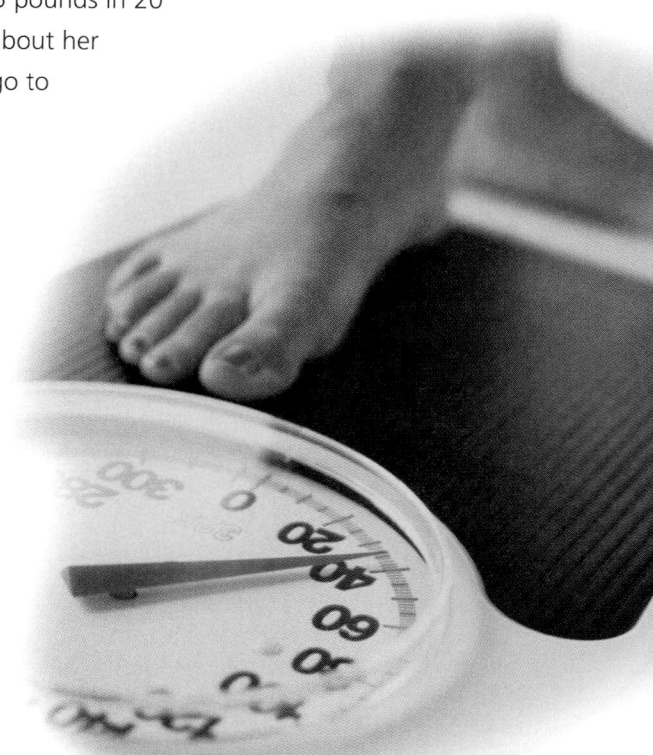

Nutrition Connection

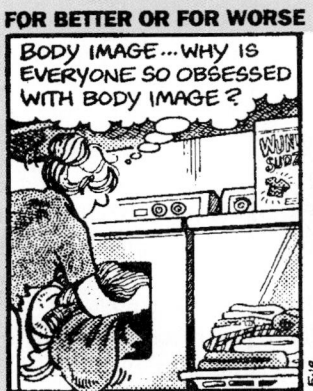
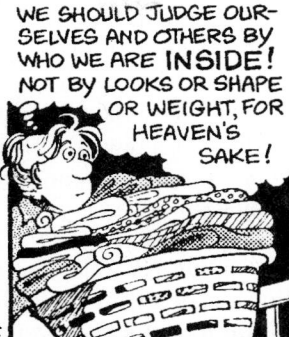
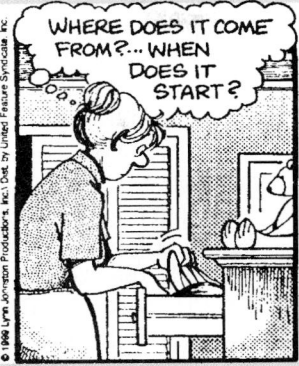
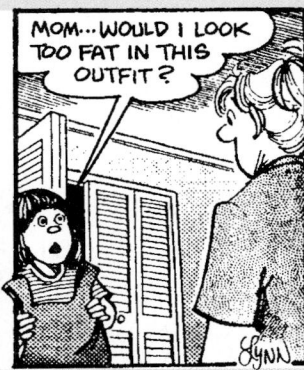

Concern with body image often starts early in life. Why do you think this is so? What recent societal trends have fostered this concern? Are some people more vulnerable, based on genetics and environment? This chapter provides some answers.

FOR BETTER OR FOR WORSE ©United Features Syndicate. Reprinted by Permission.

From Ordered to Disordered Eating Habits

Eating—a completely instinctive behavior for animals—serves an extraordinary number of psychological, social, and cultural purposes for humans. Eating practices may take on religious meanings; signify bonds among cultural, ethnic, and family groups; and be a means to express hostility and affection, prestige, and class values. Similarly, providing, preparing, and distributing food may be a means of expressing love or hatred, or even power, in family relationships.

In our society, we are bombarded daily with images of the ideal body. Dieting is promoted to achieve this ideal body—eternally young and acceptable to those around us. Television programs, billboard advertisements, magazine pictures, movies, and newspapers tell us that an ultra-slim body will bring happiness, love, and even success. This is despite the fact that much of society is becoming fatter. In response, some of us take this to the other extreme—the pathological pursuit of weight control or weight loss.

Not comparing the media images with our own is hard. Not everyone can look like a fashion model. People who are overly susceptible to these messages, for genetic, psychological, and physical reasons, may be more likely than others to develop eating disorders in response.

Given the multiple functions associated with normal eating and the media bombardment about ideal body image, it is not surprising that some people progress from typical responses to hunger and satiety cues, to obsessive weight loss, and then to a full-blown eating disorder, often associated with unusual and strange rituals.

■ Food: More Than Just a Source of Nutrients

From birth, we link food with personal and emotional experiences. As infants, we associate milk with security and warmth, so the bottle or breast becomes a source of comfort as well as food. Even when older, some people continue to derive comfort and great pleasure from food. This is both a biological and a psychological phenomenon. Food can be a symbol of comfort, but eating can also stimulate the release of

Progression from Ordered to Disordered Eating

Attention to hunger and satiety signals; limitation of energy intake to restore weight to a healthful level

Some disordered eating habits begin as weight loss is attempted, such as very restricted eating

Clinically evident eating disorder recognized

endorphins Natural body tranquilizers that may be involved in the feeding response and function in pain reduction.

disordered eating Mild and short-term changes in eating patterns that occur in relation to a stressful event, an illness, or a desire to modify one's diet for a variety of health and personal appearance reasons.

eating disorder Severe alterations in eating patterns linked to physiological changes. The alterations are associated with food restricting, binge eating, purging, and fluctuations in weight. They also involve a number of emotional and cognitive changes that affect the way a person perceives and experiences his or her body.

bulimia nervosa An eating disorder in which large quantities of food are eaten at one time (binge eating) and then purged from the body by vomiting, or misuse of laxatives, diuretics, or enemas. Alternate means to counteract the caloric excess use are fasting and excessive exercise. The use of nervosa refers to the person's disgust with one's body.

binge-eating disorder An eating disorder characterized by recurrent binge eating and feelings of loss of control over eating that has lasted at least 6 months. Binge episodes can be triggered by frustration, anger, depression, anxiety, permission to eat forbidden foods, and excessive hunger.

certain neurotransmitters (e.g., serotonin) and *natural opioids* (including **endorphins**), which produce a sense of calm and euphoria in the human body. Thus, in times of great stress some people turn to food for a druglike, calming effect.

Food is also used as a reward or a bribe. Haven't you heard or spoken something similar to the following comments?

You can have your dessert if you eat five more bites of your vegetables.
You can't play until you clean your plate.
I'll eat the broccoli if you let me watch TV.
If you love me, you'll eat what I fixed for dinner.

On the surface, using food as a reward or bribe seems harmless enough. Eventually, however, this practice encourages both caregivers and children to use food to achieve unstated goals. Food may then become much more than a source of nutrients. Regularly using food as a bargaining chip can contribute to abnormal eating patterns. Carried to the extreme, these patterns can lead to **disordered eating**.

This disordered eating can be defined as mild and short-term changes in eating patterns that occur in relation to a stressful event, an illness, or even a desire to modify the diet for a variety of health and personal appearance reasons. The problem may be no more than a bad habit, a style of eating adapted from friends or family members, or an aspect of preparing for athletic competition. While disordered eating can lead to weight loss or weight gain and to certain nutritional problems, it rarely requires in-depth professional attention. If, however, disordered eating becomes sustained, distressing, or starts to interfere with everyday activities, it may require professional intervention.

■ Overview of Anorexia Nervosa and Bulimia Nervosa

Given the common practice of dieting in North America, it can sometimes be difficult to tell where disordered eating stops and an **eating disorder** begins. Indeed, many eating disorders get their start from a simple diet. Eating disorders then go on to involve physiological changes associated with food restricting, binge eating, purging, and fluctuations in weight. They also involve a number of emotional and cognitive changes that affect the way a person perceives and experiences his or her body, such as feelings of distress or extreme concern about body shape or weight. Eating disorders are not due to a failure of will or behavior; rather, they are real, treatable medical illnesses in which certain maladaptive patterns of eating take on a life of their own.

The main types of eating disorders are anorexia nervosa and **bulimia nervosa.** A third type, **binge-eating disorder,** has been suggested but has not yet been approved as a formal psychiatric diagnosis. More than 5 million people in North America have one of these disorders; females outnumber males 5 to 1. Eating disorders frequently develop during adolescence or early adulthood (85% of the time), but some reports indicate their onset can occur during childhood or later in adulthood. Eating disorders frequently co-occur with other psychological disorders such as depression, substance abuse, and anxiety disorders. *People who suffer from eating disorders can experience a wide range of physical health complications, including serious heart conditions and kidney failure, which may even lead to death.* Recognition of eating disorders as important and treatable diseases, therefore, is critical.

Currently, about 5% of women in North America develop a form of anorexia nervosa or bulimia nervosa in their lifetimes. This section provides a brief description of the characteristics and diagnoses of these two disorders which primarily afflict those of college age and younger. Detailed discussion of these and related disorders, including treatment, then follows.

Anorexia nervosa is characterized by extreme weight loss, a distorted body image, and an irrational, almost morbid, fear of obesity and weight gain. Anorexic patients irrationally believe they are fat, even though others constantly comment on their thin physique. Some anorexics realize they are thin but are habitually haunted by certain areas of their bodies that they believe to be fat (such as thighs, buttocks, and stomach)

(Fig. 12.1). The discrepancy between actual and perceived body shape is an important gauge of the severity of the disease.

The term *anorexia* implies a loss of appetite; however, denying one's appetite more accurately describes the behavior of people with anorexia nervosa. By rough estimate, approximately 1 in 100 girls between the ages of 12 and 18 years in North America suffers from anorexia nervosa. This high number may be due to the tendency for these females to blame themselves for the weight gain seen at that age. It happens less commonly among adult women and African-American women. Men account for only approximately 10% of the cases of anorexia nervosa, partly because the ideal image conveyed for men is big and muscular.

Bulimia nervosa (*bulimia* means "great [ox] hunger") is characterized by episodes of binge eating followed by attempts to purge the excess energy taken up by the body by vomiting or misuse of laxatives, diuretics, or enemas. Fasting and excessive exercise also may be used to compensate for the caloric excess. People with this disorder may be difficult to identify because they keep their binge-purge behaviors secret, and their symptoms are not obvious. About 3% or more of adolescent and college-age women suffer from bulimia nervosa. About 10% of the cases occur in men, especially athletes, who participate in sports that require achieving lower weights to fit weight classes, such as boxers, wrestlers, and jockeys. Other activities that may foster eating disorders in men include swimming, dancing, and modeling.

Specific criteria are used by clinicians to diagnose eating disorders. Some characteristics are listed in Table 12.1. People may also exhibit some symptoms of eating disorders but not enough to enable a medical worker to diagnose one of the two diseases. And, as suggested in the diagnostic criteria, some people show characteristics of both anorexia nervosa and bulimia nervosa because the diseases overlap considerably (Fig. 12.2). About half of the women diagnosed as having anorexia nervosa eventually develop bulimic symptoms. As shown in Table 12.1, bulimic characteristics can be seen in anorexia nervosa, which blurs the distinction. Still, appreciating the differences between the disorders helps in understanding various approaches to prevention and treatment.

Do you know someone who is at risk of these eating disorders? If so, suggest that the person seek a professional evaluation because, the sooner treatment begins, the better. However, do not try to diagnose eating disorders in your friends or family members. Only a professional can exclude other possible diseases and correctly evaluate the diagnostic criteria required to make a diagnosis of anorexia nervosa or bulimia nervosa. Once an eating disorder is diagnosed, immediate treatment is advisable. As a friend, the best you can do is to encourage an affected person to seek professional help. Note that such help is commonly available at student health centers and student guidance/counseling facilities on college campuses.

There are no simple causes of eating disorders, and there are no simple treatments. Stress may have an especially strong role in the development of eating disorders. An underlying commonality seems to be the lack of appropriate coping mechanisms as individuals begin to reach adolescence and young adulthood, coupled with dysfunctional family relationships.

■ Is There a Genetic Connection to Eating Disorders?

A few research studies have investigated the possible link between genetic factors and the development of eating disorders. These studies have involved a comparison of identical twins with fraternal twins and the incidence of eating disorders. In general, these studies have shown that identical twins have a higher likelihood of eating disorders among themselves than do fraternal twins. This indicates that genetics may have a strong role in development, since identical twins share the same DNA; however, these studies have not ruled out the impact of the environmental influences in eating disorder development. Identifying genes that cause eating disorders eventually could help in tailoring prevention efforts to those who are at risk, but affected individuals would still need the same counseling that is part of therapy today.

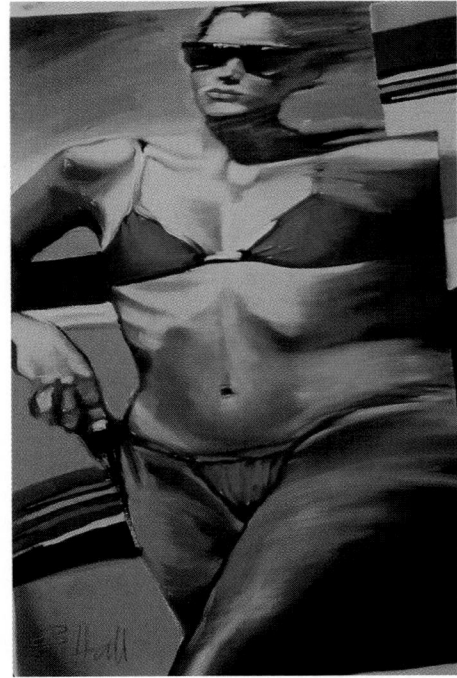

Figure 12.1 Self-image can be ever changing and deceiving. For people with eating disorders, the difference between the real and desired body images may be too difficult to accept. See the website 4women.gov/bodyimage/help.htm for details.

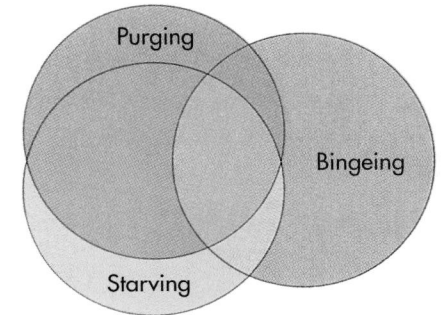

Figure 12.2 The overlap of eating disorders. A combination of binge eating, purging, and/or starving can be found in various cases of both anorexia nervosa and bulimia nervosa.

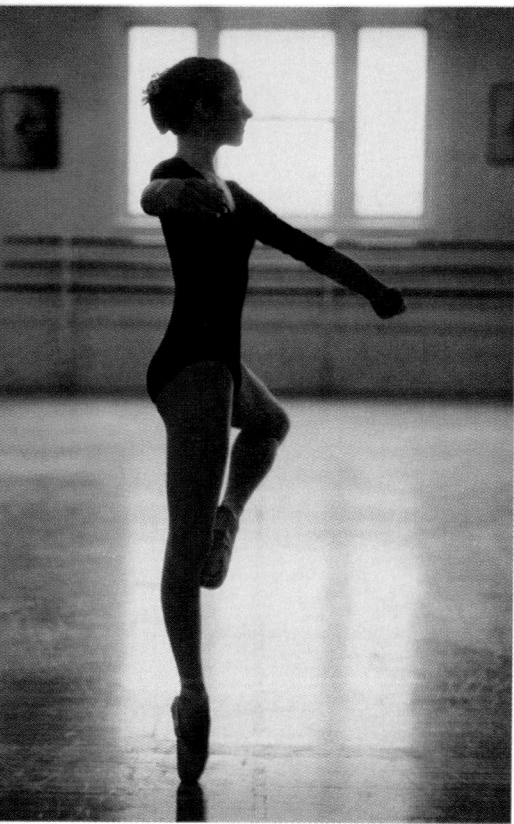

Eating disorders are commonly seen in people who must maintain low body weight, such as ballet dancers.

Table 12.1 Typical Characteristics of Anorexic and Bulimic Persons

Anorexia Nervosa	Bulimia Nervosa
• Rigid dieting causing dramatic weight loss, generally to less than 85% of what would be expected for one's age (or BMI of 17.5 or less)	• Secretive binge eating; generally not overeating in front of others
• False body perception—thinking "I'm too fat," even when extremely underweight; relentless pursuit of control	• Eating when depressed or under stress
• Rituals involving food, excessive exercise, and other aspects of life	• Bingeing on a large amount of food, followed by fasting, laxative or diuretic abuse, self-induced vomiting, or excessive exercise (at least twice a week for 3 months)
• Maintenance of rigid control in lifestyle; security found in control and order	• Shame, embarrassment, deceit, and depression; low self-esteem and guilt (especially after a binge)
• Feeling of panic after a small weight gain; intense fear of gaining weight	• Fluctuating weight resulting from alternate bingeing and fasting (±10 pounds or 5 kilograms)
• Feelings of purity, power, and superiority through maintenance of strict discipline and self-denial	• Loss of control; fear of not being able to stop eating
• Preoccupation with food, its preparation, and observing another person eat	• Perfectionism, "people pleaser"; food as the only comfort/escape in an otherwise carefully controlled and regulated life
• Helplessness in the presence of food	• Erosion of teeth, swollen glands
• Lack of menstrual periods after what should be the age of puberty for at least 3 months	• Purchase of syrup of ipecac, a compound sold in pharmacies that induces vomiting
• Possible presence of bingeing and purging practices	

Those who exhibit only one or a few of these characteristics may be at risk but probably do not have either disorder. They should, however, reflect on their eating habits and related concerns and take appropriate action, such as seeking a careful evaluation by a physician.

The Nutrition Issue at the end of this chapter adds further insight into this topic, as it reviews some sociological aspects of these disorders. This helps you further understand how the disorders develop and why some people are more susceptible than others. As is true for many health problems, both nature and nurture play a role.

Anorexia Nervosa

A person with anorexia nervosa may use the disorder to gain attention from the family, sometimes in hopes of holding the family together.

Anorexia nervosa evolves from a dangerous mental state to an often life-threatening physical condition. People suffering from this disorder think they are fat and intensely fear obesity and weight gain. They lose much more weight than is healthful. Although food is entwined in this disease, it stems more from psychological conflict.

Depression is commonly found in conjunction with an eating disorder. In fact, a study done in the 1940s at the University of Minnesota found that depression and obsessional behaviors developed in the subjects during a 6-month period of restricted calorie intake. These abnormal behaviors did not reverse immediately after refeeding but, rather, took many weeks to return to normal (see Chapter 17 for details).

About 7% of people with anorexia die within 10 years of diagnosis—from suicide, heart ailments, and infections. About one quarter of those with anorexia nervosa recover within 6 years, whereas the rest simply exist with the disease or go on to develop another form of eating disorder. The longer someone suffers from this eating disorder, the poorer the chances for complete recovery. A young patient with a brief episode and a cooperative family has a better outlook than those without these factors. Prompt and vigorous treatment with close follow-up improves the chances for success.

Anorexia nervosa may begin as a simple attempt to lose weight. A comment from a well-meaning friend, relative, or coach suggesting that the person seems to be gaining weight or is too fat may be all that is needed. The stress of having to maintain a certain weight to look attractive or competent on a job can also lead to disordered eating. Physical changes associated with puberty, the stress of leaving childhood, or the loss of a friend may serve as another trigger for extreme dieting. Leaving home for boarding school or college or starting a job can reinforce the desire to appear more "socially acceptable." Still, looking "good" does not necessarily help people deal with anger, depression, low self-esteem, or past experiences with sexual abuse. If these issues are behind the disorder and are not resolved as weight is lost, the individual may intensify efforts to lose weight "to look even better," rather than work through unresolved psychological concerns.

During adolescence, a period of turbulent sexual and social tensions, teenagers seek—and are often expected—to establish separate and independent lives. While declaring independence, they seek acceptance and support from peers and parents and react intensely to how they think others perceive them. At the same time, their bodies are changing, and much of the change is beyond their control. In response to the adolescent's or teenager's lack of control and coping mechanisms, dieting may start and then lead to a failure to gain appropriate weight-for-height. This may not be readily identified as a problem because the child has not actually lost any weight. Stunting (failure to grow in height) may also occur if inadequate calories are ingested during a period of growth. If anorexia develops before puberty, sexual maturation and menstruation may be delayed.

Teens with chronic illnesses, such as type 1 diabetes or asthma, are at even greater risk for disordered eating. Any evidence of poor weight gain/maintenance or excessive fitness among these individuals needs to be investigated as possible disordered eating.

Extreme dieting is the most important predictor of an eating disorder. (Adolescents expressing concern about their weight should be advised to focus on exercise, which does not appear to impart a risk for subsequent problems.) Once dieting begins, a person developing anorexia nervosa does not stop. The result is long periods of rigidly self-enforced semistarvation, practiced almost with a vengeance, in a relentless pursuit of control. Anorexia nervosa may eventually lead to bingeing on large amounts of food in a short time, then purging. Purging occurs primarily through vomiting, but laxatives, diuretics, and enemas are also used. Thus, a person with anorexia nervosa may exist in a state of semistarvation or may alternate periods of starvation with periods of bingeing and purging.

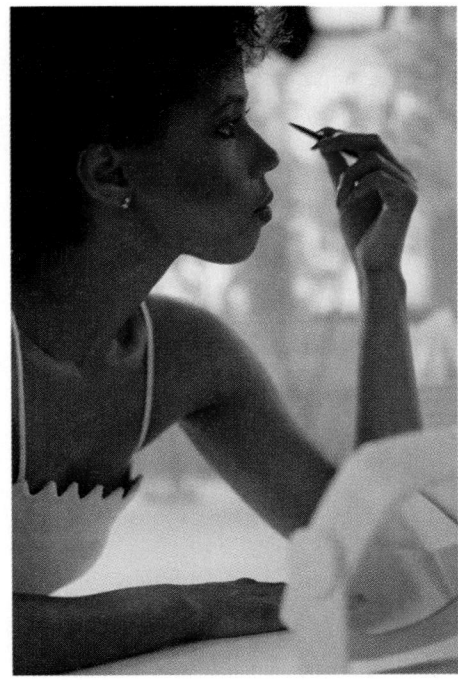

Concern over appearance begins early in life; a focus on a healthful outlook with regard to body weight should also begin at this time.

*B*y severely restricting energy intake for long periods, adolescent girls and young adult women greatly compromise their nutritional status, impair their reproductive systems, and retard growth. The harm produced by milder, shorter periods of diet restriction is not clear. Evidence, however, suggests that even moderate diet restriction, if continued, contributes to the risks for various anemias, later pregnancy complications and low-birthweight infants, and permanently reduced bone mass.

Another Bite

*R*ecently, a 19-year-old patient at the Ohio State University Hospitals was admitted on an emergency basis at a body weight of 60 pounds. She had lost 55 pounds in the previous 6 months and was at great risk of impending death. Upon interview, she said she started dieting and could not stop. She was transferred out-of-state to a clinic specializing in eating disorders.

■ Profile of the Typical Person with Anorexia Nervosa

A person with anorexia nervosa refuses to eat enough food to maintain an acceptable weight. This refusal is the hallmark of the disease, whether or not other practices, such as binge-purge cycles, appear. The most typical anorexic person is a white female from the middle or upper socioeconomic class. Perhaps her mother also has distorted views of desirable body shape and acceptable food habits. The girl is often described by parents and teachers as responsible, meticulous, and obedient.

She is competitive and often obsessive. Her parents set high standards for her. At home, she may not allow clutter in her bedroom. Physicians note that, after a physical examination, she may fold her examination gown very carefully and clean up the examination room before leaving. Even though such behavior may seem obvious, only a skilled professional can tell the difference between anorexia nervosa and other adolescent complaints, such as delayed puberty, fatigue, and depression.

A common thread underlying many—but not all—cases of anorexia nervosa is conflict within the family structure, typically manifested by an overbearing mother and an emotionally absent father. When family expectations are always too high—including those regarding body weight—resulting frustration leads to fighting. Overinvolvement, rigidity, overprotection, and denial are typical daily transactions of such families.

Often, the eating disorder allows an anorexic person to exercise control over an otherwise powerless existence (Fig. 12.3). Losing weight may be the first independent success the person has had. People with anorexia evaluate their self-worth almost entirely in terms of self-control. Issues of control are central to the development of anorexia nervosa. Some sexually abused children develop anorexia nervosa, believing that if they control their appetite for food, sexual relations, and human contact, they will feel in control and competent and will eliminate shameful feelings. Moreover, food restriction, which arrests development and shuts down sexual impulses, may be a strategy to prevent future victimization and guilt feelings in such cases. Often anorexic persons feel hopeless about human relationships and socially isolated because of their dysfunctional families. They substitute the world of food, eating, and weight for the world of human relationships.

■ Early Warning Signs

A person developing anorexia nervosa exhibits important warning signs. At first, dieting becomes the life focus. The person may think, "The only thing I am good at is dieting. I can't do anything else." This innocent beginning often leads to very abnormal self-perceptions and eating habits, such as cutting a pea in half before eating it. Other habits include hiding and storing food and or spreading food around a plate to make it look as if much has been eaten. An anorexic person may cook a large meal and watch others eat it while refusing to eat anything. Anorexics may also exercise compulsively to the point that it is obsessive and driven. It can interfere with life activities or occur at inappropriate times or settings—for example, doing squats while brushing teeth.

As the disorder progresses, the range of foods may narrow and be rigidly divided into safe and unsafe ones, with the list of safe foods becoming progressively shorter. For people developing anorexia nervosa, these practices say, "I am in control." These people may be hungry, but they deny it, driven by the belief that good things will happen by just becoming thin enough. It becomes a question of willpower.

Soon people with anorexia become irritable and hostile and begin to withdraw from family and friends. School performance generally crumbles. They refuse to eat out with family and friends, thinking, "I won't be able to have the foods I want to eat," or "I won't be able to throw up afterward."

Parents may not consider a teenager mature enough to make decisions. If the teen disagrees and the situation is very tense, she may turn to purging or starving as a way to show her power: "You may try to control my life, but I can do anything I want with my body."

In the words of one young woman, "I couldn't get angry, because it would be like destroying someone else, like my mother. It felt like she would hate me forever, I got angry through anorexia nervosa. It was my last hope. It's my own body and this was my last-ditch effort."

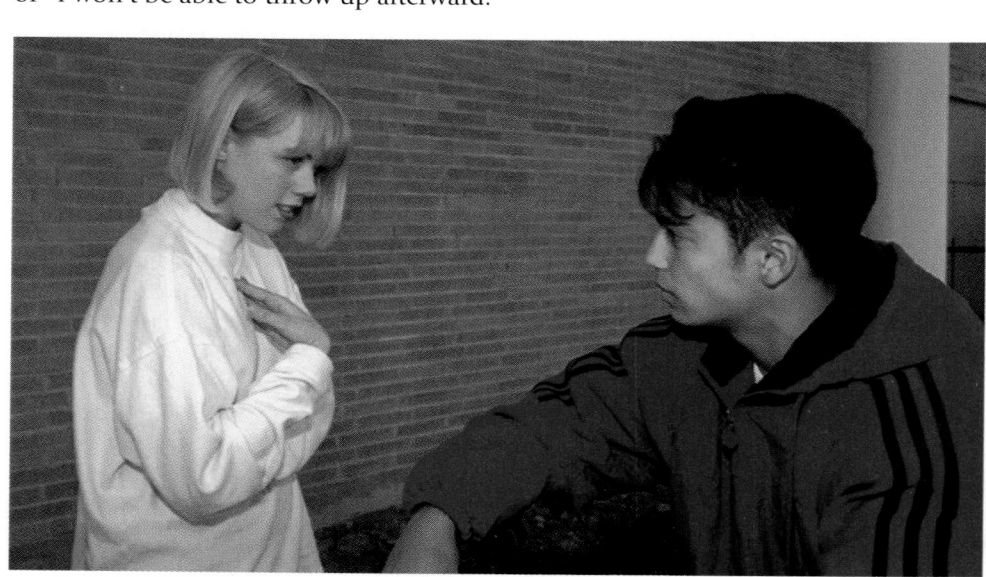

Figure 12.3 Conflict and physical changes are a common part of adolescence and may ultimately trigger an eating disorder.

Anorexic persons see themselves as rational and others as irrational. They also tend to be excessively critical of themselves and others. Nothing is good enough. Because it cannot be perfect, life appears meaningless and hopeless. A sense of joylessness colors everything.

As stress increases in the person's life, sleep disturbances and depression are common. Many of the psychological and physical problems associated with anorexia nervosa arise from insufficient energy intake, as well as deficiencies of nutrients, such as thiamin and vitamin B-6. For the latter reason, a multivitamin and mineral supplement is typically prescribed in therapy. For a female, the combination of problems—coupled with lower and lower body weight and fat stores—causes menstrual periods to cease. This may be the first sign of the disease that a parent notices and represents the hallmark of the disease.

Ultimately, an anorexic person eats very little food; 300 to 600 kcal daily is not unusual. In place of food, the person may consume up to 20 cans of diet soft drinks and chew many pieces of sugarless gum each day.

▪ Physical Effects of Anorexia Nervosa

Rooted in the emotional state of the victim, anorexia nervosa produces profound physical effects. The anorexic person often appears to be skin and bones. Body weight less than 85% of that expected is one clinical indicator of anorexia nervosa. This percentage can be calculated using the Metropolitan Life Insurance tables (see Appendix G), but it is important to note that body build and weight history should also be used when estimating an appropriate weight. BMI is a more reliable indicator of the degree of malnourishment; generally, a BMI of 17.5 or less indicates a severe case (review Chapter 10 for more on BMI). For children under age 18, growth charts should be used to assess weight status (see Chapter 14).

This state of semistarvation disturbs many body systems, as it forces the body to conserve as much energy as possible (Fig. 12.4). This attempt to conserve energy results in the most physical effects. Thus, many complications can be ended by returning to a healthy weight, provided the duration of the insult has not been too long. Following are predictable effects caused by hormonal responses to semistarvation:

- Lowered body temperature and cold intolerance caused by loss of fat insulation
- Slower metabolic rate caused by decreased synthesis of the thyroid hormones
- Decreased heart rate as metabolism slows, leading to easy fatigue, fainting, and an overwhelming need for sleep. Other changes in heart function may also occur, including loss of heart tissue itself.
- Iron-deficiency anemia from a deficient nutrient intake, which leads to further weakness
- Rough, dry, scaly, and cold skin from a deficient nutrient intake, iron-deficiency anemia, and estrogen deficiency. The skin may also show multiple bruises because of the loss of protection from the fat layer normally present under the skin.
- Low white blood cell count caused by a deficient nutrient intake. This condition increases the risk of infection, one cause of death in people with anorexia nervosa.
- Abnormal feeling of fullness or bloating, which can last for several hours after eating
- Loss of hair caused by a deficient nutrient intake
- Appearance of lanugo—downy hairs on the body that trap air, reducing heat loss and in turn replacing some insulation lost with the fat layer
- Constipation from semistarvation and laxative abuse
- Low blood potassium caused by a deficient nutrient intake, loss of potassium from vomiting, and use of some types of diuretics. This increases the risk of heart rhythm disturbances, another leading cause of death in anorexic people.

Critical Thinking

Jennifer is an attractive 13-year-old. However, she's very compulsive. Everything has to be perfect—her hair, her clothes, even her room. Since her body is beginning to mature, she's quite obsessed with having perfect physical features as well. Her parents are worried about her behavior. The school counselor told them to look for certain signs that could indicate an eating disorder. What might those signs be?

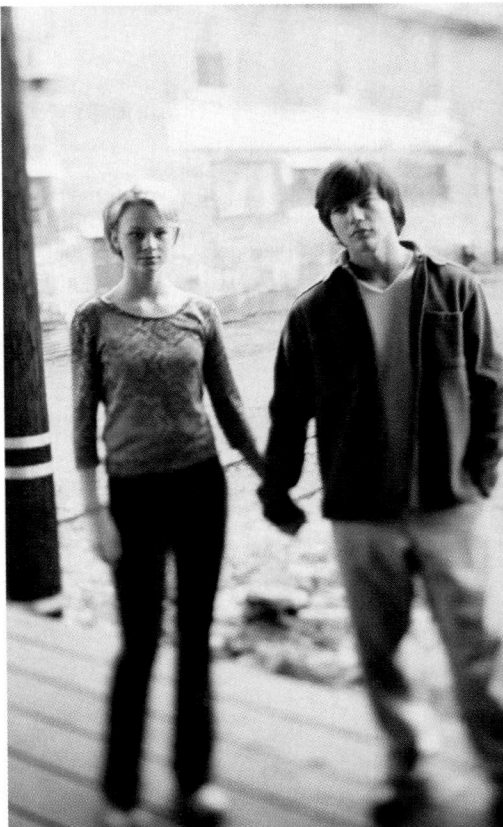

Anorexia nervosa occurs much more frequently in young women than in young men.

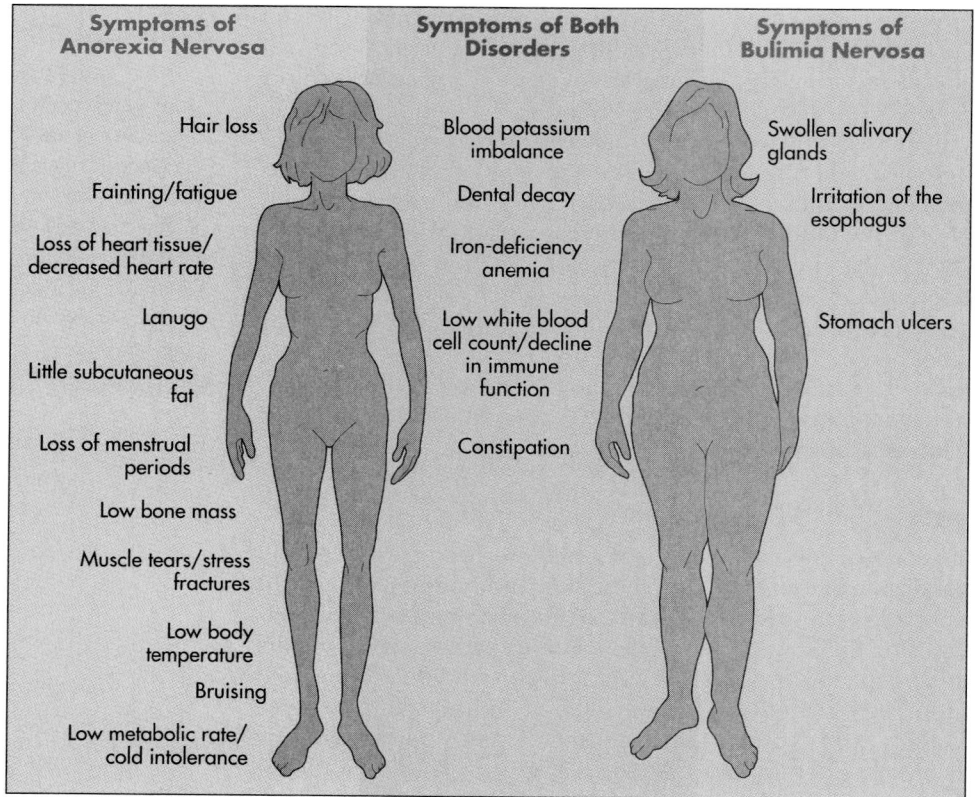

Figure 12.4 Signs and symptoms of eating disorders. A vast array of physical effects are associated with anorexia nervosa and bulimia nervosa. This figure contains many, but is not an exhaustive list of all potential consequences. These physical effects can also serve as warning signs that a problem exists. Professional evaluation is then indicated.

- Loss of menstrual periods because of low body weight, low body fat content, and the stress of the disease. Accompanying hormonal changes cause a loss of bone mass and increase the risk of osteoporosis later in life.
- Changes in neurotransmitter function in the brain, which leads to depression
- Eventual loss of teeth caused by acid erosion from frequent vomiting. Until vomiting ceases, one way to reduce this effect on teeth is to rinse the mouth with water right away and brush the teeth as soon as possible. Loss of teeth (along with low bone mass) can be lasting signs of the disease, even if the other physical and mental problems are resolved.
- Muscle tears and stress fractures in athletes because of decreased bone and muscle mass

A person with this disorder is psychologically and physically ill and needs help.

Erika Goodman, former dancer with the Joffrey Ballet, is now in her 50s and is crippled from osteoporosis resulting from years of restricting food intake in order to maintain a low body weight. This led to the irregular or absent menstrual periods for many years.

Concept Check

Anorexia nervosa is an eating disorder characterized by semistarvation. It is found primarily—but not exclusively—in adolescent girls, starting at or around puberty. People with anorexia dwindle essentially to skin and bones but still believe they are fat. Semistarvation produces hormonal and other changes, which lower body temperature, slow the heart rate, decrease immune response, stop menstrual periods, and contribute to hair, muscle, and bone loss. It is a very serious disease, which often produces lifelong consequences and may be fatal.

■ Treatment of Anorexia Nervosa

People with anorexia often sink into shells of isolation and fear. They deny that a problem exists. Frequently, their friends and family members meet with them to confront the problem in a loving way. This is called an *intervention*. They present evidence of the problem and encourage immediate treatment. Treatment then requires a multidisciplinary team of experienced physicians, registered dietitians, psychologists, and other health professionals working together. An ideal setting is an eating disorders clinic in a medical center. Outpatient therapy generally begins first. This may be extended to 3 to 5 days per week. Day hospitalization (6–12 hours) is another option, as is total hospitalization. This hospitalization is necessary once a person falls below 75% of expected weight, experiences acute medical problems, and/or exhibits severe psychological problems or suicidal risk. Still, even in the most skilled hands and using the finest facilities, efforts may fail. This tells us that the prevention of anorexia nervosa is of utmost importance.

Once a medical team has gained the cooperation and trust of an anorexic patient, the team attempts to work together to restore a sense of balance, purpose, and future possibilities. As previously stated, anorexia nervosa is usually rooted in psychological conflict. However, a person who has been barely existing in a state of semistarvation cannot focus on much besides food. Dreams and even morbid thoughts about food will interfere with therapy until sufficient weight is regained.

Nutrition Therapy

The first goal of nutrition therapy is to gain the patient's cooperation and trust, in order to increase oral food intake. Ideally, weight gain must be enough to raise the metabolic rate to normal and reverse as many physical signs of the disease as possible. Food intake is designed first to minimize or stop any further weight loss. Then the focus shifts to restoring appropriate food habits. After this, the expectation can be switched to slow weight gain. A range of 2 to 3 pounds per week is appropriate. Tube feeding and/or total parenteral nutrition support is used only if immediate renourishment is required, as this can cause the patient to distrust medical staff.

Patients need considerable reassurance during the refeeding process because of uncomfortable effects, such as bloating, increase in body heat, and increase in body fat. This is a frightening process because these changes can lead to the patient feeling out of control. Monitoring for rapid changes in electrolytes and minerals in the blood, especially potassium, phosphorus, and magnesium, is critically important during the process of incorporating more food into the diet.

In addition to helping patients reach and maintain adequate nutritional status, the registered dietitian on the medical team also provides accurate nutrition information throughout treatment, promotes a healthy attitude toward food, and helps the patient learn to eat based on natural hunger and satiety. Therapy with many anorexic persons can be frustrating for a dietitian because many of those affected are knowledgeable regarding the calorie and fat gram content of most food products. The focus should be on helping these patients identify healthy and adequate food choices that promote weight gain to achieve and maintain a clinically-estimated goal weight (e.g., BMI of 20 or more). The medical team also should assure patients that they will not be abandoned after gaining weight.

Because excessive energy expenditure prevents weight gain, professionals must work with anorexic patients to help them moderate their activity. At many treatment centers, patients are placed on moderate bed rest in the early stages of treatment to help promote weight gain.

Experienced professional help is the key. An anorexic patient may be on the verge of suicide and near starvation. Today, suicide is the most common cause of death in people with anorexia nervosa. In addition, anorexic people are often very clever and resistant. They may try to hide weight loss by wearing many layers of clothes, putting coins in their pockets, and drinking numerous glasses of water.

A young woman in a self-help group for those with anorexia nervosa explained her feelings to the other group members: "I have lost a specialness that I thought it gave me. I was different from everyone else. Now I know that I'm somebody who's overcome it, which not everybody does."

Psychological and Related Therapy

Once the physical problems of anorexic patients are addressed, the treatment focus shifts to the underlying emotional problems that led to excessive dieting and other symptoms of the disorder. To heal, these patients must reject the sense of accomplishment associated with an emaciated body and begin to accept oneself at an increased body weight. If therapists can discover reasons for the disorder, they can develop strategies for restoring normal weight and eating habits by resolving psychological conflicts. Education about the medical consequences of semistarvation is also helpful. A key aspect of psychological treatment is showing affected individuals how to regain control of some facets of their lives and cope with tough situations. As eating evolves into a normal routine, they then can turn to previously neglected activities.

Therapists may use **cognitive behavior therapy,** which involves helping the person confront and change irrational beliefs about body image, eating, relationships, and weight. Underlying issues that may be the cause for the disease, such as sexual abuse, must be identified and addressed by the therapist.

Family therapy often is important in treating anorexia nervosa, especially for younger patients who still live with their families. It focuses on the role of the illness among family members, the reactions of individual family members, and ways in which their subconscious behavior might contribute to the abnormal eating patterns. Therapy includes all family members involved with the behavior problem. Frequently, a therapist finds family struggles at the heart of the problem. As the disorder resolves, patients must relate to family members in new ways to gain the attention previously tied to the disease. For example, the family may need to help the young person ease into adulthood and accept its responsibilities as well as its advantages.

Self-help groups for anorexic (and bulimic) people, as well as their families and friends, represent nonthreatening first steps into treatment. People can also attend to get a sense of whether they really do have an eating disorder.

Medications are generally not effective in treating the primary symptoms of anorexia nervosa. Fluoxetine (Prozac) may stabilize recovery in patients with anorexia who have attained 85% of their expected body weight. Prozac works by prolonging serotonin activity in the brain, which in turn regulates mood and feelings of satiety. A variety of other pharmacologic agents may have some role in treating mood changes, anxiety, or psychotic symptoms associated with anorexia nervosa but have limited value in patients unless weight gain is also achieved. Food is the drug of choice for treating anorexic patients.

With professional help, many people with anorexia nervosa can lead normal lives. They then do not have to depend on unusual eating habits to cope with daily problems. Although they may not be totally cured, they do recover a sense of normality in their lives. No set answers or approaches exist, because each case is different. Establishing a strong relationship with either a therapist or another supportive person is an especially important key to recovery. Once anorexic patients feel understood and accepted by another person, they can begin to build a sense of self and exercise some autonomy. Then they can progress to substituting healthy relationships with others for a relationship with food, emphasizing alternative coping mechanisms.

Scenario *Follow-Up*

Sarah does have the characteristics to be diagnosed with anorexia nervosa because she refuses to maintain a healthy body weight-for-height, is at a weight below 85% of that expected, has a distorted view of her appearance, and has had no menstrual periods for over 3 consecutive months.

Sarah would need to be hospitalized initially, due to her low BMI of 13.8. While in the hospital, her treatment would most likely consist of moderate bed rest to promote weight gain and an intake of 1000 to 1600 kcal initially, which is then increased by increments of about 100 to 200 kcal every few days until an acceptable rate of weight gain is achieved.

cognitive behavior therapy Psychological therapy in which the person's assumptions about dieting, body weight, and related issues are challenged. New ways of thinking are explored and then practiced by the person. In this way, the person can learn new ways to control disordered eating behaviors and related life stress.

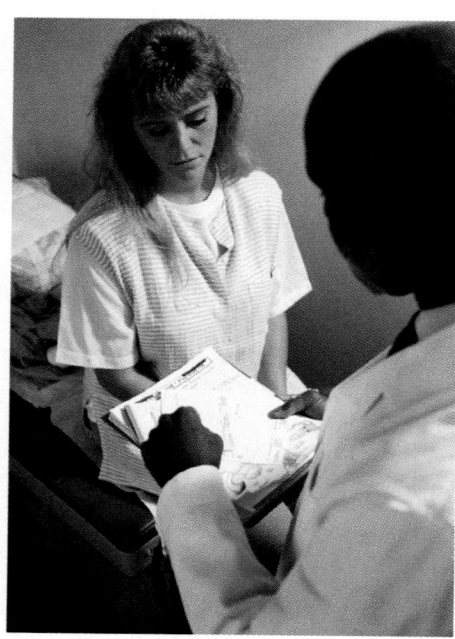

Early treatment for an eating disorder, such as anorexia nervosa, improves chances of success.

The goal is to achieve a body weight that is at least 90% of an expected weight for her age, such as a BMI of at least 19. This weight goal should also allow for resumption of menstrual periods. The physician would likely prescribe a multivitamin and mineral supplement, along with supplements of calcium as needed to make sure intake is in the range of 1200-1500 milligrams. This will correct vitamin and mineral deficiencies that exist, and the calcium will contribute to bone maintenance. A team of health professionals, most likely consisting of a physician, registered dietitian, and psychologist, would provide therapy. Sarah's cooperation would be the most important element for therapy to be successful. She needs to realize she has a problem and that she needs help, and she must be willing to accept the assistance these professionals are willing to offer. The team, especially the psychologist, may use cognitive behavior therapy to help Sarah improve her self-image.

Sarah's outlook for recovery is not good, unless she realizes she has a problem. Even if she is willing to accept the therapy and counseling, a relapse is likely to occur. Only about 50% of anorexia nervosa patients have been found to fully recover from the disease. Since Sarah's disordered eating habits have been in place for about 6 years, her problem is deep-rooted. The chances of recovery are greater if a vigorus treatment program is reinforced with close follow-up.

Singer Karen Carpenter's death from complications of anorexia nervosa in 1983 increased awareness of the serious nature of this disease. Currently, the average time for recovery from anorexia nervosa is 7 years; many insurance companies cover only a fraction of the estimated $150,000 cost of such treatment.

Concept Check

*T*o relieve the semistarved condition of most anorexic patients, the initial treatment focuses on moderately increased food intake and slow weight gain. Once this is accomplished, psychotherapy can begin to uncover the causes of the disease and help patients develop the skills needed to return to a healthy life. Family therapy can be an important tool in treatment, whereas medications have a limited role.

Bulimia Nervosa

Bulimia nervosa involves episodes of binge eating followed by various means to purge the food. This eating disorder was first described in the medical literature in 1979 and classified as a clinical psychiatric disorder in 1980. It is most common among young adults of college age, although some high school students are also at risk. Susceptible people often have genetic factors and lifestyle patterns that predispose them to becoming overweight, and many try frequent weight-reduction diets as teenagers. Like people with anorexia nervosa, those with bulimia nervosa are usually female and successful. Unlike anorexics, however, they are usually at or slightly above a normal weight. Females with bulimia nervosa are also more likely to be sexually active than those with anorexia nervosa.

The person with bulimia nervosa may think of food constantly. In contrast to the anorexic person, who turns away from food when faced with problems, the bulimic person turns toward food in critical situations. Also, unlike those with anorexia nervosa, people with bulimia nervosa recognize their behavior as abnormal. These people often have very low self-esteem and are depressed. Approximately half of the people with bulimia nervosa have major depression. Lingering effects of child abuse may be one reason for these feelings. Many bulimic persons report that they have been sexually abused. The world sees their competence, while inside they feel out of control, ashamed, and frustrated.

Bulimic people tend to be impulsive, which may be expressed as stealing, drug and alcohol abuse, self-mutilation, or attempted suicide. Some experts have suggested that part of the problem may actually arise from an inability to control responses to impulse and desire. Some studies have demonstrated that bulimic people tend to come from disengaged families—ones that are loosely organized. Roles for family members are not clearly defined. Too little protection is provided for family members, rules are very loose, and a great deal of conflict exists. Anorexic people in comparison tend to have families so actively engaged that roles may be too well defined.

Bingeing and purging (via vomiting) was evident in pre-Christian Roman times, but was practiced in a group setting. The eating disorder bulimia nervosa is generally practiced in private.

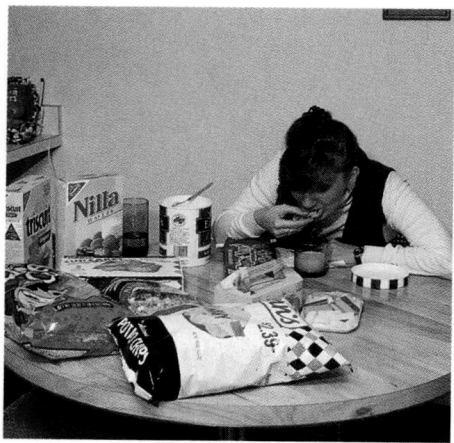

Figure 12.5   The binge-purge cycle can lead to a sense of helplessness.

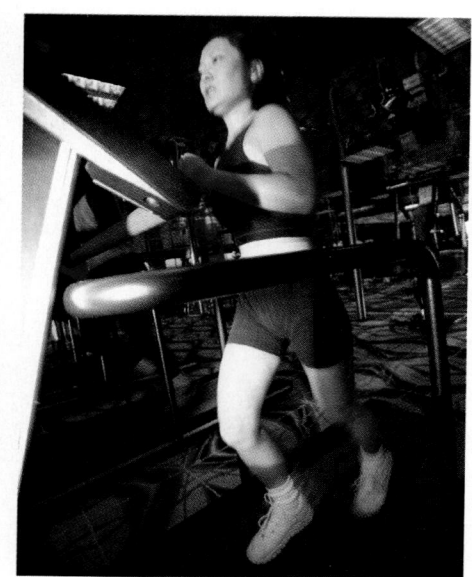

Excessive exercising can be one component of bulimia if it is used as a way to offset the calorie intake from a binge. Exercise is considered excessive when it is done at inappropriate times or settings, or when a person does it despite injury or other medical complications.

■ Typical Behavior in Bulimia Nervosa

Many people with bulimic behavior are probably never diagnosed. The strict diagnostic criteria specify that, in order to be classified as having bulimia nervosa, a person must binge and purge at least twice a week for 3 months. People with bulimia nervosa lead secret lives, hiding their abnormal eating habits. Moreover, it is impossible to recognize people with bulimia nervosa simply from their appearance. Because most diagnoses of bulimia nervosa are based on self-reports, current estimates of the number of cases are probably low. The disorder, especially in its milder forms, may be much more widespread than commonly thought.

Among sufferers of bulimia nervosa, bingeing often alternates with attempts to rigidly restrict food intake. Elaborate food rules are common, such as avoiding all sweets. Thus, eating just one cookie or donut may cause bulimic persons to feel they have broken a rule. Then the objectionable food must be eliminated. Usually, this leads to further overeating, partly because it is easier to regurgitate a large amount of food than a small amount. For intake to qualify as a binge, an atypically large amount of food must be consumed in a short time, and the person must exhibit a lack of control over this behavior.

Binge-purge cycles may be practiced daily, weekly, or at longer intervals. A special time is often set aside. Most binge eating occurs at night, when other people are less likely to interrupt, and usually lasts from ½ to 2 hours. A binge can be triggered by a combination of hunger from recent dieting, stress, boredom, loneliness, and depression. It often follows a period of strict dieting and thus can be linked to intense hunger. The binge is not at all like normal eating; once begun, it seems to propel itself. The person not only loses control but generally doesn't even taste or enjoy the food that is eaten during a binge (Fig. 12.5). This separates the practice from simple overeating.

Most commonly, bulimic people consume cakes, cookies, ice cream, and similar high-carbohydrate convenience foods during binges because these foods can be purged relatively easily and comfortably by vomiting. In a single binge, foods supplying up to 3,000 kcal or more may be eaten. Purging follows in hopes that no weight will be gained. However, even when vomiting follows the binge, 33% to 75% of the food energy taken in is still absorbed, which causes some weight gain. When laxatives or enemas are used, about 90% of the energy is absorbed, as these act in the large intestine, beyond the point of most nutrient absorption. The common belief of bulimic persons that purging soon after bingeing will prevent excessive energy absorption and weight gain is clearly a misperception.

Early in the onset of bulimia nervosa, sufferers often induce vomiting by placing their fingers deep into the mouth. They may inadvertently bite down on these fingers. The resulting bite marks around the knuckles are a characteristic sign of this disorder. Once the disease is established, however, a person can often vomit simply by contracting the abdominal muscles. Vomiting may also occur spontaneously.

Another way bulimic people attempt to compensate for a binge is by engaging in excessive exercise to expend a large amount of energy. Some bulimic people try to estimate the amount of energy eaten in a binge and then exercise to counteract this energy intake. This practice, referred to as "debting," represents an effort to control their weight.

People with bulimia nervosa are not proud of their behavior. After a binge, they usually feel guilty and depressed. Over time, they experience low self-esteem and feel hopeless about their situation (Fig. 12.6). Compulsive lying and drug abuse can further intensify these feelings. Bulimic people caught in the act of bingeing by a friend or family member may order the intruder to "get out" and "go away." Sufferers gradually distance themselves from others, spending more and more time preoccupied by and engaging in bingeing and purging.

Anxiety

Bingeing

Guilt

Fear of
fat gain

Loss of fear
of fat gain

Purging

Figure 12.6 Bulimia nervosa's vicious
cycle of obsession.

■ Health Problems Stemming from Bulimia Nervosa

The vomiting that many bulimic sufferers induce is the most physically destructive method of purging. Indeed, the majority of health problems associated with bulimia nervosa arise from vomiting:

- Repeated exposure of teeth to the acid in vomit causes demineralization, making the teeth painful and sensitive to heat, cold, and acids. Eventually, the teeth may severely decay, erode away from fillings, and finally fall out. Dental professionals are sometimes the first health professionals to notice signs of bulimia nervosa (Fig. 12.7). Until vomiting ceases, it is important to rinse the mouth with water after a vomiting episode, especially before brushing the teeth.
- Blood potassium can drop significantly with regular vomiting or the use of certain diuretics. This can disturb the heart's rhythm and even produce sudden death.
- Salivary glands may swell as a result of infection and irritation from persistent vomiting.
- Stomach ulcers and bleeding and tears in the esophagus develop in some cases.
- Constipation may result from frequent laxative use.
- Ipecac syrup, sometimes used to induce vomiting, is toxic to the heart, liver, and kidneys. It has caused accidental poisoning when taken repeatedly.

Overall, bulimia nervosa is a potentially debilitating disorder that can lead to death, usually from suicide, low blood potassium, or overwhelming infections.

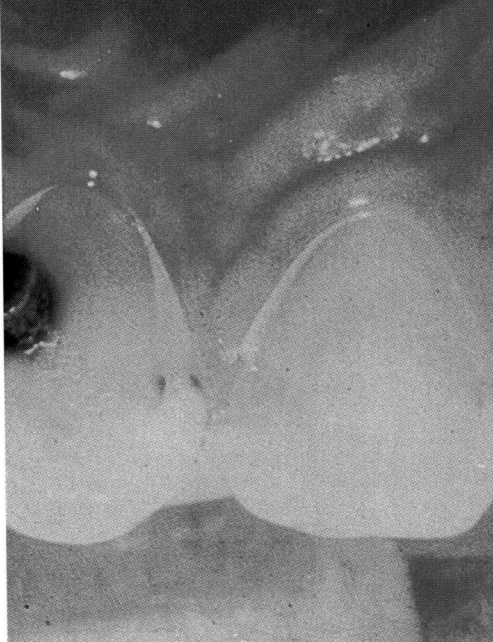

Figure 12.7 Excessive tooth decay is common in bulimic patients.

Thoughts of a Bulimic Woman

I am wide awake and immediately out of bed. I think back to the night before, when I made a new list of what I wanted to get done and how I wanted to be. My husband is not far behind me on his way into the bathroom to get ready for work. Maybe I can sneak onto the scale to see what I weigh this morning before he notices me. I am already in my private world. I feel overjoyed when the scale says that I stayed the same weight as I was the night before, and I can feel that slightly hungry feeling. Maybe it will stop today; maybe today everything will change. What were the projects I was going to get done?

We eat the same breakfast, except that I take no butter on my toast, no cream in my coffee, and never take seconds (until Doug gets out the door). Today I am going to be really good, and that means eating certain predetermined portions of food and not taking one more bite than I think I am allowed. I am very careful to see that I don't take more than Doug. I judge myself by his body. I can feel the tension building. I wish Doug would hurry up and leave so I can get going!

As soon as he shuts the door, I try to get involved with one of the myriad responsibilities on my list. I hate them all! I just want to crawl into a hole. I don't want to do anything. I'd rather eat. I am

alone; I am nervous; I am no good; I always do everything wrong anyway; I am not in control; I can't make it through the day, I know it. It has been the same for so long. I remember the starchy cereal I ate for breakfast. I am into the bathroom and onto the scale. It measures the same, but I don't want to stay the same! I want to be thinner! I look into the mirror. I think my thighs are ugly and deformed looking. I see a lumpy, clumsy, pear-shaped wimp. There is always something wrong with what I see. I feel frustrated, trapped in this body, and I don't know what to do about it.

I float to the refrigerator knowing exactly what is there. I begin with last night's brownies. I always begin with the sweets. At first I try to make it look like nothing is missing, but my appetite is huge and I resolve to make another batch of brownies. I know there is half of a bag of cookies in the bathroom, thrown out the night before, and I polish them off immediately. I take some milk so my vomiting will be smoother. I like the full feeling I get after downing a big glass. I get out six pieces of bread and toast one side of each in the broiler, turn them over and load them with pats of butter, and put them under the broiler again until they are bubbling. I take all six pieces on a plate to the television and go back for a bowl of

cereal and a banana to have along with them. Before the last piece of toast is finished, I am already preparing the next batch of six more pieces. Maybe another brownie or five, and a couple of large bowls full of ice cream, yogurt, or cottage cheese.

My stomach is stretched into a huge ball below my rib cage. I know I'll have to go into the bathroom soon, but I want to postpone it. I am in never-never land. I am waiting, feeling the pressure, pacing the floor in and out of the rooms. Time is passing. Time is passing. It is getting to be time. I wander aimlessly through each of the rooms again, tidying, making the whole house neat and put back together. I finally make the turn into the bathroom. I brace my feet, pull my hair back and stick my finger down my throat, stroking twice, and get up a huge pile of food. Three times, four times, and another pile of food. I can see everything come back. I am so glad to see those brownies because they are so fattening. The rhythm of the emptying is broken and my head is beginning to hurt. I stand up feeling dizzy, empty, and weak. The whole episode has taken about an hour.

From Hall L, Cohn L: Bulimia—a guide to recovery, Carlsbad, CA, 1992, Gurze Books.

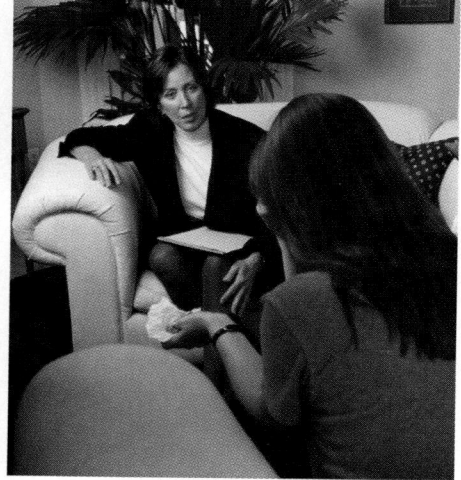

Bulimia nervosa affects many college students. Counselors are aware of this and are available to help.

■ Treatment of Bulimia Nervosa

Therapy for bulimia nervosa, as for anorexia nervosa, requires a team of experienced clinicians. These patients are less likely than those with anorexia to enter treatment in a state of semistarvation. However, if a bulimic patient has lost significant weight, this must be treated before psychological treatment begins. Although clinicians have yet to agree on the best therapy for bulimia nervosa, they generally agree that treatment should last at least 16 weeks. Hospitalization may be indicated in cases of extreme laxative abuse, regular vomiting, substance abuse, and depression, especially if physical harm is evident.

The first goal of treatment for bulimia nervosa is to decrease the amount of food consumed in a binge session in order to decrease the risk of esophageal tears from related purging by vomiting. A decrease in the number of this type of purges will also decrease damage to the teeth.

The primary aim of psychotherapy is to improve patients' self-acceptance and help them to be less concerned about body weight. Cognitive behavior therapy is generally used. Psychotherapy helps correct the all-or-none thinking typical of bulimic persons—"If I eat one cookie, I'm a failure and might as well binge." A patient may be asked to analyze the statement as a scientist would do when testing assumptions. In this way, patient and therapist together examine the validity of food and weight beliefs. The premise of this therapy is that, if abnormal attitudes and beliefs can be altered, normal eating will follow. In addition, the therapist guides the person in establishing food habits that will minimize bingeing: avoiding fasting, eating regular meals, and using alternative methods—other than eating—to cope with stressful situations. Group therapy is often useful to foster strong social support. One goal of therapy is to help bulimic persons accept as normal some depression and self-doubt.

Although pharmacological agents should not be used as the sole treatment for bulimia nervosa, studies indicate that some medications may be beneficial in conjunction with other therapies. Fluoxetine (Prozac) is the only antidepressant that has been approved by FDA for use in the treatment of bulimia nervosa, but physicians also may prescribe other forms of antidepressants and related medications.

Nutritional counseling has two main goals: correcting misconceptions about food and re-establishing regular eating habits. Patients are given information about bulimia nervosa and its consequences. Avoiding binge foods and not constantly stepping on a scale may be recommended early in treatment. The primary goal, however, is to develop a normal eating pattern. To achieve this goal, some specialists encourage patients to develop daily meal plans and keep a food diary in which they record food intake, internal sensations of hunger, environmental factors that precipitate binges, and thoughts and feelings that accompany binge-purge cycles. Keeping a food diary not only is an accurate way to monitor food intake but also may help identify situations that seem to trigger binge episodes. With the help of a therapist, patients can develop alternative coping strategies.

In general, the focus is not on stopping bingeing and purging per se but on developing regular eating habits. Once this is achieved, the binge-purge cycle should stop by itself. Patients are discouraged from following strict rules about healthy food choices, because this simply mimics the typical obsessive attitudes associated with bulimia nervosa. Rather, encouraging a mature perspective on nutrient intake—that is, regular consumption of moderate amounts of a variety of foods balanced among the food groups—helps patients overcome this disorder.

Setting time limits for the completion of meals and snacks is important for people with eating disorders. Many bulimic persons eat very quickly, reflecting their difficulties with satiety. Suggesting that the patient put his or her utensil down after each bite is a behavioral technique that a therapist might try with a recovering bulimic person. (In comparison, many anorexic persons eat in an excessively slow manner—for example, taking 1 hour to eat a muffin because it was cut into tiny, bite-size pieces.)

People with bulimia nervosa must recognize that it is a serious disorder that can have grave medical complications if not treated. Because relapse is likely, therapy should be long term. Note that those with bulimia nervosa need professional help because they can be very depressed and are at a high risk for suicide. About 50% of people with bulimia nervosa recover completely from the disorder. Others continue to struggle with it to varying degrees for the rest of their lives. This fact underscores the need for prevention because treatment is difficult.

The binge-purge cycle can create an initial state of euphoria in the person. Giving up this euphoria has been equated to giving up an addiction. Still, it is important to do so.

Concept Check

Bulimia nervosa is characterized by episodes of binge eating followed by purging, usually by vomiting. Vomiting is very destructive to the body, often causing severe dental decay, stomach ulcers, irritation of the esophagus, and blood potassium imbalances. Treatment using nutrition counseling and psychotherapy attempts to restore normal eating habits, to help the person correct distorted beliefs about diet and lifestyle, and to find tools to cope with the stresses of life. Medications, such as fluoxetine (Prozac), can aid recovery when added to this regimen.

Other Examples of Disordered Eating: Female Athlete Triad, Binge-Eating Disorder, and Baryophobia

female athlete triad A condition characterized by disordered eating, lack of menstrual periods, and osteoporosis.

baryophobia A disorder of young children and young adults characterized by stunted growth. It results from parental underfeeding in an attempt to prevent the development of obesity and heart disease.

A female high school athlete recently admitted to a 3-year struggle with anorexia nervosa and bulimia nervosa. Even after her athletic performance declined and she suffered a related sports injury, which sidelined her for a year and required surgery, she continued to think that controlling both her weight and eating behaviors would make her the best—academically and physically. This example demonstrates several important points about eating disorders: certain groups of people are at greater risk for developing eating disorders; these people are often high achievers and are very careful about concealing their eating disorder; and eating disorders such as the female athlete triad, bulimia nervosa, and anorexia nervosa frequently overlap.

In recent years, three other eating disorders—**female athlete triad**, binge-eating disorder, and **baryophobia**—have been recognized as requiring professional treatment. Although these disordered eating patterns share some characteristics with anorexia nervosa and bulimia nervosa, each has distinctive qualities.

▪ Female Athlete Triad

Women participating in appearance-based and endurance sports are at risk of developing an eating disorder. A study of college-age female athletes found that 15% of swimmers, 62% of gymnasts, and 32% of all varsity athletes exhibited disordered eating patterns. Estimates of eating disorders for college women not involved in competitive sports are much lower.

In addition to disordered eating, college women athletes tend to experience irregular menstruation more frequently than other college women. Disordered eating, particularly food restriction and stress, can precipitate this, causing women to have less dense and weaker bones than normal because of lower estrogen concentrations in the blood. Some of these young women have bones equivalent to those of 50- to 60-year-olds, making them overly susceptible to bone and stress fractures during both sports and general activities. Much of the bone loss is irreversible.

The American College of Sports Medicine (ACSM) has named the syndrome female athlete triad because it consists of three parts: disordered eating, lack of menstrual periods, and osteoporosis (Fig. 12.8). The ACSM has issued a call to teachers, coaches, health professionals, and parents to educate female athletes about the triad and its health consequences.

Many coaches/trainers and even some health professionals wrongly believe that loss of menstrual periods is a normal consequence of a high level of physical activity. However, this loss of menstrual periods has negative consequences on the body, such as fragile bones, as just mentioned. Correcting menstrual irregularities by increasing caloric intake should help normalize hormone levels and increase bone mineral density. During therapy, a physician may prescribe a multivitamin and mineral supplement as well as calcium supplements as needed to maintain an intake of 1200–1500 milligrams, as mentioned for treatment of anorexia nervosa in the answer to the Real Life Scenario.

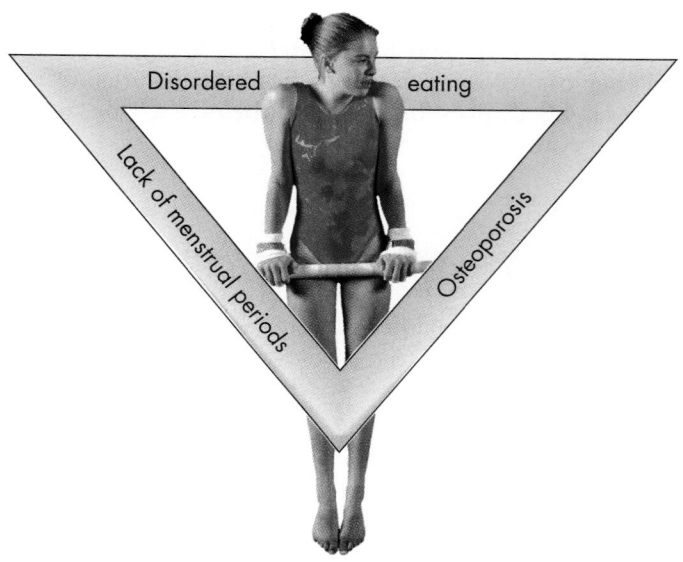

Figure 12.8 The female athlete triad occurs when the athlete has disordered eating, lack of menstrual periods, and osteoporosis. Stress fractures and recurrent fatigue also occur. This triad often is seen in appearance-related sports, such as gymnastics. Long-term health is at risk; thus, early treatment is most beneficial.

Those exhibiting symptoms should seek treatment from a multidisciplinary team of health professionals. Involving the coach or trainer in therapy is usually a key factor in the success of the treatment plan. Suggestions for treatment are as follows:

- Reduce preoccupation with food, weight, and body fat.
- Gradually increase meals and snacks to an appropriate amount.
- Achieve an appropriate weight-for-height.
- Establish regular menstrual periods.
- Decrease training time and/or intensity by 10% to 20%.

*I*t is often difficult to get female athletes to accept this advice. They can have a single-minded approach to their sport, while ignoring future health consequences.

Another Bite

*T*he tragic case of Christy Henrich illustrates why anyone at risk for the female athlete triad should seek professional help. As a young teenager, Christy weighed 95 pounds and was 4 feet 11 inches tall. She showed promise as a gymnast but was told that she was too fat to excel in gymnastics. Christy continued her training but often starved herself, some days consuming just an apple and frequently purging by vomiting. Her success in gymnastics continued, but at age 22 her weight had fallen to 52 pounds, and she died from the effects of long-term semistarvation.

■ Binge-Eating Disorder

In 1994, binge-eating disorder, commonly called *compulsive overeating*, was formally recognized by the American Psychiatric Association. The typical characteristics for this disorder are listed in Table 12.2. Generally, it can be defined as binge-eating episodes not accompanied by purging (as typifies bulimia nervosa) at least two times per week for at least 6 months. Today health-care professionals recognize this condition as a complex and potentially serious problem.

Approximately 30% to 50% of subjects in organized weight-control programs have binge-eating disorder, whereas among the general North American population about 1% to 2% have this disorder. However, many more people in the general population are likely to have less severe forms of the disorder that do not meet the formal criteria for diagnosis. The number of cases of binge-eating disorder is far greater than that of

Table 12.2 Some Characteristics of Binge-Eating Disorder

A. Recurrent episodes of binge eating, an episode being characterized by both of the following:

   (1) Eating, in a discrete period of time (e.g., within any 2-hour period), an amount of food that is definitely larger than most people would eat during a similar period of time in similar circumstances

   (2) A sense of lack of control during the episodes (e.g., a feeling that one can't stop eating or control what or how much one is eating)

B. During most binge episodes, at least three of the following occur:

   (1) Eating much more rapidly than usual

   (2) Eating until feeling uncomfortably full

   (3) Eating large amounts of food when not feeling physically hungry

   (4) Eating alone because of being embarrassed by how much one is eating

   (5) Feeling disgusted with oneself, depressed, or very guilty after overeating

C. Marked distress regarding binge eating

D. The binge eating occurs, on average, at least 2 days a week for 6 months.

E. The behavior does not occur only during the course of bulimia nervosa or anorexia nervosa.

Based on information from the *Diagnostic and Statistical Manual of Mental Disorders,* Fourth Edition (DSM-IV-TR). American Psychiatric Association, Washington DC, 2000.

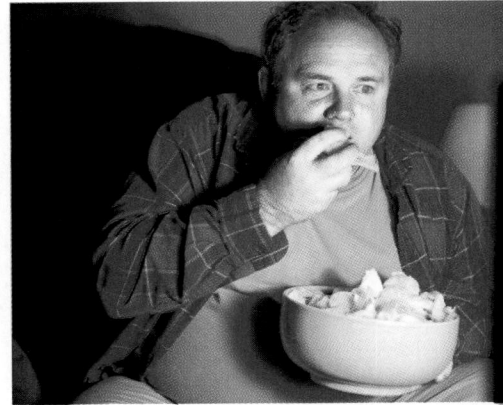

Binge-eating disorder is seen in both men and women.

either anorexia nervosa or bulimia nervosa. This disorder is also more common among the severely obese and those with a long history of frequent restrictive dieting.

Development and Characteristics of Binge-Eating Disorder

Individuals with binge-eating disorder (about 40% of whom are males) often perceive themselves as hungry more often than normal. They usually started dieting at a young age, began bingeing during adolescence or in their early 20s, and did not succeed in commercial weight-control programs. Almost half of those with severe binge-eating disorder exhibit clinical depression.

Typical binge eaters isolate themselves and eat large quantities of a favorite food. Stressful events and feelings of depression or anxiety can trigger this behavior. Giving themselves permission to eat a forbidden food can also precipitate a binge. Other triggers include loneliness, anxiety, self-pity, depression, anger, rage, alienation, and frustration. They sometimes binge on whatever is easy to eat in large amounts—noodles, rice, bread, leftovers. Characteristically, however, binge eaters consume foods that carry the social stigma of "junk" or "bad" foods—ice cream, cookies, sweets, potato chips, and similar snack foods.

In general, people engage in binge eating to induce a sense of well-being and perhaps even numbness, usually in an attempt to avoid feeling and dealing with emotional pain and anxiety. They eat without regard to biological need and often in a recurrent, ritualized fashion. Some people with this disorder eat food continually over an extended period, called *grazing*; others cycle episodes of bingeing with normal eating. For example, someone with a stressful or frustrating job might come home every night and graze until bedtime. Another person might eat normally most of the time but find comfort in consuming large quantities of food when an emotional setback occurs.

Spreading one's dietary intake into numerous, small meals (grazing) over a day does not pose a problem if overall energy intake remains appropriate.

Although people with anorexia nervosa and bulimia nervosa exhibit persistent preoccupation with body shape, weight, and thinness, binge eaters do not necessarily share these concerns. Thus, neither purging nor prolonged food restriction is characteristic of binge-eating disorder. Some physicians classify binge-eating disorder as an addiction to food, involving psychological dependence. The person becomes attached to the behavior itself and has a drive to continue it, senses only limited control over it, and needs to persist at it despite negative consequences. Food is used to reduce stress, produce feelings of power and well-being, avoid feelings of intimacy with others, and avoid life problems. Note that obesity and binge eating are not necessarily linked. Not all obese people are binge eaters, and, although obesity may result from trying to numb emotional pain with food, it is not necessarily an outcome.

Binge-eating disorder is most likely to develop in people who never learned to express and deal appropriately with their feelings. Rather than face their problems, they turn to food. They continue to do the things that perpetuate the experiences of frustration, anger, and pain. For example, people who regularly become frustrated because they don't assert themselves when necessary may eat to forget their frustration rather than learn to deal with this inhibition and practice assertiveness. The frustration will continue because they never attack the basic problem. Binge eating makes them feel they cannot control the behavior pattern and therefore cannot control their lives. Worse, the binge eating usually increases feelings of guilt, embarrassment, and shame.

People with binge-eating disorder may come from families with alcoholism or may have suffered sexual abuse. Members of such dysfunctional families often do not know how to deal effectively with emotions. They cope by turning to substances. Family members learn to cover up dysfunctional patterns for the alcoholic person and to nurture him or her at the expense of each other and their own needs.

Often, people who practice binge eating have been shaped by families who do not address and express feelings in healthful ways. The parents nurture and comfort their children with food rather than engage in healthy exchanges of self-disclosure of feelings and potential solutions. Members of such families learn to eat in response to emotional needs and pain instead of hunger. Those who regularly practice binge eating may grow up nurturing others instead of themselves, avoiding their own feelings and taking little time for themselves. Not knowing how to satisfy their personal and emotional needs in more healthful ways, people in these families turn to food.

For some people, frequent dieting beginning in childhood or adolescence is a precursor to binge-eating disorder. During periods when little food is eaten, they get very hungry and obsessive about food. When allowed to eat more food, they feel driven to eat in a compulsive, uncontrolled way. The pattern of periods of strict dieting alternating with binge eating may continue over time.

Help for the Person with Binge-Eating Disorder

Those with binge-eating disorder must learn to eat in response to hunger—a biological signal—rather than in response to emotional needs or external factors (such as the time of day or the simple presence of food). Counselors often direct binge eaters to record their perceptions of physical hunger throughout the day and at the beginning and end of every meal. These people must learn to respond to a prescribed amount of fullness at each meal. They should initially avoid weight-loss diets because feelings of food deprivation can lead to more disruptive emotions and a greater sense of unmet needs. Diets are likely to encourage more intense problems, such as extreme hunger. Many people with binge-eating disorder may experience difficulty in identifying personal emotional needs and expressing emotions. Because this problem is a common predisposing factor in binge eating, communication issues should be addressed during treatment. Binge eaters often must be helped to recognize their own buried emotions in anxiety-producing situations, and then encouraged to share them with their therapist or therapy group. Learning simple but appropriate phrases to say to oneself can help stop bingeing when the desire is strong.

Self-help groups, such as Overeaters Anonymous, aim to help recovery from binge-eating disorder. The treatment philosophy parallels that of Alcoholics Anonymous. Overeaters Anonymous attempts to create an environment of encouragement and accountability to overcome this eating disorder. Dietary advice typically ranges from avoiding restraint in eating to limiting binge foods. Some experts feel that learning to eat all foods—but in moderation—is an effective goal for binge eaters. This practice can prevent the feelings of desperation and deprivation that come from limiting particular foods. Antidepressants, such as fluoxetine (Prozac), and other types of medications also have been found to help reduce binge eating in these individuals by decreasing depression. Overall, people who have this disorder are usually unsuccessful in controlling it on their own. Professional help is advised.

■ Baryophobia

Some children and young adults who grow more slowly and have a shorter stature than normal may suffer from baryophobia (literally, "the fear of becoming heavy"). Inadequate growth in children usually results from disease—commonly, a hormonal or other metabolic abnormality. In the absence of a recognized disease in such children, the possibility of baryophobia should be investigated.

This disorder occurs when children are given the same low-fat, high-carbohydrate diet that adults follow. Adults do this in an attempt to prevent children from developing obesity or cardiovascular disease later in life. Today's parents and caregivers, themselves frequently harassed by weight problems, may be determined that the children in their care will avoid such ordeals. Although these caregivers are well intended, such severely restricted diets are detrimental to children because they don't supply enough energy to sustain an adequate growth rate. In young adults, low-energy diets may be self-imposed to avoid a perceived risk of obesity.

Because this disorder results largely from lack of appropriate nutrition information leading to poor food choices, nutritional counseling to caregivers and young adults is the most effective response. They need to be informed about the nutrient requirements and normal weight-gain patterns for the relevant age group. This counseling will show caregivers that including some sweets and medium-fat foods in a child's diet is appropriate (see Chapter 14). The diet can still minimize saturated fat and cholesterol intake, a more important focus in a diet designed to reduce the risk of cardiovascular disease. Supplying adequate carbohydrate, protein, fat, and other nutrients is the key to promoting growth in both height and weight during childhood and the young-adult years, and it can be done in a healthful manner.

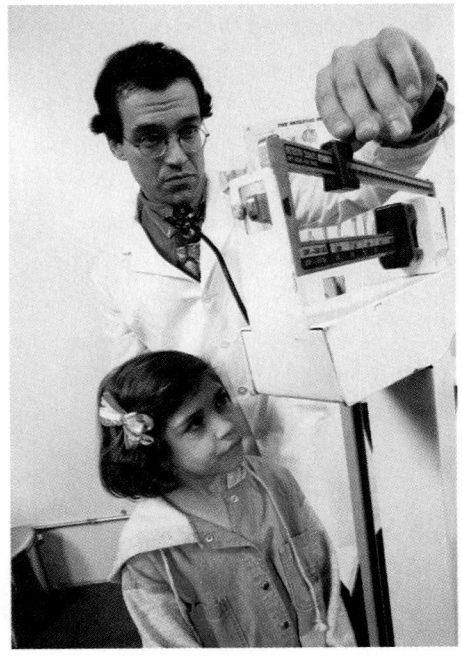

A slowdown in gains in weight and height for one's predicted age can be a sign of baryophobia. If noted, this and other causes deserve further scrutiny.

Critical Thinking

Tom, a high school teacher, is concerned about eating disorders. He wants to try to prevent young adults from falling into the discouraging traps of anorexia nervosa and bulimia nervosa. What are some of the topics and issues he should discuss with students in his health classes?

Not only is treatment of eating disorders far more difficult than prevention, these disorders also have devastating effects on the entire family. For this reason, caregivers and health-care professionals alike must emphasize the importance of an overall healthful diet and moderation, as opposed to restriction and perfection.

Prevention of Eating Disorders

A key to developing and maintaining healthful eating behavior is to realize that some concern about diet, health, and weight is normal. It is also normal to experience variation in what we eat, how we feel, and even how much we weigh. For example, it is not abnormal to experience some minimal weight change (up to 2 to 3 pounds) throughout the day and even more over the course of a week. A large weight fluctuation or ongoing weight gain or weight loss is more likely to indicate that a problem is present. If you notice a large change in your diet, how you feel, or your body weight, it is a good idea to consult your personal physician. Treating physical and emotional problems early helps lead you to peace of mind and good health.

With a view to society as a whole, many people begin to form opinions about food, nutrition, health, weight, and body image prior or during puberty. Parents, friends, and professionals working with young adults should consider the following advice for preventing eating disorders:

- Discourage restrictive dieting, meal skipping, and fasting.
- Provide information about normal changes that occur during puberty.
- Correct misconceptions about nutrition, healthy body weight, and approaches to weight loss.
- Carefully phrase weight-related recommendations and comments, and use them with caution.
- Don't overemphasize numbers on a scale. Instead, primarily promote healthful eating irrespective of body weight.
- Encourage normal expression of disruptive emotions.
- Encourage children to eat only when they're hungry.
- Teach the basics of proper nutrition and regular physical activity in school and at home.
- Provide adolescents with an appropriate, but not unlimited, degree of independence, choice, responsibility, and self-accountability for their actions.
- Increase self-acceptance and appreciation of the power and pleasure emerging from one's body.
- Enhance tolerance for diversity in body weight and shape, and personal food choices.
- Build respectful environments, supportive relationships.
- Encourage coaches to be sensitive to weight and body-image issues among athletes.
- Emphasize that thinness is not necessarily associated with better athletic performance.

Our society as a whole can benefit from a fresh focus on healthful food practices and a healthful outlook toward food and body weight.

Concept Check

*T*he female athlete triad consists of disordered eating, amenorrhea, and osteoporosis, particularly those in appearance-related and endurance sports. Parents, coaches, teachers, and health professionals need to initiate efforts to prevent and treat this problem. Grazing and food bingeing without purging are two behaviors characteristic of binge-eating disorder. Emotional disturbances are often at the root of this eating disorder. Treatment addresses deeper emotional issues and endorses avoiding food deprivation and restrictive diets, while restoring more normal eating behaviors. Baryophobia is a condition in which children are underfed by parents in an attempt to limit risk of future disease, such as obesity or cardiovascular disease. Growth failure—lack of expected weight and height gains—can result if nutrient intake is not increased to an appropriate amount.

Books and Organizations to Help You Understand More About Eating Disorders

Along with the technical articles in the references, you can gain more insight into eating disorders from the following sources designed for the lay public:

Books

Andersen A, Cohn L, Holbrook T: *Making weight: Men's conflicts with food, weight, shape, and appearance.* Carlsbad, CA: Gurze Books, 2000.

Barnhill J, Taylor N: *If you think you have an eating disorder.* New York: Dell, 1998.

Berg FM: *Women afraid to eat. Breaking free in today's weight obsessed world.* Hettinger, ND: Healthy Weight Network, 2000.

Costin C: *The eating disorder sourcebook.* Chicago: RGA, 1996.

Gilbert SD, Commeford MC: *The unofficial guide to managing eating disorders.* Foster City, CA: IDG, 2000.

Gordon, RA: *Eating disorders: Anatomy of a social epidemic.* Malden, MA: Blackwell, 2000.

Nash JD: *Binge no more: Your guide to overcoming disordered eating.* Oakland, CA: New Harbinger, 1997.

Robert-McComb JL: *Eating disorders in women and children: Stress management and prevention.* Boca Raton, FL: CRC Press, 2001.

Siegel M, Brisman J, Weinshel M: *Surviving an eating disorder. Strategies for families and friends.* New York: HarperCollins, 1998.

Organizations and Self-Help Groups

Academy for Eating Disorders, 6728 McClean Village Dr., McLean, VA 22101; 703-556-9222; www.acadeatdis.org

American Anorexia Bulimia Association, 165 West 46th St., #1108, New York, NY 10036; 212-575-6200; www.aabainc.org/home.html

Eating Disorders Awareness and Prevention (EDAP), 603 Stewart St., Suite 803, Seattle, WA 98101; 206-382-3587 or 800 931-EDAP; www.edap.org

Harvard Eating Disorders Centers, 356 Boylston St., Boston, MA 02116; 617-236-7766; www.hedc.org

The National Eating Disorders Organization, 6655 South Yale Ave., Tulsa, OK 74136; 918-481-4044; www.laureate.com

The National Institute of Mental Health has recently published a concise review of eating disorders (www.nimh.nih.gov/publicat/eatingdisorder.pdf).

Summary

1. Anorexia nervosa is most common among high-achieving, perfectionist girls from families marked by conflict, high expectations, rigidity, and denial. The disorder usually starts with dieting in early puberty and proceeds to the near-total refusal to eat. Early warning signs include intense concern about weight gain and dieting, as well as abnormal food habits, such as cooking food that they won't allow themselves to eat.

2. Anorexic persons become irritable, hostile, overly critical, and joyless; they tend to withdraw from family and friends. Eventually, anorexia nervosa can lead to numerous physical effects, including a profound decrease in body weight and body fat, a fall in body temperature and heart rate, iron-deficiency anemia, a low white blood cell count, hair loss, constipation, low blood potassium, and the loss of menstrual periods. Those with anorexia nervosa are physically very ill.

3. Treatment of anorexia nervosa includes increasing food intake to support slow weight gain. Psychological counseling attempts to help patients establish regular food habits and to find means of coping with the life stresses that led to the disorder. Hospitalization may be necessary, as well as use of certain medications.

4. Bulimia nervosa is characterized by secretive bingeing on large amounts of food at one sitting and then purging by vomiting or misuse of laxatives, diuretics, or enemas. Alternately fasting and excessive exercise may be used. Both men and women are at risk. Vomiting as a means of purging is especially destructive to the body; it can cause severe tooth decay, stomach ulcers, irritation of the esophagus, low blood potassium, and other problems. Bulimia nervosa poses a serious health problem and is associated with significant risk of suicide.

5. Treatment of bulimia nervosa includes psychological as well as nutritional counseling. During treatment, bulimic persons learn to accept themselves and to cope with problems in ways that do not involve food. Regular eating patterns are developed as these patients begin to plan meals in an informed, healthful manner. Certain medications can be a helpful addition to the regimen.

6. The female athlete triad consists of disordered eating, loss of menstrual periods, and osteoporosis and is particularly common in appearance-related and endurance sports. If not corrected, this disorder eventually leads to decreased athletic performance and general health problems.

7. Binge-eating disorder, which is more widespread than either anorexia nervosa or bulimia nervosa, is most common among people with a history of frequent, unsuccessful dieting. Binge eaters typically either practice grazing (i.e., eating continually over extended periods) or bingeing without purging. Emotional disturbances are often at the root of this disordered form of eating. Treatment addresses deeper emotional issues, discourages food deprivation and restrictive diets, and helps restore normal eating behaviors. Certain medications may be a useful addition to this therapy.

8. Baryophobia is a condition in which children are underfed by caregivers in an attempt to limit the risk of future disease, such as obesity or cardiovascular disease. Growth failure—in weight and height gains—can result if nutrient intake is not increased to appropriate amounts.

Study Questions

1. What are the typical characteristics of a person with anorexia nervosa? What may influence a person to begin rigid, self-imposed dietary patterns?

2. List the detrimental physical and psychological side effects of bulimia nervosa. Describe important goals of the psychological and nutrition therapy used to treat bulimic patients.

3. What is the current thinking concerning medication use for anorexia nervosa and bulimia nervosa?

4. Explain the role of excessive exercise in eating disorders.

5. How might parents significantly contribute to the development of an eating disorder? Suggest an attitude that a parent or an adult friend of yours displayed that may not have been conductive to developing a normal relationship to food.

6. Based on your knowledge of good nutrition and sound dietary habits, answer the following questions:
   a. How can repeated bingeing and purging lead to significant nutrient deficiencies?
   b. How can significant nutrient deficiencies contribute to major health problems in later life?
   c. A friend asks you, the nutrition expert, if it is okay to "cleanse" the body by eating only grapefruit for a week. What is your response?

7. How, in your opinion, has society contributed to the development of various forms of disordered eating? Provide an example.

8. List the three symptoms that constitute the female athlete triad. What is the major health risk associated with loss of menstrual periods in the female athlete?

9. How does binge-eating disorder differ from bulimia nervosa? Describe the factors that contribute to the development and treatment of binge-eating disorder.

10. Describe the common characteristics of a parent of a child with baryophobia.

Further Readings

1. ADA Reports: Position of the American Dietetic Association: Nutrition intervention in the treatment of anorexia nervosa, bulimia nervosa, and eating disorders not otherwise specified (EDNOS). *Journal of the American Dietetic Association* 101:810, 2001.
   Eating disorders are complex and serious illnesses, as described in detail in this article. To be effective in treating individuals who suffer from these illnesses, the expert interaction between professionals in many disciplines is required. The term Eating Disorders Not Otherwise Specified (EDNOS) used in the title includes individuals who do not meet all the criteria for anorexia nervosa or bulimia nervosa, but still exhibit some of the characteristics. This includes people who practice bulimia nervosa but do not consume large amounts of food, and people with binge-eating disorder. To simplify the chapter, this psychiatric classification was not included.

2. American Psychiatric Association: Practice guidelines for the treatment of patients with eating disorders (revision). *American Journal of Psychiatry* 157 (suppl): 4, 2000.
   People with eating disorders display a broad range of symptoms that occur along a continuum from between those of anorexia nervosa and those of bulimia nervosa. The care of these people requires a comprehensive array of approaches to provide the best chance of treatment success.

3. Anderson AE: Recognizing eating disorders, *Nutrition & the M.D.*, p.1, August 1998.
   The ultimate goal for health professionals should be to prevent eating disorders and to free adolescents from the burden of an unnecessary drive for thinness, in turn replacing this cultural insanity with healthy habits of eating and exercise. Detection and treatment of eating disorders are discussed.

4. Becker AE and others: Eating disorders. *The New England Journal of Medicine* 340:1092, 1999.
   All facets of eating disorders, from detection to treatment, are reviewed. This is an excellent reference for more in-depth knowledge of eating disorders. All those with eating disorders should be evaluated and treated for medical complications of the disease at the same time psychotherapy and nutritional counseling are undertaken.

5. Chidley E: Eating disorders, nature or nurture? *Today's Dietitian*, p. 29, February 1999.
   Various studies have shown correlations between genetics and eating disorder development. This new knowledge however is not going to change current therapy. We know that cognitive behavior therapy works for bulimia, and the fact that there are some genes that increase risk for developing the disease isn't going to change that practice.

6. Faine M, Mobley C: Case problem: Balancing nutrition advice with dental care in patients with anorexia and bulimia. *Journal of the American Dietetic Association* 99(10):1291, 1999.
   Extensive loss of tooth enamel is common in people with bulimia nervosa. The authors provide a detailed description of therapy for a patient who presented with an eating disorder and dental health problems.

7. Fairburn CG and others: Risk factors for anorexia nervosa: Three integrated case-control comparisons. *Archives of General Psychiatry* 56:468, 1999.
   Perfectionism and negative self-evaluation are common personality traits associated with an eating disorder.

8. Halmi KA: A 24-year-old with anorexia nervosa. *Journal of the American Medical Association* 279:1992, 1998.
   An in-depth case study of a patient with anorexia nervosa is presented; it focuses on understanding of the psychological aspect of the disease. Also summarized are the causes, disease patterns, clinical course, and treatment of anorexia nervosa.

9. Hobart JA, Smucker DR: The female athlete triad. *American Family Physician* 61(11):3357, 2000.
   The importance of the physician in detecting female athlete triad during a preparticipation sports physical exam is discussed. The author provides helpful hints in obtaining important information from the patient during the exam. Many patients may benefit from a treatment plan that involves consultation with subspecialists. The involvement of a psychiatrist or psychologist and a registered dietitian who specialize in the management of the female athlete triad may allow for prompt improvement.

10. Krowchuk CP and others: Problem dieting behaviors among young adolescents. *Archives of Pediatric & Adolescent Medicine* 152:884, 1998.
    There is a relationship between dieting behaviors in adolescents development of an eating disorder. Younger adolescents trying to lose weight typically engage in a variety of problem dieting and weight loss behaviors that can compromise health and may be associated with eating disorders.

11. Mehler PS: Diagnosis and care of patients with anorexia nervosa in primary care settings. *Annals of Internal Medicine* 134:1048, 2001.
    Stress is an important cause of the loss of menstrual periods in anorexia nervosa. Thus, reducing stress is an important goal of psychotherapy in this disorder.

12. Richards L: Body image and eating disorders: Not just women's issues. *Today's Dietitian*, p. 30, November 2001.
    Men also are at risk of eating disorders. Treatment is often directed at a man's desire to be seen as athletic, and should include other men in any group therapy.

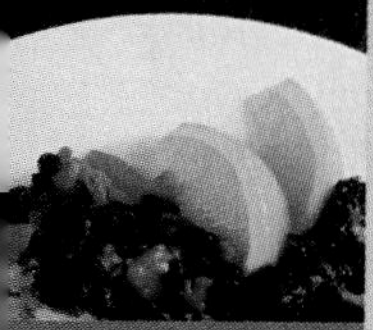

I. *Assessing Risk of Developing an Eating Disorder*

British investigators have developed a five-question screening tool called the SCOFF Questionnaire for recognizing eating disorders:[†]

1. Do you make yourself *S*ick because you feel full?

2. Do you lose *C*ontrol over how much you eat?

3. Have you lost more than *O*ne stone (about 13 pounds) recently?

4. Do you believe yourself to be *F*at when others say you are thin?

5. Does *F*ood dominate your life?

Two or more positive responses suggest an eating disorder.

1. After completing this questionnaire, do you feel that you might have an eating disorder or the potential to develop one?

   _____

   _____

2. Do you think some of your friends might have an eating disorder?

   _____

   _____

3. What counseling and education resources exist in your area or on your campus to help with a potential eating disorder?

   _____

   _____

4. If a friend has an eating disorder, what do you think is the best way to assist him or her in getting help?

   _____

   _____

[†]Morgan JF and others: The SCOFF Questionnaire, *British Medical Journal* 319:1467, 1999.

II. *Helping Prevent Eating Disorders*

You have been asked to speak to a junior high school class about eating disorders. What are four major points that you would make to help prevent disordered eating in this population?

1. _____

2. _____

3. _____

4. _____

Here are points you may consider:

1. Extreme thinness is oversold in the media. Extremely low weight (i.e., BMI of less than 18.5) is generally not healthy.

2. Self-induced vomiting is dangerous. Damage to the teeth, stomach, and esophagus often results.

3. Loss of menstrual periods is a sign of illness. It is important to see a physician about this. Bone deterioration is a common result.

4. The treatment of eating disorders in early phases aids success. These diseases are difficult to treat once firmly established.

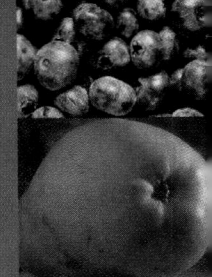

Eating Disorders: A Sociological Perspective

One of the many criteria we use to evaluate ourselves is body image. We identify our bodies with our selves and judge them as we think others see us, knowing that our appearance affects their opinions of us.

Early in life, we develop images of "acceptable" and "unacceptable" body types. Of all the attributes that constitute attractiveness, many people view body weight as the most important, partly because we can control our weight somewhat. Fatness is the most dreaded deviation from our cultural ideals of body image, the one most criticized and shunned, even among schoolchildren. Females, in particular, are likely to diet because they feel strongly about what is acceptable in both size and weight.

Changing Times

The cultural ideal of the "full-bodied" woman did not survive into the twentieth century in Western society, although it is still in fashion in many nonindustrialized countries, where a large body is a sign of wealth. Over the course of the twentieth century, the ideal female body form in North America became progressively thinner. A thin waist with modest hips is now the overriding cultural "gold standard," at least as exemplified by models. Our passion for thinness may have its roots in the Victorian era, which specialized in denying "unpleasant" physical realities, such as appetite and sexual desire. Flappers of the 1920s cemented a trend for thinness (Fig. 12.9). Even as the ideal gradually moved toward a thinner, more angular body shape, the average weight among the general female population increased.

(a)	(b)	(c)	(d)

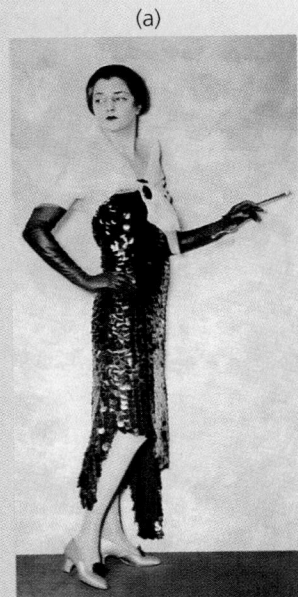 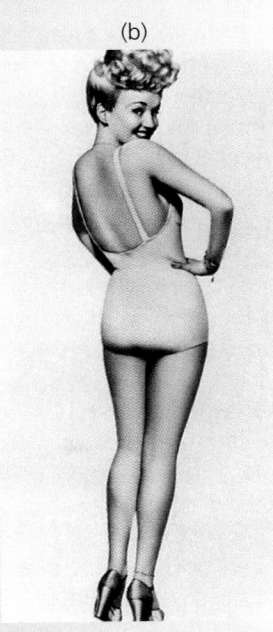 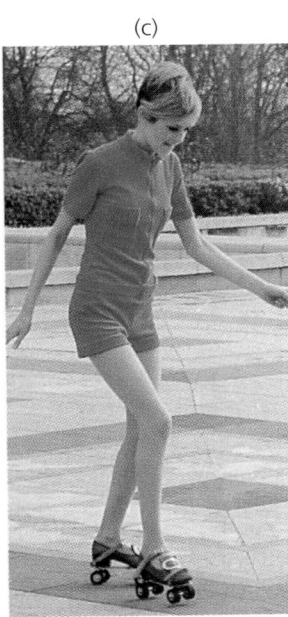 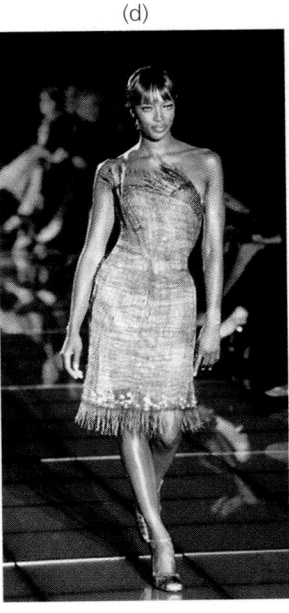

Figure 12.9 The changing views of body weight. American society has imposed varying stereotypes for body weight, especially for women. (a) The svelte flapper of the 1920s. (b) The "thin but curvaceous" look of the 1940s. (c) Ultra-thin was in during the 1960s. (d) At the turn of this new century, women's fashion is trending toward the image of the muscularly fit with little evidence of body fat.

continued

Thinness As an Indicator of Competence

Unfortunately, many North Americans today view obesity as a failure of control, willpower, competence, and productivity. At stake are social acceptance and even access to scarce resources, such as good jobs and an attractive spouse. Whether we like it or not, in today's society our appearance says a lot about us, even though the way we were raised and our genetic background are beyond our control. A prevailing myth is that thin people are more competent, energetic, and forceful than obese people.

Mixed Messages and Social Trends

Despite the pressure for thinness, our society is filled with mixed messages. Half the advertisements in women's magazines may describe diets or feature emaciated models; the other half displays tasty foods. Movie and television stars are almost always perfect physical specimens. Nevertheless, television advertisements encourage us to visit our local quick-service restaurant. There you can buy a hamburger, French fries, and large soft drink, totaling approximately 1200 kcal or more—about the amount of energy our daily basal metabolism uses—without even leaving the car.

In the past several decades, divorce, alcohol abuse in families, child abuse, school- and work-related stress, socioeconomic changes, and crowded urban conditions have all increased. These changes in our family and social environments encourage children, adolescents, and adults alike to find a release from the pressure. Many find relief in food, which sets the stage for the development of an eating disorder.

Internalizing the Thinness Ideal

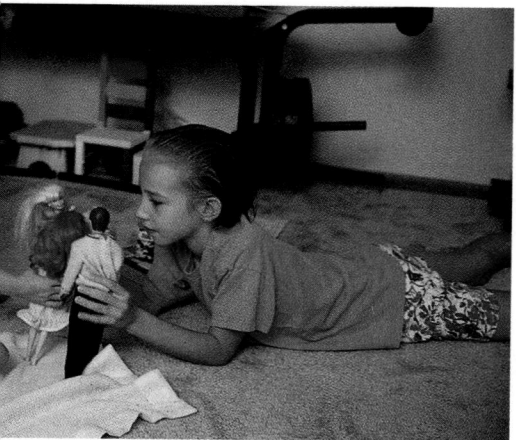

Children's dolls often portray an extremely thin and distorted body shape.

Eating disorders are usually only a symptom of significant emotional trauma or psychological stress in a person's life. When psychiatrists are able to dig deeper, they find that eating disorders mask serious questions of self-worth, family struggles, and sometimes fears of puberty and the future. The real illnesses are not the eating disorders—though they eventually contribute to poor health—but, rather, the way people feel about themselves. When people internalize the social value favoring thinness and can't meet that goal, their negative self-image is reinforced.

Researchers have linked this preference for a lean body type to the recent surge in eating disorders. As the more full-figured woman (earth mother) was displaced by the ultra-thin woman, the number of eating disorders increased, along with our society's preoccupation with obesity. The cultural pressures toward thinness seem to be stretching the physiological capabilities of many women (and men). For example, researchers surmise that the theoretical body fat content of the "Barbie doll" would not allow for menstruation.

Glimmers of Hope

Because eating disorders stem in part from certain cultural values, changing these values might reduce the pressures predisposing some people to various types of disordered eating behavior. Feminists, for example, assert that true liberation means being free to find one's natural weight. Women who combine careers and motherhood are saying that they have more important things to worry about; some fashion leaders are tolerating more curves; "plus" size models have begun to appear; exercise programs are encouraging regular brisk walking, rather than mostly jogging. Writers, therapists, and registered dietitians are working to help women accept their bodies, as noted in the "size acceptance" approach discussed in Chapter 10.

What is the difference between people who can accept themselves—even with a few more pounds than the glamorous people have—and those who chronically diet and feel dissatisfied? Perhaps it is the willingness to recognize that satisfaction comes from within, not from the mirror or the approval of others. The challenge facing many North Americans is achieving a healthy body weight without excessive dieting. This means adopting and maintaining sensible eating habits, a physically active lifestyle, and realistic and positive attitudes and emotions while practicing creative ways to handle stress.

chapter *13*

Pregnancy and Breastfeeding

*P*regnancy can be a very special time for a couple. Along with the responsibility of shaping a child's health and personality comes the prospective exhilaration of watching the child develop and grow. Those involved often feel an overriding desire to produce a healthy baby, which can pique new interest in nutrition and health information. They usually want to do everything possible to maximize their chances of having a robust, lively newborn.

Despite these possibilities, the infant mortality rate in North America is higher than that seen in many other industrialized nations. In the United States, about 7.2 of every 1000 infants per year die before their first birthday, while in Canada it is close to 6.1. Compare that to Sweden at roughly 3. Teenage mothers are at the highest risk. These are alarming statistics for two countries that have such a high per capita expenditure for health care compared to many other countries in the world.

Producing a healthy baby is not just a matter of luck. True, some aspects of fetal and newborn health are beyond our control. Still, conscious decisions about social, health, and nutritional factors significantly affect the baby's health and future. Then choosing to breastfeed the infant adds further benefit. Let's examine the practices that build toward having a healthy baby.

Check out the **Contemporary Nutrition: Issues and Insights Online Learning Center** *www.mhhe.com/wardlawcont5 for quizzes, flash cards, other activities, and web links designed to further help you learn about nutrition for pregnant and breastfeeding women.*

Chapter Objectives

Chapter 13 is designed to allow you to:

1. List major changes that occur in the body during pregnancy and the altered nutrient needs associated with each change.

2. List factors that may interfere with a successful pregnancy outcome, and specify the optimal weight gain during pregnancy for the normal adult woman.

3. Plan an adequate, balanced diet for the pregnant woman and the breastfeeding woman using the Food Guide Pyramid as a basis.

4. Identify the nutrients that may need to be supplemented during pregnancy and explain the reason for each.

5. Explain how many of the typical discomforts of pregnancy can be minimized by diet changes.

6. Describe the process of breastfeeding and list some advantages of breastfeeding for the mother and infant.

7. Describe the disease fetal alcohol syndrome and its outcomes in an infant.

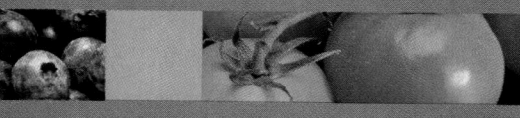

Refresh Your Memory

As you begin your study of nutrition in pregnancy and breastfeeding in Chapter 13, you may want to review:

- Typical fortification in ready-to-eat breakfast cereals in Chapter 2

- The immune system in Chapter 3

- The components of the macro-nutrient classes—carbohydrates, proteins, and lipids—in Chapters 4–6, especially omega-3 fatty acids

- Causes and effects of ketosis in Chapter 4

- Sources of alcohol in Chapter 7

- The food sources of folate in Chapter 8, and calcium, iron, and zinc in Chapter 9

- The calculation of body mass index (BMI) in Chapter 10.

Real Life Scenario

Tracey and her husband of 4 years have decided that they are ready to prepare for Tracey's first pregnancy. Tracey has been reading everything she can find on pregnancy because she knows that her prepregnancy health is important to the success of her pregnancy.

She just turned 25. She knows to avoid alcohol, especially because she could become pregnant and not find that out right away. Alcohol is particularly toxic to the growing fetus in the first weeks of pregnancy. She is not a smoker, doesn't take any medications, and limits her coffee intake to 6 cups a day.

Based on her reading, she has decided to breastfeed her infant and has already checked out childbirth classes. She has modified her diet to include some extra protein, along with more fruits and vegetables. Recently, she started a running program 5 days a week, and she plans to continue running throughout her pregnancy. She has also started taking a multivitamin and mineral supplement.

Tracey and her husband think that they have covered all the key areas of prepregnancy care. List a few positive attributes of her current practices you support. Can you identify some potential problems and what information they may have missed?

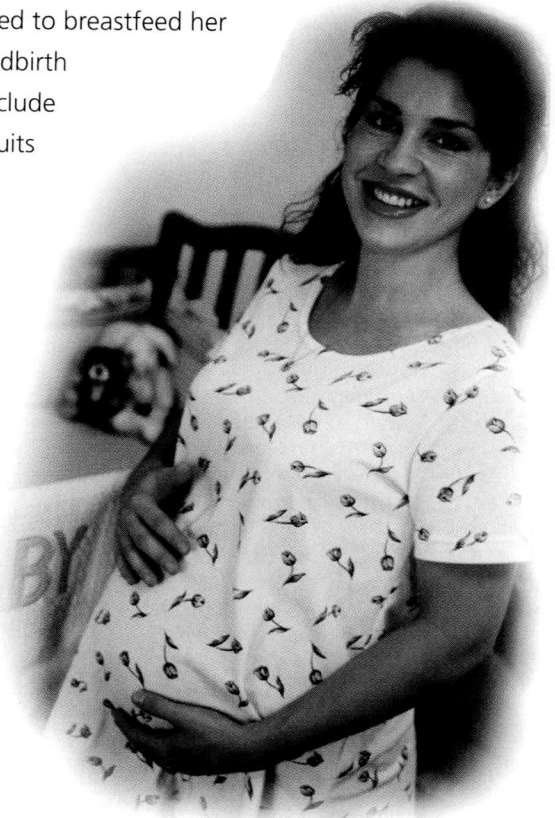

Nutrition Connection

For Better or For Worse® by Lynn Johnston

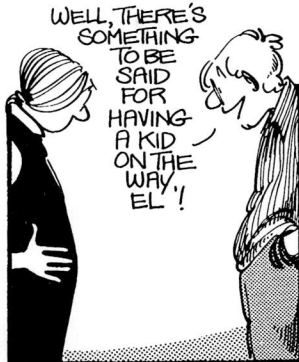
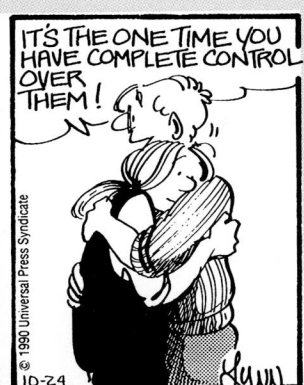

Which diet and lifestyle habits contribute to a successful pregnancy? Which are likely harmful? Why should a woman begin to prepare for pregnancy months before conception of her new baby? This chapter provides some answers.

FOR BETTER OR FOR WORSE ©United Features Syndicate. Reprinted by Permission.

Planned Pregnancy

Pregnancy deserves planning because many practices or conditions of the mother that can harm the developing fetus are modifiable, such as the following:

- Alcohol consumption
- Use of certain medications, such as heavy use of aspirin
- Use of illegal drugs, such as cocaine or marijuana
- Job-related hazards and stresses
- Smoking
- Inadequate diet, such as too little iron, zinc, and synthetic folic acid
- Excess vitamin A intake and megadose use of other nutrient supplements
- Heavy caffeine use
- Lack of medical treatment with HIV-positive status or AIDS
- Poor control of ongoing diabetes or hypertension

Women need to pay attention to these risks in the months before conception. This precaution is necessary because women often do not suspect they are pregnant during the first few weeks after conception and may not seek medical attention until after the first 2 to 3 months.

Still, even without fanfare, the child-to-be grows and develops daily. For that reason, the health and nutrition habits of a woman who is trying to become pregnant—or has the potential to become pregnant—are particularly important. Although some aspects of fetal and newborn health are beyond control, a woman's conscious decisions about social, health, and nutritional factors affect her infant's health and future. Much research suggests that an adequate vitamin and mineral intake at least 8 weeks before conception and during pregnancy can help prevent birth defects such as neural tube defects. This problem has been linked in part to a folate deficiency (see

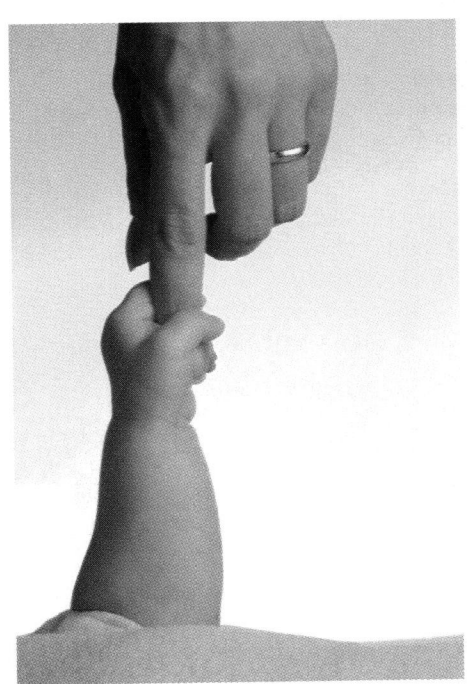

Attention to diet and lifestyle in pregnancy is worth the time and effort.

Figure 13.1 The fetus in relationship to the placenta. The placenta is the organ through which nourishment flows to the fetus.

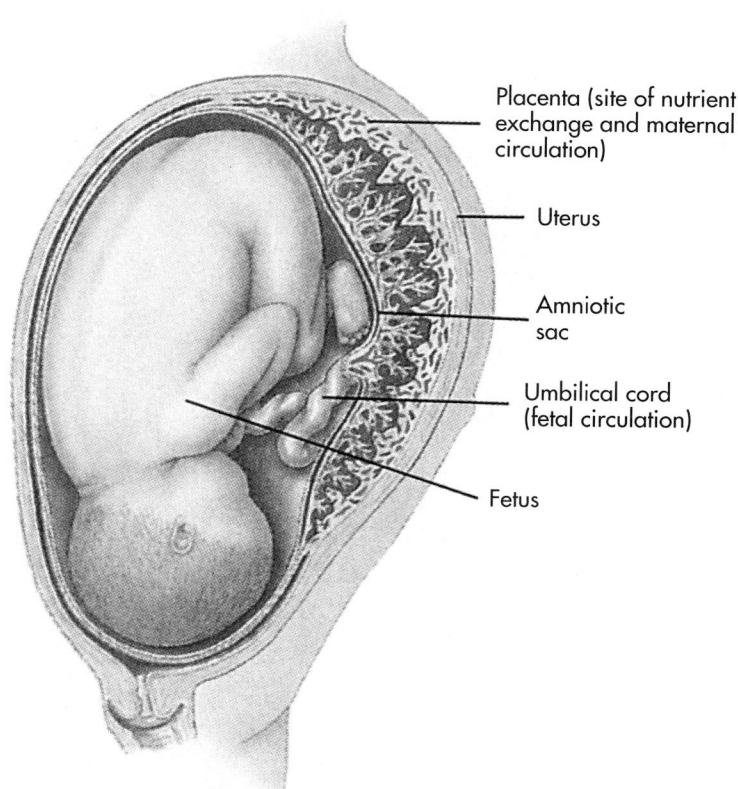

Placenta (site of nutrient exchange and maternal circulation)

Uterus

Amniotic sac

Umbilical cord (fetal circulation)

Fetus

Chapter 8). In addition, about 50% of pregnancies are unplanned. For these reasons, parents should be aware of the role nutrition plays in the development of a healthy infant both before and during pregnancy.

embryo In humans, the developing in utero offspring from about the beginning of the third week to the end of the eighth week after conception.

ovum The egg cell from which a fetus eventually develops if the egg is fertilized by a sperm cell.

placenta An organ that forms in pregnant women. Through this organ, oxygen and nutrients from the mother's blood are transferred to the fetus, and fetal wastes are removed. The placenta also releases hormones that maintain the pregnant state.

zygote The fertilized ovum; the cell resulting from the union of an egg cell (ovum) and sperm until it divides.

trimesters Three 13- to 14-week periods into which the normal pregnancy of 37 to 41 weeks is divided somewhat arbitrarily for purposes of discussion and analysis. Development of the embryo and fetus, however, is continuous throughout pregnancy, with no specific physiological markers demarcating the transition from one trimester to the next.

Prenatal Growth and Development

For 8 weeks after conception, a human **embryo** develops from an **ovum** into a **fetus.** For about another 32 weeks, the fetus continues to develop. When its body finally matures, the infant is born. Until birth, the mother nourishes it via a **placenta,** an organ that forms in her uterus. The placenta separates the blood supply of the mother from the blood supply of the fetus. Nutrients pass from the mother's blood through the placenta to accommodate the growth and development of the fetus (Fig. 13.1).

■ Early Growth—The First Trimester Is a Very Critical Time

In the formation of the human organism, egg and sperm first unite, producing the **zygote** (Fig. 13.2). From this point, the reproductive process occurs very rapidly:

- Within 30 hours—zygote divides in half to form 2 cells.
- Within 4 days—cell number climbs from 64 to 128 cells.
- At 14 days—the group of cells is called an embryo.
- Within 35 days—heart is beating, embryo is $\frac{1}{30}$ of an inch (8 millimeters) long, eyes and limb buds are clearly visible.
- At 8 weeks—the embryo is known as a fetus.
- At 13 weeks (end of first trimester—most organs are formed, and the fetus can move.

For purposes of discussion, the duration of pregnancy—normally, 37 to 41 weeks from the mother's last menstrual period—is commonly divided into three periods, called **trimesters.** Growth begins in the first trimester with a rapid increase in cell

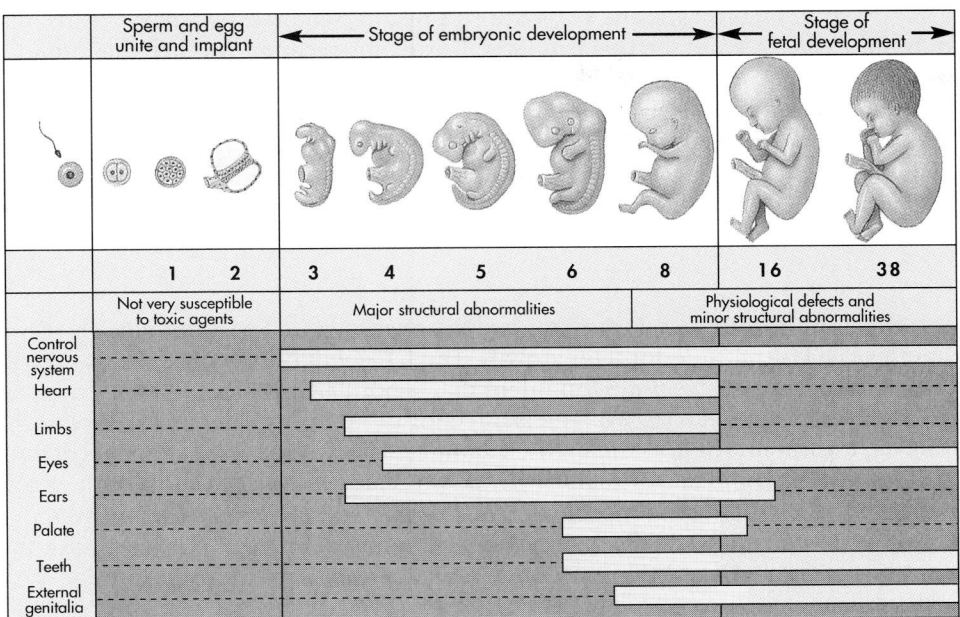

Figure 13.2 Vulnerable periods of fetal development are indicated with yellow bars. The yellow shading indicates the time of greatest risk to the organ. The most serious damage to the fetus from exposure to toxins is likely to occur during the first 8 weeks after conception, two-thirds of the way through the first trimester. As the chart shows, however, damage to vital parts of the body—including the eyes, brain, and genitals—can also occur during the last months of pregnancy.

number. This type of growth dominates embryonic and later fetal development. The newly formed cells then begin to grow larger. Further growth and development then involve mostly an increase in cell number with some increase in cell size. By the end of 13 weeks—the first trimester—most organs are formed and the fetus can move (Fig. 13.2).

Nutritional deficiencies and other insults transmitted through the mother to the embryo or fetus—for example, injuries caused by medications and other drugs, high intakes of preformed vitamin A, radiation, or trauma—can alter or arrest the current phase of development (review Fig. 13.2). The effects may last a lifetime. The most critical time for these problems to happen is during the first trimester. Most **miscarriages** (more correctly termed **spontaneous abortions**) occur at this time. Currently, about one-half or more of all pregnancies either fail to attach to the uterine wall or undergo spontaneous abortions, often so early that a woman does not even realize she was pregnant. The early spontaneous abortions usually result from a genetic defect or fatal error in fetal development.

A woman should avoid substances that may harm the developing fetus, especially during the first trimester. This holds true for the time when a woman is trying to become pregnant. As previously mentioned, she is unlikely to be aware of her pregnancy for at least a few weeks. In addition, the fetus develops so rapidly during the first trimester that if an essential nutrient is not available, the fetus may be affected even before evidence of the deficiency appears in the mother.

For this reason, the quality of one's nutritional intake is more important than quantity during the first trimester. In other words, women should consume the same amount of food, but the foods should be more nutrient dense. Although some women lose their appetite and feel nauseated during the first trimester, they should be careful to meet nutrient needs.

Second Trimester

By the beginning of the second trimester, a fetus weighs about 1 ounce. Arms, hands, fingers, legs, feet, and toes are fully formed. The fetus has ears and begins to form tooth sockets in its jawbone. Organs continue to grow and mature, and, with a stethoscope, physicians can detect the fetus's heartbeat. Most bones are distinctly evident through the body. Eventually, the fetus begins to look more like an infant. It may suck its thumb and kick strongly enough to be felt by the mother.

spontaneous abortion Any cessation of pregnancy and expulsion of the embryo or nonviable fetus as the result of natural causes, such as a genetic defect or developmental problem; also called miscarriage.

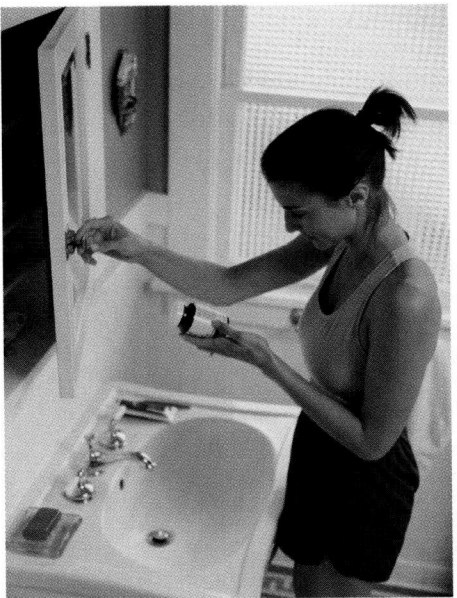

The time to begin thinking about prenatal nutrition is actually before becoming pregnant. This includes making sure that any supplemental use of preformed vitamin A does not exceed 100% of the Daily Value (1000 micrograms RAE or 5000 IU).

Although a mother's decisions, practices, and precautions during pregnancy contribute to the health of her fetus, she cannot guarantee her fetus good health because some genetic and environmental factors are beyond her control. She and others involved in the pregnancy should not hold an unrealistic illusion of control.

gestation The period of intrauterine development of offspring, from conception to birth; in humans, gestation lasts for about 40 weeks after the woman's previous menstrual period (range of 37 to 41 weeks).

Critical Thinking

Alexandra wants to have a baby. She has read that it is very important for the woman to be healthy during the pregnancy. However, Jane, her sister, tells her that, actually, the time to begin to assess her nutritional and health status is before she becomes pregnant. What additional information should Jane have given Alexandra?

A goal of Healthy People 2010 is to reduce low-birth-weight and preterm births each year by one-third.

As shown in Figure 13.2, the fetus can still be affected by exposure to toxins, but not to the degree seen in the first trimester. During the second trimester, the mother's breast weight increases by approximately 30% due to the deposition of 2 to 4 pounds of fat for lactation. Consequently, undernutrition in the second trimester has a greater effect on the mother than on the fetus. For example, if the mother does not meet her nutritional requirements during this time, her ability to successfully breastfeed her infant may be affected, as fat stored during pregnancy helps serve as an energy reserve for lactation.

Third Trimester

By the beginning of the third trimester, a fetus weighs about 2 to 3 pounds. The third trimester is a crucial time for fetal growth. The fetus will double in length and will multiply its weight by five times. An infant that is born after about 26 weeks of **gestation** has a good chance of survival if it is cared for in a nursery for high-risk newborns. However, the infant will not contain the vitamin (mainly vitamin E), mineral (mainly iron and calcium), and fat stores normally accumulated during the last month of gestation. This and other medical problems, such as a poor ability to suck and swallow, complicate nutritional care for preterm infants. Note also that infants will use the stores of the mother to obtain needed iron. If the mother is not meeting her iron needs, she can be severely depleted after delivery.

At 9 months, the fetus weighs about 7 to 9 pounds (3 to 4 kilograms) and is about 20 inches (50 centimeters) long (Fig. 13.3). A soft spot in the forehead indicates where the skull bones (fontanels) are growing together. The bones finally close by the time the baby is about 12 to 18 months of age.

Definition of a Successful Pregnancy

To define a successful pregnancy, one common criterion is the protection of the mother's physical and emotional health, so that she can return to her prepregnancy health status. As for the infant, two widely accepted criteria are (1) a gestation period longer than 37 weeks and (2) a birth weight greater than 5.5 pounds (2.5 kilograms). Sufficient lung development, which is likely to have occurred by 37 weeks' gestation, is critical to the survival of a newborn. The longer the gestation, the greater the ultimate birth weight and maturation and, hence, fewer medical problems are likely to occur.

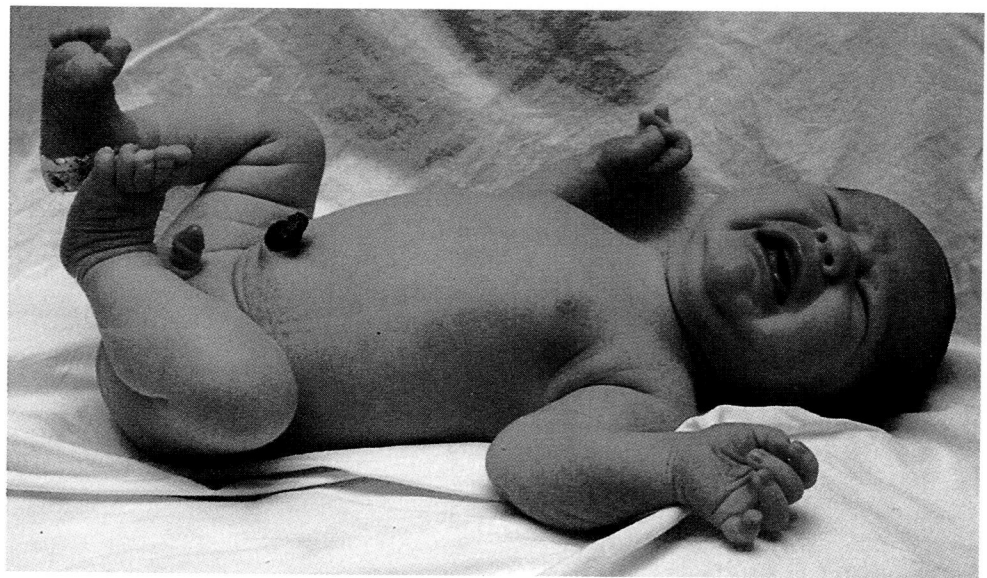

Figure 13.3 A healthy 1-week-old baby. At birth, a baby usually weighs about 7.5 pounds and is 20 inches long.

Low-birth-weight infants are those weighing less than 5.5 pounds (2.5 kilograms) at birth. Most commonly, low birth weight is associated with **preterm** birth. Full-term and preterm infants who weigh less than the expected weight for their duration of gestation, the result of insufficient growth, are described as **small for gestational age (SGA).** Thus, a full-term infant weighing less than 5.5 pounds at birth is SGA but not preterm, whereas a preterm infant born at 30 weeks' gestation is probably low birth weight without being SGA. Infants who are SGA are more likely than normal-weight infants to have medical complications, including problems with blood glucose control, temperature regulation, and growth and development in the early weeks after birth. Currently, hospital-related costs of caring for low-birth-weight newborns total more than $2 billion per year in the United States, ranging from $20,000 to $200,000 per child. Compare this with an average hospital-related cost of $5800 for a normal delivery and an average of $800 for preventive prenatal care.

The newborn's quality of life must also be considered in rating the success of a pregnancy. Overall, prospective parents should strive toward producing a baby who is born healthy, on time, and with the mental, physical, and physiological capabilities to take advantage of whatever life offers, while also protecting the mother's health.

Nutrition is one key to a successful pregnancy. Eating healthfully is vital during pregnancy to ensure the health of both the offspring and the mother. Fetal organs and body parts begin to develop very soon after conception. Again, the first trimester (13 weeks) is an especially critical period, when poor nutrition or drug use can result in birth defects.

low birth weight (LBW) Referring to any infant weighing less than 5.5 pounds (2.5 kilograms) at birth; most commonly results from preterm birth.

preterm An infant born before 37 weeks of gestation; also referred to as premature.

small for gestational age (SGA) Referring to infants who weigh less than the expected weight for their length of gestation. This corresponds to less than 5.5. pounds (2.5 kilograms) in a full-term newborn. A preterm infant who is also SGA will most likely develop some medical complications.

Concept Check

Adequate nutrition, especially meeting folic acid needs from a synthetic source starting 8 weeks before pregnancy begins, is vital both before and during pregnancy to help ensure the optimal health of both the mother and her offspring. Organs and body parts in the offspring begin to develop very soon after conception. The first trimester is a critical period when inadequate nutrient intake or alcohol and drug use can result in birth defects.

Infants born after 37 weeks of gestation who weigh more than 5.5 pounds (2.5 kilograms) have the fewest medical problems at birth. To reduce infant and maternal medical problems or death, those involved with the pregnancy should take the steps necessary to allow the mother to carry the baby in her uterus for the entire 9 months and contribute to adequate growth. Good nutrition and health practices aid in this goal.

Studies from Britain suggest that small for gestational age infants are likely to develop diabetes, hypertension, and high blood cholesterol during later adult years. Reduced growth of the liver and muscles during gestation is one possible reason. This increase in health risk is especially true if the infant also fails to gain enough weight in the first year of life.

Effect of Nutrition on the Success of Pregnancy

Is this attention to nutrition worth the effort? Yes; evidence shows that the effort is justified. Extra nutrients and energy are used for fetal growth, as well as the changes in the mother's body to accommodate the fetus. Her uterus and breasts grow, the placenta develops, her total blood volume increases, the heart and kidneys work harder, and stores of body fat increase.

Although it is difficult to specify what degree of poor nutrition will affect each pregnancy, a daily diet containing only 1000 kcal has been shown to greatly retard fetal growth and development. Increased maternal and infant death rates seen in famine-stricken areas of Africa supply further evidence (see Chapter 17).

Genetic background can explain very little of the observed differences in birth weight in North America. Both environmental factors and nutritional factors are more important. The worse the nutritional condition of the mother at the beginning of pregnancy, the more valuable a good prenatal diet and/or use of prenatal supplements are in improving the course and outcome of her pregnancy.

In the 1950s, physicians commonly recommended that women restrict weight gain to between 15 and 18 pounds. At times, they also recommended severe energy and salt restrictions to keep the baby small, in the hopes of easing labor and avoiding complications. Few of these practices were based on sound research, and we know now that many of these recommendations can actually harm the mother and fetus.

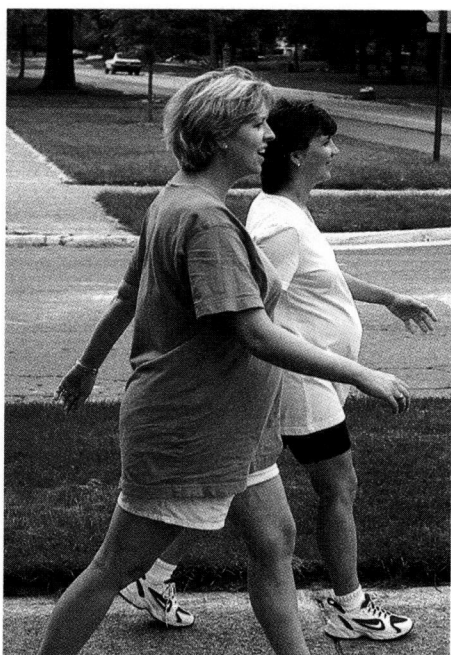

Walking, cycling, swimming, and light aerobics are all suitable exercises during pregnancy.

The American College of Obstetrics and Gynecology suggests the following guidelines for physical activity during pregnancy:

1. Do not allow heart rate to exceed 140 beats per minute.
2. Avoid exercising in hot, humid weather.
3. Discontinue exercise that causes discomfort or overheating.
4. Drink plenty of liquids to avoid dehydration and overheating (>100°F).
5. After about the fourth month, don't exercise while lying on your back.
6. Avoid an abrupt decrease in exertion. In other words, don't just stop and stand around after a hard workout; rather, continue exercising but at a slow pace, gradually reducing pulse rate.

■ Increased Nutrient Needs to Support Pregnancy

It is important to understand that pregnancy is a time of increased nutrient needs, not restrictions as was once thought. It is equally important to recognize the need for individual assessment and counseling of mothers-to-be, as the nutritional and health status of each woman is different. Still, there are some general principles that are true of most women with regard to increased nutrient needs.

■ Increased Energy Needs

An average pregnancy requires approximately 300 extra kcal daily during the second and third trimesters. Energy needs during the first trimester are essentially the same as for the nonpregnant woman. An example of such a 300-kcal increase includes six whole-wheat crackers, 1 ounce of cheese, and ½ cup of nonfat milk, or 1 cup of low-fat yogurt and an orange. Although she may "eat for two," the pregnant woman must not double her normal energy intake. She will want to seek the best-quality foods to ensure the best possible health for her child. Note that many vitamin and mineral needs are increased by 20% to 50% during pregnancy, whereas energy needs during the second and third trimesters represent only about a 15% increase, based on adding 300 kcal to an intake of 2000 kcal per day by nonpregnant women.

Adequate energy intake is easy to achieve and can be assessed by appropriate weight gain throughout the pregnancy. However, to obtain the necessary vitamins and minerals without increasing her energy intake too much, a pregnant woman needs to seek nutrient-dense foods.

If a woman is active during pregnancy, she can add the extra energy she uses to the energy allowance for pregnancy. Her greater body weight requires more energy for activity. Women can continue most activities during pregnancy, except certain calisthenics, such as deep knee bends, scuba diving, downhill skiing, weight lifting, and contact sports (such as hockey). Walking, cycling, swimming, and light aerobics are generally advised, although it is not advised that normally inactive women begin an intense exercise program during pregnancy. Because many women find that they are inactive during the later months, partly because of their increased size, an extra 300 kcal in their daily diet is usually enough.

Women with high-risk pregnancies, such as those with premature contractions, may need to restrict their physical activity. To ensure optimal health for both herself and her infant, a pregnant woman should first consult her physician about physical activity and possible limitations.

■ Recommended Weight Gain

Adequate weight gain for a mother is one of the best predictors of pregnancy outcome. According to the National Academy of Sciences, a woman of normal weight (based on BMI) should follow a diet that allows for approximately 2 to 4 pounds (0.9 to 1.8 kilograms) of weight gain during the first trimester, and then a subsequent weight gain of 0.75 to 1 pound (0.3 to 0.5 kilograms) weekly during the second and third trimesters. Total weight gain goal normally averages about 25 to 35 pounds (11.5 to 16 kilograms). Adolescents and African-American women, who often have smaller babies, are strongly advised to aim for the greater amount. Women carrying twins should gain 35 to 45 pounds, and women carrying triplets should gain 50 pounds (23 kilograms).

For women at a low BMI, the goal increases to 28 to 40 pounds (12.5 to 18 kilograms) (Table 13.1). The goal decreases to 15 to 25 pounds (7 to 11.5 kilograms) for a woman at a high BMI, and less than 15 pounds (7 kilograms) for an obese woman. Figure 13.4 shows why the typical recommendation begins at 25 pounds.

A weight gain of between 25 and 35 pounds has repeatedly been shown to yield optimal health for both mother and fetus if gestation lasts at least 38 weeks. The weight gain should yield a birth weight of 7.5 pounds (3.5 kilograms). Although

Table 13.1 Recommended Weight Gain in Pregnancy Based on Prepregnancy Body Mass Index (BMI)

BMI Category	Total Weight Gain*	
	(pounds)	(kilograms)
Low (BMI less than 19.8)	28–40	12.5–18
Normal (BMI 19.8 to 25.9)	25–35	11.5–16
High (BMI 26 to 29)	15–25	7–11.5
Obese (BMI greater than 29)	no more than 15	no more than 7

*The listed values are for singleton pregnancies. For women of normal BMI who are carrying twins, the range is 35 to 45 pounds (16 to 20 kilograms). Adolescents within 2 years of **menarche** and African-American women should strive for gains at the upper end of the ranges; short women (less than 62 inches) should strive for gains at the lower end of the ranges.

Reprinted with permission from *Nutrition During Pregnancy and Lactation,* Copyright 1992 by the National Academy of Sciences. Courtesy of the National Academy Press, Washington, DC.

menarche The onset of menstruation. Menarche usually occurs around age 13, 2 or 3 years after the first signs of puberty start to appear.

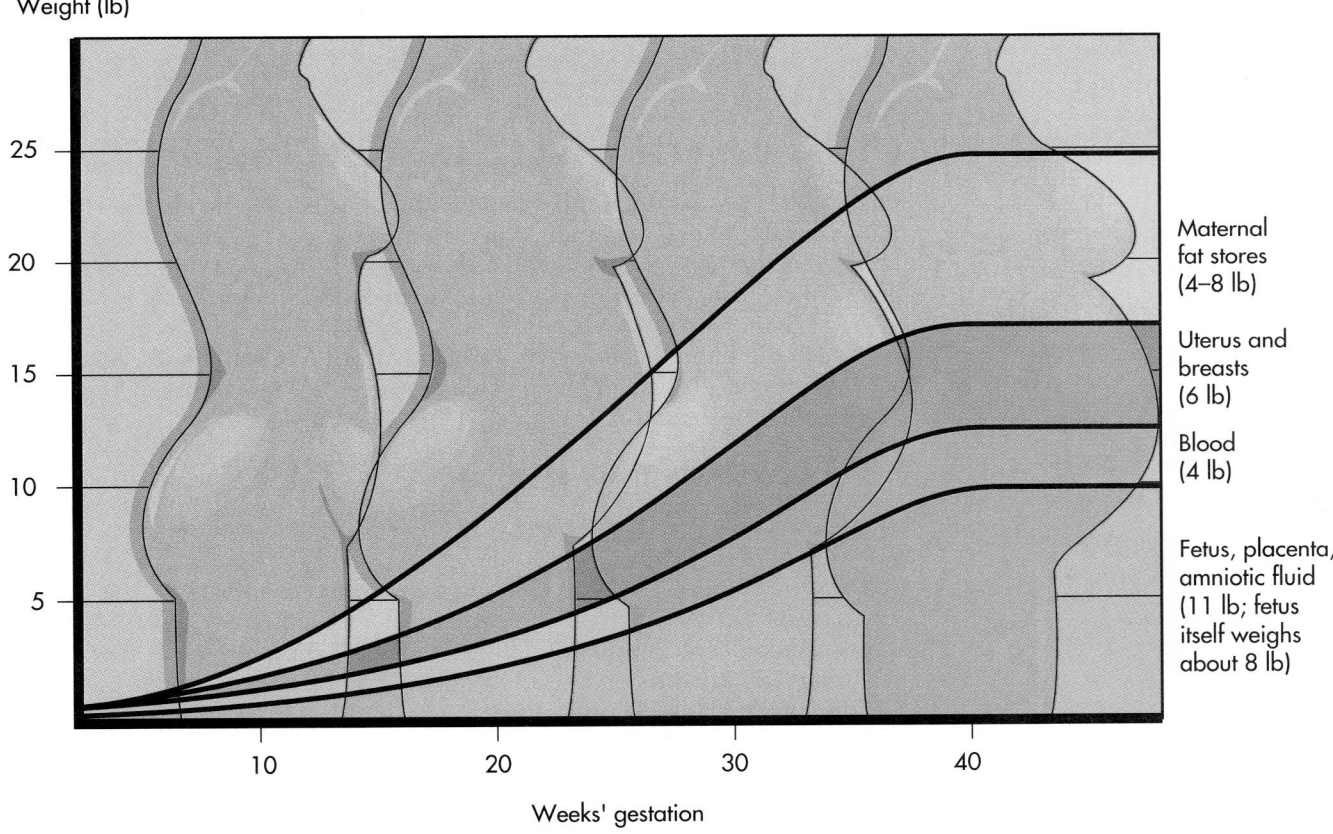

Figure 13.4 The components of weight gain in pregnancy. A weight gain of 25 to 35 pounds (lb) is recommended for most women. Note that the various components total about 25 pounds.

some extra weight gain during pregnancy is usually not harmful, it can set the stage for creeping obesity during the childbearing years if the mother does not return to about her prepregnancy weight. This is especially true if the woman intends to have more than one child.

Weight gain during pregnancy, especially in the teenage years, requires regular monitoring that approximately follows the pattern shown in Figure 13.4. Infant birth weights improve if the mother's weight gain meets the ranges previously mentioned. Keeping weekly records of a pregnant woman's weight gain helps assess how much to

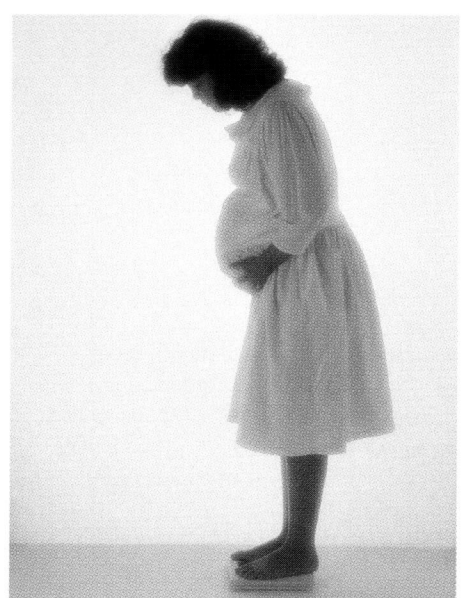

Weight gain should be carefully monitored during pregnancy.

During pregnancy, women in North America are more likely to gain excess weight and make poor food choices than to eat too little. Usually, the problem is how to limit weight gain. Excessive weight gain increases risk for complications during pregnancy and encourages excess fetal growth, which makes birth trauma more likely. Loose, accommodating maternity clothes and fluid retention can mask true weight gain during pregnancy.

Healthy People 2010 has set a goal of increasing the number of pregnancies that begin with optimum folate status, to 80% from the current estimate of 21%, thus reducing the occurrence of neural tube defects.

adjust her food intake. Weight gain is a key issue in prenatal care and a concern of many mothers. Inadequate weight gain can cause many problems. If a woman deviates from the desirable pattern, she should be warned of this and counseled on how to make the appropriate adjustment.

For example, if a woman begins to gain too much weight during her pregnancy, she should not be encouraged to lose weight to get back on track. Even if a woman gains 35 pounds in the first 7 months of pregnancy, she must still gain more during the last 2 months. Weight loss is never advised. She should simply slow the increase in weight to parallel the rise on the prenatal weight gain chart. In other words, the sources of the unnecessary food energy should be found and minimized. Alternately, if a woman has not gained the desired weight by a given point in pregnancy, she shouldn't be encouraged to gain the needed weight rapidly. Instead, she should slowly gain a little more weight than the typical pattern to meet the goal by the end of the pregnancy.

Another Bite

With regard to other weight-related issues, pregnant women who are obese are at an increased risk of hypertension and diabetes during pregnancy. The need for surgery and other complications during delivery likewise increase. Thus, these pregnancies require careful monitoring.

■ Increased Protein and Carbohydrate Needs

The RDA for protein increases by 10 to 15 grams daily, depending on age. A glass of milk alone contains 8 grams. Many nonpregnant women already eat the recommended 60 grams of protein per day and therefore don't need to increase protein intake. However, all women should check to make sure they are actually eating enough protein. Carbohydrate needs are at least 100 grams daily. This amount prevents ketosis, which can harm the fetus (see the later Nutrition Insight on the effects of this and various other health factors on pregnancy outcome). Most women already consume almost twice this amount.

■ Increased Vitamin Needs

Vitamin needs generally increase by up to 30% for the B-vitamins, except vitamin B-6 (45%) and folate (50%).

The extra amount of vitamin B-6 and other B vitamins (except folate) needed in the diet is easily met via wise food choices, such as a serving of a typical ready-to-eat breakfast cereal and some animal protein. Folate needs, however, often merit specific diet planning. Because the synthesis of DNA requires folate, this nutrient is especially crucial during pregnancy. Ultimately, both fetal and maternal growth depend on an ample supply of folate. Red blood cell formation, which requires folate, increases during pregnancy. Serious folate-related anemia can result if intake is inadequate. The RDA for folate increases during pregnancy to 600 micrograms per day. This amount is based on dietary folate equivalents, so both natural and synthetic sources can contribute to folate needs. Folate deficiency at conception and thereafter has been associated with birth defects—specifically, neural tube defects, such as spina bifida. Still, about half of these birth defects arise from genetic and other reasons unrelated to folate intake.

Increasing folate intakes to meet the 600 micrograms per day recommendation for a pregnant woman can be achieved by choosing foods rich in folate, such as ready-to-eat breakfast cereals (look for 50% to 100% of the Daily Value) and enriched grains. Use of a multivitamin and mineral or prenatal supplement is also possible.

Women who have previously given birth to an infant with a neural tube defect should consult their physician about the need for folate supplementation; an intake of 4 milligrams per day is advocated in the weeks before the start of the next pregnancy, but must be taken under a physician's supervision.

Meeting folate needs during pregnancy may be a problematic practice for women who have taken oral contraceptives for extended periods because this can inhibit folate absorption. A recent history of an inadequate diet or oral contraceptive use necessitates careful attention to folate intake during pregnancy. Ideally, the woman would begin a synthetic folic acid-rich diet (or take a supplement containing folic acid) approximately 8 weeks before conception.

▪ Increased Mineral Needs

Mineral needs generally increase during pregnancy, especially the need for iodide and iron.

Pregnant women need extra iodide (total of 220 micrograms per day) for prevention of goiter. The extra iron (total of 27 milligrams per day) is needed to synthesize the greater amount of hemoglobin needed during pregnancy and to provide iron stores for the fetus. Typical iodide intakes suffice if the woman uses iodized salt. However, women often need a supplemental iron source, especially if they start the pregnancy with low iron stores or don't regularly consume iron-fortified foods, such as ready-to-eat breakfast cereals containing about 100% of the Daily Value for iron. Generally this will indicate the need for a prenatal supplement or an iron supplement. Because iron supplements decrease appetite and can cause nausea and constipation, taking them between meals or just before going to bed is best. Milk, coffee, or tea also should not be consumed with an iron supplement because these have substances that interfere with iron absorption. Eating foods rich in vitamin C (about 75 milligrams in the meal) along with nonheme iron–containing foods helps increase iron absorption. Pregnant women who are not anemic may wait until the second trimester, when pregnancy-related nausea generally lessens, to start iron supplementation.

Severe iron-deficiency anemia in pregnancy, especially in the first half of pregnancy, may lead to preterm delivery, low birth weight, and increased risk for fetal death in the first weeks after birth. And, as previously mentioned, the fetus will deplete the mother's iron stores, especially in late pregnancy. In other words, an inadequate iron intake may actually be more harmful to the mother than to the fetus.

The RDA for zinc during pregnancy is 11 milligrams per day, 35% higher than that for nonpregnant women. The protein foods in the diet of a healthy pregnant woman should supply this much zinc. Conditions such as cereal-based diets, high doses of supplemental iron, smoking, and alcohol abuse can reduce the amount of zinc available to the fetus. Women with these conditions may be given more zinc during pregnancy (approximately 25 milligrams per day, about two times the RDA). This is the amount contained in a typical prenatal supplement.

▪ Another Bite

*I*t is a common myth that women instinctively know what to eat during pregnancy. These cravings of the last two trimesters are often related to hormonal changes in the mother, or family traditions. Such "instinct" cannot be trusted, however, based on observations that some women crave nonfood items such as laundry starch and soil (clay), part of what is called **pica.** This practice can be extremely harmful to the mother and the fetus. Overall, though women may have a natural instinct to consume the right foods in pregnancy, humans are so far removed from living by instinct that relying on our cravings to meet nutrient needs is risky. Nutritional advice by experts is more reliable.

pica The practice of eating nonfood items, such as dirt, laundry starch, or clay.

▍ Food Plan for Pregnant Women

One approach to a diet that supports a successful pregnancy is based on the Food Guide Pyramid. It includes *at least* the following:

- Two to three servings from the milk, yogurt, and cheese group (the range depends on the calcium content of other food choices)
- Three servings from the meat, poultry, fish, dry beans, eggs, and nuts group
- Three servings from the vegetable group
- Two servings from the fruit group
- Six servings from the bread, cereal, rice, and pasta group

*R*ecently, FDA warned pregnant women to avoid swordfish, shark, king mackerel, and tile fish because of possible mercury contamination. Mercury can harm the nervous system of the fetus.

Some experts recommend that trans fatty acid intake should be limited in pregnancy (and while breastfeeding). A generous intake has been linked to poor fetal growth and development.

Specifically, the servings from the milk, yogurt, and cheese group could include low-fat or nonfat versions of milk, yogurt, and cheese. These foods supply extra protein, calcium, riboflavin, and magnesium. Servings from the meat, poultry, fish, dry beans, eggs, and nuts group should include both animal and vegetable sources. Besides protein, the animal sources help provide the extra iron and zinc needed, and the vegetable sources help provide much of the extra magnesium needed during pregnancy.

The vegetable and fruit group servings provide a variety of vitamins and minerals. One serving from this combination should be a good vitamin C source, and one serving should be a green vegetable or other rich source of folate. Selections from the bread, cereal, rice, and pasta group should focus on whole-grain and enriched foods. One serving of a ready-to-eat breakfast cereal significantly contributes to meeting many vitamin and mineral needs.

Table 13.2 illustrates one daily menu based on the basic diet plan shown. This daily menu supplies about 2000 kcal but still meets the extra nutrient needs associated with pregnancy. Women who need to consume more than this—and some do for various reasons—should add more servings from the fruit and vegetable groups and the bread, cereal, rice, and pasta group to the basic plan.

■ Use of Prenatal Vitamin and Mineral Supplements

Specially formulated supplements for pregnant women are prescribed routinely by most physicians. Some are sold over the counter, while others are dispensed by prescription because of their high folate content (1 milligram), which could pose problems for others, such as older people (see Chapter 8). This routine use of prenatal supplements may exist because it is easier for physicians to prescribe supplements than to discuss diet changes. Also, some pregnant women are just not willing to change their diets to meet their increased nutrient needs, or they simply expect (or demand) this treatment. These prenatal supplements typically include the critical nutrients for pregnancy—that is, iron, zinc, and folate—and many others as well. Prenatal supplements especially may contribute to a successful pregnancy with poor women, teenagers, those with a generally deficient diet, and women carrying multiple fetuses.

There is no evidence that potential supplements cause significant health problems in pregnancy, as long as other sources of supplementary and dietary vitamin A are monitored. During pregnancy, preformed vitamin A should not exceed 3000 RAE per day (15,000 IU per day). Toxicity of vitamin A is linked with birth defects (see Chapter 8). This occurs mainly during the first trimester.

■ Pregnant Vegetarians

Women who practice either lactoovovegetarianism or lactovegetarianism generally do not face special difficulties in meeting their nutritional needs during pregnancy. Like nonvegetarian women, they should be concerned primarily with meeting iron, zinc, folate, and calcium needs.

On the other hand, when a total vegetarian (vegan) becomes pregnant, she must carefully plan a diet that includes sufficient protein, vitamin D (or sufficient sun exposure), vitamin B-6, iron, calcium, and zinc and must use a vitamin B-12 supplement. The basic vegan diet listed in Chapter 6 should be modified to include more grains, beans, nuts, and seeds to supply the necessary extra amounts of some of these nutrients. Because iron and calcium are poorly absorbed from most plant foods, iron and calcium supplements are probably necessary; however, to avoid competition for absorption, they should not be taken together. The amounts provided by typical prenatal supplements should suffice to meet iron needs but not calcium needs (only 200 milligrams of calcium are contained in a typical prenatal supplement). The prenatal supplement also fulfills vitamin D needs if sufficient sun exposure does not take place.

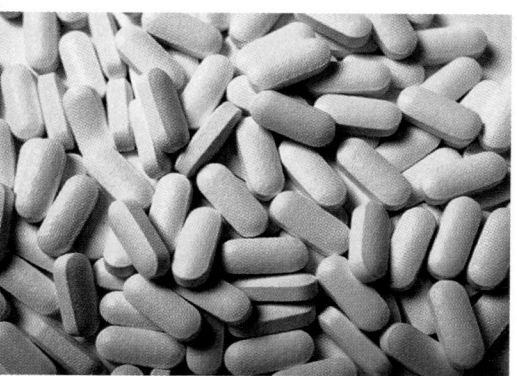

Pregnancy, in particular, is not a time to self-prescribe vitamin and mineral supplements. For example, although vitamin A is a routine component of prenatal vitamins, it is important to note that over three times the RDA has been shown to have toxic effects on the fetus.

Table 13.2 Sample 2000 kcal Daily Menu That Meets the Nutritional Needs of Most Pregnant and Breastfeeding Women

	Vitamin D	Folate	Calcium	Iron	Zinc
Breakfast					
1½ cups Quaker Toasted Oatmeal Squares cereal	✓	✓		✓	✓
½ cup orange juice		✓			
¾ cup nonfat milk	✓		✓		
Snack					
2 tablespoons peanut butter		✓		✓	✓
1 slice whole-wheat toast		✓		✓	✓
½ cup plain low-fat yogurt			✓		
½ cup strawberries					
Lunch					
1½ cups spinach salad with 1 tbsp oil and vinegar dressing		✓			
½ tomato					
1 slice whole-wheat toast		✓		✓	✓
1 ounce provolone cheese			✓		
Snack					
4 whole-wheat crackers		✓		✓	✓
1 cup nonfat milk	✓		✓		
Dinner					
3 ounces lean hamburger, broiled (with condiments)				✓	✓
½ cup baked beans		✓		✓	✓
1 hamburger bun		✓		✓	
½ sliced tomato					
¾ cup cooked broccoli		✓			
1 teaspoon soft margarine	✓				
Iced tea (milk if a teenager)					
Snack					
Nutri-Grain® Bar		✓	✓	✓	✓

This diet meets nutrient needs for pregnancy and lactation. The vitamin- and mineral-fortified breakfast cereal used in this example makes an important contribution to meeting nutrient needs, such as for synthetic folic acid (400 micrograms per cup, which equals 680 dietary folate equivalents). If more food energy is needed, 1 cup of nonfat milk, 1 slice of whole-wheat bread, and 5 baby carrots would increase intake to 2200 kcal.

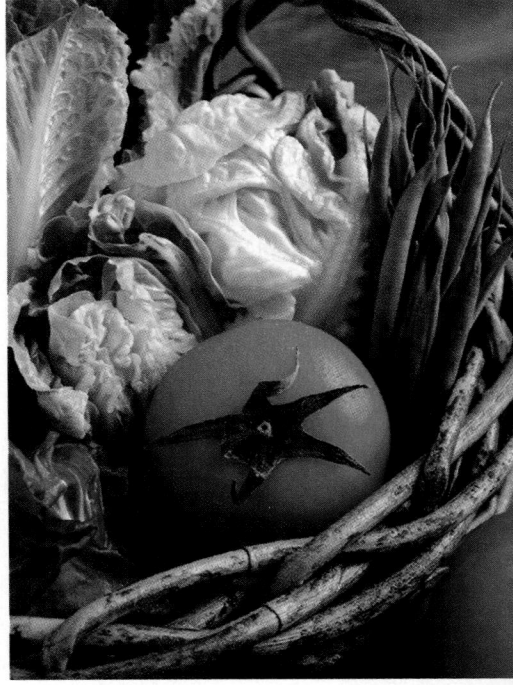

A salad each day provides many nutrients for the prenatal diet.

Concept Check

*E*nergy needs increase by an average of about 300 kcal per day during the second and third trimesters of pregnancy. Weight gain should be slow and steady up to a total of 25 to 35 pounds for a woman of normal weight (BMI 19.8 to 25.9). Protein, vitamin, and mineral needs all increase during pregnancy. Vitamin B-6, folate, iron, iodide, calcium, and zinc are nutrients of particular concern. A pregnant woman's diet should be varied and generally include more milk products than a prepregnancy diet. Prenatal supplemental vitamins and minerals are commonly prescribed but may not be necessary, depending on one's diet and current health status. Taking too many supplements—especially vitamin A—can be hazardous to the fetus.

Effects of Nutritional and Other Factors on Pregnancy Outcome

In North America, about 11 of every 100,000 live births end in the mother's death. The infant mortality rate is even higher: for each 100,000 live births, about 600 to 700 infants die within the first year. The infant death rate among African-Americans in the United States is more than double the rates among Whites and Hispanics. Such discomforting statistics can be attributed largely to the current number of teenage pregnancies and inadequate prenatal care, as well as marginal nutritional health among poor pregnant women.

Beyond the Nutrients

Many nutrition-related factors also affect the health of mother and fetus.

Low Socioeconomic Status

A constellation of characteristics that lead to poverty, inadequate health care, poor health practices, lack of education, and unmarried status is associated with problems in pregnancy. Currently, in the United States about 25% of all births are to unwed mothers, many of whom are poor.

Closely Spaced Births

Siblings born in succession with less than a year between them are more likely to be born with low birth weights than are those further apart in age. In one study, the risks of low birth weight, preterm birth, or small size for gestational age was 30% to 40% higher for infants conceived less than 6 months apart compared to those conceived 18 to 23 months apart. This danger is especially prevalent among African-American women.

Teenage Pregnancy

About half a million teenagers give birth in the United States each year, accounting for about 13% of all births. In Canada the comparable statistics are about half that amount. Teenage pregnancy poses special health problems for both the mother and child. Young women continue maturing into physical adulthood for 5 years after the onset of menstrual periods **(menarche).** Because the average age for menarche is 13 years in North America, a woman younger than 18 years is not as physically ready to be pregnant as she will be later.

Pregnant teens frequently exhibit a variety of other risk factors that can complicate pregnancy and pose a risk to the fetus. For instance, teenagers are more likely than older women to be underweight at the beginning of pregnancy and to gain fewer than 16 pounds during pregnancy. In addition, their bodies generally lack the maturity needed to safely carry a pregnancy. Sixteen percent of low-birth-weight infants are born to teenage mothers. This occurrence takes place, even with adequate prenatal care. Furthermore, the specific needs of pregnant teenagers vary according to their own growth patterns, body build, and physical activity habits. Thus, it is difficult to estimate their nutrient needs. Overall, mothers who are between the ages of 25 and 34 have the best pregnancy outcomes. Teenage pregnancy should be avoided.

Advanced Maternal Age

The risks of low birth weight and preterm delivery increase modestly, but progressively, with maternal age. Given close monitoring, however, a woman older than age 35 has an excellent chance of producing a healthy infant. Most women in this age group exhibit typical pregnancy-related problems, which usually are manageable under close medical supervision.

Inadequate Prenatal Care

Inadequate, absent, or delayed prenatal care can allow maternal nutritional deficiencies to deprive a fetus of needed nutrients. Chronic diseases, such as hypertension or diabetes, increase the risk of fetal damage. Without prenatal care, a woman is three times more likely to give birth to a low-birth-weight baby—one who will be 40 times more likely to die during the first 4 weeks of life than a normal-birth-weight infant. (The ideal time to start prenatal care is before conception.) Still, about 20% of women in the United States receive no prenatal care in the first trimester—a critical time to change habits.

Lifestyle Factors

Smoking, alcohol consumption, use of some medications, and illegal drug use (such as cocaine and marijuana) in pregnancy all lead to harmful effects. The Nutrition Issue at the end of this chapter reviews one effect of alcohol—fetal alcohol syndrome. The nicotine in cigarette smoke constricts blood vessels and is linked to preterm birth and low birth weight. Smoking also appears to increase the risk of birth defects, sudden infant death, and childhood cancer. Problem drugs include aspirin (when used heavily), hormone ointments, nose drops, rectal suppositories, and medications prescribed for previous illnesses. One goal of *Healthy People 2010* is 100% abstinence from alcohol, cigarettes, and illicit drugs by pregnant women.

Prenatal Ketosis

Ketosis is not desirable for the growing fetus. Ketone bodies are thought to be poorly used by the fetal brain, implying possible slowing of fetal brain development. Researchers oppose crash diets or fasting for more than 12 hours during pregnancy. A pregnant woman can develop significant ketosis after only 20 hours of fasting. Eating about 100 grams of carbohydrate every day prevents ketosis. Even nonpregnant women usually eat twice this amount.

Body Weight and Weight Gain

Obesity leads to an increased rate of hypertension and diabetes during pregnancy. The need for surgery and other complications during delivery likewise increase. These pregnancies require intense monitoring and are linked to an increase in risk of birth defects in the infant, primarily because the fetus can grow very large.

Inadequate weight gain, especially among underweight women, often produces infants of low birth weight. Undernourished women often have borderline vitamin and mineral intakes and need to build up body stores. They should try to reach healthy weight by the end of the first trimester. The recommendation for underweight women is to gain more weight (28 to 40 pounds total) than a woman at healthy weight. Overweight

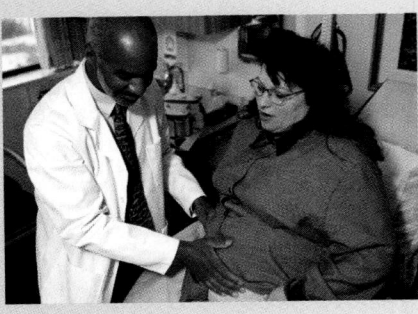

Overweight women pose a major pregnancy risk and need close monitoring by a physician.

women who try to avoid weight gain during pregnancy may rob both themselves and their fetuses of essential nutrients. Also, for efficient protein metabolism during pregnancy, enough carbohydrate and fat are needed to meet energy needs.

Caffeine Consumption

Research on the effects of caffeine consumption by pregnant women has produced some provocative findings. Caffeine decreases the absorption of iron and may reduce blood flow through the placenta, and studies have shown that the fetus is unable to detoxify caffeine. The risk of spontaneous abortion has been shown to increase in the first trimester and early in the second trimester with heavy caffeine consumption (greater than 500 milligrams per day). About 5 cups of coffee per day contain this amount of caffeine (see Appendix I). In addition, as caffeine intake increases, so does the risk of delivering a low-birth-weight infant. Heavy caffeine use during pregnancy may also lead to caffeine withdrawal symptoms in the newborn. Finally, high caffeine intake often occurs in women who also smoke. In this case, it is the smoking that is the greater contributor to low birth weight.

Although more research is needed, it is advisable to limit caffeine intake to 300 milligrams per day. This amount is found in 2–3 cups of coffee, 4 cups of tea, or 6 caffeinated soft drinks. Limiting intake from over-the-counter medicines containing caffeine and chocolate is also important. Some researchers advocate complete avoidance of caffeine during pregnancy in order to reduce the risk of spontaneous abortions, birth defects, and underweight infants.

Aspartame Use

Phenylalanine, a component of aspartame (Nutrasweet and Equal), causes concern for some pregnant women. High amounts of phenylalanine in maternal blood disrupt fetal brain development if the mother has a disease known as *phenylketonuria* (see Chapter 4). If the mother does not have this condition, however, it is unlikely that the baby will be affected by aspartame use. Some experts still recommend caution with regard to aspartame, but total abstinence is hardly warranted, based on current knowledge.

Listeria and Other Infections

Infection by the bacterium *Listeria monocytogenes* causes mild flulike symptoms, such as fever, headache, and vomiting, about 7 to 30 days after exposure. However, pregnant women, newborn infants, and people with depressed immune function may suffer more severe symptoms, including spontaneous abortion and serious blood infections. In these high-risk people, 25% of infections may be fatal.

Because unpasteurized milk, soft cheeses made from raw milk (brie, camembert, feta, and blue cheeses), and raw cabbage can be sources of *Listeria* organisms, it is especially important that pregnant women and other people at high risk avoid these products. Experts advise consuming only pasteurized milk products and cooking meat, poultry, and seafood thoroughly to kill this and other foodborne organisms. It is unsafe in pregnancy to eat any raw meats or other raw animal products. Chapter 16 covers foodborne illness, such as *Listeria* infections, in more detail.

Toxoplasmosis is another infection that causes birth defects. Pregnant women should limit exposure to the organism that causes toxoplasmosis by avoiding contact with cat feces (have someone else clean the cat's litter box), and avoiding contact with kittens, bird feces, and garden soil, and by not eating raw or undercooked meat.

Many of the risk factors described in this Nutrition Insight are avoidable. The goal of a reduction in maternal and infant deaths requires that more attention be paid to these problems.

*W*omen with acquired immune deficiency syndrome (AIDS) may pass the virus that causes this disease to the fetus during pregnancy or the birth process. About 1 in 3 infected newborns will develop AIDS symptoms and die within just a few years. Studies show that these odds of mother-infant transmission can be cut significantly if the woman begins taking the drug zidovudine (AZT) or a related medication by the fourteenth week of pregnancy. Thus, screening pregnant women for AIDS and treating those with AIDS using appropriate medications are currently advocated.

■ Prenatal Care and Counseling

Education, an adequate diet, and early and consistent prenatal medical care maximize the chances of producing a healthy baby and avoiding the risks just covered, such as X-ray exposure, smoking, vitamin A supplements, medicines, illegal drugs, and alcohol use. If diabetes or hypertension is present or developing, it must be carefully controlled to minimize complications in the pregnancy.

Again, women should receive these examinations and counseling strategies before becoming pregnant. Certainly, they should begin early in pregnancy. Many potential problems that develop associated with pregnancy can be diagnosed and quickly treated medically.

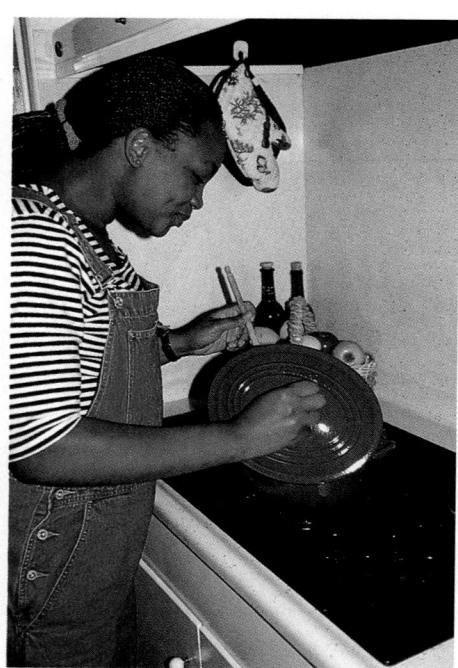

Attention to one's diet is especially important in pregnancy.

Food habits cannot be predicted from income, education, or lifestyle. Although some women already have good dietary habits, most can benefit from nutritional advice. All should be reminded of habits that may harm the growing fetus, such as severe dieting or fasting. By focusing on appropriate prenatal care, good nutrient intake, and proper health habits, as well as using common sense, parents give their fetus—and, later, infant—the very best chance of thriving.

Several U.S. government programs exist to reduce infant mortality by providing high-quality health care and foods. These are designed to alleviate the effects of poverty and insufficient education. An example of such a program is the Special Supplemental Nutrition Program for Women, Infants, and Children (WIC). This program offers health assessments and foods (or vouchers for foods) that supply high-quality protein, calcium, iron, and vitamins A and C to pregnant women, infants, and children (to age 5 years) from low-income populations.

On the WIC program, participants' diets have improved markedly, as has the likelihood that women will have healthy babies. This program is credited with decreasing the cases of iron-deficiency anemia and low-birth-weight infants within the population it serves. Studies have estimated that every dollar spent on the prenatal component of WIC saves about $3 in public health expenditures for the care of low-birth-weight babies.

The WIC program is available in all areas of the United States and has a staff trained to help women have healthy babies. More than 7 million women, infants, and young children are currently enrolled in the program. Many eligible pregnant women are not taking advantage of this program.

Scenario *Follow-Up*

From a dietary standpoint, Tracey is smart to take a close look at her protein intake because needs will increase slightly during pregnancy. More fruits and vegetables will provide some fiber to help prevent constipation, which is common in the later stages of pregnancy. These foods also supply folate, and her use of a multivitamin and mineral supplement provides an ample amount of synthetic folic acid (100% of the Daily Value yields 680 dietary folate equivalents). Still, she should discuss this supplement use with her physician and would probably eventually benefit more from a prenatal supplement if she chooses to continue to use a supplement, as this will have more iron than will an over-the-counter multivitamin and mineral supplement. Her diet may not have enough calcium, so she should pay as much attention to consuming some extra calcium as she does for protein. Avoiding alcohol is a smart move.

Many experts would say that she is consuming too much caffeine and would be wise to cut down to 1 to 2 cups of coffee per day, or possibly even eliminate coffee altogether. Her exercise routine is probably too vigorous if she hasn't already been practicing regular running. Tracey should not begin a new exercise routine upon becoming pregnant unless it is at a moderate pace, such as brisk walking or stationary biking.

▌ Concept Check

Infants born after 37 weeks of gestation and weighing more than 5.5 pounds (2.5 kilograms) have the fewest medical problems at birth. Individual mothers and whole societies can attempt to reduce infant and maternal death and medical problems by limiting the factors that increase the risk of having a preterm or small for gestational age infant. Such contributing factors, besides an inadequate diet in general, include low socioeconomic status; closely spaced births; obesity; inadequate or absent prenatal care; cigarette smoking; alcohol consumption; illegal drug use such as cocaine and marijuana; teenage pregnancy; inadequate prenatal weight gain; heavy caffeine use; *Listeria* exposure; and prenatal ketosis. Adequate nutrition can reduce the risk of many medical problems in pregnancy.

Physiological Changes That Can Cause Discomfort in Pregnancy

During pregnancy, the fetus's needs for oxygen, nutrients, and excretion increase the burden on the mother's lungs, heart, and kidneys. Although a mother's digestive and metabolic systems work very efficiently, some discomfort accompanies the changes her body undergoes to accommodate the fetus.

■ Heartburn, Constipation, and Hemorrhoids

Hormones produced by the placenta relax muscles in both the uterus and the intestinal tract. This often causes heartburn as stomach acid slips up into the esophagus (see Chapter 3). When this occurs, the woman should avoid lying down right after eating, eat less fat so that foods pass more quickly from the stomach into the small intestine, and avoid spicy foods she can't tolerate. She should also consume liquids between meals to decrease stomach volume and pressure. Women with more severe cases may need antacids or related medications.

Constipation often results as the intestinal muscles relax during pregnancy. It is especially likely to develop late in pregnancy, as the fetus competes with the GI tract for space in the abdominal cavity. To offset these discomforts, a woman should perform regular exercise and consume more fluid, dietary fiber, and dried fruits, such as prunes (dried plums). These practices can help prevent constipation and a problem that frequently accompanies it, hemorrhoids. Straining during elimination can lead to hemorrhoids, which are already more likely to occur during pregnancy because of other body changes. A reevaluation of the need and dose of iron supplementation also should be considered, as this practice is linked to constipation (especially intakes greater than 120 milligrams per day).

■ Edema

Placental hormones cause various body tissues to retain fluid during pregnancy. Blood volume also greatly expands during pregnancy. The extra fluid normally causes some swelling (edema). There is no reason to restrict salt severely or use diuretics to limit mild edema. However, the edema may limit physical activity late in pregnancy and occasionally require a woman to elevate her feet to control the symptoms. Overall, edema generally spells trouble only if hypertension and the appearance of protein in the urine accompany fluid retention (see later section on pregnancy-induced hypertension).

■ Morning Sickness

About 50% of pregnant women experience nausea during the early stages of pregnancy. This nausea may be related to the increased sense of smell induced by pregnancy-related hormones circulating in the bloodstream. Although commonly called "morning sickness," pregnancy-related nausea may occur at any time and persist all day. It is often the first signal to a woman that she is pregnant. To help control mild nausea, pregnant women can try the following: avoiding nauseating foods, such as fried or greasy foods; cooking with windows open to dissipate nauseating smells; eating soda crackers or dry cereal before getting out of bed; avoiding large fluid intakes early in the morning; and eating smaller, more frequent meals. Because the iron in prenatal supplements triggers nausea in some women, changing the type of supplement used or postponing use until the second trimester may provide relief in some cases. If a woman thinks her prenatal supplement is related to morning sickness, she should discuss switching to another supplement with her physician.

Overall, whether it is broccoli or soda crackers or lemonade, if a food sounds good to a pregnant woman with morning sickness, she should eat it and eat when she can, while also striving to follow her prenatal diet. If she has a great deal of difficulty in following her diet, she should alert her physician to this and follow the advice given.

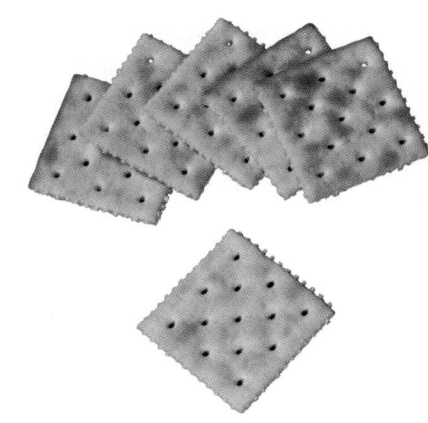

A few crackers between meals can help lessen morning sickness.

Usually, nausea stops after the first trimester; however, in about 10% to 20% of cases, it can continue throughout the entire pregnancy. In cases of serious nausea, the preceding practices offer little relief. When appetite is severely reduced or vomiting persists, medical guidance is warranted. Hospitalization may be needed if the mother exhibits significant dehydration or weight loss.

∎ Anemia

physiological anemia The normal increase in blood volume in pregnancy that dilutes the concentration of red blood cells, resulting in anemia; also called *hemodilution*.

To supply fetal needs, the mother's blood volume expands to approximately 150% of normal. The amount of red blood cells expands only 20% to 30% above normal and occurs more gradually. This leaves proportionately fewer red blood cells in a pregnant woman's bloodstream. The lower ratio of red blood cells to total blood volume is a condition known as **physiological anemia.** It is a normal response to pregnancy, rather than the result of inadequate nutrient intake. If during pregnancy, however, iron stores and/or dietary iron intake are not sufficient to meet needs, any resulting iron-deficiency anemia requires medical attention.

∎ Gestational Diabetes

gestational diabetes A high blood glucose concentration that develops during pregnancy and returns to normal after birth; one cause is the placental production of hormones that interfere with the regulation of blood glucose by insulin.

Hormones synthesized by the placenta interfere with the action of insulin. This antagonism can precipitate **gestational diabetes,** often beginning in weeks 20 to 28, particularly in women who have a family history of diabetes or who are obese. In North America, gestational diabetes develops in about 4% of pregnancies; however, it increases to 7% in the Caucasian population. Today, pregnant women often are screened at 24 to 28 weeks for elevated blood glucose concentration 1 hour after consuming about 75 grams of glucose. If gestational diabetes is detected, a special diet distributing carbohydrate intake throughout the day is recommended. Insulin injections are sometimes needed; regular physical activity is also helpful. Although gestational diabetes often disappears after the infant's birth, it is linked to the development of diabetes later in the mother's life, especially if she fails to maintain healthy body weight. Proper control of both gestational diabetes and diabetes present in the mother before pregnancy is extremely important. If not treated, the primary risks are that the fetus can grow quite large. The fetus will produce too much insulin and this will cause increased fetal growth. The pregnancy may result in a cesarean section due to the size of the fetus. Other concerns are the potential need for early delivery, increased risk of birth trauma and malformations, and low blood glucose in the infant at birth.

∎ Pregnancy-Induced Hypertension

pregnancy-induced hypertension A serious disorder that can include high blood pressure, kidney failure, convulsions, and even death of the mother and fetus. Although its exact cause is not known, meeting nutrient needs and obtaining prenatal care may prevent or limit its severity. Mild cases are known as *preeclampsia;* more severe cases are called *eclampsia* (formerly called *toxemia*).

Pregnancy-induced hypertension is a high-risk disorder that occurs in about 6% to 8% of pregnancies. In its mild forms, it is also known as *preeclampsia* and, in severe forms, as *eclampsia*. Early symptoms include a rise in blood pressure, excess protein in the urine, edema, changes in blood clotting, and nervous system disorders. Very severe effects, including convulsions, can occur in the second and third trimesters. If not controlled, eclampsia eventually damages the liver and kidneys, and both the mother and fetus may die. The population most at risk for this disorder is women over age 35 and those who have had multiple-birth pregnancies. A family history in the mother or father also increases risk, as does a generally inadequate diet, such as too little calcium.

Pregnancy-induced hypertension resolves once the pregnancy ends, making delivery the most reliable treatment for the mother. However, since the problem often begins before the fetus is ready to be born, physicians in many cases must use treatments to prevent the worsening of the disorder. Bed rest and magnesium sulfate are the most common treatment methods, although the effectiveness of these treatments varies and is often disappointing. Several other treatments such as various hypertension medications are under study, but no definite proof exists for success with any one approach.

Concept Check

Heartburn, constipation, hemorrhoids, nausea and vomiting, edema, anemia, and gestational diabetes are possible discomforts and complications of pregnancy. Changes in food habits can often ease these problems. Pregnancy-induced hypertension, with high blood pressure and kidney failure, can lead to severe complications or even death of both the mother and fetus if not treated.

Breastfeeding

Before the 1900s, if a mother didn't breastfeed (nurse) her infant, a substitute nursing mother (wet-nurse) was hired to do it. Formula feeding was fraught with complications, primarily because people did not know the importance of sterilizing formulas against bacteria. Nor did people know much about the nutritional needs of infants. During the early 1900s, the technology of formulas based on cow's milk and methods of feeding improved. From the 1920s and especially in the 1940s, when women worked in armament factories during World War II, more and more babies were fed formula. Throughout the 1950s and early 1960s, interest in breastfeeding further waned. In the 1970s, breastfeeding enjoyed a resurgence, which has since leveled off.

Healthy People 2010 has set a goal of 75% of women nursing their infants at time of hospital discharge, 50% breastfeeding for 6 months, and 25% still breastfeeding at 1 year. The American Dietetic Association and the American Academy of Pediatrics (as well as corresponding Canadian organizations) recommend breastfeeding exclusively for the first 4 months and preferably 6 months, with the continued combination of breastfeeding and infant foods until 1 year. The World Health Organization goes beyond that to recommend breastfeeding for at least 2 years, supplemented with other foods. Surveys show, however, that only about 55% of North American mothers now nurse their infants in the hospital, and at 4 and 6 months only 33% and 20% are still breastfeeding their infants, respectively. Thus, many women are leaving the hospital breastfeeding, but there is a large dropoff, especially after 2 weeks.

Women who choose to breastfeed usually find it an enjoyable, special time in their lives and their relationship with their new infant. Bottle feeding with an infant formula is also safe for infants, as discussed in Chapter 14, but does not equal the benefits derived from human milk in all aspects. If a woman doesn't nurse her child, breast weight returns to normal very soon after birth.

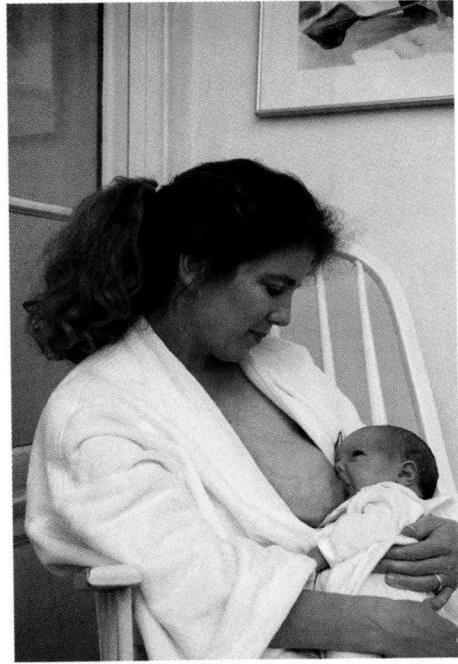

Breastfeeding fosters a closeness and bonding between the mother and the infant.

▪ Ability to Breastfeed

In most cases, problems encountered in breastfeeding are due to a lack of appropriate information, because almost all women are physically capable of nursing their children (see later section on medical conditions precluding breastfeeding for exceptions). Anatomical problems in breasts, such as inverted nipples, can be corrected during pregnancy. Breast size is no indication of success in breastfeeding, and this generally increases during pregnancy. Most women notice a dramatic increase in the size and weight of their breasts by the third or fourth day of breastfeeding. If these changes don't occur, a woman needs to speak with her physician or a lactation consultant.

Breastfed infants must be followed closely over the first days of life to ensure that the process is proceeding normally. Monitoring is especially important with a mother's first child, because the mother will be inexperienced with the process of breastfeeding. Mothers and healthy infants are commonly discharged from the hospital 1 to 2 days after delivery, whereas 20 years ago they stayed in the hospital for 3 or 4 days or longer. One result of such rapid discharge is a decreased period of infant monitoring by health-care professionals. Incidents have been reported of infants developing dehydration and blood clots soon after hospital discharge when breastfeeding did not proceed smoothly. Careful monitoring in this first week by a physician or lacatation consultant is advised.

Information on many of the benefits of breastfeeding can be found at www.4woman.gov./Breastfeeding/ index.htm, sponsored by the U.S. Surgeon General.

Figure 13.5 The anatomy of the breast. Many types of cells form a coordinated network to produce and secrete human milk.

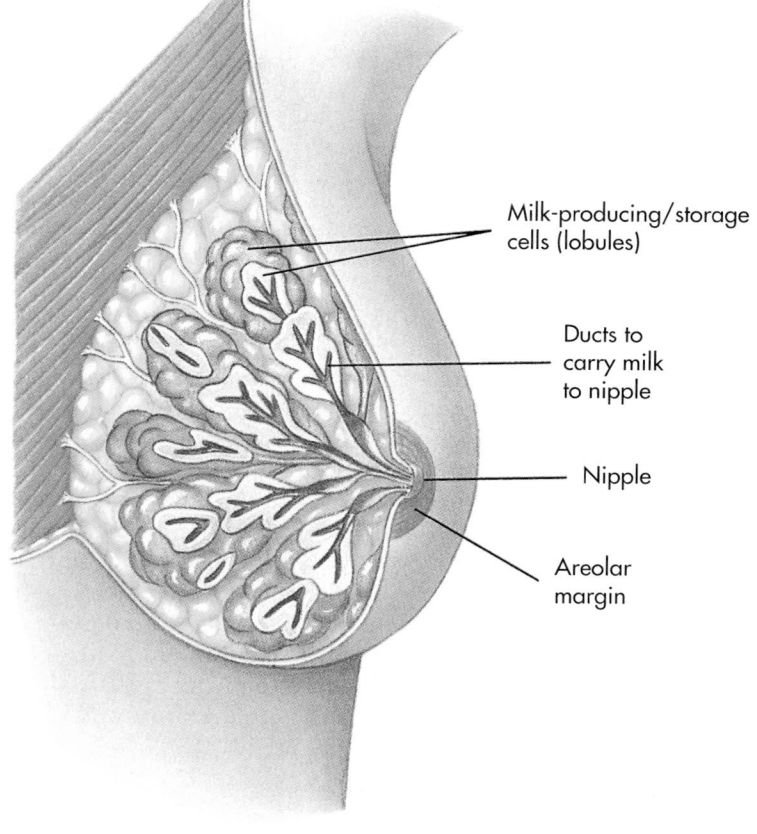

Milk-producing/storage cells (lobules)

Ducts to carry milk to nipple

Nipple

Areolar margin

First-time mothers who plan to breastfeed should learn as much as they can about the process early in their pregnancy. Interested women should learn the proper technique, what problems to expect, and how to respond to them. Overall, breastfeeding is a learned skill, and mothers need knowledge to nurse safely, especially with the first child.

▪ Production of Human Milk

lobules Saclike structures in the breast that store milk.

prolactin A hormone secreted by the mother that stimulates the synthesis of milk.

During pregnancy, cells in the breast form milk-producing **lobules** (Fig. 13.5). Hormones from the placenta stimulate these changes in the breast. After birth, the mother produces more **prolactin** hormone to maintain the changes in the breast and; therefore, the ability to produce milk. During pregnancy, breast weight increases by about 1 to 2 pounds.

The hormone prolactin also stimulates the synthesis of milk. Suckling stimulates prolactin release. Milk synthesis then occurs as an infant nurses. The more the infant suckles, the more milk is produced. Milk production closely parallels infant demand. Because of this fact, even twins can be nursed. Demand is the driving force for milk production.

Most protein found in human milk is synthesized by breast tissue. Some proteins also enter the milk directly from the mother's bloodstream. These proteins include immune factors and enzymes. Fats in human milk come from the mother's diet, and some are synthesized by breast tissue. The sugar galactose is synthesized in the breast, whereas glucose enters from the mother's bloodstream. Together, these sugars form lactose, the main carbohydrate in human milk.

▪ Let-Down Reflex

let-down reflex A reflex stimulated by infant suckling that causes the release (ejection) of milk from milk ducts in the mother's breasts; also called the milk ejection reflex.

oxytocin A hormone secreted by the posterior part of the pituitary gland. It causes contraction of the musclelike cells surrounding the ducts of the breasts, and the smooth muscle of the uterus.

An important brain-breast connection—the **let-down reflex** (also called the milk ejection reflex)—is necessary for breastfeeding. The brain releases the hormone **oxytocin** to allow the breast tissues to let down (release) the milk from storage sites (Fig. 13.6).

It travels to the nipple area. A tingling sensation signals the let-down reflex shortly before milk flow begins. If the let-down reflex doesn't operate, little milk is available to the infant. The infant then gets frustrated, and this can frustrate the mother. It is important that the woman not give up at this point.

The let-down reflex is easily inhibited by nervous tension, a lack of confidence, and fatigue. Mothers should be especially aware of the link between tension and a weak let-down reflex. They need to find a relaxed environment where they can breastfeed.

After a few weeks, the let-down reflex becomes automatic. The mother's response can be triggered just by thinking about her infant or seeing or hearing another one. At first, however, the process can be a bit bewildering. Because she cannot measure the amount of milk the infant takes in, a mother may fear that she is not adequately nourishing the infant.

As a general rule, a well-nourished breastfed infant should (1) have six or more wet diapers per day after the second day of life, (2) show a normal weight gain, and (3) pass at least one or two stools per day that look like lumpy mustard. In addition, softening of the breast during the feeding helps indicate that enough milk is being consumed. Parents who sense their infant is not consuming enough milk should consult a physician immediately because dehydration can develop rapidly.

It generally takes 2 to 3 weeks to fully establish the feeding routine: Infant and mother both feel comfortable, the milk supply meets infant demand, and initial nipple soreness disappears. Establishing the breastfeeding routine requires patience, but the rewards are great. The adjustments are easier if supplemental formula feedings are not introduced until breastfeeding is well established, after at least 3 to 4 weeks. Then a supplemental bottle or two of infant formula per day is fine.

Parents need not be concerned that breastfed infants grow a bit more slowly after about 3 months of age than formula-fed infants, based on increases in body weight. The infant's physician is the best judge of whether the rate of growth of the breastfed infant is satisfactory. Essentially, the difference is of no consequence, in part because some of it is related to increased fat deposition.

■ Nutritional Qualities of Human Milk

Human milk is very different in composition from cow's milk. Unless altered, cow's milk should not be used in infant feeding until the infant is 12 months old because cow's milk is too high in minerals and protein, does not contain enough carbohydrate to meet infant needs, and may trigger the development of diabetes in infants with a genetic predisposition to the disorder. In addition, the major protein in cow's milk, casein, is harder for an infant to digest than the major proteins in human milk, lactalbumin and other whey proteins. Finally, certain compounds in human milk presently under study show other possible benefits for the infant, such as improved vision and nervous system development. These factors, such as the omega-3 fatty acids typically found in fish (see following discussion of mature milk), are not present in cow's milk or infant formulas, but will be added in the near future (see Chapter 14).

Colostrum

The first fluid made by the human breast is **colostrum.** This thick, yellowish fluid may leak from the breast during late pregnancy and is produced in earnest for a few days to a week after birth. Colostrum contains antibodies and immune-system cells, some of which pass unaltered through the immature GI tract of the infant into the bloodstream. The first few months of life is the only time we can readily absorb whole proteins across the GI tract. These immune factors and cells protect the infant from some gastrointestinal diseases and other infectious disorders, compensating for the infant's own immature immune system during the first few months of life.

Colostrum facilitates the passage of **meconium,** a stool produced during fetal life. One component of colostrum, the *Lactobacillus bifidus* **factor,** encourages the growth of *Lactobacillus bifidus* bacteria. These bacteria limit the growth of potentially toxic

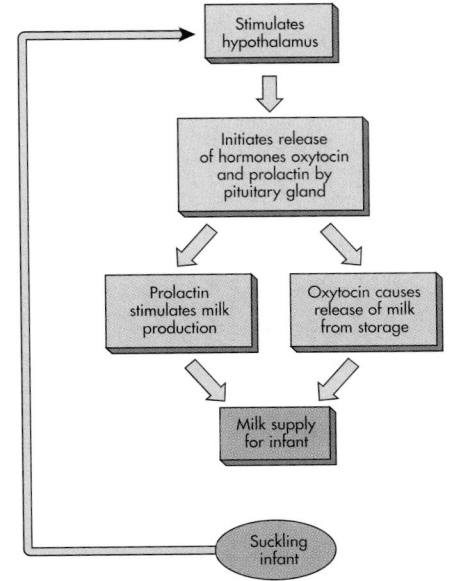

Figure 13.6 The let-down reflex—from suckling infant to human milk secretion from the breast.

*D*isposable diapers can absorb so much urine that it is difficult to judge when they are wet. A strip of paper towel laid inside a disposable diaper makes a good wetness indicator. Or cloth diapers may be used for a day or two to assess whether nursing is supplying sufficient milk.

colostrum The first fluid secreted by the breast during late pregnancy and the first few days after birth. This thick fluid is rich in immune factors and protein.

meconium The first thick, mucuslike stool passed by the infant after birth.

Lactobacillus bifidus factor A protective factor secreted in the colostrum that encourages growth of beneficial bacteria in the newborn's intestines.

bacteria in the intestine. Overall, breastfeeding promotes the intestinal health of the breastfed infant in this way.

Mature Milk

Human milk composition gradually changes until several days after delivery, when it achieves the normal composition of mature milk. Human milk looks very different from cow's milk. (Table 14.1 in the next chapter provides a direct comparison.) Human milk is thin and almost watery in appearance and often has a slightly bluish tinge. Its nutritional qualities are quite impressive.

Human milk's main protein forms a soft, light curd in the infant's stomach, easing digestion. Other human milk proteins bind iron, reducing the growth of iron-requiring bacteria. Many of these types of bacteria cause diarrhea. Still other proteins offer the important immune protection already noted.

The fat in human breast milk is high in linoleic acid and cholesterol, which are needed for brain development. Breast milk also contains long-chain omega-3 fatty acids, as just noted.

Human milk even changes in fat composition during each feeding. The consistency of milk released initially (about 60% of the volume) resembles that of skim milk. The next amount (about 35% of the total volume) has a greater fat proportion, similar to whole milk. Finally, the hindmilk (about 5% of the total) is essentially like cream and is usually released 10 to 20 minutes into the feeding. The overall energy content of human milk is about the same as that of infant formulas (67 kcal per 100 milliliters). Babies need to nurse long enough (e.g., a total of 20 or more minutes) to get the energy in the rich hindmilk to be satisfied between feedings and to grow well.

Human milk also allows for adequate hydration of the infant, provided the baby is exclusively breastfed. A question commonly asked is whether the infant needs additional water, if stressed by hot weather, diarrhea, vomiting, or fever. Providing up to 4 ounces of water a day from a bottle to young breastfed infants is fine. Note, however, that greater amounts of supplemental water can lead to brain disorders, low blood sodium, and other problems. Thus, extra water may be given, but only with a physician's guidance.

■ Food Plan for Women Who Breastfeed

Nutrient needs for a breastfeeding mother change to some extent from those of the pregnant woman (see the inside cover of this book). These include decreases in folate and iron needs and an increase in the need for energy, vitamins A, E, and C, riboflavin, copper, chromium, iodide, magnanese, selenium, and zinc. The diet for breastfeeding women can be the same as that for pregnant women, except teenagers generally should have about 4 servings from the milk, yogurt, and cheese group (review Table 13.2). As in pregnancy, a serving of a highly fortified ready-to-eat breakfast cereal or a typical multivitamin and mineral supplement is advised to meet extra nutrient needs.

A reasonable approach for a breastfeeding woman is to eat a balanced diet that supplies at least 1800 kcal per day, has a moderate fat content, includes a variety of dairy products, fruits, vegetables, and grains, and fish intake at least twice a week (or use fish oil capsules to receive 900 milligrams of omega-3 fatty acids). The woman should drink fluids every time the infant nurses, because drinking to quench thirst encourages ample milk production (a total of 8 to 12 cups per day). If a woman restricts her energy intake too severely, the quantity of milk also decreases. This is not a time to crash diet. More than two alcoholic drinks a day also decreases milk output, as does smoking. Finally, the same warning to avoid fish with possible mercury contamination given to pregnant women apply to the breastfeeding mother. The woman may also want to avoid peanuts, as the passage of peanut allergens into breastmilk is thought to put the infant at risk of such an allergy.

Milk production requires approximately 800 kcal every day. The RDA for energy during lactation is an extra 500 kcal daily above prepregnancy recommendations. The

Most substances the mother ingests are secreted into her milk. For this reason, she should limit intake of or avoid all alcohol and caffeine and check all medications with a pediatrician. Some mothers believe that some foods, such as garlic and chocolate, flavor the breast milk and upset the infant. If a woman notices a connection between a food she eats and the infant's later fussiness, she could consider avoiding that food. However, she might experiment again with it later, as infants become fussy for other reasons. Some researchers, on the other hand, feel that the passage of flavors from the mother's diet into her milk affords an opportunity for the infant to learn about the flavor of the foods of its family long before solids are introduced. These researchers suspect that bottle-fed infants are missing significant sensory experiences that until recent times in human history were common to all infants.

difference between energy needs and intake—about 300 kcal—should contribute to gradual loss of the extra body fat accumulated during pregnancy, especially if breastfeeding is continued for 6 months or more and the woman performs some physical activity. This shows how practical the link is between pregnancy and breastfeeding. Weight loss of 1 to 4 pounds per month in the nursing mother is appropriate. Milk output decreases at significantly greater rates of weight loss, as occur with severe dieting when energy intake is less than about 1500 kcal per day.

Concept Check

Recognition of the importance of breastfeeding has contributed to its greater popularity during the past 20 years. Almost all women have the ability to breastfeed. The hormone prolactin stimulates breast tissue to synthesize milk. Some components of human milk come directly from the mother's bloodstream. Infant suckling triggers a let-down reflex, which releases the milk. The more an infant nurses, the more milk is synthesized. The nutrient composition of human milk is very different from that of cow's milk and changes as the infant matures. The first fluid produced, colostrum, is rich in immune factors. The diet for breastfeeding is generally similar to that for pregnancy, except for additional fluids, as well as 4 servings from the milk, yogurt, and cheese group for teenage mothers in general.

■ Pros and Cons of Breastfeeding

As noted already, the vast majority of women are capable of breastfeeding, and infants benefit from it. The many benefits are listed in Table 13.3. Nonetheless, a woman's decision to nurse depends on a variety of factors, some of which may make breastfeeding impractical or undesirable for a woman. Mothers who don't want to breastfeed their infants should not feel compelled to do so. Breastfeeding provides distinct advantages, but none so great that a woman who decides to bottle-feed should feel she is significantly penalizing her infant.

Table 13.3 Attributes of Breastfeeding

Infant
- Bacteriologically safe
- Always fresh and ready to go
- Provides antibodies while infant's immune system is still immature, as well as other substances that contribute to maturation of the immune system
- Contributes to maturation of gastrointestinal tract via *Lactobacillus bifidus* factor; decreases development of diarrhea and respiratory disease
- Reduces risk of food allergies and intolerances, as well as other allergies
- Establishes habit of eating in moderation, thus decreasing risk of obesity later in life by about 20%
- Contributes to proper development of jaws and teeth for better speech development
- Decreases ear infections
- Facilitates bonding (psychological attachment) with mother
- May enhance nervous system development (by providing omega-3 fatty acids) and eventual learning ability
- May reduce the risk of later development of hypertension

Mother
- Contributes to earlier recovery from pregnancy due to a quicker return of the uterus to the prepregnancy state
- Decreases the risk of ovarian and premenopausal breast cancer
- Lessens the economic strain of purchasing formula
- Facilitates bonding (psychological attachment) with infant

Advantages Of Breastfeeding

Human milk is tailored to meet infant nutrient needs for the first 4 to 6 months of life. The possible exceptions are the relative lack of fluoride, iron, and vitamin D. Infant supplements, used under the guidance of a pediatrician, can supply these and are generally recommended. Some sun exposure also helps compensate for the gap in vitamin D nutriture, but will likely not be enough for dark-skinned (e.g., African-American) infants, as they synthesize less vitamin D from typical sun exposure. Supplemental vitamin D is advised (see Chapter 14). Fluoride may be found in the household water supply. If it is not present in adequate amounts or the child is not receiving tap water, a fluoride supplement after 6 months of age should be considered and a dentist consulted. Vitamin B-12 supplements are recommended for the breast-fed infant whose mother is a complete vegetarian (vegan).

Frozen human milk should not be thawed in a microwave. The heat can destroy immune factors in the milk and create hot spots, which may scald the infant's tongue.

Fewer Infections   Breastfeeding reduces the general risk of infections to the infant. This is partially because of the antibodies in human milk that an infant can use. Breastfed infants also have fewer ear infections (otitis media) because they do not sleep with a bottle in the mouth. Experts strongly discourage allowing infants to sleep with a bottle in their mouths (or continuing to breastfeed as the infant sleeps). When that happens, milk pools in the infant's mouth, backs up through the throat, and eventually settles in the ears, creating a growth medium for bacteria. Infant ear infections are a common problem. By avoiding them, parents can decrease discomfort for the infant, avoid related trips to the doctor, and prevent possible hearing loss. Tooth decay from nighttime bottles is another likely consequence (see Chapter 14).

Fewer Allergies and Intolerances   Breastfeeding also reduces the chances of allergies, especially in allergy-prone infants (see the Nutrition Issue in Chapter 14). The key time to attain this benefit from breastfeeding is during the first 4 to 6 months of an infant's life. Breastfeeding for even just the first few weeks is beneficial. A longer commitment than 4 to 6 months is better, but the first few months are most critical. Another benefit of breastfeeding is that infants are better able to tolerate human milk than formulas. Formulas must occasionally be switched several times until caregivers find the best one for the infant.

Convenience and Cost   Breastfeeding frees the mother from the time and expense involved in buying and preparing formula and washing bottles. Human milk is ready to go and sterile. This allows the mother to spend more time with her baby. On the other hand, if the child is bottle-fed, the mother may be free to do other things while others feed the baby.

Barriers to Breastfeeding

Widespread misinformation, return to jobs, and social reticence all serve as barriers to breastfeeding.

Misinformation   Probably the major barriers to breastfeeding are misinformation, such as one's breasts are too small, and lack of role models. One positive note has been the widespread increase in the availability of lactation consultants over the past several years. These consultants are a valuable source for new mothers in the adjustment to breastfeeding. If a woman is interested in breastfeeding, she should also talk to women who have done it successfully. Experienced mothers can be an enormous help to the first-time mother. The first-time mother should find a friend she can call on for advice. In almost every community, a group called La Leche League offers classes in breastfeeding and advises women who have problems with it (800-LALECHE or www.lalecheleague.org). Other resources are breastfeeding.com and breastfeeding.org.

Return to an Outside Job Working outside the home can complicate plans to breastfeed. One possibility after a month or two of breastfeeding is for the mother to regularly express and save her own milk. She can express milk by breast pump or manually into a sterile plastic bottle or nursing bag (used in a disposable bottle system). Saving human milk requires careful sanitation and rapid chilling. It can be stored in the refrigerator for 1 day and be frozen for 1 month. There is a knack to learning how to express milk, but the freedom can be worth it, because it allows others to feed the infant the mother's milk. A schedule of expressing milk and using supplemental formula feedings is most successful if begun after 1 to 2 months of exclusive breastfeeding. After 1 month or so, the baby is well adapted to breastfeeding and probably feels enough emotional security and other benefits from nursing to drink both ways.

Some women can juggle both a job and breastfeeding, but others find it too cumbersome and decide to formula-feed. A compromise—balancing some breastfeedings, perhaps early morning and night, with formula-feedings during the day—is possible. However, too many supplemental formula feedings decrease milk production.

Social Concerns Another barrier for some women is embarrassment about nursing a child in public. Historically, our society has stressed modesty and has discouraged public displays of breasts—even for as good a cause as nourishing babies. Women who feel reticent should be reassured that with appropriate clothing, they can nurse quite discreetly.

Medical Conditions Precluding Breastfeeding Breastfeeding may be ruled out by certain medical conditions in either the infant or mother. For example, infants with the disease galactosemia can't break down galactose, the major sugar in breast milk. These infants do not grow well if nursed and often suffer from vomiting and diarrhea. If left untreated, the infants ultimately develop liver disease, cataracts, and mental retardation. A special infant formula free of galactose must be used. Breastfeeding may also be detrimental to infants with phenylketonuria; the high concentration of phenylalanine in breast milk may overwhelm the impaired ability of these infants to metabolize this amino acid, leading to production of toxic products.

Mothers who take certain medications, which pass into the milk and adversely affect the nursing infant, may be advised to avoid breastfeeding. In addition, a woman in North America and other developed countries who has a serious chronic disease (such as tuberculosis, AIDS or HIV-positive status, or certain forms of hepatitis) or who is being treated with chemotherapy medications should not breastfeed. A final group can include immature mothers and those with mental problems.

B reastfeeding mothers should get their physician's permission before embarking on a vigorous exercise program. Breastfeeding women must also take care to drink plenty of fluids before and after workouts and should avoid exercising when fatigued.

▌ Another Bite

*T*hough the concerns of some women with regard to environmental contaminants in human milk are legitimate, the benefits from human milk are very well established, and the risks from environmental contaminants are still largely theoretical. Thus, it is probably best to continue with what has been shown to work until sufficiently strong research data contradict it. A few measures a woman could take to counteract some known contaminants and toxins are to (1) avoid freshwater fish from polluted waters, (2) carefully wash and peel fruits and vegetables, (3) remove the fatty edges of meat, as this is where pesticides concentrate, and (4) limit exposure to toxins such as fumes from nail polish remover, paint thinner, gasoline, and dry-cleaning solutions. In addition, a woman should not try to lose weight rapidly while nursing (more than 1 pound per week), because contaminants stored in fat tissue might then enter her bloodstream and affect her milk. If a woman questions whether her milk is safe, especially if she has lived in an area known to have a high concentration of toxic wastes or environmental pollutants, she should consult her local health department.

◼ Can a Preterm Infant Be Breastfed?

There is no clear-cut answer to whether a woman can breastfeed a preterm infant. In some cases, human milk is the most desirable form of nourishment, depending on weight and length of gestation. If so, it must usually be expressed from the breast and fed through a tube. This type of feeding demands great maternal dedication. Fortification of the milk with such nutrients as calcium, phosphorus, sodium, and protein is often necessary to match an infant's rapid growth. In other cases, special feeding problems may prevent the use of human milk or necessitate supplementing it with formula. Sometimes total parenteral nutrition support is the only option. Working as a team, the pediatrician, neonatal nurses, and registered dietitian must guide the parents in this decision.

Concept Check

Human milk supplies most of an infant's nutritional needs for the first 6 months, although supplementation with vitamin D, iron, and fluoride may be needed. Breastfeeding is less expensive and often more convenient than formula feeding. Compared with formula-fed infants, breastfed infants have fewer intestinal, respiratory, and ear infections and are less susceptible to allergies and food intolerances. Despite the advantages of breastfeeding, misinformation, a return to work, and social reticence may dissuade a mother from breastfeeding. A combination of breastfeeding and formula feeding is possible when a mother is regularly away from the infant and is not able to express and store her milk for later use. Breastfeeding is not desirable if a mother has certain diseases or must take medication potentially harmful to the infant. The preterm infant, depending on its condition, may benefit from consuming human milk.

Summary

1. Adequate nutrition is vital during pregnancy to ensure the well-being of both the infant and mother. Poor maternal nutrition and use of some medications, especially during the first trimester, can cause birth defects. Growth retardation and altered development can also occur if these insults happen later in pregnancy.
2. Infants born preterm (before 37 weeks gestation) usually have more medical problems at and following birth than do normal infants.
3. A woman typically needs an additional 300 kcal per day during the second and third trimesters of pregnancy to meet her energy needs. A better measure of meeting energy needs is weight gain. This should occur slowly, reaching a total of 25 to 35 pounds in a woman of healthy weight.
4. Protein, vitamin, and mineral needs increase during pregnancy. Extra servings from the milk, yogurt, and cheese group and the meat, poultry, fish, dry beans, eggs, and nuts group of the Food Guide Pyramid are recommended. A supplement containing folate and iron, in particular, is sometimes needed. Folate nutriture especially should be adequate at the time of conception. Any supplement use needs to be guided by a physician, as an excess intake of vitamin A and other nutrients during pregnancy can have harmful effects on the fetus.
5. The factors that contribute to poor pregnancy outcome include inadequate health care in general and prenatal care in particular,

teenage pregnancy, closely spaced births, smoking, alcohol consumption, illegal drug use (such as cocaine and marijuana), insufficient carbohydrate intake (less than 100 grams per day), obesity, heavy caffeine use, and various infections, such as *Listeria* and AIDS.
6. Gestational diabetes, heartburn, constipation, nausea, vomiting, edema, and anemia are all possible discomforts and complications of pregnancy. Nutrition therapy can help minimize some of these problems.
7. Almost all women are able to nurse their infants. The nutrient composition of human milk is very different from that of unaltered cow's milk and is much more desirable. Colostrum, the first fluid produced by the human breast, is very rich in immune factors. Mature milk is rich in the protein lactalbumin and in lactose.
8. For the infant, the advantages of breastfeeding over formula feeding are numerous, including fewer intestinal, respiratory, and ear infections and fewer allergies and food intolerances. Moreover, breastfeeding is also less expensive and possibly more convenient for the mother than formula feeding. However, an infant can be adequately nourished with formula if the mother chooses not to breastfeed. Breastfeeding is not desirable if the mother has certain diseases or must take medication that is potentially harmful to the infant. Likewise, breastfeeding is not advised for infants with certain medical conditions, including some preterm infants.

Study Questions

1. What historical evidence established the importance of nutrition in pregnancy outcome?
2. Provide three key pieces of advice for parents seeking to maximize their chances of having a healthy infant. Why did you identify those specific factors?
3. Outline current weight-gain recommendations for pregnancy. What is the basis for these recommendations?
4. How is the Food Guide Pyramid adapted to meet the increased nutrient needs of pregnancy?
5. Why does teenage pregnancy receive so much attention these days? At what age do you think pregnancy is ideal? Why?
6. Give three reasons why a woman should give serious consideration to breastfeeding her infant.
7. Describe the physiological mechanisms that stimulate milk production and release. How can knowing about these help mothers nurse successfully?
8. What guidelines can a woman use to determine whether her breastfed infant is receiving sufficient nourishment?
9. How should the basic food plan suitable for pregnancy be modified during breastfeeding?
10. Where can new mothers go for help in establishing successful breastfeeding?

Further Readings

1. ADA Reports: Position of the American Dietetic Association: Breaking barriers to breastfeeding. *Journal of the American Dietetic Association* 101:1213, 2001.
   Exclusive breastfeeding for 6 months and breastfeeding with complementary foods for at least 12 months is the ideal feeding pattern for infants. Increases in initiation and duration are needed to realize the health, nutritional, immune-related, psychological, economical, and environmental benefits of breastfeeding.

2. Artal R, Sherman C: Exercise during pregnancy: Safe and beneficial for most. *The Physician and Sportsmedicine* 27:51, 1999.
   Regular, moderate exercise may ease pregnancy and subsequent labor. Moderate exercise does not significantly affect length of gestation or birth weight.

3. Committee on Adolescents: Adolescent pregnancy—Current trends and issues: 1998. *Pediatrics* 103:516, 1999.
   The factors most associated with negative pregnancy results in teenagers are low prepregnancy weight and height, previous pregnancies, and poor pregnancy weight gain. Social factors associated with poor outcomes include poverty, unmarried status, limited education, drug use, and inadequate prenatal care.

4. Godfrey KM, Barker DJP: Fetal nutrition and adult disease. *American Journal of Clinical Nutrition* 71(Suppl):1344S, 2000.
   Fetal undernutrition in middle and late pregnancy can lead to reduced fetal growth, especially in some organs, such as the liver and kidneys. This fetal undernutrition has been linked to disordered cholesterol metabolism and cardiovascular disease, insulin resistance, hypertension, and increased blood coagulation in adulthood.

5. King JC: Physiology of pregnancy and nutrient metabolism. *American Journal of Clinical Nutrition* 71(Suppl):1218S, 2000.
   The energy needed for basal metabolism during pregnancy depends on maternal prepregnant nutritional status and on fetal size. When energy needs are not met, fetal growth may suffer. Efforts to achieve good maternal nutritional status preconception, as well as throughout gestation, best ensure a healthy outcome for fetal growth and development.

6. Kjos SL, Buchanan TA: Gestational diabetes mellitus. *The New England Journal of Medicine* 341:1750, 1999.
   An increase from 4% to 7% of gestational diabetes has been seen in the U.S. Caucasian population in recent years. Women with gestational diabetes have a 17% to 63% risk of developing type 2 diabetes within 5 to 16 years after the pregnancy. The careful monitoring of blood pressure, weight gain, and urinary protein excretion is recommended, particularly during the second half of pregnancy.

7. Lawrence RA: A 35-year-old woman experiencing difficulty with breastfeeding. *Journal of the American Medical Association* 285:73, 2001.
   This article provides much advice for successful breastfeeding. One key is careful follow-up immediately after birth. The American Academy of Pediatrics recommends an assessment 48 hours after discharge regarding the success of ongoing breastfeeding, at least by telephone, and visits to the office by the mother and infant within 7 days. It also is important to instill confidence in the mother regarding her ability to nurse her infant. She should also consume no less than 1800 kcal per day and include extra water and other fluids.

8. Pipkin FB: Risk factors for preeclampsia. *The New England Journal of Medicine* 344:926, 2001.
   The high incidence of preeclampsia in many developing countries suggests that an inadequate diet may be a risk factor. The dietary inadequacies that have been proposed include calcium, zinc, vitamins C and E, and omega-3 fatty acids. Thus, recommendations for a sensibly balanced diet during pregnancy should be part of routine care.

9. Scholl TO, Johnson WG: Folic acid: Influence on the outcome of pregnancy. *American Journal of Clinical Nutrition* 71(Suppl):1295S, 2000.
   Poor dietary folic acid intake and low circulating concentrations of folic acid in pregnant women increase the risk of adverse birth outcomes. Supplementation studies likewise suggest that some women—most likely poor women—may benefit from receiving additional folic acid before, as well as during, pregnancy.

10. Scholl TO, Reilly T: Anemia, iron and pregnancy outcome. *Journal of Nutrition* 130:443S, 2000.
    When maternal anemia is diagnosed before midpregnancy, it is associated with increased risk of preterm delivery. Maternal anemia detected during the later stages of pregnancy often reflects the expected (and necessary) expansion of maternal plasma volume. Thus, this anemia in the later stages of pregnancy is not associated with the same increased risk of preterm delivery.

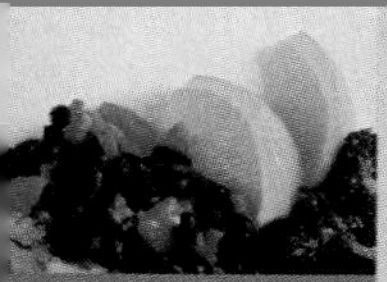

I. Targeting Nutrients Necessary for Pregnant Women

This chapter mentioned that pregnant women may have difficulty meeting their increased needs for folate, vitamin D, iron, calcium, and zinc. List five foods rich in each of these nutrients next to the appropriate heading. Refer to Chapters 8 and 9 if necessary.

Nutrient	Foods		Nutrient	Foods
Folate	_____		Calcium	_____
	_____			_____
	_____			_____
	_____			_____
	_____			_____
	_____			_____
Vitamin D	_____		Zinc	_____
	_____			_____
	_____			_____
	_____			_____
	_____			_____
	_____			_____
Iron	_____			_____
	_____			
	_____			
	_____			
	_____			
	_____			

1. Foods rich in more than one of these nutrients would be especially valuable for pregnant women. Write on the line any foods you listed that are good sources of more than one of these critical nutrients.

_____

2. The need for folate, vitamin D, iron, calcium, and zinc increases during pregnancy. For which of these nutrients can pregnant women usually obtain adequate intakes from dietary sources?

_____

Which of these nutrients are commonly taken in supplement form during pregnancy? Why might it be hard for pregnant women to meet their increased needs for these nutrients from food alone?

_____

_____

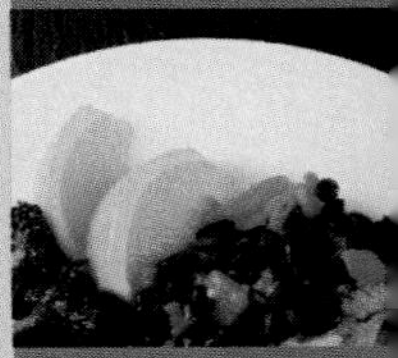

II. Putting Your Knowledge About Nutrition and Pregnancy to Work

A college friend tells you that she is newly pregnant. You are aware that this friend usually likes to eat the following foods for her meals:

Breakfast
Skips this meal, or eats a granola bar
Coffee

Lunch
Sweetened yogurt
Bagel with cream cheese
Occasional piece of fruit
Regular caffeinated soda

Snack
Chocolate candy bar

Dinner
Pizza, macaroni and cheese, or eggs with toast
Seldom eats a salad or vegetable
Regular caffeinated soda

Snacks
Pretzels or chips
Regular caffeinated soda

1. Using your software, or Appendix A, evaluate your friend's diet for protein, iron, folate, calcium, and zinc. How does her intake compare with the recommended amounts for pregnancy?

_____

_____

_____

2. Now redesign her diet and make sure that her intake meets pregnancy needs for protein, folate, calcium, and zinc. (Hint: Fortified foods, such as a ready-to-eat breakfast cereal, are generally nutrient-rich foods, which can more easily help meet one's needs.) Increase the iron content as well, but it still may be below the RDA for pregnancy.

_____

_____

_____

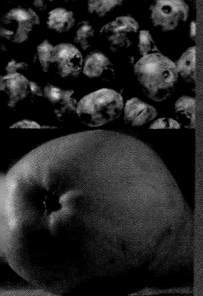

Although much is known about diagnosing and treating some learning problems in children, many causes remain elusive. One particular question haunts many mothers: Did something happen while I was pregnant that created a learning disability in my child? This question leads directly to the topic of alcohol use during pregnancy, since alcohol is the most common damaging substance to which fetuses are exposed.

Conclusive evidence shows that large amounts of alcohol harm the fetus, especially when associated with binge drinking (for a woman, consumption of four or more alcoholic drinks at one sitting). Binge drinking is especially perilous during the first 12 weeks of pregnancy, as this is when critical early developmental events take place in the womb. Scientists don't know whether pregnant women must eliminate alcohol use entirely to avoid risk of damage to the fetus; but until a safe level can be established, women are advised not to drink any alcohol during pregnancy or when there is a chance pregnancy might occur.

When a pregnant woman drinks more alcohol than she can metabolize, the excess reaches the embryo (and, at later stages, the fetus), which has no means of detoxifying it. Women with chronic alcoholism produce children with a recognizable pattern of malformations called **fetal alcohol syndrome (FAS).** A diagnosis of FAS is based mainly on poor fetal and infant growth, physical deformities (especially of facial features), and mental retardation (Fig. 13.7). The infant is frequently irritable and may develop hyperactivity and a short attention span. Limited hand-eye coordination is common. Defects in vision, hearing, and mental processing often develop over time.

The range of abnormalities from alcohol exposure varies from the severe effects associated with FAS to reduced birth weight, behavioral effects, growth retardation, and hampered learning ability in infants born to women who report only social drinking. The latter condition, termed **fetal alcohol effects (FAE),** is not marked by telltale facial abnormalities. For this reason, parents may not suspect the presence of subtle defects caused by alcohol, even when they exist. FAE can devastate learning potential.

In North America up to 30 per 10,000 infants exhibiting FAS are born each year; the incidence of FAS also has increased since the late 1970s. Many more infants are born annually with FAE. Today, 1 in 29 pregnant women reported drinking the equivalent of at least a glass of wine a day.

fetal alcohol syndrome (FAS) A group of irreversible physical and mental abnormalities in the infant that result from the mother's consuming alcohol during pregnancy.

fetal alcohol effect (FAE) Hyperactivity, attention deficit disorder, poor judgment, sleep disorders, and delayed learning as a result of being prenatally exposed to alcohol.

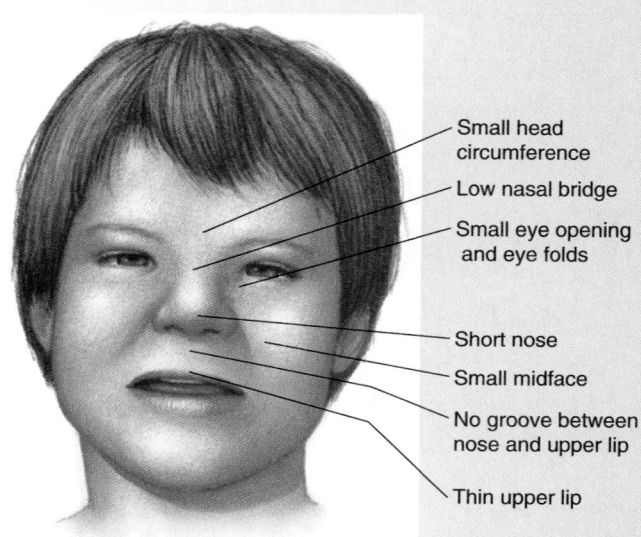

Small head circumference

Low nasal bridge

Small eye opening and eye folds

Short nose

Small midface

No groove between nose and upper lip

Thin upper lip

Figure 13.7 Fetal alcohol syndrome. Milder forms of alcohol-induced changes in the fetus and the infant are known as *fetal alcohol effects.* The facial features shown are typical of affected children. Additional abnormalities in the brain and other internal organs accompany fetal alcohol syndrome but are not immediately apparent from simply looking at the child.

Alcohol use is, in fact, the leading cause of preventable birth defects and mental retardation in North America and in the Western world as a whole.

Exactly how alcohol causes these defects is not known. One line of research suggests that alcohol, or products produced by the metabolism of alcohol (acetaldehyde), cause faulty migration of cells in the brain during early stages of development or block the action of certain neurotransmitters in the brain. In addition, inadequate nutrient intake, reduced nutrient and oxygen transfer across the placenta, cigarette smoking commonly linked to alcohol intake, drug use, and possibly other factors contribute to the overall result. Furthermore, it is not known how much alcohol it takes to produce these adverse effects. Again, for this reason, many authorities—including the U.S. Surgeon General and the American Medical Association—believe it is best that mothers-to-be avoid alcohol altogether. In other words, there is no safe drinking.

Abstinence is especially important during the first trimester, when key growth and development occur. Alcohol reaches the fetal blood at the same concentration as the mother's blood within 15 minutes of her drinking. However, the effect on the fetus may be up to 10 times greater. For example, just one bout of binge drinking can arrest and alter cell division during critical phases of fetal development. The fetus then may develop an irreversible defect.

Physical damage to the embryo (and later the fetus) results more from first-trimester drinking because the basic structures of tissues and organs develop during this period. Emotional and learning problems stem more from third-trimester drinking because this is when critical further development of the brain occurs. And, throughout the pregnancy, alcohol interferes with growth. Overall, mothers who drink at least one to two drinks a day throughout pregnancy are much more likely to have growth-retarded infants, and mothers who drink only in late pregnancy are more likely to give birth to preterm infants.

Because alcohol has the capacity to adversely affect each stage of fetal development, the earlier in pregnancy that drinking ceases, the greater the potential for improved outcome. The best course is to consider alcohol an indulgence that must be eliminated from the time of conception until after pregnancy. Currently about half of all women in North America are drinking at the time of conception (i.e., before learning they are pregnant). One step in the right direction is the mandated warnings about drinking during pregnancy that appear on all alcoholic beverage containers in the United States.

Pregnancy lasts only 9 months. In contrast, parents may spend a lifetime caring, often at great expense (estimated at $1.4 million in the United States), for their offspring needlessly handicapped by FAS or FAE. Keep in mind that fetal alcohol syndrome is a completely preventable disease.

Pregnant women should recognize that many cough syrups contain alcohol. Cases have been reported of infants with FAS born to mothers who consumed generous amounts of such cough syrups but no other alcoholic beverages.

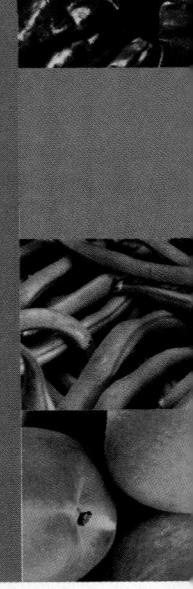

chapter *14*

Nutrition from Infancy Through Adolescence

Chapter Outline

As humans grow through early years into adulthood, our needs for energy and nutrients change. Infants need more energy, protein, vitamins, and minerals per pound of body weight than do adults to support their tremendous growth and development. As growth tapers, children need and eat proportionately less. The erratic eating behaviors of young children pose major challenges for parents and other caregivers. In turn, childhood becomes an important time to establish healthful habits, including those related to food choice and physical activity.

The family wields a subtle but important influence over the child. Thus, education designed to change children's eating behaviors must be directed simultaneously at the main caregivers. They usually determine what foods are purchased and how they are prepared. To help children adopt a lifelong healthy dietary intake, parents and caregivers should provide a variety of foods at home, limit take-out food, and introduce new foods regularly. Maintaining a healthful eating pattern should continue as children grow into teenagers. In exploring all these stages of life, this chapter looks at the key role nutrients play and how food choices should be tailored to meet those needs.

Check out the **Contemporary Nutrition: Issues and Insights Online Learning Center** www.mhhe.com/wardlawcont5 *for quizzes, flash cards, other activities, and web links designed to further help you learn about issues surrounding nutrition from infancy through adolescence.*

Chapter Objectives

Chapter 14 is designed to allow you to:

1. Describe the extent to which nutrition affects infant growth and physiological development.

2. Outline basic diet guidelines to meet the basic nutritional needs for normal growth and development for an infant and discuss some do's and don'ts associated with infant feeding.

3. List several challenges parents must face in dealing with childhood eating habits.

4. List the nutrients often found to be lacking in the diet of infants, toddlers, preschoolers, and teenagers and make recommendations to remedy the problems.

5. Describe the serious nature and overall treatment plans for obesity and type 2 diabetes in childhood.

6. Distinguish between food allergies and intolerances and provide recommendations for treating both.

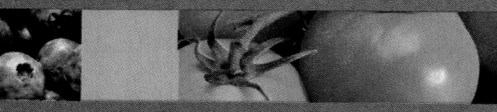

Refresh Your Memory

As you begin your study of nutrition from infancy through adolescence in Chapter 14, you may want to review:

- The Food Guide Pyramid and Dietary Guidelines in Chapter 2

- Diagnosis and treatment of type 2 diabetes in Chapter 4

- Common sources of saturated fat and trans fat in Chapter 5

- Vegetarianism in the Nutrition Issue in Chapter 6

- Rich sources of calcium, iron, and zinc in Chapter 9

- The concept of body mass index (BMI) and the treatment of obesity in Chapter 10

- The benefits of regular physical activity in Chapter 11

- Anorexia nervosa and other eating disorders in Chapter 12

Real Life Scenario

amon is a 7-month-old boy who has been taken to a clinic for a routine checkup. On examination, he was found to be moderately underweight based on age and body length. His physician was concerned with his weight status, so she scheduled a follow-up appointment in 3 months. At the 3-month visit, Damon appeared sluggish and was now even more underweight.

A registered dietician interviewed Damon's 16-year-old mother to collect dietary intakes. His intake over the last 24 hours, according to his mother, consisted of two bottles of formula, three bottles of Kool-aid, and a hot dog. His mother was still in school, and at night she often left Damon with a neighbor so she could go out for a few hours. Thus, she was not aware of all that he ate, since much of her time was spent away from him.

What problems do you think are present in Damon's diet? What potential dangers await Damon if his health status continues to follow this current lagging weight-gain trend?

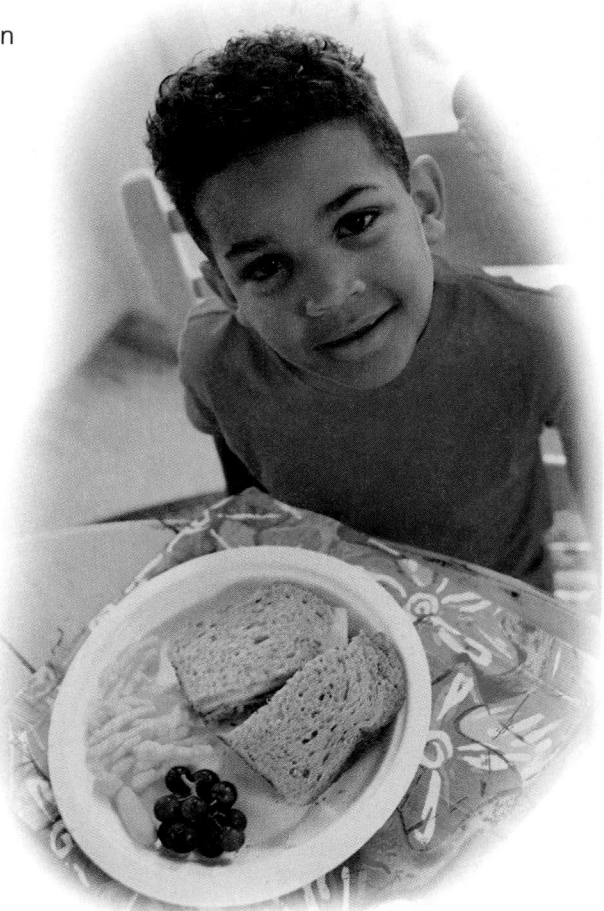

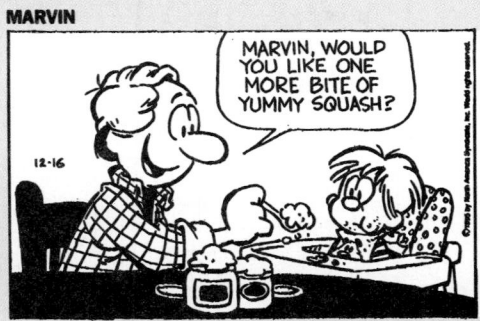
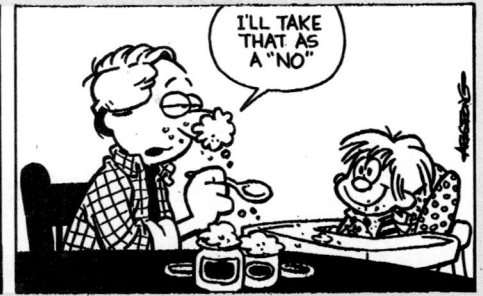

MARVIN

At what age should an infant be fed solid foods? Which foods are most appropriate for those early stages of solid food introduction? Which foods should not be fed to infants? Why? This chapter provides some answers.

MARVIN © Reprinted with special permission of King Features Syndicate, Inc.

Nutrition and Child Health—An Introduction

Current trends in nutrition and overall health among children and adolescents in North America have shown both positive and negative results. On a positive note, more children are receiving vaccinations than ever before, fewer teenagers are giving birth, and the poverty rate for children in the United States has fallen to a point equal to that of 1980. (Currently, 18% of U.S. children live in poverty.) In contrast to this good news, the number of children and teenagers with obesity and type 2 diabetes is rising, and physical activity in general is on the decline as more time is spent sitting in front of computer screens and television sets. Low calcium intakes are also receiving much attention, as soft drinks have replaced much of the milk that children and teenagers used to consume on a daily basis. This chapter will look at these trends, especially their effects on nutrition and overall health in this age group.

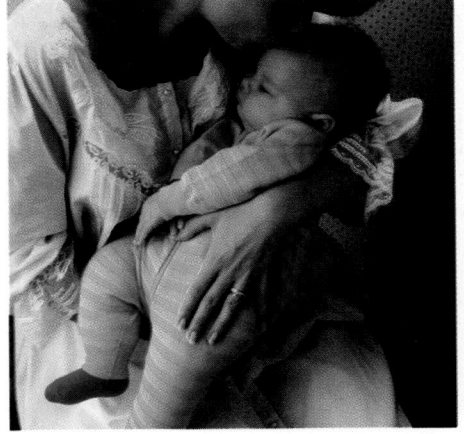

Infant Growth and Nutrition Needs

During **infancy** a child's attitudes toward foods and the whole eating process begin to take shape. If parents and other caregivers practice good nutrition and are flexible, they can lead an infant into lifelong healthful food habits. Such an infant has a good chance of starting life with the nutrients needed to support brain and body growth spurts and of developing a willingness to try new foods. However, these physical and psychological advantages alone don't guarantee that a child will thrive.

Children also need specific attention focused on them; they need to grow in a stimulating environment and they need a sense of security. For example, children hospitalized for growth failure gain weight more quickly when loving care accompanies needed nutrients.

■ The Growing Infant

All babies seem to do is eat and sleep. There's a good reason for this. An infant's birth weight doubles in the first 4 to 6 months and triples within the first year (Fig. 14.1).

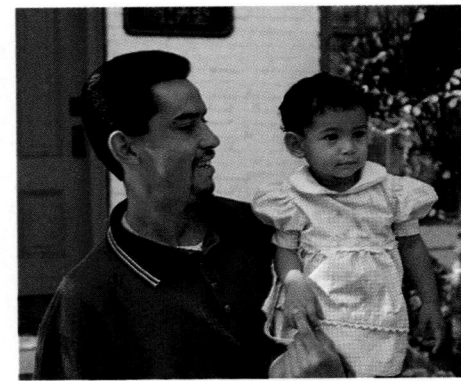

Children benefit from the love and attention of adults.

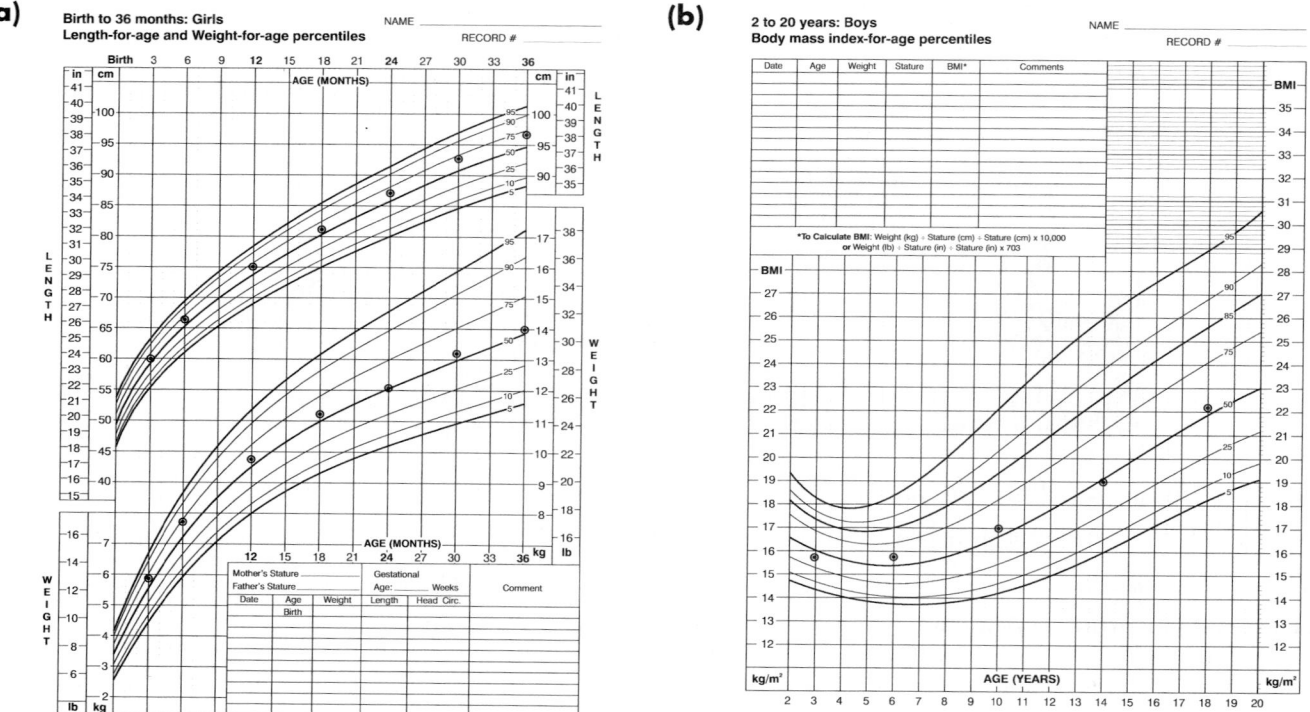

(a) Birth to 36 months: Girls
Length-for-age and Weight-for-age percentiles

(b) 2 to 20 years: Boys
Body mass index-for-age percentiles

Figure 14.1 Growth charts for assessment of children in the growing years. The growth of a youngster is plotted to show how the charts are used in health-care settings. (a) Growth charts used to assess length (height) and weight in young girls. A certain weight and length (height) correspond to a percentile value, which is a ranking of the person among 100 peers. (b) Growth charts used to assess weight-for-height relationships in boys ages 2 to 20 years. Today, these charts, for older children and adolescents typically utilize BMI for the evaluation.
Source: Developed by the National Center for Health Statistics in collaboration with the National Center for Chronic Disease Prevention and Health Promotion (2000). www.cdc.gov/growthcharts. Revised November 21, 2000.

infancy Earliest stage of childhood—from birth to 1 year.

Never again is growth so rapid. Such rapid growth requires a lot of both nourishment and sleep. After the first year, growth is slower, it takes 5 more years to double the weight seen at 1 year. An infant also increases in length in the first year by 50% and then continues to gain height throughout the preschool and teen years. These gains are not necessarily continuous—spurts of growth alternate with plateaus. Height is essentially complete by age 19, although increases of several inches may occur in the early 20s. Head size in proportion to total height shrinks from one-fourth to one-eighth during the climb from infancy to adulthood.

The human body needs a lot more food to support growth and development than to merely maintain itself once growth ceases. When nutrients are missing at critical phases of growth and development, growth slows and may even stop. From observations of Egyptian mummies, we see that infants were about the same size in 300 B.C. as they are today. However, adult mummies are much smaller than adults today. Furthermore, the suits of armor in museum collections of the Middle Ages typically would not fit modern adults. The average height of North American men in 1700 was approximately 5 feet, 8 inches, whereas today it is approximately 5 feet, 10 inches. This suggests that people of earlier times generally ate nutrient-poor diets, which did not support the growth we typically experience today.

In countries of the developing world today, about one-third of the children under 5 years of age are short and underweight for their ages. Poor nutrition—called *under-nutrition*—is at the heart of the problem. This occurs to a lesser extent in North America, but is still possible. The undernourished children are simply smaller versions of nutritionally fit children. In poorer countries, when breastfeeding ceases, children are often fed a high-carbohydrate, low-protein diet. This diet supports some growth but does not allow children to attain their genetically predetermined potential for height. To grow, children must consume adequate amounts of energy, protein, calcium, iron, zinc, and other nutrients.

Infant development follows a pattern in which body water reduces from about 70% at birth to 60% at 1 year. The latter is also the proportion typical in adults. By age 1, an infant's body nitrogen content (and thus protein content) has increased from 2% of body weight at birth to 3%, indicating the infant has synthesized much new lean tissue.

■ Effect of Undernutrition on Growth

As with the fetus in utero, the long-term effects of nutritional problems in infancy and childhood depend on the severity, timing, and duration of the nutritional insult to cell processes.

The single best indicator of a child's nutritional status is growth, particularly weight gain in the short run and length (height) in the long run. Mild zinc deficiencies in North American children have been linked to poor growth. Improving the diets of these children then leads to improved growth. Overall, eating a poor diet as an infant or a child hampers the cell division that occurs at that critical stage. Following an adequate diet later usually won't compensate for lost growth, as the hormonal and other conditions needed for growth will not likely be present. In addition, growth ceases in girls and boys when the skeleton reaches it final size. Growth plates at the ends of the bones fuse at different ages, beginning around 14 years of age in girls and 15 years of age in boys. The final stages of this process end at about 19 years of age in girls and 20 years of age in boys. Furthermore, muscles can increase in diameter later in life but the growth is constrained by the length of the bone.

For these reasons, a 15-year-old Central American girl who is 4 feet, 8 inches tall cannot attain the adult height of a typical North American girl simply by eating better. Girls experience their peak rate of growth before the onset of their menstrual periods. Once the time for growth ceases (in women this is about 5 years after they start menstruating), a sufficient nutrient intake helps maintain health and weight but does not make up for all lost growth.

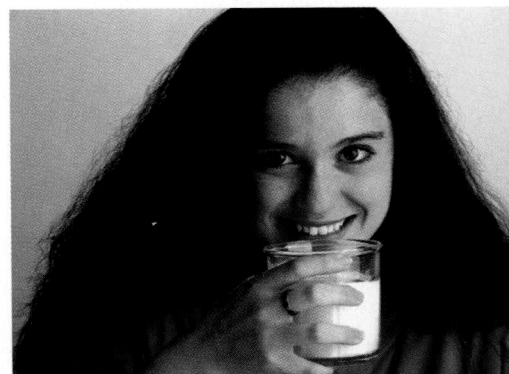

Milk is a nutrient-dense source of protein, calcium, zinc, and other nutrients to support growth. It is especially challenging to meet calcium needs in childhood without regular dairy product consumption (see Chapter 9 for alternative sources of calcium).

■ Assessment of Infant Growth and Development

Health professionals assess a child's increases in height and weight by comparing them with typical growth patterns recorded on charts. You can download the latest growth charts at www.edc.gov/nchs/data/ad314.pdf. The typical charts contain seven or nine **percentile** divisions, which represent 96% of children (review Fig. 14.1). A percentile represents the rank of the person among 100 peers matched for age and gender. If a young boy, for example, is at the 90th percentile height for age, he is shorter than 10 and taller than 89. A child at the 50th percentile is considered average. Fifty children will be taller than this child; 49 will be shorter. It is important to note that these charts were based primarily on observations of formula-fed infants. Breastfed infants may lag behind these typical patterns but eventually catch up in terms of height.

Individual growth charts are available for both males and females, for ages ranging from 0 to 36 months and 2 to 20 years. Height for age, weight for age, weight for height, and head circumference can be plotted. Body mass index (BMI) is the weight for height standard generally used in the latter age range (review Fig. 14.1b). Infants and children should have their growth assessed during regular health checkups. It takes 1 to 3 years for an infant to establish his or her own genetic percentile. Once this figure is established, such as length (height) for age, the child's measurement should then track along that percentile. If the child's growth doesn't keep up with its length-for-age percentile, the physician needs to investigate whether a medical or nutritional problem is impeding the predicted growth. Inappropriate weight gain—too little or too much—should also be investigated.

percentile Classification of a measurement of a unit into divisions of 100 units.

*C*hildren under 2 to 3 years of age are measured with knees unflexed and while lying on their backs, so the term length *is used rather than* height. *Height is measured once the child can stand erect.*

Infants born preterm may catch up in growth in 2 to 3 years. This requires that the child jump up in the percentiles. If this occurs—especially in length for age—it is usually no cause for alarm. On the other hand, jumping percentiles in weight-for-height can be disturbing if the child approaches the 80th to 90th percentiles. A child at the 85th percentile or above for BMI is considered at risk for overweight. At or above the 95th percentile, the child is considered overweight. At the 95th percentile, the diagnosis of obesity can also be established if the physical exam of the child indicates he or she is truly overfat. This is generally the case at this percentile.

Another Bite

*T*he brain grows faster in infancy than at any other time of life. To accommodate the growth, an infant's head circumference must be very large in proportion to the rest of the body. The rapid growth stops at about 18 months of age. The rest of the body eventually grows to reach a typical proportion to head size. In early physical checkups, a health professional usually measures the head circumference as another means of assessing growth, especially brain growth. How nutritional status affects brain development and intelligence quotient (IQ) is difficult to measure because scientists haven't figured out how to separate the effects of nature from those of nurture. However, studies from Central America suggest that IQ after age 5 years relates more closely to the amount of schooling a child receives than to nutritional intake during childhood.

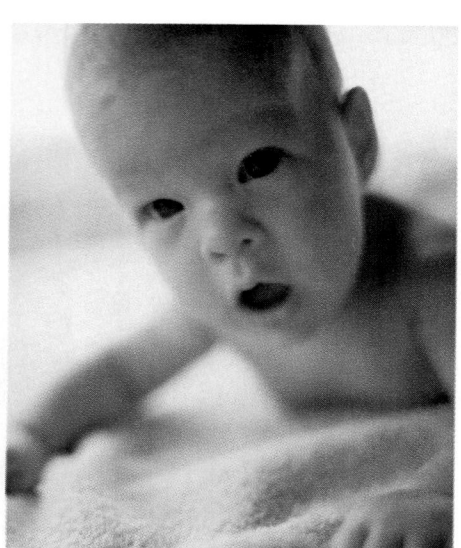

Brain growth is faster in infancy than in any other stage of life.

■ Adipose (Fat) Tissue Growth

Since 1970, researchers have speculated that overfeeding during infancy may increase adipose tissue cell numbers. Today, we know that adipose cells can also increase as adulthood obesity develops (see Chapter 10). Still, if energy intake is limited during infancy to keep down the number of adipose cells, the growth of other organ systems may also be severely retarded. Special concern revolves especially around proper brain and nervous system development. In addition, most obese infants become normal-weight preschoolers without excessive diet restrictions. For these reasons, it's unwise to restrict diet, and especially fat intake, before 2 years of age. About 40% of energy intake from fat is recommended until that age, but a recent study showed one can feed an infant about 35% of energy as fat and still provide for normal growth and development. Without adequate calories and essential nutrients, however, infants are unlikely to attain their potential adult height.

■ Failure to Thrive

Occasionally, an infant doesn't grow much in the first few months. Physical problems that may contribute to retarded growth range from poor oral cavity development, infections, and heart irregularities to constant diarrhea associated with intestinal problems. However, more than half the infants who fail to thrive have no apparent disease. Instead, the usual cause is poor infant-parent interaction. This stems from misinformation, lack of a parent role model, or apathy about the child's welfare. In general, the problems often arise from the parents' inexperience, rather than intentional negligence. A physician should determine the actual cause.

Infants not only need cuddling, they also respond to voices and eye contact, especially at feeding times. New parents need to appreciate the importance of these practices to their infant's well-being. Some parents also may be overcommitted to maintaining a lean child in the hope of preventing future obesity, as discussed in Chapter 12. The result, even though the intention was good, can be failure to thrive.

Children older than 2 years are less likely to experience failure to thrive because they can often get food for themselves. Younger children, for the most part, are limited to what caregivers provide.

Concept Check

Growth occurs rapidly during infancy: Birth weight doubles in about 4 to 6 months and triples within the first year. Lean tissue increases, and the percentage of body water falls during the first year. Undernutrition in childhood can irreversibly inhibit growth and maturation, so that an individual never attains his or her full genetic potential for height. Infant and child growth is assessed by tracking body weight, length (height), and head circumference over time. Body mass index (BMI) is generally used to assess weight for height after 2 years of age. It is not desirable for infants to become obese, although no evidence strongly indicates that obese infants become obese adults. However, severe restriction of energy intake is not recommended for infants because it may slow the growth of organ systems. When infants do not grow properly, their failure to thrive may stem from physical disorders or inadequate care, including inappropriate feeding practices.

■ Infant Nutritional Needs

Infants' nutritional needs vary as they grow, and these differ from adult needs in both amount and proportion. Initially, human milk or infant formula (generally using heat-treated cow's milk as a base) supplies needed nutrients. Solid foods are not needed until after 4 to 6 months. Even after solid foods are added, the basis of an infant's diet for the first year is still human milk or infant formula. Because of the critical importance of adequate nutrition in infancy and the difficulties encountered in feeding some infants, more time is spent in this chapter on this developmental period than on the later periods of childhood.

Energy

Infants need about 45 to 50 kcal per pound of body weight daily (98–108 kcal per kilogram, depending on age) to supply them with adequate energy. This amounts to about 700 kcal daily at 6 months of age. Based on body weight, this is two to four times more energy than adults need. Infants need an easy way to consume this amount of energy. Either human milk or infant formula is ideal for the first few months. Both are high in fat and supply about 650 kcal per quart of fluid (about 700 kcal per liter; Table 14.1). Later, human milk or infant formula, supplemented by solid foods, can provide even more energy.

The infant's high energy needs are primarily driven by its rapid growth and high metabolic rate. The high metabolic rate is caused in part by the ratio of the infant's body surface to its weight. More body surface allows more heat loss from the skin; the body must use extra energy to replace that heat.

Protein

Daily protein needs vary in infancy from 0.7 to 1 gram of protein for each pound of body weight (1.6–2.2 grams per kilogram, depending on age). About half of total protein intake should come from essential (indispensable) amino acids. Both goals are satisfied by either human milk or infant formula. Excess nitrogen and minerals supplied by high-protein diets or cow's milk would exceed the ability of an infant's kidneys to excrete the resulting metabolic waste products, adding stress to the infant's kidney function.

In North America, infant protein deficiency is unlikely, except in cases of mistaken feeding practices, such as when an infant's formula is excessively diluted with water. Protein deficiency may also be induced by elimination diets used to detect food **allergies** (hypersensitivities). As foods are eliminated from the diet, infants may not be offered enough protein to compensate for the high-protein sources no longer present (see the Nutrition Issue at the end of the chapter).

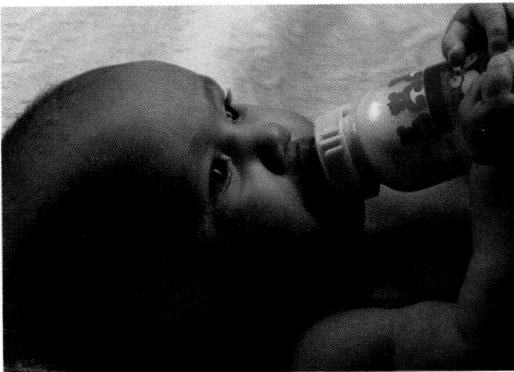

Infants who are formula-fed should remain on formula until 1 year of age. The formula should be iron fortified to reduce the risk of developing iron-deficiency anemia.

allergy A hypersensitive immune response that occurs when immune bodies produced by us react with a protein we sense as foreign (an antigen).

Table 14.1 Composition of Human and Cow's Milk and Infant Formulas Per Liter

Milk or formula	Energy (kcal per liter)	Protein (grams per liter)	Fat (grams per liter)	Carbohydrate (grams per liter)	Minerals* (grams per liter)
Milk					
Human milk	750	11	45	70	2
Cow's milk, whole	670	36	36	49	7
Cow's milk, skim	360	36	1	51	7
Casein/whey-based formulas					
Similac	680	14	36	71	3
Enfamil	670	15	37	69	3
Carnation	670	16	34	73	3
Soybean protein-based formulas					
ProSobee	670	20	35	67	4
Isomil	680	16	36	68	4
Predigested protein					
Nutramigen	670	19	26	89	1
Alimentum	680	18	37	68	1
Transition formulas/beverages†					
Similac Toddler's Best	670	25	33	75	3
Enfamil Next Step	670	17	33	74	3
Carnation Follow-Up	670	17	27	88	3

*Calcium, phosphorus, and other minerals
†For use after 6 months of age or later (see label)

Fat

As already mentioned, infants and children up to 2 years of age should consume about 40% of their energy from fat. About half the energy supplied by both human milk and infant formula comes from fat. Essential fatty acids should make up at least 3% of total energy, which is the case for human milk. Fats are an important part of the infant's diet because they are energy-dense and vital to the development of the nervous system. As a concentrated energy source, fat helps resolve the potential problem of the infant's high energy needs and small stomach capacity. Again, prior to age 2 years, there is no need to greatly restrict fat intake below 35% of calorie intake (Fig. 14.2).

Vitamins of Special Interest

Vitamin K is routinely given by injection to all infants at birth. This dose lasts until the infant's intestinal bacteria are established and begin to synthesize vitamin K. Formula-fed infants receive the rest of the vitamins they need from the formula. Breastfed infants, especially dark-skinned ones, (e.g., African-Americans), generally require a vitamin D supplement if they are not exposed to much sunlight or if the mother has poor vitamin D status. (Sunlight exposure on human skin activates synthesis of vitamin D; see Chapter 8.) Breastfed infants whose mothers are total vegetarians (vegans) should receive a vitamin B-12 supplement. As well, infants who drink goat's milk need a dietary supplement of folate because this milk doesn't supply a sufficient amount of this essential nutrient. Goat's milk is also low in iron, vitamin C, and vitamin D, making it a poor choice for human infants.

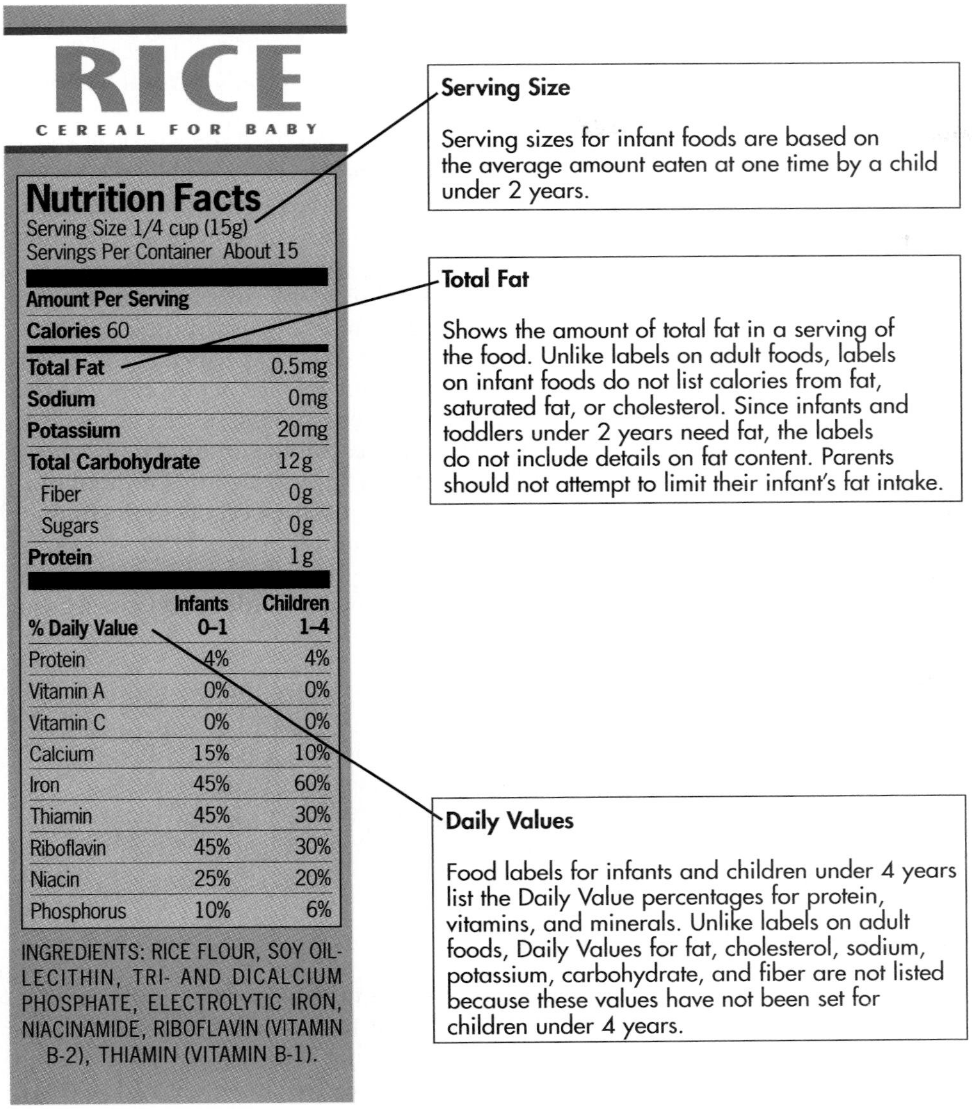

RICE
CEREAL FOR BABY

Nutrition Facts
Serving Size 1/4 cup (15g)
Servings Per Container About 15

Amount Per Serving

Calories 60	
Total Fat	0.5mg
Sodium	0mg
Potassium	20mg
Total Carbohydrate	12g
Fiber	0g
Sugars	0g
Protein	1g

% Daily Value	Infants 0–1	Children 1–4
Protein	4%	4%
Vitamin A	0%	0%
Vitamin C	0%	0%
Calcium	15%	10%
Iron	45%	60%
Thiamin	45%	30%
Riboflavin	45%	30%
Niacin	25%	20%
Phosphorus	10%	6%

INGREDIENTS: RICE FLOUR, SOY OIL-LECITHIN, TRI- AND DICALCIUM PHOSPHATE, ELECTROLYTIC IRON, NIACINAMIDE, RIBOFLAVIN (VITAMIN B-2), THIAMIN (VITAMIN B-1).

Serving Size

Serving sizes for infant foods are based on the average amount eaten at one time by a child under 2 years.

Total Fat

Shows the amount of total fat in a serving of the food. Unlike labels on adult foods, labels on infant foods do not list calories from fat, saturated fat, or cholesterol. Since infants and toddlers under 2 years need fat, the labels do not include details on fat content. Parents should not attempt to limit their infant's fat intake.

Daily Values

Food labels for infants and children under 4 years list the Daily Value percentages for protein, vitamins, and minerals. Unlike labels on adult foods, Daily Values for fat, cholesterol, sodium, potassium, carbohydrate, and fiber are not listed because these values have not been set for children under 4 years.

Figure 14.2 The labels on infant foods, like those on adult foods, contain a Nutrition Facts panel. However, the information provided on infant food labels differs from that on adult food labels, especially with respect to total fat, saturated fat, and cholesterol intake (see Fig. 2.5 for a comparison).

Minerals of Special Interest

The iron stores with which children are born are generally depleted by the time birth weight doubles, in 4 to 6 months. The American Academy of Pediatrics recommends that, to maintain a desirable iron status, formula-fed infants should be given an iron-fortified formula from birth. These experts also discourage the use of low-iron infant formulas, which are sometimes prescribed to treat infants with various GI tract problems. Breastfed infants need solid foods to supply extra iron at about 6 months of age. The need for iron is a major consideration in deciding when to introduce solid foods. Some physicians recommend liquid iron supplements from birth or by 1 month of age for breastfed infants. Iron deficiency anemia can lead to poor cognitive development in infants.

Infants need adequate amounts of zinc and iodide to support growth. Human milk and infant formula adequately supply these needs when they supply enough energy to meet needs. In addition, clinicians recommend fluoride supplements to aid tooth development for breastfed infants after 6 months of age. The same holds true for formula-fed infants if the water supply used in home formula preparation—either tap or bottled water—doesn't contain fluoride. Note that formula manufacturers use fluoride-free water in formula preparation. Parents should consult their dentist for advice on the infant's need for fluoride.

Critical Thinking

Tatiana has been breastfeeding her baby exclusively since he was born 7 months ago. When she and her husband took the baby for his checkup, they were told that he was anemic. They were very surprised, since they thought that human milk contained all the nutrients the baby needed for the first year of life. How might you explain the baby's anemia?

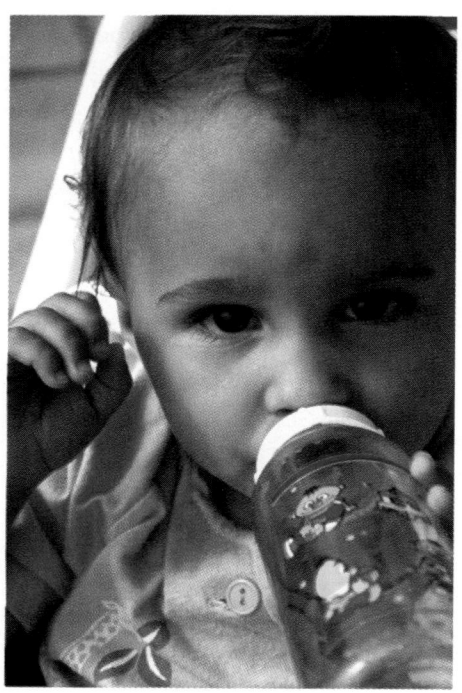

Supplemental fluids should be limited to 4 ounces per day unless the infant's physician prescribes a larger amount.

*S*oy-based formulas account for about 25% of the infant formula used in the United States. There is some concern over the use of soy milk in infant feeding because of the isoflavone content. Isoflavones may cause hormonal disruption, developmental delay in boys, and precocious puberty in girls. Currently, the American Academy of Pediatrics states that soy formulas are safe but should be used only when breastfeeding or use of typical milk-based formulas are not appropriate, such as confirmed allergies to milk, lactose intolerance, parents who insist on strict vegan diets, or certain other diagnosed health problems.

Water

An infant needs about 2 ounces of water and other fluids combined per pound of body weight (about 150 milliliters per kilogram). Infants typically consume enough human milk or formula to supply this amount. In hot climates, however, supplemental water may be necessary. Furthermore, any conditions that lead to water loss—diarrhea, vomiting, fever, and too much sun—can lead to the need for supplemental water.

Infants are easily dehydrated, a condition that has serious effects if not remedied. Dehydration can result in rapidly decreasing kidney function, and the infant may then require hospitalization for rehydration. Special fluid-replacement formulas containing electrolytes such as sodium and potassium are available in supermarkets and pharmacies to treat dehydration. A physician should guide any use of these products.

Note that in some stores, bottled water products marketed specifically for infants may be placed alongside infant formulas and electrolyte-replacement solutions. This placement may give parents and caregivers the mistaken impression that bottled water products are an appropriate feeding supplement or substitute for fluid replacement for infants; they are not and should not be used for such purposes. It is important to also remember also that excessive fluid can also be harmful, especially to the brain.

Overall, it is best to limit supplemental fluids to about 4 ounces (120 milliliters) per day, unless the physician thinks that a greater need exists because of disease or other conditions. In sum, extremes in fluid intake—either too little or too much—can lead to health problems.

Concept Check

*M*ost nutrient needs in the first 6 months are met by human milk or infant formula. Breastfed infants may need vitamin D and iron supplements, and formula-fed infants and breastfed infants may need fluoride supplements after 6 months of age. Infants usually receive enough water from the human milk or formula they drink.

■ Formula Feeding for Infants

Breastfeeding was covered in detail in Chapter 13. Let's now focus on formula feeding. You'll recall that a major advantage of breastfeeding is the provision of immune protection to the infant. Another advantage of breastfeeding is the supply of very-long-chain fatty acids (those typically found in fish such as docosahexaenoic acid [DHA]). DHA is found in high concentrations in the retina of the eye and the brain. Some research suggests that formula-fed infants are at a disadvantage, as DHA is not added at this time to commercial formulas in the United States. However, the addition of DHA to formulas has recently been approved by FDA, and should be available to consumers in the United States in the near future. Overall, in areas of the world where high standards for water purity and cleanliness are common, formula feeding is a safe alternative for infants but is not as beneficial as breastfeeding.

Formula Composition

Infants cannot tolerate cow's milk as such because of its high protein and mineral content. Cow's milk reflects the greater growth needs of calves. Thus, cow's milk must be altered to be safe for infant feeding. It is important to note that goat's milk, sweetened condensed milk, and evaporated milk also are inappropriate substances for infants. Altered forms of cow's milk, known as infant formulas, were first available commercially in 1931. Since 1980, they have been required to conform to strict federal guidelines for nutrient composition and quality. Formulas generally contain lactose and/or sucrose for carbohydrate, heat-treated proteins from cow's milk, and vegetable oils for fat (see Table 14.1). Soy protein-based formulas are available for infants who can't tolerate lactose or the types of proteins found in cow's milk. If the soybean-based formula is not tolerated, the next step is to try a formula in which the proteins have been broken down into peptides and amino acids, such as Nutramigen or Alimentum. A variety of other specialized formulas also are available for specific medical conditions. In any case, it is important to use an iron-fortified formula.

Some transition formulas/beverages have been introduced for older infants and toddlers (review Table 14.1). Some of these products are intended for use after 6 months of age if the infant is consuming solid foods, whereas others are intended for use only by toddlers. These transition products are lower in fat than human milk or standard infant formulas; their iron content is higher than that of cow's milk, and their overall mineral content is generally more like that of human milk than cow's milk. According to the manufacturers, the advantages of these transition formulas/beverages over standard formulas for older infants and toddlers include reduced cost and better flavor. Parents should consult their physician with regard to use of these products.

Formula Preparation

In the 1950s, it was common to prepare a day's supply of bottles and then sterilize them in boiling water for about 30 minutes. Today, bottles are often prepared one at a time. Some infant formulas even come in ready-to-feed form. These are poured into a clean bottle and fed immediately. Room-temperature formula is acceptable for many infants. Otherwise, to warm a bottle of formula, a caregiver can run hot water over it or place it briefly in a pan of simmering water. Note that infant formulas should not be heated in a microwave oven because hot spots may develop, which can burn the infant's mouth and esophagus.

Powdered and concentrated fluid formula preparations are more commonly used than ready-to-feed varieties. All utensils used in preparing formula from these preparations should be washed and thoroughly rinsed. Powdered or concentrated formulas are poured into a bottle to which clean, cold water is added (following label directions) and then mixed. The formula is then warmed, if desired, and fed immediately to the infant. Hot water from the faucet should not be used to make formula, since it poses a risk for high lead content (see Chapter 16). Cold water poses much less risk.

Refrigerating diluted formula for 1 day is safe. However, formula left over from a feeding should be discarded because it will be contaminated by bacteria and enzymes in the infant's saliva. If well water is used, it should be boiled before making formula for at least the infant's first 3 months of life, and it should be analyzed for excessive concentration of naturally occurring nitrates, which can lead to a severe form of anemia. Note that if nitrates are high in municipal water systems, consumers will be warned (such as in a local newspaper) not to use the water for making infant formula until the concentration falls to a safe amount. This problem with nitrates typically occurs in the summer, when these wash from fertilized farm fields into local rivers after heavy rains. Boiling tapwater is also advised by some groups, based on evidence that even municipal water may contain microbes that can harm the vulnerable, such as infants (see Chapter 9).

Feeding Technique

Because infants swallow a lot of air along with either formula or human milk, it's important to burp an infant after either 10 minutes of feeding or 1 to 2 ounces (30 to 60 milliliters) from a bottle and again at the end of feeding. Spitting up a bit of milk is normal at this time. Once fed, infants should be placed on their backs. Infants should not be placed on their stomachs because this sleeping position has been linked to sudden infant death syndrome (SIDS). The "back to sleep campaign," started in 1994 in the United States, has reduced SIDS by 40%; however, plagiocephaly, otherwise known as flat-head syndrome, has increased as a result. Infant skulls are soft and can take on a different form. Flat-head syndrome can occur if an excessive amount of an infant's life is spent on his or her back, or against a highchair/car seat. In response to this concern, the American Academy of Pediatrics

*N*ot even all formula-like products are designed for infant use. A 5-month-old girl was admitted to a hospital in Arkansas with symptoms of heart failure, rickets, inflamed blood vessels, and possible nerve damage after being fed Soy Moo (a soy beverage sold in health stores) since 3 days of age. The symptoms suggest severe vitamin deficiencies. Parents should consult a physician when choosing an appropriate infant formula.

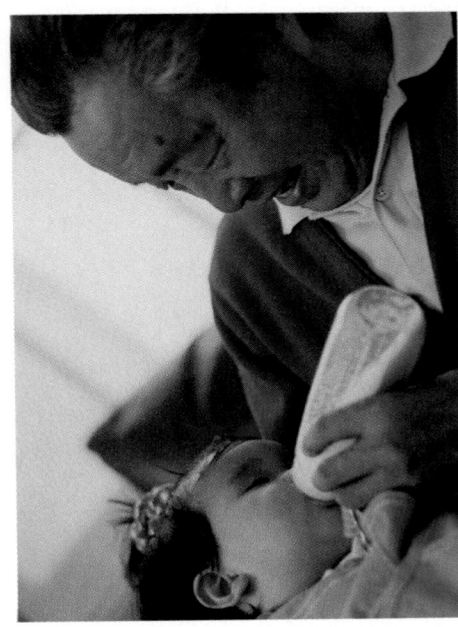

Careful attention during feeding allows the caregiver to notice the infant's signal as to when the feeding should cease.

has recommended periodic repositioning of a sleeping infant's head and allowing for time on his or her stomach while awake.

When the infant begins acting full, bottle-feeding should be stopped, even if some milk is left in the bottle. Common cues that signal that an infant has had enough include turning the head away, being inattentive, falling asleep, and becoming playful. Generally, the infant's appetite is a better guide than standardized recommendations concerning feeding amounts. Breastfeeding infants usually have had enough to eat after about 20 minutes. Although it's difficult to tell how much milk breastfed infants are getting, they also give signs when full. By carefully observing bottle-feeding or nursing infants and responding to their cues appropriately, caregivers not only can be assured that the infants' energy needs are being met but also can foster a climate of trust and responsiveness.

■ Development of Feeding Skills in Older Infants

By 6 to 7 months the infant has learned to grab and transfer objects from one hand to the other. At about this time, teeth begin to appear, and the infant begins to handle finger foods with some dexterity. Dry toast, sliced in strips, offers hours of enjoyment.

By age 7 to 8 months, infants can push food around on a plate and play with a drinking cup, can hold a bottle, and self-feed a cracker or piece of toast. In mastering these manipulations, infants develop self-confidence and self-esteem. It's important that parents be patient and support these early feeding attempts, even though they appear inefficient.

At around 10 months of age, infants practice in earnest self-feeding finger foods and drinking from a cup. Feeding time is often very messy. Food is used as a means to explore the environment. By the first birthday, their bodies have developed sufficiently to accommodate crawling, probably walking, and self-feeding. Although attempts at feeding are still erratic, developing children take great pride in doing more things independently. As children drink from a cup more frequently, fewer bottle feedings and/or breastfeedings are necessary. The added mobility of walking should naturally lead to gradual weaning from the bottle or breast.

■ Introduction of Solid Foods at 4 to 6 Months of Age

The time to introduce solid foods into an infant's diet hinges on a few important factors:

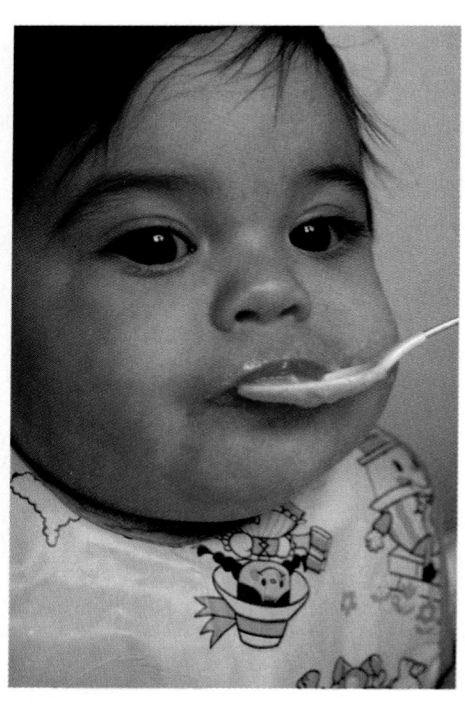

In the early stages of solid food introduction, these foods complement rather than replace human milk or infant formula in the diet.

1. *Nutritional need.* Iron stores are exhausted by about 6 months of age. Either solid foods or iron supplements are then needed to supply iron if the child is breastfed or fed a formula not supplemented with iron. Iron, however, is not the only nutrient that is low in human milk (and unfortified infant formulas). Vitamin D may also deserve attention, as previously mentioned. Still, before 4 to 6 months, it's unnecessary to add solid foods.

2. *Physiological capabilities.* Infants cannot readily digest starch before 3 months. As they age, their digestive capabilities increase. Kidney function likewise is quite limited until about 4 to 6 weeks of age. Until then, waste products from amounts of dietary protein or minerals are difficult to excrete.

3. *Physical ability.* Three markers indicate that a child is ready for solid foods: (1) the disappearance of the extrusion reflex (thrusting the tongue forward and pushing food out of the mouth), (2) head and neck control, and (3) the ability to sit up with support. These usually occur around 4 to 6 months of age, but they vary with each infant.

4. *Allergy prevention.* An infant's intestinal tract can readily absorb whole proteins from birth until 4 to 5 months of age. Thus, early exposure to many types of proteins—particularly proteins in cow's milk and egg whites—may predispose a child to future allergies and other health problems because some types of

these proteins may be absorbed intact. For this reason, it's best to minimize the number of different types of proteins in a child's diet, especially during the first 3 months.

With these considerations in mind—nutritional need, physiological and physical readiness, and allergy prevention—the American Academy of Pediatrics recommends that solid foods not be introduced until about 6 months of age and that infants receive no unaltered cow's milk before 1 year.

In general, a child starting solid foods should weigh at least 13 pounds (6 kilograms) and should be drinking more than 32 ounces (1 liter) of formula daily or breastfeeding more than 8 to 10 times within 24 hours. This description generally applies to 6-month-old infants and to some 4-month-old infants.

Before 4 to 6 months, infants are not physically mature enough to consume much solid food. Attempts to push down solid foods have sometimes led to forcefeeding with a feeder (a giant syringe) or mixing infant cereal with milk and putting it in a bottle. Even if these are traditional alternatives in your family, there is no reason to carry on these practices. The inconvenience alone should make one consider whether all the effort is worth it. This practice is unnecessary nutritionally, tedious, and possibly dangerous for the infant because it increases the risk of allergies and choking or inhaling food when crying. Even so, many children are already eating solids before 4 months of age. Only occasionally does a rapidly growing infant—one who consumes more than 32 ounces (1 liter) of formula daily—need solid foods at 4 months to meet high energy needs.

Solid Foods That Should Be Fed First

Before 6 months of age, the first solid foods should be iron-fortified cereals. A good idea is to offer foods after some breastfeeding or formula feeding, when the edge has been taken off the infant's hunger. This practice aids in early spoon-feeding. Rice cereal is the best cereal to begin with because it's least likely to cause allergies. After the age of 6 months, the first food is not such an important issue. Some pediatricians may recommend lean ground (strained) meats for more absorbable forms of iron. Although yogurt and cottage cheese are also well tolerated and their consistencies make them good candidates for early foods, they are not good sources of iron.

Start with teaspoon amounts of a single-ingredient food item, such as rice cereal, and increase the serving size gradually. Once the new food has been fed for about a week without ill effects, another food can be added to the infant's diet. At first, this can be another type of cereal or perhaps a cooked and strained (blended) vegetable, meat, fruit, or egg yolk. It is best to add vegetables before fruits. If fruits are offered first, the infant will prefer the sweet taste and likely resist vegetables. Build each feeding step on the previous step, making sure to add only a single ingredient each time.

Waiting about 7 days between news foods is important because it can take that long for evidence of an allergy or intolerance to develop. Symptoms to look for are diarrhea, vomiting, a rash, or wheezing. If one or more of these symptoms appear, the suspected problem food should be avoided for several weeks and then reintroduced in a small quantity. If the problem continues, a physician should be consulted.

It's important not to introduce mixed foods until each component of the mixed food has been given separately. Otherwise, if an allergy or intolerance develops, it will be difficult to identify the offending food. Note that many babies outgrow food sensitivities in childhood. Some foods that commonly cause an allergic response in infants are egg whites, chocolate, nuts, and cow's milk. It's best not to introduce these foods in infancy.

A variety of strained foods is available for infant feeding. Investigate these and other foods intended for infants the next time you're in a supermarket. Single-food items are more desirable than mixed dinners and desserts, which are less nutrient dense. Most brands have no added salt, but some fruit desserts contain a lot of added sugar.

Parents may believe that the early addition of solid foods will help the infant sleep through the night. This achievement is a developmental milestone; the amount of food consumed by the infant is irrelevant.

Typical Solid Food Progression, Starting at 6 Months*

Week 1	Rice cereal
Week 2	Add strained carrots
Week 3	Add applesauce
Week 4	Add oat cereal
Week 5	Add cooked egg yolk
Week 6	Add strained chicken
Week 7	Add strained peas
Week 8	Add plums

*Extending the rice cereal step for a month or so is advised if solid food introduction begins at 4 months of age. Note also that, if at any point signs of allergy or intolerance develop, substitute another, similar food item.

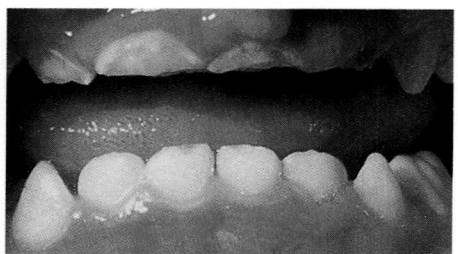

Figure 14.3 Early childhood caries. An extreme example of tooth decay probably resulting from often putting the child to bed with a bottle. The upper teeth have decayed almost all the way to the gum line. This disorder was formerly called nursing bottle syndrome.

early childhood caries Tooth decay that results from formula or juice (and even human milk) bathing the teeth as the child sleeps with a bottle in his or her mouth. The upper teeth are mostly affected as the lower teeth are protected by the tongue; formerly called nursing bottle syndrome.

As an alternative, plain foods from the table—vegetables, fruits, and meats (no seasoning added)—can be ground up in an inexpensive plastic baby food grinder/mill. Another option is to pureé a larger amount of food in a blender, freeze it in ice-cube portions, store in plastic bags, and defrost and warm as needed. Careful attention to cleanliness is necessary. Infant foods made at home should be ground before seasonings are added to please the rest of the family. The infant doesn't notice the difference if salt, sugar, or spices are omitted. It's best to introduce infants to a variety of foods, so that by the end of the first year the infant is consuming many foods—milk, meats, fruits, vegetables, and grains.

As early as possible, by about 8 months or so, juices and formulas should be offered in a cup. A heavy cup with a wide, flat bottom aids success. Drinking from a cup helps prevent **early childhood caries** (Fig. 14.3). As an infant drinks continually from a bottle, the carbohydrate-rich fluid bathes the teeth, providing an ideal growth medium for bacteria. Bacteria on the teeth then make acids, which dissolve tooth enamel. Infants should never be put to bed with a bottle or placed in an infant seat with a bottle propped up. When children are allowed to do this, fluid (even milk) pools around the teeth, increasing the likelihood of dental caries. Again, infants need careful attention when being fed. Propping up a bottle does not constitute careful attention.

Getting a baby out of the bedtime-bottle habit is difficult. Determined caregivers can either wince through a few nights of their baby's crying or slowly wean the baby away from the bottle with either a pacifier or water (for a week or so).

In the first attempts to introduce solid foods, just getting the food into the infant's mouth proves to be a challenge. The caregiver must proceed slowly. Initially, table foods supplement—rather than replace—formula or human milk. These infants control the situation by signaling when they are hungry and when they have had enough to eat. Self-feeding skills require coordination and can develop only if the infant is allowed to practice and experiment. At 9 to 10 months, the infant's desire to explore, experience, and play with food can also hinder feeding. Presenting new foods for several consecutive days can aid in an infant's acceptance of that food.

Caregivers need to relax and take this phase of infant development in stride. Sloppy, friendly mealtimes actually make for good memories.

Another Bite

*T*o ease efforts in feeding solid foods, consider the following tips:

- Use a baby-sized spoon; a small spoon with a long handle is best.
- Hold the infant comfortably on the lap, as for breastfeeding or bottle feeding, but a little more upright to ease swallowing. When in this position, the infant expects food.
- Put a small dab of food on the spoon tip and gently place it on the infant's tongue.
- Convey a calm and casual approach to the infant, who needs time to get used to food.
- Expect the infant to take only two or three bites of the first meals. Anything more than that is real success.

By the end of the first year, finger-feeding becomes more efficient, drinking from a cup improves, and chewing is easier as more teeth erupt. Foods in the diet begin to resemble a balanced diet, such as a Food Guide Pyramid pattern (Table 14.2). Still, experimentation and unpredictability are to be expected.

What Not to Feed an Infant

Following are several foods and practices to avoid when feeding an infant:

- *Honey and corn syrup.* These products may contain spores of **Clostridium botulinum.** The spores can eventually develop into bacteria in the stomach and lead to a foodborne illness known as *botulism.* This can be fatal in children under 1 year old (see Chapter 16).
- *Very salty and very sweet foods.* Infants don't need a lot of sugar or salt added to their foods. They enjoy bland foods much more than do adults.
- *Excessive infant formula or human milk.* After 6 to 8 months, solid foods should play a greater role in satisfying an infant's increasing appetite. The main reason to switch is that solid foods contain considerably more iron than do human milk, cow's milk, and low-iron formulas. About 24 to 32 ounces (¾ to 1 liter) of human milk or formula daily is ideal after 6 months, with food supplying the rest of the infant's energy needs.
- *Foods that tend to cause choking.* These foods include hot dogs (unless finely cut into sticks, not coin shapes), candy, whole nuts, grapes, coarsely cut meats, raw carrots, popcorn, and peanut butter. Caregivers should not allow younger children to gobble snack foods during playtime and should supervise all meals.
- *Cow's milk, especially low-fat or nonfat cow's milk.* Beyond 2 years, children can drink fat-reduced or 1% milk, because by then they are consuming enough solid foods to supply energy and fat needs. Before that age, the amount of fat-reduced, 1%, or nonfat milk needed for energy needs would supply too many minerals. That could overwhelm the kidneys' ability to excrete the excess. The lower fat intake might also harm nervous system development. The American Academy of Pediatrics strongly urges parents not to give children under age 2 fat-reduced, 1%, or nonfat milk.
- *Feeding excessive amounts of juice, especially apple or pear juice.* The fructose and sorbitol contained in these juices can lead to diarrhea (sometimes called toddlers diarrhea), because they are slowly absorbed. Also, if fruit juice or related drink

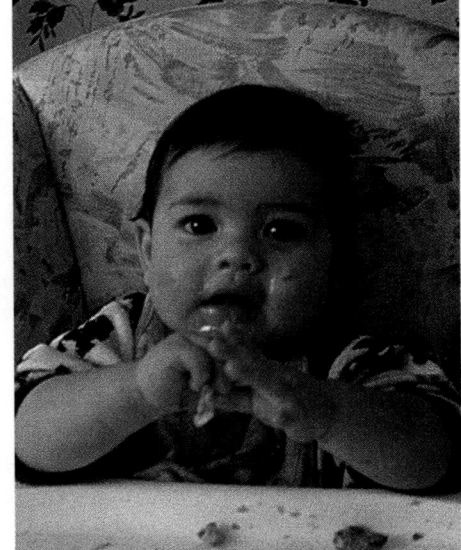

Early feeding attempts should be encouraged, even though they're messy.

*E*gg whites also should not be fed to children before 1 year of age to help prevent the development of allergies.

Table 14.2 Sample Daily Menu for a 1-Year-Old Child*

Breakfast	Snack
1–2 tbsp applesauce ¼ cup Cheerios ½ cup whole milk	½ oz cheddar cheese 4 wheat crackers ½ cup whole milk
Snack	**Dinner**
½ hard-cooked egg ½ slice wheat toast with ½ tsp margarine ½ cup orange juice	1 oz hamburger (crumbled) 1–2 tbsp mashed potatoes with ½ tsp margarine 1–2 tbsp cooked carrots (cut in strips, not coins) ½ cup whole milk
Lunch	**Snack**
1 oz roasted chicken, minced 1–2 tbsp rice with ½ tsp margarine 1–2 tbsp cooked peas ½ cup whole milk	½ banana 2 oatmeal cookies (no raisins) ½ cup whole milk

Nutritional analysis	
Total energy (kcal)	1100
% energy from:	
Carbohydrate	40%
Protein	19%
Fat	41%

*This diet is just a start. A 1-year-old may need more or less food. In those cases, serving sizes should be adjusted. The milk can be fed by cup; some can be put into a bottle if the child has not been fully weaned from the bottle. The juice should be fed in a cup.

Dietary Guidelines for Infant Feeding

*I*n response to various controversies surrounding infant feeding, the American Academy of Pediatrics has issued a number of statements concerning infant diets. The following guidelines are based on these statements:

- *Build to a variety of foods.* For the first months of life, human milk is all an infant needs. When the infant is ready, start adding new foods, one at a time. During the first year, the goal is to teach an infant to enjoy a variety of nutritious foods. A lifetime of healthy eating habits begins with this important first step.
- *Pay attention to your infant's appetite to avoid overfeeding or underfeeding.* Feed infants when they are hungry. Never force an infant to finish an unwanted serving of food. Watch for signs that indicate hunger or fullness.

- *Infants need fat.* Although fat is the cause of many adult health problems, it's an essential source of energy for growing infants. Fat also helps the nervous system develop.
- *Choose fruits, vegetables, and grains, but don't overdo high-fiber foods.* Although many adults benefit from higher-fiber diets, they are not good for infants. They are bulky, filling, and often low in energy. The natural amounts of fiber and nutrients in fruits, vegetables, and grains are appropriate as part of a healthy infant diet.
- *Infants need sugars in moderation.* Sugars are an additional source of energy for active, rapidly growing infants. Foods such as human milk, fruits, and juices are natural sources of sugars and other nutrients as well.

Foods that contain artificial sweeteners should be avoided; they don't provide the energy growing infants need.
- *Infants need sodium in moderation.* Sodium is a necessary mineral found naturally in almost all foods. As part of a healthy diet, infants need sodium for their bodies to work properly.
- *Choose foods containing iron, zinc, and calcium.* Infants need good sources of iron, zinc, and calcium for optimum growth in the first 2 years. These minerals are important for healthy blood, proper growth, and strong bones.

In essence, there is no evidence that very restrictive diets during infancy have positive effects, whereas their hazards are well documented.

---

products are replacing formula or milk in the diet, the infant may not be receiving adequate amounts of calcium and other minerals that are essential for bone growth. In fact, studies have shown a link between excessive amounts of fruit juice and failure to thrive, GI tract complications, obesity, short stature, and poor dental health. Thus, these substances would be used sparingly. Infants over the age of 6 months can usually safely consume up to 6 ounces of juice in the course of a day, with no more than 2 to 4 ounces at a time.

Scenario *Follow-Up*

Damon's diet is inadequate for a 10-month-old infant because it still lacks enough of the nutritious foods his growing body needs to support weight gain. These foods include iron-fortified cereal, puréed infant foods, and appropriate table foods. Damon should stay on the infant formula until 1 year of age and should not be given sugary drinks, nor should these drinks be fed by bottle if used. Damon needs a more energy-dense diet containing a healthful variety of solid foods to provide him with enough calories and essential nutrients to grow and develop.

Concept Check

*I*nfant formulas generally contain lactose or sucrose, heat-treated proteins from cow's milk, and vegetable oil. Formulas may or may not be fortified with iron. Sanitation is very important in preparing and storing formula. Solid foods should not be added to an infant's diet until the child is both ready for and needs solid food, usually at about 4 to 6 months of age. The first solid food can be iron-fortified infant cereals, with very gradual additions of other foods—one at a time each week. Some foods to avoid giving infants in the first year are honey, cow's milk (particularly fat-reduced, 1%, or nonfat milk), egg whites, very salty or sweet foods, foods that may cause the child to choke, and excessive amounts of fruit juice or related products (e.g., fruit drinks).

A Summary of Infant Feeding Recommendations

Breastfed Infants

- Breastfeed for 1 year or longer, if possible. Introduce infant formula if and when breastfeeding ceases before 1 year of age.
- Add iron-fortified cereal at about 6 months of age.
- Investigate the need for fluoride, iron, and vitamin D supplements.
- Provide a variety of basic, soft foods after 6 months of age, advancing to a varied diet.

Formula-Fed Infants

- Use infant formula for the first year of life, preferably an iron-fortified type.
- Add iron-fortified cereal at about 6 months of age.
- Investigate the need for a fluoride supplement if the water supply is not fluoridated.
- Provide a variety of basic, soft foods after 6 months, advancing to a varied diet.

■ Health Problems Related to Infant Nutrition

Parents, other caregivers, and clinicians should be alert for a variety of potential health problems related to infant nutrition, so that corrective action can be taken quickly. In some cases, such problems stem from inappropriate feeding practices and inadequate nutrient intakes, including the following:

- Diet providing insufficient iron
- Absence from the diet of an entire food group of the Food Guide Pyramid (or other related pyramid) as solid foods are introduced and become the main source of nutrients
- Drinking raw (unpasteurized) milk, which may be contaminated with bacteria or viruses
- Drinking goat's milk, which is low in folate, iron, vitamin C, and vitamin D; if used, it must be pasteurized and given in conjunction with a balanced vitamin and mineral supplement
- Failure to begin drinking from a cup by 1 year of age
- Continuing to feed from a bottle past 18 months of age
- Intake of supplemental vitamins or minerals above 100% of the appropriate RDA or other nutrient standard
- Drinking large amounts of fruit juice after 6 months of age, as a substitute for infant formula or human milk (recall that fruit juice is not to be fed before 6 months of age)

Now let's look more closely at four common infant health problems that cause concern for caregivers: colic, diarrhea, milk allergy, and iron-deficiency anemia. Parents and other caregivers usually need to consult with a physician in dealing with these conditions. The website of the American Association of Pediatrics (www.aap.org) can also provide useful information.

Colic

The first time an otherwise healthy, well-fed infant has a lengthy, unexplained crying spell, most parents panic. Repeated crying episodes that last 3 or more hours and don't respond to typical remedies—such as feeding, holding, or changing diapers—are characteristics of infants who develop **colic**. Colic affects about 10% to 30% of all infants, so it is neither uncommon nor abnormal. Colicky infants typically cry during the late afternoon and early evening, and their nighttime sleeping is almost always disturbed by crying spells. In addition, these infants frequently pass gas rectally, clench their fists, draw up their legs, hold their body straight, and want to be held. The only good news is that colic usually goes away after a few months.

Colic generally occurs in the absence of any physical problem in the infant. It tends to be most common in "temperamental" infants—those who are more sensitive, more irritable, more intense, less adaptable, and less consolable than average for their age. In addition, a lack of harmonious interaction between parents and the infant may contribute to the problem. Some researchers have speculated that immature central nervous system mechanisms may cause colic.

Parents can do several things to help reduce excessive crying. For instance, many infants tend to become quiet and alert when held snugly to the shoulder. Parents should also check to see whether the infant is tired or bored or wants to suckle. Some infants can be calmed by rhythmic sounds or movement or with pacifiers.

Breastfeeding of colicky infants should continue. The breastfeeding mother's temporary decrease or cessation in consumption of dairy products, caffeine, chocolate, and vegetables such as broccoli and onions may help reduce colic in her infant. Formula-fed infants with severe colic are sometimes helped by changing from a standard formula to a soy-based or predigested protein formula (see Table 14.1). In addition, physicians may prescribe medications to calm colicky infants and reduce gas buildup.

Diarrhea

Diarrhea in infants, characterized by numerous loose stools per day, results from various causes, including bacterial and viral infections. In the United States, about

colic Sharp abdominal pain that generally occurs in otherwise healthy infants and is associated with periodic, inconsolable crying spells.

500 infants die each year of simple dehydration resulting from diarrhea, and about 210,000 are hospitalized for this disorder. Typical symptoms include dry mouth or tongue, few or no tears when crying, no wet diapers for 3 hours or more, irritability and listlessness, and sunken eyes and cheeks. To prevent dehydration, infants with diarrhea should be given plenty of fluids, under the supervision of a physician. Specialized electrolyte-replacement fluids, such as Pedialyte, may be recommended for very short-term use. These contain glucose, sodium, potassium, chloride, and water.

Once diarrhea subsides, a bottle-fed infant may be switched to a soy-based, lactose-free formula for a few days. This allows time for the intestine to produce sufficient lactase enzyme to digest the large amount of lactose typically found in formulas. A breastfed infant should continue at the breast for the duration of the diarrhea. If solid foods are consumed, the physician may also prescribe a BRAT diet (bananas, rice, applesauce, toast) diet for short-term use; this is not a nutritionally adequate diet for long-term use.

Milk Allergy

Cow's milk contains more than 40 proteins that can cause allergic reactions in infants. Although some of these proteins are inactivated by heating (scalding) milk, others are very heat stable. A true milk allergy develops in about 1% to 3% of formula-fed infants. Such infants may experience vomiting, diarrhea, blood in the stool, constipation, and other symptoms. If milk allergy is suspected, a formula-fed infant can be switched to a soy-based formula. In 20% to 50% of cases, however, the use of soy formula provides only temporary relief because the soy protein eventually triggers an allergic reaction in some infants. In such cases a predigested-protein formula is necessary (review Table 14.1). If the child is breastfeeding, the mother may experiment with eliminating cow's milk from her diet. Fortunately, such an allergy seldom lasts beyond 3 years of age.

Iron-Deficiency Anemia

Iron-deficiency anemia typically occurs in older infants who consume few solid foods and whose diets are dominated by cow's milk, which contains little iron and causes intestinal bleeding in young infants. Iron stores are then quickly depleted by the daily need to synthesize new red blood cells. The best way to prevent iron-deficiency anemia is to feed an iron-fortified formula beginning at birth, if formula is used. Then start an infant on iron-fortified cereals and meats at about 6 months, and limit formula to 16 to 25 ounces (500 to 750 milliliters) daily at this age. If anemia does develop, medicinal iron is used under a physician's guidance.

Feeding Preterm Infants

Preterm infants are fed either human milk or a specially designed formula. Total parenteral nutrition may also be required in the initial phase of hospitalization. As noted in Chapter 13, nutrients may be added to human milk to increase its protein, mineral, and energy content. Preterm infants must be fed immediately because their bodies store little fat or carbohydrate. The body composition of a full-term infant includes about 12% fat, whereas the composition of a very preterm infant can include as little as 2% fat.

Concept Check

Colic is commonly associated with inconsolable crying. Switching to an infant formula made with soy or predigested proteins may reduce colic. It may also be helpful for breastfeeding mothers to decrease or avoid intake of dairy products, caffeine, chocolate, and certain vegetables, under a physician's guidance. Diarrhea requires additional fluids to prevent dehydration. Infants allergic to proteins in standard cow's milk formula can be switched to an infant formula containing soy protein or predigested protein. Introducing iron-containing solid foods at an appropriate time and avoiding use of cow's milk during the first year can generally prevent iron-deficiency anemia in infants.

Preschool Children: Nutrition Concerns

The rapid growth rate that characterized infancy tapers off quickly during the subsequent few years. The average annual weight gain is only 4.5 to 6.6 pounds (2 to 3 kilograms), and the average annual height gain is only 3 to 4 inches (7.5 to 10 centimeters) between the ages of 2 and 5. As a toddler's growth rate tapers off, eating behavior changes. For example, the decreased growth rate leads to a decreased appetite compared with infants.

Because of the reduced appetite of preschool children, planning a diet that meets their nutrient needs poses a challenge to caregivers. Choosing nutrient-dense foods is particularly important with children who eat relatively little. This is a good time to emphasize some whole grains, fruits, and vegetables without increasing fat and simple sugar intake. A whole-grain breakfast cereal with limited fat and sugar is an excellent choice. There is no need to decrease fat or simple sugar intake severely, but fatty and sweet food choices should not overwhelm more nutritious ones.

The preschool years are the best time for a child to start a healthful pattern of living and eating, focusing on regular physical activity and nutritious foods (Fig. 14.4). Parents and other caregivers are role models: If they eat a variety of foods, the children will eat a variety of foods. One possible policy is the one-bite rule: Within reason, children should take at least one bite or taste of the foods presented to them. For snacks, parents should select several possibilities of acceptable choices and allow children to choose one; responsibility for food choice ideally should start early.

■ How to Help a Child Choose Nutritious Foods

Adults can encourage young children to eat nutritious, well-balanced meals by serving new foods and repeating exposure to them. If a child observes adults and older children eating and enjoying a food, there's a good chance that, most of the time, he

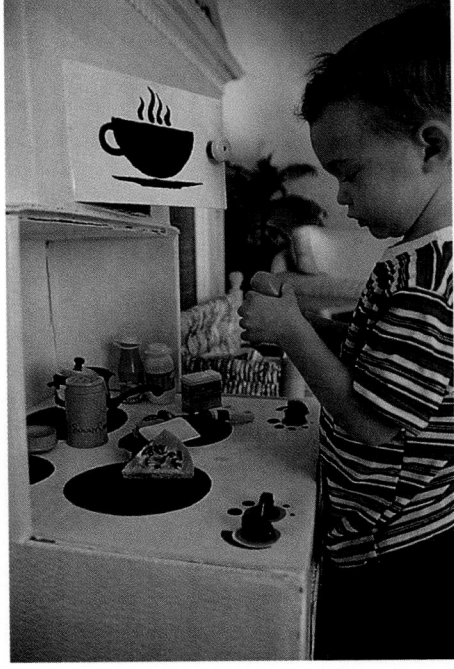

Interest in food starts early in life.

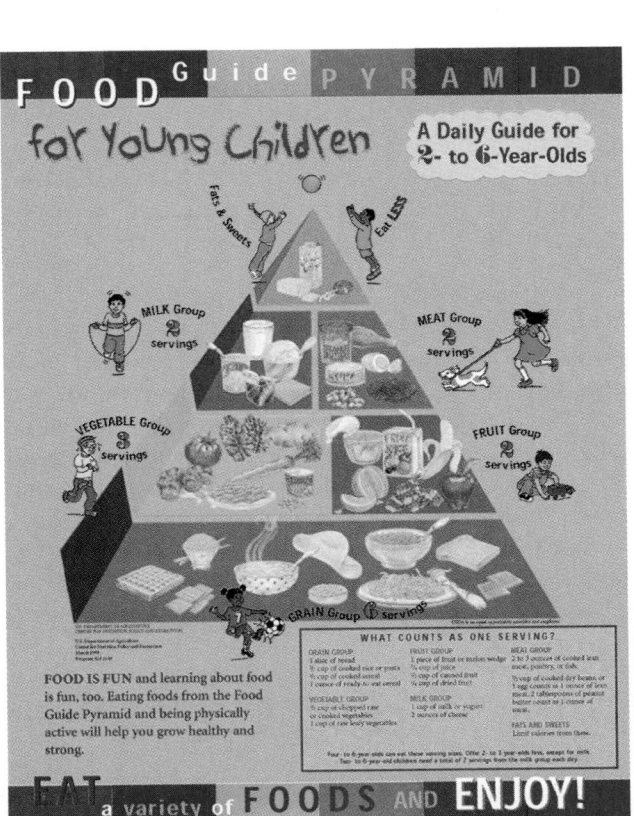

Figure 14.4 USDA has created a Food Guide Pyramid for children ages 2 through 6 years. The pyramid base recommends that young children consume six servings a day of grains such as bread, cereal, rice, and pasta; three servings of vegetables; and two servings each of fruit, milk, and meat. The pyramid is designed to be very child-friendly, showing foods children will recognize in appealing graphic format. It also emphasizes the importance of physical activity for good health by featuring many children playing actively around the pyramid to symbolize how eating and activity work hand-in-hand. The booklet accompanying this pyramid can be downloaded at www.usda.gov/cnpp.

or she will eventually accept it. The dinner hour is a good time for children to experience new foods and to develop their own food preferences. Preschool children especially tend to be wary of new foods. One reason is that they have more taste buds and their taste buds are more sensitive than those of adults. In addition, they have a general distrust of unfamiliar foods. If adults can be patient and persevere, children will build good food habits. Above all, the dinner table should not become a battleground, and using one food as a bribe to eat another—for example, a piece of pie for peas—is strongly discouraged.

Perseverance with children is critical, because it takes effort and commitment to guide them into liking a variety of foods. Be ready for some surprises. Also, if left to their own devices, preschool children would find a few foods they like and eat them every day. However, by constantly being introduced to new foods, children at this age can expand their nutritional choices, develop an experimental approach, and learn to appreciate a variety of foods. It may take 10 to 15 exposures, but eventually children will accept most foods. A positive outlook by the caregivers helps a lot.

Children generally like certain foods—especially those with crisp textures and mild flavors—and familiar foods. Young children are especially sensitive to hot-temperature foods and tend to reject them.

Parents and other caregivers play a central role in teaching by example. Children more readily learn good table manners alongside others who practice them. The harmony that comes from working at being polite creates a positive environment for learning good nutrition habits. Preschoolers eventually develop skill with spoons and forks and can even use dull knives. However, it's still a good idea to serve some finger foods. A goal should be to make mealtime a happy, social time, sharing enjoyment of healthful foods. A regular family meal daily—whether breakfast, lunch, or dinner—is an appropriate setting for children to learn about healthful eating and to build good eating habits.

▮ Childhood Feeding Problems

Tensions between parents, or between parents and children, especially during meal times, often contribute to eating problems. Getting to the root of family problems and creating a more harmonious family atmosphere are important steps toward resolving many childhood feeding problems. In addition, many parents must be educated as to what to expect of a preschool child and what food-related goals to set. Let's consider some typical complaints and concerns of parents, the causes of the problems, and suggestions for correcting them.

"My Child Won't Eat As Much or As Regularly As He Did As an Infant."

This behavior is typical of preschoolers, because their growth rate slows after infancy; thus, they don't need as much food. Parents often need reminding that a 3-year-old can't be expected to eat as voraciously as an infant or to eat adult-size portions. Table 14.3 shows a general food plan, based on the Food Guide Pyramid, that is appropriate for preschool and school-age children. Until about 5 years of age, serving sizes in the vegetable group, fruit group, and meat, poultry, fish, dry beans, eggs, and nuts group can be estimated as about 1 tablespoon per year of life. The same restriction does apply to cereals or milk. For example, a 3-year-old would eat 3 tablespoons of meat, 3 tablespoons of green beans, and 3 tablespoons of mashed potatoes at dinner.

Normal-weight children have a built-in feeding mechanism, which adjusts hunger to regulate food intake at each stage of growth. If a child is developing and growing normally and the caregiver is providing a variety of healthful foods, all can be confident the child isn't starving. Caregivers should avoid nagging, forcing, and bribing.

Appetite also varies with activity level and general health. An initial symptom of a sick child is poor appetite. Picky eating is also just another indication of a child's

*T*wo-year-olds commonly prefer particular foods, but parents needn't worry about this. A child may switch from one specific food focus (often called a jag) to another with equal intensity, (older infants may also act this way). If the caregiver continues to offer choices, the child will soon begin to eat a wider variety of foods again, and the specific food focus will disappear as suddenly as it appeared.

Table 14.3 Food Plan for Preschool and School-Age Children Based on the Food Guide Pyramid

Food Group	No. of Servings	Age 1–2	Approximate Serving Size* Age 3–4	Age 5–6	Age 7–12
Milk, yogurt (cups), and cheese (oz)	3	½–¾ cup or 1 ounce	¾ cup or 1½ ounces	1 cup or 2 ounces	1 cup or 2 ounces
Meat, poultry, fish, dry beans, eggs, and nuts	2 or more	1 ounce or 1–2 tbsp	1½ ounces or 3–4 tbsp	1½ ounces or ½ cup	2 ounces or ½ cup
Vegetables	3 or more	1–2 tbsp	3–4 tbsp	½ cup	½ cup
Fruit	2 or more	1–2 tbsp or ½ cup juice	3–4 tbsp or ½ cup juice	½ cup or ½ cup juice	½ cup or ½ cup juice
Bread, cereal, rice, and pasta	6 or more	½ slice or ½ cup	1 slice or ½ cup	1 slice or ¾ cup	1 slice or ¾ cup

*Use as a starting point. Increase serving size as energy yields dictate, but maintain variety in the diet by making sure all food groups are still appropriately represented.
Adapted from Food and Nutrition Service, U.S. Department of Agriculture: *Meal pattern requirements and offer versus serve manual,* FNS-265, 1990.

striving toward independence and his or her strong desire to establish routines. Asserting himself or herself about food preferences is a relatively easy way for the child to do this, as this may worsen if parents are too restrictive.

Parents should also be reminded that food likes and dislikes change rapidly in childhood and are influenced by food temperature, appearance, texture, and taste. Sometimes children object to having foods mixed, as in stews and casseroles, even if they normally like the ingredients separately.

In addition, parents should recognize that this is an important age for children to explore the world around them. Even good eaters are sometimes more interested in exploring than eating. There's room for occasional indulgences, a skipped meal or two, or once-in-a-while "less than ideal" choices. It's eating and lifestyle habits over the course of a month and lifetime that matter. Children master their eating when adults provide opportunities to learn, give support for exploration, and limit inappropriate behavior.

The foods that pose a risk for choking in infants also do so in young children.

"My Child Is Always Snacking, Yet She Never Finishes Her Meal."

Children have small stomachs. Offering them six or so small meals succeeds better than limiting them to three meals each day. Sticking to three meals a day offers no special nutritional advantages; it's just a social custom. Snacking is fine, as long as good dental habits are practiced. When we eat isn't nearly so important as what we eat. If nutritious snacks are readily available, these would be good to offer at mid-morning or midafternoon when the child becomes hungry (Table 14.4). Fruits and vegetables (fresh, frozen, or juice) and whole-grain breads and crackers are good snack choices. Working parents should make sure their children are provided with nutritional snacks to tide them over until dinnertime.

When a child refuses to eat, it's best not to overreact. Doing so may give the child the idea that eating is a means of getting attention or manipulating a scene. Most children don't starve themselves to any point approaching physical harm. When children refuse to eat, have them sit at the table for a while; if they still aren't interested in eating, remove the food and wait until the next scheduled meal or snack.

"My Child Never Eats Vegetables."

Children generally eat enough fruit but not an adequate amount of vegetables. Everyone dislikes certain foods. Again, the one-bite policy can be encouraged, including for vegetable servings, and guidelines can be set to discourage fussing over unfamiliar foods. Children eventually learn that they can eat some of a food they don't

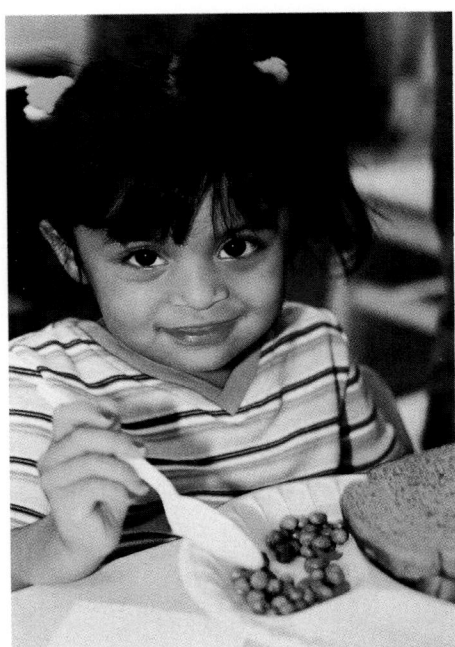

Childhood is an ideal time to begin to enjoy healthful foods.

Table 14.4 Ideas for Nutritious Snacks and Beverages

Snack	Serving Suggestion	Snack	Serving Suggestion	Snack	Serving Suggestion
Fresh raw vegetables	Serve with a dip of cottage cheese or yogurt blended with dried buttermilk dressing.	Ready-to-eat cereals	Use brands low in sugar and containing fiber; serve with raisins.	Parfait	Make with yogurt, fruit, and granola.
Celery	Spread with peanut butter and sprinkle on raisins, shredded carrots, or finely chopped nuts.	Pita bread	Place sliced meat, cheese, lettuce, and tomato in open pocket.	Gelatin	Add fruit or vegetable juice, vegetables, fruits, or cottage cheese.
Bananas	Dip in sweetened yogurt or spread with peanut butter and roll in coconut, chopped nuts, or granola.	English muffins or pita bread	Top with spaghetti sauce, grated cheese, meats; broil or bake and cut in fourths.	Frozen fruit cubes	Freeze puréed applesauce or fruit juice into cubes.
Sliced apples or crackers	Serve with a dip of peanut butter, honey, nuts, raisins, and coconut.	Potato skins	Sprinkle with shredded cheese, broil, and top with yogurt and bacon bits.	Fruit fizz	Add club soda to juice instead of serving soft drinks.
Bagels	Spread with cream cheese or peanut butter and top with chopped bananas, crushed pineapple, or shredded carrots.	Canned chili with beans	Heat and top with onions, lettuce, and tomato; use as dip for Italian or French bread, biscuits, or cornbread.	Fruit shake	Blend milk with fresh fruit (bananas, berries, or a peach) and a dash of cinnamon or nutmeg.
Quick bread or muffins	Make with carrots, zucchini, pumpkin, bananas, nuts, dates, raisins, lemons, squash, or berries.	Kabobs	Make with any combination of fruit, vegetables, and sliced or cubed cooked meat (remove toothpicks before serving).	Yogurt frost	Combine fruit juice and yogurt; add fresh fruit, if desired.
Flour tortilla	Spread with refried beans or canned chili with beans, sprinkle with grated cheese and broil; top with chili sauce.	Popcorn	Serve plain or make 3 quarts and sprinkle with ¼ cup grated cheese and ½ tsp garlic or onion salt.	Hot chocolate	Make hot chocolate or cocoa with milk chocolate and a dash of cinnamon.
				Seeds	Choose shelled sunflower seeds.
				Fish	Put tuna salad on crackers.
				Canned soup	Serve a cup of vegetable or minestrone; nice on a cold winter day.

particularly like without first gagging, choking, and yelling, "Oh, gross!" It takes time for a child to become enthusiastic about a new food; however, with continual exposure and a positive role model, chances are the child may even grow to like it.

Children cannot and should not be forced to eat. They need to develop independence and identities separate from their parents. In other words, children have to choose for themselves—a practice that should be encouraged. No one food is an essential part of a diet. Hunger is still the best means for getting a child to eat. It may be effective to feed children vegetables at the start of a meal, when they are hungriest. Offer new foods with familiar ones. A platter of raw or lightly cooked carrots, broccoli, green and red peppers, cabbage, and mushrooms eaten as a snack with friends can do a lot to remedy a vegetable problem. A 4- or 5-year-old child can safely eat raw vegetables without fear of choking. Recall that children often are more sensitive than adults to strong flavors and odors. Nutritious dips "sell" vegetables to many children. Vegetables may acquire more appeal when children help prepare them. And, as with any food, it is important to remember that children have likes and dislikes, too.

■ Do Children Need a Multivitamin and Mineral Supplement?

Major scientific groups, such as the American Dietetic Association, believe that a multivitamin and mineral supplement is unnecessary for healthy children; it's better to emphasize good foods. Ready-to-eat breakfast cereals are especially helpful in closing any gap between current vitamin and mineral intake and needs. Two minerals of particular concern are iron and zinc. These may be lacking in children's diets because they consume such small portions of rich sources, such as animal protein foods. In addition, since the current Dietary Guidelines for Americans suggest that children over age 2 years follow a diet low in saturated fat and cholesterol, rich sources of iron and zinc may be lacking in their diets. To compensate, parents can search for a whole-grain breakfast cereal that the child likes that also has at least 25% of the Daily Value for iron and zinc. (This will supply a significant increase in intake of both nutrients since the Daily Values are based on the higher needs of adults.) If that's not possible, especially for a child who is ill or has a very erratic food preference pattern or appetite, the child can be given a multivitamin and mineral supplement not exceeding 100% of Daily Values on the label, especially if these conditions persist. Diets for children who eat totally vegetarian fare should focus also on protein and vitamin B-12.

If current childhood feeding practices are to become more healthful, the focus should be on the bottom half of the Food Guide Pyramid (or related pyramid) shown in Chapter 2, including whole grains, fruits, and vegetables. Caregivers can model this behavior by ordering from the salad bar more often and ordering French fries less often at quick-service restaurants. Children do not need to be severely restricted but, rather, should modify food habits with small changes. Some easy diet changes to begin with are bagels instead of doughnuts, nonfat frozen yogurt instead of ice cream, fat-reduced or 1% milk instead of whole milk, fruit instead of crackers and cheese for snacks, and air-popped popcorn instead of chips.

■ Nutritional Problems in Preschool Children

Three nutrition-related problems found in preschool children are iron-deficiency anemia, constipation, and dental caries. Proper diet can help correct or relieve these conditions substantially.

Iron-Deficiency Anemia

Childhood iron-deficiency anemia is most likely to appear in children between 1 and 2 years of age. It can lead to decreases in both stamina and learning ability because the oxygen supply to cells decreases. Another effect is lowered resistance to disease. Fortunately, childhood anemia is fairly uncommon in North America, probably because of children's use of iron-fortified breakfast cereals. Also deserving of credit in the United States is the Special Supplemental Nutrition Program for Women, Infants, and Children (WIC), sponsored by the federal government. This program emphasizes the importance of iron-fortified formulas and cereals and distributes them—along with nutrition education—to low-income parents of infants and preschool children considered to be at nutritional risk.

The best way to prevent iron-deficiency anemia in children is to regularly provide them foods that are adequate sources of iron. Iron-fortified breakfast cereals and a few ounces of lean meat are convenient means of adding more iron into a child's diet. The high proportion of heme iron in many animal foods allows the iron to be more readily absorbed than is iron from plant foods. Consuming a rich vitamin C source along with the less readily absorbed iron in plants and supplements aid absorption.

Chapter 4 noted that it's unlikely that the use of sugar is the cause of hyperactivity or antisocial behavior in most children.

Constipation

Constipation may be associated with another disease, some young children experience constipation that is unrelated to any medical condition. When presented with a constipated child, a physician first has to rule out a medical cause, such as intestinal blockage. And, although the most common gastrointestinal symptom that reflects intolerance to cow's milk is diarrhea, chronic constipation may also result. This possibility should be investigated by the physician. Treatment for constipation generally consists of first using medications to induce a bowel movement. The promotion of regular bowel habits then follows, with any further use of medications directed by the physician. Several months to years of supportive intervention may be required for effective treatment.

*E*xcessive fruit juice and fruit drink use is another potential problem in preschool (and later adolescent) years. The American Academy of Pediatrics recommends no more than 4 to 6 ounces per day for children 1 to 6 years (and 8 to 12 ounces per day for ages 7 to 18 years).

Dietary interventions include eating more dietary fiber and drinking more fluids. Foods to emphasize for dietary fiber are fruits, vegetables, whole-grain breads and cereals, and beans. The current daily dietary fiber goal for children between ages 3 and 18 years is the child's age plus 5 grams. After age 18 years, typical adult recommendations are appropriate (review Chapter 4). Accompanying fluid recommendations are 5 cups per day for toddlers and up to 9 cups per day for older children.

Dental Caries

A proper diet goes a long way in reducing the risk for dental caries in young children. Earlier it was mentioned that infants are prone to early childhood caries, which can lead to excessive tooth decay. The following tips can help reduce dental problems in children:

- Begin oral hygiene when teeth start to appear.
- Seek early pediatric dental care.
- Drink fluoridated water.
- Use small amounts of fluoridated toothpaste twice daily.
- Snack in moderation.
- Have a dentist apply tooth sealants if needed.
- Avoid sticky, high-sugar snacks, especially between meals.
- If toddlers or preschoolers chew gum, sugarless gum is the best choice, as this has been shown to reduce the incidence of dental caries.

Chapters 4 and 9 provide a fuller description of diet and dental health. If needed, these discussions will aid in putting this list of recommendations into perspective.

■ Modifications of Childhood Diets to Reduce Future Disease Risk

Earlier chapters covered the role of diet in development of cardiovascular disease and hypertension and the recommendations concerning diet to reduce the risk for these diseases. Parents sometimes wonder whether similar diet modifications are appropriate and beneficial during childhood.

Diets Designed to Limit Cardiovascular Disease for Children 2 Years of Age and Older

The development of atherosclerosis begins in childhood. As a result, many experts recommend screening for blood cholesterol in children whose families have histories of early development of cardiovascular disease or high blood cholesterol and treating children found to have high blood cholesterol with appropriate diet and drug therapy, as discussed in Chapter 5. With regard to diet, children in the United States currently derive about 33% of their energy from fat, with about 13% of energy from saturated fat. The latest advice from the National Cholesterol Education Program in the United States is that a diet to reduce cardiovascular disease risk can include up to 35% of calories as fat (range of 25% to 35%) as long as saturated fat intake is no more than 7% of calories, cholesterol intake does not exceed 200 milligrams per day, and weight loss is not needed. Trans fat intake should also be minimal. An emphasis on plant oils such as canola oil as a major source of fat in the diet helps meet the goals of reduced saturated fat, trans fat, and cholesterol intake. If weight loss is needed (typically not the case in childhood), dietary fat intake should probably be somewhat lower, following the 30% or less of calories recommended by the American Heart Association to aid in that goal. In general, it's unnecessary to discourage children from consuming nutrient-dense foods, such as milk and animal proteins, just because they contain some animal fat. The overriding message is moderation in these and other fat sources, while especially limiting saturated fat and trans fat intake.

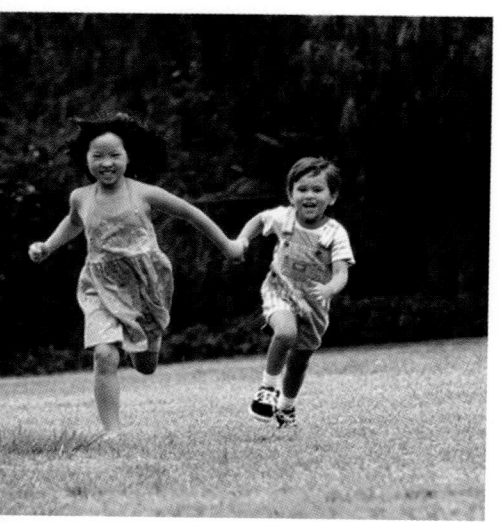

Children benefit from opportunities to be physically active. This contributes to cardiovascular health. The current goal is about 60 minutes of such activity each day.

Salt-Restricted Diets

Scientific data neither confirm nor refute the notion that eating less salt (sodium) reduces the risk of future hypertension. Moderation in salt consumption does help build good health habits for the future—especially if the person later develops hypertension and needs to eat even less salt. If children become accustomed to less salt, they'll be less inclined to eat very salty foods as adults. This reduction in salt also contributes to better calcium retention in the body, as covered in Chapter 9. If a child with hypertension does not respond to diet and lifestyle therapy, typical anti-hypertensive medications may be used, but at lower doses than adults require.

■ Vegetarianism in Childhood

Vegetarian diets pose several risks for young children. These include the possibility of developing iron-deficiency anemia, a deficiency of protein and vitamin B-12, and rickets. During the first few years of life, children also may not consume enough energy when following a bulky vegetarian diet. But these known pitfalls are easily avoided by informed diet planning (see the Nutrition Issue in Chapter 6). Diets for children who eat totally vegetarian fare should focus on protein, vitamin B-12, iron, and zinc content, with additional emphasis on vitamin D (or regular sun exposure) and calcium. Some of these dietary inadequacies can be compensated for by increasing oils, nuts, seeds, and fortified soy milk in the diet. Use of a balanced multivitamin and mineral supplement is also appropriate.

Concept Check

*T*he rapid growth rate of an infant's first year slows during the toddler and preschool years (ages 1 to 5). As a child's appetite decreases, adults need to serve nutrient-dense foods and allow the child to decide how much to eat. Sudden shifts in food preferences are to be expected. Snacking is fine if attention is given to the selection of healthful foods and good dental hygiene. Multivitamin and mineral supplements are generally not needed—a plan following the Food Guide Pyramid that include a serving of a fortified breakfast cereal should meet nutrient needs. Children need plenty of iron-rich food to prevent iron-deficiency anemia, as well as zinc for growth. Adequate dietary fiber and fluid help prevent constipation. Developing heart-healthy habits after the age of 2 years is advocated by some experts, but highly restrictive diets are not appropriate during childhood. Diets for children who eat totally vegetarian fare should focus on meeting needs for protein, vitamin D (or regular sun exposure), vitamin B-12, calcium, iron, and zinc.

▎ School-Age Children: Nutrition Concerns

In general, the nutritional concerns and goals applicable to school-age children are the same as those discussed in relation to preschoolers. The Food Guide Pyramid (or a related pyramid) continues to be a good basis for diet planning, with an emphasis on moderating fat intake and ensuring adequate iron, zinc, and calcium intake. The only difference is that serving size increases as energy needs increase (review Table 14.3). Now let's look at several nutritional issues of particular concern during the school-age years.

■ Breakfast, Fat Intake, and Snacks

Once children enter school, their eating patterns become more scheduled, and the consumption of regular meals—especially breakfast—becomes an important focus. A fortified ready-to-eat breakfast cereal is typically the greatest source of iron, vitamin A, and folate for children ages 2 to 18. Although there is controversy over the true benefit of breakfast for cognitive ability, children who eat breakfast likely meet their needs for vitamins and minerals compared to children who do not eat breakfast. To influence morning test performance, it currently appears that breakfast must be eaten within a few hours of a test; the rise in blood glucose is thought to change performance.

*I*n a recent survey, 17% of children aged 10 years old said they skip breakfast.

Breakfast menus need not be limited to traditional fare. A little imagination can spark the interest of the most reluctant child. Instead of conventional breakfast foods, parents can offer leftovers from dinner—pizza, spaghetti, soups, yogurt topped with trail mix, chili with beans, or sandwiches, for starters.

There is general agreement that diets of school-age children should include a variety of foods from each major group, not necessarily excluding any specific food because of its fat content. Overemphasis on fat-reduced diets during childhood has been linked to an increase in eating disorders and encourages an inappropriate "good food," "bad food" attitude.

School-age children are exposed to many outside influences—other children and their eating habits, snack machines, and television, just to name a few. Parents lose some of their influence during this time. Thus, it is very important that good nutritional habits are established before school age. Steering children toward healthful foods, in school and at home, is likely to be more successful if children are exposed to nutrition education. Since children spend much of their younger years in school, it is a great place to learn about positive, healthy eating habits. Such education can help children understand why eating a proper diet will make them feel more energetic, look better, and work more efficiently. One survey of schoolchildren highlighted the need for nutrition education. On the day of the survey, 40% of the children ate no vegetables, except for potatoes or tomato sauce; 20% ate no fruits; and 75% snacked at least twice. Some 36% of the students ate at least four different types of snack foods. Another study showed that only 2% of about 3,300 children 2 to 19 years old had met their recommended servings from all five Food Guide Pyramid groups. Clearly, the diets of many school-age students can stand general improvement, particularly with regard to fruit, vegetable, whole grain, and dairy choices. Drinking minimal amounts of sugared soft drinks is also advised.

▪ Type 2 Diabetes

Type 2 diabetes is generally thought of as an adult condition. As reviewed in the Nutrition Issue in Chapter 4, it frequently occurs in overweight people who are older than 40. However, recently physicians have noted an increase in the frequency of the disease among children (and teenagers). This is primarily due to the rise in obesity in this age group, coupled with little physical activity. Up to 85% of children with the disease are overweight at diagnosis. Experts are currently calling for the screening of fasting blood glucose in at-risk children every 2 years, starting at age 10 or the onset of puberty. Besides obesity and a sedentary lifestyle, risk factors include having a first- or second-degree relative with the disease, or belonging to an ethnic (non-Caucasion) population. Appropriate diet and physical activity interventions should be implemented, along with the use of medications when necessary (see Chapter 4). An adequate intake of low-glycemic index fruits, vegetables, and whole grains is especially recommended.

▪ Obesity

In North America, about 25% to 30% of school-age children place above the 85th percentile for BMI and are considered at risk for or overweight, and the number of cases is currently increasing, especially in minority populations. Obesity is generally diagnosed when a child reaches the 95th percentile for BMI and a physical exam indicates the child is truly overfat. This usually is the case for a child that reaches this degree of BMI. In the short run, ridicule, embarrassment, and possibly depression and short stature linked to early puberty are the main consequences of such obesity. In the long run, significant health problems associated with obesity, such as cardiovascular disease, type 2 diabetes, and hypertension usually don't appear until adulthood. However, an increase in these health-related complications has been noted in children. Childhood obesity is a serious health threat, since about 40% of obese children (and about 80% of obese adolescents) become obese adults. Significant weight gain generally begins either between ages 5 and 7, during puberty, or during the teenage years.

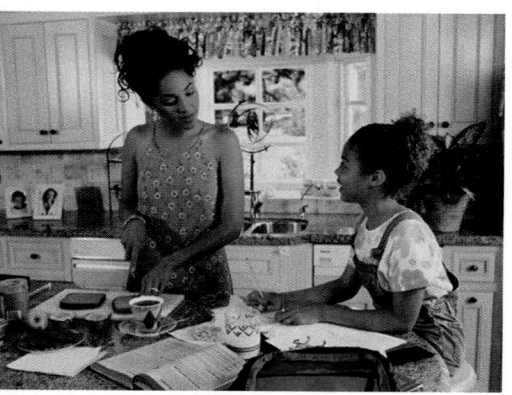

Nutrition education ideally begins in the home as parents and other caregivers provide a healthy, well-balanced diet.

Current research points to many potential causes of childhood obesity. Recall the nature versus nurture discussion in Chapter 10. Some infants are born with lower metabolic rates; they use energy more efficiently and in turn can more easily save energy intake for fat storage. Thus childhood obesity is linked to heredity. Obesity in children also has a correlation to sibling and maternal obesity. Studies also suggest, though, that this genetic link accounts for only one-third of individual differences in body weight.

Researchers believe that although diet is still an important factor, inactivity is the key to the increase in childhood obesity. The TV generation now glues itself to the tube for an average of 24 hours a week; many children spend another 10 hours or so playing computer and video games. And three out of every five children agaed 12 to 17 have a TV in their bedroom. The American Academy of Pediatrics recommends a limit of 14 hours of TV and computer time per week. In addition, excessive snacking, overreliance on quick-service restaurants, parental neglect, lack of safe areas to play, latchkey conditions, and high-fat/high-energy food choices also contribute to childhood obesity.

The initial approach in treating an obese child is to assess how much physical activity he or she engages in. If a child spends much free time in sedentary activities (such as watching television or playing video games), more physical activities should be encouraged. Both the U.S. federal government and health professionals recommend about 60 minutes or more of moderate to intense physical activity per day for children and adolescents. An overall active lifestyle will help children not only to attain a healthy body weight but also to keep a similar body height-weight relationship later in life. An increase in physical activity won't just happen; parents need to plan for it. Two good ideas are getting the family together for a brisk walk after dinner and finding an after-school sport the child enjoys.

Moderation in energy intake is important, especially paying careful attention to high-fat and high-energy foods, such as sugared soft drinks and high-fat milk. The focus should be on more nutrient-dense foods and healthy snacks.

Resorting to a weight-loss diet is usually not necessary. As a start, it's best to emphasize changing habits that allow for weight maintenance. Children have an advantage over adults in dealing with obesity; their bodies can use stored energy for growth. Thus, if weight gain can be moderated, increases in height and resulting lean body tissue may reduce the percentage of body weight accounted for as stored fat, yielding a more healthful weight-to-height ratio. This is one reason why it's desirable to treat obesity in childhood. Further growth can contribute to success.

If a child is still obese after attaining ultimate adult height, a weight-loss regimen may be necessary. This is especially appropriate after the adolescent growth spurt but may be considered starting at 8 years of age. Weight loss should be gradual, perhaps ½ pound per week. If weight loss is necessary in young children, the child should be watched closely to ensure that the rate of growth continues to be normal. The child's energy intake shouldn't be so low that gains in height diminish.

Obese children often need to find a new way to relate to foods, especially snack foods. An important family rule could be that children are allowed to eat only while sitting at the dining table or in the kitchen. This could stop endless hours of snacking in front of the television and make all family members more conscious of when they are eating. It also might be helpful to put portions of snack foods on plates, rather than allow snacking to go on indefinitely, as often happens when children eat directly from a full box of crackers or cookies.

A child's self-esteem is extremely fragile. Obesity itself affects the child's psyche. Humiliation doesn't work; it only makes the child feel worse. Support, admiration, and encouragement of the child's efforts at weight control are more effective and should be emphasized.

Finally, it is important to understand that not all children are designed to look like society's ideal. In other words, some children simply weigh more than others. A healthful lifestyle with plenty of physical activity and nutritious foods remains the key concern.

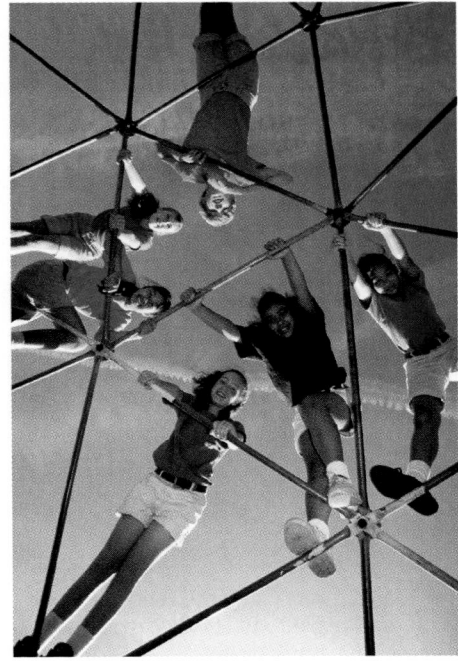

Regular physical activity is an important part of prevention and treatment of weight problems in childhood.

To get kids involved in exercise, new physical education classes have been introduced into schools. These classes provide lifelong fitness lessons, such as in rock climbing, in-line skating, and recreational jogging. These classes help promote activity because they take the focus away from teams and competition, which often discourage and embarrass kids who lack athletic talent.

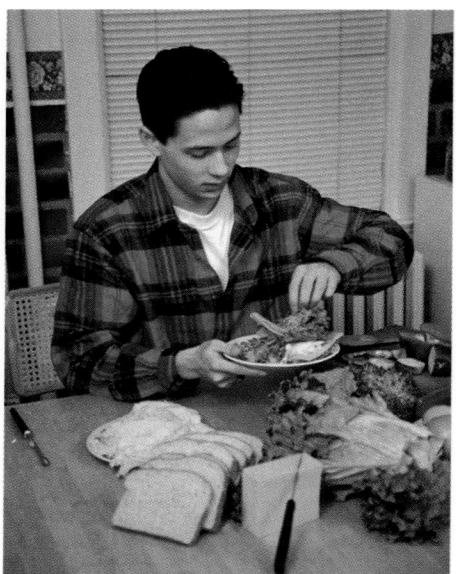

The teenage years are noted for snacking. With reasonable food choices, teenagers can have healthful diets.

A strictly vegetarian diet must be monitored for adequate energy, protein, iron, vitamin B-12, calcium, and vitamin D. This becomes particularly important in teenagers, as their diets are often already compromised.

The school-age child is advised to follow the Food Guide Pyramid (or a related pyramid), moderating choices high in fat and simple sugars. Breakfast is an important meal to refuel the body for a new school day and to help ensure fulfilling nutrient needs for the day. Attention to regular physical activity and healthy diet should help prevent/treat childhood obesity and type 2 diabetes and build a desirable lifestyle pattern for later life.

Teenage Years: Nutrition Concerns

Most girls begin a rapid growth spurt between the ages of 10 and 13, and most boys experience rapid growth between the ages of 12 and 15. Nearly every organ in the body grows during these periods. Most noticeable are increases in height and weight and development of secondary sexual characteristics. Girls usually begin menstruating (reach menarche) during this growth spurt, and they grow very little beyond 5 years after menarche. Early-maturing girls may begin their growth spurt as early as age 7 to 8, whereas early-maturing boys may begin growing by age 9 to 10.

During the growth spurt, girls gain about 10 inches (25 centimeters in height) and boys gain about 12 inches (30 centimeters). Girls also tend to accumulate both lean and fat tissue, whereas boys tend to gain mostly lean tissue. This growth spurt provides about 50% of ultimate adult weight and about 15% of ultimate adult height (review Fig. 14.1).

As the growth spurt begins, teenagers begin to eat more. However, peer pressure often dictates the food choices that teens make. Eating what is healthy is not always consistent with eating what is popular. If teens choose nutritious food, they can take advantage of their increased hunger and easily satisfy their nutrient needs. As with older age groups, the Food Guide Pyramid can provide the basis for meeting these nutrient needs, with the major difference being servings of milk and milk products (Table 14.5).

▮ Nutritional Problems and Concerns of Teens

Anorexia nervosa and bulimia nervosa were covered in detail in Chapter 12. Other nutritional problems are more common during the teen years. A survey of high school students showed that only a little over 25% had eaten 5 servings of fruits and vegetables on the previous day. At the same time, they are consuming more salt (sodium) and saturated fat than recommended. Another concern is that many teenage girls stop

Table 14.5 Food Plan for Teenagers Based on the Food Guide Pyramid*

Food Category	Minimum Number of Daily Servings†
Milk, yogurt, and cheese (preferably low fat or nonfat)	3
Meat, poultry, fish, dry beans, eggs, and nuts	2–3
Vegetables	3–5
Fruit	2–4
Bread, cereal, rice, and pasta (preferably whole grain; otherwise, enriched or fortified)	6–11
Fats, oils, and sweets	Use sparingly

*Here we define "teenager" as a person who has some gain in height in the past year and is at least 12 years old. This food plan is applicable through age 18 years.
†Use same serving size as for adults (see Table 2.6 in Chapter 2).

drinking milk, so they may not consume enough calcium to allow for maximal mineralization of bones through their early 20s. Most young women who don't consume enough calcium are likely to develop osteoporosis later, as discussed in Chapter 9.

The Adequate Intake for calcium for both males and females between ages 9 and 18 years is 1300 milligrams per day, compared with 800 milligrams per day for younger children. Three servings per day from the milk, yogurt, and cheese group are recommended for all teenagers and young adults to meet calcium needs.

A further concern is iron deficiency. Iron-deficiency anemia sometimes appears in girls after they start menstruating (menarche) and in boys during their growth spurt. About 10% of teenagers have low iron stores or related anemia. Teens who strive to forge an identity by adopting dietary patterns unfamiliar to their families—vegetarianism, for example—may not know enough about the alternate diet pattern to keep from developing health problems, such as iron-deficiency anemia. It's important that teenagers choose good food sources of iron, such as lean meats, whole grains, and enriched cereals. Teenage girls, particularly those with heavy menstrual flows, need to eat good sources of iron (or regularly consume a multivitamin and mineral supplement). Iron-deficiency anemia is a highly undesirable condition for a teen. It can produce increased fatigue and decreased ability to concentrate and learn. School and physical performance may suffer.

> *Drinking soft drinks in place of milk causes many teenagers to have inadequate calcium intake. Because soft drinks are rich in phosphorus, this practice produces an imbalance in the intakes of calcium and phosphorus, a pattern that fails to promote optimal bone development, and it has been linked to increased bone fractures in this age group.*

Another Bite

Acne is a common teen concern—about 80% of teens experience it. Although it's popularly believed that eating nuts, chocolate, and pizza can make acne worse, scientific studies have failed to show a strong link between any dietary factor and acne. It is important to note that many acne medications contain analogs of vitamin A. Although these treatments can be quite effective, the close supervision of a physician is crucial as these vitamin A analogs can be toxic. Vitamin A itself is no help in treating acne, and excess amounts of vitamin A or related analogs can cause birth defects. Thus, girls taking vitamin A medications should not become pregnant.

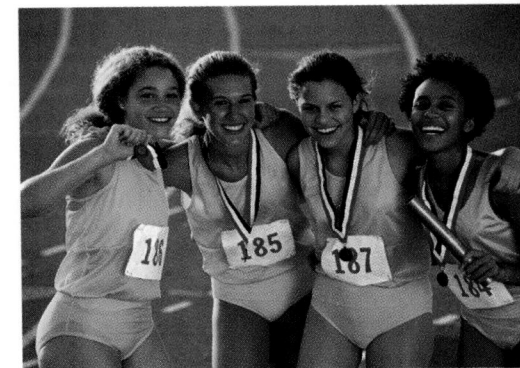

An active lifestyle coupled with a healthy diet should be part of the teen years.

■ A Closer Look at the Diets of Teenage Girls

Teenagers in general are apt to adopt fad diets, eat away from home or miss meals completely, and snack a lot. Teenage girls especially are very concerned with weight gain, appearance, and social acceptance. U.S. government statistics reveal that female students were significantly more likely to report currently trying to lose weight (44%) than male students (15%). Moreover, 27% of female students who considered themselves the right weight report they are currently trying to lose weight. It is important to inform teenage girls that weight gain in the form of increased body fat is to be expected in the adolescent growth spurt.

In an attempt to reach personal goals, teenage girls may eat dangerously little, select just a few items, and frequently skip meals altogether. If their limited food choices then consist of French fries, sugared soft drinks, and pastries, little room is left for foods that are rich nutrient sources. Another common practice among teenage girls is having a fat phobia, focusing primarily on foods that are fat-free. However, many teens may not realize that some fat is essential for body functions, thus emphasizing the need for some fat in the diet. This concept is discussed in Chapter 5. The diets of teenage girls often lack adequate sources of folate, calcium, zinc, and vitamins A, C, and E. The possibility for this should be assessed and corrective action then implemented. Diet changes, fortified foods, and a multivitamin and mineral supplement are possible corrective measures. Routinely, experts recommend diet changes first. The common use of diet pills and the increasing number of anorexia nervosa and bulimia nervosa cases further add to nutritional problems in this age group.

> *Alcoholism, a significant health problem that may have its roots in the teen years, is covered in detail in Chapter 7. Smoking—another habit that compromises health—also often begins in the teen years and is currently increasing in this age group. Some of this is in an attempt to control body weight—not an advisable method.*

■ Helping Teens Eat More Nutritious Foods

Teenagers face a variety of challenges. They pursue their independence, experience identity crises, seek peer acceptance, and worry about physical appearance. All of these factors affect food choice. Teens are constantly bombarded with a mixed message. The media directs advertisements for high-fat and high-sugar foods at teens, while at the same time the media also "sells" the importance of having a "perfect body." Potato chips and French fries make up more than one-third of the vegetable servings consumed by teens. Additionally, many schools offer French fries on a regular basis, and soft drink machines can be found in school hallways and cafeterias, in turn competing with the school lunch.

Teens often don't think about the long-term benefits of good health. They have a hard time relating today's actions to tomorrow's health outcomes. Many teenagers tend to think they can just change habits later—there's no hurry.

Still, healthful teen food habits don't have to include giving up favorite foods. Small portions of fatty foods can complement larger portions of nonfat and low-fat dairy products, lean meats, vegetable proteins, fruits, vegetables, and whole grain products. An example is a plain hamburger with a garden salad (minimize the amount of regular dressing or use a low-fat variety), a small order of French fries or chili, and a medium diet soft drink.

■ Overcoming the Teenage Mind-Set

One strategy for working with teenage boys is to stress the importance of nutrition and physical activity for physical development—especially muscular development—and for fitness, vigor, and health. With teenage girls, one approach is to help them understand how to choose nutrient-dense foods and activities that lead to better health while maintaining a healthy weight. For teenagers, it's more effective to focus on the benefits of healthful foods and regular physical activity they can reap right now than to talk about health hazards that may or may not happen later.

■ Are Teenage Snacking Practices Harmful?

Teens often obtain one-fourth to one-third of all their energy and major nutrients from snacks. Unfortunately, studies have found just what you might expect—that teens snack mostly on potato and corn chips, cookies, candies, and ice cream. Key reasons for snacking include an opportunity to get out and socialize with friends, accessibility, hunger, and celebration of a special event. Teenagers can obtain many nutrients from snacking. Even quick-service restaurants offer some good food choices. By choosing wisely and eating in moderation, teens can eat at quick-service restaurants and still consume a very healthful diet. Snacks and quick-service restaurants themselves are not the problem; poor food choices are.

Poor dietary habits formed during teenage years often continue into adulthood, giving rise to an increased risk of chronic diseases, such as cardiovascular disease, osteoporosis, and some types of cancer. Getting this message across to teenagers is an important and challenging task for parents and health professionals.

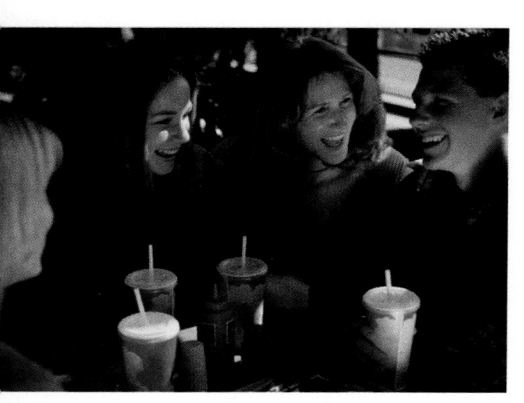

One way to reduce calorie intake in a restaurant is to choose diet soft drinks in place of regular soft drinks. This will greatly reduce sugar intake in the meal or snack, especially considering the large serving sizes typically offered.

Concept Check

A second period of rapid growth occurs during the teen years. Girls generally start this growth spurt earlier than boys. The Food Guide Pyramid (or related pyramid) should guide meal planning. Common nutritional problems in these years arise from poor food choices and include inadequate calcium intake in girls, iron-deficiency anemia, and generally excessive intakes of salt (sodium) and saturated fat. A plan to correct these nutritional problems should be put into place. Because changes occur so rapidly during these years, and in so many areas—psychological, social, and physical—it may be difficult to stress the importance of nutrition to teenagers. Moderation in fat and sugar intake are goals to consider when choosing snacks.

Summary

1. Growth is very rapid during infancy; birth weight doubles in 4 to 6 months, and length increases by 50% in the first year. An adequate diet, especially in terms of energy, as well as the nutrients protein and zinc, is essential to support normal growth. Undernutrition can cause irreversible changes in growth and development. Growth in infants and children can be assessed by measuring body weight, height (or length), and head circumference over time. Growth charts have recently been revised to include a more valid measurement for determining children's growth, body mass index (BMI).

2. Nutrient needs in the first 6 months can be met by human milk or iron-fortified infant formula. Supplementary vitamin D and iron may be needed in the first 6 months for breastfed infants, and many infants may need supplemental fluoride after 6 months of age.

3. Infant formulas generally contain lactose or sucrose, heat-treated proteins from cow's milk, and vegetable oil. These formulas may or may not be fortified with iron. Sanitation is very important when preparing and storing formula.

4. Most infants don't need solid foods before about 4 to 6 months of age. Solid food should not be added to an infant's diet until the nutrients are needed, the GI tract can digest complex foods, the infant has the physical ability to control tongue thrusting, and the risk of developing food allergies has decreased.

5. The first solid food given should be iron-fortified infant cereals or ground meats. Other single foods can be added gradually, at the rate of about one each week. Some foods to avoid giving infants in the first year include honey, cow's milk (especially fat-reduced varieties), very salty or sweet foods, or foods that may cause choking.

6. Introducing iron-containing solid food at the appropriate time and not offering cow's milk until 1 year of age can generally prevent iron-deficiency anemia in late infancy.

7. A slower growth rate in preschool years underlies the importance of children's eating nutrient-dense foods and reducing their food serving sizes. Choosing iron-rich foods, such as lean red meats, is important at this age. Portion sizes at meals of 1 tablespoon of each food for each year of life is a good rule of thumb for vegetables, fruits, and meats.

8. Preschoolers should be given some leeway in determining serving size and should be encouraged to try new foods. Highly restrictive diets designed to reduce the risk of cardiovascular disease or hypertension are not recommended for preschoolers or older children, unless prescribed by a physician.

9. Obese children and adolescents are more likely to become obese adults and, so, incur greater health risks. Parents can provide healthful food choices, and children should control portion sizes. When controlled early through diet and exercise interventions, a problem of obesity (and type 2 diabetes) may correct itself as the child continues to grow in height.

10. During the adolescent growth spurt, both boys and girls have increased needs for iron and calcium. Inadequate calcium intake by teenage girls is a major concern because it can set the stage for development of osteoporosis later in life. Teenagers generally should moderate their intake of saturated fat-rich, salt-rich, and sugar-rich foods—especially snacks and quick-service foods, which they often consume in abundance—and perform regular physical activity.

Study Questions

1. List two factors that limit "catch-up" growth in adulthood when a nutrient-deficient diet has been consumed throughout childhood.

2. Describe how you would assess whether an 8-month-old infant is consuming a healthful diet.

3. Outline three key factors that help determine when to introduce solid foods into an infant's diet.

4. A 3-month-old infant is brought to a clinic with failure to thrive. What are two possible explanations?

5. List three reasons why preschoolers are noted for fussy eating. For each, describe an appropriate parent response.

6. What three factors are likely to contribute to obesity in a typical 10-year-old child?

7. Compare the guidelines for infant feeding summarized in the chapter with the Dietary Guidelines for children over 2 and adults discussed in Chapter 2. Which guidelines are similar? Do any contradict each other? If so, why?

8. Describe three pros and cons of snacking. What is the basic advice for healthful snacking from childhood through the teenage years?

9. Which two nutrients are of particular interest in planning diets for teenagers? Why does each deserve to be singled out?

10. List three nutrients of concern for a teenage vegetarian.

Further Readings

1. ADA Reports: Position of the American Dietetic Association: Dietary guidance for healthy children aged 2 to 11 years. *Journal of American Dietetic Association* 99:93, 1999.
Children older than 2 years of age should gradually adopt a diet by the age of 5 that reflects a lifelong healthy, nutrient-rich dietary pattern. The health status of U.S. children generally has improved over the past three decades; however, the number of children who are overweight has more than doubled.

2. Bellizzi MC, Dietz WH: Workshop on childhood obesity: Summary of the discussion. *American Journal of Clinical Nutrition* 70:173S, 1999.
Early identification of childhood obesity is key in preventing obesity and health-related complications in later adulthood. Body mass index in children 2 years and older is favorable to other methods for assessing weight status.

3. Berenson GS and others: Association between multiple cardiovascular risk factors and atherosclerosis in children in young adults. *New England Journal of Medicine* 338:1650, 1998.
As the number of cardiovascular risk factors increases in children, so does the severity of atherosclerosis. Interventions related to the risk factors, such as prevention of smoking, weight control, encouragement of physical exercise, and a moderate fat diet—if undertaken early in life, retard the development of atherosclerosis.

4. Cohen AR: Choosing the best strategy to prevent childhood iron deficiency. *Journal of the American Medical Association* 281:2247, 1999.
Although there has been a decline in the prevalence of childhood iron deficiency in the United States, studies indicate that children who were diagnosed with the problem between the ages of 1 and 2 years were behind their peers in both mental and motor development. Targeted screening of iron status is important in younger children.

5. Formanek RF: Food allergies: When food becomes the enemy. *FDA Consumer*, p. 10, July–August, 2001.
Food allergy patterns in adults differ somewhat from those in children. The most common foods to cause allergies in adults are shellfish, peanuts, walnuts, and other tree nuts, fish, and eggs. In children, eggs, milk, peanuts, soy, and wheat are the main culprits. The article discusses both the diagnosis and treatment of food allergies.

6. Fomon SF: Feeding normal infants: Rationale for recommendations. *Journal of the American Dietetic Association* 101:1002, 2001.
Breastfed infants should receive a daily supplement of iron and vitamin D, while formula-fed infants should receive iron-fortified formulas. Solid foods should not be introduced before 4 months of age. Iron-fortified cereals are the best solid foods to first introduce, but children with a strong family history of allergies may benefit from soft-cooked red meats as the first foods. Cow's milk should not be fed before one year of age.

7. Ganley T, Sherman C: Exercise and children's health: A little counseling can pay lasting dividends. *The Physician and Sportsmedicine* 26(2):85, 2000.
Despite the growing epidemic of childhood obesity and related health complications, nearly half of the children in the United States are not involved in regular activity sufficient for cardiovascular fitness. It is important for children—with the help of parents—to find activities that are interesting, enjoyable, and appropriate for their age and physical abilities. The goal of safe, enjoyable exercise is readily attainable by virtually all youngsters.

8. Ludwig DS, Ebbeling CB: Type 2 diabetes mellitus in children: Primary care and public health considerations. *Journal of the American Medical Association* 286:1427, 2001.
There has been a recent increase in type 2 diabetes in children. This is largely due to the increase in obesity in this population. Type 2 diabetes carries enormous, long-term public health implications. A healthful diet that includes low-glycemic index foods, such as fruits, vegetables, and whole grains, and a physically active lifestyle should be emphasized for these children, and other children in general. Weight loss is also generally indicated.

9. McBean LD, Miller GD: Enhancing the nutrition of America's youth. *Journal of the American College of Nutrition* 18:563, 1999.
Today, children's diets are out of balance with the Food Guide Pyramid recommendations. Dietary guidance should be conducive to consuming a variety of helpful foods in moderation, not food restrictions, and encouraging physical activity in children.

10. Neumark-Sztainer D and others: Factors influencing food choices of adolescents: Findings from focus-group discussions with adolescents. *Journal of the American Dietetic Association* 99:929, 1999.
Nutritional needs during adolescence are higher than at any other time in life due to the increased need for growth and development. Thus, adolescents should strive to make nutritious choices regarding their diet. One approach could be nutrition education to make it "cool" to eat healthfully.

11. Patton S: Connecting with overweight kids. *Today's Dietitian*, p. 36, September 2001.
Educational activities to help overweight children should include information on how to set limits, identify problem situations, and what to do in the problem situations. The influence of social changes and the media should also be discussed, and specific goals set for the children should utilize some fun activities.

12. Schardt D: Food allergies. *Nutrition Action Healthletter*, p. 10, April 2001.
Since there is no treatment or cure for food allergies, the only way to avoid allergic reactions is to avoid the offending foods. Allergies to peanuts, nuts, and seafood seldom disappear. Food intolerances on the other hand—except for those caused by sulfites—are not as serious a health problem.

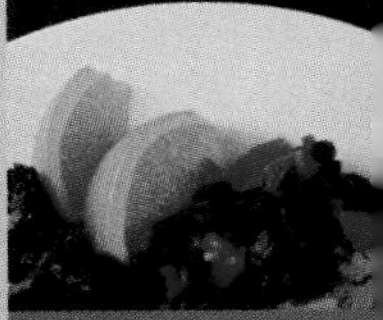

I. Getting Young Bill to Eat

Bill is 3 years old, and his mother is worried about his eating habits. He absolutely refuses to eat vegetables, meat, and dinner in general. Some days he eats very little food. He wants to eat snacks most of the time. His mother wants him to eat a sit-down lunch and dinner to make sure he gets all the nutrients he needs. Mealtime is a battle because Bill says he isn't hungry, but his mother wants him to eat everything served on his plate. He drinks five or six glasses of whole milk per day because that is the one food he likes.

When his mother prepares dinner, she makes plenty of vegetables, boiling them until they are soft, hoping this will appeal to Bill. Bill's dad waits to eat his vegetables last, regularly telling the family that he eats them only because he has to. He also regularly complains about how dinner has been prepared. Bill saves his vegetables until last and usually gags when his mother orders him to eat them. Bill has been known to sit at the dinner table for an hour until the war of wills ends. Bill's mother serves casseroles and stews regularly because these are her best dishes. Bill likes to eat breakfast cereal, fruit, and cheese and regularly requests these foods for snacks. However, his mother tries to deny his requests, so he will have an appetite for dinner. Bill's mother comes to you and asks you what she should do to get Bill to eat.

Analysis

1. List four mistakes Bill's parents are making that contribute to Bill's poor eating habits.

_____

_____

_____

_____

2. List four strategies they might try to promote good eating habits in Bill.

_____

_____

_____

_____

continued

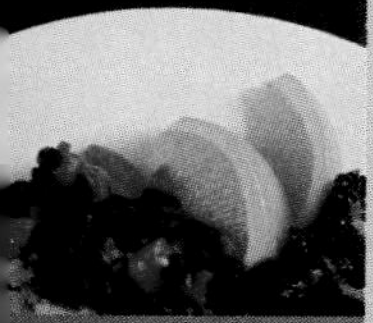

II. *Evaluating a Teen Lunch*

The following are two typical teen lunches and nutritional information for each:

	Meal 1	Meal 2	Nutrient Needs for Teens
	2 slices cheese pizza	1 hamburger with condiments	
	1 milk chocolate candy bar	30 French fries	
	20 fl oz cola	20 fl oz cola	
kcal	990	1000	Males: 3000 Females: 2200
Protein	32	20	Males: 59 Females: 44
Vitamin C (milligrams)	5	18	Both genders: 45–75
Vitamin A (micrograms RAE)	300	10	Males: 900 Females: 700
Iron (milligrams)	3	4	Males: 11 Females: 15
Calcium (milligrams)	545	100	Both genders: 1300

1. Keeping in mind that meals should meet about one-third of nutrient needs, what are the shortcomings and excesses of these meals? Given the nutritional information, compare these meals with one-third the RDA for calories, protein, vitamin C, vitamin A, and iron and the Adequate Intake for calcium?

_____

_____

_____

_____

2. How would you change these meals to improve balance and to meet the nutrient needs listed in part II above? (Hint: Use your software program or Appendix A.)

_____

_____

_____

3. Reflect on your food choices as a teenager. Do you think your meal choices were balanced and varied? Why or why not? What could you have done to improve your nutritional habits at that time?

_____

_____

_____

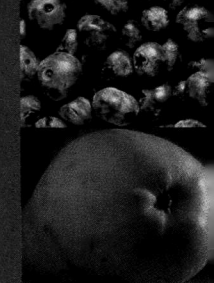

Food Allergies and Intolerances

Adverse reactions to foods—indicated by sneezing, coughing, nausea, vomiting, diarrhea, hives, and other rashes—are broadly classed as food allergies (also called *hypersensitivities*) or **food intolerances.** Allergies involve responses of the immune system designed to eliminate foreign proteins, called **allergens.** The symptoms experienced by susceptible people, such as rapid increase in heart rate and shortness of breath, are the result of this battle. In contrast, the symptoms of food intolerances do not result from a true allergic reaction. Rather, food intolerances are caused by an individual's inability to digest certain food components or by the direct effect of a food component or contaminant on the body. Let's examine each process, first allergies and then intolerances, so you can learn how to reduce the risk of becoming a victim of the food you eat.

Food Allergies: Symptoms And Mechanism

Allergic reactions to foods are quite common and occur more frequently in females than males. Food allergies occur most frequently during infancy and young adulthood. Experts estimate that up to about 2% of adults and up to about 6% of children are allergic to certain foods. Three types of reactions may occur after ingestion of problem foods by susceptible people:

- *Classic*—itching, reddening skin, asthma, swelling, choking, and a runny nose
- *GI tract*—nausea, vomiting, diarrhea, intestinal gas, bloating, pain, constipation, and indigestion
- *General*—headache, skin reactions, tension and fatigue, tremors, and psychological problems

Any reaction that is milder than these distinct allergic ones is referred to as a **food sensitivity.**

Allergic reactions vary not only in the body system affected but also in their duration, ranging from seconds to a few days. A generalized, all-systems reaction is called **anaphylactic shock.** This severe allergic response results in low blood pressure and respiratory and GI tract distress. It can be fatal. Overall, allergic reactions result in 30,000 emergency room visits and 150 to 200 deaths per year. A person who is extremely sensitive to a food may not be able to touch the food or even be in the same room where it is being cooked without responding to it. Although any food can trigger anaphylactic shock, the most common culprits are peanuts (actually a legume, not a nut), tree nuts (walnuts, pecans, etc.), shellfish, milk, eggs, soybeans, wheat, and fish. For a small number of people, avoiding foods such as peanuts or shellfish is a matter of life and death.

Almost all food allergies are caused by proteins in milk (also look for casein on the label), eggs (also look for albumin on the label), corn, nuts, peanuts, seafood, soy products, and wheat. Other foods frequently identified with adverse reactions include meat and meat products, fruits, and cheese.

Testing for a Food Allergy

The diagnosis of a food allergy can often be a difficult task (Table 14.6). It requires the participation of a skilled physician. The first step in determining whether a food allergy is present is to record in detail a history of symptoms, time from ingestion to onset of symptoms, most recent reaction, quantity and nature of food needed to produce a reaction, and food suspected of causing a reaction. A family history of allergic diseases can also help, as allergic reactions tend to run in families. A physical examination may reveal evidence of an allergy, such as skin diseases and asthma. Various diagnostic tests can rule out other conditions.

continued

food intolerance An adverse reaction to food that does not involve an allergic reaction.

allergen A foreign protein, or antigen, that induces excess production of certain immune system antibodies; subsequent exposure to the same protein leads to allergic symptoms. Whereas all allergens are antigens, not all antigens are allergens.

food sensitivity A mild reaction to a substance in a food that might be expressed as light itching or redness of the skin.

People with a history of serious allergic reactions should carry a self-administered form of epinephrine, such as EpiPen.

The American Academy of Allergy and Immunology has a 24-hour toll-free hot line (800-822-2762) to answer questions about food allergies and to help direct people to specialists who treat the problem. Free information on food allergies is available by writing to The Food Allergy Network, 4744 Holly Ave., Fairfax, VA 22030. The telephone number is 800-929-4040; the website is www.foodallergy.org.

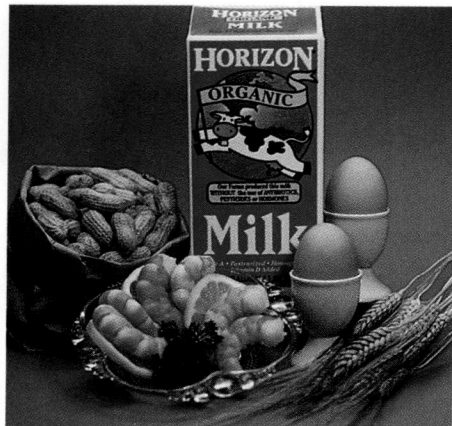

Eggs, wheat, milk, nuts, and seafood pose the greatest risk for food allergies in childhood.

Table 14.6 Assessment Strategies for Food Allergies

History	Includes description of symptoms, time between food ingestion and onset of symptoms, duration of symptoms, most recent allergic episode, quantity of food required to produce reaction, suspected foods, and allergic diseases in other family members
Physical examination	Look for signs of an allergic reaction (rash, itching, intestinal bloating, etc.)
Skin test	Place a sample of the suspected allergen under the skin and watch for an inflamatory reaction
RAST test	Determine presence of antibodies in blood that bind to antigens tested
Elimination diet	Establish a diet lacking the suspected offending foods and stay on it for 1 to 2 weeks or until symptoms clear
Food challenge	Add back small amounts of excluded foods one at a time, as long as anaphylactic shock is not a possible consequence

Perhaps the best laboratory test for determining which compounds a person is allergic to is the RAST test. This test estimates the blood concentration of antibodies that binds certain food-borne antigens. Skin tests can also be used; a drop of antigen is placed under the skin where it has been scratched or punctured. If a person is allergic to the test antigen, a red eruption will develop.

The next step is to eliminate from the diet for 1 to 2 weeks all tested compounds that appear to cause allergic symptoms, plus all other foods suspected of causing an allergy based on the person's food history. The person generally starts out eating foods to which almost no one reacts, such as rice, vegetables, noncitrus fruits, and fresh meats and poultry. If symptoms are still present, the person can more severely restrict the diet or even use special formula diets that are hypoallergenic.

elimination diet A restrictive diet that systematically tests foods that may cause an allergic response by first eliminating them for 1 to 2 weeks and then adding them back one at a time.

Once a diet is found that causes no symptoms, called an **elimination diet,** foods that are known not to trigger anaphylactic shock can be added back one at a time. Doses of ½ to 1 teaspoon (2.5 to 5 milliliters) are given at first. The amount is increased until the dose approximates usual intake. This should be done using a double-blind approach (review Chapter 1), especially when the reaction has a psychological component or when symptoms are vague or ill-defined. Dried foods can be encapsulated and then given to the person. Any reintroduced food that causes significant symptoms to appear is identified as an allergen for the person.

■ Treating Food Allergies

Once potential allergens are identified, the best treatment is to avoid them, especially for people with zero tolerance. Careful reading of food labels is essential for many allergic people and advisable for all. A major challenge for the clinician treating a person with a food allergy is to make sure that what remains in the diet can still provide essential nutrients. The small food intake of children permits less leeway in removing the offending foods that may contain numerous nutrients. A registered dietitian can help guide the diet-planning process to ensure that what remains of the food choices still meets nutrient needs or to guide supplement use, if that is necessary.

If an allergy-prone woman is pregnant or breastfeeding, she should avoid offending foods—such as eggs, shellfish, and peanuts—because allergens can cross the placenta during pregnancy. Allergens are also secreted in her milk. She should work with her physician and registered dietitian to make sure she still consumes an adequate diet. In addition, when food allergies are common in the family, women are advised to breastfeed their infants exclusively for 6 months. Human milk contains factors that play a role in maturation of the small intestine. Formula-fed infants, especially those on formulas based on cow's milk, have a greater risk for developing allergies. Breastfeeding, thus, should continue for as long as possible, preferably to 1 year.

prognosis A forecast of the course and end of a disease.

The **prognosis** for food allergies that first appear before 3 years of age is good. About 80% of young children with food allergies outgrow them before 3 years. Parents should be made aware of this and certainly not assume the allergy will be long-lived. Food allergies diagnosed after 3 years of age, however, are often more long-lived, but not always. In these cases, about 33% of people outgrow their food allergies within 3 years. For others, the condition may be prolonged; some food allergies can last a lifetime, such as those for peanuts, tree nuts, and shellfish. Periodic reintroduction of offending foods in some cases can be tried every 6 to 12 months or so to see whether the allergic reaction has decreased. If no symptoms appear, tolerance to the food has developed.

Food Intolerances

Food intolerances are adverse reactions to food that do not involve allergic mechanisms. Generally, larger amounts of an offending food are required to produce symptoms of an intolerance than to trigger allergic symptoms. Common causes of food intolerances include:

- Constituents of certain foods (e.g., red wine, tomatoes, pineapples) that have a druglike activity, causing physiological effects such as changes in blood pressure
- Certain synthetic compounds added to foods, such as sulfites, food-coloring agents, and monosodium glutamate (MSG)
- Food contaminants, including antibiotics and other chemicals used in the production of livestock and crops, as well as insect parts not removed during processing
- Toxic contaminants resulting from ingestion of improperly handled and prepared foods containing *Clostridium botulinum*, *Salmonella* bacteria, or other foodborne microbes (see Chapter 16)
- Deficiencies in digestive enzymes, such as lactase (see Chapter 4)

Almost everyone is sensitive to one or more of these causes of food intolerance, many of which produce GI tract symptoms.

Sulfites, which are added to foods and beverages as antioxidants, cause flushing, spasms of the airways, and a loss of blood pressure in susceptible people. Wine, dehydrated potatoes, dried fruits, gravy, soup mixes, and restaurant salad greens commonly contain sulfites. A reaction to MSG may include an increase in blood pressure, numbness, sweating, vomiting, headache, and facial pressure. MSG is commonly found in Chinese food and many processed foods (e.g., soups). A reaction to tartrazine, a food-coloring additive, includes spasm of the airways, itching, and reddening skin. Tyramine, a derivative of the amino acid tyrosine, is commonly found in "aged" foods, such as cheeses and red wines. This natural food constituent can cause high blood pressure in people taking monoamine-oxidase inhibitor medications, which may be prescribed for mental depression.

The basic treatment for food intolerances is to avoid specific offending components. However, total elimination often is not required because people generally are not as sensitive to compounds causing food intolerances as they are to allergens. For instance, a slight amount of sulfites in a glass of wine may be tolerable, whereas a large amount from a chef's salad may cause a reaction.

chapter 15

Nutrition During Adulthood

Chapter Outline

*E*ating is one of our great pleasures. Guided by common sense and moderation, eating well is also a means to good health. Most of us want a long, productive life, free of illness, yet many people from early middle age onward suffer from cardiovascular disease, hypertension and strokes, type 2 diabetes, osteoporosis, and other chronic diseases. We can slow the development of, and in some cases even prevent, these diseases by pursuing a diet that works against them. This action is most profitable if we begin early and continue throughout adulthood. We serve ourselves best—as individuals and as a nation—by striving to maintain vitality even in the later decades of life. This concept was first explored in Chapter 1 and is discussed again in this chapter, along with the special nutrition needs of older persons.

Keep in mind that present day-to-day health practices can significantly influence health during later life. Although genetics does play a role, as discussed in Chapter 3, many of the health problems that occur with age are not inevitable; they result from disease processes that influence physical health. Much can be learned from healthy older people whose attention to a healthy diet and physical activity—along with a little luck— keeps them active and vibrant well beyond typical retirement years. Successful aging is the goal. Age quickly or slowly—it is partly your choice.

Check out the **Contemporary Nutrition: Issues and Insights Online Learning Center** www.mhhe.com/wardlawcont5 *for quizzes, flash cards, other activities, and web links designed to further help you learn about nutrient needs in adulthood.*

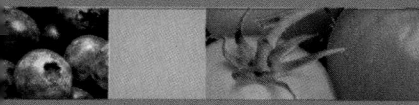

Refresh Your Memory

*As you begin your study of adult
nutrition issues in Chapter 15, you may
want to review:*

- Implications of the 1994 Dietary
Supplement Health and Education
Act in terms of what nutrients and
related compounds can be sold
today in the United States without
FDA approval in Chapter 1

- The effect of genetics on health in
Chapter 3

- The various body systems covered in
Chapter 3

- The sources of dietary fiber and
sugar in Chapter 4

- Recommendations for alcohol intake
in Chapter 7

- The dietary sources of vitamin D, the
various B-vitamins, and calcium in
Chapters 8 and 9

- Recommendations for salt intake in
Chapter 9

- Definition of healthy body weight in
Chapter 10

- The benefits of regular physical
activity in Chapter 11

Real Life Scenario

Frances is a 78-year-old woman who suffers from macular degeneration,
osteoporosis, and arthritis. Since her husband died 1 year ago, she has
moved from their family house to a small one-bedroom apartment. Her
eyesight is progressively getting worse, making it hard to go to the grocery store or
even to cook for herself (for fear of burning herself). She is often lonely; her only son
lives 1 hour away and works two jobs, but he visits her as often as he can. Frances
has lost her appetite and, as a result, often skips meals throughout the week. She has
resorted to eating mostly cold foods that are simple to prepare but at the same time
is seriously limiting diet variety and palatability. She is slowly losing weight as a result
of her dietary changes and loss of appetite.

Her typical diet usually consists of a
breakfast that may include 1 slice of
wheat toast with margarine,
honey, and cinnamon and 1 cup
of hot tea. If she has lunch, she
normally has ½ can of peaches, ½
of a turkey and cheese
sandwich, and ½ glass of water.
For dinner, she might have ½ of a
tuna fish sandwich made with
mayonnaise and 1 cup of iced
tea. Occasionally, she includes
one or two cookies at bedtime.

What services do you think
are available that could help
Frances improve her diet and
possibly increase her appetite?
What other convenience foods
could be included in her diet to
make it more healthful and more
varied?

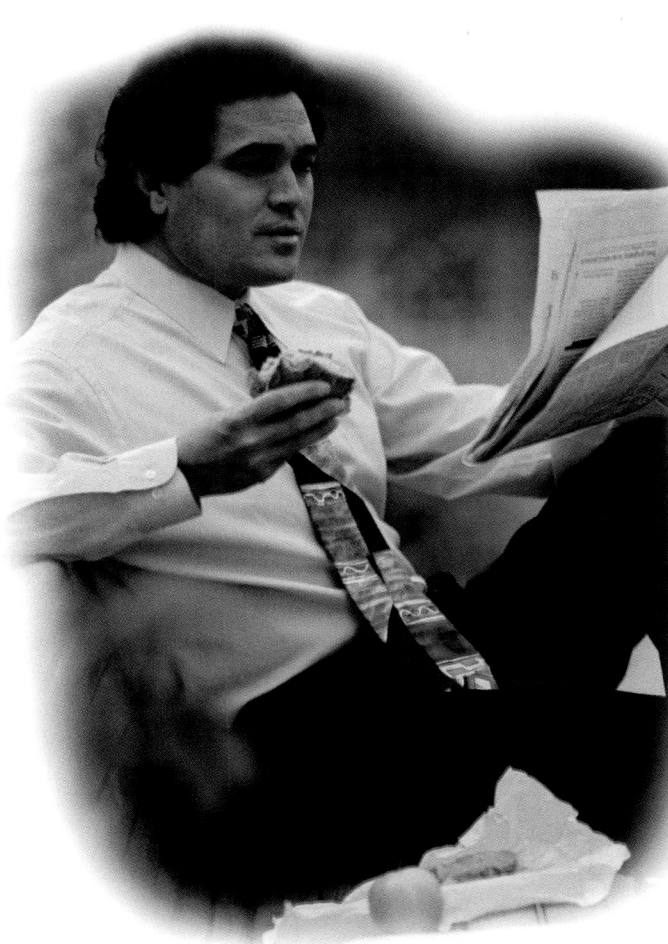

Nutrition Connection

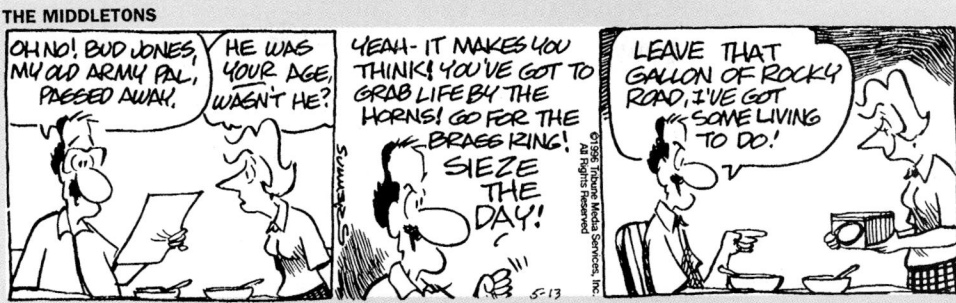

THE MIDDLETONS

Is a decline in health inevitable as we age? Which diet and lifestyle interventions have been shown to slow (or reverse) the aging process? Which nutrition problems are typically seen in older adults? How should one compensate for these? This chapter provides some answers.

Nutrition and Adulthood—An Introduction

Many adults in North America today are doing what is within their control to achieve a healthy lifestyle, such as a healthful diet and body weight and a regimen of regular physical activity. Coupled with avoidance of tobacco products; limitation of or other adaptation to stress; adequate sleep; adequate fluid intake; maintaining friendships and optimism; lifelong learning; keeping blood cholesterol, blood glucose, and blood pressure under control; and consultation with healthcare professionals on a regular basis, these actions contribute to a healthful, long life. Overall, the key to maximizing health throughout life is to establish harmony among one's physical, mental, psychological, and social states (see Part I in the Rate Your Plate section at the end of this chapter).

From a nutritional point of view, one's adult years are divided into four stages: ages 19 to 30, 31 to 50, 51 to 70, and beyond 70 years of age. The two intervals encompassing ages 19 to 50 can be seen as young adulthood; 51 to 70 then would be middle adulthood; and beyond 70 years of age would be older adulthood.

Nutritional needs change throughout these intervals. For example, calcium needs increase after age 50 for males and females. Vitamin B-12 needs also change after age 50, in that one should consume foods fortified with crystalline vitamin B-12 or take a multivitamin and mineral supplement containing vitamin B-12. Recall from Chapter 8 that this latter advice stems from the fact that about 10% to 30% of older people may malabsorb food-bound vitamin B-12 because of reduced acid production by the stomach. Vitamin D needs also change. Adults over age 70 need three times more vitamin D than they did when they were ages 19 to 50, and they need 50% more than they did during ages 51 to 70. In response to this increase in vitamin D needs for people over age 70, nutrition experts at Tufts University have suggested a modification of the Food Guide Pyramid to include a supplemental vitamin D source for this age group. This is especially important if a person does not receive regular sun exposure, such as would be in the case of winter months in New England and Canada (see Chapter 8). Other such changes suggested by these experts for the Food Guide Pyramid will be mentioned in the section "Nutrient Needs in Middle and Older Adulthood."

Attention to healthy nutrition and overall lifestyle habits is important at all ages. Providing dietary advice for adults ages 19 to 50 years is the focus of the beginning of this chapter. The chapter will then look at additional recommendations for adults 51 and older.

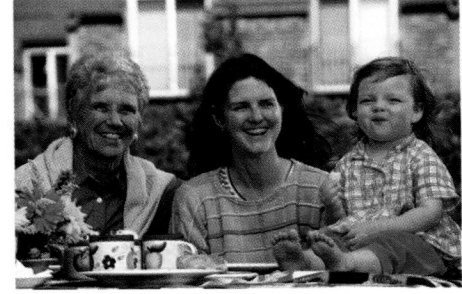

As we age, our nutrient needs change. For example, vitamin D needs are higher for older stages of adulthood than for younger stages or for childhood.

Keep in mind that extending life without delaying onset of chronic disease prolongs suffering in many cases. In addition, the greater number of disabled years is a great cost to all North Americans. For these reasons, prolonging life without compressing the number of disabled years is called the "failure of success."

*A*ppendix B reviews diet planning guidelines issued by the Canadian government for Canadians. In addition, Chapter 1 discussed Healthy People 2010, a U.S. federal agenda aimed at disease prevention and health promotion.

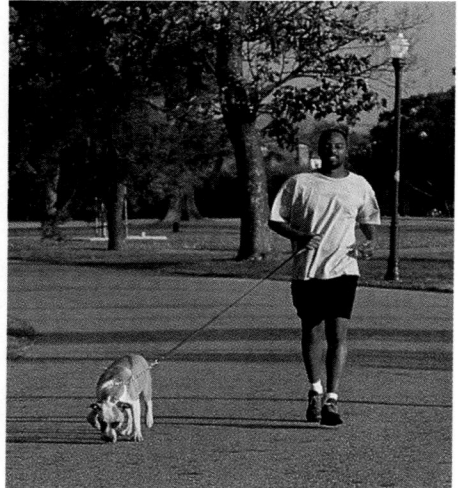

Many adults find that regular physical activity adds an important dimension to their lives. The Dietary Guidelines for Americans recommend that men over 40 and women over 50 years of age obtain physician approval before beginning a program of vigorous physical activity. This is especially important for people with evidence of cardiovascular disease, hypertension, or diabetes.

Figure 15.1 Using the tools provided by the Food Guide Pyramid and Dietary Guidelines for Americans is one way for adults to plan a healthy diet. Chapter 16 provides more information on food safety issues. They will help you implement that Dietary Guideline.

A Diet for the Adult Years

One diet approach that optimizes long-term nutritional health emphasizes low-fat and nonfat dairy products, some lean meats and fish, plant proteins, a rich variety of fruits and vegetables, and generous amounts of whole-grain breads and cereals. The Food Guide Pyramid, combined with the Dietary Guidelines for Americans discussed in Chapter 2, is one blueprint for this diet.

Figure 15.1 depicts those two tools for diet design. The practices recommended can accommodate many cultural dietary patterns (see the Nutrition Issue in Chapter 2). They are broad enough to allow you to include all the foods you enjoy in an eating plan—you just may have to eat some foods less frequently than others or in smaller portions, depending on your health needs and preferences. Moderation, rather than elimination, should be your overriding consideration.

Beyond the general recommendations shown in Figure 15.1, adults should moderate use of cured and smoked foods because they are likely to increase the risk of certain forms of cancer (see Chapter 8). Obtaining adequate fluoride to promote dental health and drinking plenty of fluids is also important. In addition, women of childbearing age need to eat iron-rich foods, primarily to avoid developing iron-deficiency anemia. With regard to nutrient supplements, some younger adults especially benefit from a multivitamin and mineral supplement to meet specific nutrient needs. For example, especially women who could become pregnant are advised to consume foods fortified with synthetic folic acid or to take a supplement containing it, in addition to consuming folate-rich foods. This practice reduces the risk of some serious birth defects. Adults who seldom eat dairy products or other rich sources of calcium need a calcium supplement, and adults who eat no animal foods need to take a supplement containing vitamin B-12. Use of a vitamin E supplement (200 milligrams; about 400 IU) could also be considered for adults in general, but there is no consensus on this recommendation. In addition, sometimes vitamins or minerals are prescribed for meeting nutrient needs for various medical purposes. For example, pregnant women or those with heavy menstrual periods may be advised to take an iron supplement. Still, supplements of some nutrients, such as vitamin A and selenium, can be harmful if taken in large amounts. As well, because foods contain many substances that promote health, one should

Let the pyramid guide your food choices.

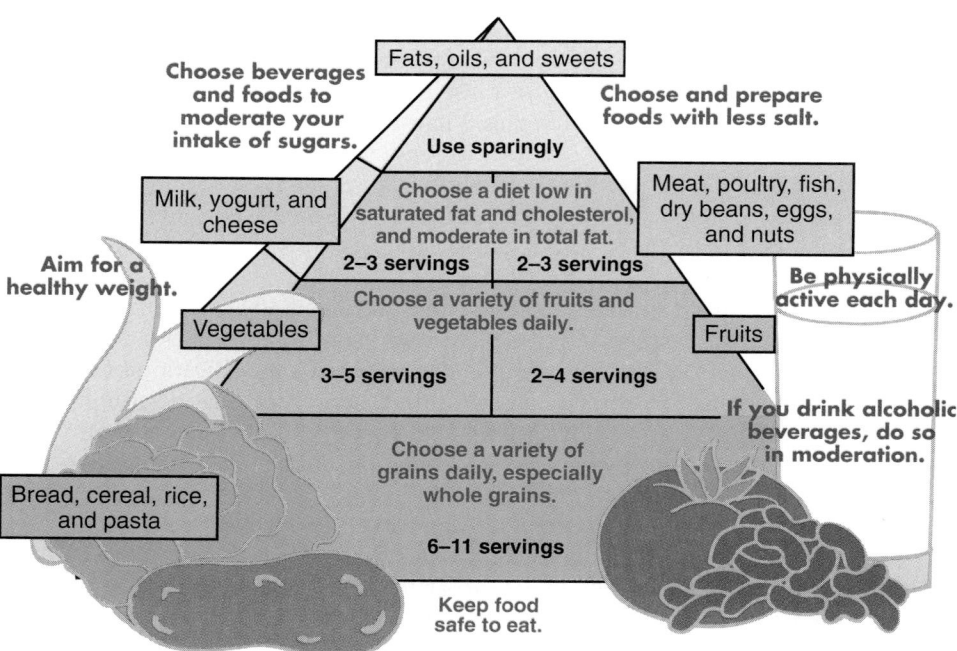

Choose beverages and foods to moderate your intake of sugars.

Fats, oils, and sweets

Choose and prepare foods with less salt.

Use sparingly

Milk, yogurt, and cheese

Choose a diet low in saturated fat and cholesterol, and moderate in total fat.

Meat, poultry, fish, dry beans, eggs, and nuts

Aim for a healthy weight.

2–3 servings   2–3 servings

Be physically active each day.

Choose a variety of fruits and vegetables daily.

Vegetables   Fruits

3–5 servings   2–4 servings

If you drink alcoholic beverages, do so in moderation.

Choose a variety of grains daily, especially whole grains.

Bread, cereal, rice, and pasta

6–11 servings

Keep food safe to eat.

always use the Food Guide Pyramid (or related pyramid) as a starting point when planning a diet, rather than depending mostly on supplements to meet nutrient needs.

■ Are Adults Following Current Dietary Recommendations?

In general, adults in North America are trying to follow many of the diet recommendations listed. Since the mid-1950s, they have consumed less saturated fat as more people substitute nonfat and low-fat milk for cream and whole milk. They eat more cheese, however, which is usually a concentrated form of saturated fat. Since 1963, they have eaten less butter, fewer eggs, less animal fat, and more vegetable fats and oils and fish. These changes generally follow the recommendations to reduce the intake of saturated fat and cholesterol and, instead, to emphasize unsaturated fat. Today, animal breeders are raising much leaner cattle and hogs than those produced in 1950, which helps. Our demand for chicken, a relatively lean source of animal protein, has skyrocketed.

Other aspects of the average adult diet are more mixed. The latest nutrition survey of eating habits in the United States shows that the major contributors of energy to the adult diet are white bread, beef, milk, doughnuts, cakes and cookies, soft drinks, chicken, cheese, salad dressing, mayonnaise, margarine, and sugars/syrups/jams. If the trend in diets were truly toward decreasing sugar and saturated fat intake, and increasing dietary fiber intake, many of these foods would not appear at the top of the list.

A list incorporating this book's suggestions for improvement would stress low-fat and nonfat milk and yogurt, whole-wheat bread and whole-grain cereals, lean meat, salmon and tuna, peanuts and other nuts, kidney and pinto beans, oranges, carrots, broccoli, and romaine lettuce with tomatoes and Italian dressing.

The overriding consideration should be quality and length of life and the impact dietary changes might have on them. Adulthood is the key time to learn more about risk factors for chronic diseases and to do something about each one, when possible.

■ A Note of Caution

Not all nutrition and health researchers agree with the blanket guidelines set by major health and science institutions, as noted in Chapter 2. Some scientists do not think that general recommendations for the public can be justified for sugar, salt, and cholesterol. Rather, they believe that this advice needs to be individualized.

Although it can be argued that individualized dietary recommendations for some nutrients and other dietary constituents are best, that approach is generally too costly for the nation and therefore impractical. More global recommendations are appropriate if they benefit most people while not hampering the health of others. Not all people will benefit equally—for example, a reduction in salt intake—but no one is likely to be harmed. The dietary change may simply cause some inconvenience and necessitate the formation of new eating habits for some people. Nevertheless, we should all consider the general dietary advice, personalizing this when possible under the guidance of our health-care advisers.

Nutrient supplements can complement, but should not substitute for a more comprehensive plan to maintain health as one ages.

Critical Thinking

The "fountain of youth" remains a mystery. Many people believe a source exists that can stop the aging process, allowing youth to remain. However, Neil, a history student, asserts that the fountain of youth is not a place or a particular thing but, rather, a combination of diet and lifestyle. How can he justify this claim?

Concept Check

A basic plan to promote health and prevent disease includes eating a balanced, varied diet; performing regular physical activity; and limiting or abstaining from alcohol intake. More specific Dietary Guidelines for Americans direct people to eat a variety of foods; maintain healthy weight; choose a diet low in saturated fat and cholesterol and moderate in total fat; choose a diet with plenty of vegetables, fruits, and grain products; use sugars only in moderation; and use salt only in moderation. Recommendations also include warnings against relying primarily on nutrient supplements to meet nutrient needs, but in some cases these especially can provide a healthful addition to a diet. Some scientists believe that these many guidelines do not necessarily constitute an individual "prescription."

▮ Middle and Older Adulthood

How long do your family members generally live? Of those who died early in adulthood, can you pinpoint some causes? Do you plan to live longer than your parents did or will? How long will that be? Some basic statistics can help you predict this.

▮ Life Span

Life span refers to the maximal number of years humans live. As far as we know, this hasn't changed in recorded time. The longest human life documented to date is 122 years for a woman and 113 years for a man. One's genes play a key role in determining longevity, but environment is also important. Note also by comparison that the domestic dog has a life span of 20 years; a rat, 5 years.

▮ Life Expectancy

Life expectancy is the time an average person born in a specific year, such as 2002, can expect to live. Currently, life expectancy in North America is about 73 years for men and about 80 years for women, with a span of "healthy years" of about 64. Furthermore, if you survive to the age of 80, you can tack on another 7 to 10 years of life expectancy.

Worldwide, the highest average life expectancy is 82 years for women and 76 years for men in Japan. Researchers suggest that a diet based on rice, fish, vegetable protein sources, fruits, vegetables, and small amounts of meat contributes to this record longevity (see the Nutrition Insight).

Life expectancy hasn't always been this long; for primitive humans, it was about 20 to 35 years. It increased to 40 years in Medieval England and increased to 49 years by the turn of the twentieth century. During the last 80 years, life expectancy for nearly all people has increased, mainly because of changes in the principal causes of death.

In the early 1900s, infectious diseases were the first three causes of death. Vaccines and antibiotics have tremendously lowered death from disease. The decline in infant and childhood deaths, coupled with better diets and health care, has allowed more people to age first into maturity and then into older years. Now the principal causes of death in Western societies are related to cardiovascular diseases and cancer (review Table 1.1).

Historically, the trend in the United States, Canada, and other developed nations has been toward an ever older population. For example, during Colonial times, half of the U.S. population was over 16 years of age. By 1990, half were over 33. By 2050, half of the U.S. population could be over 43, and approximately 20% will be 65 years and older, twice as many as reach 65 today. This age—65 years—is arbitrarily listed as a dividing line for the beginning of later life because one can currently qualify for full Social Security benefits in the United States. The time at which old age occurs, however, varies for each person, according to health and independence.

Among the older population, the group constituting those aged 85+ years is the fastest growing segment. Between 1997 and 2050, the population aged 85+ years in the United States is expected to increase from 3.4 million to 19 million. This is the first time in history North America and other Western nations will need to accommodate such a large population of older people. The associated expense will be enormous if a large percentage need special care because of ill health. Even more amazing, 1 million or more people in the U.S. alone could be over 100 years old in 2050.

B *esides having other long-lived family members, people who live to 100 years generally:*
- Do not smoke or drink heavily
- Gain little weight in adulthood
- Eat many fruits and vegetables
- Perform daily physical activity
- Challenge their minds
- Have a positive outlook
- Maintain close friendships
- Are (or were) married (especially true for men)

O *f all the people who have ever lived to age 65, more than half are now alive.*

▮ The Graying of North America

This "graying" of North America poses some problems. Today, although people older than age 65 account for 13% of the U.S. population, they account for more than 25% of all prescription medications used, 40% of acute care hospital stays, and 50% of the federal health budget. Hip fractures alone cost the nation about $10 billion per year. Of older persons, 85% have nutrition-related problems, such as cardiovascular disease, type 2 diabetes, hypertension, and osteoporosis.

Postponing these chronic diseases for as long as possible will help control health-care costs. The more independent, healthy years people live, the better life can be for them and the less they burden the health-care system, which will increasingly have to scramble to accommodate a growing older population. Keep in mind that aging is not a disease. Furthermore, diseases that commonly accompany old age—osteoporosis and atherosclerosis, for example—are not an inevitable part of aging. Many can be prevented or managed, for the most part. Some people do die of old age, not as a direct result of disease.

▪ What Actually Is Aging?

One view of aging describes it as processes of slow cell death, beginning soon after fertilization. When we are young, aging is not apparent because the major metabolic activities are geared toward growth and maturation. We produce plenty of active cells to meet physiological needs. During late adolescence and adulthood, the body's major task is to maintain cells. Inevitably, though, cells age and die. Eventually, as more cells die, the body can't adjust to meet all physiological demands. Body functioning begins to decrease (Fig. 15.2). Still, organs usually retain enough **reserve capacity** that, for a long time, the body shows no outward disease. Although no symptoms appear, subclinical disease may develop, and, if the disease is allowed to progress unchecked, organ function and then body function eventually deteriorate noticeably.

The aging process is clearly illustrated by changes for many people in the function of the enzyme lactase. For some people, lactase activity in the small intestine slows during childhood. Generally, however, clear symptoms of this decline—gas and bloating after milk consumption—do not appear until adulthood. Although lactase output decreases in these cases, perhaps from birth, enough enzyme is present to digest the lactose consumed until adulthood.

Cells age probably because of automatic cellular changes and environmental influences. Even in the most supportive of environments, cell structure and function inevitably change. Eventually, cells lose their ability to regenerate the internal parts they need, and they die. This inevitable dying off of deteriorating cells is actually beneficial, as researchers have concluded it likely prevents diseases such as cancer.

Unfortunately, there are still consequences to this natural cell progression, because as more and more cells in an organ system die, organ function decreases. For example, **kidney nephrons** are continually lost as we age. In some people, this loss leads to eventual kidney failure, but most of us maintain sufficient kidney function throughout life. Again, in aging, there is first a reduction in reserve capacity. Only after that is exhausted does actual organ function noticeably decrease.

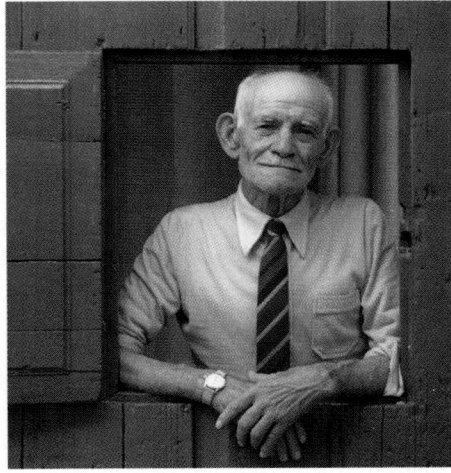

A diet based on vegetables, fruits, pasta, and olive oil as a source of fat—and with a small amount of alcohol in the form of red wine—provides southern Italians with many healthy years of life. Their active lifestyle is an additional contributing factor.

reserve capacity The extent to which an organ can preserve essentially normal function despite decreasing cell number or cell activity.

kidney nephrons The units of kidney cells that filter wastes from the bloodstream and deposits them into the urine.

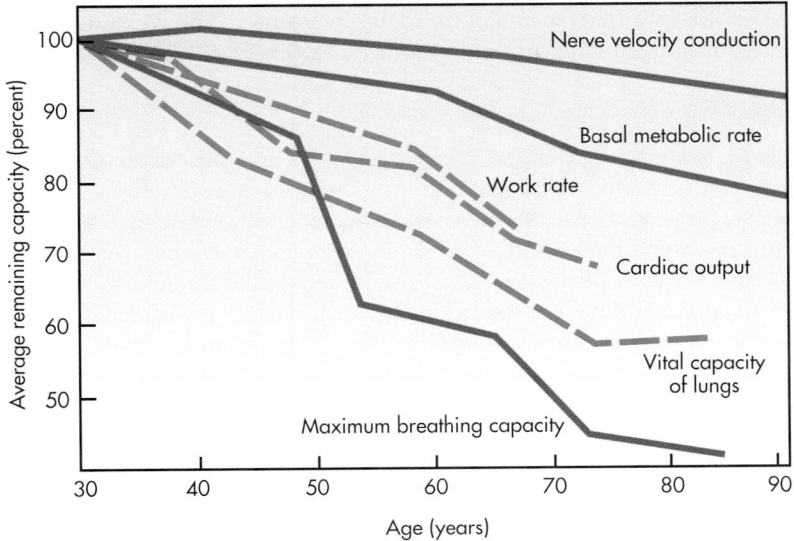

Figure 15.2 Declines in physiological function seen with aging. The decline in many body functions is especially evident in sedentary people.

Table 15.1 Current Hypotheses About the Causes of Aging

Errors occur in copying the genetic blueprint (DNA)

Once sufficient errors in DNA copying accumulate, a cell can no longer synthesize the major proteins needed to function and it therefore dies.

Connective tissue stiffens

Parallel protein strands, found mostly in connective tissue, chemically bond and cross-link to each other. The bonding decreases flexibility in key body components, altering organ function (e.g., joints and arteries stiffen).

Electron-seeking compounds damage cell parts

Electron-seeking free radicals can break down cell membranes and proteins. One way to prevent some damage from these compounds is to consume adequate amounts of vitamins E and C, selenium, and carotenoids.

Hormone function changes

The blood concentration of many hormones, such as testosterone in men and estrogen in women, falls during the aging process. Replacement of these and other hormones is possible; research is ongoing (see the Nutrition Insight).

Glycosylation of proteins

Blood glucose, when chronically elevated, attaches to (glycates) various blood and body proteins. This decreases protein function and can encourage immune system attack on such altered proteins. Such problems are typical of people with poorly controlled diabetes.

The immune system loses some efficiency

The immune system is most efficient during childhood and young adulthood, but with advancing age it is less able to recognize and counteract foreign substances, such as viruses, that enter the body. Nutrient deficiencies, particularly of protein, vitamin E, vitamin B-6, and zinc, also hamper immune function (see Chapter 3).

Autoimmunity develops

Autoimmune reactions occur when white blood cells and other immune bodies fail to distinguish between substances normally present in the body and invading foreign proteins. White blood cells and other immune bodies then begin to attack body tissues in addition to foreign proteins. Many diseases, including some forms of arthritis, involve this autoimmune response.

Death is programmed into the cell

Each human cell can divide only about 50 times. Once this number of divisions occurs, the cell automatically succumbs. This degradation occurs by design, probably as a way for the body to regulate cell number. One mechanism for this limitation is that DNA shortens in length with every cell division. Recall from Chapter 8 that cancer cells defeat this shortening, in turn allowing for immortal growth.

Excess energy intake speeds body breakdown

Underfed animals, such as spiders, mice, and rats, live longer. Scientists have yet to pinpoint the exact mechanisms that allow for life extension in calorie-restricted animals (see the Nutrition Insight).

The causes of this aging of the body are still a mystery. Most likely, aging results from an interaction of genetic background and the changes listed in Table 15.1. Even very healthy people have a shortened life expectancy if they are exposed to sufficient environmental stress, such as radiation and certain chemical agents like industrial solvents. Because cell aging and diseases such as cancer are aggravated by environmental factors, it makes good sense to avoid such risks as excessive sunlight exposure and hazardous chemicals. Again, as has been stressed, we have some control over how quickly we age. You can obtain a free fact sheet on aging by going to the website for the National Institute on Aging at www.nih.gov/nia or by calling (800) 222-2225.

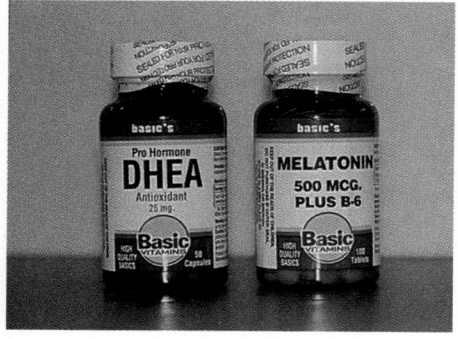

As discussed in the Nutrition Insight, a variety of products are advocated to slow aging. No research to date supports such effectiveness in humans.

Concept Check

Although life span has not changed, life expectancy has increased dramatically over the past century. In many societies, this means an increasing proportion of the North American population is, and will be, over 65 years of age. Avoiding continually rising health-care costs and maximizing satisfaction with life require postponing and minimizing chronic illness. Aging begins early in life and probably results from both automatic cellular changes and environmental influences. Some current hypotheses of aging suggest these possible causes: errors in DNA copying accumulate, connective tissue stiffens, damaged cell components build up, electron-seeking free radical compounds break down cell parts, hormonal and immune systems don't function well, and autoimmune responses and high blood glucose damage key body compounds. Researchers are also studying the possibility that excess energy intakes may be a factor in premature death. Diet can play a role in slowing some of these processes.

Tinkering with the March of Time—What Works to Slow Aging?

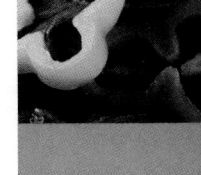

Effective Interventions

Healthy Diet

As noted in the chapter, some of the longest-lived peoples of the world live in Japan, especially on the island of Okinawa. Researchers suggest that a diet based on rice, fish, vegetable protein sources (including soy), fruits, vegetables, tea, herbs for seasoning, and limited meat, salt, and alcohol contributes to this record longevity in Japan. In addition, these people consume a modest amount of calories compared to energy expenditure such that they remain lean throughout life (BMI≈21). Use of supplements to correct nutrient deficiencies also has been shown to improve the span of healthy years in older people in the United States (see later section on Nutrient Needs of Middle and Older Adulthood).

Spartan Energy Intake

For many years, scientists have known that underfed animals live longer. All other nutrient needs are met, but calories are restricted. Scientists have not yet pinpointed the exact mechanism that allows for life extension in calorie-restricted animals, but they speculate that modified glucose use, decreased free-radical damage, changes in gene function, less cell metabolism, and a variety of other factors contribute to longer life. Researchers are currently studying rhesus monkeys that are on a 30% lower energy intake than typical rhesus monkeys. Though the calorie-restricted monkeys have lower blood pressure, blood cholesterol, and triglycerides, and high HDL-cholesterol after 17 years, it is too soon to analyze the full implications of this severe restriction. On the downside, the monkeys have the same appetite as typical monkeys, making them somewhat desperate for food; their bone density is reduced; and their reproductive ability is in question.

Like the rhesus monkeys, humans housed in Biosphere II (conducted outside Tucson, Arizona) had to follow a limited diet because they overestimated their ability to grow their own food. They experienced declines in body weight, blood pressure, blood cholesterol, and blood glucose on the spartan 1800 kcal diets. These parameters remained at the low end of healthy values. It is unknown whether adults in general would voluntarily restrict themselves to this degree in order to obtain the same health benefits.

Aerobic and Strength-Training Physical Activity

Older adults who exercise regularly to their capacity add from months to years to their life. From simple brisk walking to water aerobics and light weightlifting—any activity is helpful. Physical activity increases muscle strength and mobility, improves mental outlook, eases daily tasks that require some strength, improves sleep and balance, slows bone loss, and increases joint movement, reducing injuries. It also decreases the risk of cardiovascular disease, type 2 diabetes, hypertension, decline in mental function, depression, and some forms of cancer. However, when older adults stop their resistance (weight-training) and aerobic exercise programs, gains in muscle strength and many other health-related parameters are quickly lost. This illustrates the importance of regular physical activity throughout life.

After obtaining their physician's approval to get started, older people can seek out programs to begin strength and aerobic training at community recreation or cardiac rehabilitation centers or the local YMCA or YWCA. Most of these organizations have qualified trainers who can help set up a program. Dumbbells are inexpensive and, thus, ideal for performing weight training at home. Chapter 11 provides some general advice on this topic, including advice for warm-up, stretching, and cooldown activities. Overall, much of what we associate with aging in terms of physical health results from long-standing sedentary lifestyles.

Experimental Medical Therapies

Growth Hormone

A fall in growth hormone concentration is also being investigated as a potentially treatable hormonal cause of aging. Growth hormone is secreted by the pituitary gland and stimulates protein synthesis in cells, such as muscle cells, as well as produces various other effects in the body. However, replacing growth hormone has wide-ranging, unpredictable effects and is very costly. Growth hormone should be used only under physician supervision; it is routinely used in children who secrete abnormally low amounts. Studies so far support the hypothesis that growth hormone-related loss of lean body mass plays a role in aging. Still, once treatment with growth hormone in adults is stopped, gains in lean body mass are lost.

The risks and benefits of this treatment probably will be known within 2 or 3 years, but it could take another 5 to 10 years to determine the best dosage. Growth hormone therapy has been associated with significant adverse side effects, such as **carpal tunnel syndrome,** breast development in men, swollen ankles and legs, and possibly hypertension, diabetes-like symptoms, and certain forms of cancer. All of these problems may limit its clinical usefulness in older people. Growth hormone is currently available only by prescription.

Testosterone

Testosterone concentration declines with age. This decline in testosterone is linked to a decline in muscle strength. Studies support the concept that a subgroup of older males may benefit from testosterone therapy. Postmenopausal women, especially those who have undergone surgical menopause, may also be candidates for testosterone therapy if estrogen therapy alone does not reduce menopausal symptoms. Note that there are some side effects with use, such as masculinizing effects in women, a decline in HDL-cholesterol in the blood, and prostate gland enlargement. Treatment is still in the experimental phase and currently is not generally recommended due to possible side effects.

continued

Dubious, Unregulated, and Potentially Dangerous Interventions

DHEA

The hormone *dehydroepiandrosterone (DHEA)*, produced by the adrenal glands (located on top of the kidneys), circulates at extremely high concentration in young adults and falls after the age of 30. This change has led to speculation that DHEA decline plays a role in aging. However, the physiological function of this steroid hormone is unclear, and long-term effects of using products containing this hormone are also unknown. Unfortunately, many adults do not know that DHEA can cause acne, irritability, fall in HDL-cholesterol in the blood, insomnia, masculinization of women, prostate gland enlargement, and possibly prostate and breast cancer. Until long-term studies ensure the safety of DHEA, extreme caution should accompany any use of this still mysterious hormone. Note that many adult men show prostate gland enlargement, making DHEA use for them a very risky proposition.

Melatonin

Production of the hormone melatonin declines after puberty. Melatonin is known for its ability to induce sleep; the production of melatonin is highest at night and falls during the day. It was once thought that this hormone decreases with age, but new research has shown that melatonin production remains relatively constant during aging, with variations from person to person. Currently, little is known about the long-term effects of this treatment on humans; there is evidence that it reduces ovulation in women. In fact, French, British, and Canadian governments have banned its sale. Overall, until it is shown to be safe and effective, it is premature to take melatonin preparations in the hope of slowing the aging process.

Coenzyme Q-10

Coenzyme Q-10, compound used in energy metabolism, is very popular in Japan and is also sold in the United States. Early studies were promising in showing that the enzyme worked as an antioxidant, slowed aging, and treated heart failure, but the studies were small and short term. The latest research casts doubt on any benefits from Coenzyme Q-10. The body produces much Coenzyme Q-10, and it is widely distributed in the food supply.

In summary, there is no pill that substitutes for a healthy diet and regular physical activity. Some medical interventions look promising for selected persons; physician monitoring is crucial in all cases.

Effects of Aging on Nutritional Health

Adults over age 50 vary more in health status among themselves than do persons in any other age group. This means that chronological age is not useful in predicting physical health status (physiological age). Among people aged 70 and over, some are totally independent, healthy people, whereas others are frail and require almost total care. To predict the nutritional problems of an older person, it is necessary to know the extent of physiological change caused by aging and whether the person shows early warning signs for long-term poor nutrition. As you examine how aging affects body systems and how these changes contribute to nutritional health, note the suggested ways to lessen health risks (Table 15.2).

Other Factors That Influence Nutrient Needs in Aging

Medications and old age often go together. Medications can improve health and quality of life, but some of them also profoundly affect nutrient needs at all ages, including the later years. Two-thirds of older adults take prescription drugs; one-half of the older adult population regularly take multiple prescription drugs. Many drugs affect appetite or the absorption of nutrients. Often, people must take medications for long periods. They should make sure to work with their physician and pharmacist to coordinate all medications taken. Pharmacists can advise when to take drugs—with or between meals—for maximum effectiveness.

Drug-related nutritional problems include (1) increased need for potassium when certain types of diuretics increase excretion from the body and (2) changes in appetite caused by antidepressant agents or certain antibiotics. Blood loss from the long-term use of aspirin or aspirin-like medications depletes iron reserves and can lead to anemia. People who must take one or more medications for more than just a few weeks should closely watch their diets, eat nutrient-dense foods, and possibly take nutrient supplements to counteract the effects of certain medications. A physician should supervise this last practice, because some supplements can interfere with the function

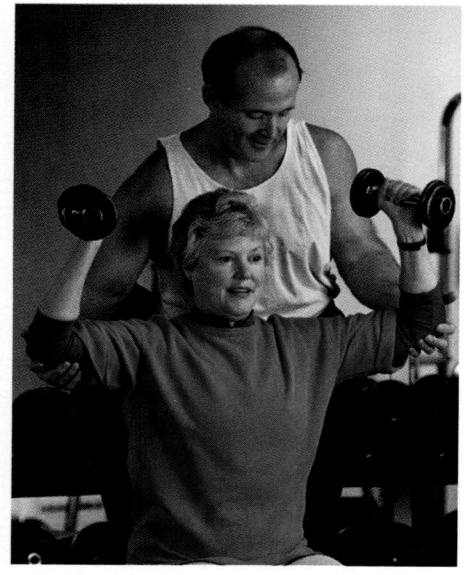

Older people benefit from both aerobic and strength-training (resistance) exercises. Strength-training especially helps reverse some of the decline in daily function associated with the muscle loss typically seen in older adulthood.

Table 15.2 Typical Physiological Changes Experienced by Older Adults and Recommended Diet Lifestyle Responses

Change	Recommended Response
Decrease in appetite and food intake	Monitor weight and strive to eat enough to maintain healthy weight; consider liquid meal replacement products such as Boost and Ensure (liquid and bar form)
Decline in sense of taste and smell	Vary the diet and experiment with herbs and spices
Loss of teeth	Work with a dentist to maximize chewing ability; modify food consistency as necessary; provide energy dense snacks
Decreased sense of thirst	Consume about 8 cups of fluid each day, and watch for evidence of dehydration (e.g., minimal urine output or dark color)
Constipation	Consume 20 to 30 grams of dietary fiber daily, choosing primarily fruits, vegetables, and whole grains; meet fluid needs (see Chapter 4)
Decline in lactase production	Limit milk serving size at each use; consume yogurt or cheese; use reduced-lactose or lactose-free products; seek other calcium sources (see Chapter 9 for ideas)
Iron-deficiency anemia	Include some lean meat and iron-fortified foods in the diet; ask physician to monitor blood iron status
Decline in liver function	Consume alcohol in moderation, if at all; avoid excess vitamin A consumption
Decline in insulin function	Maintain healthy body weight and perform regular physical activity
Decline in kidney function	Modify protein and other nutrients in diet when advised by physician
Decline in immune function	Meet nutrient needs, especially protein, vitamin E, vitamin B-6, and zinc, and perform regular physical activity
Decline in lung function	Don't smoke tobacco products; perform regular physical activity
Decline in vision	Consume fruits, vegetables, and whole grains regularly to gain the potential benefits of carotenoids, as well as vitamins C and E and the mineral zinc (wear sunglasses as well in sunny conditions and don't smoke)
Decrease in lean tissue	Meet nutrient needs (such as protein) and perform regular physical activity, including some resistance (strength-training) activity (see Chapter 11)
Increase in fat stores leading to obesity	Watch overeating; perform regular physical activity (see Chapter 10)
Decrease in cardiovascular function	Keep blood lipids and blood pressure within desirable range, using diet changes and medications when needed (see Chapters 5 and 9); stay physically active; remain in a healthy body weight range (see Chapter 10)
Decrease in bone mass	Meet nutrient needs, especially calcium and vitamin D (regular sun exposure helps meet needs for vitamin D), perform regular physical activity, and women should consider use of approved osteoporosis medications at menopause (see Chapter 9)
Decrease in mental function	Strive for lifelong learning; perform regular physical activity; obtain adequate sleep; follow a healthy dietary pattern

What is seen as the physiological changes associated with aging is the sum of natural processes and lifestyle practices. By adopting practices that minimize a decline in body function in the adult years, we invest in our future health. (The first Rate Your Plate activity outlines one comprehensive approach to healthful aging.)

of certain medications. For example, vitamin K can reduce the activity of oral anticoagulants (see Chapter 8).

■ Depression in Older Adults

Depression occurs in about 20% of nursing home residents. In contrast, it occurs in only 5% to 10% of older adults who reside outside of nursing homes. Depression—combined with isolation and loneliness as family and friends die, move away, or become less mobile—frequently contributes to apathetic eating and weight loss. People living alone do not necessarily make poor food choices, but they often consume less energy, in part by skipping meals. Older men are especially prone to this habit. About one-third of all older people not in nursing homes live alone. Depression can be a downward spiral in which poor appetite produces weakness, which leads to even poorer appetite (Fig. 15.3). In older adults, the resulting poor nutritional state can produce further mental confusion and increased isolation and loneliness.

If depression is left untreated, it is estimated that 15% of the cases may be fatal (suicide). Depression also may be a sign of an underlying illness, which is another

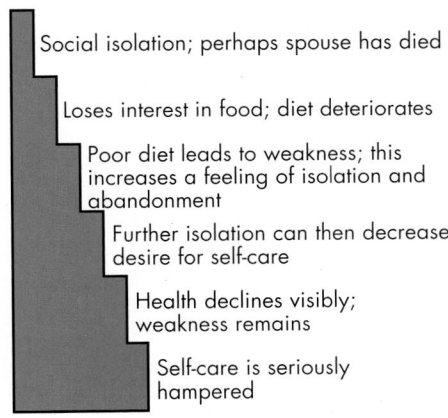

Social isolation; perhaps spouse has died

Loses interest in food; diet deteriorates

Poor diet leads to weakness; this increases a feeling of isolation and abandonment

Further isolation can then decrease desire for self-care

Health declines visibly; weakness remains

Self-care is seriously hampered

Figure 15.3 The decline of health often seen in older adults. This decline needs to be prevented whenever possible.

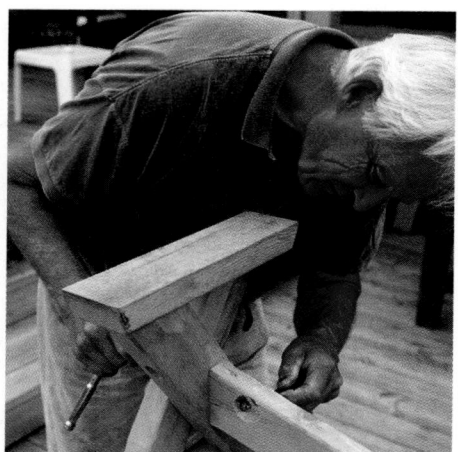

Aging is no reason to withdraw from life. Learning and practicing new skills throughout life contribute to overall health.

*F*ormer president Jimmy Carter recommends that older adults stay connected to life to maximize health. This can include volunteering one's services and helping one's friends in their later years.

Ten Warning Signs of Alzheimer's Disease

1. Recent memory loss that affects job performance
2. Difficulty performing familiar tasks
3. Problems with language
4. Disorientation to time and place
5. Faulty or decreased judgment
6. Problems with abstract thinking
7. Tendency to misplace things
8. Changes in mood or behavior
9. Changes in personality
10. Loss of initiative

reason that early detection is important in older adults. Depression is often treatable, but medication alone will not help those who are experiencing major life changes, such as the death of a spouse. Adequate social support also is essential.

∎ Alcoholism in Older Adults

Alcoholism is a problem in the older population, and about 17% of adults older than age 60 in North America are substance abusers. Many older people experience increased stressors, such as the loss of a spouse, loneliness, depression, or chronic diseases. Approximately two-thirds of these alcohol abusers turn to alcohol much earlier in life and simply continue the habit. About one-third begin the habit later in life, due to a variety of factors—more free time, social events centered around drinking, loneliness, or depression. Some of the symptoms of alcoholism in older persons include trembling hands, sleep problems, memory loss, and unsteady gait; these can be easily overlooked simply because they are similar to symptoms of old age.

Older adults become intoxicated on a smaller amount of alcohol than when younger because they metabolize alcohol more slowly. And even small amounts of alcohol can react negatively with various medications that many older persons take routinely. In addition to having adverse effects on the liver, drinking large amounts of alcohol increases the risk of hemorrhagic stroke and may worsen hypertension in older adults. Since drinking large amounts of alcohol produces adverse effects, people over the age of 65 should limit alcohol consumption to no more than one drink per day. Recall from Chapter 7 that one drink per day is defined as 5 ounces of wine, 12 ounces of beer, or 1.5 ounce shot of 80-proof liquor.

Another Bite

*T*he disease known as Alzheimer's often takes a terrible toll on the mental and eventual physical health of older people. In general terms, Alzheimer's disease is best described as a progressive brain disorder marked by an inability to remember, reason, or understand what is going on. Age is the primary risk factor. Scientists propose causes, including altered cell development and altered brain proteins, as well as high blood pressure, high blood cholesterol, and high blood homocysteine. Three medications are approved for minimizing Alzheimer's symptoms, but they show only limited benefits. Dietary concerns revolve around making sure the person eats enough food to maintain healthy weight and overall nutrient needs and observation of the person's meals to make sure meal habits do not pose a health risk (e.g., holding food in one's mouth or forgetting how to swallow). Warning signs of Alzheimer's disease are listed in the margin. Preventive measures for Alzheimer's disease focus on lifelong learning. Experimental therapies currently in clinical trials, include megadoses of vitamin E (2000 IU), estrogen replacement in women, and use of ibuprofen and related pain medications. To find out more about Alzheimer's disease, you can go to the website for the Alzheimer's Association at www.alz.org, or call (800) 272-3900. You can also call the National Institute on Aging's Alzheimer's Disease Education and Referral Center at (800) 428-4380.

Concept Check

*N*utritional problems common to aging adults relate to both the process of chronic diseases and the normal decrease in organ function that occurs with time. All of these organ systems and functions can decrease as we age: appetite; sense of taste, smell, thirst, hearing, and sight; digestion and absorption; liver, gallbladder, pancreatic, kidney, lung, and heart function; and the immune system. In addition, bone mass and muscle mass gradually decrease, the latter largely because of a deficient diet and inactivity. Appropriate dietary changes and regular physical activity can often help reduce the impact of these results of aging.

■ Nutrient Needs in Middle and Older Adulthood

The latest RDAs and related standards for nutrients and energy include a category for both men and women who are 51 to 70 years of age and more than 70 years of age. Because the lifestyle of an active older person can differ considerably from that of a nursing home resident, establishing nutrient needs during these wide age ranges is problematic.

Do Nutrient Needs Change in Later Life?

Only during the past few years has much research focused on the question of whether nutrient needs change. Because RDAs and related standards apply only to healthy people, many older people—for example, those who have ulcers or are heavy aspirin users—are not covered by these standards. Indeed, it is particularly tricky to develop nutrient standards that are valid for most older people because so many are ill and/or regularly take medication.

A well-planned diet that follows the Food Guide Pyramid can meet all nutrient needs for healthy older people within about 1600 to 1800 kcal, except for probably vitamin D, vitamin B-12, folate, and calcium. It would take at least 3 servings from the milk, yogurt, and cheese group for calcium—a recommendation that most older people would find difficult to meet. Calcium-fortified foods can help when necessary (see Chapter 9 for details) (Fig. 15.4). Meeting the folate and vitamin B-12 standard also is aided by use of fortified foods, such as ready-to-eat breakfast cereals. The use of a balanced multivitamin and mineral supplement is especially helpful for meeting vitamin D needs if the person does not receive regular sun exposure. Any supplement used should be low in or free of iron. Currently, many nutrition experts recommend this practice of taking a daily multivitamin and mineral supplement for older adults. If rich calcium sources are not consumed, the person would also need a calcium supplement, as typical multivitamin and mineral supplements contain little calcium (about 200 milligrams). As noted in Chapter 8, providing more calcium than that would greatly increase the pill size. Finally, use of a vitamin E supplement (200 milligrams; about 400 IU) could be employed.

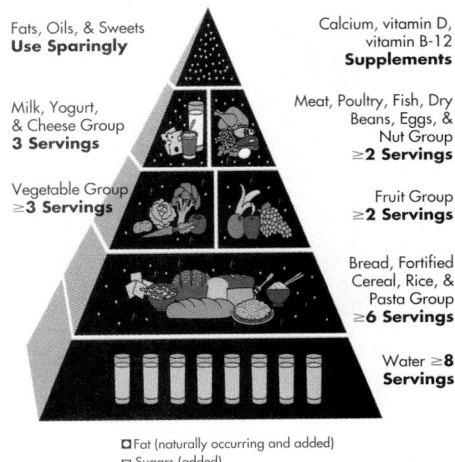

Tufts University's Modified Food Pyramid for 70+ Adults

Fats, Oils, & Sweets **Use Sparingly**

Calcium, vitamin D, vitamin B-12 **Supplements**

Milk, Yogurt, & Cheese Group **3 Servings**

Meat, Poultry, Fish, Dry Beans, Eggs, & Nut Group **≥2 Servings**

Vegetable Group **≥3 Servings**

Fruit Group **≥2 Servings**

Bread, Fortified Cereal, Rice, & Pasta Group **≥6 Servings**

Water **≥8 Servings**

☐ Fat (naturally occurring and added)
☑ Sugars (added)
▨ Fiber (should be present)

These symbols show fat, added sugars, and fiber in foods.

Figure 15.4 Nutrition experts at Tufts University recently suggested a modification of the Food Guide Pyramid to include vitamin D, vitamin B-12, and calcium supplements for adults over 70 years of age. Other changes suggested were at least 3 servings from the milk, yogurt, and cheese group and at least 8 servings of water (or other fluids). The use of a supplement to help meet vitamin D, vitamin B-12, and calcium needs is especially helpful for older people who require such a low energy intake that they are not able to consume enough food to supply these nutrients.

Another Bite

Women after menopause have iron needs that are the same as men, as they no longer lose iron in menstruation. Recall from Chapter 9 that men should not take a supplement containing iron unless they have evidence of iron-deficiency anemia, as they consume enough iron and it can easily accumulate to toxic amounts in the body. This advice now applies to women, as they experience minimal iron loss in the postmenopausal state.

Planning a Diet for People in Their Later Years

To supply energy needs for males age 51 and older, the 1989 RDAs suggest 2300 kcal; for females, the recommendation is 1900 kcal. (These values are based on a 170-pound, 68-inch tall man and a 143-pound, 63-inch tall woman.) Studies show that older men eat closer to 1800 to 2100 kcal, whereas women eat about 1300 to 1600

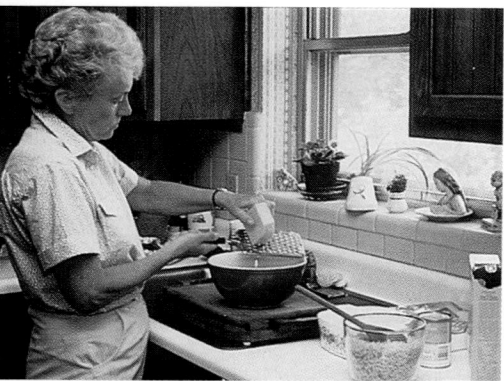

Cooking for just one or two people can be challenging in one's older years. Consuming half of what is prepared and freezing the other half is one tip.

kcal. Furthermore, surveys indicate that many older adults are consuming less protein and calcium than are needed.

A good practice would be to decrease fat and sugar consumption to increase the diet's nutrient density and to make sure dietary fiber intake is adequate. In addition, some protein should come from lean meats to help meet protein needs.

Fluid needs are about 8 cups (about 2 liters) per day. A high-fiber diet especially requires attention to fluid needs. Fiber intake should be slowly increased to about 30 grams per day, with each serving of fiber accompanied by a glass of water (or other fluid).

Singles of all ages face logistical problems with food: Purchasing, preparing, storing, and using food with minimal waste are challenging. Economy packages of meats and vegetables are normally too large to be useful for a single person. Many singles live in small dwellings, some without kitchens and freezers. Creating a diet to accommodate a limited budget and facilities and a single appetite requires special considerations. Following are some practical suggestions for diet planning for singles:

- If one owns a freezer, cook large amounts, divide into portions, and freeze.
- Buy only what one uses; small containers may be expensive, but letting food spoil is also costly.
- Ask the grocer to break open a family-sized package of wrapped meat or fresh vegetables and separate it into smaller units.
- Buy only several pieces of fruit—perhaps a ripe one, a medium-ripe one, and an unripe one—so that the fruit can be eaten over a period of several days.
- Keep a box of dry milk—handy to add nutrients to recipes for baked foods and other foods for which this addition is acceptable.

Nutritional deficiencies and protein-energy undernutrition have been identified among some aging populations, particularly those in nursing homes or long-term care facilities and those who are hospitalized. These nutritional problems increase the risk for many diseases, including bed sores (pressure ulcers), and compromise recovery from illness and surgery. Friends, relatives, and health-care personnel should look for poor nutrient intake in all older people, including those who live in nursing home settings. About 40% of North American adults now age 65 will spend some time in a nursing home. Family members have a unique opportunity to make sure nutrient needs are met by looking for weight maintenance based on regular, healthful meal patterns. If problems arise in instituting a healthful diet, registered dietitians can offer professional and personalized advice.

Surveys show that the majority of older adults like most vegetables, despite misconceptions that they do not like broccoli (because it forms gas) or tomatoes (because they contain too much acid). By the time we reach adulthood, our eating habits reflect regional tastes, social class, ethnic group, and life experiences. There is no generic food list for older people.

Overall, good nutrition benefits older adults in many ways. Meeting nutrient needs delays the onset of some diseases; improves the management of some existing diseases; hastens recovery from many illnesses; can increase mental, physical, and social well-being; and often decreases the need for and length of hospitalization. A variety of strategies can promote healthful eating in later life (Table 15.3). These should focus on presenting nutritious, tasty foods in a pleasant environment.

Obtaining enough food may be difficult for some older persons, especially if they are unable to drive and relatives do not live close enough to help with cooking or shopping. Older persons tend to see asking for help as a symbolic loss of independence. Pride, or fear of being victimized by those they hire, may stand in the way of much needed help. In these cases, friends can be a big help. Special transportation arrangements may also be available through a local transit company or taxi service.

Many eligible older people are missing meals and are poorly nourished simply because they don't know of available programs to help them. Irregular meal patterns

Table 15.3 Guidelines for Healthful Eating in Later Years

- Eat regularly; small, frequent meals may be best. Use nutrient-dense foods as a basis for each menu.
- Find out which convenience foods and labor-saving devices can be of help.
- Try new foods, new seasonings, and new ways of preparing foods. Don't use just convenience foods and canned goods.
- Keep some easy-to-prepare foods on hand for times when you feel tired.
- Have a treat occasionally, perhaps an expensive cut of meat or a favorite fresh fruit.
- Eat in a well-lit or sunny area; serve meals attractively; use foods with different flavors, colors, shapes, textures, and smells.
- Arrange things so that food preparation and clean-up are easier.
- Eat with friends, relatives, or at a senior center when possible.
- Share cooking responsibilities with a neighbor.
- Use community resources for help in shopping and other daily care needs.
- Stay physically active.
- If possible, take a walk before eating to stimulate appetite.
- When necessary, chop, grind, or blend hard-to-chew foods. Softer, protein-rich foods can be substituted for meat when poor dental function limits normal food intake. Prepare soups, stews, cooked whole-grain cereals, and casseroles.
- If your feeding movements are limited, cut the food ahead of time, use utensils with deep sides or handles, and obtain more specialized utensils if needed.

To learn about meal programs for senior citizens in your area, call the Administration on Aging's Elder Care Locator, 800-677-1116. For general information on programs for older persons, visit the following websites: National Institute on Aging, *www.nih.gov/nia/;* American Geriatrics Society, *www.americangeriatrics.org/;* and Administration on Aging, *www.aoa.dhhs.gov/.*

and weight loss, often caused by difficulties in preparing food, are warning signs that undernutrition may be developing. An effort should be made to identify poorly nourished people and inform them of community services.

Community Nutrition Services for Older People

Health-care advice and services for older people can come from clinics, private practitioners, hospitals, and health maintenance organizations. Home health-care agencies, adult day-care programs, adult overnight-care programs, and **hospice units** (for the terminally ill) can supply daily care.

The Nutrition Screening Initiative, a nutrition checklist for health-care workers, family members, and older persons, can be used as a tool to increase health and nutrition awareness and to plan related education of older persons (Fig. 15.5). The Nutrition Screening Initiative incorporates the acronym "DETERMINE" (see margin). Overall, professionals in the just-mentioned organizations should try to identify older people whose health needs require extra attention.

Nutrition programs for those age 60 and over in the United States offer congregate meal programs, which provide lunch at a central location, and home-delivered meals (often known as Meals-on-Wheels if sponsored by the local private or public agencies). About 2.3 million older adults are served each year. Currently about half of the meals use the home-delivered method.

The U.S. federal government sets specific standards for home-delivered meals and for those served in congregate feeding centers. The meals are designed to provide one-third of the nutrient needs. The social aspect often improves appetite and general outlook.

Still, congregate meal programs generally provide one meal a day (some provide more) and usually not every day of the week. The problem with home-delivered

DETERMINE:
- **D**isease
- **E**ating poorly
- **T**ooth loss or mouth pain
- **E**conomic hardship
- **R**educed social contact and interaction
- **M**ultiple medications
- **I**nvoluntary weight loss or gain
- **N**eed for assistance with self care
- **E**lder at an advanced age

hospice units A facility offering care that emphasizes comfort and dignity in death.

Figure 15.5 A nutrition checklist for older adults.
Reprinted with permission by the Nutrition Screening Initiative, a project of the American Academy of Family Physicians, the American Dietetic Association, and the National Council on Aging, Inc., and funded in part by a grant from Ross Products Division, Abbott Laboratories.

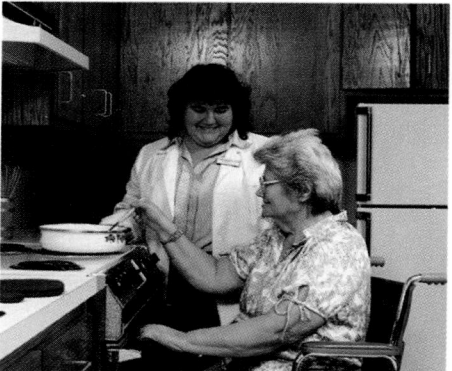

Help is available in most communities to assist older adults in daily tasks. This, in turn, helps older adults meet nutrient needs.

A Nutrition Test for Older Adults

Here's a nutrition check for anyone over age 65. Circle the number of points for each statement that applies. Then compute the total and check it against the nutritional score.

1. The person has a chronic illness or current condition that has changed the kind or amount of food eaten. (2 points)
2. The person eats fewer than two full meals per day. (3 points)
3. The person eats few fruits, vegetables, or milk products. (2 points)
4. The person drinks 3 or more servings of beer, liquor, or wine almost every day. (2 points)
5. The person has tooth or mouth problems that make eating difficult. (2 points)
6. The person does not have enough money for food. (4 points)
7. The person eats alone most of the time. (1 point)
8. The person takes three or more different prescription or over-the-counter drugs each day. (1 point)
9. The person has unintentionally lost or gained 10 pounds within the last 6 months. (2 points)
10. The person cannot always shop, cook, or feed himself or herself. (2 points)

Nutritional score:

0–2: Good. Recheck in 6 months.

3–5: Marginal. A local agency on aging has information about nutrition programs for the elderly. The National Association of Area Agencies on Aging can assist in finding help; call (800) 677-1116. Recheck in 6 months.

6 or more: High risk. A doctor should review this test and suggest how to improve nutritional health.

meals is that the one or two meals delivered may never be eaten, and, if not eaten on delivery and left at room temperature, they may become unsafe to eat later. Thus, these programs can help older adults but probably don't meet all their nutritional needs.

In addition to congregate and home-delivered meals, federal commodity distribution is available in some areas of the United States to low-income older people. Food stamps can benefit older people whose incomes are below the poverty level (see Chapter 17 for details on these programs). Food cooperatives and a variety of clubs and social organizations provide additional aid.

Concept Check

Specific nutrient requirements for older adults are only now being extensively studied. Diet plans should be modified for decreased physical abilities, the presence of drug-nutrient interactions, possible depression, and economic constraints. Particular attention should be paid to the opportunity for sun exposure and intake of the vitamins D, B-6, E, folate, and B-12, as well as the minerals calcium and zinc and dietary fiber. A nutrient-dense diet helps meet these needs. Carefully planned multivitamin and mineral supplement use can also help. In the United States, many nutrition services—such as congregate and home-delivered meals—are available to help aging population obtain a healthful diet.

Scenario Follow-Up

Frances could contact a local government office that offers congregate meal programs at a central location. She could inquire about location and available transportation to the site. This would give her social contact with other older persons, which is probably an important element that is missing in her life. This could help alleviate her loneliness. She could also request Meals-on-Wheels (if available) to provide one hot meal a day. One hot meal a day that is prepared for her may be just what she needs to help stimulate her appetite. She could also have groceries delivered to her home if her budget could withstand the extra cost. Other convenience foods that could be included in her diet include milk, assorted nuts, peanut butter, breakfast cereals, canned chicken or deli meats, yogurt, sliced cheese, cottage cheese, calcium-fortified orange juice, canned or frozen fruits and vegetables, and some fresh fruits and vegetables that do not require preparation, such as prewashed lettuce and bananas. A further possibility is a liquid nutritional supplement, such as a can of Ensure, or a nutrition bar, such as an Ensure bar.

Two other websites for organizations that focus on issues surrounding age are:

www.ilcusa.org
www.aging-institute.org.

Summary

1. Although scientists disagree as to the best diet recommendations for the general public, most agree on some general principles, including those laid out by the Food Guide Pyramid and Dietary Guidelines for Americans. Such authorities recommend that individuals eat a variety of foods; balance the food eaten with physical activity to maintain or improve weight; choose a diet with plenty of grain products, vegetables, and fruits; choose a diet low in saturated fat and cholesterol; choose a diet moderate in sugars; choose a diet moderate in salt; and moderate or avoid alcoholic beverage intake. Regular physical activity is also important. In addition, recommendations to reduce cancer risk emphasize moderation in the use of cured and smoked meats.

2. Although maximum life span hasn't changed, life expectancy has increased dramatically over the past century. For many societies, this means that an increasing proportion of the population is over 65 years of age. As health-care costs rise, the goal of delaying disease becomes even more important for all of us.

3. Aging begins before birth. Cell aging probably results from automatic cellular changes and environmental influences, such as DNA damage. Add to this list damage caused by electron-seeking free-radical compounds, high blood glucose, hormonal changes, and alterations in the immune system as possible causes.

4. Nutritional problems of older adults are related to the presence of chronic diseases and to the normal decreases in organ function that occur with time. These include loss of teeth, lessened sensitivity to taste and smell, changes in gastrointestinal tract function, and deterioration in cardiovascular and bone health. Although disease affects nutritional state, the reverse is also true. Undernutrition adversely affects immune function, allowing for infection.

5. Scientists are only now beginning extensive study of specific nutrient needs for older people. Diet plans should be based on a nutrient-dense approach and individualized for existing health problems, decreased physical abilities, presence of drug-nutrient interactions, possible depression, and economic constraints. Specific nutrients, such as protein, vitamin D, vitamin E, vitamin B-6, folate, vitamin B-12, zinc, and calcium, along with dietary fiber, often deserve special attention in diet planning. A multivitamin and mineral supplement can be used to help meet needs.

6. Health-care workers and family members should use available options for the procurement of food for the elderly, especially for those who are nutritionally compromised. Most communities have congregate or home-delivered meal systems, food stamps, and other provisions for those who qualify.

Study Questions

1. List four of the Dietary Guidelines for Americans and give an example of why each one may be difficult for the elderly to implement. What are some solutions to these barriers?

2. What is the difference between life span and life expectancy? As life expectancy increases, what consequence affects the entire population?

3. Name three hormones that decline with aging and the functions of each.

4. Describe two hypotheses proposed to explain the causes of aging, and note evidence for each in your daily life experiences.

5. List four organ systems that can decline in function in later years, along with a diet/lifestyle response to help cope with the decline.

6. Defend the recommendation for regular physical activity during late adulthood, including some resistance activity (weight training).

7. How might the nutritional needs of older people differ from those of younger people? How are their needs similar? Be specific.

8. What three resources in a community are widely available to aid older adults in maintaining nutritional health?

9. Describe some early warning signs of Alzheimer's disease and note some of the nutritional implications as this disease advances.

10. List four warning signs of undernutrition in older people that are part of the acronym DETERMINE. Briefly justify the inclusion of each.

Further Readings

1. ADA Reports: Position of the American Dietetic Association: Nutrition, aging, and the continuum of care. *Journal of the American Dietetic Association* 100:580, 2000.

   As the baby boomer population grows older, nutrition professionals need to focus more on developing successful interventions that will influence the proper nourishment of older adults, such as initiating nutrition screening of older adults and working with other health professionals to expand services to older persons. Multiple factors that influence nutritional status in older adults include medical problems, medications, housing, the availability of transportation, dental health, current diet modifications, and income.

2. Alzheimer's disease: Glimmers of hope. *Consumer Reports on Health*, p. 1, April 2000.

   Scientists are currently testing at least 50 new drugs in humans for the treatment of Alzheimer's disease. For people who have the disease, important precautions for caretakers are to monitor all medication used, arrange for the treatment of other health problems, reduce clutter and chaos, having calming conversations, and take walks together.

3. Anti-aging therapies. *Mayo Clinic Health Letter* 17(5):1, 1999.

   Despite tempting claims, there is no product proven to prevent or reverse aging. This includes DHEA and melatonin. Anyone considering a so-called anti-aging product should speak with a physician first. The physician can help one decide whether the potential benefits of a product outweigh any risks.

4. Barrett S, Herbert V: Alternative nutrition therapies. In Shils ME and others (eds.): *Modern nutrition in health and disease.* 9th ed. Baltimore MD: Williams & Wilkins, 1999.

   When someone feels better after using a product or procedure, it is natural to credit whatever was done. This can be misleading, however, because most ailments resolve spontaneously, and even those that persist can have symptoms that wax and wane. In addition, taking action for a problem often temporarily relieves symptoms via the placebo effect. People unaware of these facts often give undeserved credit to "alternative" methods of medical treatment.

5. Christensen D: Making sense of centenarians. *Science News* 159:156, 2001.

   The most important factors with regard to longevity can be found in a person's lifestyle: what foods they eat, how much they exercise, what social networks they have, and how well they handle stress. No more than 30% of the variation in lifespan between those individuals who live 100 years or more and those that do not is due to genetic differences.

6. Christmas C, Andersen RA: Exercise and older patients: Guidelines for the clinician. *Journal of the American Geriatric Society* 48:321, 2000.

   The goal for older persons is to exercise for 30 minutes with moderate intensity more days than not. Stretching and warm-up activities are particularly important in this age group. Including strength training on a regular basis further contributes to physical health.

7. Live longer, feel younger. *Consumer Reports on Health*, p. 1, March 1999.

   It is never too late to improve physical or mental health, even if one is already ailing, by adopting healthy habits. Exercise is particularly useful, since it can ward off sickness, strengthen the body, sharpen the mind, and lift the spirits.

8. Mar C, Bent S: An evidence-based review of the 10 most commonly used herbs. *Western Journal of Medicine* 171:168, 1999.

   The most popular herbal supplements include echinacea, St. John's Wort, ginkgo biloba, garlic, saw palmetto, ginseng, and valerian. People should be advised to avoid using a wide variety of herbs at one time because herb-herb interactions are poorly understood. The starting dose for each herb should be the lowest in which desired effects occur. Long-term use of herbal products should be discouraged because long-term effects are unknown.

9. McBean LD and others: Healthy eating in later years. *Nutrition Today* 36 (4): 192, 2001.

   Older adults are a diverse, heterogeneous group with unique nutritional needs and health risks. Practical dietary and lifestyle advice tailored to this growing segment of the population can help them age successfully and ensure their quality of life. Healthful food choices, including high-quality, nutrient-dense foods, adequate hydration, and regular physical activity, are critical components of successful aging.

10. Miller KE and others: The geriatric patient: A systematic approach to maintaining health. *American Family Physician* 61:1089, 2000.

    A nutritional health screening for older persons should consider whether an illness or a condition has made the person change that type or amount of food consumed. Other problems include eating fewer than two meals a day, consuming few fruits, vegetables, or milk products; consuming three or more alcoholic drinks a day; experiencing tooth loss; not having enough income to buy the food needed; eating alone most of the time; taking three or more different prescription drugs daily; losing or gaining 10 pounds in the past six months without particularly trying to do so; and not always being physically able to shop and feed oneself.

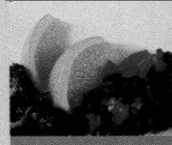

I. Am I Aging Healthfully?

Take Control of Your Aging by Dr. William B. Malarkey (Wooster Book Co., Wooster OH, 1999) includes a plan that incorporates various diet and lifestyle factors that are associated with successful aging. Indicate the degree to which you are following such a plan (or alternatively fill this out with a parent or another older relative in mind).

Physical: Do you eat a well-balanced diet, exercise on a regular basis, remain free of illness, abstain from smoking, refrain from drinking alcohol excessively, and experience refreshing sleep?

_____

_____

_____

Intellectual: Are you analytical, do you read regularly, do you learn new things each day, do you engage your mental ability at work (or at school), and do you often reflect on your life?

_____

_____

_____

Emotional: Are you at peace, do you like who you are, are you optimistic, and do you laugh and relax regularly?

_____

_____

_____

Relational: Are you a good listener, do you feel supported by friends, do you attend social functions, do you talk with family members often, and do you feel close to coworkers (or fellow students)?

_____

_____

_____

Spiritual: Do you appreciate nature, give to or serve others, meditate or seek religious worship, and feel life has meaning?

_____

_____

_____

The more of these factors that you include in your life, the more well rounded is your plan for maintaining overall health. Any one of the five areas in which you are not achieving success should show you characteristics to work on in the future.

continued

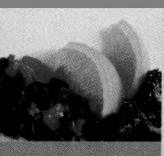

II. Helping Older Adults Eat Better

During their lifetimes, most people usually eat meals with families or loved ones. As people reach their older ages, many of them are faced with living and eating alone. In a study of the diets of 4400 older adults in the United States, one man in every five living alone and over age 55 ate poorly. One of four women between the ages of 55 and 64 years followed a low-quality diet. These poor diets can contribute to deteriorating mental and physical health. Consider the following example of the living situation of an older adult.

Neal, a 70-year-old man, lives alone in a home in a local suburban area. His wife died 1 year ago. He doesn't have many friends; his wife was his primary confidante. His neighbors across the street and next door are friendly, and Neal used to help them with yard projects in his spare time. Neal's health has been good, but he has had trouble with his teeth recently. His diet has been poor, and in the past 3 months his physical and mental vigor have deteriorated. He has been slowly lapsing into a depression and, so, keeps the shades drawn and rarely leaves his house. Neal keeps very little food in the house because his wife did most of the cooking and shopping and he just isn't that interested in food.

If you were one of Neal's relatives and learned of Neal's situation, what six things could you do or suggest to help improve his nutritional status and mental outlook? Look back into the chapter to get some ideas.

1. _____

2. _____

3. _____

4. _____

5. _____

6. _____

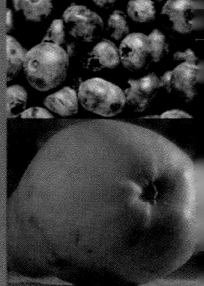

Complementary and Alternative Medicine Practices

Consumer interest in complementary and alternative medicine (CAM) (also called complementary care and integrative medicine) is growing; about 34% of people recently surveyed in the United States used alternative medical practices in the past year, and most of the associated expenses for these often expensive products and services (about $4 billion per year) were paid out-of-pocket. Interest in herbal supplements, however, is currently waning, likely because many people have tried them but have not experienced enough benefit to justify the cost. The majority of the consumers did not discuss the practice with their primary care physician.

Given the phenomenal advances in medicine over the past decades, what brings people in such numbers and with such affinity to embrace alternative therapies? It may be that many people assume that natural substances are gentler forms of therapy, lacking the harsher side effects of some pharmacological medicines. People may also seek complementary medicine because standard medical treatments didn't work, standard medical treatments had too many adverse effects, they simply wanted to actively participate in treatment, or they wanted to combat poor doctor communication. The majority of alternative medicine consumers have illnesses for which conventional medicine cannot offer a cure, such as arthritis, terminal stages of AIDS, and stress-related conditions. These people will almost certainly benefit from the reassurance, hope, and relief that comes with being in a healing situation.

In many instances, self-prescription or healing rituals involve the participants' optimism, commitment, attention, and high expectations for improvement. The mind is a powerful component of a treatment situation, which is proven in many trials as a placebo effect in which a person takes a "sugar pill" but believes that he or she is being treated with a real medication and subsequently feels and reacts better. It is likely that most alternative or natural treatments of the past probably have no intrinsic therapeutic value beyond the benefit of the placebo effect. And, besides the powerful placebo effect, there are many possible reasons that a folk remedy works, such as the natural ups and downs of symptoms, the remission of disease, the possibility that the remedy contains the effective dose of a pharmaceutical medicine or is adulterated with medicines not listed on the label, and the denial of symptoms or misrepresentation of effectiveness by people who believe the remedy is effective.

In truth, little scientific evidence is available for physicians and health-care professionals to decipher the positive and negative aspects of natural therapies. Indeed, Western medicine is based on accurate scientific knowledge, which serves as a protective device to prevent harm. On the other hand, alternative therapies often involve **folk medicine** and weak scientific evidence (due to lack of large research trials). Still, health professionals should be aware of the scientific knowledge that does or does not exist on some alternative therapies, since clients will likely express interest in these therapies. Many clients wish physicians would take the time to explain (in simple terms) the nature of the problem; to acknowledge nutritional influences on health, rather than just recommend drugs and surgery as the only approaches for treating illness; to answer questions intelligently about dietary supplements; to be sensitive to mind-body interactions; and to respect questions about alternative practices.

To date, few complementary and alternative therapies have been subjected to scientific scrutiny, and many of the practices are based on presumptions that are unconvincing at best, yet some of the therapies (e.g., acupuncture and chiropractic therapies) show promise in the treatment of certain conditions. The National Institutes of Health has created the following seven categories of complementary and alternative therapies:

1. Mind-body interventions: the use of the mind, such as hypnosis, meditation, biofeedback, and yoga, to enhance health. Integrative medicine teaches health-care providers to focus on

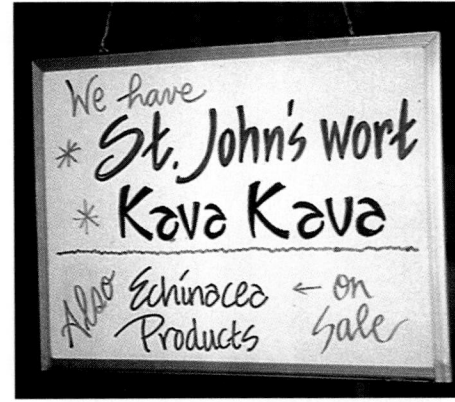

Some herbal products are effective for treating specific medical problems. Follow label instructions carefully, if used. Note potential side effects listed, as well as who should not use the product.

folk medicine A medical treatment based on the beliefs, traditions, or customs of a particular society or ethnic/cultural group.

continued

chelation The use of medicinal compounds, such as ethylenediaminetetraacetic acid (EDTA), to bind metals and other constituents in the blood.

aromatherapy The use of the vapors of essential oils extracted from flowers, leaves, stalks, fruits, and roots for therapeutic purposes.

*A*nother concern regarding use of herbal and related supplements is the actual content of the active ingredient(s) in the product. Recently, many of these products have been tested by independent laboratories and found to contain either less than or more than the stated label content (see the website consumerlabs.com for details).

the subtle yet complex interactions of mind, body, spirit, community, and environment. *Ayurveda* is a natural healing process from India, which includes eating healthful, fresh foods and taking medicinal herbs suited to one's particular mind-body type.

2. Bioelectrical magnetic therapies: the use of electrical currents or magnetic fields to promote healing, such as the use of electrical currents to help heal broken bones

3. Alternative systems of medical practice: the use of medicine from another culture, such as Native American medicine and Chinese medicine (for example, acupuncture). Acupuncture likely works by stimulating sensory nerves leading to the spinal cord. This leads to a reduction in pain. Acupuncture also may be effective for treating people who experience nausea and vomiting following surgery or chemotherapy, nausea that accompanies pregnancy, pain experienced after certain dental procedures, and recovery from a drug addiction. Typically, a course of treatments should end after 10 sessions if it is not showing benefit. FDA recently announced that acupuncture is no longer considered experimental. However, a qualified, certified practitioner must use sterile needles intended for single use and made from nonreactive materials.

4. Manual healing methods: the use of the hands to promote healing, such as chiropractic or osteopathic manipulation or massage. FDA recognizes the effectiveness of chiropractic care for the treatment of acute low back pain.

5. Pharmacologic and biologic treatments: the use of various substances to treat specific medical problems. This includes **chelation** therapy.

6. Herbal medicine: the use of plants as medicines to treat or prevent disease. By definition, an herb is any plant or part of a plant that is used primarily for medicinal purposes. This includes **aromatherapy.** Dosage forms include capsules, tablets, extracts or tinctures, powders, dried herbs, teas, creams, and ointments. In March 1999, FDA established regulations that require the labels of such supplements to include name, quantity, dosage per day, and ingredient amounts.

7. Diet and nutrition: the use of foods, vitamins, and minerals to prevent illness and treat disease

The following are a few practical tips on using complementary and alternative medicine practices:

- We often tend to believe what we hear or what close acquaintances tell us. This well-meaning advice does not substitute for scientific verification of safety and effectiveness when it comes to health practices.
- The U.S. federal government provides little regulation regarding nutrient supplements or remedies. "Let the buyer beware" is prudent advice to follow when using these products. Knowledgeable, professional guidance is needed.
- Fraudulent claims for diet- and health-related remedies have always been a part of our culture. It is important to scrutinize carefully the credentials and motives of anyone providing medical or health advice. Phony credentials and bogus practitioners are widespread.
- If it sounds too good to be true, it probably is. The medical community gains nothing by holding back effective cures from the public, despite what the alternative practitioners may say.

Vitamin and Herbal Supplements Are Regulated Loosely by FDA

Unless FDA has evidence that a supplement is inherently dangerous or marked with illegal claims, FDA will not regulate it closely. FDA is, in fact, prevented from doing so by the Proxmire Amendment to the 1938 Food, Drug, and Cosmetic Act, along with follow-up legislation—the Dietary Supplement Health and Education Act (DSHEA), which was passed in 1994 (and reviewed in Chapter 1). FDA requires a standardized Supplement Facts label on herbs and other related supplements. These labels must list the ingredients, the percent of Daily Value if applicable, common name of the plant, the part of the plant that was used, how much is present in each pill, and a suggested daily dose (Fig. 15.6). It is permissible for the labels on such products to claim a benefit related to a classic nutrient-deficiency disease, describe how a nutrient affects human body structure or function, and claim that general well-being results from consumption of the ingredient(s).

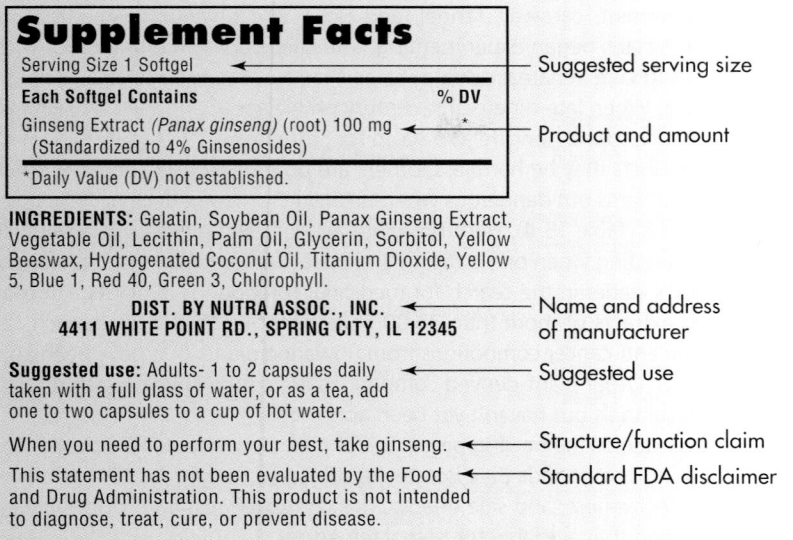

Supplement Facts

Serving Size 1 Softgel ← — Suggested serving size

Each Softgel Contains	% DV
Ginseng Extract *(Panax ginseng)* (root) 100 mg ← * — Product and amount	
(Standardized to 4% Ginsenosides)	

*Daily Value (DV) not established.

INGREDIENTS: Gelatin, Soybean Oil, Panax Ginseng Extract, Vegetable Oil, Lecithin, Palm Oil, Glycerin, Sorbitol, Yellow Beeswax, Hydrogenated Coconut Oil, Titanium Dioxide, Yellow 5, Blue 1, Red 40, Green 3, Chlorophyll.

DIST. BY NUTRA ASSOC., INC. ← — Name and address
4411 WHITE POINT RD., SPRING CITY, IL 12345 — of manufacturer

Suggested use: Adults- 1 to 2 capsules daily ← — Suggested use
taken with a full glass of water, or as a tea, add
one to two capsules to a cup of hot water.

When you need to perform your best, take ginseng. ← — Structure/function claim

This statement has not been evaluated by the Food ← — Standard FDA disclaimer
and Drug Administration. This product is not intended
to diagnose, treat, cure, or prevent disease.

Figure 15.6 Supplement Facts label on an herbal product. Any nutrients or other food constituents would also be listed if contained in the product.

Dietary Supplement Claims

Although structure/function claims do not have to be approved by FDA, they must have evidence that their marketing statements are truthful and not misleading. In addition, the labels of products bearing such claims must prominently display in boldface type the following disclaimer: **"This statement has not been evaluated by the Food and Drug Administration. This product is not intended to diagnose, treat, cure, or prevent any disease."** Despite this statement, consumers may mistakenly assume FDA has carefully evaluated the products.

Practice the following when evaluating dietary supplement claims:

1. Examine product labels carefully. A product is not likely to do something that is not specifically claimed on its label or package insert (legally part of the label). Be skeptical of any product promotion not clearly stated on the label, such as:
   - Testimonials about personal experience
   - Dramatic results (rarely true)
   - Lack of evidence from supporting studies made by other scientists
   - Statements that particular foods can cure specific diseases or that many harmful foods should be eliminated from the diet
   - Claims that only natural foods should be eaten because modern processing methods strip the nutritional value from foods
   - Warnings that stress greatly increases the need for nutrients
2. Examine the background and scientific credentials of the individual, organizations, or publication making the nutritional claim. Usually, a reputable author is one whose educational background or present affiliation is with a nationally recognized university or medical center that offers programs or courses in the field of nutrition, medicine, or another certified health profession.
3. Note the size and duration of any study cited in support of a nutrition claim. The larger it is and the longer it went on, the more dependable its findings. Check out the group studied; a study of men or women in Sweden may be less relevant than one of men or women of southern European, African, or Hispanic descent, because it involves more than one ethnicity. Keep in mind that "contributes to," "is linked to," or "is associated with" does not mean "causes." In addition, one study may not prove anything; many studies are needed to verify or strengthen the association or finding.

Critical Thinking

Jamila went to her local pharmacy yesterday to look for a product to help her stay awake while studying. On the shelves she found a dietary supplement claiming to be a Chinese herbal remedy for sleepiness and fatigue. She thought that since a pharmacy carried the product, it should be safe, and work as indicated on the label.

Is she correct in these assumptions? Are there specific risks associated with taking such herbal remedies?

A Closer Look at Herbal Therapy

Throughout history, healers have gone to the garden, forest, and sea to seek herbal remedies. Largely by trial and error, these healers have found the leaves and seeds of various herbs, roots, and barks to possess medicinal properties. As early as the second century B.C., the Egyptians use

continued

*I*nformation in this chapter primarily refers to statistics and laws that apply to the United States. Other people in North America face the same general food-safety risks described in the chapter, but the actual laws and agencies that oversee food safety differ. These laws and agencies (such as the Canadian Food Inspection Agency) are discussed in Appendix B.

toxins Poisonous compounds produced by an organism that can cause disease.

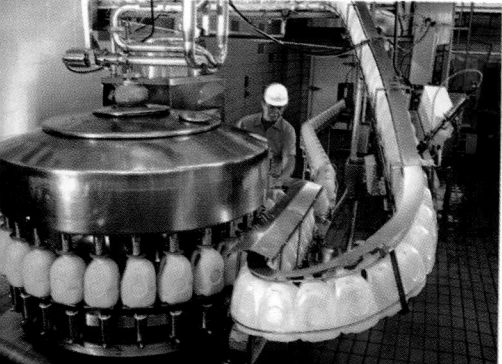

Food contaminated in a central plant can go on to produce illness in people in surrounding states or even across the nation. In the case of juices, it is important that they are pasteurized to reduce risk of foodborne illness.

- Infants and children
- Older adults
- Those with liver disease, diabetes, or HIV infection (and AIDS)
- Cancer patients
- Pregnant women
- People taking immunosuppresant agents

As you can see, foodborne illness has the greatest effect on the most vulnerable people in terms of health status (estimated to be about 30 million people in the United States alone). Some of these bouts of foodborne illness coupled with the ongoing health conditions, are lengthy and lead to food allergies, seizures, blood poisoning (from **toxins** or microbes in the bloodstream), or other illnesses.

Because foodborne illness often results from the unsafe handling of food at home, we each bear some responsibility for preventing foodborne illness. Usually, you can't tell by taste, smell, or sight that a particular food contains harmful microorganisms, so you might not even be aware that food has caused your distress. In fact, your last case of diarrhea may have been caused by something you ate (Table 16.1).

■ Why Is Foodborne Illness So Common?

The risk of contracting foodborne illness is high because—in addition to problems from consumers' mishandling of food—recent trends have added new causes. First, there is greater consumer interest in eating foods of animal origin raw or undercooked. In addition, more people receive medication that suppresses their ability to combat foodborne infectious agents. Another factor is the continuing increase in the number of older adults in the population.

Furthermore, the food industry tries whenever possible to increase the shelf life of food products; however, a longer shelf life at room temperature allows more time for bacteria in foods to multiply. Some bacteria grow even at refrigeration temperatures. Partially cooked—and some fully cooked—products pose a particular risk because refrigerated storage may only slow, not prevent, bacterial growth.

The risk of illness from foodborne microorganisms increases as more of our foods are prepared in centralized kitchens outside the home. Supermarkets have become major food processors over the past decade and now offer a variety of prepared foods from specialty meat shops, salad bars, and bakeries. With the increasing number of two-income families, more people are looking for convenient, easy-to-prepare, nutritious foods. Supermarkets offer entrées that can be served immediately or reheated. The foods are usually prepared in central kitchens or processing plants and shipped to individual stores. If a food product is contaminated in the central kitchen or processing plant, patrons of stores over a wide area can suffer foodborne illness.

The centralization of food production by the food-processing industry also adds to the risk of foodborne illness. For example, a malfunction in an ice cream plant in Minnesota in 1994 resulted in 224,000 suspected cases of *Salmonella* bacterial infections, linked to use of contaminated ice cream mix. In 1987, lettuce shredded in a Texas plant and then placed in large plastic bags was the cause of the largest *Shigella* bacterial outbreak ever reported in the United States. At least 347 people became ill. The nutrients released when the lettuce was shredded, coupled with the moist environment provided by the plastic bags, allowed growth and reproduction of the organism.

A survey showed that only 13% of restaurants in the United States implement the voluntary FDA Food Code for cooking temperatures for meat, eggs, fish, and poultry. It is no surprise, then, that in 1993 at least 4 people died and 700 became ill in Washington and surrounding western states after eating at a chain of quick-service restaurants. The source of the problem was undercooked hamburger contaminated with the bacterium *E. coli* 0157:H7. Overall, the growth of large-scale food production and distribution technologies has introduced new and different foodborne risks.

Still another cause of increased foodborne illness in North America is greater consumption of ready-to-eat foods imported from foreign countries. In the past, food

Table 16.1 Some Examples of Cases of Foodborne Illness

Bacteria

- A previously healthy 5-month-old girl suddenly died at home from contact with a pet iguana infected with *Salmonella*. Unpasteurized juice products were recalled after 57 cases of *Salmonella* illness were reported in California and Colorado. Eight people became ill from *Salmonella* after consuming tiramisu, a dessert that contains raw eggs.
- Six persons were reported ill from a *Shigella* infection after eating chopped, uncooked parsley that was served on chicken sandwiches and in coleslaw. A cruise ship had to return to port when more than 600 people developed shigellosis and one person died.
- The first documented foodborne illness caused by *Listeria* organisms in North America occurred in commercially prepared coleslaw. Later, incidents that involved 48 deaths were associated with soft, Mexican-style cheeses. A listeriosis outbreak associated with undercooked hot dogs and cold cuts resulted in more than 82 illnesses and 17 deaths in 19 states. Recently 14.5 million pounds of ready-to-eat meat and poultry products were recalled because of possible *Listeria* contamination.
- The first community outbreak in the United States of *E. coli* 0111:H8 sickened 58 teenagers at a cheerleading camp in Texas. Suspected sources of infection included the camp salad bar and a communal water barrel. One of the largest *E. coli* 0157:H7 outbreaks on record infected more than 1000 people in upstate New York at a county fair. The bacterium was found in infected well water. It killed a 79-year-old man and a 4-year-old girl, and it required 10 other children to undergo kidney dialysis. Six adults and a 2-year-old child were killed after an *E. coli* outbreak from contaminated drinking water in Canada. The bacteria entered the water supply from animal manure after flooding from a heavy storm. In northeastern Oklahoma, five children were infected with *E. coli* after consuming unpasterized apple cider. Recently 25 million pounds of hamburger had to be recalled because of potential *E. coli* 0157:H7 contamination.
- A man in Arkansas developed botulism after eating stew that was cooked and then kept at room temperature for 3 days. He spent 49 days in the hospital—42 of them on mechanical ventilation. Another recent case involved a man who ate hard-boiled eggs that were left in a pickling solution at room temperature for 7 days.
- Since 1992, 17 people in Florida have died of *Vibrio vulnificus* infections after eating raw oysters.
- A teenage boy and his father experienced abdominal pain, vomiting, and diarrhea within 30 minutes of eating 4-day-old homemade pesto. The pesto had been reheated and left out a number of times during the 4-day period. It was apparently contaminated with *Bacillus cereus*. As a result, the boy died of liver failure.

Viruses

- An estimated 6 million oysters from Louisiana were bathed with the *Norwalk virus* after ships with ill crew members dumped their sewage overboard. By the time the outbreak was recognized, an estimated 20,000 to 30,000 people had become ill. Another outbreak of the virus was attributed to an infected bakery worker, who stirred a vat full of buttercream frosting with his bare hand and arm. In Florida, 83 fraternity members caught the virus from the fraternity house ice machine. During the Gulf War, the Norwalk virus was one of the most common causes of gastroenteritis among U.S. troops.

Parasites

- A group attending a dinner banquet developed diarrhea after 3 to 9 days of eating green onions, which was the likely cause of the outbreak. Eight of 10 stool specimens obtained from the group with foodborne illness were positive for *Cryptosporidium*. Food workers at the restaurant reported they did not consistently wash green onions before using them to prepare food or serving them to patrons.
- Guatemalan raspberries have been associated with approximately 1000 cases of *Cyclospora* in the United States and Canada. Authorities speculate that contaminated water caused the outbreak. The United States has banned this source of the fruit until further precautions can be taken.

Risks from Seafood

- Four adults became ill with scrombroid fish poisoning after eating tuna-spinach salad at a restaurant in Pennsylvania.
- An outbreak of Ciguatera fish poisoning involved 17 crew members of a cargo ship that caught, cooked, and ate a barracuda in the Bahamas. All 17 men became ill with nausea, vomiting, abdominal cramps, and diarrhea within hours of eating the fish. Within 2 days, all of the men suffered from muscle pain and weakness, dizziness, and numb or itchy feet, hands, and mouth.

imports were mostly raw products processed here under strict sanitation standards. Now, however, we import more processed foods—such as cheese from France and seafood from Asia—some of which are contaminated. U.S. authorities are currently reexamining inspection procedures for these imports.

The use of antibiotics in animal feeds is increasing the severity of cases of foodborne illness. This use encourages bacteria to develop resistant strains, those that can grow even if exposed to typical antibiotic medicines. This issue currently is receiving considerable attention.

Finally, more cases of foodborne disease are reported now because scientists are more aware of the roles of various players in the process. In addition, physicians are more likely to suspect foodborne contaminants as a cause of illness. Every decade the list of microorganisms suspected of causing foodborne illness lengthens (Table 16.2). Furthermore, we now know that food, besides serving as a good growth medium for some microorganisms, simply transmits many others as well. Seafood is receiving greater scrutiny and surveillance by FDA as a cause of foodborne illness. In addition,

When traveling to developing countries, it is recommended that you "boil it, peel it, or don't eat it." Ironically, up to 70% of our fruits and vegetables during certain seasons comes from these countries. In other words, you do not have to travel to acquire traveler's diarrhea. In response, we should carefully inspect and wash produce, as we would in a foreign country.

A seafood hot line is also available through the American Seafood Institute. For free information on the purchase, preparation, and nutritional value of seafood products, call 1-800-328-3474 between 9 A.M. and 5 P.M. Eastern time on weekdays.

irradiation A process in which radiation energy is applied to foods, creating compounds (free radicals) within the food that destroy cell membranes, break down DNA, link proteins together, limit enzyme activity, and alter a variety of other proteins and cell functions that can lead to food spoilage. This process does not make the food radioactive.

aseptic processing A method by which food and container are simultaneously sterilized; it allows manufacturers to produce boxes of milk that can be stored at room temperature.

This is the Radura, the international label denoting prior irradiation of the food product.

FDA is conducting a $500,000 campaign to educate U.S. consumers about the risks of eating raw oysters. For more information about these risks, contact FDA's Seafood Hotline at 1-800-FDA-4010.

Food Preservation—Past, Present, and Future

For centuries, salt, sugar, smoke, fermentation, and drying have been used to preserve food. Ancient Romans used sulfites to disinfect wine containers and preserve wine. In the age of exploration, European adventurers traveling to the New World preserved their meat by salting it. Most preserving methods work on the principle of decreasing water content. Bacteria need abundant stores of water to grow; yeasts and molds can grow with less water, but some is still necessary. Adding sugar or salt decreases water available to these microbes by binding to it. The process of drying drives off free water.

Decreasing the water content of some high-moisture foods, however, causes them to lose essential characteristics. To preserve such foods—cucumber pickles, sauerkraut, milk (yogurt), and wine—fermentation has been a traditional alternative. Selected bacteria are used to ferment or pickle foods. The fermenting bacteria make acids and alcohol, which minimize the growth of other microorganisms.

Today we can add pasteurization, sterilization, refrigeration, freezing, **irradiation**, canning, and chemical preservatives to the list of food preservation techniques. An additional method of food preservation—**aseptic processing**—simultaneously sterilizes the food and package separately before the food enters the package. Liquid foods, such as fruit juices, are especially easy to process in this manner. With aseptic packaging, boxes of sterile milk and juices can remain on supermarket shelves, free of microbial growth, for many years.

Food irradiation is also a method used to treat food. It uses minimal doses of radiation in order to control pathogens such as *E. coli* 0157:H7 and *Salmonella*. Even though FDA has permitted irradiation of certain food products for more than a decade, the history of the technology goes back nearly a century, including scientific research, evaluation, and testing. The radiation used does not make the food radioactive. The rays essentially pass through the food, and no radioactive residues are left behind. However, the energy is strong enough to break chemical bonds, destroy cell walls and cell membranes, break down DNA, and link proteins together. Irradiation thereby controls growth of insects, bacteria, fungi, and parasites in foods.

FDA recently approved the use of irradiation for raw red meat to reduce risk of *E. coli* and other infectious microorganisms. Other additions to the approved list are shell eggs and seeds. Prior to this, the only animal products so treated were pork and chicken. Irradiation also extends the shelf life of spices, dry vegetable seasonings, meats in general, and fresh fruits and vegetables. Due to recent *Listeria* bacteria outbreaks, manufacturers are petitioning the U.S. government for permission to irradiate processed meats, such as hot dogs.

Irradiated food, except for dried seasonings, must be labeled with the international symbol, the Radura, and a statement that the product has been treated by irradiation. Foods treated this way are safe in the opinion of FDA and many other health authorities, including the American Academy of Pediatrics. Although the demand for irradiated foods has yet to get off the ground in the United States, other countries, including Japan, France, Italy, and Mexico, all use food irradiation technology widely. Certain consumer groups continually try to block its use in the United States, claiming that irradiation diminishes the nutritional value of food and that it can lead to the formation of harmful compounds. Similar claims were once made about pasteurization. Many speculate that consumers will eventually accept the process, just as they did with pasteurization during the late nineteenth century. Keep in mind also that, even when foods, especially meats, have been irradiated, it is still important to follow basic food-safety procedures, as later contamination in food preparation is possible.

Foodborne Illness: When Undesirable Microorganisms Alter Foods

Most (about 75%) of the verifiable cases of foodborne illness are caused by specific toxin-producing bacteria, viruses, and other microbes. Bacteria specifically cause health problems either directly by invading the intestinal wall and producing an *infection* via a toxin contained in the organism, or indirectly by producing a toxin that is secreted into the food, which later harms us (called an *intoxication*). The main way to distinguish an infectious route from an intoxication is time: If symptoms appear in 4 hours or less, it is an intoxication.

Many types of bacteria cause foodborne illness, such as *Bacillus, Campylobacter, Clostridium, Escherichia, Listeria, Vibrio, Yersinia, Salmonella,* and *Staphylococcus,* (review Table 16.2). Because each teaspoon of soil contains about 2 billion bacteria, we are constantly at risk for foodborne illness. Luckily, only a small number of all bacteria actually pose a threat. In addition, experts speculate that about 80% of cases of foodborne illness go undiagnosed because they result from viral causes, such as the Norwalk virus, and there is no easy way to test for these pathogens. A website coordinating the U.S. efforts on food safety is www.foodsafety.gov. Another useful website is www.ama-assn.org/foodborne.

■ General Rules for Preventing Foodborne Illness

You can greatly reduce the risk of foodborne illness by following some very important rules. It's a long list, because many risky habits need to be addressed.

Purchasing Food

- When shopping, select frozen foods and perishable foods last, such as meat, poultry, or fish. Always have these products put in separate plastic bags, so that drippings don't contaminate other foods in the shopping cart. Don't let groceries sit in a warm car; this allows bacteria to grow. Get the perishable foods home and promptly refrigerate or freeze.
- Don't buy or use food from damaged containers that leak, bulge, or are severely dented or buy or use food from jars that are cracked or have loose or bulging lids. Don't taste or use food that has a foul odor or spurts liquid when the can is opened; the deadly *Clostridium botulinum* toxin may be present.
- Purchase only pasteurized milk and cheese (check the label). This is especially important for pregnant women because highly toxic bacteria and viruses that can harm the fetus thrive in unpasteurized milk.
- Purchase only the amount of produce needed for a week's time. The longer you keep fruits and vegetables, the more time is available for bacteria to grow.
- When purchasing precut produce, avoid those that look slimy, brownish, or dry; these are signs of improper holding temperatures.

Preparing Food

- Thoroughly wash hands with hot, soapy water before and after handling food. This practice is especially important when handling raw meat, fish, poultry, and eggs, after using the bathroom, after playing with pets, or after changing diapers.
- Make sure counters, cutting boards, dishes, and other equipment are thoroughly cleaned and rinsed before use. Be especially careful to use hot, soapy water to wash surfaces and equipment that have come in contact with raw meat, fish, poultry, and eggs as soon as possible to remove *Salmonella* bacteria that may be present.
- If possible, cut foods to be eaten raw on a clean cutting board reserved for that purpose. Then clean this cutting board using hot, soapy water. If the same board must be used for both meat and other foods, cut any potentially contaminated items, such as meat, last. After cutting the meat, wash the cutting board thoroughly.

The World Health Organization's Golden Rules for Safe Food Preparation

1. Choose foods processed for safety.
2. Cook food thoroughly.
3. Eat cooked foods immediately.
4. Store cooked foods carefully.
5. Reheat cooked foods thoroughly.
6. Avoid contact between raw and cooked foods.
7. Wash hands repeatedly.
8. Keep all kitchen surfaces meticulously clean.
9. Protect foods from insects, rodents, and other animals.
10. Use pure water.

The USDA recently simplified these rules into four actions as a part of their Fight BAC!

Program (check out www.fightbac.org)

1. Clean. Wash hands and surfaces often.
2. Separate. Don't cross-contaminate.
3. Cook. Cook to proper temperatures.
4. Chill. Refrigerate promptly.

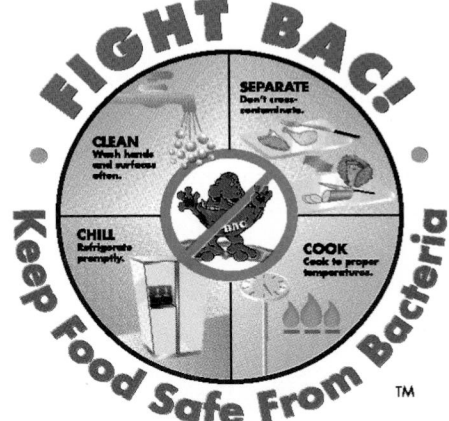

Food safety logo of USDA.

A goal of Healthy People 2010 *is to reduce the number of cases of* foodborne illness from Campylobacter, E. coli, Listeria, *and* Salmonella *by 50%.*

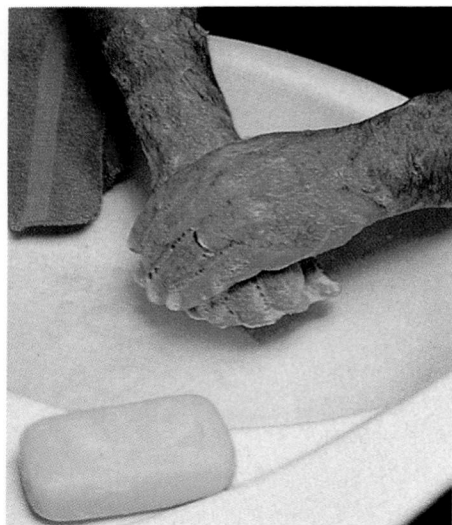

Washing hands thoroughly (for about 45 seconds) with hot water and soap should be the first step in food preparation. The 4 "F's" of food contamination are fingers, foods, feces, and flies. Handwashing especially combats the fecal and finger routes.

USDA recommends cutting boards with unmarred surfaces made of easy-to-clean, nonporous materials, such as plastic, marble, or glass. If you prefer a wooden board, reserve it for a specific purpose; for example, set it aside for cutting raw meat and poultry. Then keep a separate wooden cutting board for chopping produce and slicing bread to prevent these products from picking up bacteria from raw meat. Note that many foods are served raw, so any bacteria clinging to them are not destroyed.

Furthermore, USDA recommends that all cutting boards be replaced when they become streaked with hard-to-clean grooves or cuts, which may harbor bacteria. In addition, cutting boards should be sanitized once a week in a solution of 2 teaspoons chlorine bleach per quart of water. Flood the board with the solution, let it sit a few minutes, and then rise thoroughly.

- When thawing foods, do so in the refrigerator for 1 to 3 days, under cold running water, or in a microwave oven. Also, cook foods immediately after thawing under cold water or in the microwave. Never let frozen foods thaw unrefrigerated all day or night. Also, marinate food in the refrigerator.
- Avoid coughing or sneezing over foods, even when you're healthy. Cover cuts on hands with a sterile bandage. This helps stop *Staphylococcus* from entering food.
- Carefully wash fresh fruit and vegetables under running water to remove dirt and bacteria clinging to the surface, using a vegetable brush if the skin is to be eaten. People have become ill from *Salmonella* that was introduced from melons used in making a fruit salad and from oranges used for fresh-squeezed orange juice. The bacteria were on the outside of the melons and oranges.
- Completely remove moldy portions of food or don't eat the food. *When in doubt, throw the food out.* Mold growth is prevented by properly storing food at cold temperatures and using the food promptly.
- Use refrigerated ground meat and patties in 1 to 2 days and frozen meat and patties within 3 to 4 months.

Cooking Food

- Cook food thoroughly, especially beef, fish, and pork (160°F [71°C]), poultry (180°F [82°C]), eggs (until the yolk and white are hard), and alfalfa sprouts and other types of sprouts. Cooking is by far the most reliable way to destroy foodborne bacteria, such as toxic strains of *E. coli*, whereas freezing only halts growth. FDA does not recommend that eggs be prepared sunny-side-up or over-easy for consumption. Restaurants must now include an advisory on menus stating that an increased risk of foodborne illness is associated with eating undercooked eggs. As long as restaurants provide this warning on their menus, however, they are allowed to cook eggs to any temperature requested by the consumer. Still, a good general precaution is to eat no raw animal products. USDA answers questions about the safe use of animal products (800-535-4555, 10 A.M. to 4 P.M. weekdays, Eastern time).

Seafood also poses a risk of foodborne illness. Properly cooked fish should flake easily and be opaque or dull and firm. If it's translucent or shiny, it's not done.

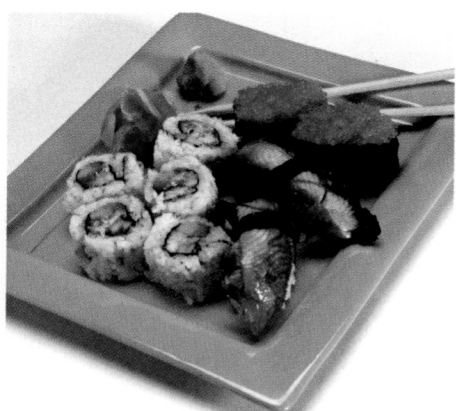

Sushi, like all raw fish or meat dishes, is a high-risk food. For maximum protection from foodborne illness, animal foods should be cooked thoroughly before eating.

Another Bite

Raw fish dishes, such as sushi, can be safe for most people to eat if they are made with very fresh fish that has been commercially frozen and then thawed. The freezing is important to eliminate potential health risks from parasites. FDA recommends that the fish be frozen to an internal temperature of −10°F for 7 days. If you choose to eat uncooked fish, purchase the fish from reputable establishments that have high standards for quality and sanitation. People at high risk for foodborne illness would be wise to avoid raw fish products.

- Cook stuffing separately from poultry (or wash poultry thoroughly, stuff immediately before cooking, and then transfer the stuffing to a clean bowl immediately after cooking). Make sure the stuffing reaches 165°F (74°C). Again, *Salmonella* is the major concern with poultry.
- Once a food is cooked, consume it right away, or cool it to below 41°F (5°C) within 2 hours. If it is not to be eaten immediately, in hot weather (85°F and above) make sure this cooling is done within 1 hour. Do this by separating the food into as many shallow pans as needed to provide a large surface area. Be careful not to recontaminate cooked food by contact with raw meat or juices from hands, cutting boards, dirty utensils, or in other ways.
- Serve meat, poultry, and fish on a clean plate—never the same plate that was used to hold the raw product. For example, when grilling hamburgers, don't put cooked items on the same plate that was used to carry the raw product out to the grill.
- Cook food completely at the picnic site, with no partial cooking in advance.

Storing and Reheating Cooked Food

- Keep hot foods hot and cold foods cold. Hold food below 41°F (5°C) or above 140°F (60°C) (Fig. 16.1). Foodborne microorganisms thrive in more moderate temperatures (60°F to 110°F [16°C to 43°C]). Some microorganisms can even grow in the refrigerator. Again, don't leave cooked or refrigerated foods, such as meats and salads, at room temperature for more than 2 hours (or 1 hour in hot weather) because that gives microorganisms an opportunity to grow. Store dry food at 60°F to 70°F (16°C to 21°C).
- Reheat leftovers to 165°F (74°C); reheat gravy to a rolling boil to kill *Clostridium perfringens* bacteria, which may be present. Merely reheating to a good eating temperature isn't enough to kill sufficient bacteria.
- Store peeled or cut-up produce, such as melon balls, in the refrigerator.
- Make sure the refrigerator stays below 41°F (5°C). Either use a refrigerator thermometer or keep it as cold as possible without freezing milk and lettuce.

Microorganisms that cause foodborne illness commonly enter food through cross-contamination—from one source to another—and grow in temperatures favorable to them, as occurred at a large gathering where turkey franks were contaminated with bacteria. When the franks were later added to a salad, it too became contaminated, causing foodborne illness. Potential sources of cross-contamination are dirty kitchen towels and sponges. It's essential to practice sanitary food-handling procedures when preparing any food.

Scenario *Follow-Up*

Aaron likely contracted *Clostridium perfringens,* based on the fact that he had diarrhea but did not vomit, and the symptoms occurred about 8 hours after consuming the contaminated food (review Table 16.2). Spores of *Clostridium perfringens* are typically present in meat. Thorough cooking will kill any of the live bacteria present, but the product still may contain spores. These can later develop into bacteria if the product is kept in a warm setting for a few hours. The Argentine beef likely contained spores of *Clostridium perfringens.* The bacteria that later formed produced a toxin as the product sat in the car and on the buffet table. Ideally, this product should have remained at room temperature for no longer than 1 hour. Thus, soon after Aaron and his wife took it out of the oven, it should have been separated into a few smaller pans to speed cooling and then refrigerated because they knew it was not going to be served within 1 to 2 hours. Before leaving, they could have recombined the dish into one clean pan. Once they arrived at the party, the dish again should have been refrigerated and then thoroughly reheated when it was time to eat. Overall, it is risky to leave perishable items such as meat, fish, poultry, eggs, and dairy products at room temperature for more than 1 to 2 hours.

*T*o reduce the risk of bacteria surviving during microwave cooking,

- Cover food with glass or ceramic when possible to decrease evaporation and heat the surface.
- Stir and rotate food at least once or twice for even cooking. Then, allow microwaved food to stand, covered, after cooking is completed to help cook the exterior and equalize the temperature throughout.
- Use the oven temperature probe or a meat thermometer to check that food is done. Insert it at several spots.
- If thawing meat in the microwave, use the oven's defrost setting. Ice crystals in frozen foods are not heated well by the microwave oven and can create cold spots, which later cook more slowly.

Figure 16.1 Effects of temperature on microbes that cause foodborne illness. Adapted from *Temperature Guide to Food Safety: Food and Home Notes.* No. 25, Washington DC, June 20, 1977, USDA

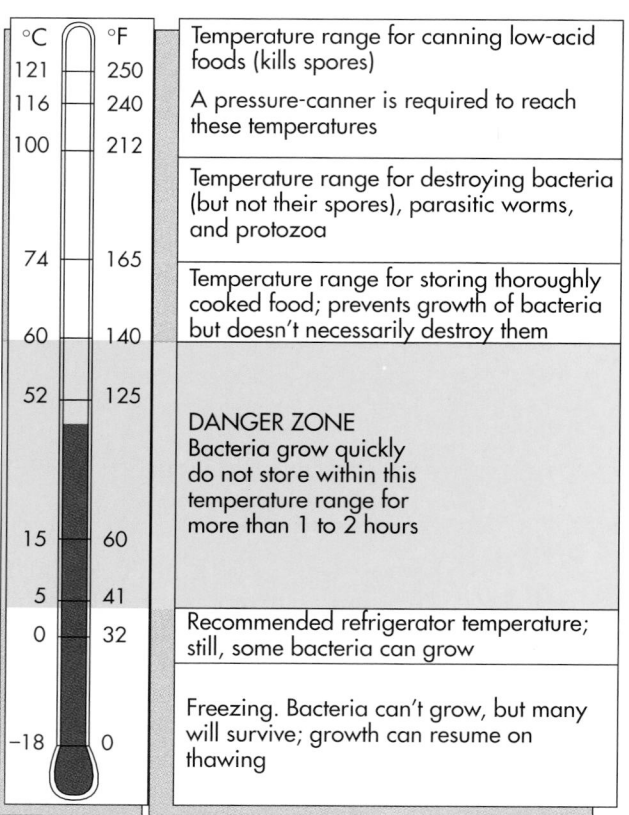

°C	°F	
121	250	Temperature range for canning low-acid foods (kills spores)
116	240	A pressure-canner is required to reach these temperatures
100	212	
		Temperature range for destroying bacteria (but not their spores), parasitic worms, and protozoa
74	165	
		Temperature range for storing thoroughly cooked food; prevents growth of bacteria but doesn't necessarily destroy them
60	140	
52	125	DANGER ZONE Bacteria grow quickly do not store within this temperature range for more than 1 to 2 hours
15	60	
5	41	
0	32	Recommended refrigerator temperature; still, some bacteria can grow
−18	0	Freezing. Bacteria can't grow, but many will survive; growth can resume on thawing

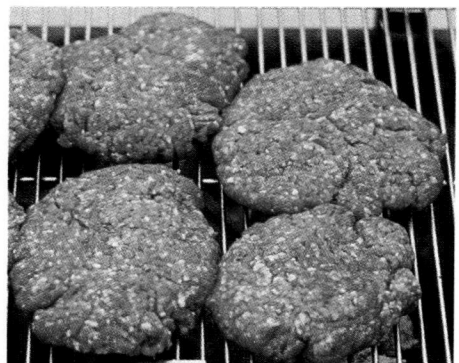

Cook hamburgers until they are brown throughout, the juices run clear, and the inside is hot. This protects against *E. coli* foodborne illness if the bacteria are present.

As one final precaution, watch for safe food-handling techniques when you eat out. Check that foods in a salad bar are iced; custard and pudding pies are chilled; hot foods served on a hot food bar are, in fact, hot; and vending machines are checked regularly, especially those containing sandwiches and milk. Send back any meat, poultry, seafood, or fish that does not appear thoroughly cooked. Food stored and served in dormitory cafeterias should also be properly handled.

Critical Thinking

Diana had a party at her house for her son's birthday. While cleaning up after the kids went home, she realized she had forgotten to put away the potato salad and coleslaw and decided to discard it. However, her husband, Tim, wanted her to just refrigerate it. "After all," he reasoned, "it was only left out for a couple of hours." Why was Diana right in wanting to throw the leftover unrefrigerated food away?

Concept Check

*B*acteria and the toxins they produce pose the greatest risk for foodborne illness. In the past, the addition of sugar and salt to foods, as well as smoking and drying, were used to prevent the growth of microorganisms. Today, we know that ensuring cleanliness, keeping hot foods hot and cold foods cold, and cooking foods thoroughly offer additional protection from foodborne illness. Commercial processes, such as pasteurization and irradiation, do the same. Treat all raw animal products, cooked food, and raw fruits and vegetables as potential sources of foodborne illness.

Thoroughly cook all meat and poultry to reduce the risk of foodborne illness from *Campylobacter,* and *Salmonella.* In addition, always separate raw meats and poultry products from cooked foods. To prevent foodborne intoxication from *Staphylococcus* organisms, cover cuts on hands and avoid sneezing on foods. To avoid intoxication from *Clostridium perfringens,* rapidly cool leftover foods and thoroughly reheat them. To avoid intoxication from *Clostridium botulinum,* carefully examine canned foods. Overall, don't allow cooked food to stand for more than 1 to 2 hours at room temperature. For other causes of foodborne illness, precautions already mentioned generally apply as well. In addition, thoroughly cook fish and other seafood; consume only pasteurized dairy products; wash all fruits and vegetables; and thoroughly wash your hands with soap and water before and after preparing food and after using the bathroom.

Food Additives

By the time you see a food on the market shelf, it usually contains substances added to make it more palatable or increase its nutrient content or shelf life. Manufacturers also add some substances to foods to make them easier to process. Other substances may have accidentally found their way into the foods you buy. All of these extraneous substances are known as **additives,** and, although some may be beneficial, others, such as sulfites, may be harmful for some people. All purposefully added substances must be evaluated by FDA.

■ Why Are Food Additives Used?

Most additives are used to limit food spoilage. Food additives, such as potassium sorbate are used to maintain the safety and acceptability of foods by retarding the growth of microbes implicated in foodborne illness.

Additives are also used to combat some enzymes that lead to undesirable changes in color and flavor in foods but don't cause anything as serious as foodborne illness. This second type of food spoilage occurs when enzymes in a food react to oxygen—for example, when apple and peach slices darken or turn rust color as they are exposed to air. Antioxidants are a type of preservative that retards the action of oxygen-requiring enzymes on food surfaces. These preservatives are not necessarily novel chemicals. They include vitamins E and C and a variety of sulfites.

Without the use of some food additives, it would be impossible to safely produce massive quantities of foods and distribute them nationwide or worldwide, as is now done. Despite consumer concerns about the safety of food additives, many have been extensively studied and proved safe when FDA guidelines for their use are followed.

■ Intentional Versus Incidental Food Additives

Food additives are classified into two types: **intentional food additives** (directly added to foods) and **incidental food additives** (indirectly added as contaminants). Both types of agents are regulated by FDA in the United States. Currently, more than 2800 different substances are intentionally added to foods. As many as 10,000 other substances enter foods as contaminants. This includes substances that may reasonably be expected to enter food through surface contact with processing equipment or packaging materials.

■ The GRAS List

In 1958, all food additives used in the United States and considered safe at that time were put on a **generally recognized as safe (GRAS)** list. The U.S. Congress established the GRAS list because it believed manufacturers did not need to prove the safety of substances that were already generally regarded as safe by knowledgeable scientists. Since that time, FDA has been responsible for proving that a substance does not belong on the GRAS list.

Since 1958, some substances on the list have been reviewed. A few, such as cyclamates, failed the review process and were removed from the list. The additive red dye #3 was banned because it is linked to cancer. Many chemicals on the GRAS list have not yet been rigorously tested, primarily because of expense. These chemicals have received a low priority for testing, mostly because they have long histories of use without evidence of toxicity or because their chemical forms do not suggest they are potential health hazards.

■ Are Synthetic Chemicals Always Harmful?

Nothing about a natural product makes it inherently safer than a synthetic product. Many synthetic products are simply laboratory copies of chemicals that also occur in nature (see the discussion in Chapter 17 on biotechnology for some examples). Moreover, although human endeavors contribute some toxins to foods, such as synthetic pesticides and industrial chemicals, nature's poisons are often even more potent and widespread. Some cancer researchers suggest that we ingest at least 10,000 times more (by weight) natural toxins produced by plants than we do synthetic pesticide residues. This comparison doesn't make synthetic chemicals any less toxic, but it does lend perspective.

Consider vitamin E, which is often added to food to prevent rancidity of fats. This chemical is safe when used within certain limits. However, high doses have been associated with health problems, such as interfering with vitamin K activity in the body (see Chapter 8). Thus, even well-known chemicals we are comfortable using can be toxic in some circumstances and at some concentrations.

∎ Tests of Food Additives for Safety

Food additives are tested under FDA scrutiny for safety on at least two animal species, usually rats and mice. Scientists determine the highest dose of the additive that produces *no observable effects* in the animals. These doses are proportionately much higher than humans are ever exposed to. The maximum dosage is then divided by at least 100 to establish a margin of safety for human use. This 100-fold margin is used because it is assumed that we are at least 10 times more sensitive to food additives than are laboratory animals and that any one person might be 10 times more sensitive than another. This very broad margin essentially ensures that the food additive in question will cause no harmful health effects in humans. In fact, many synthetic chemicals are probably less dangerous at these low doses than the natural compounds in apples or celery.

One important exception applies to the schema for testing intentional food additives: If an additive is shown to cause cancer, even though only in very high doses, no margin of safety is allowed. The food additive cannot be used, because it would violate the **Delaney Clause** in the 1958 Food Additives Amendment. This clause prohibits intentionally adding to foods a compound that was introduced after 1958 and causes cancer. Evidence for cancer could come from either laboratory animal or human studies. Very few exceptions to this clause are allowed; the few are discussed regarding curing and pickling agents in Table 16.3.

Recently, the value of animal cancer tests has been questioned. Research suggests that when rats are fed massive doses of chemicals, as they typically are in the tests, it may be the dose itself, rather than the chemical action, that causes cancer. The scientific community is currently debating which is the best method to test additives to evaluate cancer risk in humans. Nevertheless, until a better method is established, we are left with our current ban on the intentional addition of chemicals that cause cancer.

Incidental food additives are another matter altogether. FDA cannot simply ban various industrial chemicals, pesticide residues, and mold toxins from foods, even though some of these contaminants can cause cancer. These products are not purposely added to foods. FDA sets an acceptable level for these substances. Basically, an incidental substance found in a food cannot contribute to more than one cancer case during the lifetimes of 1 million people. If a higher risk exists, the amount of the compound in a food must be reduced until the guideline is met.

∎ Approval for a New Food Additive

Today, before a new food additive can be added to foods, FDA must approve its use. Besides rigorously testing an additive to establish its safety margins, manufacturers must give FDA information that (1) identifies the new additive, (2) gives its chemical composition, (3) states how it is manufactured, and (4) specifies laboratory methods used to measure its presence in the food supply at the amount of intended use.

*N*ote that this 100-fold margin of safety is over 30 times than that for vitamin A.

Delaney Clause A clause to the 1958 Food Additives Amendment of the Pure Food and Drug Act in the United States that prevents the intentional (direct) addition to foods of a compound that has been shown to cause cancer in laboratory animals or humans.

*S*ugar, salt, corn syrup, and citric acid constitute 98% of all additives (by weight) used in food processing.

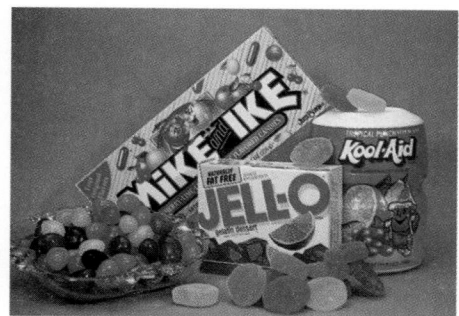

Color additives make some foods more desirable. Their use must be noted on the label so people sensitive to certain varieties can avoid that substance.

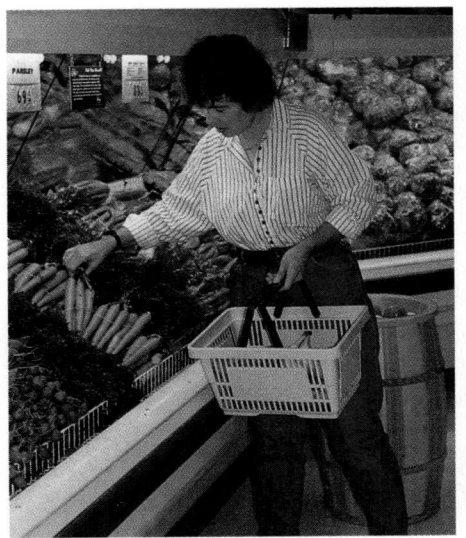 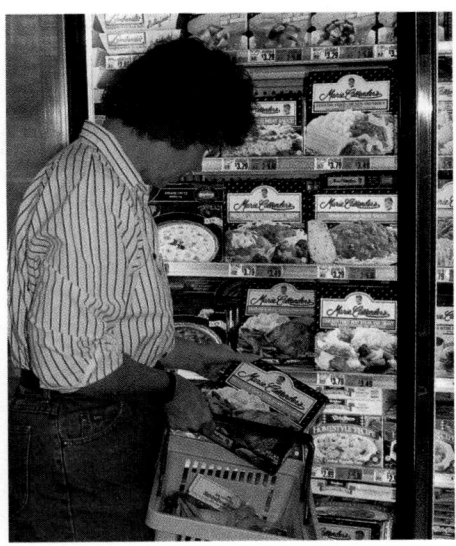

Figure 16.2 Depending on food choices, a diet can be either (a) essentially free of or (b) contain food additives. For most of us, this specific concern regarding food choice is not worth worrying about.

Manufacturers must also offer proof that the additive will accomplish its intended purpose in a food, that it is safe, and that it is to be used in no higher amount than needed. Additives cannot be used to hide defective food ingredients, such as rancid oils; to deceive customers; or replace good manufacturing practices. A manufacturer must establish that the ingredient is necessary for producing a specific food product.

■ Common Food Additives

Table 16.3 lists common food additives. Some serve the general function of **preservatives:** acidic or alkaline agents, antioxidants, antimicrobial agents, curing and pickling agents, and **sequestrants.** This table helps you to understand exactly why these are used and to learn more about the specific substances used.

In general, if you consume a variety of foods in moderation, the chances of food additives jeopardizing your health are minimal. Pay attention to your body. If you suspect an intolerance or a sensitivity, consult your physician for further evaluation. Remember that in the short run, you are more likely to suffer either from foodborne illness due to poor food-handling practices that allow bacteria to grow in food, or from the consumption of raw animal foods, than from consuming additives. Excess energy, saturated fat, salt, and other potential "problem" nutrients in our diets pose the greatest long-term risk.

Critical Thinking

Recognizing that Joseph is taking a nutrition class, his roommate ask him, "What is more risky: the bacteria that can be present in food or the additives listed on the label of my favorite snack cake?" How should Joseph respond? On what information should he base his conclusions?

preservatives Compounds that extend the shelf life of foods by inhibiting microbial growth or minimizing the destructive effect of oxygen and metals.

sequestrants Compounds that bind free metal ions. By so doing, they reduce the ability of ions to cause rancidity in foods containing fat.

Another Bite

*I*f you are bewildered or concerned about all the additives creeping into your diet, you can easily avoid most of them by emphasizing unprocessed whole foods (Fig. 16.2). However, no evidence shows that this will necessarily make you healthier, nor can you avoid all additives, since some are used even on whole foods, such as with pesticides. It amounts to a personal decision. Do you have confidence that FDA and food manufacturers are adequately protecting your health and welfare, or do you want to take more personal control by minimizing your intake of compounds not naturally found in foods?

Soft drinks are typical sources of alternative sweeteners for many of us. Moderate use of these products generally poses no health risk in most people.

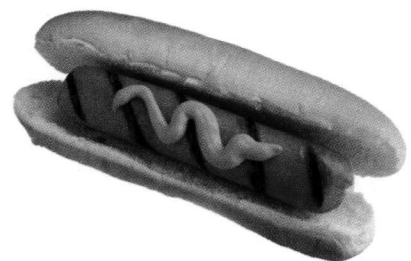

Cured meats derive their pink color from nitrates. The National Cancer Institutes advises consuming these foods in moderation, as the nitrates/nitrites present some cancer risk, such as colon cancer.

You might wonder why, if nitrates and nitrites form chemical substances that can cause cancer, they aren't banned by the Delaney Clause. In the United States, USDA regulates the use of chemicals in meats. The laws that govern USDA regulation of foods are separate from those that govern FDA regulation. Because of this, the Delaney Clause does not apply to USDA actions. Currently USDA sees no clear threat to public safety from the regulated use of nitrates and nitrites in meats, so no action has been taken.

Table 16.3 Common Food Additives—Sources and Related Health Concerns

Food Additives	Attributes	Health Risks
Acidic or alkaline agents, such as calcium lactate and sodium hydroxide	Acids impart a tart taste to soft drinks, sherbets, and cheese spreads, inhibit mold growth, and lessen discoloration and rancidity. They also reduce the risk of botulism in naturally low-acid vegetables, such as canned beets. Alkaline agents neutralize acids produced during fermentation, and so improve flavor	No known health risks when used properly
Alternative sweeteners, such as saccharin, sucralose, ascesulfame potassium, and aspartame	Sweeten foods without adding more than a few calories	Moderate use of these alternative sweeteners is considered safe (except for aspartame in people with the disease PKU)
Anticaking agents, such as calcium silicate, magnesium stearate, and silicon dioxide	Absorb moisture to keep table salt, baking powder, or powdered sugar and powdered food products free-flowing and prevent caking and lumping	No know health risks when used properly
Antimicrobial agents, such as sodium benzonate, sorbic acid, and calcium propionate	Inhibit mold and fungal growth	No known health risks when used properly
Antioxidants, such as BHA (butylated hydroxyanisole), BHT (butylated hydroxytolune), alpha-tocopherol (vitamin E), ascorbic acid (vitamin C), and sulfites	Delay food discolorations from oxygen exposure Reduce rancidity from the breakdown of fats Maintain the color of luncheon meats Prevent the formation of cancer-causing nitrosamines	Sulfites can cause an allergic reaction in about 1 in every 100 people. Symptoms include difficulty breathing, wheezing, hives, diarrhea, abdominal pain, cramps, and dizziness. Salad bars, dried fruit, and wine are typical sources of sulfites
Color additives, such as tartrazine	Make foods more appealing	Tartrazine (FD&C yellow number 5) can cause allergic symptoms such as hives and nasal discharge in some people, especially those allergic to aspirin. FDA requires manufacturers to list all forms of synthetic colors on the labels of foods that contain them
Curing and pickling agents, such as **nitrates** and nitrites	Act as preservatives, especially to prevent the growth of *Clostridium botulinium;* often used in conjunction with salt	Nitrate and nitrite consumption from both cured foods and that found naturally in some vegetables has been associated with synthesis of nitrosamines. Some nitrosamines are cancer-causing agents, particularly for the stomach, esophagus, and colon. Thus, the National Cancer Institute advises consuming these foods in moderation

Table 16.3 Common Food Additives—Sources and Related Health Concerns (concluded)

Food Additives	Attributes	Health Risks
Emulsifiers, such as monoglycerides and lecithins	Suspend fat in water to improve uniformity, smoothness, and body of foods, such as baked goods, ice cream, and mayonnaise	No known health risks when used properly
Fat replacements, such as Paselli SA2, Dur-Low, Oatrim, Sta-Slim 143, Stellar, and Olean	Limit calorie content of foods by reducing some of the fat content	Generally no known health risks when used properly. Olean can cause gastrointestinal upset and diarrhea at intakes greater than 20 grams per day
Flavor and flavoring agents, such as natural and artificial flavors	Impart more flavor to foods	No known health risks when used properly
Flavor enhancers, such as monosodium glutamate (MSG)	Help bring out the natural flavor of foods, such as meats	Some people (especially infants) are sensitive to the glutamate portion of MSG and after exposure experience flushing, chest pain, facial pressure, dizziness, sweating, rapid heart rate, nausea, vomiting, increase in blood pressure, and headache. Those so affected should look for glutamate on food labels, and isolated protein, yeast extract, bullion, and soup stock
Humectants, such as glycerol, propylene glycol, and sorbitol	Retain more moisture, texture, and fresh flavor in foods such as candies, shredded coconut, and marshmallows	No known health risk when used properly
Leavening agents, such as yeast, baking powder, and baking soda	Introduce carbon dioxide into food products	No known health risk when used properly
Maturing and bleaching agents, such as bromates, peroxides, and ammonium chloride	Shorten the time needed for maturation of flour to become usable for baking products	No known health risk when used properly
Nutrient supplements, such as vitamin A, vitamin D, and potassium iodide	Enhance the nutrient content of foods such as margarine, milk, and ready-to-eat breakfast cereals	No known health risk if intake from such supplementaion combined with other food intake does not exceed the Upper Level set for a particular nutrient (iron may be one exception; see Chapter 8)
Stabilizers and thickeners, such as pectins, gums, gelatins, and agars	Impart a smooth texture and uniform color flavor to candies, ice cream, and other frozen desserts, chocolate milk, and beverages containing alternative sweeteners. Prevent evaporation and deterioration of flavorings used in cakes, puddings, and gelatin mixes	No known health risk when used properly
Sequestrants, such as EDTA and citric acid	Bind free ions, helping preserve food quality by reducing ability of ions to cause rancidity in products containing fat	No known health risk when used properly

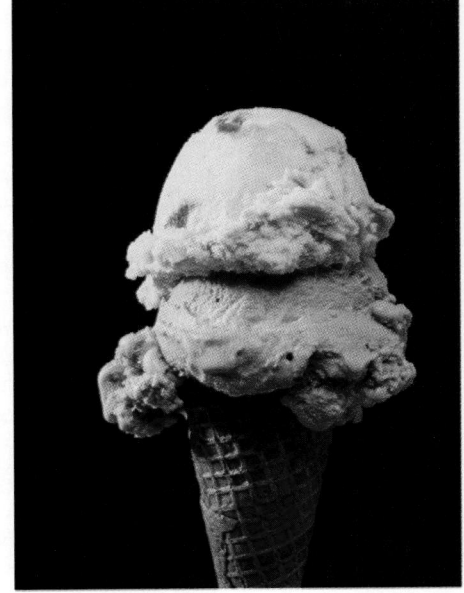

Emulsifiers improve the texture of foods such as ice cream, baked goods, and cookies.

Caffeine—Is There an Ax to Grind?

Why all the controversy over a cup of coffee? Can't we come to one definite conclusion? Researchers have spent a great deal of time on the study of caffeine, the substance of greatest concern in the favorite beverage of many of us. So why do recommendations change from year to year?

Many factors complicate the study of caffeine intake, not the least of which is the memory of study participants. On average, we consume 75% of our caffeine intake as coffee, 15% as tea, 10% as soft drinks, and 2% as chocolate. But researchers need a more detailed picture of individuals' specific habits, so they ask people to remember consumption patterns from 10 years ago or more. Do you remember how many cans of soft drinks you drank a day 10 years ago? Do you remember all the sources of caffeine you consumed, or how many cups of regular versus decaf coffee you drank 3 years ago?

Another factor that complicates research is that heavy coffee drinkers often have other deleterious health habits such as heavy alcohol consumption and smoking. In addition, smokers are likely to drink more coffee because their blood is cleared of caffeine faster than are nonsmokers. Are the health consequences found in heavy coffee drinkers due to caffeine, or is it possible that these other harmful habits are the true cause? In addition, caffeine is not often consumed by itself. With the recent popularity of trendy coffee shops that serve everything from mocha java to flavored lattes, it is difficult to separate caffeine intake from cream, sugar, alternative sweeteners, and flavorings. So what is the conscientious coffee drinker to think? Let's explore the myths and facts of caffeine intake as it is known today.

Caffeine does not accumulate in the body and is normally excreted within several hours following consumption. Caffeine can cause anxiety, increased heart rate, insomnia, increased urination, diarrhea, and gastrointestinal upset in high doses. In addition, those already suffering from ulcers may experience irritation due to increased acid production; those who have anxiety or panic attacks may find that caffeine worsens the

symptoms; and those prone to heartburn may find that caffeine worsens this symptom because it relaxes sphincter muscles in the esophagus. Some people need very little caffeine to feel such effects, and the dosage for children is likely even lower than that for adults.

Withdrawal symptoms are also very real. Former coffee drinkers may experience headache, nausea, and depression for a short time after discontinuing use. These symptoms can be expected to peak at 20 to 48 hours following the last intake of caffeine. Symptoms hold true even for those trying to quit as little as one cup of coffee a day. Slow tapering of use over a few days is recommended to avoid this problem.

Are there more serious consequences of consuming caffeine regularly? It has been hypothesized that caffeine consumption can lead to certain types of cancer, such as pancreatic and bladder cancers. The association of caffeine with cancer has not been supported in recent literature. At this time it appears that there is no major connection between caffeine and cancer. If fact, regular coffee consumption has been linked to a decreased risk of colon cancer.

The limelight also has been drawn away from caffeine with regard to cardiovascular disease and coffee consumption. Heavy use does increase blood pressure for a short period of time. Coffee consumption also has been linked to increased LDL-cholesterol and triglycerides. This association was found to be caused by cafestol and kahweol, two oils in ground coffee, as noted in Chapter 5. However, since 1975, filtered and instant coffees have become popular, and these products do not contain the harmful oils. When researchers correct for tobacco use in coffee drinkers, no distinct correlation is seen between filtered or instant coffee consumption and increased risk for cardiovascular disease. It is prudent, though, to limit the amount of coffee from French coffee presses and from espresso, as these beverages are not filtered.

Women are thought to be at higher risk for a variety of deleterious effects with caffeine consumption, including

osteoporosis, and birth defects and miscarriages in their offspring. It is true that heavy caffeine use increases the amount of calcium excreted in urine. For this reason, it is important that heavy coffee drinkers check their diets for adequate calcium sources. Some studies do show a higher likelihood for miscarriages in women consuming more than 500 milligrams of caffeine per day (Appendix H lists the caffeine content of foods). FDA warns women to consume caffeine in moderation.

In contrast to these possibly harmful effects of caffeine consumption, many people are convinced of the benefits of a "cup of joe." Though some women testify to the idea that caffeine improves premenstrual symptoms, currently no study proves this theory. Some weight-loss drugs previously contained caffeine, under the assumption that it made the drugs more effective. FDA has since banned this use as it was found to be ineffective. Some newer research findings suggest caffeine may reduce the risk of developing headaches, cirrhosis of the liver, some forms of kidney stones, gallbladder stones, and some nerve-related diseases. You may have heard that caffeine can improve physical performance. This has been shown in highly trained athletes; recall that use of large amounts of caffeine is banned in international events (review Chapter 11). For those who are below professional status, though, no benefit has been shown. Also keep in mind that coffee will not "sober up" a person who is drunk.

Though the debate over caffeine will likely continue as long as North Americans drink coffee, current research does not support many of the concepts previously thought of as fact. These studies are, in fact, reinforcing the idea of moderation—the equivalent of about two to three cups of coffee per day. Remember that there are no good or bad foods, but anything in excess can have damaging effects, caffeine and coffee included, and more so in some people than others. A prudent dose of caffeine is 200–300 milligrams per day, which corresponds to about three cups of coffee (again, review Appendix H). One cup of North American coffee contains about 100 milligrams of caffeine.

Substances That Occur Naturally in Foods and Can Cause Illness

Foods contain a variety of naturally occurring substances that can cause illness. Here are some of the more important examples:

Safrole—found in sassafras, mace, and nutmeg; causes cancer

Solanine—found in potato shoots and green spots on potato skins; inhibits the action of neurotransmitters

Mushroom toxins—found in some species of mushrooms such as aminita; can cause stomach upset, dizziness, hallucinations, and other neurological symptoms. The more lethal varieties can cause liver and kidney failure, coma, and even death. FDA regulates commercially grown and harvested mushrooms. These are cultivated in concrete buildings or caves. However, there are no systematic controls on individual gatherers harvesting wild species, except in Michigan and Illinois

Avidin—found in raw egg whites; binds the vitamin biotin in a way that prevents its absorption, so a biotin deficiency may ultimately develop over the long term

Thiaminase—found in raw fish, clams, and mussels; destroys the vitamin thiamin

Tetrodotoxin—found in puffer fish; causes respiratory paralysis

Protease inhibitors—found in raw soybeans; inhibits digestive enzymes

Oxalic acid—found in spinach, strawberries, sesame seeds, and other foods; binds calcium and iron in the foods, and so limits absorption of these nutrients

Herbal teas—containing senna or comfrey; can cause diarrhea and liver damage

People have coexisted for centuries with these naturally occurring substances and have learned to avoid some of them and limit intake in other cases. Today, they pose little health risk. Farmers know potatoes must be stored in the dark, so that solanine won't be synthesized. Furthermore, we've developed cooking and food-preparation methods to limit the potency of other substances, such as thiaminase. Spices are used in such small amounts that health risks don't result. Nevertheless, it's important to understand that some potentially harmful chemicals in foods occur naturally.

Environmental Contaminants in Food

A variety of environmental contaminants can be found in foods. Table 16.6 in the Nutrition Issue lists ways to limit pesticide residues in the diet. Aside from pesticide residues and products of fungal growth, other potential contaminants that deserve attention are listed in Table 16.4.

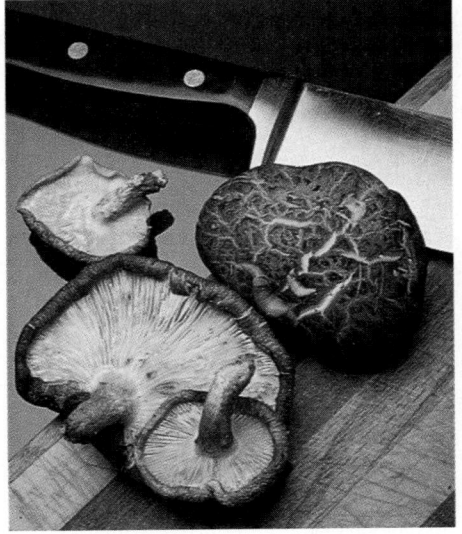

When hunting wild mushrooms, know what you are looking for. Many varieties contain deadly toxins.

*G*enetic alteration of foods such as corn and soybeans has recently created concern, especially in Europe. FDA considers genetically-altered products safe if approval for human use has been granted (see Chapter 17 for details).

Table 16.4 Potential Environmental Contaminants in Our Food Supply

Chemical Substance	Sources	Toxic Effects	Preventive Measures
Lead	Lead-based paint chips and related dust in older homes Occupational exposure (e.g., radiator repair) Lead caps on wine bottles Fruit juices and pickled vegetables stored in galvanized or tin containers or leaded glass Some types of solder used in joining copper pipes (mostly in older homes) Mexican pottery dishes Koo Soo herbal remedies	Anemia Kidney disease Nervous system damage (tiredness and changes in behavior are symptoms) Reduced learning capacity in childhood	Avoid paint chips and related dust in older homes; regular cleaning of these homes is also important (see www.hud.gov/offices/lead/index.cfm) Meet iron and calcium needs to reduce lead absorption Wipe the inside and outside neck of wine bottles before use if the bottle has a lead cap Store fruit juices and pickled vegetables in glass or plastic or waxed paper containers Let water run 1 minute or so if off for more than 2 hours, and use only cold water for cooking; do not soften drinking water
Dioxin	Trash-burning incinerators Bottom-feeding fish from the Great Lakes Animal fats from animals exposed to such contamination via water or soil	Abnormal reproduction and fetal/infant development Immune suppression Cancer (to date only clearly shown in laboratory animals)	Pay attention to warnings of dioxin risks from local fish; if risk exists, limit intake as suggested on the fishing license Consume a variety of fish from local waters rather than mostly one specific species
Mercury	Swordfish, shark, king mackerel, and tilefish	Reduced fetal/child development and birth defects; toxic to nervous system	Consume these sources no more than once per week; pregnant women should avoid these species of fish
Urethane	Alcoholic beverages such as sherry, bourbon, sake, and fruit brandies	Cancer (to date only clearly shown in laboratory animals)	Avoid generous amounts of typical sources
Polychlorinated biphenyls (PCBs)	Fish from the Great Lakes and Hudson River Valley (e.g., coho salmon)	Cancer (to date only clearly shown in laboratory animals), as well as a potential for liver, immune, and reproductive disorders	Pay attention to warnings of PCB contamination from local fish; if risk exists, limit intake as suggested on the fishing license or on state advisories

■ Protection from Environmental Toxins in Foods

To reduce exposure to environmental toxins that cause disease can be present in foods, find out which foods pose a risk. In addition, emphasize variety and moderation in food selection. The presence of mercury in swordfish or shark may concern you, but it's normally not a health risk unless your diet is dominated by these fish. The small amount of mercury in most swordfish or shark isn't harmful if you're exposed to it infrequently. Note also that tips provided in Table 16.6 in the Nutrition Issue also apply to reducing exposure to environmental contaminants.

Concept Check

A general program to minimize exposure to environmental contaminants includes knowing which foods pose greater risks and consuming a wide variety of foods in moderation.

Summary

1. Bacteria and other microorganisms in food pose the greatest risk for foodborne illness. In the past, salt, sugar, smoke, fermentation, and drying were used to protect against foodborne illness. Today, careful cooking, pasteurization, and keeping hot foods hot and cold foods cold, and thorough hand washing provide additional insurance.

2. Major causes of foodborne illness are the bacteria *Campylobacter jejuni, Salmonella, Shigella, Staphylococcus aureus,* and *Clostridium perfringens.* In addition, such bacteria as *Clostridium botulinum, Listeria monocytogenes, Yersinia enterocolitica,* and *Escherichia coli* have been found to cause illness, as have viruses such as the Norwalk virus.

3. To protect against bacteria, cook susceptible foods thoroughly. In addition, cover cuts on the hands, do not sneeze or cough on foods, avoid contact between raw meat or poultry products and other food products, rapidly cool and thoroughly reheat leftovers, and use pasteurized dairy products.

4. Cross-contamination commonly causes foodborne illness. It occurs particularly when bacteria on raw animal products contact foods that can support bacterial growth. Because of the risk of cross-contamination, no perishable food should be kept at room temperature for more than 1 to 2 hours (depending on the environmental temperature), especially if it may have come in contact with raw animal products.

5. Treatment for foodborne illness usually requires drinking lots of fluids, avoiding touching food while diarrhea is present, washing hands thoroughly, and getting bed rest. Botulism, hepatitis A infec-

tions, and trichinosis are types of foodborne illness that require prompt medical attention.

6. Food additives are used primarily to extend shelf life by preventing microbial growth and the destruction of food components by oxygen, metals, and other substances. Food additives are classified as those intentionally added to foods and those that incidentally appear in foods. An intentional additive is limited to no more than one-one-hundredth of the greatest amount that causes no observed symptoms in animals. The Delaney Clause allows FDA to ban the use of any intentional food additive under its jurisdiction in the United States that causes cancer.

7. Antioxidants, such as BHA, BHT, vitamins E and C, and sulfites, prevent oxygen and enzyme destruction of food products. Emulsifiers suspend fat in water, improving the uniformity, smoothness, and body of foods such as ice cream. Common preservatives include sodium benzoate and sorbic acid, which prevent bacterial growth. Sequestrants bind metals and thus prevent spoilage of food from metal contamination.

8. Toxic substances occur naturally in a variety of foods, such as green potatoes, raw fish, mushrooms, raw soybeans, and raw egg whites. Cooking foods limits their toxic effects in some cases; others are best to avoid, such as toxic mushroom species and the green parts of potatoes.

9. A variety of environmental contaminants can be found in foods. It is helpful to know which foods pose risks and act accordingly to reduce exposure.

Study Questions

1. Identify three major classes of microorganisms that are responsible for foodborne illness.

2. Which kinds of foods are most likely to be involved in foodborne illness? Why are they targets for contamination?

3. What three trends in food purchasing and production have led to a greater number of cases of foodborne illness in recent years?

4. Why is thoroughly cooking food an important practice for reducing the risk of foodborne illness?

5. List four techniques other than thorough cooking that are important in preventing foodborne illness.

6. Define the term *food additive,* and give examples of four intentional food additives. What are their specific functions in foods? What is their relationship to the GRAS list?

7. Describe the federal process that governs the use of food additives, including the Delaney Clause.

8. Put into perspective the benefits and risks of using additives in food. Point out an easy way to reduce the consumption of food additives. Do you think this is worth the effort in terms of maintaining health? Why or why not?

9. Describe four recommendations for reducing the risk of toxicity from environmental contaminants.

10. Read the Nutrition Issue before answering the following question. How do various U.S. federal agencies work together to maintain the safety of food?

Further Readings

1. Bender J and others: Foodborne disease in the 21st century: What challenges await us. *Postgraduate Medicine* 106(2):109, 1999.

The factors that contribute to an increasing incidence of foodborne disease include diet, the global distribution of foods, the expansion of commercial food services, and new methods of large-scale food production. Critical aspects to help reduce the risk for disease include improved surveillance, community education, the use of preventive strategies, and ionizing radiation.

2. Bren L: Trying to keep mad cow disease out of U.S. herds. *FDA Consumer*, p. 12, March–April 2001.

No cases of Mad Cow disease in humans has been identified in the United States. FDA and USDA are aggressively enforcing regulations to minimize the risk on the introduction of Mad Cow disease in the U.S. herds.

3. Daniels R: Home food safety. *Food Technology* 52(2):54, 1998.

Currently, 99% of households do not meet food safety standards. And, since proper preparation at home is the last chance people have to protect themselves, raising public awareness of home food safety is an important issue. For the general public, key efforts include avoiding cross-contamination, washing hands, cooking to appropriate temperature, and cooling of foods properly.

4. Faley D: Dangers of lead still linger. *FDA Consumer*, p. 16, January/February 1998.

Although the percentage of potentially harmful blood lead concentrations has dropped dramatically in the past 20 years, lead is still a problem. Sources include lead paint in older housing, in the soil where leaded gasoline was once used, at some work sites, and occasionally in drinking water, ceramic ware, and a number of other products.

5. Food-borne antibiotic-resistant *Campylobacter* infections. *Nutrition Reviews* 57:224, 2000.

In modern breeding of food animals, large amounts of antibiotics are used for a variety of reasons, including growth promotion. This has caused foodborne bacterial pathogens to become resistant to antibiotics and has caused an increase in related sickness and death among humans. Well-coordinated international programs are needed to reduce the worldwide use of antibiotics in food animals.

6. Food safety guide. *Nutrition Action Healthletter*, p. 3, October 1999.

This article discusses the major causes of foodborn illnesses and precautions to take to prevent infections. Some ways to avoid contracting a foodborne illness are to marinate and defrost food in the refrigerator, not eat raw shellfish, discard cracked eggs, and wash fresh fruits and vegetables. These and other precautions should be taken in order to protect against harmful microbes.

7. Formanek R: Food for thought. *FDA Consumer*, p. 13, September–October 2001.

North Americans enjoy one of the safest food supplies in the world. Despite this fact, diseases caused by food are responsible for an estimated 76 million cases of GI tract illnesses and 5000 deaths per year in the United States alone. Therefore, vigilance against foodborne illness should be an important consideration for everyone. The main consumer messages are: keep hands and cooking surfaces clean, cook food to proper temperatures, refrigerate food promptly, and separate food to avoid cross-contamination.

8. Medeiros LC and others: Identification and classification of consumer food-handling behaviors for food safety education. *Journal of the American Dietetic Association* 101:1326, 2001.

Foodborne illness is a major cause of economic burden, human suffering, and death in the United States. Each year more than 1 in 4 people in the United States become infected with some form of foodborne illness. Some new recommendations for preventing foodborne illness are heating lunch meat steaming hot to 165°F before eating if one is pregnant, immunocompromised, or of advanced age. Avoiding raw sprouts is also important.

9. New findings on caffeine and your health. *Tufts University Health & Nutrition Letter* 19(1) (March), 2001.

Coffee use has been linked to a decreased risk of headaches, colon cancer, and some nerve disorders. Up to three cups of coffee per day is a safe intake for men and women.

10. Pesticide residues: Cause for concern? *Health News* p. 3, April 15, 1999.

Since there's no firm evidence that eating produce with pesticide residues is unhealthy, consumers should not let the pesticide controversy scare them away from eating plenty of fruits and vegetables. Still, to be on the safe side, we should carefully rinse all fruits and vegetables under cold, running water before consumption.

11. *Residue monitoring 1999.* Washington, DC: Food and Drug Administration Pesticide Program, Food and Drug Administration, 1999.

Based on FDA's Total Diet Study comprising 3500 different foods purchased from stores throughout the United States, only 0.8% of foods had pesticide residues exceeding EPA allowances. For imported products, 3.5% had pesticide residues exceeding EPA allowances. Otherwise, pesticide residues were either undetectable (about 60% of the time) or within allowable amounts for over 99% of domestic products and about 97% of imported products.

12. Safe food 2000 quiz. *Nutrition Action Healthletter*, p. 10, November 2000.

About half of all foodborne illness cases occur because of practices in the home. This quiz challanges you to discover unsafe food practices in your daily life; such as whether it is safe to eat raw hot dogs.

13. Woteki CE and others: Keep food safe to eat: Healthful food must be safe as well as nutritious. *Journal of Nutrition* 131:502S, 2001.

Food safety education is a critical part of the overall strategy to reduce the incidence of foodborne illness. New technologies such as radiation are important risk management strategies. Inclusion of food safety in the Dietary Guidelines for Americans should go a long way toward ensuring that the public is aware of the importance of this issue.

I. Can You Spot the Improper Food-Safety Practices?

In this chapter you learned the following facts: (1) foodborne illness strikes up to 76 million U.S. citizens each year; (2) about 5000 deaths each year in the United States are caused by foodborne organisms.

Carefully preparing foods to prevent foodborne illness can minimize its occurrence for most of us. Read the following excerpt and find the food-safety violations that could contribute to this risk.

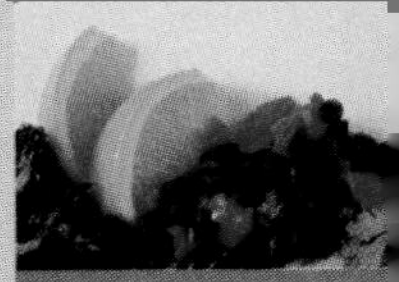

A Local Health Department Inspector Gives the Following Account of His Visit to a Local Diner

As I walked through the kitchen of the Morningside Diner, I noticed that all food handlers washed their hands thoroughly with hot, soapy water before handling the food, especially after handling raw meat, fish, poultry, or eggs. Before preparing raw foods, they also thoroughly washed the cutting boards, dishes, and other equipment. As they used their cutting boards after cutting foods, they wiped them with a damp rag and used them again to cut more food.

When preparing fresh fruits and vegetables, they washed them but were careful to leave a little dirt on for fear of washing important nutrients from the outside. The cooks generally cooked meats to an internal temperature of 180°F (82°C). However, to preserve the flavor, pork was cooked to an internal temperature of 140°F (60°C). Some cooked foods to be served later were cooled to below 41°F (5°C) within 2 hours, and foods like beef stew were cooled in shallow pans.

The diner served canned foods, even when the cans were dented. When leftovers were reheated, they were raised to an internal temperature of 150°F (66°C) and served immediately. Food handlers took great care to remove moldy portions of food. The cooks prepared stuffing separately from the poultry. The temperature of refrigerators was approximately 45°F (7°C).

1. List the violations of food-safety practices that could contribute to foodborne illness.

_____

_____

_____

_____

2. If you were writing a report describing ways to correct these practices, what would you say?

_____

_____

_____

_____

_____

continued

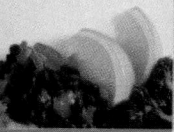

II. Take a Closer Look at Food Additives

Evaluate a food label of a convenience food item either in the supermarket or one you have available.

1. Write out the list of ingredients.

_____

_____

_____

_____

2. Identify the ingredients that you think may be food additives.

_____

_____

_____

_____

3. Based on the information available in this chapter, what are the functions of these food additives?

_____

_____

_____

_____

4. How might this food product differ without these ingredients?

_____

_____

_____

_____

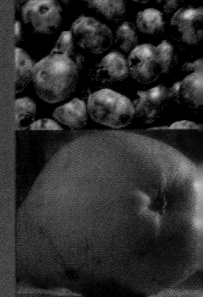

Pesticides used in food production produce both beneficial and unwanted effects. Most health authorities believe that the benefits greatly outweigh the risks. Pesticides help ensure a safe and adequate food supply and help make foods available at reasonable cost. However, sentiment is growing nationwide that pesticides pose avoidable health risks. Consumers have come to assume that synthetic is dangerous and organic is safe. Some researchers believe this sentiment is grounded in fear and fueled by unbalanced reports. Other researchers say concern about pesticides is valid and overdue.

Most concern about pesticide residues in food appropriately focuses on chronic rather than acute toxicity because the amounts of residue present, if any, are extremely small. These low concentrations found in foods are not known to produce adverse effects in the short term, although harm has been caused by the high amounts that occasionally result from accidents or misuse. For humans, pesticides pose a danger mainly in their cumulative effects, so their threats to health are difficult to determine. However, growing evidence, including the problems of the contamination of underground water supplies and destruction of wildlife habitats, indicates that North America would likely be better off if we could reduce our use of pesticides. Both the U.S. federal government and many farmers are working toward that end.

One of the problems with pesticides is that they create new pests because they destroy the spiders, wasps, and predatory beetles that naturally keep most plantfeeding insect populations in check. The brown plant hopper, which recently plagued Indonesian rice fields was not a serious problem before heavy pesticide use began in the early 1970s. In the United States, such major pests as spider mites and the cotton bollworm were merely nuisances until pesticides decimated their predators.

What Is a Pesticide?

U.S. federal law defines a pesticide as any substance or mixture of substances intended to prevent, destroy, repel, or mitigate any pest. The built-in toxic properties of pesticides lead to the possibility that other, nontarget organisms, including humans, might also be harmed. The term *pesticide* tends to be used as a generic reference to many types of products, including insecticides, **herbicides,** fungicides, and rodenticides. A pesticide product may be chemical or bacterial, natural or synthetic. For agriculture, EPA allows about 10,000 pesticide uses, involving some 300 active ingredients. About 1.2 billion pounds of pesticides are used each year in the United States, much of which is applied to agricultural crops.

Once a pesticide is applied, it can turn up in a number of unintended and unwanted places. It may be carried in the air and dust by wind currents, remain in soil attached to soil particles, be taken up by organisms in the soil, decompose to other compounds, be taken up by plant roots, enter groundwater, or invade aquatic habitats. Each is a route to the food chain; some are more direct than others.

Why Use Pesticides?

In the United States alone, pests destroy nearly $20 billion of food crops yearly, despite extensive pesticide use. The primary reason for using pesticides is economic—the use of agricultural chemicals increases production and lowers the cost of food, at least in the short run. Many farmers believe they would have a tough time staying in business without pesticides. Quick and direct, pesticides help protect farmers from ruinous losses caused by a sudden pest outbreak.

Consumer demands also have changed over the years. At one time, we wouldn't have thought twice about buying an apple with a worm hole; we simply took it home, cut out the wormy part, and ate the apple. Today, consumers find worm holes less acceptable, so farmers rely more and more on pesticides to produce cosmetically attractive fruits and vegetables. On the practical side, pesticides can protect against the rotting and decay of fresh fruits and vegetables. This is helpful because our food distribution system doesn't usually permit consumer purchase

continued

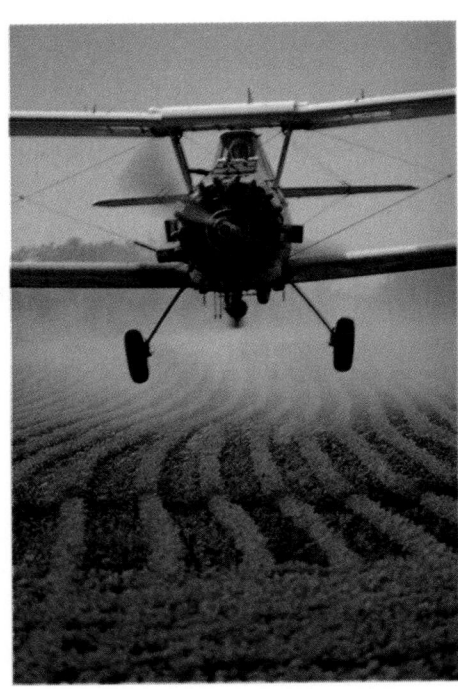

Pesticides use poses a risk-versus-benefit question. Each side has points that deserve to be considered. Rural communities, where exposure is more direct, experience the greatest short-term risk.

within hours of harvest. Also, food grown without pesticides can contain naturally occurring organisms that produce carcinogens at concentrations far above current standards for pesticide residues. For example, fungicides help prevent the carcinogen aflatoxin (caused by growth of a fungus) from forming on some crops. Thus, although some pesticides may improve the appearance of food products, others help keep some foods fresher and safer to eat.

Regulation of Pesticides

The responsibility for ensuring that residues of pesticides in foods are below amounts that pose a danger to health is shared by FDA, EPA, and the Food Safety and Inspection Service of USDA in the United States. Table 16.5 lists the roles of various food protection agencies. FDA is responsible for enforcing pesticide tolerances in all foods except meat, poultry, and certain egg products, which are monitored by USDA. A newly proposed pesticide is exhaustively tested, perhaps over 10 years or more, before it is approved for use. EPA must decide both that the pesticide causes no unreasonable adverse effects on people and the environment and that benefits of use outweigh the risks of using it. However, there is concern about older chemicals registered before 1970, when less stringent testing conditions were permitted. EPA is now asking chemical companies to retest the old compounds using more rigorous tests. Unfortunately, inadequate funding at EPA has hampered the review of older pesticides. The slow pace of this retesting has angered the critics of pesticide use. When weighing whether to approve or cancel a pesticide, EPA considers how much more it would cost the farmer to use an alternative pesticide or process

Table 16.5 U.S. Agencies Responsible for Monitoring the Food Supply

Agency Name	Responsibilities	Methods	How to Contact
United States Department of Agriculture (USDA)	• Enforces wholesomeness and quality standards for grains and produce (while in the field), meat, poultry, milk, and eggs and egg products	• Inspection • Grading • "Safe Handling Label"	www.usda.gov/fsis or www.nal.usda.gov/fnicfoodborne/foodborn.htm or call 1-800-535-4555
Bureau of Alcohol, Tobacco, and Fire Arms (ATF)	• Enforces laws on alcoholic beverages	• Inspection	www.atf.treas.gov
Environmental Protection Agency (EPA)	• Regulates pesticides • Establishes water quality standards	• Approval required for all U.S. pesticides • Sets pesticide residue limits in food	www.epa.gov
Food and Drug Administration (FDA)	• Ensures safety and wholesomeness of all foods in interstate commerce (except meat, poultry, and processed egg products) • Regulates seafood • Controls product labels	• Inspection • Food sample studies • Sets standards for specific foods	www.fda.gov or call 1-800-FDA-4010
Centers for Disease Control and Prevention (CDC)	• Protects food safety	• Responds to emergencies concerning foodborne illness • Surveys and studies environmental health problems • Directs/enforces quarantines • National programs for prevention and control of foodborne and other diseases	www.cdc.gov
The National Marine Fisheries Service or NOAA Fisheries	• Domestic and international conservation and management of living marine resources	• Voluntary seafood inspection program • Can use mark to show federal inspection	www.nmfs.noaa.gov
State and local governments	• Milk safety • Monitors food industry within their borders	• Inspection of food-related establishments	Government pages of telephone book

and whether cancellation would decrease productivity. After determining the dollar cost to the farmer, EPA then looks at costs to processors and consumers. Once a pesticide is approved for use, it must follow the margin of safety provisions required of food additives (see the section on testing food additives for safety).

How Safe Are Pesticides?

Dangers from exposure to pesticides through food depend on how potent the chemical toxin is, how concentrated it is in the food, how much and how frequently it's eaten, and the consumer's resistance or susceptibility to the substance. Pesticide use is clearly associated with declining water quality. Accumulating information also links pesticide use to increased cancer rates in farm communities. For rural counties in the United States, the incidence of lymph, genital, brain, and digestive tract cancers increases with higher-than-average pesticide use. Respiratory cancer cases increase with greater insecticide use. In tests using laboratory animals, scientists have found that some of the chemicals present in pesticide residues cause birth defects, sterility, tumors, organ damage, and injury to the central nervous system. Some pesticides persist in the environment for years.

Still, some researchers argue that the cancer risk from pesticide residues is hundreds of times less than the risk from eating such common foods as peanut butter, brown mustard, and basil. Plants manufacture their own toxic substances to defend themselves against insects, birds, and grazing animals (including humans). When plants are stressed or damaged, they produce even more of these toxins. Because of this, many foods contain naturally occurring chemicals considered toxic, and some are even carcinogenic. Other scientists argue that if natural carcinogens are already in the food supply, then we should reduce the number of added carcinogens whenever possible. In other words, we should do what we can to decrease the problem.

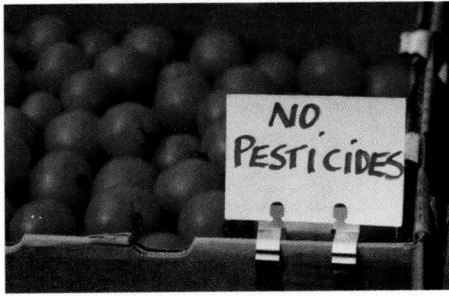

Fruits and vegetables grown without use of pesticides are available, and may bear an "organic" label (see Table 2.11 in Chapter 2 for rules regarding the use of the term "organic" on food labels). These products generally are more expensive than those grown using pesticides. Consumers need to decide if the potential benefits of the products are worth the extra cost.

The Risks of Pesticides to Children

Any discussions of pesticides and associated health risks must focus on children. They are not simply small adults in a biological sense. Children face a higher risk from pesticide exposure than do adults for several reasons.

1. Their exposure is greater; children eat more food in proportion to their body weight than do adults.
2. Children consume more foods that are potential sources of pesticide residues than do adults. For example, they eat more fruit.
3. Exposure at an early age carries a greater risk than does exposure later in life; residues can accumulate to toxic amounts over a longer period. Also, cancer has more time to develop.
4. Physiological susceptibility to the effects of carcinogens and other toxins in pesticides may be greater; the cells in children are dividing rapidly, and the enzyme systems that detoxify chemicals are not fully developed.

Until recent years, EPA did not consider these factors in risk calculations. However, the recent Food Quality Protection Act now requires EPA to look at age-related consumption data for the approval of new pesticides. Although children are at greater risk from pesticides, the magnitude of that risk and how best to calculate it are open to debate. Overall, experts stress the value of including fruits and vegetables in children's diets and caution parents not to change their children's diets to avoid these foods. Carefully washing fresh fruits and vegetables and consuming a wide variety are sufficient recommendations. Peeling fruits and vegetables is another option. A final general precaution is to keep children away from lawns, gardens, and flower beds that have recently been treated with pesticides and herbicides.

Tests of the Amounts of Pesticides in Foods

FDA tests thousands of raw products each year for pesticide residues. (A pesticide is considered illegal in this case if it is not approved for use on the crop in question or if the amount used exceeds the allowed tolerance.) The latest FDA study showed no residues in about 60% of

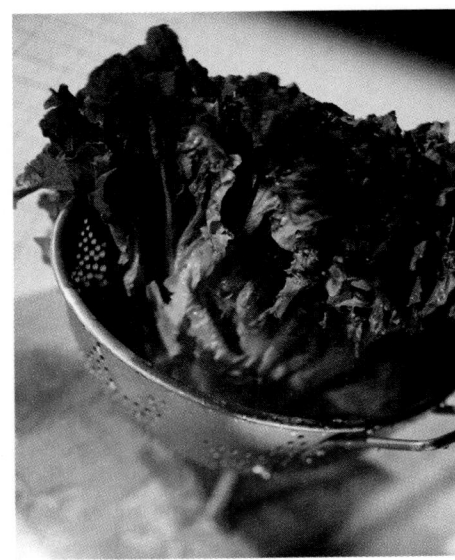

Rinsing fruits and vegetables under running water is advised to reduce pesticide exposure.

continued

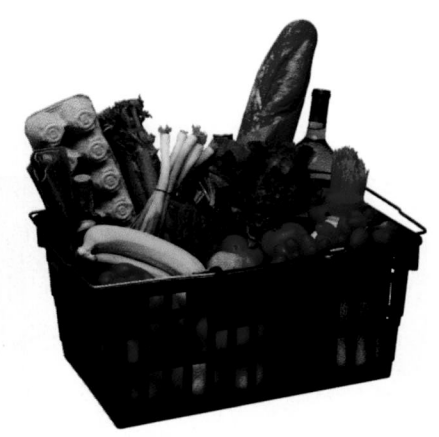

FDA's yearly evaluation of a "market basket" of typical foods shows that pesticide content is minimal in most foods.

samples. Less than 1% of domestic and about 3% of import samples had residues that were over tolerance. These findings continue to support previous FDA studies over the past 20 years that pesticide residues in foods are generally well below EPA tolerances, and they confirm the safety of the food supply relative to pesticide residues.

Residues sometimes appear on the wrong crops or in excessive amounts because of contamination from nearby farms via wind or water. When a problem is identified, FDA takes steps to make sure it's corrected and that the tainted food in question never reaches the consumer. However, of 600 pesticides available on international markets, many are not even detected by any of FDA's multiresidue tests. This has raised concern by pesticide critics with regard to imported foods. Better tests that detect single residues are less frequently used because of cost.

Personal Action

We often take risks in our own lives, but we prefer to have a choice in the matter after weighing the pros and cons. For instance, we can choose not to immunize a child, but we do so with the understanding that the child might get sick. We can also choose to risk cancer from smoking or to avoid that risk, or we can drive recklessly. In regard to pesticides in food, however, someone else is deciding what is acceptable and what is not. Our only choice is whether to buy or avoid pesticide-containing foods. In reality it's almost impossible to avoid pesticides entirely, because even organic produce often contains traces of pesticides, probably as the result of cross-contamination from nearby farms.

Short-term studies of the effects of pesticides on laboratory animals cannot pinpoint long-term cancer risks precisely. It should be clearly understood, however, that the presence of minute traces of an environmental chemical in a food doesn't mean that any adverse effect will result from eating that food.

FDA and other scientific organizations believe that the hazards are comparatively low and in the short run are less than the hazards of foodborne illness created in our own kitchens. We can't avoid pesticide risks entirely, but we can limit exposure by following some simple advice (Table 16.6).

We can also encourage farmers to use fewer pesticides to reduce exposure to our foods and water supplies, but we'll have to settle for produce that isn't perfect in appearance. Are you concerned enough about pesticides on food to change your shopping habits or take more political action?

Table 16.6 What You Can Do to Reduce Dietary Exposure to Pesticides

FDA's sampling and testing show that pesticide residues in foods do not pose a health hazard. Nevertheless, if you want to reduce dietary exposure to pesticides, follow this advice from the Environmental Protection Agency:

- Thoroughly rinse and scrub (with a brush if possible) fruits and vegetables. Peel them, if appropriate—although some nutrients will be peeled away.
- Remove the outer leaves of leafy vegetables, such as lettuce and cabbage.
- Trim fat from meat, poultry, and fish, remove skin (which contains most of the fat) from poultry and fish, and discard fats and oils in broths and pan drippings. Residues of some pesticides in feed concentrate in the animals' fat.
- When fishing, throw back the big fish—the little ones have had less time to take up and concentrate pesticides and other harmful residues. In addition, pay attention to any warnings by local authorities (and the fishing license) about the high risk for contamination in specific waters or species of fish.

Adapted from Food and Drug Administration: Safety first: Protecting America's food supply, *FDA Consumer,* p. 26, November 1988.

Undernutrition Throughout the World

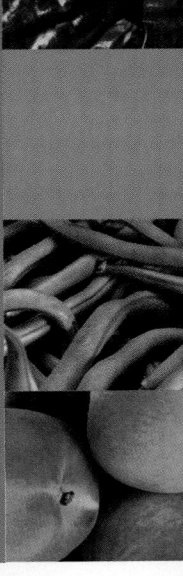

Chapter Outline

*T*he images are both vivid and heartrending. Emaciated children with enormous eyes and stomachs, too weak to cry, stare at us from news photos and television screens. Of the nearly 12 million children under 5 who die each year in developing countries, 55% of the deaths are attributable to undernutrition.

Today, nearly one in six people worldwide is chronically undernourished—too hungry to lead a productive, active life. Over the past 10 years, this problem has even worsened. Throughout the world the problems of poverty and undernutrition are widespread and growing.

The majority (two-thirds) of undernourished people live in Asia. However, the largest increases in numbers of chronically hungry people currently occur in eastern Africa, particularly in Ethiopia, Sudan, Rwanda, Burundi, Sierra Leone, Kenya, Somalia, and Tanzania. Their eyes haunt us.

This chapter examines the problem of undernutrition and the conditions that create it, as well as some possible solutions. If we are to eradicate undernutrition, we all have to understand the problem and assume responsibility for supplying some answers. It is important to recognize that many political leaders and citizens worldwide contribute directly and indirectly to the economic and social destruction that spawns hunger.

*Check out the **Contemporary Nutrition: Issues and Insights Online Learning Center** www.mhhe.com/wardlawcont5 for quizzes, flash cards, other activities, and web links designed to further help you learn about issues surrounding world hunger.*

Chapter Objectives

Chapter 17 is designed to allow you to:

1. Define and characterize the terms *hunger, malnutrition,* and *undernutrition.*

2. Evaluate the consequences of undernutrition during critical periods in a person's life.

3. Examine undernutrition in the United States and highlight several programs established to combat this problem.

4. Examine undernutrition in the developing world and evaluate the major obstacles that hinder a solution.

5. Outline some possible solutions to undernutrition in the developing world.

6. List the worldwide effects of AIDS.

7. Consider how biotechnology may help solve the food shortage/distribution problem in the developing world.

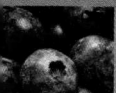 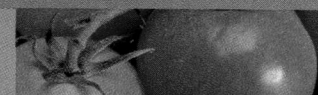

Refresh Your Memory

As you begin your study of world hunger in Chapter 17, you may want to review:

- Immune system function in Chapter 3

- The health effects of protein-energy malnutrition in Chapter 6

- The role of vitamin A and rich food sources in Chapter 8

- The roles of iron, zinc and iodide, and rich food sources in Chapter 9

- The advantage of breastfeeding to infants in Chapter 13

- Methods to monitor the adequacy of growth in Chapter 14

Real Life Scenario

*J*amal traveled during spring break with his church group to Guatemala. During their week-long stay, they were to help build shelters for people in the village in which a large fire had destroyed most of the housing a few weeks before. Jamal noticed that many of the children in the village are short, much shorter than the children in his neighborhood. Mothers in the village stated that their children often have diarrhea and are ill. Jamal also noticed that the children are not as lively as he would expect.

A nurse at the local health clinic pointed out that these children generally do not have enough to eat and that health problems are rampant. She hoped that the recent fire would spur the Guatemalan government to send supplies to the village, particularly food and medicines.

Should Jamal have been surprised by widespread disease and general listlessness of the children in the Guatemala village? What nutrients are likely to be deficient in the diets of these children, in turn contributing to their poor health status?

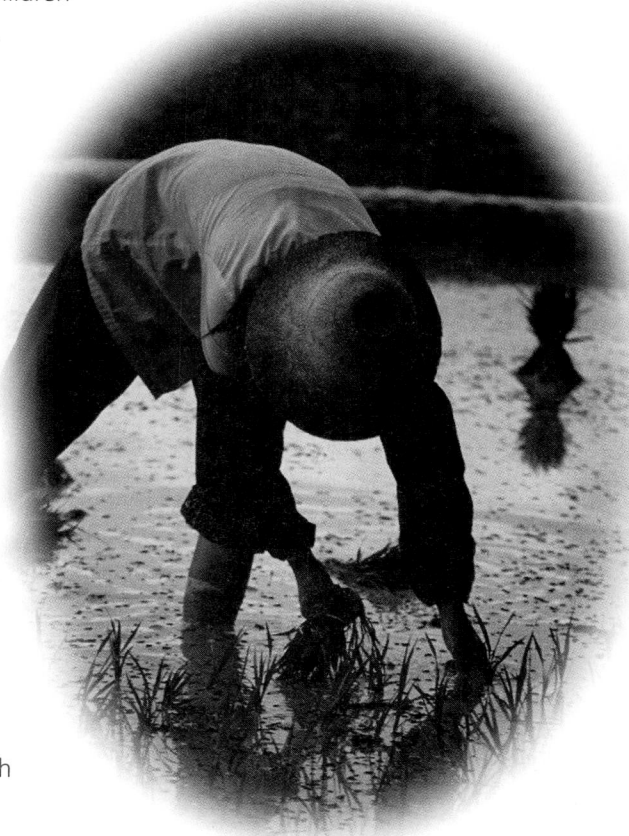

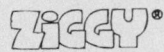utrition Connection

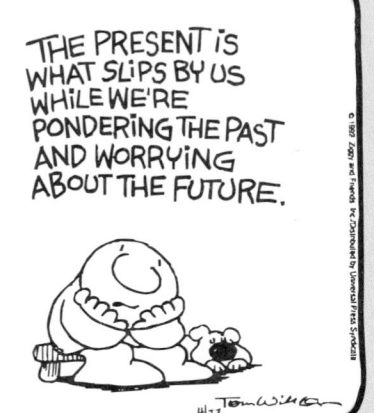

THE PRESENT IS WHAT SLIPS BY US WHILE WE'RE PONDERING THE PAST AND WORRYING ABOUT THE FUTURE.

Millions of people worldwide die each year from health problems related to undernutrition. War and environmental catastrophe combine today with the global threat of AIDS as important causes. Why must we act today to stem this tide of undernutrition? Why is Ziggy's concern an important one? This chapter provides some answers.

World Hunger: A Continuing Plague

In November 1974, the United Nations World Food Conference proclaimed its bold objective "that within a decade no child will go to bed hungry, that no family will fear for its next day's bread, and that no human being's future and capacities will be stunted by malnutrition." Today, this promise remains unfulfilled: Uncertainty regarding from where one's next meal will come remains a daily experience for one in seven people in the developing world (830 million to 1.1 billion) and one in ten households in the United States.

The famines that occurred in Ethiopia in the 1980s elicited widespread public support for immediate aid to the victims. Still, far from ending, hunger remains frequently in the news. The past 3 years of extended drought have once again left many people in Ethiopia without crops, livestock, and food. Civil wars and droughts in many parts of the world have brought millions of people to the brink of starvation. About two-thirds of these people live in Africa. Relief aid has been arriving but often with too little, too late. The deadly combination of political corruption, administrative ineptness, war, and poor weather has also led to increasing hunger in Bangladesh, Afghanistan, Haiti, the Philippines, Indonesia, Guinea, North Korea, and Cambodia.

We must face the reality that the United Nations' members have yet to meet their pledge to elevate 3 billion people (half of the world's population) out of abject poverty (living on less than $2 per day). We also have to consider that 45% of the world's income currently goes to the 12% of the world's people who live in the rich industrial nations such as the United States and Canada.

World Hunger Today

Let's begin our look at the problem of world hunger today by first defining some key words.

Hunger is the physiological state that results when not enough food is eaten to meet energy needs. It also describes an uneasiness, a discomfort, a weakness, or a pain caused by lack of food. If hunger is not relieved, the resulting medical and social costs of undernutrition are high—preterm births and mental retardation, inadequate

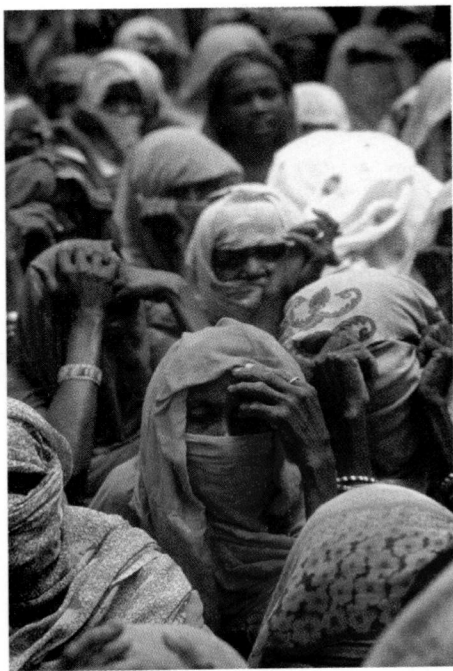

Every year crises that develop worldwide put many people at risk of undernutrition.

*A*bout 2 billion people in the world are infected with tuberculosis and are at risk of developing an active case of the disease. Tuberculosis kills 70% of the people who develop active cases. Undernutrition and HIV/AIDS makes matters even worse. The worst burden of tuberculosis worldwide occurs in India, China, Russia, South Africa, and Brazil.

Table 17.1 The Realities of Undernutrition

- Nearly one in six people worldwide is chronically undernourished—too hungry to lead a productive, active life. This includes one-third of the world's children.
- About 55,000 people die of hunger each day—two-thirds of them children.
- Three million newborns in the developing world die in the first week of life.
- Over half of all children who die each year in developing countries do so from causes that could be prevented at low cost.
- At least 250,000–500,000 children are permanently blinded each year simply from lack of vitamin A. About 100 million–140 million children are deficient in vitamin A.
- Residents in developed countries spend more money on pet food, perfumes, and cosmetics than it would take to provide basic education, water and sanitation, health care, and nutrition for all those now deprived of it.
- About 50 million people worldwide have developed brain damage from maternal iodide deficiency; currently, 2 billion people are at risk for iodide deficiency.
- Women in poor countries average up to four times more births than women in North America.
- Every day the world produces about 2400 kcal for each person, generally meeting average energy needs. A daily intake less than 2100 kcal would not likely sustain an older child or adult.
- Poor women in developing countries face a 50 to 200-fold increased risk of death in pregnancy, compared with women in North America.
- In many developing countries, life expectancy of the population is one-half to two-thirds of that in North America.
- Almost half of the world's people earn less than $200 a year—many use 80% to 90% of that income to obtain food. About $2000 to $3000 of income each year is needed for a person to reach the life expectancy seen in North America.
- Of the 6 billion people on earth, more than 1 billion drink contaminated water. In India alone, 300,000 children die each year from drinking polluted water.
- About 3 billion people in the world live without proper sanitation, such as reliable toilet facilities.
- About 1 billion people in the world have iron deficiency.
- Developing countries have 95% of the over 40 million AIDS cases worldwide.
- Developing countries bear 93% of the world's disease burden but expend only 11% of the world's health-care resources.

growth and development in childhood, poor school performance, decreased work output in adulthood, and chronic disease (Table 17.1). Symptoms of chronic hunger are found not only among people in the developing world but also among many people living at or below the poverty level in North America. Of any industrialized country, the United States has the largest number of children living in poverty (12 million under the age of 19). About one out of every six children in the United States goes hungry or is at risk for inadequate food.

Malnutrition is a condition of impaired development or function caused by either a long-term deficiency or an excess in energy and/or nutrient intake, the latter representing the state of overnutrition described in Chapter 2. When food supplies are low and the population is large, undernutrition is common, leading to nutritional deficiency diseases, such as goiter (from an iodide deficiency) and xerophthalmia (eye problems caused by poor vitamin A intake). However, when the food supply is ample or overabundant, incorrect food choices coupled with an excessive intake can lead to overnutrition-related chronic diseases, such as type 2 diabetes.

Undernutrition is the most common form of malnutrition among the poor in both developing and developed countries. Currently, about half of the 4 million African children under 5 years of age who die annually are undernourished. Undernutrition is also the primary cause of specific nutrient deficiencies that can result in muscle wasting, blindness, scurvy, pellagra, beriberi, anemia, rickets, goiter, and a host of other problems (Table 17.2).

The most critical micronutrients missing from diets worldwide are iron, vitamin A, vitamin B-12, and iodide. About 1 billion people, mostly in the developing world, are

Table 17.2 Effects of Nutrient-Deficiency Diseases That Commonly Accompany Undernutrition

Disease and Key Nutrient Involved	Typical Effects	Foods Rich in Deficient Nutrient	Where the Problem Currently Still Exists
Xerophthalmia Vitamin A	Blindness from chronic eye infections, retarded growth, dryness and keratinization of epithelial tissues	Liver, fortified milk, sweet potatoes, spinach, greens, carrots, cantaloupe, apricots	Asia, Africa
Rickets Vitamin D	Poorly calcified bones, bowed legs, other bone deformities	Fortified milk, fish oils, sun exposure	Asia and Africa where religious dress codes prevent women and children from receiving adequate sun exposure; older adults in developed nations
Beriberi Thiamin	Nerve degeneration, altered muscle coordination, cardiovascular problems	Sunflower seeds, pork, whole and enriched grains, dried beans	Areas of famine in Africa
Ariboflavinosis Riboflavin	Inflammation of tongue, mouth, face and oral cavity, nervous system disorders	Milk, mushrooms, spinach, liver, enriched grains	Areas of famine in Africa
Pellagra Niacin	Diarrhea, dermatitis, dementia	Mushrooms, bran, tuna, chicken, beef, peanuts, whole and enriched grains	Areas of famine in Africa
Scurvy Vitamin C	Delayed wound healing, internal bleeding, abnormal formation of bones and teeth	Citrus fruits, strawberries, broccoli	Areas of famine in Africa
Iron deficiency anemia Iron	Reduced work output, retarded growth, increased health risk in pregnancy	Meats, seafood, broccoli, peas, bran, whole-grain and enriched breads	Worldwide
Goiter Iodide	Enlarged thyroid gland in teenagers and adults, possible mental retardation, cretinism	Iodized salt, saltwater fish	South America, Eastern Europe, Africa

Often two or more nutrition-deficiency diseases are found in an undernourished person in the developing world. This separate discussion of nutrients just makes it easier to see the important role of each nutrient.

affected with iron deficiency. This impairs the cognitive development of children and likely is a permanent result if the iron deficiency is prolonged in early infancy. It is estimated that 20 million people worldwide show brain damage from preventable maternal iodide deficiency. Although severe vitamin A deficiency, which causes blindness, is on the decline, up to 250 to 500 thousand preschool children are still affected by it. This vitamin deficiency also raises the risk for other diseases, such as measles. The United Nations International Children's Fund reports that the lives of 1 million to 3 million children could be saved annually in the developing world if vitamin A supplements were provided a few times a year. The annual cost per child would be about 6 cents.

Of the 6 billion people in the world, up to 3 billion may be affected by some form of micronutrient malnutrition and experience episodes of food shortages. Death and disease from infections, particularly those causing acute and prolonged diarrhea or acute lower respiratory disease, increase dramatically when the infections are

famine An extreme shortage of food, which leads to massive starvation in a population; often associated with crop failures, war, and political unrest.

M ore than 3 million people may have perished in the great famine of 1943 in Bengal, India. In 1974, another 1.5 million from that region starved in the country of Bangladesh. China suffered an almost unbelievable famine from 1959 to 1961—estimates of mortality range from 16 million to 64 million.

superimposed on a state of chronic undernutrition. Chronic undernutrition leaves many people in the developing world in a continual state of depressed immune function. Diarrhea alone is the number one killer of children in developing countries, responsible for over 2 million deaths of children under 5 years of age.

Protein-energy malnutrition (PEM) is a form of undernutrition caused by an extremely deficient intake of energy or protein generally accompanied by an illness. The typically dramatic results of PEM—kwashiorkor and marasmus—were described in Chapter 6. This chapter focuses on the more subtle effects of a chronic lack of food.

Famine is not the same thing as chronic hunger. Although both result from poverty and a lack of food, famine is the extreme form of chronic hunger. Periods of famine are characterized by large-scale loss of life, social disruption, and economic chaos that slows food production. As a result of these extreme events, the affected community experiences a downward spiral characterized by human distress; sales of land, livestock, and other important farm assets; migration; division and impoverishment of the poorest families; crime; and the weakening of customary moral codes, as seen in Sudan and Rwanda. In the midst of all this, undernutrition rates soar; infectious diseases, such as cholera, spread; and many people die.

Special efforts are needed to eradicate the fundamental causes of famine. Causes vary by region and decade, but the most common underlying cause is crop failure. The most obvious causes of crop failure are bad weather, war, and civil strife, or all three. War, in fact, deserves a special focus; this will be specifically addressed in an upcoming section on war and political/civil unrest.

▮ Critical Life Stages When Undernutrition Is Particularly Devastating

Prolonged undernutrition is detrimental to health at all stages of life but is particularly critical during some periods of growth and old age (Fig. 17.1).

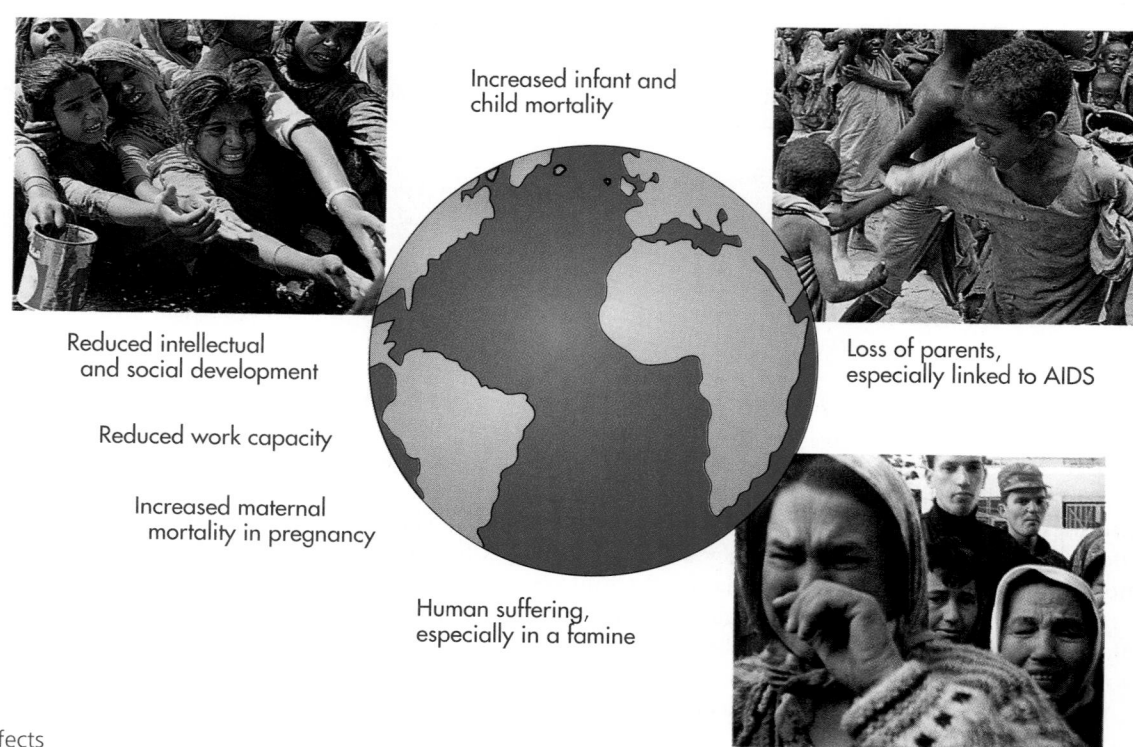

Increased infant and child mortality

Reduced intellectual and social development

Reduced work capacity

Increased maternal mortality in pregnancy

Human suffering, especially in a famine

Loss of parents, especially linked to AIDS

Exploitation of women in general

Figure 17.1 Undernutrition affects many aspects of human health and humanity in general.

Pregnancy

The period when undernutrition poses the greatest health risk is during pregnancy. A pregnant woman needs extra nutrients to meet both her own needs and those of her developing fetus. Nourishing the fetus may deplete stores of maternal nutrients. Maternal iron-deficiency anemia is one possible consequence (see Chapter 13).

In Africa, women give birth, on average, to more than six live babies. Coupled with chronic undernutrition, these high birth rates create a 1 in 20 chance that a woman will die from pregnancy-related causes. In contrast, North American women face a risk of 1 death in about 8000 births from pregnancy-related causes. No other social indicator, including literacy, life expectancy, and infant mortality, betrays a wider gap between the developing and industrialized worlds.

Fetal and Infant Stages

The fetus faces major health risks from undernutrition during gestation. To support growth and development of the brain and other body tissues, a growing fetus requires a rich supply of protein, vitamins, and minerals. When these needs are not met, the infant is often born before 37 weeks of gestation, well before the 40 weeks of gestation that is considered ideal. The consequences of preterm birth include reduced lung function and a weakened immune system. These conditions not only compromise health but also increase the likelihood of premature death. Long-term problems in growth and development can result if the infant survives. In extreme cases, low-birth-weight babies (about 5.5 pounds [2.5 kilograms] or less) face 5 to 10 times the normal risk of dying before the age of 1 year, primarily because of reduced lung development as noted in Chapter 13. When low birth weight is accompanied by other physical abnormalities, medical intervention can cost $200,000 or more. These costs can only be met in developed countries.

In the United States, low birth weight accounts for more than half of all infant deaths and for 75% of deaths of babies under 1 month of age. Currently, about 7% of infants born in the United States have low birth weights. The comparable Canadian statistic is closer to 6%. Worldwide, more than 30 million infants are born with low birth weight.

Childhood

Early childhood, when growth is rapid, is another period when undernutrition is extremely risky. The central nervous system—including the brain—is particularly vulnerable because of rapid growth from conception through early childhood. After the preschool years, brain growth and development slow dramatically until maturity, when they cease. Nutritional deprivation, especially in early infancy, can lead to permanent brain impairment. If more is not done, it is projected that ongoing undernutrition could leave more than 1 billion children with mental impairment by 2020.

In general, poor children experience more nutritional deprivation and overall illness and are more severely affected than other children. Stunted growth is an obvious effect, seen in about one-third of children under 5 years of age worldwide. In addition, iron-deficiency anemia is much more common among poor children than children from less deprived families. This deficiency can lead to fatigue upon exertion, reduced stamina, stunted growth, impaired motor development, and learning problems. Undernutrition in childhood can also weaken resistance to infection because immune function decreases when such nutrients as protein, vitamin A, and zinc are very low in a diet. Clearly, undernutrition and illness have a cyclical relationship. Not only does undernutrition cause illness, but illness worsens undernutrition, particularly by diarrhea and infectious diseases. For this reason, many children in developing countries are dying from the combination of malnutrition and infection. Conversely, when adequate nutrients are restored to children's diets, improvements in health can be obvious.

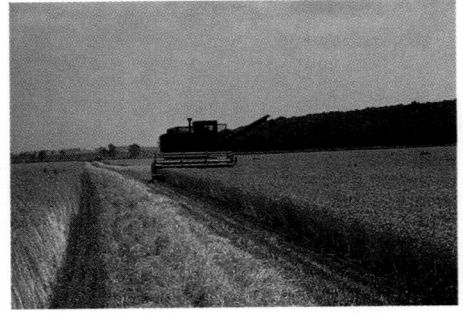
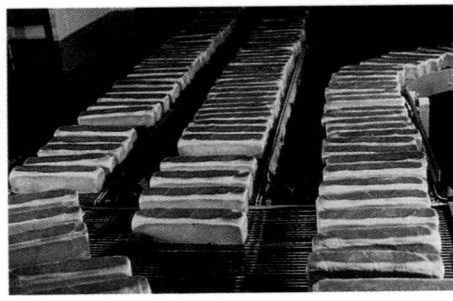

The bounty of food we enjoy in North America relies on our rich agricultural resources. Many developing countries do not have such resources to employ.

About 30% of children in developing countries show evidence of growth failure.

Later Years

Older adults are also at risk for undernutrition. They often require nutrient-dense foods, in amounts depending on their state of health and degree of physical activity. Because many of them have fixed incomes and incur significant medical costs, food often becomes a low-priority item. In addition, older adults are often unable to take care of all their own needs, are sometimes isolated, and may be depressed—all important factors that influence food intake (see Chapter 15).

Another Bite

*I*n the 1940s, a group of researchers led by Dr. Ansel Keys maintained 32 previously healthy men on a diet averaging about 1600 kcal daily for 6 months. During this time, the men lost an average of 24% of their body weight. After about 3 months, the participants complained of fatigue, muscle soreness, irritability, and hunger pains. They exhibited a lack of ambition and self-discipline and poor concentration. They were often moody and depressed. They became less able to laugh heartily, sneeze, and tolerate heat. Heart rate and muscle tone also decreased. When the men were permitted to eat normally again, the desire for more food and a feeling of fatigue continued, even after 12 weeks of rehabilitation. Full recovery required about 8 months.

The effects of undernutrition in poor countries are probably even greater than this research indicated because the participants in this study had adequate vitamin and mineral intakes. In addition, the inhabitants of poorer countries must contend with recurrent infections, poor sanitary conditions, extreme weather conditions, and regular exposure to extremely infectious diseases. They require greater amounts of certain nutrients—especially iron—to combat rampant parasite and other infections, which compounds the problem. Deficiencies in both iron and zinc can lead to reduced immune function and thereby increase the risk of disease caused by infections such as diarrhea, pneumonia, and dysentery.

■ General Effects of Semistarvation

In the initial stages, the results of undernutrition from semistarvation are often so mild that physical symptoms are absent and blood tests do not usually detect the slight metabolic changes. Even in the absence of clinical symptoms, however, undernourishment may affect reproductive capacity, resistance to and recovery from disease, physical activity and work output, and lead to lassitude and behavior problems. Recall from Chapter 2 that, as tissues continue to be depleted of nutrients, blood tests eventually detect biochemical changes, such as a drop in blood hemoglobin concentration. Physical symptoms, such as body weakness, appear with further depletion. Finally, the full-blown symptoms of the predominating deficiency are recognizable, such as when edema accompanies a protein deficiency.

In general, when a few people in a population develop a severe deficiency, this represents only the tip of the iceberg. Typically, a much greater number have milder degrees of undernutrition. These deficiencies should not, therefore, be dismissed as trivial, especially in the developing world. It is becoming clear that combined deficiencies of specific vitamins and the minerals iron and zinc can seriously reduce work performance, even when they don't cause obvious physical symptoms. This resulting state of ill health, in turn, diminishes the ability of individuals, communities, and even whole countries to perform at peak levels of physical and mental capacity, creating a dearth in human resources (Fig. 17.2).

*H*unger reduces energy and strength; it diminishes concentration. Hunger reduces a child's ability to learn. Hunger hurts businesses when workers are more concerned about their next meal than the task at hand. Hunger among older adults makes chronic health conditions worse and can cause others. Hunger is patient, quiet, and persistent, and its effects can be widespread.

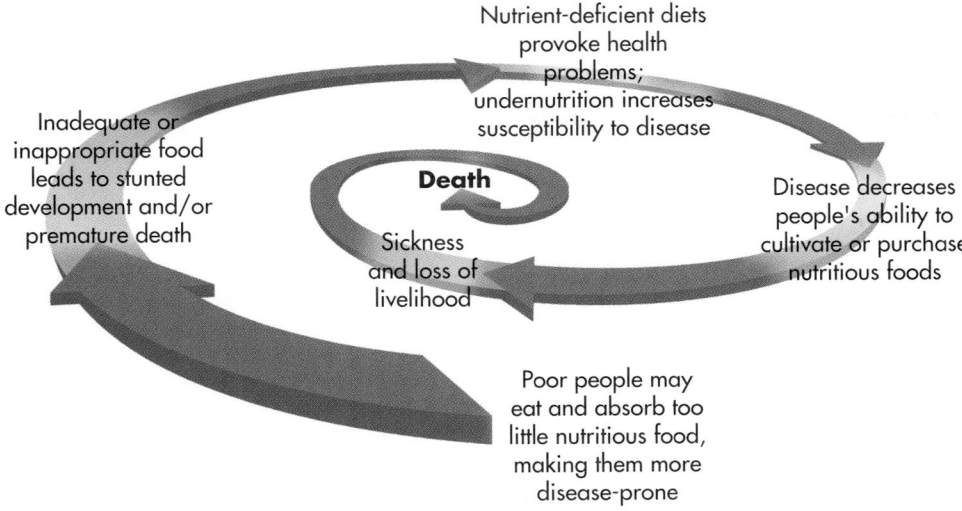

Nutrient-deficient diets provoke health problems; undernutrition increases susceptibility to disease

Inadequate or inappropriate food leads to stunted development and/or premature death

Death

Sickness and loss of livelihood

Disease decreases people's ability to cultivate or purchase nutritious foods

Poor people may eat and absorb too little nutritious food, making them more disease-prone

Figure 17.2 The downward spiral of poverty and illness can ultimately end in death (based on World Food Program graphic).

Scenario Follow-Up

Jamal should not be surprised that the children in the village were often sick and listless. Vitamin A, iron, iodide, and zinc deficiencies contribute to poor growth and depressed immune function. One or more of these deficiencies is likely seen in many children in the village. The diets of these children may also be marginal in protein and calories, further contributing to poor growth and overall health. We know from many nutrition intervention studies that the provision of more calories, protein, vitamin A, iron, iodide, and zinc—along with other micronutrients—can reverse some of this disease pattern and improve health. Still, we know that many children throughout the world exist in a stunted and immune-depressed state associated with their chronically deficient diets.

Concept Check

Hunger is the uneasiness and pain that results when insufficient food is eaten to meet energy needs. Chronic hunger leads to undernutrition, which can cause growth failure in children and weakness in adults. Risk of infection increases, and nutrient-deficiency diseases result. The primary cause of undernutrition is poverty. The critical periods for undernutrition occur during pregnancy, infancy, childhood, and old age. Chronic undernutrition causes decreased work performance and motivation and compromises immune function. The adverse effects in pregnancy and infancy are quite dramatic, as evidenced by mortality rates much higher than those of healthy populations.

Undernutrition in the United States

About 31 million (11%) of people in the United States live at or near the poverty level, currently estimated at about $17,050 annually for a family of four (Table 17.3). These poor include about 16% of all children; children, in fact, comprise about 37% of the poor.

Currently, 8% of Caucasians are poor, 24% of African-Americans are poor, and 23% of Hispanics are poor. Many Native Americans are also poor, as are 11% of Asian-Americans. (Many Native Americans in Canada also live in poverty.)

Critical Thinking

While studying early childhood development, Nakia was surprised to learn that some children in the United States are undernourished. What evidence might Nakia observe in children that would suggest undernourishment?

Table 17.3 The Realities of Poverty and Undernutrition in the United States

- About 7% of infants born in the United States are low birth weight. This accounts for more than half of all infant deaths and for 75% of deaths of babies under 1 month of age.
- The infant mortality rate in the United States is higher than that of 24 other industrialized countries. Teenage pregnancy contributes to infant mortality because young mothers frequently don't meet their nutrient needs.
- Single-parent families constitute about 25% of all families with children. The poverty rate (60%) for the approximately 14 million children in such families is five times higher than that for children in two-parent families.
- About 31 million people in the United States live at or near the poverty level. These poor include about 16% of all children; children, in fact, comprise 37% of the poor. Hunger frequently accompanies poverty.
- A family of four in the United States at the bottom 20% of households has an average income of $17,196. Contrast that to the average earnings of the top 20% of households: $79,375.
- In the United States, an estimated 12 million people, or 6.5% of all adults, have experienced homelessness sometime during their lives. An episode of homelessness nearly always lasts for at least 1 week and often for a month or more.
- The Food Stamp program for low-income people provides each household with $170 per month. About 1 person in 16 currently participates in this program.
- Second Harvest, the largest U.S. food bank, estimates that 23 million people, or more than 1 person in 10, rely on food depositories and soup kitchens to feed themselves and their families. Most of these people, the organization reports, are workers who have lost their jobs.
- Food thrown out in U.S. cafeterias, supermarkets, and restaurants could feed 49 million people per year.

Undernutrition in North America is a much more subtle problem than in developing countries. To the untrained eye, undernourished children may just seem skinny, when, in fact, their growth is being stunted by insufficient nutrients. It is also possible that poverty-stricken children in this country are overweight. This is because quick-service restaurants provide cheap, accessible food, and, consequently, the poor often eat a diet high in fat and calories.

The poor often face difficult choices: whether to buy groceries for the family or pay this month's rent; whether to have dental work done or pay the current utility bill; whether to replace clothes the children have outgrown or pay for transportation to apply for a job. Food is one of the few flexible items in a poor person's budget. Rents are fixed, utility costs aren't negotiable, the price of medical care and prescription drugs can't be bargained down, and bus drivers won't accept less than the going rate to transport riders. A person can always eat less, however. The short-term consequences may be less dramatic than having the utilities shut off. The long-term cumulative effects, however, are disturbing.

In sheer numbers, undernutrition in the United States is a troubling problem. Its existence is all the more disturbing because, although the threat of undernutrition for most people in the United States was virtually eliminated in the 1970s, it reemerged and spread rapidly in the 1980s. The fact that undernutrition and hunger remain today indicates that their roots are mainly political and socioeconomic, rather than technical. Clearly, U.S. society is productive enough to generate the resources required to feed all its citizens. (In the developing world, far more factors complicate this problem.)

■ Helping the Hungry in the United States: An Historical Perspective

Until the twentieth century, individuals and a wide variety of charitable, often church-related organizations, provided most of the help to poor, undernourished people in the United States. Few early efforts distributed direct cash payments to poor people because these were thought to reduce recipients' motivation to improve their circumstances or change behavior, such as excessive drinking, that contributed to their poverty. Beginning in the early 1900s, the involvement of local, county, and state governments in providing assistance to the poor has steadily increased.

Depression Era to the Mid-1970s

The Great Depression of the 1930s marked a decisive change. Studies at the time documented both undernutrition and the existence of widespread pellagra (niacin deficiency) and rickets (vitamin D deficiency). In response, the federal government

Table 17.4 Some Current Federally Subsidized Programs That Supply Food for People in the United States

Program	Eligibility	Description
Food Stamps	Low income; employment generally necessary	Coupons or Electronic Benefit Transfer (debit) cards are given to purchase food at grocery stores; the amount is based on size of household and income.
Emergency Food System	Low income	Food stamps are issued on 24-hour notice for 1 month while eligibility for further use of the program can be investigated.
Commodity Supplemental Food Program	Certain low-income populations, such as pregnant women and young children	USDA surplus foods are distributed by county agencies.
Special Supplemental Nutrition Program for Women, Infants, and Children (WIC)	Low-income pregnant/lactating women, infants, and children less than 5 years old at nutritional risk	Coupons are given to purchase milk, cheese, fruit juice, cereal, infant formula, and other specific food items at grocery stores.
School Lunch	Low income	Free or reduced-price lunch is distributed by the school; meal follows USDA pattern based on the Food Guide Pyramid; cost for the child depends on family income. In schools without a lunch program, special milk program may be available.
School Breakfast	Low income	Free or reduced-price breakfast is distributed by the school; meal follows USDA pattern; cost for the child depends on family income.
Child Care Food Program	Child enrolled in organized child-care program; income guidelines are the same as those for the School Lunch program	Reimbursement is given for meals supplied to children at the site; meals must follow USDA guidelines based on the Food Guide Pyramid.
Congregate Meals for the Elderly	Age 60 or over (no income guidelines)	Free noon meal is furnished at a site; meal follows specific pattern based on one-third of nutrient needs.
Home-Delivered Meals	Age 60 or over, homebound	Noon meal is delivered at no cost or for a fee, depending on income, at least 5 days a week. Sometimes other meals for later consumption are delivered at the same time; private organizations that sponsor these programs often refer to them as "Meals on Wheels."
Summer Food Service Program	Low income	Free, nutritious meals and snacks are given to a group of children in a low-income area at a central site, such as a school or a community center during long school vacations.

sponsored soup kitchens and other programs that distributed food commodities throughout the country. During World War II, a large percentage of the men rejected for the draft for physical reasons were found to have been undernourished 10 to 12 years earlier, during the Depression era. This practical demonstration of the long-term detrimental effects of childhood undernutrition led the U.S. Congress to enact legislation setting up the School Lunch program in 1946.

In the 1950s, it was assumed that all in the United States had enough to eat. Nevertheless, occasional reports of undernutrition surfaced, mostly among the truly destitute: migrant workers, Native Americans, African-Americans in the South, unemployed minorities in general, and some older people.

After observing extensive hunger and poverty during his presidential campaign in the 1960s, John F. Kennedy revitalized the Food Stamp program, which actually had begun two decades earlier, and expanded commodity distribution programs. The Food Stamp program for low-income people allows recipients to use food stamps to purchase food and seeds—but not tobacco, cleaning items, alcoholic beverages, and nonedible products—at stores authorized to accept them. Each participating household receives about $170 per month, on average. Currently about 18 million people in the United States participate in this program (Table 17.4).

The presence of undernutrition in the United States raises a broad question for the society at large: Where can people in such situations turn when their own resources fail? The responsibility for helping those in need could lie with federal, state, and local governments; religious groups; charitable organizations; and, in many cases, with the individuals themselves. All can be part of the solution.

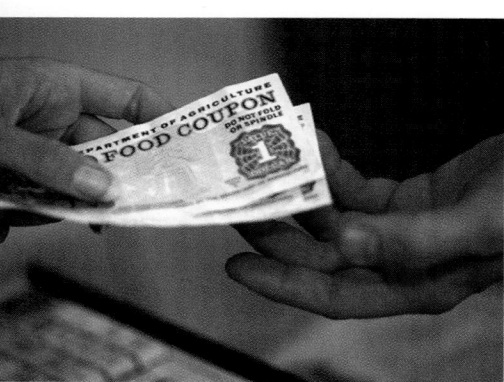

The Food Stamp program is part of the social safety net in the United States.

*O*ne goal of Healthy People 2010 *is to increase food security among* U.S. households from the current 88% to 94%.

The U.S. Congress established the school breakfast program in 1965 as politicians were made aware of the number of children coming to school hungry. School breakfast and lunch programs still enable low-income students—6.5 million for breakfast and 26 million for lunch—to receive meals free or at reduced cost if certain income guidelines are met (under $22,945 to $32,653, respectively, for annual income of a family of four). In the same year, the U.S. Congress funded group noontime (called *congregate*) meals and home-delivered meals for all citizens over 60 years of age, regardless of income. Both remain active programs, serving about 1 million meals each day, but they still do not reach all who need help. In addition, in 1972 the Special Supplemental Nutrition Program for Women, Infants, and Children (WIC) was authorized. This program provides food vouchers and nutrition education to low-income pregnant and lactating women and their young children. Today, it serves about 7 million people.

Political and social awareness of hunger and undernutrition in the late 1960s was spurred on by the book *Hunger USA* and a resulting television documentary, *Hunger in America*, shown in May 1968. The film graphically demonstrated that hunger exists in all areas and ethnic groups in the United States. The response was dramatic. Between 1969 and 1971, some already large federal food programs were expanded and others were created. For example, the Food Stamp program served only 2 million people in 1968, but by 1971 it was serving 11 million. The School Lunch program, which served only 2 million poor children before 1970, was serving 8 million children by 1971. Soon after, the School Breakfast program, a pilot program for children living in impoverished areas, became available nationally. And, as just mentioned, in 1972 the Special Supplemental Nutrition Program for Women, Infants, and Children (WIC) began.

A Reevaluation for Our Times

The first official recognition that widespread hunger had reappeared in the United States came from a conference of mayors in 1982. Why was there a sudden increase in hungry people in the United States? First, unemployment in the United States rose in early 1980. Second, the eligibility and funding for federal food assistance programs, such as the Food Stamp program and the School Lunch and Breakfast programs, were tightened and reduced, respectively. Overall, the safety net of the previous decade became more porous: Hunger and related food insecurity has thus continued to be a problem in the United States.

USDA defines this food insecurity as not having enough food, enough money to buy food, or experiencing concern over having enough food. Food insecurity includes limiting or reducing food intake, cutting or skipping meals, or feeding children a less than nutritious diet, without resorting to unusual strategies to obtain food (e.g., stealing or scavenging). About 10% of households in the United States fall into this category. In contrast, food security means household members had access at all times to enough food for an active, healthy life.

Privately funded programs have stepped in to take an important role in augmenting state and federal efforts to combat hunger and related food insecurity in the United States. There are currently more than 180 food banks, 23,000 food pantries, and 3300 soup kitchens helping to cope with this problem. A recent survey found that slightly more than two of every three people requesting such emergency food assistance were members of families—children and their parents. Second Harvest, the largest domestic hunger-relief organization in the United States, has recently merged with Food Chain, a leader in food-rescue programs. Second Harvest estimates that more than 1 in 12 of all people in the United States rely on food depositories and soup kitchens to feed themselves and their families, and the number is on the rise. Nearly 40% of people asking for help lived in families with at least one working adult.

■ Socioeconomic Factors Related to Undernutrition

In the United States today, persistent hunger and food insecurity are largely associated with two interrelated conditions: poverty and homelessness. Thus, the economic, social, and political changes that lead to an increase in the number of poor or homeless people also tend to intensify the problem.

Poverty

Although highly trained people are quite competitive in the increasingly global economy, there is a glut of unskilled manual labor available throughout the world. Many families have suffered economic hardship caused by massive layoffs in U.S. manufacturing industries, which began in the late 1980s and continued in the 1990s as the economy became more global. Furthermore, many jobs created in the 1980s were in the service sector, such as quick-service restaurants. When one or both parents have one of these low-paying jobs—even full-time—their families may still be at or below the poverty level. Note that parents in most poor families do work; nearly two in three families contain at least one worker.

Another primary factor contributing to poverty has been the dramatic increase in the number of single-parent families in the United States, the result of high rates of divorce and out-of-wedlock births. Currently, single-parent families constitute about 4 million. The poverty rate (40%) for the approximately 19 million children in single-parent families is five times higher than the rate for those in two-parent families.

Some observers believe that many publicly funded assistance programs have actually provided an incentive for poor, single women to have more children: The more children they have, the more welfare and other assistance benefits they receive. The new welfare reform laws reflect this thinking by requiring able-bodied adults to get jobs, limiting future direct support to 3 years in a row and a total of 5 years in a lifetime. It is up to each state to determine how to implement this work requirement and establish exceptions, such as in the case of disability, short term downturns in the economy, or other overwhelming hardships.

Many politicians and political writers point out that we need greater wisdom in our approach to illegitimacy and single parenthood. Some suggest improving child care, teaching parenting skills, and expanding job opportunities. To a great extent, states are doing this as they help people end their dependence on welfare payments. Nationwide, the number of people on welfare rolls has fallen 60% since 1992, but recently has stabilized, and even increased slightly in some states. People remaining on welfare typically have numerous barriers to overcome if they are to support themselves and family members. There is also concern that the incomes of many people leaving welfare are still too low to meet needs because most of the jobs they find pay minimum wage. These changes in welfare laws will be reevaluated by the U.S. Congress in 2002; it is likely that the work requirement and time limits will remain in some form.

Homelessness

The economics of poverty and undernutrition have changed in one additional important way. Homelessness is much more evident now than in 1980. Families with children currently account for about 43% of the homeless. An estimated 12 million people, or 6.5% of all adults, in the United States have experienced homelessness sometime during their lives. Episodes of homelessness nearly always last for at least 1 week and often for a month or more. The estimated lifetime homelessness rate rises to about 15% of the adult population in the United States when it includes people who have moved into someone else's residence during periods when they had nowhere else to live.

Although many citizens of the United States in general are enjoying continuing prosperity, the economic status of many of the working poor has declined because

The availability of cooking facilities affects nutrient intake among the poor. Without cooking facilities, people may buy expensive foods that require no preparation. These are typically processed snack foods, which provide food energy but are often lacking in nutrients.

Homeless children suffer higher rates of many medical problems than do other children, some of which include:
Upper respiratory tract infections
Scabies and lice
Tooth decay
Ear and skin infections
Diaper rash
Eye infections
Developmental delays
Trauma-related injuries

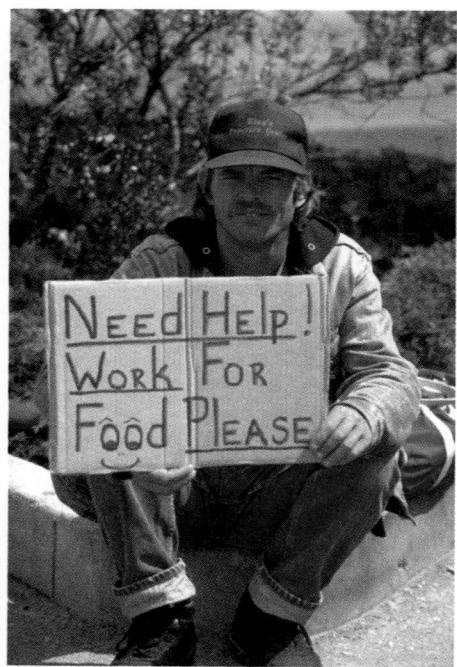

Major job layoffs in blue-collar industries have contributed to the twin problems of hunger and homelessness in the United States.

affordable housing is harder and harder for them to find. Due to the nation's rising prosperity, higher-income tenants have bid up the prices of the apartments in some cities beyond the financial resources of the poorer tenants. The U.S. government considers housing costs, which include rent and utilities, to be affordable if they consume no more than 30% of a family's income. A recent U.S. government report stated that 5.4 million low-income families pay more than half their incomes for housing or live in dilapidated units. These families, although not homeless, are likely to experience undernutrition without direct food assistance. Moreover, the continuing changes in the economic circumstances they face could force such poor families into actual homelessness, at least temporarily.

Other important causes of homelessness include the widespread release of mentally ill patients from mental institutions in the 1980s, unemployment, substance abuse, and personal crises. The abuse of alcohol and crack cocaine is another notable cause. Up to 85% of all homeless people in large cities in the United States abuse alcohol or drugs or have a mental illness. Most people with such problems are unable to find and hold employment; without support from family or friends, they and their dependents will probably become homeless.

■ Possible Solutions to Hunger in the United States

Few would argue the need to support the physically and mentally handicapped, as well as the multitude of poor children, in the United States. The debate begins when able-bodied adults are receiving public aid. Many of these people have extenuating circumstances or have dug such a deep hole for themselves financially that it is difficult to get out. It is also true that the United States has enough money and food to feed every citizen. The question is, can government programs provide a permanent solution to poverty?

Private emergency-food network systems are also important, as noted earlier, but are not sufficient to meet all food needs in the United States. Furthermore, most of the donated items are limited in nutritional value. By necessity, processed and canned grocery items predominate, rather than protein-rich foods and perishable items, such as fresh produce and milk.

Still, a long-term solution to the problem of hunger in the United States can't be achieved by the government or private agencies alone. Change also requires a cultural shift emphasizing the responsibility of all citizens to provide as best they can for themselves, their families, and the less fortunate around them. Many in the United States consider an increase in individual responsibility as a critical goal. Government programs can't easily fix poverty and the resulting hunger that stem from irresponsible individual behavior. Government programs can, however, help reduce or prevent the poverty that results largely from lack of education or opportunity.

Clearly, the victims of poverty don't deserve all the blame. The poor confront substantial difficulties: substandard education and training, poor communication skills, lack of reliable and safe child care, inability to relocate, little employment experience, and no economic reserves to fall back on during crises. Even with a strong desire for a better life, people may get discouraged and apathetic in the face of apparently insurmountable obstacles. Moreover, many of the poor are unable to meet the demands of a modern, dynamic society—in particular, older adults, sick, and disabled people, and young single mothers with children. Regardless of how repugnant government assistance appears to some people, it will probably always be necessary to some extent.

Because long-term undernutrition—especially among children—has both individual and societal consequences, all in the United States are affected by this problem, either directly or indirectly. The next few years are likely to bring further changes in both government and private assistance programs, demanding new initiatives. As the welfare system is reformed and government programs are redesigned, it is likely that some will suffer. The hope is that these new approaches will lead to long-term progress and the eventual relief of poverty and hunger.

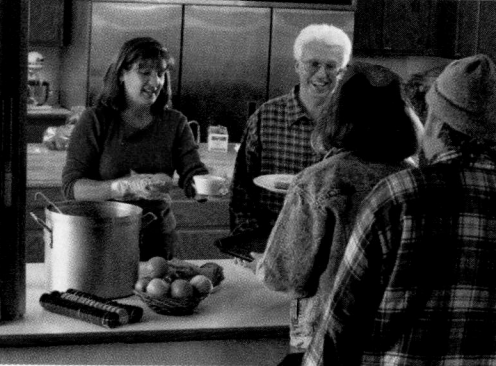

Food pantries and soup kitchens are important sources of nutrients for a growing number of people in the United States.

Concept Check

Federal programs in the United States designed to reduce hunger and undernutrition began in the 1930s, during the Great Depression. In response to reports of widespread poverty and hunger during the early 1960s, the U.S. Congress established several food assistance programs and substantially increased funding for already existing programs. Largely as a result of these federal programs, undernutrition had decreased substantially by the mid-1970s. The improvement was short-lived, and the number of people experiencing poverty, homelessness, and undernutrition grew during the 1980s and 1990s, linked to federal cutbacks in human services programs. The presence of these three interrelated problems is influenced by economic, cultural, and individual factors, as well as government policies. The serious questions about the long-term effectiveness of many government assistance programs are causing major changes in their future administration, funding mechanisms, and program design. All citizens can help reduce the problem of undernutrition.

Undernutrition in the Developing World

Undernutrition in the developing world is also tied to poverty, and any true solution must address this problem. However, these countries have a multitude of problems so complex and interrelated that they cannot be treated separately. Programs that have proved immensely helpful in the United States (and throughout the rest of North America) are only a starting point in this context. The following major obstacles challenge those seeking a solution:

- Extreme imbalances in the food/population ratio in different regions of a country
- War and political/civil unrest
- The rapid depletion of natural resources
- Cultural attitudes toward certain foods
- The disease AIDS, especially in sub-Saharan Africa and Asia
- High external debt
- Poor **infrastructure**, especially poor housing, sanitation and storage facilities, education, communications, and transportation systems

Each problem deserves individual consideration (Fig. 17.3).

infrastructure The basic framework of a system of organization. For a society, this includes roads, bridges, telephones, and other basic technologies.

■ Food/Population Ratio

Whether the earth can yield enough food for all people has been a long-standing question. As early as 1798, English clergyman and political economist, Thomas Malthus, proposed a rather pessimistic view of our prospects. He said that given the passion between the genders (which he felt should be discouraged), the population would always increase in **geometric ratio**—2, 4, 8, 16, 32, and so on. Meanwhile, at best, the food supply would increase only **arithmetically**—2, 4, 6, 8, 10, and so on. This prediction means that while the food/population ratio might begin at 2/2, eventually population will grow to 32 while food supplies will only increase to feed 10.

Malthus's proposals became the object of intense controversy in England and elsewhere, often meeting vigorous opposition. Eminent British scientists pointed out that scientific advances in agriculture would greatly increase food production. In fact, that has proved true. Nevertheless, the aptly named population explosion has undermined this progress. Overall population growth has not slowed significantly through natural checks, disease, or recent human interventions, such as birth control. In the year 1800, 1 billion people inhabited the earth. By the year 2000, this number skyrocketed to more than 6 billion. By 2050, the United Nations estimates that the world population could reach 8 to 12 billion. (The recent spread of AIDS throughout the world has put into question these future population estimates dropping the estimate to 7 to 9 billion [see the Nutrition Insight].)

geometric ratio A group of numbers wherein the division of each number by the one to the left of it yields the same answer.

arithmetic ratio A group of numbers wherein the difference between each number is the same.

By taking on the challenges of illiteracy, economic insecurity, and population growth, the developing world can begin to escape the expensive trap of humanitarian intervention and crisis management for peoples in need. Otherwise, it is likely that Malthus's gloomy prediction may soon become a fact.

Concept Check

Currently, world food production is sufficient to meet the energy needs of the world's population. Despite adequate food resources, however, undernutrition exists because of poverty, politics, and unequal distribution. In addition, projected population growth may soon overwhelm food production. Most scientists and world leaders recommend limiting population growth, especially in developing countries where birth rates are high.

■ War and Political/Civil Unrest

The recent Millennium Summit of the United Nations pledged to "spare no effort to free our peoples from the scourge of war." Against that background stands the reality that worldwide military spending has doubled over the past 20 years. In the twentieth century, deadly weapons of war took an enormous toll on civilians living in poor, politically vulnerable, war-torn nations. Although Africa has been ravaged by economic decay and famines for years, military spending in Africa more than doubled in the 1970s and held firm through the 1990s. Currently, less than one-half of 1% of the world's yearly production of goods and services is devoted to economic development assistance, whereas approximately 6% goes to military expenditures.

Civil disruptions and wars are setting back the progress of the poor and contribute to massive undernutrition. All but two of the major conflicts in 2000 took place in the developing world. War-related famine affects at least 20 million people in southern and northeastern Africa. The border war between Ethiopia and neighboring Eritrea has had a tremendous impact on government resources. A World Bank official stated that the food shortage in Ethiopia is a problem that will persist until political changes are made. Currently, 12.4 million people in Ethiopia, Eritrea, Djibouti, Kenya, and Somalia are at risk for food shortages resulting in starvation. Other conflicts continue between Congo and the Republic of Congo, as well as in Angola, where millions have been left to starve. Most of these people are without shelter, clothing, food, and any means of obtaining them. Worldwide, this entire problem is projected to worsen over the next 15 years.

Even when food is available, political divisions may impede distribution to the point that undernutrition will plague many people for years to come. Especially during emergencies, programs designed to help the poor have been undermined by poor administration, corruption, and political influence. During such political chaos, relief agencies are often caught between warring factions and those they are trying to help. This was the case in Zaire, where Rwandan refugee camps fell under the control of a militant group. The rebels controlled the food coming in the camps and would not allow relief agencies to do their work.

During the 1960s and 1970s, the problem of undernutrition in developing countries was perceived as a technical one: how to produce enough food for the growing world population. The problem is now seen as largely political: how to achieve cooperation among and within nations, so that gains in food production and infrastructure are not wiped out by war. Only a combination of approaches—finding technical solutions that may help with the problems of chronic hunger and poverty and solving political crises that push developing nations into a state of acute hunger and chaos—will help.

■ Rapid Depletion of Natural Resources

As we quickly deplete the earth's resources, population control grows increasingly critical. The productive capacity of agriculture is approaching its limits in many areas

The Nutrition Insight in this chapter discusses the impact of AIDS worldwide. Currently in the developing world, the impact of AIDS is analogous to that of ongoing war and civil strife, as it disrupts the lives of families, communities, and entire nations.

worldwide. Environmentally unsustainable farming methods undermine food production, especially in parts of the developing world.

The term **green revolution** describes a phenomenon that began in the 1960s when crop yields rose dramatically in some countries, such as the Philippines, India, and Mexico (countries in Africa did not benefit because climates were not compatible with the crops used). The increased use of fertilizers, irrigation, and the development of superior crops through careful plant breeding made this rise possible. Many of the technologies associated with the green revolution have now achieved most of their potential. For example, rice yield has not increased significantly since the release of superior varieties in 1966.

Future gains in productivity may be much harder to accomplish because of the need to farm less productive soils. Until the introduction of another superior strain of rice or other grain, developing countries will not benefit greatly from recent, more modest breakthroughs in biotechnology (see the Nutrition Issue on use of biotechnology). Actually, the green revolution was never intended to solve the world's food problems, according to Dr. Norman Borlaug, its chief architect. It was just a stopgap measure until world leaders could control population growth.

Areas of the world that remain uncultivated or ungrazed are mostly unsuited to farming: rocky, steep, infertile, too dry, too wet, or inaccessible. Much of this land is nonetheless invaluable for the crucial **ecosystem** benefits it provides, such as a depository for a wide variety of plants. This is particularly true for humid tropical areas, such as the Amazon basin rain forests.

In Africa, an area of land twice the size of New Jersey is turned into unproductive desert each year because of soil erosion. The erosion results from overgrazing by livestock, destructive farming techniques, and burning of mature rain forests. Also, the cultivation of many **cash crops** in African countries damages the land, draining the soil of vital nutrients. Then, when the land has been used up, farmers move on to other areas, leaving behind desolate land vulnerable to soil erosion. In the short run, farmers can overplow and overpump water with impressive results, but in the long run they use up natural resources on which long-term productivity depends. Soil erosion is also a problem in North America. Farmland equivalent in size to Ireland is currently lost in the United States to erosion every year. New farming techniques, such as "no till" planting, where plowing is kept to a minimum, are helping reverse this trend.

Nearly all irrigation water available worldwide is currently being used, and groundwater supplies are becoming depleted at rapid rates in many regions. The eventual water shortage this will create is projected to even increase war and civil unrest in arid areas of the world, such as Northern Africa and the Middle East. China, which has more than 20% of the world's irrigated land, as well is plagued with a growing scarcity of fresh water. Overall, in the future 3 billion people will face ongoing water shortages.

The prospects of obtaining substantially more food from the oceans are also poor. In recent years, the amount of fish caught worldwide has leveled off at about 80 million metric tons a year. Fish was once considered the poor person's protein. But, without actual farming of fish, which is becoming more common worldwide, this is unlikely to be true again.

Clearly, we can exploit the earth's resources only so far—world population probably can't continue to expand as it does today without the potential for serious famine and death. The Food and Agriculture Organization (FAO) of the United Nations works on this principle: "The fight to ensure that all people have enough nutritious food to eat is worthy of our greatest efforts, but it must be fought with the full recognition that it cannot be won unless agricultural, fishery, and forestry production returns to the earth as much as—or more than—it takes." This statement highlights the need for immediate action to protect the earth's already deteriorated environment from further destruction, if food production is to keep up with the expanding population.

green revolution This refers to increases in crop yields that accompany the introduction of new agricultural technologies in less-developed countries, beginning in the 1960s. The key technologies were high-yielding, disease-resistant strains of rice, wheat, and corn; greater use of fertilizer and water; and improved cultivation practices.

ecosystem A community in nature that includes plants, animals, and their environment.

cash crop A crop grown specifically for export, so that goods from other countries can be purchased. Cultivation of cash crops diverts agricultural resources necessary to feed a country's own citizens. Examples of cash crops are coffee, tea, cocoa, and bananas.

*I*n North America, many people shun potential foods such as horse meat, insects, and algae.

*I*n Brazil, migrants displaced by multinational land developers have flooded from the north and northeast into Rio de Janeiro and São Paulo, attracted by the prospect of jobs. There they have built shantytowns next to apartment towers and affluent suburbs, but the jobs do not materialize, and urban poverty simply replaces rural impoverishment.

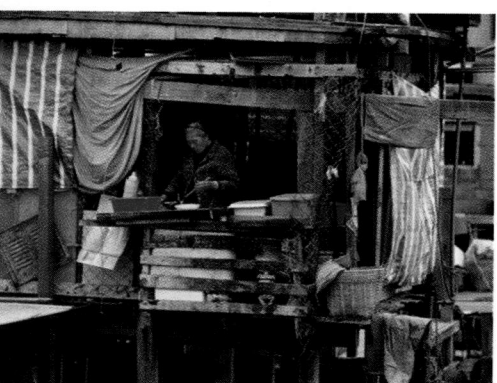

Inadequate sanitation facilities and the consumption of contaminated water cause 75% of all diseases, yet people in developing countries often lack access to a safe water supply.

■ Cultural Attitudes Toward Certain Foods

Culture affects food use, just as it does family size. In India, for example, the Hindu reverence for cattle has worsened some already significant nutrition problems. These sacred cows consume food rather than provide it; the wandering cows also damage vegetation that could otherwise feed humans. Although the cows provide milk, no attempt is made to improve milk production through selective breeding practices. In certain areas of India, a child may not be fed milk curds, because of a superstitious belief that they inhibit growth. Bananas may not be fed because they supposedly cause convulsions. These are obstacles, but not barriers, to good nutrition. Given adequate food resources, a healthful diet allowing for individual food taboos and prejudices is possible.

■ Inadequate Shelter and Sanitation

When people die from undernutrition in developing countries, other influences, such as inadequate shelter and sanitation, almost always contribute. Poor sanitation raises the risk of infection, as does undernutrition. Together these represent a lethal combination (Fig. 17.4). For example, the 1994 plague, which killed almost 5000 people and sparked the panicked exodus of another half a million in Surat, in northwest India, was linked mainly to unsanitary housing conditions.

Inadequate and deteriorating shelters threaten the lives of more than 500 million people today. Many of the 15 million annual deaths of children—half of them under 5 years old—in developing countries could be prevented by improving the standards of environmental hygiene. Urban populations of some developing countries are currently growing at an annual rate of 5% to 7%. Such a skewed population distribution will result in more poverty. The current urban explosion is the result of both high birth rates and continuing migration of people to the cities from the countryside. People go to the cities to find employment and resources the countryside can no longer provide. Worldwide, 38% of people lived in urban areas in 1975. The figure is now 50%, and is expected to reach 70% by 2050. Nine of the 10 largest cities 20 years from now will be in poor countries. Los Angeles, which is now the seventh largest city in the world, and New York, which is third, will drop far down the list.

In developing countries, the poor make up most of the urban population, and their needs for housing and community services often outstrip available governmental resources. Most of these urban poor live in overcrowded, self-made shelters, which lack a safe and adequate water supply and are only partially served by public utilities. The shantytowns and ghettos of the developing world are often worse than the rural areas the people left behind. Because the urban poor need cash to purchase food, they often subsist on diets that are even more meager than the homegrown rural fare. Making matters worse, haphazard shelters often lack facilities to protect food from spoilage or the ravages of insects and rodents. In some developing countries, food losses can amount to as much as 40% of the perishable foods.

The shift from rural to urban life takes its greatest toll on infants and children. Infants are often weaned early from the breast, partly because the mother must find employment and partly because she may be influenced by the images of sophisticated, formula-using women promoted in advertisements. Unfortunately, because infant formulas are relatively expensive, poor parents may overdilute the mixture or use too little to meet the baby's needs. Because the water supply may not be safe, the prepared formula is also likely to be contaminated with bacteria. Human milk, in contrast, is generally much more hygienic, readily available, and nutritious, and it provides infants with immunity to some ailments. Promoting breastfeeding when it is safe for a mother to breastfeed her baby is important (see the discussion of AIDS in the Nutrition Insight for further details on when it is safe to breastfeed).

Overall, the single most effective health advantage for people, wherever they live, is a safe and convenient water supply. Inadequate sanitation and the consumption of contaminated water cause 75% of all diseases and more than one-third of all deaths in developing countries. The World Health Organization (WHO) estimates that 1 billion people, about one-sixth of all people, have an unsafe and inadequate

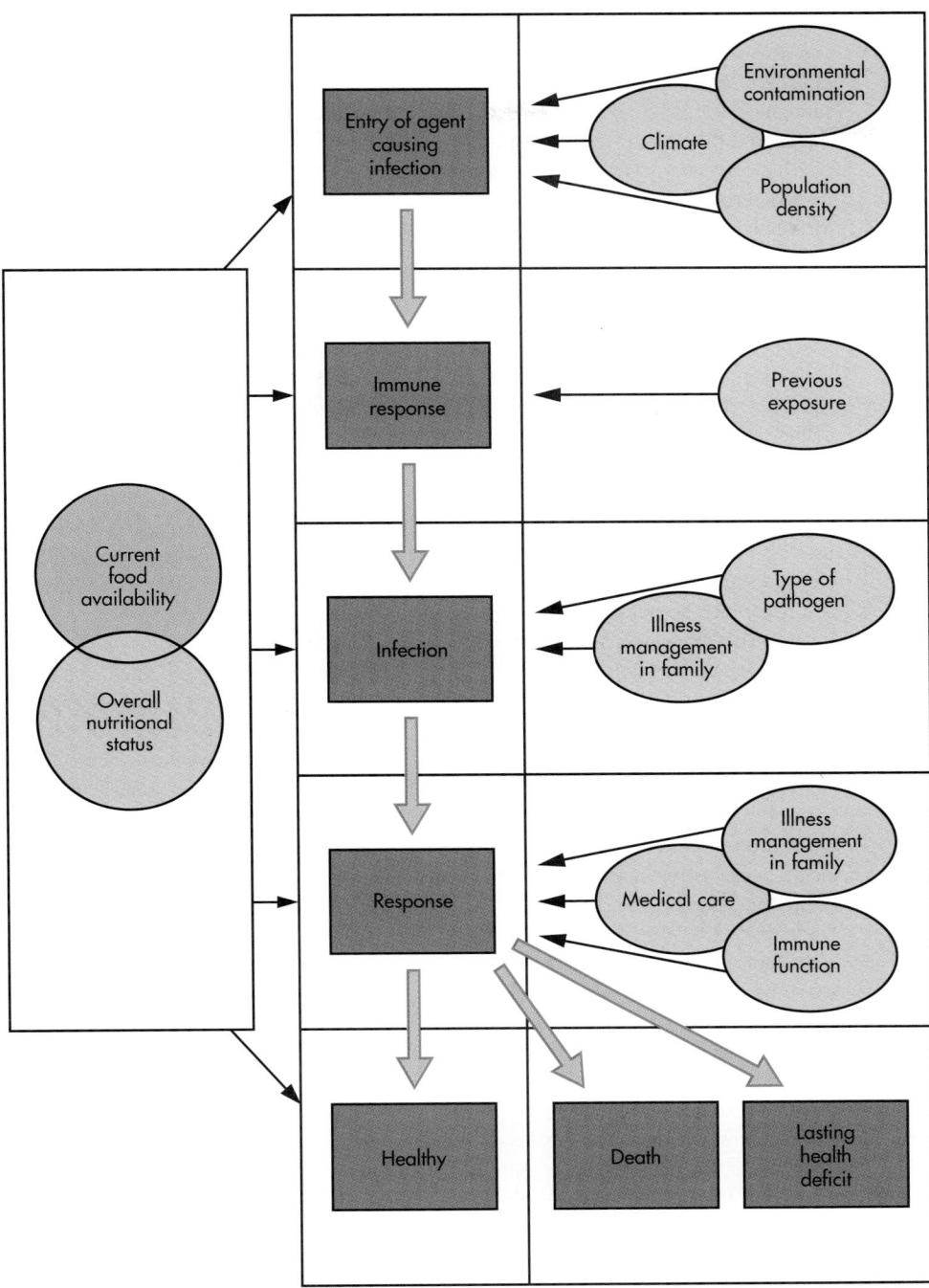

Figure 17.4 Nutritional status and overall food supply combine with a variety of environmental factors to influence the risk of infection and the ultimate outcome.

water supply. In addition, up to 90% of the diseases seen in developing countries may be attributed to contaminated water.

Poor sanitation, another example of inadequate infrastructure in the developing world, creates another critical public health problem. Human feces, rotting garbage, and associated insect and rodent infestations are commonly seen in urban areas of the developing world. Potent sources of disease organisms—human urine and feces—are two of the most dangerous substances people encounter in routine daily living. The inability to dispose of the massive numbers of dead people (and dead animals) resulting from civil wars causes additional sanitation problems. In some developing countries, diarrheal diseases account for as many as one-third of all deaths in children under 5 years of age. WHO estimates that even with improvements in housing, 3 billion people in the world still lack proper sanitation facilities.

The Impact of AIDS Worldwide

The Black Death left its grim mark on civilization by claiming the lives of approximately 25 million people in the fourteenth century. Today there are more than 40 million people around the world with **human immunodeficiency virus (HIV) infection** or **acquired immune deficiency syndrome (AIDS),** leading to an estimated 25 million deaths to date. This represents a current worldwide epidemic. Once infected with HIV, the person is said to be HIV-positive. If untreated, the viral disease progresses over the next few years, and the person develops symptoms such as diarrhea, lung disease, weight loss, and a form of cancer. The person is now said to have AIDS. In 1998, an estimated 5.8 million new HIV infections occurred worldwide—approximately 16,000 each day.

In the United States, it is estimated that 940,000 people are infected with HIV, of whom more than 200,000 are unaware of their infection. This means that as many as 1 of every 280 people in the United States may be infected. About 450,000 people in the United States have died from the disease. In more than 60 U.S. cities, AIDS is the number one killer of men ages 25 to 44. Minority populations account for more cases than do Caucasians in the United States, based on their percentage of the population. Stopping the spread of this disease is imperative for the United States, especially in minority communities. People at risk are urged to seek testing.

In Africa, particularly sub-Saharan countries, the HIV virus is rampant throughout the entire population, with this region containing nearly 70% of the world's HIV-positive people. In many villages, AIDS is creating orphans. In most areas of sub-Saharan Africa, AIDS is reducing life expectancy by one-half, especially if the person also has tuberculosis. As noted in the chapter, world population projections for the next 50 years may have to be reduced to account for the impact of AIDS in Africa and in Asia.

The AIDS virus takes the RNA it contains and converts that into DNA. The DNA is then used to direct the synthesis of the proteins by the infected cell that are needed to make new viral particles. Cells of the immune system are prime targets of the virus; it is in these cells that the new viral particles are made. The resulting dramatic fall in immune function from HIV infection is the hallmark of the disease.

The virus is transferred between people via blood contact or body secretions, including sexual secretions. It has a very limited ability to exist outside the body. Experts have blamed sexual promiscuity in some African societies, as well as sexual practices that can make it easier for the virus to enter a woman's bloodstream, for the rapid spread of the disease in that area of the world. Many people in Africa engage in unprotected sex because they can't afford condoms, or because the females cannot get their male partners to use them. Overall, 75% to 85% of all cases of HIV have been spread through sexual contact, homosexual as well as heterosexual. Intravenous drug use, via shared needles, accounts for a large number of the rest of the cases.

One drug used to treat HIV infection blocks the activity of the enzyme used by HIV to convert RNA to DNA. A common form of this drug is zidovudine (AZT). Other drugs used to treat HIV infection block specific enzymes in HIV that are needed to assemble the viral particle. These drugs are called protease inhibitors; a common form is Indinavir (Crixivan). The latest therapies can significantly slow the progress of the disease, but this requires patients to take at least three different drugs and about 14 pills each day. This costs approximately $14,000 per year, not including any unforeseen hospital stays. Once the AIDS drugs have been started, the person must continue taking the drugs. If the drugs are stopped, the virus can mutate, and the mutated virus will likely be able to resist the effects of the present drug regimen. This will then also complicate further drug therapy. As well, without treatment, the person generally dies in 4 to 5 years.

Making AIDS drugs available to people in developing countries is a major roadblock to solving the AIDS crisis in those regions. Certain drug companies and governments are working to lower the cost of AIDS drugs to developing nations. Still, in many cases, the cost will remain out of reach to many who need the drugs.

It has been suggested that developed nations step in and cover most of the costs. The United Nations is spearheading an effort to raise the $7 to $10 billion needed to fight the disease. The United States recently pledged $1.3 billion toward the effort. An open question is whether the recent "war on terrorism" will derail this effort to raise the funds needed.

The main hope for addressing the problem of AIDS in the developing world is the creation and widespread use of a vaccine against the virus. This would significantly reduce the spread to further individuals but would be of no help to those already infected with the virus. Aside from providing AIDS drugs used in the developed countries, there is currently no answer to the AIDS crisis in the developing world beyond safe sex, use of clean needles, and other behavior-linked approaches.

The devastating effects of AIDS on our civilization have been very rapid when measured by earth's scale of time, and the true costs to societies—other than the cost of human lives—have yet to emerge. The very nature of the disease is likely to wreak significant human devastation in North America and worldwide, partly because its primary route of transmission is a basic human behavior—sexual activity.

An encouraging study done in rural Uganda suggests that people with minimal amounts of HIV in their blood show a low likelihood of spreading the virus to others during unprotected sex. This is a positive finding, since treatment reduces the viral load in infected patients, which in turn might help decrease the spread of this disease. On a more pessimistic note, highly drug-resistant strains of HIV are increasing, appearing in as many as 5% of newly infected patients in the United States.

Who Is Affected?

The belief that AIDS is a novel disease affecting a limited population of homosexual males on the East and West Coasts of the United States is dangerously inaccurate. With the number of new cases per year among homosexual men dramatically decreasing, the number of new infections among heterosexuals, particularly among women, has accelerated dramatically. In fact, recent studies show that about 20% of people in some south Florida towns have HIV infections, with heterosexual contact being the main method of contracting the virus. Along with the increase in infection in women, there is an increased number of HIV-infected infants and children.

AIDS needs no passport. Heterosexually transmitted HIV flows freely in Thai sex brothels, along the truck routes of India, around Dominican Republic sugar-cane plantations, and in the copper mines of Zambia. It is likely that one-fourth of all adults in Zambia are infected with HIV. Heterosexual contact accounts for the majority of cases. A recent study warns us that 57 countries risk major HIV outbreaks. Reported HIV cases are increasing rapidly in Africa, Asia, and Russia, with an estimated 5.8 million men, women, and children becoming infected yearly worldwide.

Nutrition and AIDS

On a more individual scale, can eating a balanced diet prevent HIV or stave off AIDS? The answer is no. Consuming a balanced diet, however, helps lessen the impact of infections but does not cure the disease or make it less deadly, while poor nutritional status contributes to quicker onset of such symptoms as body wasting and fever. This ultimately leads to a quicker demise. Overall, AIDS patients should consider sufficient food an integral part of their treatment regimen.

Breastfeeding becomes an issue for mothers who test HIV-positive. Research shows that babies have a 10% chance of getting the virus from their HIV-infected mothers' milk if they breastfeed for

2 years. Many experts recommend the avoidance of breastfeeding as an intervention to prevent the transmission of the virus from mother to child. However, in many situations, nutritionally adequate breast-milk substitutes are not available, especially in an environment where infectious diseases and malnutrition are the primary causes of death during infancy. In these instances, feeding with infant formulas can increase a child's risk of illness and death, and, thus, breastfeeding is still the recommended alternative. In the end, the choice is with the mother, based on current circumstances. Some African countries are now supplying infant formulas if an HIV-positive mother chooses to use this option.

What Are the Combined Costs of AIDS?

Although human life can't be tagged with a price, the cost of AIDS research and medical care for AIDS patients, the loss of labor force for industry, and the economic hardship experienced by families of victims can be quantified. A conservative estimate for the total lifetime cost of treating HIV-related illness in just one person is $154,000. Consider those dollars, and then think about the more than 40 million people around the world who are infected.

Behind the mind-boggling statistics on AIDS are less obvious costs to businesses, families, schools and universities, and society in general. In India and Thailand, for example, a significant number of the adult male population will die of AIDS. Worker productivity will plummet because

AIDS victims produce less and demand more, especially as they waste away in the latter stages of the disease. Business productivity drops even further when relatives take time away from work and school to care for family members afflicted with AIDS. Furthermore, AIDS demands a considerable amount of family income. Hard-pressed families, who have to devote much of their income to doctors and medicines, have little left for living expenses. Other family members must struggle to keep up with daily duties because they must care for orphans left behind in the disease's wake. The number of youngsters orphaned by AIDS could more than double in the next 3 years to reach 3.7 million worldwide.

Individual and Government Response

Governments worldwide have come under fire for their slow response in fighting AIDS. Many governments of developing nations can't afford to supply AIDS counseling or treatment. More recently, governments are trying to take more responsibility in stopping the spread of AIDS, as noted earlier.

The world must act in concert to stop the spread of HIV. To do any less is to allow the problem of undernutrition to worsen throughout the world. For further information on HIV and AIDS, call the CDC national HIV/AIDS hot line at 1-800-458-5231. As well, visit the following websites:
www.aegis.com
www.thebody.com
www.aids.org

■ High External Debt

During the 1970s and through today, many developing countries became trapped in the cycle of borrowing repeatedly from foreign countries. Servicing these external debts, which now total about $2.5 trillion, has brought several countries to the verge of economic collapse. About $6 billion is owed to the United States. The external debt of Latin America represents 45% of the region's gross regional output of goods and services.

Many African nations also carry large debt burdens—currently, $350 billion. Recent drops in prices for raw commodities they export, higher prices for imported oil, and embezzlement of funds by high-ranking political officials are at the root of this problem. Although the African debts are much smaller in absolute terms than those of Brazil, Argentina, and Mexico, for example, the actual burden is greater when national incomes and export earnings are considered. Nearly half the money African nations earn from exports goes to paying off the continent's multibillion-dollar debt. As a result, African nations have had to impose cuts in domestic programs, which can cause

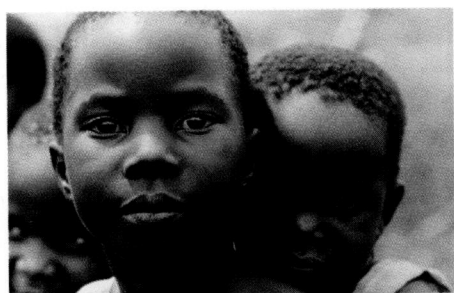

A particularly sad development of AIDS in Africa is the number of AIDS orphans, children whose parents have both died of AIDS.

widespread undernutrition in many of these poor nations, in part because these countries still need to import—and pay for—machinery, concrete, trucks, and consumer goods. To make up the difference between export income and import expenses, countries have been forced to borrow billions of dollars from international banks.

Concept Check

War and civil strife, along with a decline in the world's natural resources, contribute to the difficulty of ending undernutrition in many developing countries. In addition, inadequate housing conditions, impure water, and inadequate sanitation worldwide increase the risk for infection and disease. Infection then combines with undernutrition to compromise further the health of impoverished people. Finally, many developing countries are burdened by extremely high external debts, which severely limit their ability to implement programs to reduce undernutrition.

■ Reducing Undernutrition in the Developing World

As you have probably guessed, greatly reducing undernutrition in the developing world will be complicated and will take considerable time to accomplish. Today, it is a common practice for the more affluent nations to supply famine areas with direct food aid. However highly publicized and praised at the time, direct food aid is not a long-term solution. Although it reduces the number of deaths from famine, it can also reduce incentives for local production by driving down local prices. In addition, the affected countries may have little or no means of transporting the food to those who need it most. Furthermore, the donated foods may receive little cultural acceptance.

In the short run, there is no choice—aid must be given because people are starving. Still, improving the infrastructure for poor people, especially rural people, needs to be the long-term focus. This long-term approach is necessary because the most significant factor affecting the undernutrition of people in impoverished areas of the world is their reliance on outside sources for basic needs. Their dependence makes them constantly vulnerable.

One U.S. program that has helped improve the infrastructure of developing nations is the Peace Corps, which provides education, distributes food and medical supplies, and builds structures for local use. The aim of the Peace Corps is to improve the infrastructure and education of developing countries and thereby help create independent, self-sustaining economies around the world.

Development Tailored to Local Conditions

Recall that, in the past 40 years, world food supplies have grown faster than the population. Thus, the increase in undernutrition during this period is caused by an increase in the number of people cut off from their share of this supply. Millions of farmers are losing access to resources they need to be self-reliant. In response, careful, small-scale regional development is one option. There is a growing realization that rural people who own no land will flock to the overcrowded cities unless economic opportunities can be created as part of a plan for sustainable development.

For the most part, the solution lies in helping people meet their own needs and directing them to resources and employment opportunities, rather than simply giving them resources. Experience has shown that credit—along with training, food storage facilities, and marketing—allows rural people to participate in development to their benefit and that of their families and communities.

Impoverished women are a special concern. In addition to working longer hours than do men, they grow most of the food for family consumption and make up three-fourths of the labor force in the informal sector and an increasing proportion in the formal economy. Economic opportunities for women must be augmented. Of the

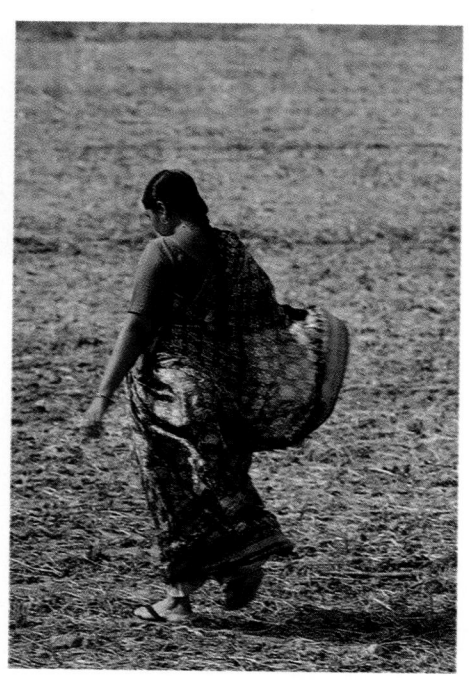
Women are receiving more attention as efforts to improve the health and welfare of the world's people evolve.

3 billion people in the world living on less than $2 a day, 70% are women. Moreover, among the developing world's 900 million illiterate people, women outnumber men 2 to 1. Thus, an important means of propelling nations out of poverty is to end the cycle of female neglect. A United Nations Conference on Women in Beijing had one critical message: Providing women with education, entrepreneurship, and political power could pay off in numerous ways, ranging from slower population growth (as mentioned earlier) and higher incomes to healthier families.

Suitable technologies for processing, preserving, marketing, and distributing nutritious local staples also need to be encouraged, so that small farmers can flourish. Education on how to use these foods to create healthful diets, such as preparing vitamin A-rich vegetables, adds further benefit. Supplementing indigenous foods with nutrients that are in short supply, such as iron, vitamin B-12, zinc, and iodide, also deserves consideration. One current program involves adding iron to sugar in various parts of the world. In addition, advances in water purification using ultraviolet light have the potential to cut energy expenditures by 20,000 times what is used now. This new method would result in a cost of 7 cents for a typical village's annual drinking water bill.

Promoting extensive landownership is a key part of the solution. Increasing the availability of food is one of the many advantages. If food resources are concentrated among a minority of people, as often happens with unequal landownership, food won't be equally distributed unless efficient transportation systems are in place. Inequitable distribution then proves a very difficult problem to resolve.

Raising the economic status of impoverished people by employing them is as important as expanding the food supply. If an increase in food supply is achieved without an accompanying rise in employment, there may be no long-term change in the number of undernourished people. Although food prices may fall with increased mechanization, use of fertilizers, and other modern technologies, these advances can also displace people from jobs.

A shipment of high-technology tractors, for example, might put local laborers out of work. From this perspective, it is of little consequence that jobs are technologically primitive by Western standards. As mentioned before, increasing both per capita income and education is necessary. That effort must include employment. Making full use of the human resources available in the developing world itself is more essential than ever.

Overemphasizing cash crops, such as coffee, tea, rubber, and cocoa—as some developing countries have done, especially in Latin America—is not likely to solve the nutritional problems of poor people. Cash crops are usually grown at the expense of food crops on the assumption that money earned from the cash crops will be used to purchase food for the families of the workers. However, this is not always the case. Food can be bought, but it may not be enough, and it is more expensive. In such a situation, poorer families are at greater risk than others, because the money earned from cash crops is often not enough to meet other basic family needs, let alone their food needs. As with poor families in North America, buying quality foods often takes a secondary position, resulting in nutritional deprivation.

■ Some Concluding Thoughts

Clearly, the developing world will have to rely largely on its own resources to finance development. For decades, countries in Africa could count on the Cold War as an economic resource. The United States and the former Soviet Union opposed each other through African proxies, pouring in money to prop up pro-Western or pro-Communist governments. Now the big powers' priorities have turned inward.

Also detrimental is the economics of drug crops, such as cocaine, marijuana, and opium. Perceiving drugs as valuable cash crops, workers often believe that the large sums of money netted from these crops—which are often more easily grown than food crops—can meet family needs and increase the standard of living. An unfortunate reality is that many workers see little or no cash earnings and become victims of their trade. Cash from drug crops often lines the pockets of criminals and

Critical Thinking

Stan has read about various relief efforts to help undernourished people in developing countries, especially the emergency food aid programs for famine-ravaged areas. Many of these efforts appear to be only temporary, and he wonders what long-range approaches might help alleviate the problem of undernutrition. What suggestions would you give Stan about possible long-term solutions for undernutrition in developing countries?

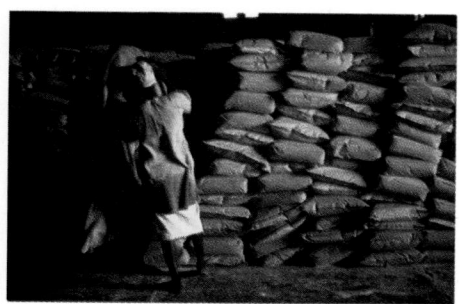

There is no doubt that food aid is important in reducing death from famine, but it isn't a long-term solution.

W ith regard to the world food supply, the current generation of young adults and the next will not likely have to face the absolute limits. Instead, they will have to make difficult choices if the outlook for future generations is to improve.

corrupt government officials and results in little incentive to initiate subsistence-level food crops that could provide employment and nourishment for many.

Today, the economic loss from undernutrition is staggering, and the amount of human pain and suffering is incalculable. With all the international relief efforts and assistance from governments and private organizations combined, we are still lacking when it comes to our battle against undernutrition.

Currently, some experts are concerned about the "marginalization" of problems in the developing world, fearing rich nations might dismiss war, disease, and famine as a way of life for poorer nations. In a recent survey, people in the United States identified world famine as less of a concern than violence, drugs, and inflation. (Currently, U.S. food aid stands at $2.4 billion.) Ultimately, however, the depletion of world resources, the massive debt incurred by poorer countries, the threat of danger to more prosperous countries nearby, and the toll taken in human lives does affect the world economy and well-being.

Leaders of rich and poor nations alike need to come to an agreement on the best possible means to serve all of the world's citizens. Perhaps if we rid ourselves of negative government policies worldwide, the task can become easier. Life is not necessarily fair, but the aim of civilization should be to make it fairer. The world has both the food and the technical expertise to end hunger. What is lacking is the political will to do so.

Concept Check

O verall, one important solution to reducing undernutrition in the developing world lies in providing sufficient employment, so that people can purchase the food their families need or provide access to land and other food production resources. Development programs must be sensitive to regional conditions to ensure that the new technologies introduced don't intensify existing problems for the poorest people.

Summary

1. Poverty is commonly linked to undernutrition. Malnutrition can occur when the food supply is either scarce or abundant. The resulting deficiency conditions and degenerative diseases contribute to poor health.

2. Undernutrition is the most common form of malnutrition in developing countries. It results from inadequate intake, absorption, or use of nutrients or food energy. Many deficiency conditions consequently appear, and infectious diseases thrive because the immune system cannot function properly.

3. The greatest risk of undernutrition occurs during critical periods of growth and development: gestation, infancy, and childhood. Low birth weight is a leading cause of infant deaths worldwide. Many developmental problems are caused by nutritional deprivation during critical periods of brain growth. People in their later years are also at greater risk.

4. Undernutrition diminishes both physical and mental capabilities. In poor countries, this is worsened by recurrent infections, unsanitary conditions, extreme weather, inadequate shelter, and exposure to diseases.

5. In the United States, famine has been nonexistent since the 1930s, but undernutrition remains. Soup kitchens, food stamps, school lunch and breakfast programs, and the Special Supplemental Nutrition Program for Women, Infants, and Children (WIC) have focused on improving the nutritional health of poor and at-risk people. When adequately funded, these programs have proved effective in reducing undernutrition. The need to reduce

out-of-wedlock pregnancies remains a national priority because single parents and their children are likely to live in poverty.

6. Multiple factors contribute to the problem of undernutrition in the developing world. In densely populated countries, food resources, as well as the means for distributing food, may be inadequate. Farming methods often encourage erosion, which deprives the soil of valuable nutrients and thereby hampers future efforts to grow food. Limited water availability limits food production. Naturally occurring devastation from droughts, excessive rainfall, fire, crop infestation, and human causes—such as urbanization, war and civil unrest, debt, and poor sanitation—all contribute to the major problem of undernutrition, as does AIDS.

7. Proposed solutions to world undernutrition must include consideration of the interaction of multiple factors, many of which are thoroughly embedded in cultural traditions. Family planning efforts, for example, may not succeed until life expectancy increases. Through education, efforts should be made to upgrade farming methods, improve crops, limit pregnancies, encourage breastfeeding when it is safe to do so, and improve sanitation and hygiene. Direct food aid is only a short-term solution. In what may appear to be a step backward, many experts recommend sustainable subsistence-level farming, away from the specialization of cash crops, to increase the economic status of poor people. Small-scale industrial development is another way to create meaningful employment and purchasing power for vast numbers of the rural poor.

Study Questions

1. Describe the difference between malnutrition and undernutrition.
2. Describe in a short paragraph any evidence of undernutrition that you saw while you were growing up, such as on television. What are/were the likely roots of these problems?
3. What do you believe are the major factors contributing to undernutrition in wealthy nations, such as the United States? What are some solutions to this problem?
4. What three points would you make to a group of seventh-grade girls concerning the economic perils of teenage pregnancy and parenting?
5. Personal responsibility is a common theme in political circles. How does this relate to the problem of undernutrition in the United States? Does it apply to all causes of the problem?
6. Outline how war and civil unrest in developing countries have worsened problems of chronic hunger over the past few years.
7. How important is population control in addressing the problem of world hunger now and in the future? Support your answer with three main points.
8. Why is solving the problem of undernutrition a key factor in the development of the full potential of developing countries? What basic nutrients are keys to the health of these people?
9. Discuss how infrastructure could influence the causes and solutions of chronic hunger in a developing nation.
10. Name three nutrients that are often lacking in the diets of undernourished people. What effects can be expected with each deficiency?

Further Readings

1. ADA Reports: Position of the American Dietetic Association: Domestic food and nutrition security. *Journal of the American Dietetic Association* 98:337, 1998.
   Aggressive action is needed to bring an end to domestic hunger and to achieve food and nutrition security for all residents of the United States. Immediate and long-range interventions are needed, including adequate program funding of federal programs and assistance from private sources.

2. ADA Reports: Position of the American Dietetic Association and Dietitians of Canada: Nutrition intervention in the care of persons with human immunodeficiency virus infection. *Journal of the American Dietetic Association* 100:708, 2000.
   Malnutrition, various forms of tissue wasting, fat accumulation, and risk of additional chronic disease have become central issues in health-care plans for patients living with HIV. Efforts to optimize nutritional status, including nutrition therapy and nutrition-related education, should be components of the total health care provided to people infected with the HIV virus.

3. Brundtland GH: Nutrition and infection: Malnutrition and mortality in public health. *Nutrition Reviews* 58(II):S1, 2000.
   The combination of malnutrition and infectious disease is deadly. These conditions arise from poverty and keep people in poverty—not just for one generation, but for many generations. Many infections are preventable. For example, when vitamin A is introduced as part of measles management, the fatality rate can be reduced by greater than 50%.

4. Ezzell C: Care for a dying continent. *Scientific American*, p. 96, May 2000.
   AIDS is destined to alter history in Africa—and, in fact, the world—to a degree not seen in humanity's past since the Black Death. It is estimated that between 20% and 25% of the population in Zimbabwe carries the virus, and an estimated 10 million children are destined to become orphaned on the continent of Africa due to the AIDS epidemic. The AIDS drugs available to many in the developed world—which cost upward of $14,000 per person per year—are unthinkable for the majority of people in Africa.

5. Food and Agriculture Organization: The state of food insecurity in the world: 2000, Food and Agriculture Organization of the United Nations, Rome Italy, 2000.
   Countries with the highest numbers and greatest depth of hunger include 18 countries in Africa, as well as Afghanistan, Bangladesh, Haiti, the Democratic People's Republic of Korea, Republic of Korea, and Mongolia. These countries face difficult problems in feeding their people due to instability and conflict, poor governance, erratic weather, poverty, agricultural failure, population pressure, and fragile ecosystems.

6. Humphrey J, Iliff P: Is breast not best? Feeding babies born to HIV-positive mothers: Bringing balance to a complex issue. *Nutrition Reviews* 59(4):119, 2001.
   Several conditions must be in place and accepted before formula feeding can replace breastfeeding in order to increase HIV-free survival for infants. Currently the proportion of sub-Saharan African women who have access to and will accept these conditions is small. Thus, at this time breastfeeding will probably benefit a greater number of African babies than will formula feeding.

7. Lappe FM and others: *World hunger: Twelve myths*, Grove Press, New York, Second edition, 1998.
   Choices determine whether we are helping to end world hunger. Only as we make our choices conscious do we become less victims of the world handed to us, and more its creators. The more we consciously align our life choices with a vision of the world we're working toward, the more powerful we become in solving this problem of world hunger.

8. Lee JS, Frongillo EA: Nutritional and health consequences are associated with food insecurity among U.S. elderly persons. *Journal of Nutrition* 131:1503, 2001.
   Older persons experiencing food insecurity have poorer dietary intakes than those who are food secure. With an increasing aging population, making sure that every older person has enough food to eat to meet his or her nutritional needs is an important way to help older adults enjoy healthy, active, and successful aging. Food insecurity among older adults is also considered ethically unacceptable.

9. Thompson L: Are bioengineered foods safe? *FDA Consumer*, p. 18, January/February 2000.
   There is no evidence that bioengineered foods pose any human health concerns or that they are in any way less safe than crops produced through traditional breeding. No matter how a new crop is created—using traditional methods or biotechnology tools—breeders must conduct field testing for several seasons to make sure the crops are safe for widespread use.

10. UNICEF: The state of the world's children 2001, United Nations Children Fund, New York, NY, 2001.
    Most brain development happens before a child reaches 3 years old. Long before many adults even realize what is happening, the brain cells of a new infant proliferate, synapses develop, and the patterns of a lifetime are established. In these early years, children develop their abilities to think and speak, learn and reason, and lay the foundation for their values and social behavior as adults.

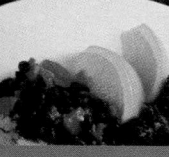

I. Fighting World Undernutrition on a Personal Level

If you want to do something about world and domestic undernutrition, the following activities are suggested. It is a noble act to try to make a difference, even if you make just one small step. As with any change in behavior, don't try to do too many things at once. Try one or two activities that represent your commitment to solving this problem.

1. Volunteer at a local soup kitchen or homeless shelter for a limited period of time (1 month, for example). What insights did you gain?

2. Coordinate the efforts of a campus organization to donate some money to a voluntary agency that does antihunger work, such as the following:

Bread for the World
802 Rhode Island Ave., NE
Washington, DC 20018

Oxfam America
115 Broadway
Boston, MA 02116

Save the Children Foundation
P.O. Box 970
Westport, CT 06881

Earth Save Foundation
1509 Suite B1 Seabright Ave.
Santa Cruz, CA 95062

Catholic Relief Services
209 W. Fayette St.
Baltimore, MD 21201

CARE
660 First Ave.
New York, NY 10016

Second Harvest
116 Michigan Ave., Suite #4
Chicago, IL 60603

3. Take a contribution for the ongoing offering of nonperishable foods at your church, mosque, or synagog, or one near you. If your church doesn't have this offering, start one.

4. Get on a food recovery program's mailing list and read its newsletters for information on upcoming fund-raisers and programs to become involved.

5. Participate in food drives organized by local grocery stores through contributing food or services. Food-drive organizers may need volunteers to transport the donations from the store to a food pantry.

6. Point, click, and fight hunger. Internet users can find information on hunger at several sites, including the following:

- Someone somewhere dies of hunger every 3.6 seconds. You can help stop the clock: go to www.thehungersite.com and click on Donate Free Food to send a meal to a needy someone. This site is affiliated with the UN World Food Program, which tracks the number of clicks and then sends a bill to one of its corporate or nonprofit sponsors.

- HungerWeb, at Brown University, offers information on hunger research, programs, mailing lists, education, and advocacy, as well as an overview of the Alan Shawn Feinstein World Hunger Program at Brown. This site contains web links to Internet sites run by the UN, U.S. AID, and the World Bank. www.netspace.org/hungerweb

- The Food and Agriculture Organization of the United Nations has worked to alleviate poverty and hunger by promoting agricultural development, improved nutrition, and the pursuit of food security. This website will keep you up-to-date on recent issues and provides an extensive list of publications related to food security. www.fao.org

- America's Second Harvest, the largest domestic hunger-relief organization, shows you how to help online and has information about the latest updates. www.secondharvest.org

- Bread for the World is a nationwide Christian citizens' movement seeking justice for the world's hungry people by lobbying our nation's decision makers. www.bread.org

- CARE is one of the world's largest private international relief and development organizations, with the goal of saving lives, building opportunity, and bringing hope to people in need. www.care.org

II. Joining the Battle Against Undernutrition

Imagine that you recently spent your summer vacation in a developing country and saw evidence of undernutrition and hunger. Then imagine that you are now asking a large corporation to support your efforts to ease hunger and suffering in this area. Develop a two-paragraph statement outlining why addressing hunger issues in this area is important. Address how you think a large corporation could assist you in your efforts.

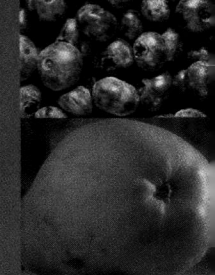

The Role of Biotechnology in Expanding Worldwide Food Availability

The ability of humans to manipulate nature has enabled us to improve the production and yield of many important foods. Traditional **biotechnology** is almost as old as agriculture. The first farmer to improve his stock by selectively breeding the best bull with the best cows was implementing biotechnology in a simple sense. The first baker to use yeast to make bread rise took similar advantage of biotechnology.

By the 1930s, biotechnology made possible the selective breeding of better plant hybrids: As a result, corn production in the United States quickly doubled. Through similar methods, agricultural wheat was crossed with wild grasses to confer more desirable properties, such as greater yield, increased resistance to mildew and bacterial diseases, and tolerance to salt or adverse climatic conditions.

Another type of biotechnology uses hormones rather than breeding. In the last decade, Canadian salmon have been treated with a hormone that allows them to mature three times faster than normal—without changing the fish in any other way. In general terms, biotechnology can be understood as the use of living things—plants, animals, bacteria—to manufacture products.

biotechnology A collection of processes that involve the use of biological systems for altering and, ideally, improving the characteristics of plants, animals, and other forms of life.

The New Biotechnology

The new biotechnology used in agriculture includes several methods that directly modify products. It differs from traditional methods because it directly changes some of the genetic material (DNA) of organisms to improve characteristics. Cross-breeding plants or animals is no longer the only tool. Development of the new process, called **genetic engineering,** began in the 1970s. The field now features a wide range of cell and subcell techniques for the synthesis and placement of genetic material in organisms (Fig. 17.5). This process of **recombinant DNA technology** allows access to a wider gene pool, and it permits faster and more accurate production of new and more useful microbial, plant, and animal species. Traditional breeding has had inconsistent results; biotechnology is more precise and provides more options of genetic material to

genetic engineering Manipulation of the genetic make up or any organism with recombinant DNA technology.

recombinant DNA technology A test tube technology that rearranges DNA sequences in an organism by cutting and rejoining DNA molecules with a series of enzymes.

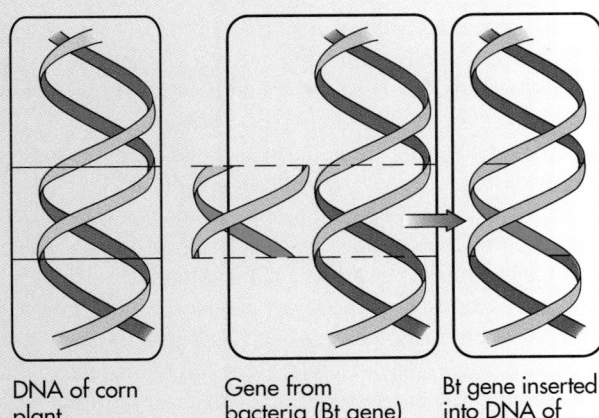

DNA of corn plant.

Gene from bacteria (Bt gene) that produces a protein toxic to the European corn borer.

Bt gene inserted into DNA of corn plant. Now the corn plant makes the Bt toxin and, so, is resistant to the European corn borer.

Figure 17.5 Biotechnology involves various techniques for transferring foreign DNA into an organism. In this diagram, a sample of DNA is cleaved out of a larger DNA fragment and inserted into the DNA of a host cell. Thus, the host cell contains new genetic information, with the potential of providing the cell with new capabilities. For corn, this means resistance to the European corn borer. The corn plant is now referred to as a genetically modified organism (GMO). In other applications, bacteria can be engineered to produce the human form of the hormone insulin and another hormone that increases milk production in cows.
Rollins Graphics

continued

genetically modified organism (GMO)
Any organism created by genetic engineering.

Fish have been genetically engineered to grow four times faster than native varieties. The final adult size is the same, however.

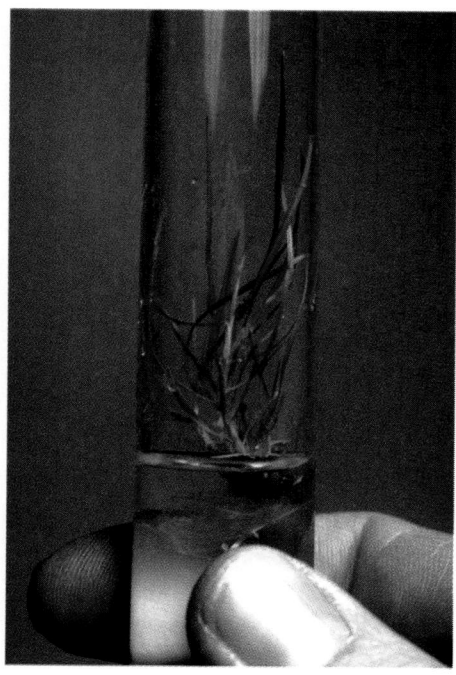

Both traditional plant breeding and biotechnology have produced high-yielding plant varieties.

GMO products are widely distributed in our food supply. Gerber Products Co. tried to introduce a line of GMO-free baby foods and found that they could not produce such products from raw materials currently available. These commonly have at least low-level GMO content.

utilize. Scientists select the traits they want and genetically engineer or introduce the gene that produces the desired trait into plants or animals, (now called a **genetically modified organism [GMO]**). It is important to note, however, the genetic engineering doesn't replace conventional breeding practices; both work together.

Already, genetic engineering at the agricultural level has allowed us to make use of new types of seeds, growth hormones, and microbial inoculants to stop pests and frost damage. Biotechnology is also used to develop drought-tolerant crops, as well as to detect *Listeria* and other microorganisms that cause foodborne illness. Scientists are engineering plants that grow without pesticides and new forms of potatoes that can last without preservatives. In addition, biotechnology can allow scientists to create fruits and grains with more or less sucrose, and greater amounts of beta-carotene and vitamins E and C. Researchers are also examining ways to modify the fatty-acid makeup of vegetable oils. Because cautious use is the order of the day, these early benefits of the new biotechnology will strike us as only subtly different. The ultimate benefits, however, could be substantial if foods eaten by indigenous people can be so enhanced.

Few consumers in the United States realize that currently about one-quarter of all corn and half of all soybeans produced in the United States have been genetically engineered in such a way to resist certain insects, in the case of corn, and to reduce pesticide use, in the case of soybeans. Some papaya plants have been genetically engineered to resist a certain virus. Corn is genetically altered by inserting a gene from the bacterium *Bacillus thurigiensis,* usually referred to as the Bt gene, in the corn DNA. The gene then allows the corn plant to make a protein that is lethal to certain caterpillars that destroy the plant. (Organic farmers even use the Bt bacteria to dust plants in order to destroy pests.) The Bt protein in the corn, which is present in the plant in very low concentrations, has no effect on humans, as it is digested along with the other proteins in corn. FDA is confident that these currently approved varieties of genetically engineered foods are safe to consume. (The controversy over use of StarLink corn in 2000 arose because this GMO corn variety was not approved for human consumption. It found its way, however, into some corn products, such as taco shells.) Foods are not currently required to state the amount of GMO content, but some manufacturers have put GMO-free labels on their products. FDA does not feel labeling of GMO products is needed because these pose no health risk. The biggest debate in the United States surrounds the potential hazards to the environment from introducing genes from one species to another. There is also a question regarding the actual reduction in pesticide use that accompanies the cultivation of some of these products; it may not be as great as was originally predicted.

Public response to use of the new biotechnology has been mixed. Even the scientific community has mixed feelings about this new technology, with supporters as convinced about the benefits as opponents are of the risks. Although the use of genetically modified organisms may reduce the need for environmentally harmful activities, such as spraying crops with insecticides, critics point out that seeds produced with natural insecticides will lead to rapid insect resistance because the insecticides are continuously being emitted. When farmers use insecticides, they use them sparingly and only when needed, in part so the insects do not become resistant.

Although the risks may appear to be momentarily negligible, they may be cumulative and therefore dangerous in the long run. In addition, will allergens, such as those found in peanuts, eggs, milk, wheat, and shellfish, be added to genetically engineered foods that previously did not contain them? Evidence that this can happen has been seen in soybeans. Note, however, that FDA carefully examines all products developed using this technology and will enforce labeling of potential allergens that may be newly present in a biotech food.

The public has long been opposed to processes perceived as harmful to the environment, such as producing unnatural products. Because food reserves are high in the United States, Canada, and Europe, some question the need to increase food production. Skepticism surrounds unnatural products, as exemplified by western Europe's ban of a growth hormone previously used in beef production. Citizens believed the increase in meat supply was not worth the perceived risks associated with the product. Both scientists and concerned consumer groups are currently studying other potentially beneficial applications of the new biotechnology. Bovine somatotropin (BST), a hormone produced by cattle, has been known since the 1930s to increase milk production when injected into dairy cattle. Today an identical BST (Posilac) produced through genetic engineering can be used to greatly increase milk yield. Because it is a protein, any BST in the milk produced would be digested and therefore inactivated. People even produce their own form of somatotropin, but its structure differs considerably from that of BST. Because cows produce BST naturally, it has always been present in their milk. Treating the animals with the proposed higher levels of BST won't increase the concentration of hormone occurring naturally in the milk, nor will it alter the milk's nutrient composition.

While FDA is still evaluating the safety of BST with respect to animals and the environment, the agency has determined that milk from treated animals is safe for human consumption. Currently about 1 in 10 dairy farms uses the product. Some critics question whether the increased milk production will stress the health of the cows, leading farmers to use more antibiotics, which can show up in milk. The public already appears to oppose BST, and the European Economic Community has banned its use.

Opponents to BST call for labeling of milk from treated cows. The biotech industry opposes labeling the milk because studies show no harmful effects from milk of BST-treated cows. FDA has not required such labeling, but such foods using genetic engineering cannot carry an "organic" label (see Table 2.11 in Chapter 2).

Again, with a surplus of milk in North America and Europe, garnering public support will be difficult. Furthermore, dairy farmers in Wisconsin and other dairy-producing regions generally oppose the introduction of the hormone, because they fear negative consumer reaction will lower milk consumption. The industry is also concerned that a sharp increase in milk output will adversely affect prices and thereby harm thousands of small dairy farms facing an already precarious economic situation.

Role of the New Biotechnology in the Developing World

Whether genetically engineered applications will help to significantly reduce undernutrition in the developing world remains to be seen. Unless price cuts accompany the increased production, only landowners and suppliers of biotechnology will enjoy the benefits. This point deserves emphasis: The person who couldn't afford a GMO papaya yesterday probably won't be able to afford one tomorrow. The same can be said for improved sweet potato seeds. As with most innovations, the more successful farmers, often those with larger farms, will adopt the new biotechnology first. Because of this, the present trend of fewer and larger farms will continue in the developing world, a trend that undermines the most pressing undernutrition issues there. Furthermore, biotechnology does not promise dramatic increases in the production of most grains and cassava, the primary food resources in the world.

Perhaps the most promising potential of genetically engineered foods is the idea of plant breeding for micronutrients. The dilemma of micronutrient undernutrition may be decreased in developing countries if farmers have access to the seeds and related plant materials that produce more of these nutrients. Greater yields for indigenous plants, such as tomatoes that tolerate high amounts of salinity in the soil, is another hopeful outcome. Still, for the developing world, the focus needs to be on providing people with resources to produce and purchase their own food, not on simply growing more food. Biotechnology is a useful tool against the complex scourge of world undernutrition, but it's no panacea. Improved crops produced by this technology will likely be able to contribute to the battle, together with political and other efforts.

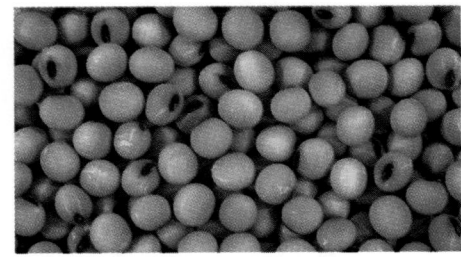

Soybeans are a common GMO food in the marketplace.

The European Economic Community is very skeptical regarding the use of genetic engineering in foods. This may be because these citizens feel they cannot rely on their governments to ensure food safety, given the problem with mad cow disease in Britain. In contrast, U.S. citizens show great confidence in FDA oversight of food safety. Activism is also much more prevalent in Europe than in the United States. In addition, Europeans feel that the benefits of using GMO varieties are gained mostly by U.S. farmers and U.S. companies, not the Europeans themselves. Currently, it is illegal to import genetically engineered foods, such as products made from genetically engineered corn or soybeans, into Europe. (The same is true for Japan.)

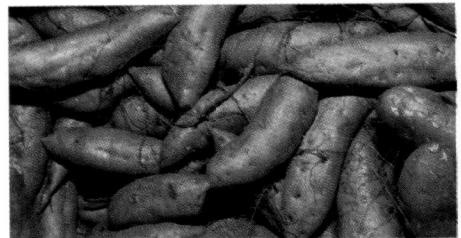

Sweet potatoes have been genetically engineered to resist a virus common in Africa. Yields are increased when these GMO sweet potatoes are grown.

Appendices

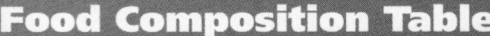
The following table of nutrient values of foods represents a small portion of the database found in the FoodWise diet analysis program available with the textbook. The nutrient data found in FoodWise is largely derived from the USDA Standard Reference and other USDA sources. Some nutrient or food component values for some foods are not included in the database because no *accurate* data values exist. The nutrient or component may in fact be present in the food, but insufficient laboratory analyses have been performed to establish an accurate value.

Name-brand foods often have missing values because manufacturers are only required to analyze for nutrients that must appear on Nutrition Facts labels and only to the level of accuracy required by the nutrition labeling regulations. All missing nutrient or food component values are clearly marked in the table. You are encouraged to refer to the Nutrition Analysis website (www.mhhe.com/nutritionanalysis) for links to nutrient data sites provided by food manufacturers and restaurants not found in Appendix A.

The following is a list of abbreviations used in the Food Composition Table:

Abbreviation Key:

Unit/Amt = Unit Amount
Wt (g) = Weight in grams
Energy (Kcal) = kilocalories
Prot (g) = Protein
Carb (g) = Carbohydrate
Fiber (g) = Dietary fiber
Fat (g) = Total fat
Mono (g) = Monounsaturated fat
Poly (g) = Polyunsaturated fat
Sat (g) = Saturated fat
Chol (mg) = Cholesterol
Cal (mg) = Calcium
Iron (mg) = Iron
Magn (mg) = Magnesium

Phos (mg) = Phosphorus
Pota (mg) = Potassium
Sodi (mg) = Sodium
Zinc (mg) = Zinc
Vit A (RE) = Vitamin A
Vit C (mg) = Vitamin C
Vit E (mg) = Vitamin E
Thia (mg) = Thiamin
Ribo (mg) = Riboflavin
Niac (mg) = Niacin
Vit B-6 (mg) = Vitamin B-6
Fol (µg) = Folate
Vit B-12 (µg) = Vitamin B-12
Wat (g) = Water

Note   g = gram
         mg = milligram
         µg = microgram

Code	Food Name	Unit/Amt	Wt (g)	Energy (Kcal)	Prot (g)	Carb (g)	Fiber (g)	Fat (g)	Mono (g)	Poly (g)
16104	Bacon, Vegetarian, Meatless	1 strip	5	15.5	0.5	0.3	0.1	1.5	0.4	0.8
18005	Bagel, Cinnamon-Raisin	1 mini bagel 2.5" dia	46	126.0	4.5	25.4	1.1	0.8	0.1	0.3
18003	Bagel, Egg	1 bagel 3.5" dia	64	177.9	6.8	33.9	1.5	1.3	0.3	0.4
18007	Bagel, Oatbran	1 bagel 3.5" dia	64	163.2	6.8	34.1	2.3	0.8	0.2	0.3
918008	Bagel, Oatbran, toasted, mini/small sizes	1 mini bagel 2.5" dia	46	126.0	5.3	26.4	1.7	0.6	0.0	0.0
18001	Bagel, Plain/Onion/Poppy/Sesame, enriched	1 bagel 3.5" dia	64	176.0	6.7	34.2	1.5	1.0	0.1	0.4
918801	Leavening Agent, Baking Powder	1 tsp	4	12.5	1.5	1.5	1.5	0.0	0.0	0.0
924037	Bean Burrito	8.0 oz	224	463.7	20.0	64.0	1.5	14.3	0.0	0.0
16115	Bean Flour, Soy, fullfat, raw	1 cup	85	370.6	29.4	29.9	8.2	17.6	3.9	9.9
16118	Bean Flour, Soy, lowfat	1 cup	88	327.4	40.9	33.4	9.0	5.9	1.3	3.3
16112	Bean Sauce, Fermented Soy Product, Miso	½ cup	138	284.3	16.3	38.6	7.5	8.4	1.9	4.7
16114	Bean Sauce, Fermented Soy Product, Tempeh	½ cup	83	165.2	15.7	14.1	0.0	6.4	1.4	3.6
16123	Bean Sauce, Soy & Wheat (Shoyu)	1 tbsp	15	8.0	0.8	1.3	0.1	0.0	0.0	0.0
16424	Bean Sauce, Soy & Wheat (Shoyu) low sodium	1 tbsp	15	8.0	0.8	1.3	0.1	0.0	0.0	0.0
16008	Beans, Baked w/franks, canned	1 cup	256	363.5	17.3	39.4	17.7	16.8	7.2	2.1
16011	Beans, Baked w/pork & tom sauce, canned	1 cup	227	222.5	11.7	44.0	10.9	2.3	1.0	0.3
16006	Beans, Baked, Plain or Vegetarian, canned	1 cup	254	236.2	12.2	52.1	12.7	1.1	0.1	0.5
16018	Beans, Black Turtle Soup, mature seeds, canned	1 cup	253	230.2	15.3	41.9	17.5	0.7	0.1	0.3
16054	Beans, Broadbeans (Fava) mature seeds, canned	½ cup	94	66.7	5.1	11.7	3.5	0.2	0.0	0.1
16026	Beans, Great Northern, mature seeds, canned	½ cup	131	149.3	9.7	27.5	6.4	0.5	0.0	0.2
16029	Beans, Kidney, mature seeds, canned	½ cup	128	103.7	6.7	19.0	4.5	0.4	0.0	0.2
16070	Beans, Lentils, mature seeds, boiled w/o salt	½ cup	99	114.8	8.9	19.9	7.8	0.4	0.1	0.2
16081	Beans, Mung, mature seeds, boiled w/o salt	½ cup	52	54.6	3.7	10.0	4.0	0.2	0.0	0.1
16039	Beans, Navy, mature seeds, canned	½ cup	91	102.8	6.9	18.6	4.6	0.4	0.0	0.2
16044	Beans, Pinto, mature seeds, canned	½ cup	113	97.2	5.5	17.2	5.2	0.9	0.2	0.3
16103	Beans, Refried, canned (includes USDA Commodity)	½ cup	126	118.4	6.9	19.6	6.7	1.6	0.7	0.2
16111	Beans, Soy, mature seeds, dry roasted	½ cup	144	648.0	57.0	47.1	11.7	31.1	6.9	17.6
16162	Beans, Soy, Tofu, Mori-Nu, silken, firm	¼ block	84	52.1	5.8	2.0	0.1	2.3	0.5	1.2
16164	Beans, Soy, Tofu, Mori-Nu, silken, lite firm	¼ block	84	31.1	5.3	0.9	0.0	0.7	0.1	0.4
16161	Beans, Soy, Tofu, Mori-Nu, silken, soft	¼ block	84	46.2	4.0	2.4	0.1	2.3	0.4	1.3
16132	Beans, Soy, Tofu, Nigari, Fuyu, salted & fermented	¼ block	84	97.4	6.8	4.3	0.0	6.7	1.5	3.8
913524	Beef Brisket, All Grades, lean (½"trim) braised	3.5 oz	100	241.0	29.4	0.0	0.0	12.8	0.0	0.0
913522	Beef Brisket, All Grades, lean&fat (½"trim) braised	3.5 oz	100	391.0	23.0	0.0	0.0	32.4	0.0	0.0
924324	Beef Burgundy, frz (Le Menu)	7.5 oz	213	315.2	25.1	12.3	0.0	18.5	0.0	0.0
924246	Beef Chop Suey	1 cup	250	300.0	26.0	12.5	1.3	17.0	0.0	0.0
924222	Beef Chow Mein/LaChoy	¾ cup	120	60.0	6.0	5.0	2.0	1.0	0.6	0.0
924022	Beef Goulash	7.5 oz	213	213.0	13.2	21.7	0.0	8.1	0.0	0.0
13326	Beef Liver, braised	3.5 oz	100	161.0	24.4	3.4	0.0	4.9	0.7	1.1
13327	Beef Liver, pan fried	4.0 oz	119	258.2	31.8	9.3	0.0	9.5	1.9	2.0
924002	Beef Pot Pie, frz (Banquet)	7.0 oz	198	485.1	19.8	36.8	1.7	28.3	12.2	7.0
924034	Beef Stroganoff, frz (Stouffers)	4.0 oz	142	200.2	15.6	5.8	0.0	12.8	0.0	0.0
913512	Beef, All Cuts, All Grades, lean (½"trim) ckd	3.5 oz	100	222.0	30.4	0.0	0.0	10.2	0.0	0.0
13012	Beef, All Cuts, All Grades, lean (¼"trim) ckd	3.5 oz	100	216.0	29.6	0.0	0.0	9.9	4.2	0.3
913504	Beef, All Cuts, All Grades, lean&fat (½"trim) ckd	3.5 oz	100	349.0	25.0	0.0	0.0	26.9	0.0	0.0
13004	Beef, All Cuts, All Grades, lean&fat (¼"trim) ckd	3.5 oz	100	305.0	25.9	0.0	0.0	21.5	9.2	0.8
13366	Beef, All Cuts, Select, lean (0"trim) ckd	3.5 oz	100	201.0	29.9	0.0	0.0	8.1	3.4	0.3
924108	Beef, Corned Beef Hash	3.5 oz	100	184.0	8.5	8.5	1.2	12.7	5.8	0.6
924325	Beef, Creamed Chipped	4.0 oz	113	174.0	9.3	8.0	0.0	11.6	4.6	0.6
13347	Beef, Cured Corned Beef Brisket, cooked	3.5 oz	100	251.0	18.2	0.5	0.0	19.0	9.2	0.7
13418	Beef, Eye of Round, All Grades, lean (0"trim) roasted	100	166.0	29.0	0.0	0.0	4.7	2.0	0.2	1.7
13300	Beef, Ground, extra lean, pan fried, medium	4.0 oz	119	303.5	29.7	0.0	0.0	19.5	8.6	0.7
13305	Beef, Ground, lean, broiled, medium	3.5 oz	100	272.0	24.7	0.0	0.0	18.5	8.1	0.7
13307	Beef, Ground, lean, pan fried, medium	3.5 oz	100	275.0	24.2	0.0	0.0	19.1	8.3	0.7
13312	Beef, Ground, regular, broiled, medium	3.5 oz	100	289.0	24.1	0.0	0.0	20.7	9.1	0.8
13314	Beef, Ground, regular, pan fried, medium	4.0 oz	119	364.1	28.5	0.0	0.0	26.8	11.8	1.0
13315	Beef, Ground, regular, pan fried, welldone	4.0 oz	119	340.3	32.1	0.0	0.0	22.5	9.9	0.8
14177	Beverage Mix, Chocolate Flavor, dry mix, prep w/milk	8.0 oz	224	190.4	7.4	26.0	1.1	7.4	2.2	0.3
14317	Beverage Mix, Chocolate Malt Milk Flavor Powder, no added nutrients	¾ oz (3 heaping tsp)	21	78.8	1.1	18.4	0.2	0.8	0.2	0.1
14316	Beverage Mix, Chocolate Malt Powder, fort, prep w/milk	8.0 oz	224	190.4	7.6	24.6	0.2	7.4	2.2	0.3
14318	Beverage Mix, Chocolate Malted Milk Powder, no added nutrients, prep w/milk	8.0 oz	224	192.6	7.6	25.3	0.2	7.6	2.2	0.3
14245	Beverage Mix, Eggnog, dry, prep w/milk	8.0 oz	224	215.0	6.7	32.0	0.7	6.9	2.0	0.3
14310	Beverage Mix, Natural Malt Powder, fortified, prep w/milk	8.0 oz	224	194.9	8.3	24.0	0.0	7.4	2.1	0.3
14351	Beverage Mix, Strawberry Flavor, dry, prep w/milk	8.0 oz	224	197.1	6.7	27.6	0.0	6.9	2.0	0.3
14006	Beverage, Alcoholic, Beer, Light	12.0 oz	360	100.8	0.7	4.7	0.0	0.0	0.0	0.0
14003	Beverage, Alcoholic, Beer, Regular	12.0 oz	360	147.6	1.1	13.3	0.7	0.0	0.0	0.0
914008	Beverage, Alcoholic, Bloody Mary, prep from recipe	5.0 oz	148	115.4	0.7	4.9	0.4	0.1	0.0	0.0
914870	Beverage, Alcoholic, Champagne	3.5 oz	103	72.1	0.2	2.6	0.0	0.0	0.0	0.0
14414	Beverage, Alcoholic, Coffee Liqueur 53 proof	1.5 oz	52	174.7	0.1	24.3	0.0	0.2	0.0	0.1
14009	Beverage, Alcoholic, Daiquiri, canned	6.8 oz	209	261.3	0.0	32.8	0.0	0.0	0.0	0.0

Sat (g)	Chol (mg)	Cal (mg)	Iron (mg)	Magn (mg)	Phos (mg)	Pota (mg)	Sodi (mg)	Zinc (mg)	Vit A (RE)	Vit C (mg)	Vit E (mg)	Thia (mg)	Ribo (mg)	Niac (mg)	Vit B-6 (mg)	Fol (µg)	Vit B-12 (µg)	Wat (g)
0.2	0.0	1.2	0.1	1.0	3.5	8.5	73.3	0.0	0.5	0.0	0.3	0.2	0.0	0.4	0.0	2.1	0.0	2.4
0.1	0.0	8.7	1.7	12.9	46.0	68.1	148.1	0.5	0.0	0.3	0.1	0.2	0.1	1.4	0.0	41.4	0.0	14.7
0.3	15.4	8.3	2.5	16.0	53.8	43.5	323.2	0.5	21.1	0.4	0.0	0.3	0.2	2.2	0.1	56.3	0.1	20.9
0.1	0.0	7.7	2.0	19.8	70.4	73.6	324.5	0.6	0.0	0.1	0.1	0.2	0.2	1.9	0.0	51.8	0.0	21.1
0.2	0.1	6.0	1.5	28.5	81.4	100.7	250.7	1.0	0.0	0.0	0.1	0.1	0.2	1.3	0.1	16.1	0.0	12.8
0.1	0.0	47.4	2.3	18.6	61.4	64.6	341.8	0.6	0.0	0.0	0.0	0.3	0.2	2.9	0.0	56.3	0.0	20.9
0.0	0.0	8.5	0.7	0.0	70.0	76.0	5.0	0.3	0.0	0.0	0.0	0.6	0.2	1.5	0.2	156.5	0.0	0.0
0.0	0.0	275.7	1.6	103.4	265.1	634.9	1387.7	0.0	0.0	0.0	0.0	0.0	0.0	0.0	0.0	0.0	0.0	0.0
2.5	0.0	175.1	5.4	364.7	419.9	2137.8	11.1	3.3	10.2	0.0	1.7	0.5	1.0	3.7	0.4	293.3	0.0	4.4
0.9	0.0	165.4	5.3	201.5	521.8	2261.6	15.8	1.0	3.5	0.0	0.2	0.3	0.3	1.9	0.5	360.8	0.0	2.4
1.2	0.0	91.1	3.8	58.0	211.1	226.3	5032.9	4.6	12.4	0.0	0.0	0.1	0.3	1.2	0.3	45.5	0.0	57.2
0.9	0.0	77.2	1.9	58.1	171.0	304.6	5.0	1.5	57.3	0.0	0.0	0.1	0.1	3.8	0.2	43.2	0.8	45.6
0.0	0.0	2.6	0.3	5.1	16.5	27.0	857.3	0.1	0.0	0.0	0.0	0.0	0.0	0.5	0.0	2.3	0.0	10.7
0.0	0.0	2.6	0.3	5.1	16.5	27.0	500.0	0.1	0.0	0.0	0.0	0.0	0.0	0.5	0.0	2.3	0.0	10.7
6.0	15.4	122.9	4.4	71.7	266.2	601.6	1100.8	4.8	38.4	5.9	1.2	0.1	0.1	2.3	0.1	76.8	0.0	177.5
0.9	15.9	127.1	7.4	79.5	265.6	681.0	998.8	13.3	27.2	7.0	1.2	0.1	0.1	1.1	0.2	51.1	0.0	165.0
0.3	0.0	127.0	0.7	81.3	264.2	751.8	1008.4	3.6	43.2	7.9	1.3	0.4	0.2	1.1	0.3	60.7	0.0	184.5
0.2	0.0	88.6	4.8	88.6	273.2	779.2	971.5	1.4	0.0	6.8	0.0	0.4	0.3	1.6	0.1	153.8	0.0	191.4
0.0	0.0	24.4	0.9	30.1	74.3	227.5	425.8	0.6	0.9	1.7	0.0	0.0	0.0	0.9	0.0	30.7	0.0	75.5
0.2	0.0	69.4	2.1	66.8	178.2	459.8	5.2	0.9	0.0	1.7	0.0	0.2	0.1	0.6	0.1	106.5	0.0	91.6
0.1	0.0	34.6	1.6	39.7	134.4	329.0	444.2	0.7	0.0	1.5	0.0	0.1	0.1	0.6	0.1	63.0	0.0	99.8
0.1	0.0	18.8	3.3	35.6	178.2	365.3	2.0	1.3	1.0	1.5	0.1	0.2	0.1	1.0	0.2	179.0	0.0	68.9
0.1	0.0	14.0	0.7	25.0	51.5	138.3	1.0	0.4	1.0	0.5	0.3	0.1	0.0	0.3	0.0	82.6	0.0	37.8
0.1	0.0	42.8	1.7	42.8	121.9	262.1	407.7	0.7	0.0	0.6	0.3	0.1	0.1	0.4	0.1	56.7	0.0	64.1
0.2	0.0	48.6	1.6	30.5	104.0	274.6	332.2	0.8	2.3	1.0	1.1	0.1	0.1	0.3	0.1	68.0	0.0	87.6
0.6	10.1	44.1	2.1	41.6	108.4	336.4	376.7	1.5	0.0	7.6	0.0	0.0	0.0	0.4	0.2	13.9	0.0	95.7
4.5	0.0	201.6	5.7	328.3	934.6	1964.2	2.9	6.9	2.9	6.6	0.0	0.6	1.1	1.5	0.3	294.6	0.0	1.2
0.3	0.0	26.9	0.9	22.7	75.6	163.0	30.2	0.5	0.0	0.0	0.2	0.1	0.0	0.2	0.0	0.0	0.0	73.4
0.1	0.0	30.2	0.6	8.4	68.0	52.9	71.4	0.3	0.0	0.0	0.1	0.0	0.0	0.1	0.0	0.0	0.0	76.8
0.3	0.0	26.0	0.7	24.4	52.1	151.2	4.2	0.4	0.0	0.0	0.2	0.1	0.0	0.3	0.0	0.0	0.0	74.8
1.0	0.0	38.6	1.7	43.7	61.3	63.0	2413.3	1.3	14.3	0.2	0.0	0.1	0.1	0.3	0.1	24.4	0.0	58.8
0.4	5.8	6.0	2.8	23.0	239.0	287.0	72.0	6.9	0.0	0.0	0.0	0.1	0.2	3.8	0.3	8.0	2.6	55.7
1.2	14.7	9.0	2.2	18.0	184.0	229.0	61.0	5.0	0.0	0.0	0.0	0.1	0.2	3.0	0.3	6.0	2.2	43.0
0.0	0.0	37.0	1.0	0.0	0.0	231.0	640.0	0.0	207.4	2.0	0.0	0.1	0.3	3.6	0.0	0.0	0.0	0.0
8.5	0.0	60.0	4.8	0.0	248.0	425.0	1053.0	0.0	120.0	33.0	0.0	0.3	0.4	5.0	0.0	0.0	0.0	188.5
0.4	16.0	80.0	1.4	0.0	0.0	150.0	890.0	0.0	150.0	2.0	0.0	0.1	0.1	1.2	0.0	0.0	0.0	0.0
0.0	0.0	49.0	1.7	0.0	0.0	357.0	753.0	0.0	144.4	1.0	0.0	0.0	0.2	1.7	0.0	0.0	0.0	167.2
1.9	389.0	7.0	6.8	20.0	404.0	235.0	70.0	6.1	10602.0	23.0	0.0	0.2	4.1	10.7	0.9	217.0	71.0	65.9
3.2	573.6	13.1	7.5	27.4	548.6	433.2	126.1	6.5	12767.5	27.4	0.8	0.2	4.9	17.2	1.7	261.8	133.0	66.3
7.4	39.6	27.3	3.6	0.0	140.5	314.9	561.9	3.0	795.8	5.7	0.0	0.3	0.3	4.5	0.2	27.3	0.0	0.0
0.0	56.5	33.9	1.4	0.0	0.0	270.2	795.5	0.0	8.5	0.0	0.0	0.1	0.3	2.6	0.0	0.0	0.0	105.1
0.4	4.5	8.0	3.2	27.0	245.0	352.0	65.0	7.1	0.0	0.0	0.0	0.3	0.3	4.2	0.4	9.0	2.7	57.8
3.8	86.0	9.0	3.0	26.0	233.0	360.0	67.0	6.9	0.0	0.0	0.1	0.1	0.2	4.1	0.4	8.0	2.6	59.3
1.0	12.0	10.0	2.6	21.0	193.0	287.0	59.0	5.5	0.0	0.0	0.0	0.1	0.2	3.5	0.3	7.0	2.4	46.9
8.5	88.0	10.0	2.6	22.0	203.0	313.0	62.0	5.9	0.0	0.0	0.0	0.2	0.1	3.6	0.3	7.0	2.4	51.4
3.1	86.0	8.0	3.0	26.0	231.0	354.0	66.0	6.8	0.0	0.0	0.0	0.1	0.2	4.0	0.4	8.0	2.6	60.1
4.9	155.3	34.1	5.2	0.0	172.9	517.6	672.9	5.2	0.0	0.0	9.4	0.0	0.1	5.3	0.5	17.6	0.0	0.0
6.3	29.5	118.5	0.9	0.0	158.2	173.0	809.0	0.0	81.2	0.5	0.0	0.1	0.2	0.7	0.0	0.0	0.0	81.4
6.3	98.0	8.0	1.9	12.0	125.0	145.0	1134.0	4.6	0.0	0.0	0.2	0.0	0.2	3.0	0.2	6.0	1.6	59.8
69.0		5.0	2.0	27.0	226.0	395.0	62.0	4.7	0.0	0.0	0.1	0.1	0.2	3.8	0.4	7.0	2.2	64.6
7.7	96.4	8.3	2.8	25.0	190.4	371.3	83.3	6.4	0.0	0.0	0.2	0.1	0.3	5.6	0.3	10.7	2.4	68.5
7.3	87.0	11.0	2.1	21.0	158.0	301.0	77.0	5.4	0.0	0.0	0.2	0.1	0.2	5.2	0.3	9.0	2.4	55.7
7.5	84.0	10.0	2.2	20.0	159.0	299.0	77.0	5.2	0.0	0.0	0.2	0.1	0.2	4.8	0.3	9.0	2.3	55.6
8.1	90.0	11.0	2.4	20.0	170.0	292.0	83.0	5.2	0.0	0.0	0.2	0.0	0.2	5.8	0.3	9.0	2.9	54.2
10.5	105.9	13.1	2.9	23.8	203.5	357.0	100.0	6.0	0.0	0.0	0.0	0.3	0.0	6.9	0.3	10.7	3.2	62.2
8.8	116.6	15.5	3.2	26.2	224.9	395.1	110.7	6.7	0.0	0.0	0.0	0.0	0.2	7.7	0.3	11.9	3.6	62.7
4.6	26.9	253.1	0.7	44.8	215.0	418.9	138.9	1.1	65.0	2.0	0.0	0.1	0.4	0.3	0.1	10.3	0.7	181.2
0.5	1.1	12.6	0.5	14.7	36.8	129.8	52.7	0.2	4.0	0.3	0.1	0.0	0.0	0.4	0.0	4.2	0.0	0.3
4.6	29.1	324.8	3.2	44.8	264.3	524.2	206.1	1.0	761.6	28.7	0.0	0.6	1.1	9.2	0.9	26.9	0.7	181.9
4.7	29.1	257.6	0.5	40.3	224.0	421.1	145.6	0.9	67.2	2.2	0.0	0.1	0.4	0.5	0.1	13.9	0.8	181.7
4.2	26.9	239.7	0.3	26.9	188.2	304.6	134.4	0.8	62.7	1.8	0.0	0.1	0.3	0.2	0.1	10.1	0.7	176.7
4.6	29.1	313.6	3.0	40.3	259.8	483.8	172.5	0.9	627.2	24.9	0.0	0.6	1.0	8.8	0.7	18.4	0.9	182.1
4.3	26.9	246.4	0.2	26.9	192.6	311.4	107.5	0.8	62.7	2.0	0.0	0.1	0.4	0.2	0.1	10.3	0.7	181.2
0.0	0.0	18.0	0.1	18.0	43.2	64.8	10.8	0.1	0.0	0.0	0.0	0.0	0.1	1.4	0.1	14.8	0.0	342.7
0.0	0.0	18.0	0.1	21.6	43.2	90.0	18.0	0.1	0.0	0.0	0.0	0.0	0.1	1.6	0.2	21.6	0.1	332.3
0.0	0.0	10.4	0.5	11.8	20.7	216.1	331.5	0.1	50.3	20.4	0.0	0.1	0.0	0.6	0.1	19.7	0.0	127.3
0.0	0.0	0.0	0.0	0.0	0.0	0.0	0.0	0.0	0.0	0.0	0.0	0.0	0.0	0.0	0.0	0.0	0.0	0.0
0.1	0.0	0.5	0.0	1.6	3.1	15.6	4.2	0.0	0.0	0.0	0.0	0.0	0.0	0.1	0.0	0.0	0.0	16.1
0.0	0.0	0.0	0.0	2.1	4.2	23.0	83.6	0.1	0.0	2.7	0.0	0.0	0.0	0.0	0.0	1.7	0.0	155.9

Code	Food Name	Unit/Amt	Wt (g)	Energy (Kcal)	Prot (g)	Carb (g)	Fiber (g)	Fat (g)	Mono (g)	Poly (g)
14037	Beverage, Alcoholic, Distilled Spirits (gin, rum, vodka or whisky) 80 proof	1.5 oz	42	97.0	0.0	0.0	0.0	0.0	0.0	0.0
914011	Beverage, Alcoholic, Gin and Tonic, prep from recipe	7.5 oz	225	171.0	0.0	15.8	0.0	0.0	0.0	0.0
914014	Beverage, Alcoholic, Martini, prep from recipe	2.5 oz	70	156.1	0.0	0.2	0.0	0.0	0.0	0.0
14015	Beverage, Alcoholic, Pina Colada, canned	6.8 oz	209	495.3	1.3	57.7	0.2	15.9	0.9	0.3
14027	Beverage, Alcoholic, Whiskey Sour, canned	6.8 oz	209	248.7	0.0	28.0	0.2	0.0	0.0	0.0
14084	Beverage, Alcoholic, Wine (all table)	3.5 oz	103	72.1	0.2	1.4	0.0	0.0	0.0	0.0
14115	Beverage, Alpine Spiced Cider, Instant Apple Flavor Drink Mix, h powder/Continenta	2 tbsp	8	31.6	0.0	7.9	0.0	0.0	0.0	0.0
14181	Beverage, Chocolate Syrup w/o added nutrients	2 tbsp	38	82.8	0.7	22.4	0.7	0.3	0.1	0.1
14186	Beverage, Chocolate Syrup, fortified, mixed w/milk	8.0 oz	224	168.0	7.2	20.2	0.7	7.2	2.1	0.3
14390	Beverage, Cocoa Mix w/aspartame, dry, low kcal, prep w/H₂O	8.0 oz	224	56.0	4.5	9.9	0.4	0.4	0.2	0.0
14194	Beverage, Cocoa Mix, dry, w/o added nutrients, prep w/H₂O	8.0 oz	224	112.0	3.4	24.4	2.7	1.3	0.4	0.0
14417	Beverage, Cocoa Mix, fortified, dry, prep w/H₂O	8.0 oz	224	127.7	2.0	25.8	0.9	3.1	1.1	0.1
14195	Beverage, Cocoa, Hot Cocoa Mix w/marshmallows/Carnation	2 tbsp	22	87.8	1.1	19.1	0.4	0.8	0.2	0.3
14418	Beverage, Coffee Mix w/sugar (Cappuccino) dry, prep w/H₂O	8.0 oz	224	71.7	0.4	12.5	0.0	2.5	0.1	0.0
14209	Beverage, Coffee, Brewed	6.0 oz	168	3.4	0.2	0.7	0.0	0.0	0.0	0.0
14219	Beverage, Coffee, Instant powder, decaffeinated, prep	1 rd tsp.	1.8	0.0	0.0	0.0	0.0	0.0	0.0	0.0
14215	Beverage, Coffee, Instant, prep	6.0 oz	168	3.4	0.2	0.7	0.0	0.0	0.0	0.0
14400	Beverage, Cola w/caffeine	12.0 oz	336	137.8	0.0	34.9	0.0	0.0	0.0	0.0
1057	Beverage, Eggnog	8.0 oz	254	341.9	9.7	34.4	0.0	19.0	5.7	0.9
914840	Beverage, Fruit Tea Punch	6.0 oz	168	107.5	0.0	27.0	0.0	0.0	0.0	0.0
14123	Beverage, Kiwi Strawberry Cocktail/Snapple	6.0 oz	168	80.0	0.2	19.8	0.0	0.0	0.0	0.0
14305	Beverage, Malt Beverage	6.0 oz	168	100.8	0.5	22.6	0.0	0.2	0.0	0.1
14137	Beverage, Nestea Ice Tea, Lemon Flavor	6.0 oz	168	61.7	0.0	14.3	0.0	0.5	0.0	0.0
914814	Beverage, Soft Drink, Chocolate Carbonated	12.0 oz	355	163.3	0.0	41.5	0.0	0.0	0.0	0.0
14121	Beverage, Soft Drink, Club Soda	12.0 oz	355	0.0	0.0	0.0	0.0	0.0	0.0	0.0
14166	Beverage, Soft Drink, Cola or Pepper-type, low kcal w/saccharin & caffeine	12.0 oz	355	0.0	0.0	0.4	0.0	0.0	0.0	0.0
14535	Beverage, Soft Drink, Cola, low kcal w/saccharin&aspartame, w/caffeine	12.0 oz	355	3.6	0.4	0.4	0.0	0.0	0.0	0.0
14416	Beverage, Soft Drink, Cola, w/aspartame, low kcal	12.0 oz	355	3.6	0.4	0.4	0.0	0.0	0.0	0.0
14130	Beverage, Soft Drink, Cream Soda	12.0 oz	355	181.1	0.0	47.2	0.0	0.0	0.0	0.0
914818	Beverage, Soft Drink, Diet Fruit Flavor	12.0 oz	355	3.6	0.0	0.0	0.0	0.0	0.0	0.0
914819	Beverage, Soft Drink, Diet Ginger Ale	12.0 oz	355	3.6	0.0	1.5	0.0	0.0	0.0	0.0
914820	Beverage, Soft Drink, Diet Lemon-Lime	12.0 oz	355	0.0	0.0	0.0	0.0	0.0	0.0	0.0
914887	Beverage, Soft Drink, Diet Root Beer	12.0 oz	355	0.0	0.0	0.4	0.0	0.0	0.0	0.0
14136	Beverage, Soft Drink, Ginger Ale	12.0 oz	355	120.7	0.0	30.9	0.0	0.0	0.0	0.0
14142	Beverage, Soft Drink, Grape	12.0 oz	355	152.7	0.0	39.8	0.0	0.0	0.0	0.0
14145	Beverage, Soft Drink, Lemon-Lime	12.0 oz	355	142.0	0.0	36.9	0.0	0.0	0.0	0.0
914888	Beverage, Soft Drink, Mineral H₂O	12.0 oz	355	0.0	0.0	0.0	0.0	0.0	0.0	0.0
14537	Beverage, Soft Drink, Not Cola or Pepper-type, w/saccharin, low kcal	12.0 oz	355	0.0	0.0	0.4	0.0	0.0	0.0	0.0
14150	Beverage, Soft Drink, Orange	12.0 oz	355	170.4	0.0	43.7	0.0	0.0	0.0	0.0
14153	Beverage, Soft Drink, Pepper type	12.0 oz	355	145.6	0.0	36.9	0.0	0.4	0.0	0.0
14157	Beverage, Soft Drink, Root Beer	12.0 oz	355	145.6	0.0	37.6	0.0	0.0	0.0	0.0
14376	Beverage, Tea Mix, Instant w/lemon flavor, w/saccharin, dry, prep	2 tsp	1.4	0.0	0.0	0.0	0.0	0.0	0.0	0.0
14369	Beverage, Tea Mix, Instant w/lemon, unsweetened, dry, prep	2 tsp	1.4	0.0	0.0	0.0	0.0	0.0	0.0	0.0
14367	Beverage, Tea Mix, Instant, unsweetened, dry, prep	2 tsp	1.4	0.0	0.0	0.0	0.0	0.0	0.0	0.0
14355	Beverage, Tea, Brewed	6.0 oz	240	2.4	0.0	0.7	0.0	0.0	0.0	0.0
14545	Beverage, Tea, Chamomile, Brewed	6.0 oz	240	2.4	0.0	0.5	0.0	0.0	0.0	0.0
914810	Beverage, Tea, Crystal Light	6.0 oz	240	2.4	0.1	0.4	0.0	0.0	0.0	0.0
14381	Beverage, Tea, Herbal (not chamomile) Brewed	6.0 oz	240	2.4	0.0	0.5	0.0	0.0	0.0	0.0
14549	Beverage, Tea, Instant, w/sugar, lemon-flavored, w/added Vit C, dry, prep	6.0 oz	240	81.6	0.2	20.4	0.0	0.0	0.0	0.0
914906	Beverage, Tea, sweetened, canned	12.0 oz	480	196.8	0.0	48.7	0.0	0.0	0.0	0.0
14133	Beverage, Tomato Cocktail/Bloody Mary mix, mild/Tabasco	6.0 oz	240	55.7	2.2	11.8	0.0	0.0	0.0	0.0
14429	Beverage, Water	1.0 fl oz	30	0.3	0.0	0.0	0.0	0.0	0.0	0.0
14155	Beverage, Water, Carbonated, Tonic (Quinine)	12.0 oz can or bottle	366	124.4	0.0	32.2	0.0	0.0	0.0	0.0
14384	Beverage, Water, Perrier	6.5 fl oz bottle	192	0.0	0.0	0.0	0.0	0.0	0.0	0.0
18615	Biscuit, Buttermilk Biscuit Mix, dry/Martha White	1 biscuit	41	171.4	3.0	26.4	0.0	5.9	0.0	0.0
18017	Biscuit, Mixed Grain, refrig dough	1 biscuit (2.5" dia)	44	115.7	2.7	20.9	0.0	2.5	1.3	0.4
18633	Biscuit, Pillsbury Grands Buttermilk, refrigerated dough/Pillsbury	1 biscuit	61	194.8	4.1	25.1	0.0	8.7	0.0	0.0
18009	Biscuit, Plain or Buttermilk, commercially baked	1 small (2.5" diam)	35	127.4	2.2	17.0	0.5	5.8	2.4	2.2
918011	Biscuit, Plain or Buttermilk, dry mix, prep	1 biscuit (3" dia)	57	191.0	4.2	27.6	1.0	6.9	0.0	0.0
18016	Biscuit, Plain or Buttermilk, homemade	1 medium biscuit (2.5" dia)	60	212.4	4.2	26.8	0.9	9.8	4.2	2.5
18013	Biscuit, Plain or Buttermilk, refrig dough, baked, reduced fat	1 biscuit (2.25" dia)	21	62.8	1.6	11.6	0.4	1.1	0.6	0.2
18015	Biscuit, Plain or Buttermilk, refrig dough, bkd	1 biscuit (2.5" dia)	27	93.4	1.8	12.8	0.4	4.0	2.2	0.5
20015	Bran, Corn, crude	1 tbsp	4.8	10.8	0.4	4.1	4.1	0.0	0.0	0.0
20034	Bran, Oat, ckd	1 tbsp	13.7	5.5	0.4	1.6	0.4	0.1	0.0	0.0
20060	Bran, Rice, crude	1 tbsp	7.4	23.4	1.0	3.7	1.6	1.5	0.6	0.6
20077	Bran, Wheat, crude	1 tbsp	3.5	7.6	0.5	2.3	1.5	0.1	0.0	0.1
18376	Bread Crumbs, dry, grated, seasoned	1 oz	28	102.8	4.0	19.7	1.2	0.7	0.3	0.2
18079	Bread Crumbs, Plain, grated, dry	¼ cup	27	106.7	3.4	19.6	0.6	1.5	0.6	0.3

Sat (g)	Chol (mg)	Cal (mg)	Iron (mg)	Magn (mg)	Phos (mg)	Pota (mg)	Sodi (mg)	Zinc (mg)	Vit A (RE)	Vit C (mg)	Vit E (mg)	Thia (mg)	Ribo (mg)	Niac (mg)	Vit B-6 (mg)	Fol (µg)	Vit B-12 (µg)	Wat (g)
0.0	0.0	0.0	0.0	0.0	1.7	0.8	0.4	0.0	0.0	0.0	0.0	0.0	0.0	0.0	0.0	0.0	0.0	28.0
0.0	0.0	4.5	0.0	2.3	2.3	11.3	9.0	0.2	0.0	0.9	0.0	0.0	0.0	0.0	0.0	1.1	0.0	193.1
0.0	0.0	1.4	0.1	1.4	2.1	12.6	2.1	0.0	0.0	0.0	0.0	0.0	0.0	0.0	0.1	0.0	0.0	47.3
13.7	0.0	2.1	0.1	12.5	75.2	173.5	148.4	0.4	4.2	3.1	0.0	0.0	0.0	0.2	0.0	12.5	0.0	114.7
0.0	0.0	0.0	0.0	2.1	12.5	23.0	92.0	0.1	2.1	3.3	0.0	0.0	0.0	0.0	0.0	0.0	0.0	160.7
0.0	0.0	8.2	0.4	10.3	14.4	91.7	8.2	0.1	0.0	0.0	0.0	0.0	0.0	0.1	0.0	1.1	0.0	91.6
0.0	0.0	0.0	0.0	0.0	0.0	0.0	0.1	0.0	0.0	29.0	0.0	0.0	0.0	0.0	0.0	0.0	0.0	0.0
0.2	0.0	5.3	0.8	24.7	49.0	85.1	36.5	0.3	1.1	0.1	0.0	0.0	0.0	0.1	0.0	1.5	0.0	14.1
4.4	29.1	248.6	2.3	26.9	194.9	392.0	125.4	0.8	273.3	2.0	0.0	0.1	0.5	5.6	0.1	10.3	0.7	187.7
0.3	2.2	105.3	0.9	38.1	156.8	472.6	201.6	0.6	0.0	0.0	0.0	0.0	0.2	0.2	0.1	2.7	0.3	207.0
0.7	2.2	105.3	0.4	26.9	96.3	219.5	161.3	0.5	0.0	0.4	0.0	0.0	0.2	0.2	0.0	0.0	0.4	193.5
1.9	0.0	112.0	1.9	24.6	118.7	434.6	221.8	0.3	161.3	6.5	0.0	0.2	0.2	2.1	0.0	0.0	0.4	190.8
0.3	1.3	32.3	0.2	12.8	45.5	111.5	75.5	0.2	0.0	0.0	0.0	0.0	0.1	0.1	0.0	0.9	0.1	0.4
2.1	0.0	9.0	0.2	11.2	31.4	138.9	121.0	0.1	0.0	0.0	0.0	0.0	0.0	0.4	0.0	0.2	0.0	207.4
0.0	0.0	3.4	0.1	8.4	1.7	90.7	3.4	0.0	0.0	0.0	0.0	0.0	0.0	0.4	0.0	0.2	0.0	166.8
0.0	0.0	0.1	0.0	0.1	0.1	0.6	0.1	0.0	0.0	0.0	0.0	0.0	0.0	0.0	0.0	0.0	0.0	1.8
0.0	0.0	5.0	0.1	6.7	5.0	60.5	5.0	0.1	0.0	0.0	0.0	0.0	0.0	0.5	0.0	0.0	0.0	166.3
0.0	0.0	10.1	0.1	3.4	40.3	3.4	13.4	0.0	0.0	0.0	0.0	0.0	0.0	0.0	0.0	0.0	0.0	300.4
11.3	149.1	330.2	0.5	47.0	277.9	419.6	138.2	1.2	203.2	3.8	0.6	0.1	0.5	0.3	0.1	2.3	1.1	188.9
0.0	0.0	0.0	0.0	0.0	0.0	0.0	9.1	0.0	0.0	0.0	0.0	0.0	0.0	0.0	0.0	0.0	0.0	0.0
0.0	0.0	0.0	0.0	0.0	0.0	0.0	4.2	0.0	0.0	0.0	0.0	0.0	0.0	0.0	0.0	0.0	0.0	147.8
0.0	0.0	8.4	0.1	11.8	37.0	13.4	21.8	0.0	0.0	0.0	0.8	0.0	0.1	1.9	0.0	23.5	0.0	144.5
0.0	0.0	0.0	0.0	0.0	0.0	0.0	0.0	0.0	0.0	0.0	0.0	0.0	0.0	0.0	0.0	0.0	0.0	153.2
0.0	0.0	0.0	0.0	0.0	0.0	0.0	26.6	0.0	0.0	0.0	0.0	0.0	0.0	0.0	0.0	0.0	0.0	0.0
0.0	0.0	17.8	0.0	3.6	0.0	7.1	74.6	0.4	0.0	0.0	0.0	0.0	0.0	0.0	0.0	0.0	0.0	354.6
0.0	0.0	14.2	0.1	3.6	39.1	7.1	56.8	0.2	0.0	0.0	0.0	0.0	0.0	0.0	0.0	0.0	0.0	354.3
0.0	0.0	14.2	0.1	3.6	32.0	0.0	32.0	0.3	0.0	0.0	0.0	0.1	0.0	0.0	0.0	0.0	0.0	354.3
0.0	0.0	14.2	0.1	3.6	32.0	0.0	21.3	0.3	0.0	0.0	0.0	0.1	0.0	0.0	0.0	0.0	0.0	354.3
0.0	0.0	17.8	0.2	3.6	0.0	3.6	42.6	0.2	0.0	0.0	0.0	0.0	0.0	0.0	0.0	0.0	0.0	307.8
0.0	0.0	35.5	0.0	0.0	0.0	0.0	21.7	0.0	0.0	0.0	0.0	0.0	0.0	0.0	0.0	0.0	0.0	0.0
0.0	0.0	17.8	0.0	0.0	0.0	0.0	31.6	0.0	0.0	0.0	0.0	0.0	0.0	0.0	0.0	0.0	0.0	0.0
0.0	0.0	34.5	0.0	0.0	0.0	3.9	48.3	0.0	0.0	0.0	0.0	0.0	0.0	0.0	0.0	0.0	0.0	0.0
0.0	0.0	0.0	0.0	0.0	0.0	0.0	56.6	0.0	0.0	0.0	0.0	0.0	0.0	0.0	0.0	0.0	0.0	0.0
0.0	0.0	10.7	0.6	3.6	0.0	3.6	24.9	0.2	0.0	0.0	0.0	0.0	0.0	0.0	0.0	0.0	0.0	323.8
0.0	0.0	10.7	0.3	3.6	0.0	3.6	53.3	0.2	0.0	0.0	0.0	0.0	0.0	0.0	0.0	0.0	0.0	315.2
0.0	0.0	7.1	0.2	3.6	0.0	3.6	39.1	0.2	0.0	0.0	0.0	0.0	0.1	0.0	0.0	0.0	0.0	317.7
0.0	0.0	48.1	0.0	1.8	0.0	0.0	5.5	0.0	0.0	0.0	0.0	0.0	0.0	0.0	0.0	0.0	0.0	354.8
0.0	0.0	14.2	0.1	3.6	0.0	7.1	56.8	0.2	0.0	0.0	0.0	0.0	0.0	0.0	0.0	0.0	0.0	354.3
0.0	0.0	17.8	0.2	3.6	3.6	7.1	42.6	0.4	0.0	0.0	0.0	0.0	0.0	0.0	0.0	0.0	0.0	311.0
0.2	0.0	10.7	0.1	0.0	39.1	3.6	35.5	0.1	0.0	0.0	0.0	0.0	0.0	0.0	0.0	0.0	0.0	317.4
0.0	0.0	17.8	0.2	3.6	0.0	3.6	46.2	0.2	0.0	0.0	0.0	0.0	0.0	0.0	0.0	0.0	0.0	317.0
0.0	0.0	0.0	0.0	0.0	0.0	0.2	0.1	0.0	0.0	0.0	0.0	0.0	0.0	0.0	0.0	0.0	0.0	1.4
0.0	0.0	0.0	0.0	0.0	0.0	0.3	0.1	0.0	0.0	0.0	0.0	0.0	0.0	0.0	0.0	0.0	0.0	1.4
0.0	0.0	0.0	0.0	0.0	0.0	0.3	0.0	0.0	0.0	0.0	0.0	0.0	0.0	0.0	0.0	0.0	0.0	1.4
0.0	0.0	0.0	0.0	7.2	2.4	88.8	7.2	0.0	0.0	0.0	0.0	0.0	0.0	0.0	0.0	12.5	0.0	239.3
0.0	0.0	4.8	0.2	2.4	0.0	21.6	2.4	0.1	4.8	0.0	0.2	0.0	0.0	0.0	0.0	1.4	0.0	239.3
0.0	0.0	0.0	0.0	10.1	0.0	15.1	1.0	0.0	0.0	6.1	0.0	0.0	0.0	0.0	0.0	0.0	0.0	238.9
0.0	0.0	4.8	0.2	2.4	0.0	21.6	2.4	0.1	0.0	0.0	0.0	0.0	0.0	0.0	0.0	1.4	0.0	239.3
0.0	0.0	4.8	0.0	4.8	2.4	45.6	7.2	0.1	0.0	21.6	0.0	0.0	0.0	0.1	0.0	8.9	0.0	218.9
0.0	0.0	0.0	0.0	0.0	0.0	125.3	17.3	0.0	0.0	0.0	0.0	0.0	0.0	0.0	0.0	0.0	0.0	0.0
0.0	0.0	0.0	1.7	0.0	75.2	0.0	1164.0	0.0	0.0	0.0	0.0	0.0	0.0	0.0	0.0	0.0	0.0	221.5
0.0	0.0	0.6	0.0	0.3	0.0	0.0	0.9	0.0	0.0	0.0	0.0	0.0	0.0	0.0	0.0	0.0	0.0	30.0
0.0	0.0	3.7	0.0	0.0	0.0	0.0	14.6	0.4	0.0	0.0	0.0	0.0	0.0	0.0	0.0	0.0	0.0	333.4
0.0	0.0	26.9	0.0	0.0	0.0	0.0	1.9	0.0	0.0	0.0	0.0	0.0	0.0	0.0	0.0	0.0	0.0	191.8
1.1	0.0	60.7	0.0	0.0	0.0	0.0	504.3	0.0	0.0	0.0	0.0	0.0	0.0	0.0	0.0	0.0	0.0	3.6
0.6	0.0	7.5	1.2	13.2	103.8	200.6	294.8	0.3	0.0	0.0	0.0	0.2	0.1	1.5	0.0	36.5	0.0	16.6
2.4	0.0	0.0	1.5	0.0	0.0	0.0	605.1	0.0	0.0	0.0	0.0	0.0	0.0	1.2	0.0	0.0	0.0	21.2
0.9	0.4	17.2	1.2	6.0	150.5	78.4	368.2	0.2	0.4	0.0	1.0	0.1	0.1	1.7	0.0	20.7	0.0	9.3
2.5	2.4	105.5	1.2	14.3	267.9	107.2	544.4	0.3	14.8	0.2	0.0	0.2	0.2	1.7	0.0	3.4	0.1	16.5
2.6	1.8	141.0	1.7	10.8	98.4	72.6	348.0	0.3	13.8	0.1	0.8	0.2	0.2	1.8	0.0	36.6	0.0	17.3
0.3	0.0	4.0	0.6	3.6	97.7	38.9	304.7	0.1	0.0	0.0	0.1	0.1	0.0	0.7	0.0	14.5	0.0	5.8
1.0	0.0	5.4	0.7	3.8	104.0	42.4	324.5	0.1	0.0	0.0	0.5	0.1	0.1	0.8	0.0	11.6	0.0	7.5
0.0	0.0	2.0	0.1	3.1	3.5	2.1	0.3	0.1	0.0	0.3	0.0	0.1	0.0	0.0	0.1	0.2	0.0	0.2
0.0	0.0	1.4	0.1	5.5	16.3	12.6	0.1	0.1	0.0	0.0	0.0	0.0	0.0	0.0	0.0	0.8	0.0	11.5
0.3	0.0	4.2	1.4	57.8	124.1	109.9	0.4	0.4	0.0	0.0	0.4	0.2	0.0	2.5	0.3	4.7	0.0	0.5
0.0	0.0	2.6	0.4	21.4	35.5	41.4	0.1	0.3	0.0	0.0	0.0	0.1	0.0	0.5	0.0	2.8	0.0	1.6
0.2	0.3	27.7	0.9	10.6	37.2	75.6	742.0	0.3	0.8	0.1	0.0	0.0	0.0	0.8	0.0	30.5	0.0	1.6
0.3	0.0	61.3	1.7	12.4	39.7	59.7	232.7	0.3	0.0	0.0	0.2	0.2	0.1	1.8	0.0	29.4	0.0	1.7

Code	Food Name	Unit/Amt	Wt (g)	Energy (Kcal)	Prot (g)	Carb (g)	Fiber (g)	Fat (g)	Mono (g)	Poly (g)
18080	Bread sticks, plain	1 small stick (4.25" long)	5	20.6	0.6	3.4	0.2	0.5	0.2	0.2
18085	Bread Stuffing, Corn, dry mix, prep	½ cup	100	179.0	2.9	21.9	2.9	8.8	3.9	2.7
18082	Bread Stuffing, Plain, dry mix, prep	½ cup	100	178.0	3.2	21.7	2.9	8.6	3.8	2.6
918083	Bread Stuffing, Plain, homemade	½ cup	100	168.0	3.8	22.2	0.0	7.2	0.0	0.0
918020	Bread, Banana, homemade w/vegetable shortening	½ cup	116	392.1	5.0	63.9	0.0	13.7	0.0	0.0
18021	Bread, Boston Brown, canned	1 slice	45	87.8	2.3	19.5	2.1	0.7	0.1	0.3
918023	Bread, Corn, dry mix, prep	1 piece	60	188.4	4.3	28.9	1.4	6.0	0.0	0.0
918026	Bread, Cracked Wheat, toasted	1 thin slice	18	50.9	1.7	9.7	1.1	0.8	0.0	0.0
18027	Bread, Egg	1 slice (5" x 3" x 0.5")	40	114.8	3.8	19.1	0.9	2.4	0.9	0.4
18029	Bread, French/Vienna/Sourdough	1 medium slice (4.75 x 4 x 0.5")	25	68.5	2.2	13.0	0.8	0.8	0.3	0.2
18604	Bread, Garlic, frozen/Campione	1 slice	50	181.2	4.3	22.2	2.4	8.4	0.0	0.0
18641	Bread, Hamburger Rolls/Wonder	1 roll	43	115.5	4.3	21.2	0.0	1.5	0.0	0.0
18033	Bread, Italian	1 medium slice	20	54.2	1.8	10.0	0.5	0.7	0.2	0.3
18035	Bread, Mixed Grain/7-Grain/Whole Grain	1 large slice	32	80.0	3.2	14.8	2.0	1.2	0.5	0.3
18037	Bread, Oatbran	1 slice	30	70.8	3.1	11.9	1.4	1.3	0.5	0.5
18049	Bread, Oatbran, reduced kcal	1.0 oz	28.35	57.0	2.3	11.7	3.4	0.9	0.2	0.5
18039	Bread, Oatmeal	1.0 oz	28.35	76.3	2.4	13.7	1.1	1.2	0.4	0.5
18041	Bread, Pita, White, enriched	1 small pita (4" dia)	28	77.0	2.5	15.6	0.6	0.3	0.0	0.1
18042	Bread, Pita, Whole Wheat	1 small pita (4" dia)	28	74.5	2.7	15.4	2.1	0.7	0.1	0.3
18044	Bread, Pumpernickel	1 thin slice	20	50.0	1.7	9.5	1.3	0.6	0.2	0.2
918046	Bread, Pumpkin, homemade	1 slice (3.75 x 3 x 0.5")	60	198.6	2.4	30.7	0.0	7.7	0.0	0.0
18047	Bread, Raisin, enriched	1 slice	26	71.2	2.1	13.6	1.1	1.1	0.6	0.2
18059	Bread, Rice Bran	1 slice	27	65.6	2.4	11.7	1.3	1.2	0.4	0.5
18060	Bread, Rye	1 slice	32	82.9	2.7	15.5	1.9	1.1	0.4	0.3
18064	Bread, Wheat (includes wheat berry)	1 slice	25	65.0	2.3	11.8	1.1	1.0	0.4	0.2
18066	Bread, Wheat Bran	1 slice	36	89.3	3.2	17.2	1.4	1.2	0.6	0.2
18055	Bread, Wheat, reduced kcal	1 slice	23	45.5	2.1	10.0	2.8	0.5	0.1	0.2
18069	Bread, White, commercially prep, crumbs/cubes/slices	¼ cup of crumbs	12	32.0	1.0	5.9	0.3	0.4	0.2	0.1
18057	Bread, White, reduced kcal	1 slice	23	47.6	2.0	10.2	2.2	0.6	0.2	0.1
18075	Bread, Whole Wheat, commercially prep	1 slice	29	71.3	2.8	13.4	2.0	1.2	0.5	0.3
18022	Bread/Muffins, Corn, dry mix, enriched	¼ cup of crumbs	12	50.2	0.8	8.3	0.8	1.5	0.8	0.2
908918	Breakfast Bar, Chocolate Chip	1 bar	41	198.0	6.5	20.6	1.4	10.6	5.3	1.1
908919	Breakfast Bar, Chocolate Crunch	1 bar	38	183.2	6.8	18.6	1.2	9.8	4.3	1.6
908920	Breakfast Bar, Peanut Chocolate Chip	1 bar	40	196.0	7.0	19.4	1.4	10.6	5.4	2.2
908921	Breakfast Bar, Peanut Crunch	1 bar	38	188.9	7.1	17.9	1.0	10.4	5.3	2.3
1001	Butter, Regular (with salt)	1 pat (1" sq, ⅓" high)	5	35.9	0.0	0.0	0.0	4.1	1.2	0.2
1145	Butter, Unsalted	1 tbsp	14	100.4	0.1	0.0	0.0	11.4	3.3	0.4
1002	Butter, Whipped (with salt)	1 pat (1" sq, ⅓" high)	4	28.7	0.0	0.0	0.0	3.2	0.9	0.1
18086	Cake, Angelfood, commercially prep	1 piece (¹⁄₁₂ of 12 oz cake)	29	74.8	1.7	16.8	0.4	0.2	0.0	0.1
18088	Cake, Angelfood, dry mix, prep	1 piece (¹⁄₁₂ of 10" dia)	50	128.5	3.1	29.4	0.1	0.2	0.0	0.1
918823	Cake, Apple Streusel Crumb	1 piece	52	240.2	2.0	33.0	0.3	11.0	5.0	3.0
918824	Cake, Banana	¹⁄₁₂ cake	75	249.8	3.0	36.0	0.3	11.0	0.0	0.0
18090	Cake, Boston Cream Pie, commercially prep	1 piece (⅙ of pie)	92	231.8	2.2	39.5	1.3	7.8	4.2	0.9
918093	Cake, Carrot, dry mix, prep, w/o icing	1 piece (¹⁄₁₂ of 9" dia)	70	239.4	3.6	32.7	1.4	11.0	0.0	0.0
918828	Cake, Chocolate Fudge	⅙ cake	60	310.2	30.0	40.0	0.0	15.0	5.0	6.0
918858	Cake, Chocolate Suzy Q's/Hostess	2 cakes	128	480.0	4.0	74.0	0.5	20.0	0.0	0.0
18099	Cake, Chocolate, dry mix, regular	1 package (18.5 oz)	524	2242.7	30.9	382.5	12.6	81.7	33.1	26.4
918129	Cake, Chocolate, dry mix, special dietary	1 package (8 oz)	227	874.0	7.5	176.2	0.0	22.2	0.0	0.0
18101	Cake, Chocolate, homemade, w/o icing	1 piece (¹⁄₁₂ of 9" dia)	95	340.1	5.0	50.7	1.5	14.3	5.7	2.6
918846	Cake, Cinnamon Streusel, frozen	⅛ cake	39	145.9	2.2	19.4	0.3	7.1	0.0	0.0
918851	Cake, Devil Square/LittleDeb	2 squares	62	295.1	1.9	32.9	0.5	17.3	11.3	1.3
918831	Cake, German Chocolate, frozen	⅛ cake	50	198.0	2.5	22.1	0.9	11.4	0.0	0.0
918115	Cake, Gingerbread, dry mix, prep	1.0 oz	28	86.5	1.1	14.2	0.3	2.9	0.0	0.0
918853	Cake, Ho Ho's/Hostess	2 cakes	56	240.2	2.0	34.0	0.5	12.0	0.0	0.0
918838	Cake, Pineapple Upside Down Mix	⅑ cake	68	250.2	2.0	39.0	0.7	10.0	5.0	0.0
18120	Cake, Pound, commercially prep w/butter	1 piece (¹⁄₁₀ of cake)	30	116.4	1.7	14.6	0.1	6.0	1.8	0.3
918855	Cake, Snoballs/Hostess	2 cakes	86	300.1	2.0	56.0	0.5	8.0	0.0	0.0
18133	Cake, Sponge, commercially prep	1 piece (¹⁄₁₂ of 16 oz cake)	38	109.8	2.1	23.2	0.2	1.0	0.4	0.2
918859	Cake, Twinkies/Hostess	2 cakes	86	319.9	2.0	52.0	0.5	10.0	0.0	0.0
918811	Cake, White w/chocolate icing, slice	¹⁄₁₆ cake	78	250.4	3.0	45.0	0.5	8.0	0.0	0.0
18137	Cake, White, dry mix, regular	1.0 oz	29	123.5	1.3	22.6	0.3	3.2	1.3	1.2
18140	Cake, Yellow w/chocolate icing, commercially prep	1 piece (⅛ of 18 oz cake)	64	242.6	2.4	35.5	1.2	11.1	6.1	1.4
18141	Cake, Yellow w/vanilla icing, commercially prep	1 piece (⅛ of 18 oz cake)	64	238.7	2.2	37.6	0.2	9.3	3.9	3.3
19159	Candy Bar, 3 Musketeers/M&M Mars	1 bar (.8 oz)	23	95.7	0.7	17.7	0.4	3.0	1.0	0.1
19065	Candy Bar, Almond Joy/Hershey	1.76 oz	50	233.5	2.1	29.2	2.4	13.4	3.3	0.8
19111	Candy Bar, Baby Ruth/Nestle	2.1 oz	60	288.6	4.5	39.1	1.7	12.7	3.9	2.0
19075	Candy Bar, Caramello/Hershey	1.6 oz	45	213.3	2.7	28.5	0.7	9.8	3.2	0.3
919944	Candy Bar, Chocolate Almond/Hershey	1.0 oz	28	157.1	3.2	13.9	0.4	9.8	2.8	1.3
19119	Candy Bar, Chunky	1.0 oz	28	138.6	2.5	16.0	1.3	8.2	0.1	1.2

Sat (g)	Chol (mg)	Cal (mg)	Iron (mg)	Magn (mg)	Phos (mg)	Pota (mg)	Sodi (mg)	Zinc (mg)	Vit A (RE)	Vit C (mg)	Vit E (mg)	Thia (mg)	Ribo (mg)	Niac (mg)	Vit B-6 (mg)	Fol (µg)	Vit B-12 (µg)	Wat (g)
0.1	0.0	1.1	0.2	1.6	6.1	6.2	32.9	0.0	0.0	0.0	0.1	0.0	0.0	0.3	0.0	6.1	0.0	0.3
1.8	0.0	26.0	0.9	13.0	34.0	62.0	455.0	0.2	85.0	0.8	1.4	0.1	0.1	1.2	0.0	97.0	0.0	64.9
1.7	0.0	32.0	1.1	12.0	42.0	74.0	543.0	0.3	81.0	0.0	1.4	0.1	0.1	1.5	0.0	101.0	0.0	64.8
2.1	3.2	64.0	1.6	15.0	49.0	131.0	461.0	0.3	69.0	1.7	0.0	0.2	0.1	1.6	0.1	17.0	0.0	65.2
3.4	5.8	20.9	1.6	16.2	65.0	152.0	229.7	0.4	27.8	2.0	0.0	0.2	0.2	1.7	0.2	12.8	0.1	32.2
0.1	0.5	31.5	0.9	28.4	50.4	143.1	284.0	0.2	5.0	0.0	0.3	0.0	0.1	0.5	0.0	5.0	0.0	21.2
0.7	3.1	43.8	1.1	12.0	225.6	76.8	466.8	0.4	26.4	0.1	0.0	0.1	0.2	1.2	0.1	6.6	0.1	19.1
0.1	0.4	8.5	0.5	10.3	29.9	34.6	105.3	0.2	0.0	0.1	0.1	0.1	0.0	0.6	0.1	5.4	0.0	5.4
0.6	20.4	37.2	1.2	7.6	42.4	46.0	196.8	0.3	9.2	0.0	0.2	0.2	0.2	1.9	0.0	42.0	0.0	13.9
0.2	0.0	18.8	0.6	6.8	26.3	28.3	152.3	0.2	0.0	0.0	0.1	0.1	0.1	1.2	0.0	23.8	0.0	8.6
1.4	0.0	0.0	0.5	0.0	0.0	0.0	275.0	0.0	0.0	0.0	0.0	0.0	0.0	0.0	0.0	0.0	0.0	14.3
0.4	0.0	74.8	1.0	0.0	0.0	0.0	256.3	0.0	0.0	0.0	0.0	0.0	0.0	0.0	0.0	0.0	0.0	15.0
0.2	0.0	15.6	0.6	5.4	20.6	22.0	116.8	0.2	0.0	0.0	0.1	0.1	0.1	0.9	0.0	19.0	0.0	7.1
0.3	0.0	29.1	1.1	17.0	56.3	65.3	155.8	0.4	0.0	0.0	0.2	0.1	0.1	1.4	0.1	25.6	0.0	12.1
0.2	0.0	19.5	0.9	10.5	42.3	44.1	122.1	0.3	0.0	0.0	0.2	0.2	0.1	1.4	0.0	24.3	0.0	13.2
0.1	0.0	16.2	0.9	15.6	39.4	28.9	99.5	0.3	0.0	0.0	0.1	0.1	0.1	1.1	0.0	18.7	0.0	13.0
0.2	0.0	18.7	0.8	10.5	35.7	40.3	169.8	0.3	0.6	0.0	0.2	0.1	0.1	0.9	0.0	17.6	0.0	10.4
0.0	0.0	24.1	0.7	7.3	27.2	33.6	150.1	0.2	0.0	0.0	0.0	0.2	0.1	1.3	0.0	26.6	0.0	9.0
0.1	0.0	4.2	0.9	19.3	50.4	47.6	149.0	0.4	0.0	0.0	0.3	0.1	0.0	0.8	0.1	14.0	0.0	8.6
0.1	0.0	13.6	0.6	10.8	35.6	41.6	134.2	0.3	0.0	0.0	0.1	0.1	0.1	0.6	0.0	16.0	0.0	7.6
4.1	1.9	10.8	1.0	7.8	31.8	55.2	187.8	0.2	334.2	0.6	0.0	0.1	0.1	0.8	0.0	6.6	0.0	18.5
0.3	0.0	17.2	0.8	6.8	28.3	59.0	101.4	0.2	0.0	0.0	0.1	0.1	0.1	0.9	0.0	22.6	0.0	8.7
0.2	0.0	18.6	1.0	21.6	48.1	58.1	118.8	0.4	0.0	0.0	0.2	0.2	0.1	1.8	0.1	17.6	0.0	11.1
0.2	0.0	23.4	0.9	12.8	40.0	53.1	211.2	0.4	0.3	0.1	0.1	0.1	0.1	1.2	0.0	27.5	0.0	11.9
0.2	0.0	26.3	0.8	11.5	37.5	50.3	132.5	0.3	0.0	0.0	0.1	0.1	0.1	1.0	0.0	19.3	0.0	9.3
0.3	0.0	26.6	1.1	29.2	66.6	81.7	175.0	0.5	0.0	0.0	0.2	0.1	0.1	1.6	0.1	24.8	0.0	13.6
0.1	0.0	18.4	0.7	9.0	23.5	28.1	117.5	0.3	0.0	0.0	0.0	0.1	0.1	0.9	0.0	16.3	0.0	9.9
0.1	0.1	13.0	0.4	2.9	11.3	14.3	64.6	0.1	0.0	0.0	0.1	0.1	0.0	0.5	0.0	11.4	0.0	4.4
0.1	0.0	21.6	0.7	5.3	27.8	17.5	104.2	0.3	0.2	0.1	0.0	0.1	0.1	0.8	0.0	21.9	0.1	9.9
0.3	0.0	20.9	1.0	24.9	66.4	73.1	152.8	0.6	0.0	0.0	0.2	0.1	0.1	1.1	0.1	14.5	0.0	10.9
0.4	0.2	6.8	0.3	2.9	58.7	13.6	133.3	0.1	1.4	0.0	0.2	0.1	0.0	0.4	0.0	12.6	0.0	0.9
4.2	0.0	20.0	4.5	60.0	60.0	98.0	177.0	3.0	350.0	28.0	0.0	0.3	0.0	5.0	0.4	100.0	0.6	1.9
3.9	0.0	20.0	4.5	60.0	60.0	127.0	151.0	3.0	350.0	28.0	0.0	0.3	0.0	5.0	0.4	100.0	0.6	1.7
3.0	0.0	20.0	4.5	60.0	60.0	110.0	167.0	3.0	350.0	28.0	0.0	0.3	0.0	5.0	0.4	100.0	0.6	1.4
2.8	0.0	20.0	4.5	60.0	60.0	107.0	177.0	3.0	350.0	28.0	0.0	0.3	0.0	5.0	0.4	100.0	0.6	1.5
2.5	10.9	1.2	0.0	0.1	1.2	1.3	41.3	0.0	37.7	0.0	0.1	0.0	0.0	0.0	0.0	0.2	0.0	0.8
7.1	30.6	3.3	0.0	0.3	3.2	3.6	1.5	0.0	105.6	0.0	0.2	0.0	0.0	0.0	0.0	0.4	0.0	2.5
2.0	8.8	0.9	0.0	0.1	0.9	1.0	33.1	0.0	30.2	0.0	0.1	0.0	0.0	0.0	0.0	0.1	0.0	0.6
0.0	0.0	40.6	0.2	3.5	9.3	27.0	217.2	0.0	0.0	0.0	0.0	0.0	0.1	0.3	0.0	10.2	0.0	9.6
0.0	0.0	42.0	0.1	4.0	116.0	67.5	254.5	0.1	0.0	0.0	0.0	0.0	0.1	0.1	0.0	15.0	0.0	16.5
3.0	45.0	11.0	0.8	0.0	31.0	50.0	190.0	0.0	13.0	15.0	0.0	0.1	0.1	0.9	0.0	0.0	0.0	0.0
0.0	0.0	0.0	0.0	0.0	0.0	80.0	290.0	0.0	0.0	0.0	0.0	0.0	0.0	0.0	0.0	0.0	0.0	0.0
2.2	34.0	21.2	0.3	5.5	45.1	35.9	132.5	0.1	21.2	0.2	1.0	0.4	0.2	0.2	0.0	13.8	0.1	41.8
5.0	3.4	77.0	0.9	4.9	122.5	84.0	249.2	0.2	172.9	1.7	0.0	0.1	0.1	0.8	0.1	8.4	0.8	21.6
4.0	35.0	0.0	0.0	0.0	0.0	80.0	300.0	0.0	0.0	0.0	0.0	0.0	0.0	0.0	0.0	0.0	0.0	0.0
0.0	32.0	42.0	1.6	0.0	0.0	0.0	600.0	0.0	0.0	0.0	0.0	0.0	0.1	1.0	0.0	5.0	0.0	16.2
17.1	0.0	786.0	23.6	246.3	1414.8	1729.2	4323.0	4.2	0.0	0.0	12.6	0.9	0.8	8.4	0.2	283.0	0.0	16.2
1.6	9.0	81.7	5.8	104.4	778.6	583.4	935.2	1.9	0.0	0.0	0.0	0.5	0.4	4.4	0.0	22.7	0.0	10.9
5.2	55.1	57.0	1.5	30.4	100.7	133.0	299.3	0.7	38.0	0.2	1.5	0.1	0.2	1.1	0.0	25.7	0.2	23.2
0.0	0.0	12.0	0.7	6.0	28.0	36.0	134.0	0.0	51.2	0.0	0.0	0.1	0.1	0.8	0.0	0.0	0.0	10.0
4.7	0.0	0.0	1.0	0.0	0.0	75.0	136.0	0.0	0.0	0.0	0.0	0.1	0.1	0.7	0.0	5.0	0.0	9.4
0.0	0.0	28.0	0.9	14.0	63.0	93.0	153.0	0.0	37.8	0.0	0.0	0.0	0.1	0.3	0.0	5.0	0.0	12.6
0.4	1.6	19.3	0.9	4.5	47.0	67.5	128.2	0.1	4.5	0.0	0.4	0.1	0.1	0.4	0.0	2.8	0.0	9.3
0.0	26.0	24.0	0.6	0.0	0.0	0.0	180.0	0.0	0.0	0.0	0.0	0.0	0.0	0.0	0.0	4.0	0.0	0.0
4.0	40.0	0.0	0.0	0.0	0.0	70.0	210.0	0.0	0.0	0.0	0.0	0.0	0.0	0.0	0.0	0.0	0.0	0.0
3.5	66.3	10.5	0.4	3.3	41.1	35.7	119.4	0.1	46.8	0.0	0.0	0.0	0.1	0.4	0.0	12.3	0.1	7.4
0.0	4.0	24.0	1.0	0.0	0.0*	0.0	340.0	0.0	0.0	0.0	0.0	0.0	0.1	0.0	0.0	0.0	0.0	0.0
0.3	38.8	26.6	1.0	4.2	52.1	37.6	92.7	0.2	17.5	0.0	0.1	0.1	0.1	0.7	0.0	14.8	0.1	11.3
0.0	40.0	38.0	1.1	0.0	0.0	0.0	300.0	0.0	0.0	0.0	0.0	0.1	0.1	1.0	0.0	5.0	0.0	0.0
3.0	1.0	70.0	0.7	15.0	127.0	82.0	238.0	0.2	8.0	0.0	0.0	0.1	0.1	0.8	0.0	4.0	0.1	15.8
0.5	0.0	55.7	0.4	3.2	97.7	33.9	192.6	0.1	0.0	0.1	0.6	0.1	0.1	0.3	0.0	13.9	0.1	1.2
3.0	35.2	23.7	1.3	19.2	103.0	113.9	215.7	0.4	21.1	0.0	1.5	0.1	0.1	0.8	0.0	14.1	0.1	14.0
1.5	35.2	39.7	0.7	3.8	91.5	33.9	220.2	0.2	12.2	0.0	0.0	0.1	0.0	0.3	0.0	17.3	0.1	14.1
1.5	2.5	19.3	0.2	6.7	20.9	30.6	44.6	0.1	5.5	0.1	0.1	0.0	0.0	0.1	0.0	0.0	0.0	1.3
8.7	2.0	30.5	0.7	0.0	0.0	123.0	73.0	0.0	0.0	0.0	0.0	0.0	0.0	0.0	0.0	0.0	0.0	4.8
7.4	2.4	24.6	0.1	48.0	90.6	237.6	135.6	0.8	0.0	0.0	1.1	0.1	0.1	1.7	0.0	18.6	0.0	2.9
6.3	12.2	82.8	0.3	0.0	0.0	0.0	61.7	0.0	0.0	0.0	0.0	0.0	0.0	0.0	0.0	0.0	0.0	3.3
5.7	7.5	73.8	0.5	25.3	84.0	120.2	34.8	0.5	5.1	0.0	0.0	0.0	0.1	0.1	0.0	0.0	0.0	0.0
6.5	3.1	40.0	0.4	20.4	58.2	149.5	14.8	0.5	3.1	0.1	0.0	0.0	0.1	0.5	0.0	6.2	0.1	0.8

Code	Food Name	Unit/Amt	Wt (g)	Energy (Kcal)	Prot (g)	Carb (g)	Fiber (g)	Fat (g)	Mono (g)	Poly (g)
19130	Candy Bar, Golden Almond Chocolate Bar/Hershey	3.2 oz	91	522.3	11.2	41.6	4.4	34.7	16.1	3.5
19109	Candy Bar, Kit Kat Wafer/Hershey	1.62 oz	46	236.4	3.3	29.4	0.9	11.7	3.4	0.4
19115	Candy Bar, Mars Almond/M&M Mars	1.76 oz (69 pieces)	48	224.2	3.9	30.1	1.0	11.0	5.1	1.9
19135	Candy Bar, Mars Milky Way/M&M Mars	2.1 oz	60	253.8	2.7	43.0	1.0	9.7	3.6	0.4
19142	Candy Bar, Mounds/Hershey	1.55 oz	44	209.9	1.7	25.9	2.6	11.0	1.9	0.2
19143	Candy Bar, Mr. Goodbar/Hershey	1.75 oz	50	272.5	5.4	25.9	1.8	17.5	5.9	2.4
19136	Candy Bar, Skor Toffee Candy/Hershey	1.4 oz	40	222.4	1.8	23.1	0.6	13.6	4.4	0.6
19155	Candy Bar, Snickers/M&M Mars	2.16 oz	61	292.2	4.9	36.1	1.5	15.0	6.4	3.0
19164	Candy Bar, Special Dark Sweet Chocolate/Hershey	1.45 oz bar	41	226.3	2.0	24.8	2.1	13.3	4.6	0.4
919967	Candy Bar, Summit Bar	0.75 oz bar	22	100.1	1.0	11.0	0.4	6.0	0.0	0.0
19093	Candy Bar, Symphony Milk Chocolate/Hershey	1.4 oz	40	221.2	2.9	23.2	0.8	13.1	0.0	0.0
919951	Candy Bar, Tiger Milk Bar	2.0 oz	56	249.8	9.0	35.0	29.1	8.0	0.0	0.0
19160	Candy Bar, Twix Caramel Cookie/M&M Mars	2.0 oz	57	284.4	2.6	37.4	0.6	13.9	7.6	0.5
919912	Candy, Candy Corn	¼ cup	50	182.0	0.1	44.8	0.0	1.0	0.5	0.2
19074	Candy, Caramel	1 piece (0.75" cube)	10	38.2	0.5	7.7	0.1	0.8	0.1	0.0
19071	Candy, Carob	3.0 oz	87	469.8	7.1	49.0	3.3	27.3	0.4	0.3
919901	Candy, Chocolate Caramel Turtle	0.6 oz	17	81.9	1.1	9.9	0.0	4.7	1.9	0.8
19080	Candy, Chocolate Chips, semisweet	1 cup, large chips	182	871.8	7.6	114.8	10.7	54.6	18.1	1.8
919921	Candy, Chocolate Chips/Bakers	¼ cup	44	200.6	1.7	32.0	0.7	9.0	1.6	0.3
919956	Candy, Chocolate w/cream center	1.0 oz	28	122.9	1.1	19.9	0.4	4.8	2.8	0.6
919946	Candy, Chocolate, dietetic	1 bar	56	333.8	7.2	14.0	0.0	27.8	0.0	0.0
19014	Candy, Fruit Leather, roll	1 small roll	14	49.0	0.1	11.8	0.5	0.4	0.2	0.1
919970	Candy, Fruit Roll Snack	1 large roll	21	73.1	0.2	17.7	0.5	0.6	0.3	0.1
19100	Candy, Fudge, Chocolate, homemade	1 piece	17	64.8	0.3	13.5	0.1	1.4	0.4	0.1
19103	Candy, Fudge, Vanilla, homemade	1 piece	16	59.0	0.2	13.2	0.0	0.9	0.2	0.0
19105	Candy, Goobers Chocolate Covered Peanuts/Nestle	10 pieces	10	51.3	1.4	4.9	0.6	3.4	1.5	0.5
19106	Candy, Gumdrops/Gummy Bears/Fish/Worm/Dinosaur	1 small gumdrop (0.5" dia)	3	11.6	0.0	3.0	0.0	0.0	0.0	0.0
19117	Candy, Halvah, Plain	1 bar (8 oz)	227	1064.6	28.4	137.3	10.2	48.9	18.6	19.3
19107	Candy, Hard Candy	1 lollipop (0.75" diam)	6	23.6	0.0	5.9	0.0	0.0	0.0	0.0
19108	Candy, Jellybeans	10 small	11	40.4	0.0	10.2	0.0	0.1	0.0	0.0
19140	Candy, M&M's Peanut Chocolate	1 piece	2	10.3	0.2	1.2	0.1	0.5	0.2	0.1
19141	Candy, M&M's Plain Chocolate	1 piece	0.7	3.4	0.0	0.5	0.0	0.1	0.0	0.0
19148	Candy, Peanut Brittle, homemade	1.0 oz	28	126.8	2.1	19.4	0.6	5.3	2.4	1.3
19150	Candy, Peanut Butter Cups, Reese's/Hershey	1 miniature cup	7	37.9	0.7	3.8	0.2	2.2	0.9	0.4
19126	Candy, Peanuts, milk chocolate coated	10 pieces	40	207.6	5.2	19.8	1.9	13.4	5.2	1.7
919072	Candy, Pudding Pops, Chocolate, frozen	1 pop	47	71.9	1.9	11.9	0.2	2.2	0.0	0.0
919073	Candy, Pudding Pops, Vanilla, frozen	1 pop	47	74.7	1.9	12.6	0.0	2.1	0.0	0.0
19149	Candy, Raisinets/Nestle	10 pieces	10	41.2	0.5	7.1	0.5	1.6	0.6	0.2
19127	Candy, Raisins, milk chocolate coated	10 pieces	10	39.0	0.4	6.8	0.4	1.5	0.5	0.1
19152	Candy, Rolo Caramel, milk chocolate/Hershey	1.94 oz (8 pieces)	55	226.6	2.7	29.4	0.4	11.0	3.5	0.3
919923	Candy, Semisweet Chocolate Chips/Nestle	1.0 oz	28	148.1	1.0	17.8	1.0	7.9	2.2	0.7
919947	Candy, Semisweet Chocolate/Baker	1.0 oz	28	135.0	2.0	16.3	0.5	9.0	3.2	0.4
919948	Candy, Semisweet Chocolate/Hershey	1.0 oz	28	147.0	1.2	17.5	0.5	9.2	0.0	0.0
19370	Candy, Skittles, Original Bite Size Candy/M&M Mars	2.3 oz (59 pieces)	65	263.3	0.1	58.9	0.0	2.8	1.9	0.1
919958	Candy, Sno Caps	1 oz	28	131.9	1.5	20.6	0.2	5.6	2.0	0.5
19156	Candy, Starburst Fruit Chews/M&M Mars	2.07 oz	59	233.6	0.2	49.9	0.0	4.9	2.1	1.8
919966	Candy, Taffy	0.5 oz piece	15	56.0	0.0	13.7	0.0	0.4	0.1	0.0
19112	Candy, Twizzlers Strawberry/Hershey	1 package (2.5 oz)	71	237.1	2.4	55.0	1.0	1.1	0.0	0.0
19091	Candy, York Peppermint Patty	0.39 oz, 1 sm patty	11	43.2	0.2	8.8	0.2	0.8	0.3	0.0
8053	Cereal, 100% Bran (wheat bran & barley)	1 cup	66	177.5	8.3	48.1	19.5	3.3	0.6	1.9
908912	Cereal, 100% Natural/Quaker	¼ cup	28	127.1	3.3	18.0	2.0	5.5	0.9	0.6
8153	Cereal, 40% Bran Flakes/Ralston Purina	1.0 oz, @ ¾ cup	29	94.0	3.3	23.1	4.1	0.4	0.0	0.0
8001	Cereal, All-Bran/Kellogg	½ cup	30	79.2	3.7	22.8	9.7	0.9	0.2	0.5
8006	Cereal, Bran Chex (wheat & corn)	1 cup	49	156.3	5.0	39.1	7.9	1.4	0.3	0.7
8010	Cereal, Cap'n Crunch/Quaker	¾ cup	27	107.2	1.4	23.0	0.9	1.4	0.3	0.2
8013	Cereal, Cheerios/Gen Mills	1 cup	30	109.5	3.1	22.9	2.6	1.8	0.6	0.2
8014	Cereal, Cocoa Krispies/Kellogg	¾ cup	31	120.3	1.6	27.2	0.4	0.8	0.1	0.1
8017	Cereal, Cookie Crisp, Chocolate Chip & Vanilla	1 cup	30	120.0	1.5	26.3	0.4	1.1	0.2	0.2
8019	Cereal, Corn Chex	1 single serving box (.75 oz)	21.3	83.5	1.5	18.7	0.4	0.1	0.0	0.0
8022	Cereal, Corn Flakes, low sodium	1.0 oz	28.35	113.1	2.2	25.2	0.3	0.1	0.0	0.0
8020	Cereal, Corn Flakes/Kellogg	1 cup	28	102.2	1.8	24.2	0.8	0.2	0.0	0.1
8023	Cereal, Cracklin' Oat Bran/Kellogg	¾ cup	55	225.0	4.6	40.1	6.5	7.0	3.2	0.8
8101	Cereal, Cream of Rice, prep w/o salt	1 tbsp	15.2	7.9	0.1	1.7	0.0	0.0	0.0	0.0
8109	Cereal, Cream of Wheat, Plain, Mix 'n Eat, prep	1 packet, prep	142	102.2	2.7	21.4	0.4	0.3	0.0	0.2
8103	Cereal, Cream of Wheat, Regular, prep w/o salt	1 cup	251	133.0	3.8	27.6	1.8	0.5	0.1	0.3
8259	Cereal, Crispix/Kellogg	1 cup	29	108.5	2.1	25.0	0.6	0.3	0.1	0.1
8018	Cereal, Crunchy Bran/Quaker	¾ cup	27	89.9	1.9	22.7	4.8	0.9	0.2	0.3
8244	Cereal, Fiber One/Gen Mills	1 cup	60	123.0	5.6	48.0	28.5	1.7	0.3	0.1
8030	Cereal, Froot Loops/Kellogg	1 cup	30	117.3	1.5	26.5	0.6	0.9	0.2	0.3

Sat (g)	Chol (mg)	Cal (mg)	Iron (mg)	Magn (mg)	Phos (mg)	Pota (mg)	Sodi (mg)	Zinc (mg)	Vit A (RE)	Vit C (mg)	Vit E (mg)	Thia (mg)	Ribo (mg)	Niac (mg)	Vit B-6 (mg)	Fol (µg)	Vit B-12 (µg)	Wat (g)
14.9	13.7	203.8	1.6	0.0	0.0	0.0	61.0	0.0	0.0	0.0	0.0	0.0	0.0	0.0	0.0	0.0	0.0	1.9
7.5	2.8	75.9	0.4	17.9	109.5	133.9	34.5	0.6	22.1	0.3	0.4	0.1	0.2	1.2	0.1	65.3	0.1	0.8
3.5	8.2	80.6	0.5	34.6	112.3	156.0	81.6	0.5	24.0	0.3	2.2	0.0	0.1	0.5	0.0	9.1	0.2	2.2
4.7	8.4	78.0	0.5	20.4	86.4	144.6	144.0	0.4	19.2	0.6	0.4	0.0	0.1	0.2	0.0	6.0	0.2	3.8
8.9	0.9	6.6	0.9	24.6	40.0	108.7	65.6	0.4	0.4	0.2	0.3	0.0	0.0	0.1	0.0	1.3	0.0	4.8
7.5	4.0	54.0	0.7	43.0	124.0	223.5	74.5	0.9	18.5	0.0	1.4	0.1	0.1	1.7	0.0	19.5	0.2	0.4
8.7	20.4	52.0	0.2	0.0	0.0	0.0	110.4	0.0	0.0	0.0	0.0	0.0	0.0	0.0	0.0	0.0	0.0	1.0
5.5	7.9	57.3	0.5	43.9	135.4	197.6	162.3	1.4	23.8	0.4	0.9	0.1	0.1	2.6	0.1	24.4	0.1	3.3
8.3	0.4	11.1	1.0	45.5	61.5	122.6	2.9	0.6	1.6	0.0	0.2	0.0	0.0	0.2	0.0	0.8	0.0	0.4
0.0	0.0	0.0	0.0	0.0	0.0	0.0	0.0	0.0	0.0	0.0	0.0	0.0	0.0	0.0	0.0	0.0	0.0	0.0
0.0	8.8	86.0	0.5	0.0	0.0	0.0	36.8	0.0	0.0	0.0	0.0	0.0	0.0	0.0	0.0	0.0	0.0	0.2
0.0	0.0	0.0	6.3	0.0	0.0	0.0	0.0	0.0	0.0	0.0	0.0	0.5	0.7	0.6	0.0	0.0	0.0	0.0
5.1	2.9	51.3	0.5	18.2	68.4	115.1	110.0	0.4	14.3	0.2	0.7	0.1	0.1	0.7	0.0	13.7	0.1	2.4
0.3	0.0	7.0	0.6	0.0	3.0	2.0	106.0	0.0	0.0	0.0	0.0	0.0	0.0	0.0	0.0	0.0	0.0	3.8
0.7	0.7	13.8	0.0	1.7	11.4	21.4	24.5	0.0	0.8	0.1	0.0	0.0	0.0	0.0	0.0	0.5	0.0	0.9
25.2	2.6	263.6	1.1	31.3	109.6	550.7	93.1	3.1	7.0	0.4	1.4	0.1	0.2	0.9	0.1	24.4	0.9	1.3
1.8	4.0	27.0	0.2	0.0	0.0	52.0	16.0	0.0	6.0	0.0	0.0	0.0	0.0	0.1	0.0	0.0	0.0	0.0
32.3	0.0	58.2	5.7	209.3	240.2	664.3	20.0	2.9	3.6	0.0	2.2	0.1	0.2	0.8	0.1	5.5	0.0	1.3
7.1	0.0	66.5	0.9	35.8	82.9	227.2	26.6	0.5	0.8	0.0	0.0	0.1	0.1	0.1	0.0	2.0	0.1	0.4
1.4	0.0	36.0	0.2	0.0	31.0	50.0	52.0	0.0	0.0	0.0	0.0	0.0	0.0	0.0	0.0	0.0	0.0	2.1
0.0	0.0	0.0	0.0	0.0	0.0	0.0	0.0	0.0	0.0	0.0	0.0	0.0	0.0	0.0	0.0	0.0	0.0	0.0
0.1	0.0	4.5	0.1	2.8	4.3	41.2	8.5	0.0	1.7	0.9	0.0	0.0	0.0	0.0	0.0	1.1	0.0	1.5
0.1	0.0	7.0	0.2	4.0	7.0	62.0	13.0	0.0	2.0	1.0	0.0	0.0	0.0	0.0	0.1	0.0	0.0	2.3
0.9	2.4	7.1	0.1	4.3	9.9	17.5	10.5	0.1	7.8	0.0	0.0	0.0	0.0	0.0	0.0	0.3	0.0	1.6
0.5	2.6	6.2	0.0	0.8	5.1	8.0	10.7	0.0	8.0	0.0	0.0	0.0	0.0	0.0	0.0	0.2	0.0	1.7
1.2	0.9	12.7	0.1	11.9	29.6	50.2	4.1	0.2	0.0	0.0	0.0	0.0	0.0	0.5	0.0	0.8	0.0	0.2
0.0	0.0	0.1	0.0	0.0	0.0	0.2	1.3	0.0	0.0	0.0	0.0	0.0	0.0	0.0	0.0	0.0	0.0	0.0
9.4	0.0	74.9	10.3	494.9	1377.9	424.5	442.7	9.8	0.0	0.2	6.4	1.0	0.2	6.5	0.8	147.6	0.1	8.3
0.0	0.0	0.2	0.0	0.2	0.2	0.3	2.3	0.0	0.0	0.0	0.0	0.0	0.0	0.0	0.0	0.0	0.0	0.1
0.0	0.0	0.3	0.1	0.2	0.4	4.1	2.8	0.0	0.0	0.0	0.0	0.0	0.0	0.0	0.0	0.0	0.0	0.7
0.2	0.2	2.0	0.0	1.5	4.6	6.9	1.0	0.0	0.5	0.0	0.0	0.0	0.0	0.1	0.0	0.7	0.0	0.0
0.1	0.1	0.7	0.0	0.3	1.1	1.9	0.4	0.0	0.4	0.0	0.0	0.0	0.0	0.0	0.0	0.0	0.0	0.0
1.4	3.6	8.4	0.4	14.0	31.1	58.2	126.6	0.3	13.2	0.0	0.5	0.1	0.0	1.0	0.0	19.6	0.0	0.5
0.8	0.4	5.5	0.5	6.2	14.2	24.6	22.2	0.1	1.3	0.0	0.3	0.0	0.0	0.3	0.0	3.9	0.0	0.1
5.8	3.6	41.6	0.5	37.6	84.8	200.8	16.4	0.8	0.0	0.0	1.0	0.0	0.1	1.7	0.1	3.2	0.1	0.8
0.0	0.9	66.3	0.2	9.9	52.6	105.3	77.6	0.2	15.5	0.2	0.0	0.0	0.1	0.1	0.0	1.4	0.3	30.4
0.0	0.9	60.6	0.0	5.2	47.5	64.9	49.8	0.2	24.4	0.1	0.0	0.0	0.1	0.0	0.0	2.4	0.2	30.0
0.7	0.4	10.8	0.1	4.5	14.4	51.4	3.6	0.1	0.9	0.0	0.0	0.0	0.0	0.0	0.0	0.5	0.0	0.6
0.9	0.3	8.6	0.2	4.5	14.3	51.4	3.6	0.1	0.7	0.0	0.1	0.0	0.0	0.0	0.0	0.5	0.0	1.1
6.7	9.9	84.2	0.3	21.5	82.5	136.4	96.8	0.5	20.4	0.2	0.5	0.0	0.1	0.1	0.0	2.8	0.2	11.1
5.0	0.0	10.0	1.0	0.0	30.0	99.0	4.0	0.4	0.1	0.0	0.0	0.0	0.0	0.2	0.0	3.6	0.0	0.0
5.4	0.0	11.0	1.0	41.0	57.0	116.0	1.0	1.0	1.6	0.0	0.0	0.0	0.0	0.2	0.0	1.0	0.0	0.0
5.7	0.0	9.0	0.9	0.0	43.0	92.0	5.0	0.0	2.0	0.0	0.0	0.0	0.1	0.1	0.0	1.0	0.0	0.0
0.6	0.0	0.0	0.0	0.7	1.3	3.3	10.4	0.0	0.0	43.5	0.2	0.0	0.0	0.0	0.0	0.0	0.0	2.5
3.1	0.0	38.0	0.4	0.0	40.0	71.0	20.0	0.5	6.0	0.0	0.0	0.0	0.1	0.1	0.0	0.0	0.0	0.3
0.7	0.0	2.4	0.1	0.6	4.1	1.2	33.0	0.0	0.0	31.2	0.9	0.0	0.0	0.0	0.0	0.0	0.0	4.0
0.3	1.0	0.0	0.0	0.0	0.0	1.0	13.0	0.0	5.0	0.0	0.0	0.0	0.0	0.0	0.0	0.0	0.0	0.7
0.3	0.0	5.0	0.2	0.0	0.0	0.0	175.4	0.0	0.0	0.0	0.0	0.0	0.0	0.0	0.0	0.0	0.0	11.9
0.5	0.1	1.7	0.1	0.0	0.0	14.2	2.6	0.0	0.0	0.0	0.0	0.0	0.0	0.0	0.0	0.0	0.0	1.1
0.6	0.0	46.2	8.1	312.2	801.2	652.1	457.4	5.7	0.0	62.7	1.5	1.6	1.8	20.9	2.1	46.9	6.3	2.0
3.1	0.0	43.0	0.8	31.0	101.0	134.0	14.0	0.6	0.0	0.0	0.0	0.1	0.1	0.4	0.1	12.0	0.3	0.6
0.0	0.0	13.3	4.6	69.6	161.5	169.4	270.0	1.2	384.0	15.4	0.0	0.4	0.4	5.1	0.5	102.4	1.5	0.7
0.2	0.0	105.9	4.5	128.7	294.0	341.7	60.9	3.8	225.3	15.0	0.6	0.4	0.4	5.0	0.5	90.0	1.5	1.0
0.2	0.0	29.4	14.0	69.1	173.0	216.1	345.5	6.5	10.8	26.0	0.6	0.6	0.3	8.6	0.9	173.0	2.6	1.1
0.4	0.0	5.4	4.5	9.5	28.6	34.6	208.4	3.8	3.5	0.0	0.1	0.4	0.4	5.0	0.5	100.2	0.0	0.6
0.4	0.0	55.2	8.1	32.7	114.0	88.5	284.1	3.8	375.3	15.0	0.2	0.4	0.4	5.0	0.5	99.9	0.0	1.0
0.6	0.0	4.0	1.8	11.5	29.5	60.1	210.2	1.5	225.1	15.0	0.1	0.4	0.4	5.0	0.5	93.0	0.0	0.7
0.6	0.0	5.7	4.8	8.4	24.0	29.4	206.7	3.2	0.0	0.0	0.1	0.4	0.3	5.3	0.5	105.9	1.6	0.6
0.0	0.0	2.3	6.1	3.0	8.3	17.3	232.8	0.1	10.7	11.3	0.1	0.3	0.1	3.7	0.4	75.2	1.1	0.4
0.0	0.0	12.2	0.6	3.7	13.9	20.7	2.8	0.1	10.8	0.0	0.0	0.0	0.1	0.1	0.0	2.0	0.0	0.9
0.1	0.0	1.1	8.7	3.4	10.9	25.5	297.9	0.2	210.3	14.0	0.0	0.4	0.4	4.7	0.5	98.8	0.0	0.9
2.9	0.0	24.8	2.0	76.5	186.5	254.7	195.3	1.7	253.0	16.8	0.4	0.4	0.5	5.6	0.6	152.9	0.0	2.0
0.0	0.0	0.5	0.0	0.5	2.6	3.0	0.2	0.0	0.0	0.0	0.0	0.0	0.1	0.0	0.0	0.5	0.0	13.3
0.0	0.0	19.9	8.1	7.1	19.9	38.3	241.4	0.2	376.3	0.0	0.0	0.4	0.3	5.0	0.6	100.8	0.0	116.6
0.1	0.0	50.2	10.3	10.0	42.7	42.7	2.5	0.3	0.0	0.0	0.0	0.3	0.0	1.5	0.0	45.2	0.0	218.6
0.1	0.0	3.5	1.8	7.0	26.7	35.1	240.1	1.5	225.3	15.0	0.1	0.4	0.4	5.0	0.5	87.0	0.0	0.9
0.2	0.0	20.5	7.6	14.3	35.6	56.2	253.3	3.8	3.8	0.0	0.1	0.1	0.4	5.0	0.5	100.2	0.0	0.7
0.3	0.0	117.0	9.0	136.2	336.6	433.8	285.0	2.5	0.0	18.0	0.7	0.8	0.9	10.0	1.0	199.8	0.0	2.3
0.4	0.0	3.3	4.2	8.7	20.7	31.5	140.7	3.8	211.2	14.1	0.1	0.4	0.4	5.0	0.5	90.0	0.0	0.7

Code	Food Name	Unit/Amt	Wt (g)	Energy (Kcal)	Prot (g)	Carb (g)	Fiber (g)	Fat (g)	Mono (g)	Poly (g)
8319	Cereal, Frosted Mini-Wheats, bite size/Kellogg	1 cup, bite size	55	187.0	5.2	44.8	5.9	0.9	0.2	0.6
8035	Cereal, Golden Grahams/Gen Mills	¾ cup	30	115.5	1.6	25.7	0.9	1.1	0.3	0.2
8037	Cereal, Granola (oats & wheat germ) homemade	1.0 oz	29	135.4	4.3	15.4	3.0	7.1	2.3	3.1
908038	Cereal, Grape-Nuts	1-⅓ oz box	38	135.7	4.4	31.2	3.8	0.2	0.0	0.0
8040	Cereal, Heartland Natural, Plain (oats & wheat germ)	1 cup	115	499.1	11.6	78.5	7.0	17.7	4.8	7.1
8211	Cereal, Honey Graham Oh!s/Quaker	¾ cup	27	111.8	1.4	22.7	0.7	1.9	1.1	0.3
908046	Cereal, Honeycomb	1.0 oz	28	109.5	1.6	24.9	0.8	0.5	0.0	0.0
8242	Cereal, Just Right w/crunchy nuggets/Kellogg	1 cup	109	404.4	8.4	91.2	5.6	2.9	0.5	2.1
8048	Cereal, Kix/Gen Mills	1 cup	105	400.1	6.8	90.7	2.8	2.2	0.5	0.1
8049	Cereal, Life, Plain/Quaker	1 cup	110	416.9	10.8	86.6	7.0	4.4	1.4	1.9
8050	Cereal, Lucky Charms/Gen Mills	1 cup	115	445.1	8.3	96.5	4.6	4.2	1.5	0.6
8117	Cereal, Malt-O-Meal, plain & chocolate, prep w/o salt	1 cup	30	15.3	0.5	3.2	0.1	0.0	0.0	0.0
8277	Cereal, Nature Valley Low Fat Fruit Granola/Gen Mills	1 cup	22	84.9	1.8	17.5	1.4	1.2	0.6	0.2
8043	Cereal, Nut & Honey Crunch/Kellogg	¾ cup	27	109.4	2.0	22.6	0.4	1.2	0.6	0.4
8291	Cereal, Nutri-Grain Almond and Raisin/Kellogg	1-⅓ cup	30	110.1	2.4	23.3	2.4	1.7	0.8	0.9
8292	Cereal, Nutri-Grain Wheat/Kellogg	¾ cup	32	107.2	3.2	25.6	4.0	1.1	0.3	0.7
8202	Cereal, Oatmeal Crisp w/almonds/Gen Mills	1 cup	55	218.9	5.8	42.0	4.3	4.6	2.4	1.1
8190	Cereal, Oatmeal Crisp w/apples/Gen Mills	1 cup	55	205.2	4.3	46.2	4.5	1.8	0.6	0.2
8227	Cereal, Oatmeal, Instant w/fruit & cream, prep/Quaker	3.5 oz, @ 1 cup	100	118.0	2.5	23.1	1.9	2.2	0.7	0.5
8304	Cereal, Oatmeal, Quick 'N Hearty Regular Flavor, microwave/Quaker	1 packet	29	105.9	3.8	19.1	2.4	2.1	0.7	0.7
8127	Cereal, Oats, Instant w/bran & raisins, fortified, prep	1 packet prep	195	158.0	4.9	30.4	5.5	2.0	0.0	0.0
8123	Cereal, Oats, Instant, Plain, fortified, prep	1 cup, cooked	234	138.1	5.9	23.9	4.0	2.3	0.7	0.9
8180	Cereal, Oats, Regular/Quick/Instant, ckd w/salt	1 packet, prep	158	98.0	4.1	17.1	2.7	1.6	0.5	0.6
8058	Cereal, Product 19/Kellogg	¾ cup	175	640.5	15.6	145.6	5.8	2.3	0.9	1.2
8066	Cereal, Puffed Rice/Quaker	1 cup	30	114.9	2.1	26.3	0.4	0.3	0.1	0.1
908911	Cereal, Puffed Wheat/Quaker	1 cup	14	50.0	2.4	10.5	1.0	0.2	0.0	0.1
908061	Cereal, Raisin Bran, Post	1 single serving box (1.25 oz)	35	107.5	3.3	26.5	4.9	0.7	0.0	0.0
8261	Cereal, Raisin Nut Bran/Gen Mills	1 cup	55	209.0	5.2	41.5	5.1	4.4	1.9	0.5
8287	Cereal, Raisin Squares Mini-Wheats/Kellogg	¾ cup	55	187.0	4.4	42.9	5.2	1.5	0.1	0.5
8185	Cereal, Ralston, ckd w/salt	1 cup	253	134.1	5.6	28.3	6.1	0.8	0.0	0.0
8064	Cereal, Rice Chex	1 cup	33	130.4	1.7	29.4	0.6	0.1	0.0	0.0
8065	Cereal, Rice Krispies/Kellogg	⅝ oz box	18	67.9	1.1	15.6	0.2	0.2	0.1	0.1
8156	Cereal, Rice, Puffed, fortified	0.5 oz	14.2	57.1	0.9	12.8	0.2	0.1	0.0	0.0
8067	Cereal, Special K/Kellogg	0.63 oz box	18	66.6	3.7	13.0	0.6	0.2	0.0	0.1
8070	Cereal, Sugar Frosted Flakes/Ralston Purina	1 cup	38	148.6	2.0	34.2	0.8	0.5	0.1	0.1
8074	Cereal, Tasteeos	10 pieces	1	3.9	0.1	0.8	0.1	0.0	0.0	0.0
908075	Cereal, Team	1 cup	42	164.2	2.7	36.0	0.5	0.8	0.0	0.0
8077	Cereal, Total/Gen Mills	¾ cup	30	105.3	3.0	23.9	2.6	0.7	0.1	0.1
8082	Cereal, Wheat Chex	1 cup	46	168.8	4.6	37.8	4.1	1.2	0.1	0.5
8157	Cereal, Wheat, Puffed, fortified	1 cup	12	43.7	1.8	9.6	0.5	0.1	0.1	0.1
8148	Cereal, Wheat, Shredded, small biscuit	1 single serving box (.875 oz)	24.8	88.5	2.7	19.9	2.4	0.4	0.1	0.2
8089	Cereal, Wheaties/Gen Mills	1 cup	30	110.1	3.2	23.8	2.1	0.9	0.2	0.2
924035	Cheese Blintzes	8.0 oz	227	431.3	19.2	31.2	0.0	25.6	0.0	0.0
1163	Cheese Fondue	1.0 oz	28	64.1	4.0	1.1	0.0	3.8	1.0	0.1
1150	Cheese Spread, Pasteurized Process, American w/disodium phosphate	1.0 oz	28	81.3	4.6	2.4	0.0	5.9	1.7	0.2
1161	Cheese Substitute, Mozzarella	1.0 oz	28	69.4	3.2	6.6	0.0	3.4	1.7	0.5
1004	Cheese, Blue	1.0 oz	28	98.9	6.0	0.7	0.0	8.0	2.2	0.2
1005	Cheese, Brick	1.0 oz	28	103.9	6.5	0.8	0.0	8.3	2.4	0.2
1006	Cheese, Brie	1.0 oz	28	93.4	5.8	0.1	0.0	7.8	2.2	0.2
1007	Cheese, Camembert	1.0 oz	28	83.9	5.5	0.1	0.0	6.8	2.0	0.2
1008	Cheese, Caraway	1.0 oz	28	105.3	7.1	0.9	0.0	8.2	2.3	0.2
1009	Cheese, Cheddar	1.0 oz	28	112.7	7.0	0.4	0.0	9.3	2.6	0.3
1169	Cheese, Cheddar of Colby, low-sodium	1.0 oz	28	111.4	6.8	0.5	0.0	9.1	2.6	0.3
1168	Cheese, Cheddar or Colby, low fat	1.0 oz	28	48.4	6.8	0.5	0.0	2.0	0.6	0.1
1011	Cheese, Colby	1.0 oz	28	110.2	6.7	0.7	0.0	9.0	2.6	0.3
1012	Cheese, Cottage, Creamed, large or small curd	1.0 oz or 1 tbsp	28	28.9	3.5	0.8	0.0	1.3	0.4	0.0
1013	Cheese, Cottage, Creamed, w/fruit	1.0 oz or 1 tbsp	28	34.6	2.8	3.7	0.0	1.0	0.3	0.0
1016	Cheese, Cottage, Lowfat, 1% fat	1.0 oz or 1 tbsp	28	20.3	3.5	0.8	0.0	0.3	0.1	0.0
1015	Cheese, Cottage, Lowfat, 2% fat	1.0 oz or 1 tbsp	28	25.1	3.8	1.0	0.0	0.5	0.2	0.0
1014	Cheese, Cottage, Nonfat, Uncreamed, Dry, large or small curd	1.0 oz or 1 tbsp	28	23.7	4.8	0.5	0.0	0.1	0.0	0.0
1017	Cheese, Cream	1.0 oz or 1 tbsp	28	97.7	2.1	0.7	0.0	9.8	2.8	0.4
1186	Cheese, Cream, fat free	1.0 oz or 1 tbsp	28	26.9	4.0	1.6	0.0	0.4	0.1	0.0
1018	Cheese, Edam	1.0 oz	28	99.8	7.0	0.4	0.0	7.8	2.3	0.2
1019	Cheese, Feta	1.0 oz	28	73.8	4.0	1.1	0.0	6.0	1.3	0.2
1020	Cheese, Fontina	1.0 oz	28	108.9	7.2	0.4	0.0	8.7	2.4	0.5
1022	Cheese, Gouda	1.0 oz	28	99.8	7.0	0.6	0.0	7.7	2.2	0.2
1023	Cheese, Gruyere	1.0 oz	28	115.6	8.3	0.1	0.0	9.1	2.8	0.5
1165	Cheese, Mexican, Queso Anejo	1.0 oz	28	104.4	6.0	1.3	0.0	8.4	2.4	0.3
1025	Cheese, Monterey	1.0 oz	28	104.5	6.9	0.2	0.0	8.5	2.5	0.3

Sat (g)	Chol (mg)	Cal (mg)	Iron (mg)	Magn (mg)	Phos (mg)	Pota (mg)	Sodi (mg)	Zinc (mg)	Vit A (RE)	Vit C (mg)	Vit E (mg)	Thia (mg)	Ribo (mg)	Niac (mg)	Vit B-6 (mg)	Fol (µg)	Vit B-12 (µg)	Wat (g)
0.2	0.0	0.0	15.4	55.6	159.5	186.5	1.7	1.4	0.0	0.0	0.0	0.3	0.4	4.7	0.4	110.0	1.4	2.9
0.2	0.0	14.4	4.5	9.3	36.0	52.8	274.5	3.8	225.3	15.0	0.2	0.4	0.4	5.0	0.5	99.9	0.0	0.8
1.4	0.0	23.5	1.2	51.6	134.0	156.0	7.0	1.2	1.2	0.4	3.7	0.2	0.1	0.6	0.1	24.9	0.0	1.5
0.1	0.0	3.6	10.9	25.5	95.4	126.9	264.1	0.8	503.1	0.0	0.1	0.5	0.6	6.7	0.7	134.1	2.0	1.2
4.5	0.0	74.8	4.3	147.2	416.3	385.3	293.3	3.0	6.9	1.2	0.8	0.4	0.2	1.6	0.2	64.4	0.0	4.7
0.6	0.0	12.4	4.5	12.7	41.9	45.1	177.9	3.8	301.3	12.0	0.1	0.4	0.4	5.0	0.5	100.4	0.0	0.5
0.1	0.1	4.8	2.7	9.5	27.7	32.2	157.6	1.5	370.7	0.0	0.1	0.4	0.4	4.9	0.5	98.8	1.5	0.4
0.2	0.0	28.3	32.2	67.6	210.4	239.8	669.3	1.7	744.5	0.0	4.4	0.8	0.9	9.9	1.0	202.7	2.9	3.5
0.6	0.0	152.3	28.4	32.6	147.0	143.9	920.9	13.1	1313.6	52.5	0.3	1.3	1.5	17.5	1.8	349.7	0.0	2.1
0.8	0.0	335.5	30.8	106.7	466.4	271.7	599.5	13.8	4.4	0.0	0.6	1.4	1.6	18.3	1.8	367.4	0.0	4.4
0.8	0.0	124.2	17.3	74.8	289.8	207.0	778.6	14.4	863.7	57.5	0.5	1.4	1.6	19.2	1.9	383.0	0.0	2.7
0.0	0.0	0.6	1.2	0.6	3.0	3.9	0.3	0.0	0.0	0.0	0.0	0.1	0.0	0.7	0.0	0.6	0.0	26.3
0.1	0.0	15.8	0.6	7.5	72.2	64.7	82.1	0.3	0.0	0.0	0.3	0.0	0.0	0.4	0.0	2.9	0.0	1.0
0.2	0.0	2.7	2.2	2.4	17.8	29.4	181.7	0.2	110.7	7.4	0.1	0.2	0.2	2.5	0.2	54.0	0.0	0.7
0.1	0.0	91.5	0.8	6.9	102.3	107.1	106.5	2.0	0.0	0.0	3.0	0.2	0.2	2.7	0.3	60.0	0.8	1.9
0.1	0.0	10.2	1.1	25.9	115.5	116.8	235.5	4.0	0.0	16.0	5.8	0.4	0.4	5.3	0.5	96.0	1.6	1.2
0.6	0.0	35.8	4.5	57.2	144.1	184.8	250.3	3.8	0.0	9.0	3.1	0.4	0.4	5.0	0.5	99.6	0.0	1.3
0.4	0.0	23.1	4.5	45.1	121.6	159.5	281.6	3.8	0.0	9.0	0.4	0.4	0.4	5.0	0.5	99.6	0.0	1.3
0.5	0.0	94.0	3.5	25.0	92.0	85.0	150.0	0.6	277.0	0.1	0.1	0.3	0.3	3.7	0.4	74.0	0.0	71.2
0.4	0.0	107.9	8.5	38.6	136.3	110.2	152.5	0.9	315.2	0.0	0.0	0.3	0.4	4.2	0.4	84.1	0.0	2.8
0.4	0.0	173.6	7.6	56.6	206.7	236.0	247.7	1.3	479.7	0.0	0.0	0.6	0.6	8.1	0.8	156.0	0.0	156.0
0.4	0.0	215.3	8.3	56.2	175.5	131.0	376.7	1.1	599.0	0.0	0.3	0.7	0.4	7.2	1.0	198.9	0.0	200.1
0.3	0.0	12.6	1.1	37.9	120.1	88.5	252.8	0.8	3.2	0.0	0.2	0.0	0.2	0.2	0.0	6.3	0.0	134.8
0.2	0.0	15.8	105.0	71.8	192.5	236.3	1260.0	87.5	1314.3	350.0	129.5	8.8	10.0	116.7	11.7	2275.0	35.0	6.0
0.1	0.0	2.7	0.9	9.0	35.4	34.8	1.5	0.3	0.0	0.0	0.0	0.1	0.0	1.9	0.0	3.0	0.0	1.2
0.0	0.0	3.0	0.6	19.0	47.0	53.0	1.0	0.4	0.0	0.0	0.0	0.1	0.0	1.6	0.0	4.0	0.0	0.5
0.3	0.1	16.5	5.6	59.5	146.7	215.6	228.2	1.9	463.4	0.0	0.8	0.5	0.5	6.2	0.6	123.6	1.9	3.2
0.7	0.0	73.7	4.5	53.9	162.8	218.4	245.9	1.1	0.0	0.0	2.0	0.4	0.4	5.0	0.5	99.6	0.0	2.5
0.2	0.0	18.7	16.8	47.9	159.5	259.6	3.3	1.5	0.0	0.0	0.0	0.3	0.4	5.2	0.5	110.0	1.5	5.2
0.1	0.0	12.7	1.6	58.2	146.7	154.3	475.6	1.4	0.0	0.0	0.0	0.2	0.2	2.0	0.1	17.7	0.1	217.8
0.0	0.0	4.6	9.4	8.3	32.3	38.3	275.9	0.5	2.0	17.5	0.0	0.4	0.4	5.8	0.6	116.5	1.7	0.9
0.1	0.0	1.8	1.1	8.6	23.8	23.0	193.0	0.3	135.2	9.0	0.0	0.2	0.3	3.0	0.3	63.5	0.0	0.5
0.0	0.0	0.9	4.5	3.6	13.9	16.0	0.4	0.1	0.0	0.0	0.0	0.4	0.3	5.0	0.0	2.7	0.0	0.4
0.0	0.0	2.7	5.1	10.3	29.5	31.7	145.1	2.2	130.7	8.7	0.0	0.3	0.3	4.1	0.4	54.0	0.0	0.5
0.3	0.0	4.2	1.0	2.7	9.5	23.9	246.6	0.8	503.1	20.1	0.1	0.5	0.6	6.7	0.7	2.7	2.0	0.6
0.0	0.0	0.5	0.3	1.1	4.0	3.0	7.6	0.0	13.2	0.5	0.0	0.0	0.0	0.2	0.0	3.5	0.1	0.0
0.3	0.2	6.3	12.0	11.8	65.1	71.0	259.6	0.6	556.1	22.3	0.1	0.5	0.6	7.4	0.8	6.7	2.2	1.6
0.2	0.0	258.3	18.0	32.1	210.9	96.9	198.6	15.0	375.3	60.0	23.5	1.5	1.7	20.1	2.0	399.9	7.7	0.8
0.2	0.0	17.9	13.1	58.4	181.7	173.4	308.2	1.2	0.0	24.4	0.2	0.6	0.2	8.1	0.8	162.4	2.4	1.2
0.0	0.0	3.4	3.8	17.4	42.6	41.8	0.5	0.3	0.0	0.0	0.0	0.3	0.2	4.2	0.0	3.8	0.0	0.4
0.1	0.0	9.4	1.0	32.7	87.5	89.5	2.5	0.8	0.0	0.0	0.1	0.1	0.1	1.3	0.1	12.4	0.0	1.3
0.2	0.0	54.6	8.1	31.8	95.4	104.1	222.3	0.7	225.3	15.0	0.4	0.4	0.4	5.0	0.5	99.9	0.0	1.0
0.0	436.0	336.0	4.8	0.0	0.0	312.0	246.0	0.0	313.6	0.0	0.0	0.3	2.0	3.9	0.0	0.0	0.0	0.0
2.4	12.6	133.3	0.1	6.4	85.7	29.4	37.0	0.5	31.9	0.0	0.0	0.1	0.1	0.0	0.0	2.2	0.2	17.3
3.7	15.5	157.3	0.1	8.0	245.0	67.7	455.0	0.7	52.9	0.0	0.0	0.0	0.1	0.0	0.0	2.0	0.1	13.3
1.0	0.0	170.8	0.1	11.5	163.2	127.4	191.8	0.5	122.4	0.0	0.6	0.0	0.1	0.1	0.0	3.1	0.2	13.3
5.2	21.1	147.7	0.1	6.4	108.5	71.8	390.7	0.7	63.8	0.0	0.2	0.1	0.3	0.0	0.0	10.2	0.3	11.9
5.3	26.4	188.6	0.1	6.8	126.3	38.0	156.7	0.7	84.6	0.0	0.1	0.0	0.0	0.0	0.0	5.7	0.4	11.5
4.9	28.0	51.5	0.1	5.6	52.6	42.6	176.2	0.7	51.0	0.0	0.2	0.0	0.1	0.1	0.1	18.2	0.5	13.6
4.3	20.2	108.5	0.1	5.6	97.0	52.2	235.7	0.7	70.6	0.0	0.2	0.0	0.1	0.2	0.1	17.4	0.4	14.5
5.2	26.0	188.5	0.2	6.2	137.2	26.0	193.2	0.8	80.9	0.0	0.0	0.1	0.1	0.0	0.0	5.1	0.1	11.0
5.9	29.4	202.0	0.2	7.8	143.4	27.6	173.7	0.9	77.8	0.0	0.1	0.1	0.1	0.0	0.0	5.1	0.2	10.3
5.8	28.0	196.8	0.2	7.6	135.5	31.4	5.9	0.9	80.6	0.0	0.1	0.1	0.1	0.0	0.0	5.0	0.2	10.9
1.2	5.9	116.2	0.1	4.5	135.5	18.5	171.4	0.5	17.9	0.0	0.0	0.0	0.0	0.0	0.0	3.1	0.1	17.7
5.7	26.6	191.7	0.2	7.2	127.8	35.4	169.2	0.9	77.0	0.0	0.1	0.1	0.1	0.0	0.0	5.1	0.2	10.7
0.8	4.2	16.8	0.0	1.5	36.9	23.6	113.3	0.1	13.4	0.0	0.0	0.0	0.0	0.0	0.0	3.4	0.2	22.1
0.6	3.1	13.3	0.0	1.2	29.3	18.7	113.3	0.1	10.1	0.0	0.0	0.0	0.0	0.0	0.0	2.7	0.1	20.2
0.2	1.2	17.1	0.0	1.5	37.5	23.9	113.7	0.1	3.1	0.0	0.0	0.0	0.0	0.0	0.0	3.5	0.2	23.1
0.3	2.4	19.2	0.0	1.7	42.1	26.9	113.7	0.1	5.6	0.0	0.0	0.1	0.0	0.0	0.0	3.7	0.2	22.2
0.1	1.9	8.9	0.1	1.1	29.1	9.1	3.6	0.1	2.2	0.0	0.0	0.0	0.0	0.0	0.0	4.1	0.2	22.3
6.2	30.7	22.4	0.3	1.8	29.2	33.4	82.7	0.2	107.0	0.0	0.3	0.0	0.1	0.0	0.0	3.7	0.1	15.1
0.3	2.2	51.8	0.1	3.9	121.5	45.6	152.6	0.2	78.1	0.0	0.0	0.0	0.0	0.0	0.0	10.4	0.2	21.1
4.9	25.0	204.7	0.1	8.3	150.0	52.6	270.2	1.1	70.8	0.0	0.2	0.0	0.1	0.0	0.0	4.5	0.4	11.6
4.2	24.9	137.9	0.2	5.4	94.4	17.3	312.5	0.8	35.8	0.0	0.0	0.0	0.2	0.3	0.1	9.0	0.5	15.5
5.4	32.5	154.0	0.1	3.9	97.0	17.8	224.0	1.0	81.2	0.0	0.1	0.0	0.1	0.0	0.0	1.7	0.5	10.6
4.9	31.9	195.9	0.1	8.1	153.0	33.7	229.4	1.1	48.7	0.0	0.1	0.0	0.1	0.0	0.0	5.9	0.4	11.6
5.3	30.8	283.1	0.0	10.1	169.5	22.7	94.1	1.1	84.3	0.0	0.1	0.0	0.1	0.0	0.0	2.9	0.4	9.3
5.3	29.4	190.4	0.1	7.8	124.3	24.4	316.7	0.8	17.6	0.0	0.0	0.0	0.1	0.0	0.0	0.3	0.4	10.7
5.3	24.9	209.0	0.2	7.6	124.3	22.6	150.2	0.8	70.8	0.0	0.1	0.0	0.1	0.0	0.0	5.1	0.2	11.5

Code	Food Name	Unit/Amt	Wt (g)	Energy (Kcal)	Prot (g)	Carb (g)	Fiber (g)	Fat (g)	Mono (g)	Poly (g)
1028	Cheese, Mozzarella, Part Skim Milk	1.0 oz	28	71.2	6.8	0.8	0.0	4.5	1.3	0.1
1026	Cheese, Mozzarella, Whole Milk	1.0 oz	28	78.8	5.4	0.6	0.0	6.0	1.8	0.2
1030	Cheese, Muenster	1.0 oz	28	103.1	6.6	0.3	0.0	8.4	2.4	0.2
1031	Cheese, Neufchatel	1.0 oz or 1 tbsp	28	72.8	2.8	0.8	0.0	6.6	1.9	0.2
1032	Cheese, Parmesan, grated	1.0 oz	28	127.6	11.6	1.0	0.0	8.4	2.4	0.2
1033	Cheese, Parmesan, hard	1.0 oz	28	109.8	10.0	0.9	0.0	7.2	2.1	0.2
1146	Cheese, Parmesan, shredded	1.0 oz	28	116.2	10.6	1.0	0.0	7.7	2.4	0.2
1042	Cheese, Pasteurized Process, American with disodium phosphate	1 cup, shredded	113	424.3	25.0	1.8	0.0	35.3	10.1	1.1
1043	Cheese, Pasteurized Process, Pimiento	1 cup, shredded	113	424.2	25.0	2.0	0.0	35.3	10.1	1.1
1044	Cheese, Pasteurized Process, Swiss with disodium phosphate	1 cup, shredded	113	376.9	27.9	2.4	0.0	28.3	8.0	0.7
901903	Cheese, Process, Cheez Whiz	1.0 oz	28	77.0	4.6	1.8	0.0	5.7	2.3	0.1
901901	Cheese, Process, Velveeta	1 oz	28	84.0	5.2	2.2	0.0	6.1	2.0	0.2
1035	Cheese, Provolone	1 cup, diced	132	464.0	33.8	2.8	0.0	35.1	9.8	1.0
1037	Cheese, Ricotta, Part Skim Milk	1.0 oz or 1 tbsp	15.4	21.3	1.8	0.8	0.0	1.2	0.4	0.0
1036	Cheese, Ricotta, Whole Milk	1.0 oz or 1 tbsp	15.4	26.8	1.7	0.5	0.0	2.0	0.6	0.1
1038	Cheese, Romano	1.0 oz	28	108.3	8.9	1.0	0.0	7.5	2.2	0.2
1039	Cheese, Roquefort	1.0 oz	28	103.3	6.0	0.6	0.0	8.6	2.4	0.4
1040	Cheese, Swiss	1.0 oz	108	405.8	30.7	3.7	0.0	29.6	7.9	1.0
18147	Cheesecake, commercially prep	1 piece (½ of 9" dia)	128	410.9	7.0	32.6	0.5	28.8	11.1	2.1
918149	Cheesecake, homemade	1 piece (½ of 9" dia)	99	353.4	6.7	24.9	0.0	25.7	0.0	0.0
18148	Cheesecake, no bake mix, prep	1 piece (½ of 9" dia)	142	389.1	7.8	50.4	2.7	18.0	6.4	1.1
1045	Cheesefood, Cold Pack, American	1.0 oz	28	92.7	5.5	2.3	0.0	6.8	2.0	0.2
1149	Cheesefood, Pasteurized Process, American w/disodium phosphate	1.0 oz	28	91.9	5.5	2.0	0.0	6.9	2.0	0.2
1047	Cheesefood, Pasteurized Process, Swiss	1.0 oz	28	90.5	6.1	1.3	0.0	6.8	1.9	0.2
5028	Chicken Liver, simmered	3.5 oz	100	157.0	24.4	0.9	0.0	5.5	1.3	0.9
22703	Chicken & Dumplings, canned/Sweet Sue	1 package	681	619.7	42.9	64.7	7.5	21.1	8.4	4.6
924003	Chicken A la King frz (Le Menu 10. 5 oz meal)	1 package	299	574.1	32.9	14.6	0.1	41.5	16.4	7.6
924006	Chicken Chow Mein	10.0 oz	284	289.7	35.2	11.4	3.4	14.2	5.6	4.0
924005	Chicken Chow Mein, canned	¾ cup	200	76.0	5.6	14.4	1.6	0.8	0.1	0.6
924248	Chicken Chow Mein/Chun King	¾ cup	200	200.0	13.6	28.7	0.0	3.3	0.0	0.0
924068	Chicken Egg Roll/LaChoy	3 medium	37	89.9	3.0	12.0	0.0	3.0	1.1	1.3
924043	Chicken Kiev, frozen	1 breast w/ filling	280	604.8	22.3	41.4	0.0	39.0	0.0	0.0
924051	Chicken Parmigiana	11 .5 oz	356	548.2	38.4	39.3	0.0	26.3	0.0	0.0
22527	Chicken Pie, frozen/Stouffers	1 slice	232	468.6	19.0	29.9	2.6	30.4	10.1	8.6
924007	Chicken Pot Pie	7.0 oz	198	465.3	19.6	35.8	1.5	27.7	13.2	5.6
924171	Chicken Teriyaki/LaChoy	¾ cup	120	85.2	8.0	8.0	1.0	2.0	1.1	0.4
924242	Chicken w/vegetables&pasta	9.5 oz	269	121.1	10.8	13.7	0.0	2.4	0.0	0.0
924004	Chicken&Noodles	1 cup	240	364.8	22.0	26.0	0.1	18.0	7.1	3.9
924047	Chicken&Rice	7.0 oz pkg	200	364.0	22.0	26.0	1.0	18.0	7.0	4.0
5060	Chicken, Broiler or Fryer, Breast w/skin, roasted	3.5 oz	100	197.0	29.8	0.0	0.0	7.8	3.0	1.7
5061	Chicken, Broiler or Fryer, Breast w/skin, stewed	3.5 oz	100	184.0	27.4	0.0	0.0	7.4	2.9	1.6
5063	Chicken, Broiler or Fryer, Breast, no skin, fried	3.5 oz	100	187.0	33.4	0.5	0.0	4.7	1.7	1.1
5064	Chicken, Broiler or Fryer, Breast, no skin, roasted	3.5 oz	100	165.0	31.0	0.0	0.0	3.6	1.2	0.8
5065	Chicken, Broiler or Fryer, Breast, no skin, stewed	3.5 oz	100	151.0	29.0	0.0	0.0	3.0	1.0	0.7
5037	Chicken, Broiler or Fryer, Dark Meat w/skin, roasted	3.5 oz	100	253.0	26.0	0.0	0.0	15.8	6.2	3.5
5038	Chicken, Broiler or Fryer, Dark Meat w/skin, stewed	3.5 oz	100	233.0	23.5	0.0	0.0	14.7	5.8	3.2
5044	Chicken, Broiler or Fryer, Dark Meat, no skin, fried	4.0 oz	119	284.4	34.5	3.1	0.0	13.8	5.1	3.3
5045	Chicken, Broiler or Fryer, Dark Meat, no skin, roasted	3.5 oz	100	205.0	27.4	0.0	0.0	9.7	3.6	2.3
5046	Chicken, Broiler or Fryer, Dark Meat, no skin, stewed	3.5 oz	100	192.0	26.0	0.0	0.0	9.0	3.3	2.1
5078	Chicken, Broiler or Fryer, Leg w/skin, roasted	3.5 oz	100	232.0	26.0	0.0	0.0	13.5	5.2	3.0
5079	Chicken, Broiler or Fryer, Leg w/skin, stewed	3.5 oz	100	220.0	24.2	0.0	0.0	12.9	5.0	2.9
5081	Chicken, Broiler or Fryer, Leg, no skin, fried	4.0 oz	119	247.5	33.8	0.8	0.0	11.1	4.1	2.6
5082	Chicken, Broiler or Fryer, Leg, no skin, roasted	3.5 oz	100	191.0	27.0	0.0	0.0	8.4	3.1	2.0
5083	Chicken, Broiler or Fryer, Leg, no skin, stewed	3.5 oz	100	185.0	26.3	0.0	0.0	8.1	2.9	1.9
5032	Chicken, Broiler or Fryer, Light Meat w/skin, roasted	3.5 oz	100	222.0	29.0	0.0	0.0	10.9	4.3	2.3
5033	Chicken, Broiler or Fryer, Light Meat w/skin, stewed	3.5 oz	100	201.0	26.1	0.0	0.0	10.0	3.9	2.1
5040	Chicken, Broiler or Fryer, Light Meat, no skin, fried	4.0 oz	119	228.5	39.1	0.5	0.0	6.6	2.3	1.5
5041	Chicken, Broiler or Fryer, Light Meat, no skin, roasted	3.5 oz	100	173.0	30.9	0.0	0.0	4.5	1.5	1.0
5042	Chicken, Broiler or Fryer, Light Meat, no skin, stewed	3.5 oz	100	159.0	28.9	0.0	0.0	4.0	1.4	0.9
5009	Chicken, Broiler or Fryer, meat & skin, roasted	3.5 oz	100	239.0	27.3	0.0	0.0	13.6	5.3	3.0
5010	Chicken, Broiler or Fryer, meat & skin, stewed	3.5 oz	100	219.0	24.7	0.0	0.0	12.6	4.9	2.7
5094	Chicken, Broiler or Fryer, Thigh w/skin, roasted	3.5 oz	100	247.0	25.1	0.0	0.0	15.5	6.2	3.4
5095	Chicken, Broiler or Fryer, Thigh w/skin, stewed	3.5 oz	100	232.0	23.3	0.0	0.0	14.7	5.8	3.3
5097	Chicken, Broiler or Fryer, Thigh, no skin, fried	4.0 oz	119	259.4	33.5	1.4	0.0	12.3	4.5	2.9
5098	Chicken, Broiler or Fryer, Thigh, no skin, roasted	3.5 oz	100	209.0	25.9	0.0	0.0	10.9	4.2	2.5
5099	Chicken, Broiler or Fryer, Thigh, no skin, stewed	3.5 oz	100	195.0	25.0	0.0	0.0	9.8	3.7	2.2
5103	Chicken, Broiler or Fryer, Wing w/skin, roasted	3.5 oz	100	290.0	26.9	0.0	0.0	19.5	7.6	4.1
5104	Chicken, Broiler or Fryer, Wing w/skin, stewed	3.5 oz	100	249.0	22.8	0.0	0.0	16.8	6.6	3.6
5106	Chicken, Broiler or Fryer, Wing, no skin, fried	4.0 oz	119	251.1	35.9	0.0	0.0	10.9	3.7	2.5

Sat (g)	Chol (mg)	Cal (mg)	Iron (mg)	Magn (mg)	Phos (mg)	Pota (mg)	Sodi (mg)	Zinc (mg)	Vit A (RE)	Vit C (mg)	Vit E (mg)	Thia (mg)	Ribo (mg)	Niac (mg)	Vit B-6 (mg)	Fol (µg)	Vit B-12 (µg)	Wat (g)
2.8	16.2	180.8	0.1	6.5	129.6	23.4	130.5	0.8	49.6	0.0	0.1	0.0	0.1	0.0	0.0	2.5	0.2	15.1
3.7	22.0	144.8	0.1	5.2	103.8	18.8	104.5	0.6	67.5	0.0	0.1	0.0	0.1	0.0	0.0	2.0	0.2	15.2
5.4	26.8	200.8	0.1	7.7	131.0	37.6	175.8	0.8	88.5	0.0	0.1	0.0	0.1	0.0	0.0	3.4	0.4	11.7
4.1	21.3	21.1	0.1	2.1	38.2	31.9	111.8	0.1	84.0	0.0	0.0	0.0	0.1	0.0	0.0	3.2	0.1	17.4
5.3	22.0	385.2	0.3	14.2	226.0	30.0	521.2	0.9	48.4	0.0	0.2	0.0	0.1	0.1	0.0	2.2	0.4	4.9
4.6	19.0	331.4	0.2	12.2	194.4	25.8	448.4	0.8	41.7	0.0	0.2	0.0	0.1	0.1	0.0	1.9	0.3	8.2
4.9	20.2	350.8	0.2	14.2	205.8	27.2	474.9	0.9	48.4	0.0	0.0	0.0	0.1	0.1	0.0	2.2	0.4	7.0
22.3	106.7	695.5	0.4	25.1	841.7	183.1	1616.4	3.4	327.7	0.0	0.5	0.0	0.4	0.1	0.1	8.8	0.8	44.3
22.2	106.4	694.3	0.5	25.1	840.5	182.7	1613.1	3.4	363.9	2.5	0.5	0.0	0.4	0.1	0.1	8.8	0.8	44.2
18.1	95.8	872.2	0.7	32.9	860.5	243.5	1548.4	4.1	258.8	0.0	0.8	0.0	0.3		0.0	6.7	1.4	47.8
3.1	16.0	147.0	0.1	8.0	255.0	52.0	370.0	0.7	38.6	0.0	0.0	0.0	0.1	0.1	0.0	4.0	0.2	14.5
3.6	21.0	154.0	0.1	8.0	292.0	88.0	454.0	0.6	68.6	0.0	0.0	0.0	0.1	0.0	0.0	6.0	0.3	13.0
22.5	90.9	997.8	0.7	36.4	654.9	182.6	1155.7	4.3	348.5	0.0	0.5	0.0	0.4	0.2	0.1	13.7	1.9	54.1
0.8	4.7	41.9	0.1	2.3	28.1	19.3	19.2	0.2	17.4	0.0	0.0	0.0	0.0	0.0	0.0	2.0	0.0	11.5
1.3	7.8	31.9	0.1	1.7	24.3	16.1	13.0	0.2	20.6	0.0	0.1	0.0	0.0	0.0	0.0	1.9	0.1	11.0
4.8	29.1	297.9	0.2	11.5	212.8	24.2	336.0	0.7	39.5	0.0	0.2	0.0	0.1	0.0	0.0	1.9	0.3	8.7
5.4	25.2	185.3	0.2	8.3	109.8	25.4	506.5	0.6	83.7	0.0	0.0	0.0	0.2	0.2	0.0	13.7	0.2	11.0
19.2	99.0	1037.8	0.2	38.8	653.0	119.6	280.8	4.2	273.2	0.0	0.5	0.0	0.4	0.1	0.1	6.9	1.8	40.2
12.7	70.4	65.3	0.8	14.1	119.0	115.2	265.0	0.7	186.9	0.5	2.0	0.0	0.2	0.2	0.1	23.0	0.2	58.4
2.0	8.0	57.4	1.2	7.9	95.0	101.0	280.2	0.5	317.8	0.4	0.0	0.0	0.2	0.4	0.0	11.9	0.2	40.5
9.5	41.2	244.2	0.7	27.0	332.3	299.6	539.6	0.7	140.6	0.7	0.0	0.2	0.4	0.7	0.1	42.6	0.4	62.8
4.3	17.8	139.2	0.2	8.3	112.0	101.6	270.5	0.8	56.6	0.0	0.0	0.0	0.1	0.0	0.0	1.5	0.4	12.1
4.3	17.9	160.8	0.2	8.6	211.1	78.1	446.9	0.8	61.3	0.0	0.0	0.0	0.1	0.0	0.0	2.0	0.3	12.1
4.3	22.9	202.6	0.2	7.8	147.3	79.5	434.6	1.0	68.0	0.0	0.0	0.0	0.1	0.0	0.0	1.6	0.6	12.2
1.8	631.0	14.0	8.5	21.0	312.0	140.0	51.0	4.3	4913.0	15.8	1.4	0.2	1.7	4.5	0.6	770.0	19.4	68.3
5.1	102.2	0.0	7.3	0.0	0.0	0.0	2683.1	0.0	0.0	0.0	0.0	0.0	0.0	0.0	0.0	0.0	0.0	544.1
15.7	269.7	155.0	3.0	0.0	436.9	493.0	927.5	2.2	275.8	14.6	0.0	0.1	0.5	6.6	0.3	13.4	0.0	0.0
4.7	85.2	65.9	2.8	0.0	332.8	537.3	815.6	2.4	63.6	11.4	0.0	0.1	0.3	4.9	0.5	21.6	0.0	0.0
0.1	6.4	36.0	1.0	0.0	68.0	334.4	580.0	1.0	24.0	10.4	0.0	0.1	0.1	0.8	0.1	9.6	0.0	0.0
0.0	0.0	14.6	1.1	0.0	111.1	140.9	845.5	2.2	68.6	0.0	0.1	0.1	1.6			0.0	0.0	0.0
0.6	3.0	9.0	0.8	0.0	0.0	55.0	140.0	0.0	5.0	2.0	0.0	0.1	0.1	1.1	0.0	0.0	0.0	0.0
0.0	0.0	54.3	1.5	0.0	0.0	291.1	95.0	0.0	397.4	2.5	0.0	0.2	0.2	9.0	0.0	0.0	0.0	0.0
0.0	0.0	309.7	11.2	0.0	521.5	608.8	637.2	0.0	494.1	28.5	0.0	0.3	0.3	8.5	0.0	0.0	0.0	0.0
8.8	62.6	83.5	2.5	0.0	0.0	0.0	772.6	0.0	0.0	0.0	0.0	0.0	0.0	0.0	0.0	0.0	0.0	149.4
8.8	47.8	59.7	2.6	0.0	198.0	292.7	506.9	1.7	1232.4	4.3	0.0	0.3	0.3	4.2	0.4	24.8	0.0	0.0
0.5	20.0	20.0	1.1	0.0	0.0	230.0	850.0	0.0	200.0	12.0	0.0	0.0	0.1	2.0	0.0	0.0	0.0	0.0
0.0	0.0	50.0	1.3	0.0	0.0	195.0	965.0	0.0	493.4	5.0	0.0	0.1	0.1	2.9	0.0	0.0	0.0	0.0
5.1	103.0	26.0	2.2	0.0	247.0	149.0	600.0	2.1	86.0	0.0	0.0	0.1	0.2	4.3	0.2	9.0	0.0	0.0
5.0	103.0	26.0	2.4	0.0	247.0	211.0	600.0	2.1	26.0	1.0	0.0	0.1	0.2	4.3	0.2	9.0	0.0	0.0
2.2	84.0	14.0	1.1	27.0	214.0	245.0	71.0	1.0	27.0	0.0	0.3	0.1	0.1	12.7	0.6	4.0	0.3	62.4
2.1	75.0	13.0	0.9	22.0	156.0	178.0	62.0	1.0	24.0	0.0	0.3	0.0	0.1	7.8	0.3	3.0	0.2	66.2
1.3	91.0	16.0	1.1	31.0	246.0	276.0	79.0	1.1	7.0	0.0	0.4	0.1	0.1	14.8	0.6	4.0	0.4	60.2
1.0	85.0	15.0	1.0	29.0	228.0	256.0	74.0	1.0	6.0	0.0	0.3	0.1	0.1	13.7	0.6	4.0	0.3	65.3
0.9	77.0	13.0	0.9	24.0	165.0	187.0	63.0	1.0	6.0	0.0	0.3	0.0	0.1	8.5	0.3	3.0	0.2	68.3
4.4	91.0	15.0	1.4	22.0	168.0	220.0	87.0	2.5	58.0	0.0	0.0	0.1	0.2	6.4	0.3	7.0	0.3	58.6
4.1	82.0	14.0	1.3	18.0	133.0	166.0	70.0	2.3	54.0	0.0	0.0	0.1	0.2	4.5	0.2	6.0	0.2	63.0
3.7	114.2	21.4	1.8	29.8	222.5	301.1	115.4	3.5	28.6	0.0	0.0	0.1	0.3	8.4	0.4	10.7	0.4	66.3
2.7	93.0	15.0	1.3	23.0	179.0	240.0	93.0	2.8	22.0	0.0	0.3	0.1	0.2	6.5	0.4	8.0	0.3	63.1
2.5	88.0	14.0	1.4	20.0	143.0	181.0	74.0	2.7	21.0	0.0	0.3	0.1	0.2	4.7	0.2	7.0	0.2	65.8
3.7	92.0	12.0	1.3	23.0	174.0	225.0	87.0	2.6	39.0	0.0	0.3	0.1	0.2	6.2	0.3	7.0	0.3	60.9
3.6	84.0	11.0	1.4	20.0	139.0	176.0	73.0	2.4	36.0	0.0	0.3	0.1	0.2	4.6	0.2	6.0	0.2	64.0
3.0	117.8	15.5	1.7	29.8	229.7	302.3	114.2	3.5	23.8	0.0	0.0	0.1	0.3	8.0	0.5	10.7	0.4	72.1
2.3	94.0	12.0	1.3	24.0	183.0	242.0	91.0	2.9	19.0	0.0	0.3	0.1	0.2	6.3	0.4	8.0	0.3	64.7
2.2	89.0	11.0	1.4	21.0	149.0	190.0	78.0	2.8	18.0	0.0	0.3	0.1	0.2	4.8	0.2	8.0	0.2	66.4
3.1	84.0	15.0	1.1	25.0	200.0	227.0	75.0	1.2	32.0	0.0	0.0	0.1	0.1	11.1	0.5	3.0	0.3	60.5
2.8	74.0	13.0	1.0	20.0	146.0	167.0	63.0	1.1	28.0	0.0	0.3	0.0	0.1	6.9	0.3	3.0	0.2	65.1
1.8	107.1	19.0	1.4	34.5	274.9	313.0	96.4	1.5	10.7	0.0	0.0	0.1	0.1	15.9	0.7	4.8	0.4	71.6
1.3	85.0	15.0	1.1	27.0	216.0	247.0	77.0	1.2	9.0	0.0	0.3	0.1	0.1	12.4	0.6	4.0	0.3	64.8
1.1	77.0	13.0	0.9	22.0	159.0	180.0	65.0	1.2	8.0	0.0	0.3	0.0	0.1	7.8	0.3	3.0	0.2	68.0
3.8	88.0	15.0	1.3	23.0	182.0	223.0	82.0	1.9	47.0	0.0	0.3	0.1	0.2	8.5	0.4	5.0	0.3	59.5
3.5	78.0	13.0	1.2	19.0	139.0	166.0	67.0	1.8	42.0	0.0	0.3	0.0	0.1	5.6	0.2	5.0	0.2	63.9
4.3	93.0	12.0	1.3	22.0	174.0	222.0	84.0	2.4	48.0	0.0	0.3	0.1	0.2	6.4	0.3	7.0	0.3	59.4
4.1	84.0	11.0	1.4	19.0	139.0	170.0	71.0	2.3	44.0	0.0	0.3	0.1	0.2	4.9	0.2	6.0	0.2	63.1
3.3	121.4	15.5	1.7	30.9	236.8	308.2	113.1	3.3	25.0	0.0	0.0	0.1	0.3	8.5	0.5	10.7	0.4	70.6
3.0	95.0	12.0	1.3	24.0	183.0	238.0	88.0	2.6	20.0	0.0	0.3	0.1	0.2	6.5	0.4	8.0	0.3	62.9
2.7	90.0	11.0	1.4	21.0	149.0	183.0	75.0	2.6	19.0	0.0	0.3	0.1	0.2	5.2	0.2	7.0	0.2	65.6
5.5	84.0	15.0	1.3	19.0	151.0	184.0	82.0	1.8	47.0	0.0	0.3	0.0	0.1	6.6	0.4	3.0	0.3	55.0
4.7	70.0	12.0	1.1	16.0	121.0	139.0	67.0	1.6	40.0	0.0	0.3	0.0	0.1	4.6	0.2	3.0	0.2	62.2
3.0	100.0	17.9	1.4	25.0	195.2	247.5	108.3	2.5	21.4	0.0	0.0	0.1	0.2	8.6	0.7	4.8	0.4	71.2

Code	Food Name	Unit/Amt	Wt (g)	Energy (Kcal)	Prot (g)	Carb (g)	Fiber (g)	Fat (g)	Mono (g)	Poly (g)
5107	Chicken, Broiler or Fryer, Wing, no skin, roasted	3.5 oz	100	203.0	30.5	0.0	0.0	8.1	2.6	1.8
5108	Chicken, Broiler or Fryer, Wing, no skin, stewed	3.5 oz	100	181.0	27.2	0.0	0.0	7.2	2.3	1.6
22697	Chicken, Chicken Salad Ready To Serve Sandwich Salad/Libby Spreadable	1 package	227	329.2	11.1	22.9	0.0	21.3	6.7	8.1
5277	Chicken, meat only w/broth, canned	2.5 oz	71	117.2	15.5	0.0	0.0	5.6	2.2	1.2
51608	Chicken, Nugget, breaded/Pierre product #1879	3.5 oz	100	329.0	16.8	13.3	1.1	23.4	6.9	10.4
924008	Chili con Carne	¾ cup	120	159.6	8.9	14.6	2.8	7.5	3.4	0.5
22904	Chili con carne w/beans, canned entree	1 cup	255	293.3	23.2	28.1	9.4	9.4	2.5	1.7
924243	Chili w/beans	1 package	425	909.5	30.9	90.8	11.6	52.2	28.0	2.7
16059	Chili w/beans, canned	1 cup	220	246.4	12.6	26.2	9.7	12.1	5.1	0.8
924059	Chili w/beans, homemade	1 cup	247	328.5	18.5	30.1	1.5	15.1	0.0	0.0
924056	Chili w/o Beans, homemade	1 cup	236	472.0	24.3	13.7	0.5	34.9	18.6	2.1
22720	Chili, Vegetarian Chili w/beans, canned entree/Hormel	1 cup	247	205.0	11.9	38.0	9.9	0.7	0.1	0.4
18606	Chocolate Cake, Snack Cake, Chocolate Creme Filling-Ding Dongs/Hostess	1 cup	220	1015.5	6.8	130.2	4.6	51.9	0.0	0.0
918804	Chocolate, Baking, Choco-Bake/Nestle	1 serving	80	480.0	4.0	34.0	0.0	39.4	0.0	0.0
918805	Chocolate, Baking, Hershey	1 oz	28	185.1	4.0	6.7	0.7	15.8	4.8	1.0
19146	Chocolate, Baking, M&M's Milk Chocolate Mini Baking Bits	1 oz	28	139.4	1.3	18.8	0.8	6.5	2.1	0.2
19139	Chocolate, Baking, M&M's Semisweet Chocolate Mini Baking Bits	1 serving	14.2	73.6	0.6	9.4	1.0	3.7	1.2	0.1
19124	Chocolate, Baking, Mexican, squares	1 tbsp	14	59.6	0.5	10.8	0.5	2.2	0.7	0.2
918806	Chocolate, Baking, Unsweetened Liquid	1 tablet	20	95.8	2.4	6.9	0.0	9.6	1.9	2.1
918870	Cobbler, Peach	1 oz	28	44.8	0.3	7.1	0.3	1.8	0.0	0.0
14198	Cocoa Mix, No Sugar Added Hot Cocoa Mix/Carnation	⅓ cup	100	365.0	28.7	56.2	5.0	2.8	0.9	0.1
14197	Cocoa Mix, Rich Chocolate Hot Cocoa Mix/Carnation	1 envelope	15	60.0	0.7	13.0	0.4	0.6	0.2	0.1
1105	Cocoa, Hot, homemade w/whole milk	1 envelope	28	21.6	1.1	3.3	0.2	0.7	0.2	0.0
918844	Coffee Cake, Apple, frozen	1 fl oz	31.2	100.5	1.4	14.0	0.1	4.4	0.0	0.0
918845	Coffee Cake, Blueberry, frozen	⅛ cake	50	190.0	2.6	25.1	0.6	8.9	0.0	0.0
18103	Coffee Cake, Cheese	⅙ Ring	35	118.7	2.5	15.5	0.4	5.3	2.5	0.6
918109	Coffee Cake, Cinnamon Crumb, homemade	1.0 oz	28.4	113.6	1.8	14.3	0.0	5.7	0.0	0.0
18108	Coffee Cake, Cinnamon w/crumb topping, dry mix, prep	1.0 oz	28	89.0	1.5	14.8	0.3	2.7	1.1	0.9
18104	Coffee Cake, Cinnamon w/crumb topping, enriched, commercially prep	1.0 oz	29	121.2	2.0	13.5	0.6	6.8	3.8	0.9
18106	Coffee Cake, Fruit	1.0 oz	28.4	88.3	1.5	14.6	0.7	2.9	1.6	0.4
918847	Coffee Cake, Pecan, frozen	1.0 oz	29	110.8	1.7	13.8	0.3	6.2	0.0	0.0
918843	Coffee Cake/LittleDeb	⅛ cake	40	153.6	2.0	26.8	0.0	4.2	1.6	1.6
14210	Coffee, brewed, espresso, restaurant-prep	2.0 oz	57	5.1	0.0	0.9	0.0	0.1	0.0	0.1
902912	Condiment, A-1 Sauce	6 fl oz	177	118.6	0.0	29.5	0.0	0.0	0.0	0.0
902922	Condiment, Enchilada Sauce	¼ cup	60	21.0	0.0	2.8	0.0	0.0	0.0	0.0
2055	Condiment, Horseradish, prep	1 tbsp	15	7.2	0.2	1.7	0.5	0.1	0.0	0.1
902916	Condiment, Mustard, brown	1 tsp	5	5.0	0.3	0.3	0.1	0.3	0.0	0.0
902917	Condiment, Mustard, yellow	1 tsp	5	4.0	0.2	0.3	0.1	0.2	0.0	0.0
902925	Condiment, Picante Sauce	3 tbsp	57	16.0	0.0	4.0	0.0	0.0	0.0	0.0
902918	Condiment, Pickle, Sour Relish	1 tbsp	15	16.1	0.0	3.8	0.2	0.0	0.0	0.0
902926	Condiment, Salsa	3 tbsp	43	24.9	1.0	6.0	0.0	0.0	0.0	0.0
902927	Condiment, Taco Sauce, chunky	3 tbsp	43	24.9	1.0	6.0	0.0	0.0	0.0	0.0
902928	Condiment, Taco Sauce, hot/mild	3 tbsp	43	15.1	0.0	4.0	0.0	0.0	0.0	0.0
11935	Condiment, Vege, Tomato Catsup	1 tbsp	15	15.6	0.2	4.1	0.2	0.1	0.0	0.0
11949	Condiment, Vege, Tomato Catsup, low sodium	1 tbsp	15	15.6	0.2	4.1	0.2	0.1	0.0	0.0
902919	Condiment, Worcestershire Sauce	1 tbsp	15	11.0	0.3	2.7	0.0	0.0	0.0	0.0
18150	Cookie, Animal Crackers/Arrowroot/Tea Biscuits	1 cracker	2	8.9	0.1	1.5	0.0	0.3	0.2	0.0
918153	Cookie, Brownies, dry mix, prep	1 brownie (2″ square)	33	139.6	1.4	20.4	0.9	6.6	0.0	0.0
18197	Cookie, Brownies, dry mix, prep, special dietary	1 brownie (2″ square)	22	84.5	0.8	15.7	0.8	2.4	1.0	0.2
18154	Cookie, Brownies, homemade	1 brownie (2″ square)	24	111.8	1.5	12.0	0.0	7.0	2.6	2.3
18155	Cookie, Butter, enriched, commercially prep	1 cookie	5	23.4	0.3	3.4	0.0	0.9	0.3	0.0
918861	Cookie, Capri/PepFarm	1 cookie	16	81.9	0.8	9.7	0.1	4.6	0.0	0.0
18614	Cookie, Chewy Fudge Brownie Mix, dry/Martha White	1 serving	28	114.1	1.3	23.2	0.0	1.8	0.0	0.0
18198	Cookie, Chocolate Chip, commercially prep, special dietary	1 medium cookie (1.6″ dia)	7	31.5	0.3	5.1	0.1	1.2	0.5	0.4
918162	Cookie, Chocolate Chip, dry mix, prep	1 cookie (2″ dia)	16	79.4	0.9	10.3	0.2	4.1	0.0	0.0
18159	Cookie, Chocolate Chip, enriched, commercially prep	1 large Keebler RichnChip/ PecanChipDelux	14	67.3	0.8	9.4	0.4	3.2	1.6	0.3
18378	Cookie, Chocolate Chip, homemade w/butter	1 medium cookie (2.25″ dia)	16	78.1	0.9	9.3	0.0	4.5	1.3	0.7
18158	Cookie, Chocolate Chip, lower fat, commercially prep	1 cookie	10	45.3	0.6	7.3	0.4	1.5	0.6	0.5
918164	Cookie, Chocolate Chip, refrig dough, bkd	1.0 oz	28	137.8	1.4	19.1	0.5	6.3	0.0	0.0
18160	Cookie, Chocolate Chip, soft, commercially prep	1 cookie	15	68.7	0.5	8.9	0.5	3.6	2.0	0.5
918862	Cookie, Chocolate Chip/PepFarm	2 large	64	321.3	3.2	44.2	0.0	14.7	0.0	0.0
918895	Cookie, Chocolate Coated Graham/Lance	1.8 oz	50	249.0	3.5	32.7	0.0	13.5	7.5	0.6
918854	Cookie, Chocolate Marshmallow Pie/LittleDeb	1.4 oz	39	170.0	1.5	27.1	0.0	6.2	3.3	0.7
18169	Cookie, Coconut Macaroons, homemade	1 individual pkg (2 oz pkg w/2 3″-bars	57	230.3	2.1	41.2	1.0	7.2	0.3	0.1
18170	Cookie, Fig Bar	1 cookie	16	55.7	0.6	11.3	0.7	1.2	0.5	0.4
18171	Cookie, Fortune	1 cookie	8	30.2	0.3	6.7	0.1	0.2	0.1	0.0

Sat (g)	Chol (mg)	Cal (mg)	Iron (mg)	Magn (mg)	Phos (mg)	Pota (mg)	Sodi (mg)	Zinc (mg)	Vit A (RE)	Vit C (mg)	Vit E (mg)	Thia (mg)	Ribo (mg)	Niac (mg)	Vit B-6 (mg)	Fol (µg)	Vit B-12 (µg)	Wat (g)
2.3	85.0	16.0	1.2	21.0	166.0	210.0	92.0	2.1	18.0	0.0	0.3	0.0	0.1	7.3	0.6	4.0	0.3	62.8
2.0	74.0	13.0	1.1	18.0	134.0	153.0	73.0	2.0	16.0	0.0	0.3	0.0	0.1	5.2	0.3	3.0	0.2	67.0
4.4	59.0	0.0	0.0	0.0	0.0	0.0	1062.4	0.0	0.0	0.0	0.0	0.0	0.0	0.0	0.0	0.0	0.0	167.3
1.6	44.0	9.9	1.1	8.5	78.8	98.0	357.1	1.0	24.1	1.4	0.2	0.0	0.1	4.5	0.2	2.8	0.2	48.7
4.6	39.0	36.0	2.2	24.0	225.0	211.0	697.0	2.5	0.0	0.0	2.7	0.3	0.2	6.3	0.3	29.0	0.7	44.6
2.7	13.2	38.6	2.0	0.0	151.1	279.5	637.2	2.4	14.1	3.8	0.0	0.0	0.1	1.6	0.2	19.3	0.0	0.0
2.4	28.1	76.5	3.8	63.8	221.9	698.7	1185.8	2.8	107.1	1.0	0.3	0.2	0.2	2.4	0.2	66.3	0.7	189.3
18.9	125.6	183.5	12.4	0.0	388.3	2801.1	1931.8	3.9	566.0	77.3	0.0	0.8	0.6	8.5	0.5	48.3	0.0	0.0
5.2	37.4	103.4	7.5	99.0	338.8	803.0	1148.4	4.4	74.8	3.7	1.6	0.1	0.2	0.8	0.3	49.9	0.0	166.1
0.0	0.0	79.0	4.2	0.0	311.2	575.5	1311.6	0.0	29.6	0.0	0.0	0.1	0.2	3.2	0.0	0.0	0.0	178.8
14.2	101.5	89.7	3.3	0.0	358.7	2199.5	3138.8	11.8	70.8	4.7	0.0	0.0	0.3	5.2	0.6	0.0	0.0	157.9
0.1	0.0	96.3	3.5	81.5	0.0	802.8	778.1	1.7	0.0	1.2	0.0	0.0	0.0	0.0	0.0	0.0	0.0	192.5
30.6	30.1	0.0	5.1	0.0	0.0	0.0	547.8	0.0	0.0	0.0	0.0	0.0	0.0	0.0	0.0	0.0	0.0	28.2
0.0	0.0	0.0	0.0	0.0	0.0	817.1	8.6	0.0	0.0	0.0	0.0	0.0	0.0	0.0	0.0	0.0	0.0	0.0
10.0	0.0	20.0	2.0	84.0	123.0	224.0	3.0	1.1	1.2	0.0	0.0	0.0	0.1	0.3	0.0	3.0	0.0	0.0
4.0	4.2	32.5	0.3	12.9	46.5	82.0	19.0	0.3	12.6	0.2	0.3	0.0	0.1	0.1	0.0	1.4	0.1	0.7
2.2	0.4	4.8	0.4	15.1	17.3	47.7	0.4	0.2	1.0	0.0	0.1	0.0	0.0	0.1	0.0	4.0	0.0	0.2
1.2	0.0	4.8	0.3	13.3	19.9	55.6	0.4	0.2	0.3	0.0	0.1	0.0	0.0	0.3	0.0	0.3	0.0	0.2
5.1	0.0	10.7	0.8	53.6	68.6	236.4	2.1	0.7	2.4	0.0	0.0	0.1	0.4	0.0	0.0	0.0	0.2	
0.8	0.0	2.0	0.1	0.0	4.5	24.6	44.2	0.0	26.8	7.3	0.0	0.0	0.0	0.3	0.0	0.0	0.0	0.0
1.4	19.0	823.0	2.6	180.0	900.0	1921.0	947.0	4.0	0.0	2.7	0.1	0.4	1.5	1.2	0.4	39.0	3.0	3.3
0.2	0.9	21.5	0.2	14.7	38.0	104.1	54.5	0.2	0.0	0.0	0.0	0.0	0.1	0.1	0.0	1.1	0.1	0.2
0.4	2.2	35.3	0.1	7.8	32.8	56.0	14.3	0.2	15.4	0.3	0.0	0.0	0.0	0.0	0.0	1.7	0.1	22.7
0.0	0.0	8.7	0.4	3.1	18.7	23.7	121.1	0.0	30.6	2.5	0.0	0.1	0.5	0.0	0.0	0.0	0.0	10.4
0.0	0.0	8.6	0.8	7.1	31.4	41.4	192.9	0.0	14.0	0.0	0.0	0.1	0.1	1.1	0.0	0.0	0.0	11.9
1.9	29.8	20.7	0.2	5.3	35.4	101.2	118.7	0.2	30.5	0.0	0.5	0.0	0.0	0.2	0.0	13.7	0.1	11.3
2.2	2.2	31.8	0.6	11.4	39.2	67.9	110.5	0.2	46.9	0.1	0.0	0.1	0.1	0.3	0.0	4.3	0.0	6.0
0.5	13.7	38.1	0.4	5.0	60.2	31.4	117.9	0.1	11.2	0.1	0.5	0.0	0.0	0.4	0.0	19.0	0.0	8.5
1.7	9.3	15.7	0.6	6.4	31.3	35.7	101.8	0.2	9.6	0.1	1.0	0.1	0.1	0.5	0.0	17.7	0.1	6.4
0.7	2.0	12.8	0.7	4.8	33.5	25.6	109.3	0.2	5.7	0.2	0.2	0.0	0.1	0.7	0.0	13.3	0.0	9.0
0.0	0.0	5.8	0.5	5.8	21.0	22.5	115.3	0.0	37.1	0.0	0.0	0.1	0.1	0.6	0.0	0.0	0.0	6.6
1.0	0.7	0.0	0.6	0.0	0.0	0.0	148.1	0.0	0.0	0.0	0.0	0.1	0.1	1.0	0.0	0.0	0.0	6.5
0.1	0.0	1.1	0.1	45.6	4.0	65.6	8.0	0.0	0.0	0.1	0.0	0.0	0.1	3.0	0.0	0.6	0.0	55.7
0.0	0.0	9.8	1.0	0.0	0.0	167.2	2625.5	0.0	0.0	0.0	0.0	0.0	0.0	0.0	0.0	0.0	0.0	0.0
0.0	0.0	9.8	0.6	0.0	0.0	9.8	209.3	0.0	99.1	7.0	0.0	0.0	0.0	0.4	0.0	0.0	0.0	0.0
0.0	0.0	8.4	0.1	4.1	4.7	36.9	47.1	0.1	0.0	3.7	0.0	0.0	0.0	0.1	0.0	8.6	0.0	12.8
0.0	0.0	6.0	0.1	0.0	7.0	7.0	65.0	0.0	0.0	0.0	0.0	0.0	0.0	0.0	0.0	0.0	0.0	3.9
0.0	0.0	4.0	0.1	0.0	4.0	7.0	63.0	0.0	0.0	0.0	0.0	0.0	0.0	0.0	0.0	0.0	0.0	4.0
0.0	0.0	12.0	0.2	0.0	0.0	130.0	650.0	0.0	45.0	10.0	0.0	0.0	0.1	0.5	0.0	0.0	0.0	0.0
0.0	0.0	4.3	0.2	0.0	3.2	0.0	75.0	0.0	4.7	0.0	0.0	0.0	0.0	0.1	0.0	0.0	0.0	0.0
0.0	0.0	35.0	0.2	0.0	0.0	130.0	350.0	0.0	94.0	17.0	0.0	0.0	0.3	0.7	0.0	0.0	0.0	0.0
0.0	0.0	20.0	0.7	0.0	0.0	100.0	310.0	0.0	87.0	16.0	0.0	0.0	0.2	0.7	0.0	0.0	0.0	0.0
0.0	0.0	25.0	0.2	0.0	0.0	130.0	310.0	0.0	46.0	7.0	0.0	0.0	0.0	0.5	0.0	0.0	0.0	0.0
0.0	0.0	2.9	0.1	3.3	5.9	72.2	177.9	0.0	15.3	2.3	0.2	0.0	0.0	0.2	0.0	2.3	0.0	10.0
0.0	0.0	2.9	0.1	3.3	5.9	72.2	3.0	0.0	15.3	2.3	0.2	0.0	0.0	0.2	0.0	2.3	0.0	10.0
0.0	0.0	15.0	0.9	0.0	0.0	120.0	234.0	0.0	10.2	27.0	0.0	0.0	0.0	0.0	0.0	0.0	0.0	0.0
0.1	0.0	0.9	0.1	0.4	2.3	2.0	7.9	0.0	0.0	0.0	0.0	0.0	0.0	0.1	0.0	1.7	0.0	0.1
2.8	2.0	6.3	0.6	10.9	25.7	60.7	83.2	0.2	4.3	0.0	0.0	0.0	0.0	0.5	0.0	2.6	0.0	4.3
1.1	0.0	2.6	0.3	1.3	11.4	69.1	20.7	0.0	0.0	0.0	0.4	0.0	0.0	0.2	0.0	7.5	0.0	2.9
1.8	17.5	13.7	0.4	12.7	31.7	42.2	82.3	0.2	47.8	0.1	0.0	0.0	0.0	0.2	0.0	7.0	0.0	3.0
0.6	5.9	1.5	0.1	0.6	5.1	5.6	17.6	0.0	8.4	0.0	0.0	0.0	0.0	0.2	0.0	2.0	0.0	0.2
0.0	0.0	6.0	0.3	0.0	16.0	36.0	39.0	0.0	0.0	0.0	0.0	0.0	0.0	0.2	0.0	0.0	0.0	0.2
0.4	0.0	0.0	1.1	0.0	0.0	0.0	138.3	0.0	0.0	0.0	0.0	0.0	0.0	0.0	0.0	0.0	0.0	1.2
0.3	0.0	3.2	0.2	1.5	7.6	13.9	0.8	0.0	0.0	0.0	0.2	0.0	0.0	0.2	0.0	3.2	0.0	0.4
0.4	2.1	7.5	0.3	5.8	15.2	34.1	46.9	0.1	3.0	0.0	0.0	0.0	0.0	0.3	0.0	1.3	0.0	0.6
1.0	0.0	3.5	0.4	4.3	15.1	18.9	44.1	0.1	0.0	0.0	0.4	0.0	0.0	0.4	0.0	5.9	0.0	0.6
2.3	11.2	6.1	0.4	8.8	16.0	35.4	54.6	0.2	23.5	0.0	0.0	0.0	0.0	0.2	0.0	5.3	0.0	0.9
0.4	0.0	1.9	0.3	2.8	8.4	12.3	37.7	0.1	0.0	0.0	0.0	0.0	0.0	0.3	0.0	7.0	0.0	0.4
0.6	3.2	7.8	0.7	7.6	21.3	56.0	65.0	0.2	4.8	0.0	0.0	0.0	0.1	0.6	0.0	2.0	0.0	0.8
1.1	0.0	2.3	0.4	5.3	7.5	14.0	48.9	0.1	0.0	0.0	0.0	0.0	0.0	0.2	0.0	5.9	0.0	1.7
0.0	0.0	15.0	0.8	0.0	0.0	141.0	182.0	0.0	0.0	0.0	0.0	0.0	0.0	0.3	0.0	0.0	0.0	1.3
5.4	0.0	120.0	0.1	0.0	0.0	50.0	79.0	0.0	0.0	0.0	0.0	0.1	0.1	0.6	0.0	0.0	0.0	1.0
2.2	0.0	0.0	0.7	0.0	0.0	0.0	77.0	0.0	0.0	0.0	0.0	0.0	0.1	0.0	0.0	0.0	0.0	3.9
6.4	0.0	4.0	0.4	12.0	24.5	88.9	140.8	0.4	0.0	0.0	0.2	0.0	0.1	0.1	0.1	2.3	0.0	6.0
0.2	0.0	10.2	0.5	4.3	9.9	33.1	56.0	0.1	0.6	0.0	0.2	0.0	0.0	0.3	0.0	4.3	0.0	2.6
0.1	0.2	1.0	0.1	0.6	2.8	3.3	21.9	0.0	0.1	0.0	0.0	0.0	0.0	0.1	0.0	4.4	0.0	0.6

A-16 ■ Appendices

Code	Food Name	Unit/Amt	Wt (g)	Energy (Kcal)	Prot (g)	Carb (g)	Fiber (g)	Fat (g)	Mono (g)	Poly (g)
918822	Cookie, Fudge Brownie/LittleDeb	1 brownie	57	236.0	2.7	38.6	0.0	8.0	4.5	1.5
18172	Cookie, Ginger Snaps	1 cookie	7	29.1	0.4	5.4	0.2	0.7	0.4	0.1
18609	Cookie, Golden Vanilla Wafers/Keebler	1 large (3.5" - 4" dia)	32	152.0	1.7	22.3	0.0	6.2	0.0	0.0
18174	Cookie, Graham Crackers, chocolate coated	1 cracker (2.5" square)	14	67.8	0.8	9.3	0.4	3.2	1.1	0.1
18173	Cookie, Graham Crackers, Plain/Honey/Cinnamon	1 large or 4 small rectangular piec	14	59.2	1.0	10.8	0.4	1.4	0.6	0.5
918812	Cookie, Iced Brownies w/nuts	1 ladyfinger	11	44.6	0.5	7.0	0.0	1.9	0.8	0.4
18423	Cookie, Ladyfinger/Egg Jumbo/Breakfast Treat/Anisette Sponge w/o lemon	1 ladyfinger	11	40.2	1.2	6.6	0.1	1.0	0.5	0.2
918863	Cookie, Lemon Nut/PepFarm	2 large	64	336.0	3.8	40.3	0.0	17.9	0.0	0.0
18612	Cookie, Little Debbie Nutty Bars, Chocolate Covered Wafers w/Peanut Butter	1 bar	57	312.4	4.6	31.5	0.0	18.7	0.0	0.0
18176	Cookie, Marshmallow, chocolate coated/Marshmallow Pie	1 marshmallow pie (3" dia x 0.75")	39	164.2	1.6	26.4	0.8	6.6	3.6	0.8
18177	Cookie, Molasses	1 large (3.5"-4" dia/ Archway Brand)	32	137.6	1.8	23.6	0.3	4.1	2.3	0.6
18178	Cookie, Oatmeal, commercially prep	1 cookie	18	81.0	1.1	12.4	0.5	3.3	1.8	0.5
18200	Cookie, Oatmeal, commercially prep, special dietary	1 small cookie (1.75" dia x 0.75")	13	58.4	0.6	9.1	0.4	2.3	1.0	0.9
918181	Cookie, Oatmeal, dry mix, prep	1 large cookie:3.5-4"dia Archway,Grandma	25	115.5	1.9	16.3	1.0	4.9	0.0	0.0
18377	Cookie, Oatmeal, homemade w/o raisins	1 medium cookie (1.6" dia)	7	31.3	0.5	4.6	0.0	1.3	0.5	0.4
918183	Cookie, Oatmeal, refrig dough, bkd	1 cookie (2.65" dia)	15	70.7	0.9	9.9	0.4	3.2	0.0	0.0
918809	Cookie, Oreos	3 cookies	28	100.0	2.0	16.0	0.6	4.0	3.0	0.0
918821	Cookie, Peanut Butter Brownie	1 brownie	25	120.0	3.0	16.0	0.2	5.0	3.0	1.0
18185	Cookie, Peanut Butter, commercially prep	1 cookie	15	71.6	1.4	8.8	0.3	3.5	1.9	0.8
18189	Cookie, Peanut Butter, homemade	1 cookie (3" dia)	20	95.0	1.8	11.8	0.0	4.8	2.2	1.4
918188	Cookie, Peanut Butter, refrig dough, bkd	1 cookie	12	60.4	1.1	6.9	0.1	3.3	0.0	0.0
18191	Cookie, Raisin, soft	1 cookie	15	60.2	0.6	10.2	0.2	2.0	1.1	0.3
18166	Cookie, Sandwich, Chocolate, cream filled	1.0 oz	10	47.2	0.5	7.0	0.3	2.1	0.9	0.7
18199	Cookie, Sandwich, Chocolate, cream filled, special dietary	1 cookie	10	46.1	0.5	6.8	0.4	2.2	0.9	0.8
18190	Cookie, Sandwich, Peanut Butter, regular	1 cookie	14	66.9	1.2	9.2	0.3	3.0	1.6	0.5
18201	Cookie, Sandwich, Peanut Butter, special dietary	1 cookie	10	53.5	1.0	5.1	0.0	3.4	1.5	1.2
18210	Cookie, Sandwich, Vanilla, cream filled	1 oval cookie (3-⅛ x 1.25 x ⅜")	15	72.5	0.7	10.8	0.2	3.0	1.3	1.1
918194	Cookie, Shortbread, homemade w/butter	1 medium cookie (1.5" dia)	11	60.1	0.7	6.2	0.0	3.7	0.0	0.0
18193	Cookie, Shortbread, Pecan, commercially prep	1 cookie (2" dia)	14	75.9	0.7	8.2	0.3	4.6	2.6	0.6
18192	Cookie, Shortbread, Plain, commercially prep	1 cookie (1.6" square)	8	40.2	0.5	5.2	0.1	1.9	1.1	0.3
18209	Cookie, Sugar Wafer, cream filled	1 large wafer (3.5 x 1 x 0.5")	9	46.0	0.4	6.3	0.1	2.2	0.9	0.8
18202	Cookie, Sugar Wafer, cream filled, special dietary	1 wafer	4	20.1	0.1	2.6	0.0	1.0	0.4	0.4
918207	Cookie, Sugar, homemade w/butter	1 cookie (3" diam)	14	65.9	0.8	8.4	0.0	3.3	0.0	0.0
18206	Cookie, Sugar, refrig dough, baked	1 cookie	12	58.1	0.6	7.9	0.1	2.8	1.6	0.3
18204	Cookie, Sugar/Vanilla, commercially prep	1 cookie	15	71.7	0.8	10.2	0.1	3.2	1.8	0.4
18213	Cookie, Vanilla Wafer	1 wafer	6	28.4	0.3	4.3	0.1	1.2	0.7	0.1
18212	Cookie, Vanilla Wafer, lower fat	1 large wafer	6	26.5	0.3	4.4	0.1	0.9	0.4	0.2
20018	Corn flour, degermed, unenriched, yellow	1 tbsp	7.9	29.6	0.4	6.5	0.2	0.1	0.0	0.1
924077	Corn Fritter	1 Fritter	35	132.0	2.7	13.9	1.0	7.5	0.0	0.0
13348	Corned Beef Brisket, canned	1 oz	28.35	70.9	7.7	0.0	0.0	4.2	1.7	0.2
20027	Cornstarch	1 tbsp	8	30.5	0.0	7.3	0.1	0.0	0.0	0.0
18214	Cracker, Cheese	1 cracker, (1" square)	1	5.0	0.1	0.6	0.0	0.3	0.1	0.0
18216	Cracker, Crispbread, Rye	1 crispbread, wafer or cracker	10	36.6	0.8	8.2	1.7	0.1	0.0	0.1
919977	Cracker, Goldfish/PepFarm	12 crackers	6	30.0	0.0	4.0	0.5	2.0	0.0	0.0
18218	Cracker, Matzo, Egg	1 matzo	28.35	110.8	3.5	22.3	0.8	0.6	0.2	0.1
18219	Cracker, Matzo, Whole Wheat	1 matzo	28.35	99.5	3.7	22.4	3.3	0.4	0.1	0.2
18220	Cracker, Melba Toast Rounds, Plain	1 melba round	3	11.7	0.4	2.3	0.2	0.1	0.0	0.0
18221	Cracker, Melba Toast, Rye or Pumpernickel	1 toast	5	19.5	0.6	3.9	0.4	0.2	0.0	0.1
18223	Cracker, Milk	1 cracker	11	50.1	0.8	7.7	0.2	1.7	1.0	0.2
18620	Cracker, Original Premium Saltine Crackers/Nabisco	1 serving	14	58.8	1.5	10.0	0.4	1.4	0.8	0.2
18621	Cracker, Ritz/Nabisco	1 serving	16	78.7	1.2	10.3	0.3	3.7	2.9	0.3
18224	Cracker, Rusk Toast	1 rusk	10	40.7	1.4	7.2	0.0	0.7	0.3	0.2
918808	Cracker, Rye Krisps	¼ large square	14	40.0	1.5	13.0	2.5	0.2	0.0	0.0
18425	Cracker, Saltine/Oyster/Soda/Soup, low salt	1 oyster cracker	1	4.3	0.1	0.7	0.0	0.1	0.1	0.0
18426	Cracker, Saltines/Oyster/Soda/Soup, unsalted	1 saltine	3	13.0	0.3	2.1	0.1	0.4	0.2	0.1
18230	Cracker, Sandwich, Cheese filled	1 sandwich cracker	7	33.4	0.7	4.3	0.1	1.5	0.8	0.2
18215	Cracker, Sandwich, Cheese w/peanut butter filling	1 sandwich cracker	7	33.7	0.9	4.0	0.2	1.6	0.8	0.3
18231	Cracker, Sandwich, Peanut Butter filled	1 sandwich cracker	7	34.2	0.8	4.1	0.2	1.7	0.9	0.3
18234	Cracker, Sandwich, Wheat w/peanut butter filling	1 sandwich cracker	7	34.7	0.9	3.8	0.3	1.9	0.8	0.6
18622	Cracker, Snackwell Zesty Cheese, Reduced Fat/Nabisco	1 serving	30	124.1	2.9	23.1	0.7	2.2	0.8	0.4
18229	Cracker, Standard Snack, regular	1 rectangular cracker	4	20.1	0.3	2.4	0.1	1.0	0.4	0.4
18624	Cracker, Wheat Thins, baked/Nabisco	1 serving	29	136.2	2.4	20.0	1.7	5.2	4.1	0.4
18235	Cracker, Whole Wheat	1 cracker	4	17.7	0.4	2.7	0.4	0.7	0.2	0.3

Sat (g)	Chol (mg)	Cal (mg)	Iron (mg)	Magn (mg)	Phos (mg)	Pota (mg)	Sodi (mg)	Zinc (mg)	Vit A (RE)	Vit C (mg)	Vit E (mg)	Thia (mg)	Ribo (mg)	Niac (mg)	Vit B-6 (mg)	Fol (µg)	Vit B-12 (µg)	Wat (g)
2.0	1.0	0.0	1.7	0.0	0.0	0.0	121.0	0.0	0.0	0.0	0.0	0.1	0.1	0.1	0.0	0.0	0.0	7.2
0.2	0.0	5.4	0.4	3.4	5.8	24.2	45.8	0.0	0.0	0.0	0.1	0.0	0.0	0.2	0.0	5.0	0.0	0.4
1.1	0.0	0.0	0.0	0.0	0.0	0.0	123.5	0.0	0.0	0.0	0.0	0.0	0.0	0.0	0.0	0.0	0.0	1.3
1.9	0.0	8.1	0.5	8.1	18.8	29.3	40.7	0.1	0.1	0.0	0.2	0.0	0.0	0.3	0.0	2.4	0.0	0.4
0.2	0.0	3.4	0.5	4.2	14.6	18.9	84.7	0.1	0.0	0.0	0.3	0.0	0.0	0.6	0.0	8.4	0.0	0.6
0.7	0.0	5.5	0.3	4.4	11.6	22.0	25.9	0.2	6.5	0.0	0.0	0.0	0.0	0.2	0.0	1.1	0.0	1.4
0.4	40.2	5.2	0.4	1.3	19.0	12.4	16.2	0.1	18.4	0.0	0.1	0.0	0.0	0.2	0.0	8.5	0.1	2.1
0.0	0.0	22.0	0.4	0.0	0.0	97.0	189.0	0.0	0.0	0.0	0.0	0.0	0.1	0.3	0.0	0.0	0.0	1.5
3.6	0.0	0.0	0.0	0.0	0.0	0.0	127.1	0.0	0.0	1.1	0.0	0.0	0.0	0.0	0.0	0.0	0.0	1.7
1.8	0.0	17.9	1.0	14.0	37.8	71.0	65.5	0.3	0.4	0.0	0.8	0.0	0.1	0.3	0.0	7.4	0.1	3.9
1.0	0.0	23.7	2.1	16.6	30.4	110.7	146.9	0.1	0.0	0.0	0.5	0.1	0.1	1.0	0.0	23.7	0.0	1.9
0.8	0.0	6.7	0.5	5.9	24.8	25.6	68.9	0.1	0.4	0.1	0.5	0.0	0.0	0.4	0.0	8.1	0.0	1.0
0.4	0.0	7.0	0.5	2.2	15.9	22.8	1.2	0.1	0.1	0.0	0.4	0.1	0.0	0.4	0.0	6.8	0.0	0.8
0.7	2.7	7.3	0.6	12.0	43.8	47.3	117.5	0.2	5.3	0.1	0.0	0.1	0.0	0.3	0.0	2.8	0.0	1.5
0.3	2.5	7.4	0.2	3.0	11.7	12.7	41.9	0.1	12.8	0.0	0.0	0.0	0.0	0.1	0.0	2.3	0.0	0.4
0.4	1.8	5.3	0.4	4.8	17.4	24.5	49.1	0.1	2.0	0.0	0.0	0.0	0.0	0.3	0.0	1.1	0.0	0.9
0.0	0.0	0.0	0.0	0.0	0.0	50.0	150.0	0.0	0.0	0.0	0.0	0.0	0.0	0.0	0.0	0.0	0.0	0.0
1.0	0.0	6.0	0.9	15.0	30.0	55.0	100.0	0.2	10.0	0.0	0.0	0.0	0.0	1.1	0.0	2.0	0.0	0.8
0.7	0.2	5.3	0.4	6.8	12.9	25.1	62.3	0.1	0.5	0.0	0.5	0.0	0.0	0.6	0.0	9.3	0.0	0.9
0.9	6.2	7.8	0.4	7.8	23.2	46.2	103.6	0.2	31.2	0.0	0.0	0.0	0.0	0.7	0.0	11.0	0.0	1.2
0.6	1.7	13.3	0.2	4.9	31.7	40.6	52.3	0.1	1.7	0.0	0.0	0.0	0.0	0.5	0.0	1.1	0.0	0.5
0.5	0.3	6.9	0.3	3.2	12.5	21.0	50.7	0.0	0.2	0.1	0.3	0.0	0.0	0.3	0.0	6.6	0.0	2.0
0.4	0.0	2.6	0.4	4.5	9.8	17.5	60.4	0.1	0.0	0.0	0.3	0.0	0.0	0.2	0.0	4.3	0.0	0.2
0.4	0.0	9.8	0.5	2.6	20.0	29.5	24.3	0.1	0.0	0.0	0.4	0.1	0.0	0.4	0.0	6.2	0.0	0.4
0.7	0.0	7.4	0.4	6.9	26.3	26.9	51.5	0.1	0.1	0.0	0.5	0.0	0.0	0.5	0.0	6.2	0.0	0.4
0.5	0.0	4.3	0.3	5.1	15.4	29.4	41.2	0.1	0.0	0.0	0.6	0.0	0.0	0.5	0.0	5.4	0.0	0.4
0.4	0.0	4.1	0.3	2.1	11.3	13.7	52.4	0.1	0.0	0.0	0.5	0.0	0.0	0.4	0.0	8.9	0.0	0.3
0.2	1.0	2.0	0.3	1.4	7.6	7.6	51.2	0.0	33.6	0.0	0.0	0.0	0.0	0.3	0.0	1.2	0.0	0.3
1.1	4.6	4.2	0.3	2.5	11.9	10.2	39.3	0.1	0.1	0.0	0.0	0.0	0.0	0.3	0.0	8.8	0.0	0.5
0.5	1.6	2.8	0.2	1.4	8.6	8.0	36.4	0.0	1.0	0.0	0.3	0.0	0.0	0.3	0.0	4.7	0.0	0.3
0.3	0.0	1.6	0.2	1.0	5.0	5.3	13.2	0.0	0.0	0.0	0.4	0.0	0.0	0.2	0.0	3.9	0.0	0.1
0.2	0.0	2.1	0.1	0.2	1.4	2.4	0.4	0.0	0.0	0.0	0.0	0.0	0.0	0.1	0.0	1.7	0.0	0.2
0.2	0.9	9.9	0.3	1.7	12.6	10.2	64.3	0.1	31.2	0.0	0.0	0.0	0.0	0.3	0.0	1.7	0.0	1.2
0.7	3.8	10.8	0.2	1.0	22.4	19.6	56.2	0.0	1.3	0.0	0.4	0.0	0.0	0.3	0.0	6.4	0.0	0.6
0.8	7.7	3.2	0.3	1.8	12.0	9.5	53.6	0.1	4.1	0.0	0.4	0.0	0.0	0.4	0.0	6.8	0.0	0.7
0.3	0.0	1.5	0.1	0.7	3.8	6.4	18.4	0.0	0.0	0.0	0.0	0.0	0.0	0.2	0.0	2.6	0.0	0.3
0.2	3.1	2.9	0.1	0.8	6.2	5.8	18.7	0.0	0.5	0.0	0.1	0.0	0.0	0.2	0.0	3.0	0.0	0.3
0.0	0.0	0.2	0.1	1.4	4.7	7.1	0.1	0.0	0.4	0.0	0.0	0.0	0.0	0.2	0.0	3.8	0.0	0.8
2.0	0.0	22.0	0.6	0.0	54.0	47.0	167.0	0.0	28.0	1.0	0.0	0.1	0.1	0.6	0.0	0.0	0.0	10.2
1.8	24.4	3.4	0.6	4.0	31.5	38.6	285.2	1.0	0.0	0.0	0.0	0.0	0.0	0.7	0.0	2.6	0.5	16.4
0.0	0.0	0.2	0.0	0.2	1.0	0.2	0.7	0.0	0.0	0.0	0.0	0.0	0.0	0.0	0.0	0.0	0.0	0.7
0.1	0.1	1.5	0.0	0.4	2.2	1.5	10.0	0.0	0.0	0.0	0.0	0.0	0.0	0.0	0.0	0.8	0.0	0.6
0.0	0.0	3.1	0.2	7.8	26.9	31.9	26.4	0.2	0.0	0.0	0.1	0.0	0.0	0.1	0.0	4.7	0.0	0.6
0.0	0.0	4.0	0.2	0.0	6.0	12.0	50.0	0.0	0.2	0.0	0.0	0.0	0.0	0.2	0.0	0.0	0.0	0.0
0.2	23.5	11.3	0.8	6.8	42.0	42.5	6.0	0.2	3.7	0.0	0.0	0.2	0.2	1.4	0.0	33.2	0.1	1.8
0.1	0.0	6.5	1.3	38.0	86.5	89.6	0.6	0.7	0.0	0.0	0.4	0.1	0.1	1.5	0.0	13.6	0.0	1.4
0.0	0.0	2.8	0.1	1.8	5.9	6.1	24.9	0.1	0.0	0.0	0.0	0.0	0.0	0.1	0.0	3.7	0.0	0.2
0.0	0.0	3.9	0.2	2.0	9.2	9.7	45.0	0.1	0.0	0.0	0.0	0.0	0.0	0.2	0.0	4.3	0.0	0.2
0.3	1.2	18.9	0.4	2.4	33.3	12.5	65.1	0.1	0.8	0.0	0.3	0.1	0.0	0.5	0.0	9.0	0.0	0.5
0.3	0.0	27.0	0.7	2.9	13.9	13.9	177.8	0.0	0.0	0.0	0.0	0.0	0.1	0.6	0.0	11.8	0.0	0.5
0.6	0.0	23.5	0.6	3.2	48.0	14.9	124.2	0.2	0.0	0.0	0.0	0.0	0.0	0.6	0.0	9.6	0.0	0.5
0.1	7.8	2.7	0.3	3.6	15.3	24.5	25.3	0.1	1.2	0.0	0.0	0.0	0.0	0.5	0.0	8.7	0.0	0.6
0.0	0.0	12.0	0.4	34.0	93.0	63.0	112.0	0.8	0.0	0.0	0.0	0.1	0.3	0.1	0.0	7.0	0.0	0.0
0.0	0.0	1.2	0.1	0.3	1.1	7.2	6.4	0.0	0.0	0.0	0.0	0.0	0.0	0.1	0.0	1.2	0.0	0.0
0.1	0.0	3.6	0.2	0.8	3.2	3.8	23.0	0.0	0.0	0.0	0.0	0.0	0.0	0.2	0.0	3.7	0.0	0.1
0.4	0.1	18.0	0.2	2.5	28.4	30.0	98.1	0.0	1.3	0.0	0.0	0.0	0.0	0.3	0.0	5.9	0.0	0.3
0.4	0.4	5.5	0.2	4.1	22.7	17.2	69.4	0.1	2.4	0.0	0.3	0.0	0.0	0.5	0.1	6.2	0.0	0.3
0.4	0.0	6.8	0.2	3.7	16.9	15.6	65.9	0.1	0.0	0.0	0.3	0.0	0.0	0.4	0.0	5.9	0.0	0.2
0.3	0.0	11.9	0.2	2.7	24.3	20.8	56.5	0.1	0.0	0.0	0.0	0.0	0.0	0.4	0.0	4.9	0.0	0.2
0.5	1.5	40.5	1.0	9.6	98.4	47.7	275.1	0.5	0.0	0.1	0.0	0.1	0.1	1.3	0.1	17.4	0.0	0.8
0.2	0.0	4.8	0.1	1.1	9.1	5.3	33.9	0.2	0.0	0.0	0.2	0.0	0.0	0.2	0.0	3.1	0.0	0.2
0.9	0.0	25.8	1.0	15.1	60.3	56.3	167.6	0.0	0.0	0.0	0.0	0.1	0.1	1.2	0.0	12.2	0.0	0.7
0.1	0.0	2.0	0.1	4.0	11.8	11.9	26.4	0.1	0.0	0.0	0.0	0.0	0.0	0.2	0.0	1.6	0.0	0.1

Code	Food Name	Unit/Amt	Wt (g)	Energy (Kcal)	Prot (g)	Carb (g)	Fiber (g)	Fat (g)	Mono (g)	Poly (g)
18429	Cracker, Whole Wheat, low sodium	1 cracker	4	17.7	0.4	2.7	0.4	0.7	0.2	0.3
18434	Crackers, Cheese, Cheez-its/Goldfish, low sodium	1 gold fish	0.6	3.0	0.1	0.3	0.0	0.2	0.1	0.0
18457	Crackers, Saltines, fat-free, low-sodium	3 saltines	15	59.0	1.6	12.3	0.4	0.2	0.0	0.1
1067	Cream Substitute, Nondairy, liquid w/hydrogenated vege oil and soy protein	1 tbsp	15	20.3	0.2	1.7	0.0	1.5	1.1	0.0
1069	Cream Substitute, Nondairy, powder	1 tsp	2	10.9	0.1	1.1	0.0	0.7	0.0	0.0
1058	Cream, Filled Cream, Nonbutterfat Sour Dressing, cultured	1 cup	235	417.5	7.6	11.0	0.0	38.9	4.6	1.1
1049	Cream, Half and Half	1 tbsp	15	19.6	0.4	0.6	0.0	1.7	0.5	0.1
1053	Cream, Heavy Whipping	1 tbsp	15	51.7	0.3	0.4	0.0	5.6	1.6	0.2
1052	Cream, Light Whipping	1 tbsp	15	43.9	0.3	0.4	0.0	4.6	1.4	0.1
1056	Cream, Sour, cultured	1 tbsp	12	25.7	0.4	0.5	0.0	2.5	0.7	0.1
1074	Cream, Sour, Imitation, cultured	1.0 oz	29	60.5	0.7	1.9	0.0	5.7	0.2	0.0
1055	Cream, Sour, Reduced Fat (Half and Half) cultured	2 tbsp	30	40.4	0.9	1.3	0.0	3.6	1.0	0.1
1054	Cream, Whipped Cream Topping, Pressurized	1 tbsp	3	7.7	0.1	0.4	0.0	0.7	0.2	0.0
18242	Croutons, Plain	1 cup	30	122.1	3.6	22.1	1.5	2.0	0.9	0.4
18243	Croutons, Seasoned	4 cubes	1	4.7	0.1	0.6	0.1	0.2	0.1	0.0
919168	Custard, Egg, baked, homemade	½ cup	141	148.1	7.2	15.1	0.0	6.6	0.0	0.0
19205	Custard, Egg, dry mix prep w/reduced fat (2%) milk	1 cup	266	297.9	11.2	47.1	0.0	7.4	2.4	0.5
919186	Dessert, Apple Crisp, homemade	½ cup	141	229.8	2.5	45.5	2.4	5.1	0.0	0.0
919094	Dessert, Flan (Caramel Custard) homemade	½ cup	153	220.3	6.9	34.9	0.0	6.3	0.0	0.0
902923	Dip, Jalapeno Bean	1 oz	28	33.0	1.5	2.9	0.3	1.1	0.0	0.0
18251	Donut, Cake, Chocolate w/sugar or glaze	1 small doughnut (3" dia)	42	175.1	1.9	24.1	0.9	8.4	4.7	1.0
18249	Donut, Cake, Plain w/chocolate icing	1 small doughnut (2" dia)	28	132.7	1.4	13.4	0.6	8.7	4.9	1.1
18250	Donut, Cake, Plain w/sugar or glaze	1 oz	28.35	120.8	1.5	14.4	0.4	6.5	3.6	0.8
918865	Donut, Cake/Hostess	1 doughnut	28	110.0	1.0	12.0	0.5	7.0	0.0	0.0
918866	Donut, Chocolate/Hostess	1 doughnut	28	129.9	1.0	14.0	0.5	8.0	0.0	0.0
918867	Donut, Cinnamon/Hostess	1 doughnut	28	110.0	1.0	15.0	0.5	6.0	0.0	0.0
18253	Donut, French Cruller, glazed	1 cruller (3" dia)	41	168.9	1.3	24.4	0.5	7.5	4.3	0.9
918868	Donut, Powdered Sugar/Hostess	1 mini donut	28	110.0	1.0	15.0	0.5	5.0	0.0	0.0
18254	Donut, Yeast Leavened, cream filled	1 doughnut (3.5 x 2.5" oval)	85	306.9	5.4	25.5	0.7	20.8	10.3	2.6
18256	Donut, Yeast Leavened, jelly	1 doughnut (3.5 x 2.5" oval)	85	289.0	5.0	33.2	0.7	15.9	8.7	2.0
18255	Donut/Honey Bun, Yeast Leavened, glazed	1 extra large (~ 5" dia)	122	491.7	7.8	54.0	1.5	27.8	15.7	3.5
5140	Duck, Domestic, Meat & Skin, roasted	½ duck	382	1287.3	72.5	0.0	0.0	108.3	49.3	13.9
5142	Duck, Domestic, Meat, no skin, roasted	½ duck	221	444.2	51.9	0.0	0.0	24.8	8.2	3.2
924066	Egg Foo Young/LaChoy	2 patties	120	159.6	8.0	19.0	1.0	7.0	0.8	4.0
924181	Egg Souffle w/cheese	1 cup	95	207.1	9.4	5.9	0.0	16.2	0.0	0.0
924182	Egg Souffle w/spinach, frozen/Stouffer	4.0 oz	113	141.3	6.7	9.4	0.0	8.6	0.0	0.0
901910	Egg Substitute, Country Morning	½ cup	121	173.0	14.6	1.3	0.0	12.1	0.0	0.0
1142	Egg Substitute, frozen	¼ cup	60	95.9	6.8	1.9	0.0	6.7	1.5	3.7
1143	Egg Substitute, liquid	1 tbsp	15.7	13.2	1.9	0.1	0.0	0.5	0.1	0.3
901912	Egg Substitute, Scramblend	½ cup	121	142.8	12.1	3.0	0.0	9.1	0.0	0.0
924272	Egg&Cheese Bagel, frozen/Swanson	3.6 oz	102	256.0	12.7	29.0	0.0	9.9	0.0	0.0
924323	Egg, Omelet w/bacon&onion	6.5 oz	186	364.6	17.4	12.7	0.1	27.1	0.0	0.0
924322	Egg, Omelet w/cheese	4.0 oz	113	313.0	15.9	1.3	0.0	27.1	0.0	0.0
924012	Egg, Quiche Lorraine	1 slice	176	600.2	13.0	29.0	1.0	48.0	17.8	4.1
1128	Egg, Whole, fried	1 large	46	91.5	6.2	0.6	0.0	6.9	2.7	1.3
1129	Egg, Whole, hard-cooked	1 large egg	50	77.5	6.3	0.6	0.0	5.3	2.0	0.7
1130	Egg, Whole, omelet	1 tbsp	15.2	23.1	1.6	0.2	0.0	1.7	0.7	0.3
1131	Egg, Whole, poached	large egg	50	74.5	6.2	0.6	0.0	5.0	1.9	0.7
1123	Egg, Whole, raw	1 large	50	74.5	6.2	0.6	0.0	5.0	1.9	0.7
1132	Egg, Whole, scrambled	1 large egg	61	101.3	6.8	1.3	0.0	7.4	2.9	1.3
1125	Egg, Yolk, raw, fresh	1 large egg yolk	16.6	59.4	2.8	0.3	0.0	5.1	1.9	0.7
18260	English Muffin, Mixed Grain/Granola	1 muffin	66	155.1	6.0	30.6	1.8	1.2	0.5	0.4
18258	English Muffin, Plain/Sourdough, enriched	1 muffin	57	134.0	4.4	26.2	1.5	1.0	0.2	0.5
18262	English Muffin, Raisin-Cinn/Apple Cinnamon	1 muffin	57	138.5	4.3	27.8	1.7	1.5	0.3	0.8
18264	English Muffin, Wheat	1 muffin	57	127.1	5.0	25.5	2.6	1.1	0.2	0.5
18266	English Muffin, Whole Wheat	1 muffin	66	134.0	5.8	26.7	4.4	1.4	5.1	0.7
921897	Fast Food, Apple Pie/MCD	1 pie	83	259.8	2.2	30.0	0.5	14.8	9.1	0.9
921915	Fast Food, Bean Burrito/TB	1 burrito	206	447.0	15.0	63.0	9.6	14.0	8.0	2.0
921916	Fast Food, Beef Burrito/TB	1 burrito	206	492.3	25.0	48.0	2.2	21.0	11.0	2.0
921805	Fast Food, Biscuit/MCD	1 biscuit	75	260.3	4.6	31.9	0.5	12.7	8.6	0.6
921919	Fast Food, Burrito Supreme/TB	1 burrito	255	502.4	20.0	55.0	5.8	22.0	11.0	2.0
21069	Fast Food, Burrito w/apples or cherries	1 small burrito	74	230.9	2.5	35.0	0.0	9.5	3.4	1.1
21060	Fast Food, Burrito w/beans	2 burritos	217	447.0	14.1	71.4	0.0	13.5	4.7	1.2
21061	Fast Food, Burrito w/beans & cheese	2 burritos	186	377.6	15.1	55.0	0.0	11.7	2.5	1.8
21063	Fast Food, Burrito w/beans & meat	2 burritos	231	508.2	22.5	66.0	0.0	17.8	7.0	1.2
21064	Fast Food, Burrito w/beans, cheese & beef	2 burritos	203	330.9	14.6	39.7	0.0	13.3	4.5	1.0
21066	Fast Food, Burrito w/beef	2 burritos	220	523.6	26.6	58.5	0.0	20.8	7.4	0.9
21068	Fast Food, Burrito w/beef, cheese & chili peppers	2 burritos	304	632.3	40.9	63.7	0.0	24.8	9.9	2.2
921813	Fast Food, Chicken Center Breast, extra crispy/KFC	1 piece	135	341.6	33.0	11.7	0.5	19.7	12.5	2.1

Sat (g)	Chol (mg)	Cal (mg)	Iron (mg)	Magn (mg)	Phos (mg)	Pota (mg)	Sodi (mg)	Zinc (mg)	Vit A (RE)	Vit C (mg)	Vit E (mg)	Thia (mg)	Ribo (mg)	Niac (mg)	Vit B-6 (mg)	Fol (µg)	Vit B-12 (µg)	Wat (g)
0.1	0.0	2.0	0.1	4.0	11.8	11.9	9.9	0.1	0.0	0.0	0.0	0.0	0.0	0.2	0.0	1.6	0.0	0.1
0.1	0.1	0.9	0.0	0.2	1.3	0.6	2.7	0.0	0.2	0.0	0.0	0.0	0.0	0.0	0.0	0.5	0.0	0.0
0.0	0.0	3.3	1.2	3.9	17.0	17.3	95.4	0.1	0.0	0.0	0.0	0.1	0.1	0.9	0.0	18.6	0.0	0.5
0.3	0.0	1.4	0.0	0.0	9.6	28.6	11.9	0.0	1.4	0.0	0.2	0.0	0.0	0.0	0.0	0.0	0.0	11.6
0.7	0.0	0.4	0.0	0.1	8.4	16.2	3.6	0.0	0.4	0.0	0.0	0.0	0.0	0.0	0.0	0.0	0.0	0.0
31.2	12.7	265.8	0.1	23.3	204.7	379.5	113.3	0.9	4.7	2.2	0.3	0.1	0.4	0.2	0.0	27.7	0.8	175.8
1.1	5.5	15.7	0.0	1.5	14.3	19.4	6.1	0.1	16.1	0.1	0.0	0.0	0.0	0.0	0.0	0.4	0.0	12.1
3.5	20.6	9.7	0.0	1.1	9.4	11.3	5.6	0.0	63.2	0.1	0.1	0.0	0.0	0.0	0.0	0.6	0.0	8.7
2.9	16.7	10.4	0.0	1.1	9.2	14.5	5.1	0.0	44.3	0.1	0.1	0.0	0.0	0.0	0.0	0.6	0.0	9.5
1.6	5.3	14.0	0.0	1.3	10.2	17.3	6.4	0.0	23.4	0.1	0.1	0.0	0.0	0.0	0.0	1.3	0.0	8.5
5.2	0.0	0.7	0.1	1.9	12.9	46.5	29.6	0.3	0.0	0.0	0.0	0.0	0.0	0.0	0.0	0.0	0.0	20.6
2.2	11.6	31.3	0.0	3.0	28.4	38.7	12.2	0.2	33.6	0.3	0.1	0.0	0.0	0.0	0.0	3.2	0.1	24.0
0.4	2.3	3.0	0.0	0.3	2.7	4.4	3.9	0.0	6.2	0.0	0.0	0.0	0.0	0.0	0.0	0.1	0.0	1.8
0.5	0.0	22.8	1.2	9.3	34.5	37.2	209.4	0.3	0.0	0.0	0.0	0.2	0.1	1.6	0.0	39.6	0.0	1.7
0.1	0.1	1.0	0.0	0.4	1.4	1.8	12.4	0.0	0.1	0.0	0.0	0.0	0.0	0.0	0.0	0.9	0.0	0.0
0.5	2.1	157.9	0.4	19.7	159.3	215.7	108.6	0.7	84.6	0.7	0.0	0.0	0.3	0.1	0.1	14.1	0.4	111.0
3.8	149.0	393.7	0.7	53.2	351.1	574.6	399.0	1.4	149.0	2.1	0.0	0.1	0.6	0.3	0.2	21.3	1.2	197.6
1.5	2.2	39.5	1.1	9.9	35.3	136.8	256.6	0.2	43.7	3.2	0.0	0.1	0.1	1.1	0.1	7.1	0.0	86.7
0.5	2.1	131.6	0.5	16.8	145.4	185.1	85.7	0.7	87.2	0.8	0.0	0.0	0.3	0.1	0.1	13.8	0.4	103.9
0.0	1.0	7.0	0.4	0.0	23.0	77.0	163.0	0.1	8.4	0.0	0.0	0.0	0.0	1.1	0.0	0.0	0.0	0.0
2.2	23.9	89.5	1.0	14.3	68.0	44.5	142.8	0.2	4.6	0.0	1.1	0.0	0.0	0.2	0.0	16.0	0.0	6.8
2.3	17.1	9.8	0.7	11.2	56.6	54.9	120.1	0.2	3.1	0.1	1.2	0.0	0.0	0.4	0.0	8.1	0.1	4.0
1.7	9.1	17.0	0.3	4.8	33.2	28.9	114.0	0.1	0.9	0.0	0.0	0.1	0.1	0.4	0.0	13.0	0.1	5.6
0.0	7.0	12.0	0.4	0.0	0.0	0.0	135.0	0.0	0.0	0.0	0.0	0.1	0.0	0.5	0.0	0.0	0.0	0.0
0.0	4.0	10.0	0.4	0.0	0.0	0.0	150.0	0.0	0.0	0.0	0.0	0.0	0.0	0.3	0.0	0.0	0.0	0.0
0.0	6.0	10.0	0.3	0.0	0.0	0.0	140.0	0.0	0.0	0.0	0.0	0.0	0.0	0.4	0.0	0.0	0.0	0.0
1.9	4.5	10.7	1.0	4.9	50.4	32.0	141.5	0.1	1.2	0.0	1.0	0.1	0.1	0.9	0.0	14.4	0.0	7.3
0.0	6.0	9.0	0.3	0.0	0.0	0.0	140.0	0.0	0.0	0.0	0.0	0.0	0.0	0.4	0.0	0.0	0.0	0.0
4.6	20.4	21.3	1.6	17.0	64.6	68.0	262.7	0.7	16.2	0.0	2.3	0.3	0.1	1.9	0.1	54.4	0.1	32.5
4.1	22.1	21.3	1.5	17.0	72.3	67.2	249.1	0.6	13.6	0.0	2.1	0.3	0.1	1.8	0.1	52.7	0.2	30.3
7.1	7.3	52.5	2.5	26.8	113.5	131.8	417.2	0.9	4.9	0.1	3.7	0.4	0.3	3.5	0.1	52.5	0.1	31.0
36.9	320.9	42.0	10.3	61.1	595.9	779.3	225.4	7.1	240.7	0.0	2.7	0.7	1.0	18.4	0.7	22.9	1.1	198.0
9.2	196.7	26.5	6.0	44.2	448.6	556.9	143.7	5.7	50.8	0.0	1.5	0.6	1.0	11.3	0.6	22.1	0.9	141.9
2.2	275.0	60.0	1.8	0.0	0.0	270.0	1250.0	0.0	50.0	0.0	0.0	1.2	0.1	0.0	0.0	0.0	0.0	
8.2	184.0	191.0	1.0	0.0	185.0	115.0	346.0	1.2	152.0	0.0	0.0	0.1	0.2	0.2	0.0	0.0	0.0	61.8
0.0	88.0	107.0	1.5	0.0	0.0	249.0	599.0	0.0	316.4	4.0	0.0	0.1	0.3	0.5	0.0	0.0	0.0	85.9
0.0	594.0	52.0	2.1	0.0	197.0	133.0	180.0	0.0	227.6	0.0	0.0	0.1	0.5	0.0	0.0	0.0	0.0	0.0
1.2	1.2	43.7	1.2	9.0	43.0	128.0	119.6	0.6	81.0	0.3	1.3	0.1	0.2	0.1	0.1	9.8	0.2	43.9
0.1	0.2	8.3	0.3	1.4	19.0	51.8	27.8	0.2	33.9	0.0	0.1	0.0	0.0	0.0	0.0	2.3	0.0	13.0
0.0	466.0	77.0	1.7	0.0	190.0	150.0	173.0	0.0	214.2	0.0	0.0	0.1	0.4	0.0	0.0	0.0	0.0	0.0
0.0	0.0	137.0	2.1	0.0	0.0	102.0	621.0	0.0	55.8	0.0	0.0	0.2	0.4	1.6	0.0	0.0	0.0	0.0
0.0	365.0	267.0	2.2	0.0	621.0	160.0	1148.0	0.0	141.8	2.0	0.0	0.2	0.5	1.2	0.0	0.0	0.0	0.0
0.0	328.0	245.0	1.6	0.0	0.0	128.0	398.0	0.0	0.0	0.0	0.0	0.1	0.0	0.0	0.0	0.0	0.0	0.0
23.2	285.0	211.0	1.0	0.0	276.0	283.0	653.0	2.0	328.0	0.0	0.0	0.1	0.3	0.0	0.1	17.0	0.0	0.0
1.9	211.1	25.3	0.7	5.1	89.2	60.7	162.4	0.5	114.1	0.0	0.8	0.0	0.2	0.0	0.1	17.5	0.4	31.5
1.6	212.0	25.0	0.6	5.0	86.0	63.0	62.0	0.5	84.0	0.0	0.5	0.0	0.3	0.0	0.1	22.0	0.6	37.3
0.5	53.2	6.4	0.2	1.4	22.5	15.4	41.0	0.1	28.4	0.0	0.2	0.0	0.1	0.0	0.0	4.4	0.1	11.5
1.5	211.5	24.5	0.7	5.0	88.5	60.0	140.0	0.6	95.0	0.0	0.5	0.0	0.2	0.0	0.1	17.5	0.4	37.5
1.6	212.5	24.5	0.7	5.0	89.0	60.5	63.0	0.6	95.5	0.0	0.5	0.0	0.3	0.0	0.1	23.5	0.5	37.7
2.2	214.7	43.3	0.7	7.3	103.7	84.2	170.8	0.6	119.0	0.1	0.8	0.0	0.3	0.0	0.1	18.3	0.5	44.6
1.6	212.6	22.7	0.6	1.5	81.0	15.6	7.1	0.5	96.9	0.0	0.5	0.0	0.1	0.0	0.1	24.2	0.5	8.1
0.2	0.0	129.4	2.0	27.1	53.5	103.0	274.6	0.9	0.0	0.0	0.2	0.3	0.2	2.4	0.0	52.8	0.0	26.5
0.1	0.0	99.2	1.4	12.0	75.8	74.7	264.5	0.4	0.0	0.0	0.1	0.3	0.2	2.2	0.0	46.2	0.0	24.0
0.2	0.0	83.8	1.4	8.6	39.3	118.6	254.8	0.6	0.0	0.2	0.2	0.2	0.2	2.0	0.0	46.2	0.0	22.0
0.2	0.0	101.5	1.6	21.1	61.0	106.0	217.7	0.6	0.0	0.0	0.3	0.2	0.2	1.9	0.0	31.4	0.0	24.1
8.8	0.0	174.9	1.6	46.9	186.1	138.6	420.4	1.1	0.0	0.0	0.5	0.2	0.1	2.3	0.1	27.7	0.0	30.2
4.8	6.0	11.0	0.7	0.0	6.0	39.0	240.0	0.2	0.0	11.0	0.0	0.1	0.0	0.3	0.0	5.0	0.0	0.0
4.0	9.0	144.0	2.6	0.0	253.0	495.0	1148.0	2.4	156.0	2.4	0.0	0.8	0.5	3.3	1.2	66.0	0.0	0.0
8.0	57.0	113.0	2.4	0.0	247.0	380.0	1311.0	4.4	22.0	2.2	0.0	0.3	0.5	3.7	0.2	30.0	0.0	0.0
3.4	1.0	75.0	1.3	0.0	299.0	108.0	730.0	0.3	0.0	0.0	0.0	0.2	0.1	1.7	0.0	9.0	0.0	0.0
8.0	33.0	163.0	2.5	0.0	261.0	501.0	1181.0	3.5	212.8	10.4	0.0	0.5	0.5	3.6	0.6	46.0	0.0	0.0
4.6	3.7	15.5	1.1	7.4	14.8	104.3	211.6	0.4	37.0	0.7	0.0	0.2	0.2	1.9	0.1	24.4	0.5	26.4
6.9	4.3	112.8	4.5	86.8	97.7	653.2	985.2	1.5	32.6	2.0	0.0	0.6	0.6	4.1	0.3	86.8	1.1	114.0
6.8	27.9	213.9	2.3	80.0	180.4	496.6	1166.2	1.6	238.1	1.7	0.0	0.2	0.7	3.6	0.2	74.4	0.9	100.3
8.3	48.5	106.3	4.9	83.2	140.9	656.0	1335.2	3.8	64.7	1.8	0.0	0.5	0.8	5.4	0.4	115.5	1.7	119.9
7.1	123.8	129.9	3.7	50.8	140.1	410.1	990.6	2.4	150.2	5.1	0.0	0.3	0.7	3.9	0.2	75.1	1.1	131.8
10.5	63.8	83.6	6.1	81.4	173.8	739.2	1491.6	4.7	28.6	1.1	0.0	0.2	0.9	6.4	0.3	129.8	2.0	109.1
10.4	170.2	221.9	7.8	69.9	316.2	665.8	2091.5	7.9	112.5	3.6	0.0	0.6	1.2	8.3	0.4	139.8	2.1	167.8
4.8	114.0	33.0	0.9	0.0	205.0	270.0	790.0	0.7	12.0	0.0	0.0	0.1	0.1	13.1	0.3	8.0	0.5	0.0

Code	Food Name	Unit/Amt	Wt (g)	Energy (Kcal)	Prot (g)	Carb (g)	Fiber (g)	Fat (g)	Mono (g)	Poly (g)
921867	Fast Food, Chicken Center Breast, original recipe/KFC	1 piece	115	282.9	27.5	8.8	0.1	15.3	9.0	2.0
921812	Fast Food, Chicken Drumstick, extra crispy/KFC	1 piece	69	204.2	13.6	6.1	0.5	13.9	8.0	1.7
921866	Fast Food, Chicken Drumstick, original recipe/KFC	1 piece	57	145.9	13.1	4.2	0.1	8.5	5.0	1.3
921946	Fast Food, Chicken McNuggets/MCD	1 serving	113	290.4	19.0	16.5	0.5	16.3	10.4	1.8
921884	Fast Food, Chicken Peg Legs/Long John	5 pieces	125	350.0	22.0	26.0	0.5	28.0	0.0	0.0
921876	Fast Food, Chicken Planks/Long John	4 pieces	166	456.5	27.0	35.0	1.0	23.0	0.0	0.0
921963	Fast Food, Chicken Strips/JB	4 pieces	125	348.8	29.0	28.0	0.0	14.0	5.9	0.7
921800	Fast Food, Chicken Tenders/BK	6 pieces	90	235.8	16.0	14.0	0.0	13.0	5.0	3.0
921815	Fast Food, Chicken Thigh, extra crispy/KFC	1 piece	119	405.8	20.0	14.4	0.5	29.9	18.0	4.2
921869	Fast Food, Chicken Thigh, original recipe/KFC	1 piece	104	294.3	17.9	11.1	0.1	19.7	9.0	3.1
921816	Fast Food, Chicken Wing, extra crispy/KFC	1 piece	65	254.2	12.4	9.3	0.5	18.6	11.0	2.5
921870	Fast Food, Chicken Wing, original recipe/KFC	1 piece	55	178.2	12.2	6.0	0.2	11.7	6.5	1.8
921807	Fast Food, Chicken, Hot Wings/KFC	6 pieces	119	376.0	22.4	17.3	0.5	24.1	14.0	4.1
21042	Fast Food, Chili con Carne	8 fl oz cup	253	255.5	24.6	21.9	0.0	8.3	3.4	0.5
921927	Fast Food, Chili/Wendy	1 serving	255	219.3	21.0	23.0	6.0	7.0	2.0	2.6
21070	Fast Food, Chimichanga w/beef	1 chimichanga	174	424.6	19.6	42.8	0.0	19.7	8.1	1.1
21071	Fast Food, Chimichanga w/beef & cheese	1 chimichanga	183	442.9	20.1	39.3	0.0	23.4	9.4	0.7
921951	Fast Food, Chocolate Chip Cookies/MCD	1 box	56	329.8	4.2	41.9	1.0	15.6	10.2	0.4
21043	Fast Food, Clams (shellfish) breaded, fried	1 tbsp	9.6	37.6	1.1	3.2	0.0	2.2	1.0	0.6
921896	Fast Food, Cookies, McDonaldland	1 box	56	290.1	4.2	47.1	1.0	9.2	6.8	0.5
21128	Fast Food, Corn on the Cob w/butter	1 ear	146	154.8	4.5	31.9	0.0	3.4	1.0	0.6
921044	Fast Food, Crab (shellfish) baked	1 crab	109	160.2	28.5	4.2	0.0	2.3	0.0	0.0
921045	Fast Food, Crab (shellfish) soft shell, fried	1 crab	125	333.8	11.0	31.2	0.0	17.9	0.0	0.0
21046	Fast Food, Crab Cake (shellfish)	1 cake	60	159.6	11.3	5.1	0.2	10.4	4.3	3.1
21015	Fast Food, Danish Pastry, Cheese	1 pastry	91	353.1	5.8	28.7	0.0	24.6	15.6	2.4
21016	Fast Food, Danish Pastry, Cinnamon	1 pastry	88	349.4	4.8	46.9	0.0	16.7	10.6	1.6
21017	Fast Food, Danish Pastry, Fruit	1 pastry	94	334.6	4.8	45.1	0.0	15.9	10.1	1.6
21074	Fast Food, Enchilada w/cheese	1 enchilada	163	319.5	9.6	28.5	0.0	18.8	6.3	0.8
21075	Fast Food, Enchilada w/cheese & beef	1 enchilada	192	322.6	11.9	30.5	0.0	17.6	6.1	1.4
21076	Fast Food, Enchirito w/cheese, beef & beans	1 enchirito	193	343.5	17.9	33.8	0.0	16.1	6.5	0.3
921933	Fast Food, Fish Tenders/BK	1 serving	99	267.3	12.0	18.0	0.0	16.0	7.0	4.0
921879	Fast Food, Fish, 2 pieces/Long John	2 pieces	136	651.4	30.0	53.0	1.0	36.0	0.0	0.0
921986	Fast Food, French Fries, large/Hardee	1 large	113	360.5	4.0	48.0	1.8	17.0	8.0	6.0
921984	Fast Food, French Fries, regular/Hardee	1 regular	71	230.0	3.0	30.0	1.2	11.0	5.0	4.0
921837	Fast Food, French Fries, small/DQ	1 small	71	200.2	2.0	25.0	1.0	10.0	3.0	1.0
21024	Fast Food, French Toast Sticks	5 sticks	141	513.2	8.3	57.9	2.7	29.0	12.6	9.9
21077	Fast Food, Frijoles (beans) w/cheese	8.0 oz	167	225.5	11.4	28.7	0.0	7.8	2.6	0.7
921834	Fast Food, Frozen Dessert, Freeze/DQ	1 serving, 14.0 oz	397	500.2	9.0	89.0	0.0	12.0	0.0	0.0
921835	Fast Food, Frozen Dessert, Mr Misty Freeze/DQ	1 serving, 15.0 oz	411	501.4	9.0	91.0	0.0	12.0	0.0	0.0
921841	Fast Food, Frozen Dessert, Mr Misty Kiss/DQ	1 serving 3.0 oz	89	70.3	0.0	17.0	0.0	0.0	0.0	0.0
921842	Fast Food, Frozen Dessert/DQ	1 serving 4.0 oz	113	179.7	5.0	27.0	0.0	6.0	0.0	0.0
921802	Fast Food, Ham & Cheese Sandwich	1 sandwich	230	471.5	24.0	44.0	0.5	23.0	8.0	4.0
21202	Fast Food, Hamburger, large, one meat patty w/condiments	1 sandwich	171.5	425.3	23.0	36.7	2.1	20.9	9.3	1.6
921895	Fast Food, Hot Cakes w/butter & syrup/MCD	1 serving	176	410.1	8.2	74.4	1.0	9.3	3.1	2.5
21119	Fast Food, Hot Dog w/chili, plain	1 hot dog	114	296.4	13.5	31.3	0.0	13.4	6.6	1.2
21120	Fast Food, Hot Dog w/corn flour coating, Corn Dog	1 hot dog	175	460.3	16.8	55.8	0.0	18.9	9.1	3.5
21118	Fast Food, Hot Dog, plain	1 hot dog	98	242.1	10.4	18.0	0.0	14.5	6.9	1.7
21129	Fast Food, Hush Puppies	5 hush puppies	78	256.6	4.9	34.9	0.0	11.6	7.8	0.4
921850	Fast Food, Ice Cream Cone, dipped, regular/DQ	1 regular	156	340.1	6.0	42.0	0.0	16.0	0.0	0.0
921849	Fast Food, Ice Cream Cone, dipped, small/DQ	1 small	78	190.3	3.0	25.0	0.0	9.0	0.0	0.0
921847	Fast Food, Ice Cream Cone, regular/DQ	1 regular	142	240.0	6.0	38.0	0.0	7.0	2.0	1.0
921846	Fast Food, Ice Cream Cone, small/DQ	1 small	71	139.9	3.0	22.0	0.0	4.0	1.0	1.0
921852	Fast Food, Ice Cream Parfait/DQ	1 serving	284	428.8	8.0	76.0	0.5	8.0	0.0	0.0
921853	Fast Food, Ice Cream Sandwich/DQ	1 sandwich	60	139.8	3.0	24.0	0.5	4.0	0.0	0.0
921859	Fast Food, Ice Cream Sundae, regular/DQ	1 regular	177	309.8	5.0	56.0	0.5	8.0	0.0	0.0
921858	Fast Food, Ice Cream Sundae, small/DQ	1 small	106	189.7	3.0	33.0	0.5	4.0	0.0	0.0
921823	Fast Food, Ice Cream, Banana Split/DQ	1 split	383	540.0	9.0	103.0	1.0	11.0	0.0	0.0
921824	Fast Food, Ice Cream, Buster Bar/DQ	1 bar	140	460.6	10.0	41.0	0.5	29.0	0.0	0.0
921829	Fast Food, Ice Cream, Dilly Bar/DQ	1 bar	85	210.0	3.0	21.0	0.5	13.0	0.0	0.0
921832	Fast Food, Ice Cream, Float/DQ	1 serving	397	408.9	5.0	82.0	0.0	7.0	0.0	0.0
921839	Fast Food, Ice Cream, Malt, regular/DQ	1 regular	418	760.8	14.0	134.0	0.5	18.0	0.0	0.0
921838	Fast Food, Ice Cream, Malt, small/DQ	1 small	291	520.9	10.0	91.0	0.5	13.0	0.0	0.0
21028	Fast Food, Ice Milk Cone, soft, vanilla	1 cone	103	163.8	3.9	24.1	0.1	6.1	1.8	0.4
14346	Fast Food, Milk Beverage, Chocolate Shake/MCD	1 fl oz	20.8	26.4	0.7	4.3	0.2	0.8	0.2	0.0
14428	Fast Food, Milk Beverage, Strawberry Shake	10 fl oz	283	319.8	9.6	53.5	1.1	7.9	0.0	0.0
14347	Fast Food, Shake, Vanilla/MCD	1 fl oz	20.8	23.1	0.7	3.7	0.1	0.6	0.2	0.0
21078	Fast Food, Nachos w/cheese	6-8 nachos	113	345.8	9.1	36.3	0.0	19.0	8.0	2.2
21079	Fast Food, Nachos w/cheese & jalapeno peppers	6-8 nachos	204	607.9	16.8	60.1	0.0	34.1	14.4	4.0
21080	Fast Food, Nachos w/cheese, beans, ground beef & peppers	6-8 nachos	255	568.7	19.8	55.8	0.0	30.7	11.0	5.7

Sat (g)	Chol (mg)	Cal (mg)	Iron (mg)	Magn (mg)	Phos (mg)	Pota (mg)	Sodi (mg)	Zinc (mg)	Vit A (RE)	Vit C (mg)	Vit E (mg)	Thia (mg)	Ribo (mg)	Niac (mg)	Vit B-6 (mg)	Fol (µg)	Vit B-12 (µg)	Wat (g)
3.8	93.0	36.0	1.0	0.0	205.0	267.0	672.0	0.7	12.0	0.0	0.0	0.1	0.2	11.5	0.3	8.0	0.4	0.0
3.4	71.0	13.0	0.7	0.0	100.0	147.0	324.0	1.3	8.0	0.0	0.0	0.1	0.1	3.7	0.2	6.0	0.4	0.0
2.2	67.0	21.0	1.1	0.0	95.0	125.0	275.0	1.3	6.0	1.0	0.0	0.1	0.1	3.2	0.1	4.0	0.4	0.0
4.1	65.0	13.0	1.0	0.0	283.0	302.0	520.0	0.9	0.0	0.0	0.0	0.1	0.1	9.0	0.4	11.0	0.0	0.0
0.0	0.0	0.0	0.0	0.0	0.0	0.0	0.0	0.0	0.0	0.0	0.0	0.0	0.0	0.0	0.0	0.0	0.0	0.0
0.0	0.0	0.0	0.0	0.0	0.0	0.0	0.0	0.0	0.0	0.0	0.0	0.0	0.0	0.0	0.0	0.0	0.0	0.0
6.8	68.0	0.0	0.0	0.0	0.0	0.0	748.0	0.0	0.0	0.0	0.0	0.0	0.0	0.0	0.0	0.0	0.0	0.0
3.0	46.0	18.0	0.7	24.0	236.0	200.0	541.0	0.6	19.0	0.0	0.0	0.1	0.1	7.3	0.3	10.0	0.0	0.0
7.7	129.0	49.0	1.2	0.0	170.0	217.0	688.0	1.7	26.2	0.0	0.0	0.1	0.2	6.5	0.2	9.0	1.0	0.0
5.3	123.0	65.0	1.3	0.0	170.0	220.0	619.0	1.7	20.8	0.0	0.0	0.1	0.3	5.5	0.2	9.0	1.0	0.0
4.4	67.0	18.0	0.6	0.0	77.0	90.0	422.0	0.6	6.0	0.0	0.0	0.0	0.1	3.3	0.1	5.0	0.3	0.0
3.0	64.0	48.0	1.2	0.0	75.0	85.0	372.0	0.6	11.2	0.0	0.0	0.0	0.1	3.7	0.1	4.0	0.3	0.0
5.3	148.0	0.0	0.0	0.0	0.0	0.0	677.0	0.0	0.0	0.0	0.0	0.0	0.0	0.0	0.0	0.0	0.0	0.0
3.4	134.1	68.3	5.2	45.5	197.3	690.7	1006.9	3.6	167.0	1.5	0.0	0.1	1.1	2.5	0.3	45.5	1.1	194.1
2.4	45.0	64.0	4.5	0.0	320.0	497.0	750.0	3.8	237.6	6.0	0.0	0.2	0.2	3.0	0.3	40.0	0.0	0.0
8.5	8.7	62.6	4.5	62.6	123.5	586.4	910.0	5.0	15.7	4.7	0.0	0.5	0.6	5.8	0.3	83.5	1.5	88.2
11.2	51.2	237.9	3.8	60.4	186.7	203.1	957.1	3.4	126.3	2.7	0.0	0.4	0.9	4.7	0.2	91.5	1.3	96.4
5.0	4.0	24.0	2.2	0.0	108.0	170.0	280.0	0.5	0.0	0.0	0.0	0.2	0.2	2.5	0.0	6.0	0.1	0.0
0.6	7.3	1.7	0.3	2.6	19.9	22.2	69.6	0.1	3.1	0.0	0.0	0.0	0.0	0.2	0.0	3.6	0.1	2.8
1.9	10.0	9.0	2.1	0.0	74.0	52.0	300.0	0.3	0.0	0.0	0.0	0.2	0.2	2.5	0.0	6.0	0.0	0.0
1.6	5.8	4.4	0.9	40.9	108.0	359.2	29.2	0.9	96.4	6.9	0.0	0.2	0.1	2.2	0.3	43.8	0.0	105.2
0.8	0.6	415.3	1.4	81.8	336.8	597.3	549.4	7.0	22.9	2.6	0.0	0.3	0.2	4.5	0.5	20.7	15.8	71.6
4.9	7.7	55.0	1.8	25.0	131.3	162.5	1117.5	1.1	3.8	0.8	0.0	0.1	0.1	1.8	0.2	20.0	4.5	62.3
2.2	82.2	202.2	1.1	25.2	226.8	162.0	491.4	2.1	82.2	0.2	0.0	0.1	0.1	1.2	0.1	24.6	4.4	32.0
5.1	20.0	70.1	1.8	15.5	80.1	116.5	319.4	0.6	42.8	2.6	0.0	0.3	0.2	2.5	0.1	54.6	0.2	30.8
3.5	27.3	37.0	1.8	14.1	73.9	95.9	326.5	0.5	5.3	2.6	0.0	0.3	0.2	2.2	0.1	54.6	0.2	18.4
3.3	18.8	21.6	1.4	14.1	68.6	110.0	332.8	0.5	24.4	1.6	0.0	0.3	0.2	1.8	0.1	31.0	0.2	27.3
10.6	44.0	324.4	1.3	50.5	133.7	239.6	784.0	2.5	185.8	1.0	0.0	0.1	0.4	1.9	0.4	65.2	0.7	103.1
9.0	40.3	228.5	3.1	82.6	167.0	574.1	1319.0	2.7	142.1	1.3	0.0	0.1	0.4	2.5	0.3	67.2	1.0	128.4
7.9	50.2	218.1	2.4	71.4	223.9	559.7	1250.6	2.8	133.2	4.6	0.0	0.2	0.7	3.0	0.2	59.8	1.6	121.0
3.0	28.0	0.0	0.0	0.0	0.0	0.0	870.0	0.0	0.0	0.0	0.0	0.0	0.0	0.0	0.0	0.0	0.0	0.0
0.0	27.0	0.0	0.0	0.0	0.0	0.0	1543.0	0.0	0.0	0.0	0.0	0.0	0.0	0.0	0.0	0.0	0.0	0.0
3.0	0.0	19.0	1.0	0.0	86.0	560.0	135.0	0.1	0.0	16.0	0.0	0.1	0.0	0.6	0.0	0.0	0.0	0.0
2.0	0.0	12.0	1.0	0.0	62.0	350.0	85.0	0.1	0.0	10.0	0.0	0.1	0.0	1.0	0.0	0.0	0.0	0.0
4.0	10.0	0.0	0.3	16.0	60.0	450.0	115.0	0.0	0.0	9.0	0.0	0.1	0.0	0.8	0.2	15.0	0.0	0.0
4.7	74.7	77.6	3.0	26.8	122.7	126.9	499.1	0.9	12.7	0.0	4.0	0.2	0.3	3.0	0.3	81.8	0.1	42.2
4.1	36.7	188.7	2.2	85.2	175.4	604.5	881.8	1.7	70.1	1.5	0.0	0.1	0.3	1.5	0.2	111.9	0.7	115.4
0.0	30.0	300.0	1.8	0.0	350.0	0.0	180.0	0.0	80.0	0.0	0.0	0.2	0.5	0.0	0.0	0.0	0.9	0.0
0.0	30.0	300.0	1.4	0.0	200.0	0.0	140.0	0.0	80.0	0.0	0.0	0.1	0.5	0.0	0.0	0.0	0.6	0.0
0.0	0.0	0.0	0.0	0.0	0.0	0.0	10.0	0.0	0.0	0.0	0.0	0.0	0.0	0.0	0.0	0.0	0.0	0.0
0.0	20.0	150.0	0.0	0.0	100.0	0.0	20.0	0.0	20.0	0.0	0.0	0.1	0.2	0.0	0.0	0.0	0.6	0.0
10.0	70.0	195.0	3.2	42.0	384.0	419.0	1534.0	2.4	170.0	7.0	0.0	0.9	0.4	6.0	0.3	25.0	0.6	0.0
7.9	70.3	133.8	4.1	34.3	212.7	394.5	728.9	4.8	0.0	2.6	0.0	0.3	0.3	6.5	0.2	61.7	2.6	88.8
3.7	21.0	114.0	2.1	0.0	501.0	187.0	640.0	0.7	34.6	0.0	0.0	0.3	0.3	2.8	0.1	9.0	0.2	0.0
4.9	51.3	19.4	3.3	10.3	191.5	166.4	479.9	0.8	5.7	2.7	0.0	0.2	0.4	3.7	0.0	73.0	0.3	54.5
5.2	78.8	101.5	6.2	17.5	166.3	262.5	973.0	1.3	36.8	0.0	0.0	0.3	0.7	4.2	0.1	103.3	0.4	81.7
5.1	44.1	23.5	2.3	12.7	97.0	143.1	670.3	2.0	0.0	0.1	0.0	0.2	0.3	3.6	0.0	48.0	0.5	52.9
2.7	134.9	68.6	1.4	16.4	190.3	188.0	964.9	0.4	26.5	0.0	0.0	0.0	0.0	2.0	0.1	13.3	0.2	25.2
0.0	20.0	150.0	0.7	0.0	200.0	220.0	100.0	0.7	40.0	0.0	0.0	0.1	0.3	0.0	0.1	3.0	0.6	0.0
0.0	10.0	100.0	0.4	0.0	100.0	134.0	55.0	0.5	40.0	0.0	0.0	0.0	0.1	0.0	0.0	2.0	0.4	0.0
4.0	15.0	150.0	0.7	0.0	200.0	220.0	80.0	0.7	40.0	0.0	0.0	0.1	0.3	0.0	0.1	3.0	0.6	0.0
2.0	10.0	100.0	0.4	0.0	100.0	135.0	45.0	0.5	20.0	0.0	0.0	0.0	0.2	0.0	0.0	2.0	0.4	0.0
0.0	30.0	250.0	1.4	0.0	300.0	0.0	140.0	0.0	80.0	0.0	0.0	0.1	0.4	0.4	0.0	0.0	0.9	0.0
0.0	5.0	60.0	0.0	0.0	60.0	0.0	40.0	0.0	20.0	0.0	0.0	0.0	0.1	0.4	0.0	0.0	0.1	0.0
0.0	20.0	200.0	1.1	0.0	200.0	290.0	120.0	0.9	40.0	0.0	0.0	0.1	0.3	0.3	0.1	4.0	0.6	0.0
0.0	10.0	100.0	0.4	0.0	150.0	145.0	75.0	0.5	20.0	0.0	0.0	0.0	0.2	0.2	0.0	2.0	0.4	0.0
0.0	30.0	250.0	1.8	0.0	350.0	670.0	150.0	2.1	150.0	15.0	0.0	0.1	0.5	0.4	0.8	9.0	0.9	0.0
0.0	10.0	100.0	1.1	0.0	250.0	0.0	175.0	0.0	20.0	0.0	0.0	0.1	0.2	2.0	0.0	0.0	0.4	0.0
0.0	10.0	100.0	0.4	0.0	100.0	0.0	50.0	0.0	20.0	0.0	0.0	0.0	0.2	0.0	0.0	0.0	0.2	0.0
0.0	20.0	200.0	1.1	0.0	200.0	0.0	85.0	0.0	40.0	0.0	0.0	0.1	0.3	0.0	0.0	0.0	0.6	0.0
0.0	50.0	450.0	4.5	0.0	600.0	690.0	260.0	0.1	150.0	0.0	0.0	0.3	0.8	0.8	0.2	4.0	2.1	0.0
0.0	35.0	350.0	2.7	0.0	400.0	480.0	180.0	0.1	100.0	0.0	0.0	0.2	0.6	0.4	0.1	3.0	1.2	0.0
3.5	27.8	153.5	0.2	15.5	139.1	168.9	91.7	0.6	51.5	1.1	0.4	0.1	0.3	0.3	0.1	12.4	0.2	67.4
0.5	2.7	23.5	0.1	3.5	21.2	41.6	20.2	0.1	4.8	0.1	0.0	0.0	0.1	0.0	0.0	0.7	0.1	14.9
4.9	31.1	319.8	0.3	36.8	283.0	515.1	234.9	1.0	82.1	2.3	0.0	0.1	0.6	0.5	0.1	8.5	0.9	209.7
0.4	2.3	25.4	0.0	2.5	21.2	36.2	17.1	0.1	6.7	0.2	0.0	0.0	0.0	0.0	0.0	0.7	0.1	15.5
7.8	18.1	272.3	1.3	55.4	275.7	171.8	815.9	1.8	91.5	1.2	0.0	0.2	0.4	1.5	0.2	10.2	0.8	45.7
14.0	83.6	620.2	2.4	108.1	393.7	293.8	1736.0	2.9	471.2	1.0	0.0	0.1	0.5	2.8	0.4	18.4	1.0	87.1
12.5	20.4	385.1	2.8	96.9	387.6	451.4	1800.3	3.6	469.2	4.8	0.0	0.2	0.7	3.3	0.4	38.3	1.0	142.7

Code	Food Name	Unit/Amt	Wt (g)	Energy (Kcal)	Prot (g)	Carb (g)	Fiber (g)	Fat (g)	Mono (g)	Poly (g)
21081	Fast Food, Nachos w/cinnamon & sugar	6-8 nachos	109	591.9	7.2	63.4	0.0	36.0	11.8	4.1
21130	Fast Food, Onion Rings, breaded, fried	8-9 onion rings	83	275.6	3.7	31.3	0.0	15.5	6.7	0.7
21048	Fast Food, Oysters (shellfish) battered/breaded, fried	6 oysters	139	368.4	12.5	39.9	0.0	17.9	6.9	4.6
21025	Fast Food, Pancakes w/butter & syrup	3 cakes	232	519.7	8.3	90.9	0.0	14.0	5.3	2.0
21049	Fast Food, Pizza w/cheese	1 slice (⅛ 12"-pizza)	63	140.5	7.7	20.5	0.0	3.2	1.0	0.5
21050	Fast Food, Pizza w/cheese, meat & veges	1 slice (⅛ 12"-pizza)	79	184.1	13.0	21.3	0.0	5.4	2.5	0.9
21051	Fast Food, Pizza w/pepperoni	1 slice (⅛ 12"-pizza)	71	181.1	10.1	19.9	0.0	7.0	3.1	1.2
921911	Fast Food, Pizza, Cheese Pan/PH	2 slices	205	492.0	30.0	57.0	5.0	18.0	0.0	0.0
921906	Fast Food, Pizza, Cheese, thin/PH	2 slices	148	398.1	28.0	37.0	4.0	17.0	0.0	0.0
921912	Fast Food, Pizza, Pepperoni Pan/PH	2 slices	211	540.2	29.0	62.0	5.0	22.0	0.0	0.0
921905	Fast Food, Pizza, Pepperoni, personal/PH	1 pizza	256	675.8	37.0	76.0	8.0	29.0	0.0	0.0
921907	Fast Food, Pizza, Pepperoni, thin/PH	2 slices	146	413.2	26.0	36.0	4.0	20.0	0.0	0.0
921913	Fast Food, Pizza, Super Supreme Pan/PH	2 slices	257	562.8	33.0	53.0	6.0	26.0	0.0	0.0
921908	Fast Food, Pizza, Super Supreme, thin/PH	2 slices	203	462.8	29.0	44.0	5.0	21.0	0.0	0.0
921914	Fast Food, Pizza, Supreme Pan/PH	2 slices	255	589.1	32.0	53.0	7.0	30.0	0.0	0.0
921910	Fast Food, Pizza, Supreme Personal/PH	1 pizza	264	646.8	33.0	76.0	9.0	28.0	0.0	0.0
921909	Fast Food, Pizza, Supreme, thin/PH	2 slices	200	460.0	28.0	41.0	5.0	22.0	0.0	0.0
21132	Fast Food, Potato, baked, topped w/cheese & bacon	1 potato	299	451.5	18.4	44.4	0.0	25.9	9.7	4.8
21133	Fast Food, Potato, baked, topped w/cheese & broccoli	1 potato	339	403.4	13.7	46.6	0.0	21.4	7.7	4.2
21134	Fast Food, Potato, baked, topped w/cheese & chili	1 potato	395	481.9	23.2	55.9	0.0	21.8	6.8	0.9
21131	Fast Food, Potato, baked, topped w/cheese sauce	1 potato	296	473.6	14.6	46.5	0.0	28.7	10.7	6.0
21135	Fast Food, Potato, baked, topped w/sour cream & chives	1 potato	302	392.6	6.7	50.0	0.0	22.3	7.9	3.3
21139	Fast Food, Potato, mashed	1 tbsp	15	12.5	0.3	2.4	0.0	0.2	0.1	0.0
21026	Fast Food, Potatoes, Hash Brown	1 tbsp	9	18.9	0.2	2.0	0.0	1.2	0.5	0.1
21122	Fast Food, Roast Beef Sandwich w/cheese	1 sandwich	176	473.4	32.2	45.4	0.0	18.0	3.7	3.5
21121	Fast Food, Roast Beef Sandwich, plain	1 sandwich	139	346.1	21.5	33.4	0.0	13.8	6.8	1.7
4021	Fast Food, Salad Dressing, Italian, w/salt, diet (2kcal/tsp)	1 tbsp	15	15.8	0.0	0.7	0.0	1.5	0.3	0.9
4025	Fast Food, Salad Dressing, Mayonnaise, Soybean Oil, w/salt	1 cup	220	1577.0	2.4	5.9	0.0	174.7	49.9	90.9
921983	Fast Food, Salad, Chef/Hardee	1 salad	294	241.1	22.0	5.0	0.0	15.0	5.0	1.0
921864	Fast Food, Salad, Chunky Chicken/BK	1 salad	258	141.9	20.0	8.0	0.0	4.0	1.0	1.0
21127	Fast Food, Salad, Cole Slaw	1 tbsp	8.3	12.3	0.1	1.1	0.0	0.9	0.2	0.5
921871	Fast Food, Salad, Cole Slaw/KFC	1 serving	91	119.2	1.5	13.2	1.0	6.6	2.0	3.4
921803	Fast Food, Salad, Garden/BK	1 salad	223	95.9	6.0	8.0	0.0	5.0	1.0	0.0
21140	Fast Food, Salad, Potato	1 tbsp	17.8	20.3	0.3	2.4	0.0	1.1	0.3	0.5
21083	Fast Food, Salad, Taco	1 tbsp	8.1	11.4	0.5	1.0	0.0	0.6	0.2	0.1
21084	Fast Food, Salad, Taco w/chili con carne	1 tbsp	10.9	12.1	0.7	1.1	0.0	0.5	0.2	0.1
921974	Fast Food, Sandwich, Beef & Cheddar/Arby	1 sandwich	168	490.6	24.0	51.0	0.5	21.0	11.0	5.0
921981	Fast Food, Sandwich, Big Deluxe Hamburger/Hardee	1 burger	216	499.0	27.0	32.0	0.0	30.0	12.0	5.0
921971	Fast Food, Sandwich, Big Roast Beef/Hardee	1 sandwich	134	300.2	18.0	32.0	0.5	12.0	5.0	2.0
921989	Fast Food, Sandwich, Big Twin/Hardee	1 sandwich	173	449.8	23.0	34.0	0.0	25.0	9.0	5.0
21002	Fast Food, Sandwich, Biscuit w/egg	1 biscuit	136	315.5	11.1	24.2	0.0	20.2	8.2	4.2
21003	Fast Food, Sandwich, Biscuit w/egg & bacon	1 biscuit	150	457.5	17.0	28.6	0.8	31.1	13.4	7.5
21004	Fast Food, Sandwich, Biscuit w/egg & ham	1 biscuit	192	441.6	20.4	30.3	0.8	27.0	11.0	7.7
21005	Fast Food, Sandwich, Biscuit w/egg & sausage	1 biscuit	180	581.4	19.2	41.1	0.9	38.7	16.4	4.4
21006	Fast Food, Sandwich, Biscuit w/egg & steak	1 biscuit	148	410.0	17.9	21.3	0.0	28.4	11.7	5.8
21007	Fast Food, Sandwich, Biscuit w/egg, cheese & bacon	1 biscuit	144	476.6	16.3	33.4	0.0	31.4	14.2	3.5
21093	Fast Food, Sandwich, Cheeseburger (2 patty) condiments & veges	1 burger	166	416.7	21.2	35.2	0.0	21.1	7.8	2.7
21092	Fast Food, Sandwich, Cheeseburger (2 patty) plain	1 burger	155	457.3	27.7	22.1	0.0	28.5	11.0	1.9
921969	Fast Food, Sandwich, Cheeseburger, ¼ pound/Hardee	1 burger	182	500.5	29.0	34.0	0.4	29.0	12.0	2.0
921952	Fast Food, Sandwich, Cheeseburger, Big Classic/Wendy	1 burger	295	640.2	30.0	46.0	2.0	38.0	14.0	4.0
921926	Fast Food, Sandwich, Cheeseburger, junior/Wendy	1 burger	123	300.1	17.0	31.0	0.0	13.0	0.0	0.0
21100	Fast Food, Sandwich, Cheeseburger, large (2 patty) w/condiments & vege	1 burger	258	704.3	38.0	39.7	0.0	43.7	17.4	4.7
21096	Fast Food, Sandwich, Cheeseburger, large, one meat patty, plain	1 burger	185	608.7	30.1	47.4	0.0	33.0	12.7	2.4
21089	Fast Food, Sandwich, Cheeseburger, one meat patty, plain	1 burger	102	319.3	14.8	31.8	0.0	15.1	5.8	1.5
21090	Fast Food, Sandwich, Cheeseburger, one meat patty, w/condiments	1 burger	113	294.9	16.0	26.5	0.0	14.1	5.3	1.1
21102	Fast Food, Sandwich, Chicken Filet, plain	1 sandwich	182	515.1	24.1	38.7	0.0	29.4	10.4	8.4
921934	Fast Food, Sandwich, Chicken/BK	1 sandwich	229	684.7	26.0	56.0	0.5	40.0	11.0	20.0
921979	Fast Food, Sandwich, Club/Arby	1 sandwich	252	559.4	30.0	43.0	1.0	30.0	0.0	0.0
921809	Fast Food, Sandwich, Colonel's Chicken/KFC	1 sandwich	166	481.4	20.8	38.6	1.0	27.3	12.6	8.0
921801	Fast Food, Sandwich, Croissandwich/BK	1 sandwich	144	345.6	19.0	19.0	0.5	21.0	11.0	2.0
21011	Fast Food, Sandwich, Croissant w/egg & cheese	1 croissant	127	368.3	12.8	24.3	0.0	24.7	7.5	1.4
21012	Fast Food, Sandwich, Croissant w/egg, cheese & bacon	1 croissant	129	412.8	16.2	23.6	0.0	28.4	9.2	1.8
21013	Fast Food, Sandwich, Croissant w/egg, cheese & ham	1 croissant	152	474.2	18.9	24.2	0.0	33.6	11.4	2.4
21020	Fast Food, Sandwich, English Muffin w/cheese & sausage	1 muffin	115	393.3	15.3	29.2	1.5	24.3	10.1	2.7
21021	Fast Food, Sandwich, English Muffin w/egg, cheese & Canadian bacon	1 sandwich	137	289.1	16.7	26.7	1.5	12.6	4.7	1.6
21047	Fast Food, Sandwich, Fish Filet, battered/breaded, fried	1 fillet	91	211.1	13.3	15.4	0.5	11.2	2.3	5.7
21105	Fast Food, Sandwich, Fish w/tartar sauce	1 sandwich	158	431.3	16.9	41.0	0.0	22.8	7.7	8.2
21106	Fast Food, Sandwich, Fish w/tartar sauce & cheese	1 sandwich	183	523.4	20.6	47.6	0.0	28.6	8.9	9.4
921977	Fast Food, Sandwich, Ham & Cheese/Arby	1 sandwich	154	352.7	26.0	33.0	0.5	13.0	6.0	3.0

Sat (g)	Chol (mg)	Cal (mg)	Iron (mg)	Magn (mg)	Phos (mg)	Pota (mg)	Sodi (mg)	Zinc (mg)	Vit A (RE)	Vit C (mg)	Vit E (mg)	Thia (mg)	Ribo (mg)	Niac (mg)	Vit B-6 (mg)	Fol (µg)	Vit B-12 (µg)	Wat (g)
18.2	39.2	85.0	2.9	19.6	32.7	78.5	439.3	0.6	10.9	8.0	0.0	0.2	0.4	3.9	0.2	7.6	1.7	1.1
7.0	14.1	73.0	0.8	15.8	86.3	129.5	429.9	0.3	0.8	0.6	0.3	0.1	0.1	0.9	0.1	54.8	0.1	30.8
4.6	108.4	27.8	4.5	23.6	196.0	182.1	676.9	15.6	108.4	4.2	0.0	0.3	0.3	4.4	0.0	30.6	1.0	66.7
5.9	58.0	127.6	2.6	48.7	475.6	250.6	1104.3	1.0	69.6	3.5	1.4	0.4	0.6	3.4	0.1	30.2	0.2	115.4
1.5	9.5	116.6	0.6	15.8	112.8	109.6	335.8	0.8	73.7	1.3	0.0	0.2	0.2	2.5	0.0	34.7	0.3	30.1
1.5	20.5	101.1	1.5	18.2	131.1	178.5	382.4	1.1	101.1	1.6	0.0	0.2	0.2	2.0	0.1	32.4	0.4	37.7
2.2	14.2	64.6	0.9	8.5	75.3	152.7	267.0	0.5	54.7	1.6	0.0	0.1	0.2	3.0	0.1	36.9	0.2	33.0
9.0	34.0	500.0	5.4	0.0	0.0	320.0	940.0	0.0	200.0	0.0	0.0	0.7	0.7	7.0	0.0	0.0	0.0	0.0
10.4	33.0	450.0	4.5	0.0	0.0	261.0	867.0	0.0	150.0	0.0	0.0	0.3	0.5	5.0	0.0	0.0	0.0	0.0
9.2	42.0	400.0	5.4	0.0	0.0	405.0	1127.0	0.0	250.0	4.0	0.0	0.7	0.7	8.0	0.0	0.0	0.0	0.0
12.5	53.0	0.0	0.0	0.0	0.0	408.0	1335.0	0.0	0.0	0.0	0.0	0.0	0.0	0.0	0.0	0.0	0.0	0.0
10.6	46.0	300.0	4.5	0.0	0.0	287.0	986.0	0.0	200.0	4.0	0.0	0.3	0.5	6.0	0.0	0.0	0.0	0.0
12.0	55.0	400.0	7.2	0.0	0.0	532.0	1447.0	0.0	150.0	1.0	0.0	0.9	0.8	9.0	0.0	0.0	0.0	0.0
10.3	56.0	350.0	6.3	0.0	0.0	463.0	1336.0	0.0	200.0	1.0	0.0	0.4	0.7	7.0	0.0	0.0	0.0	0.0
13.8	48.0	400.0	7.2	0.0	0.0	580.0	1363.0	0.0	200.0	9.0	0.0	0.7	0.8	9.0	0.0	0.0	0.0	0.0
11.2	49.0	0.0	0.0	0.0	0.0	487.0	1313.0	0.0	0.0	0.0	0.0	0.0	0.0	0.0	0.0	0.0	0.0	0.0
11.0	42.0	350.0	7.2	0.0	0.0	544.0	1328.0	0.0	250.0	2.0	0.0	0.4	0.7	7.0	0.0	0.0	0.0	0.0
10.1	29.9	308.0	3.1	68.8	346.8	1178.1	971.8	2.2	173.4	28.7	0.0	0.3	0.2	4.0	0.7	29.9	0.3	194.4
8.5	20.3	335.6	3.3	78.0	345.8	1440.8	484.8	2.0	278.0	48.5	0.0	0.3	0.3	3.6	0.8	61.0	0.3	237.4
13.0	31.6	410.8	6.1	110.6	497.7	1572.1	699.2	3.8	173.8	31.6	0.0	0.3	0.4	4.2	0.9	47.4	0.2	276.8
10.6	17.8	310.8	3.0	65.1	319.7	1166.2	381.8	1.9	227.9	26.0	0.0	0.2	0.2	3.3	0.7	26.6	0.2	194.6
10.0	24.2	105.7	3.1	69.5	184.2	1383.2	181.2	0.9	277.8	33.8	0.0	0.3	0.2	3.7	0.8	33.2	0.2	209.7
0.1	0.3	3.2	0.1	2.7	8.3	44.1	34.1	0.0	1.5	0.1	0.0	0.0	0.0	0.2	0.0	1.2	0.0	11.9
0.5	1.2	0.9	0.1	2.0	8.6	33.4	36.3	0.0	0.4	0.7	0.0	0.0	0.0	0.1	0.0	1.0	0.0	5.4
9.0	77.4	183.0	5.1	40.5	401.3	345.0	1633.3	5.4	45.8	0.0	0.0	0.4	0.5	5.9	0.3	63.4	2.1	76.6
3.6	51.4	54.2	4.2	30.6	239.1	315.5	792.3	3.4	20.9	2.1	0.0	0.4	0.3	5.9	0.3	57.0	1.2	67.6
0.2	0.9	0.3	0.0	0.0	0.8	2.3	118.1	0.0	0.0	0.0	0.2	0.0	0.0	0.0	0.0	0.0	0.0	12.3
26.0	129.8	39.6	1.1	2.2	61.6	74.8	1250.5	0.4	184.8	0.0	25.9	0.0	0.0	0.0	1.3	16.9	0.6	33.7
9.0	115.0	279.0	2.0	0.0	0.0	590.0	930.0	0.0	0.0	0.0	0.0	0.0	0.0	0.0	0.0	0.0	0.0	0.0
1.0	49.0	0.0	0.0	0.0	0.0	0.0	443.0	0.0	0.0	0.0	0.0	0.0	0.0	0.0	0.0	0.0	0.0	0.0
0.1	0.4	2.8	0.1	0.7	3.0	14.9	22.4	0.0	4.2	0.7	0.0	0.0	0.0	0.0	0.0	3.2	0.0	6.1
1.0	5.0	33.0	0.2	0.0	20.0	115.0	197.0	0.1	62.0	22.0	0.0	0.0	0.2	0.2	0.1	10.0	0.0	0.0
3.0	15.0	0.0	0.0	0.0	0.0	0.0	125.0	0.0	0.0	0.0	0.0	0.0	0.0	0.0	0.0	0.0	0.0	0.0
0.2	10.7	2.5	0.1	1.4	10.0	48.1	58.4	0.0	3.0	0.2	0.0	0.0	0.0	0.0	0.0	4.5	0.0	14.0
0.3	1.8	7.9	0.1	2.1	5.8	17.0	31.2	0.1	3.2	0.1	0.0	0.0	0.0	0.1	0.0	3.4	0.0	5.9
0.3	0.2	10.2	0.1	2.2	6.4	16.4	37.0	0.1	8.9	0.1	0.0	0.0	0.0	0.1	0.0	3.8	0.0	8.4
5.0	51.0	80.0	5.4	0.0	0.0	355.0	1520.0	0.0	14.2	3.0	0.0	0.1	0.3	5.0	0.0	0.0	0.0	0.0
12.0	70.0	185.0	5.0	0.0	0.0	390.0	760.0	0.0	0.0	0.0	0.0	0.0	0.0	0.0	0.0	0.0	0.0	0.0
5.0	45.0	106.0	5.0	0.0	0.0	320.0	880.0	0.0	129.6	8.0	0.0	1.0	0.2	5.2	0.0	0.0	0.0	0.0
11.0	55.0	180.0	4.0	0.0	0.0	280.0	580.0	0.0	0.0	0.0	0.0	0.0	0.0	0.0	0.0	0.0	0.0	0.0
6.2	232.6	153.7	3.1	20.4	185.0	160.5	654.2	1.1	178.2	0.0	0.0	0.3	0.3	0.7	0.1	61.2	0.7	69.5
8.0	352.5	189.0	3.7	24.0	238.5	250.5	999.0	1.6	52.5	2.7	2.1	0.1	0.2	2.4	0.1	60.0	1.0	70.0
5.9	299.5	220.8	4.6	30.7	316.8	318.7	1382.4	2.2	240.0	0.0	2.2	0.7	0.6	2.0	0.3	65.3	1.2	104.9
15.0	302.4	154.8	4.0	25.2	489.6	320.4	1141.2	2.2	163.8	0.0	2.8	0.5	0.5	3.6	0.2	64.8	1.4	77.2
8.6	272.3	137.6	5.3	25.2	225.0	306.4	888.0	2.8	190.9	0.1	0.0	0.4	0.5	3.1	0.2	56.2	1.4	77.7
11.4	260.6	164.2	2.5	20.2	459.4	230.4	1260.0	1.5	165.6	1.6	0.0	0.3	0.4	2.3	0.1	53.3	1.1	59.3
8.7	59.8	171.0	3.4	29.9	242.4	335.3	1050.8	3.5	64.7	1.7	0.0	0.3	0.3	8.1	0.2	61.4	1.9	85.0
13.0	110.1	232.5	3.4	32.6	373.6	308.5	635.5	5.0	79.1	0.0	1.2	0.2	0.4	6.0	0.2	68.2	2.3	65.7
14.0	70.0	248.0	5.0	0.0	355.0	350.0	1060.0	3.6	101.6	33.0	0.0	0.3	0.6	14.0	0.3	0.0	0.7	0.0
14.0	100.0	180.0	5.4	0.0	489.0	590.0	1370.0	9.0	87.8	2.3	0.0	0.5	0.7	11.4	0.5	31.0	0.0	0.0
0.0	45.0	0.0	0.0	0.0	0.0	220.0	745.0	0.0	0.0	0.0	0.0	0.0	0.0	0.0	0.0	0.0	0.0	0.0
17.7	141.9	239.9	5.9	51.6	394.7	596.0	1148.1	6.7	54.2	1.0	0.0	0.4	0.5	7.2	0.4	74.8	3.4	131.8
14.8	96.2	90.7	5.5	38.9	421.8	643.8	1589.2	5.6	148.0	0.0	0.0	0.5	0.6	11.2	0.3	74.0	2.5	71.5
6.5	50.0	140.8	2.4	21.4	195.8	164.2	499.8	2.4	36.7	0.0	0.0	0.4	0.4	3.7	0.1	54.1	1.0	38.0
6.3	37.3	110.7	2.4	20.3	176.3	222.6	615.9	2.1	93.8	1.9	0.5	0.2	0.2	3.7	0.1	54.2	0.9	53.9
8.5	60.1	60.1	4.7	34.6	233.0	353.1	957.3	1.9	30.9	8.9	0.0	0.3	0.2	6.8	0.2	100.1	0.4	86.1
8.0	82.0	79.0	3.3	54.0	274.0	375.0	1417.0	1.1	25.2	0.0	0.0	0.5	0.3	9.6	0.4	18.0	0.0	0.0
0.0	100.0	200.0	3.6	0.0	0.0	0.0	1610.0	0.0	0.0	0.0	0.0	0.7	0.4	7.0	0.0	0.0	0.0	0.0
5.7	47.0	46.0	1.3	0.0	0.0	0.0	1060.0	0.0	0.0	0.0	0.0	0.4	0.3	11.1	0.0	0.0	0.0	0.0
7.0	241.0	136.0	2.2	24.0	317.0	256.0	962.0	1.9	85.2	0.0	0.0	0.5	0.3	3.2	0.0	0.0	0.0	0.0
14.1	215.9	243.8	2.2	21.6	348.0	174.0	551.2	1.8	255.3	0.1	0.0	0.2	0.4	1.5	0.1	47.0	0.8	57.7
15.4	215.4	150.9	2.2	23.2	276.1	201.2	888.8	1.9	120.0	2.2	0.0	0.3	0.3	2.2	0.1	45.2	0.9	56.7
17.5	212.8	144.4	2.1	25.8	335.9	272.1	1080.7	2.2	117.0	11.4	0.0	0.5	0.3	3.2	0.2	45.6	1.0	77.7
9.9	58.7	167.9	2.3	24.2	186.3	215.1	1036.2	1.7	86.3	1.3	0.5	0.7	0.3	4.1	0.1	66.7	0.7	43.4
4.7	234.3	150.7	2.4	23.3	269.9	198.7	728.8	1.6	156.2	1.8	0.9	0.5	0.4	3.3	0.1	43.8	0.7	77.8
2.6	30.9	16.4	1.9	21.8	155.6	291.2	484.1	0.4	10.9	0.0	0.0	0.1	0.1	1.9	0.1	15.5	1.0	48.7
5.2	55.3	83.7	2.6	33.2	211.7	339.7	614.6	1.0	30.0	2.8	0.9	0.3	0.2	3.4	0.1	85.3	1.1	74.8
8.1	67.7	184.8	3.5	36.6	311.1	353.2	938.8	1.2	97.0	2.7	1.8	0.5	0.4	4.2	0.1	91.5	1.1	82.7
4.0	50.0	200.0	1.8	0.0	405.0	312.0	1655.0	2.4	40.0	24.0	0.0	1.0	0.5	6.0	0.3	26.0	0.0	0.0

Code	Food Name	Unit/Amt	Wt (g)	Energy (Kcal)	Prot (g)	Carb (g)	Fiber (g)	Fat (g)	Mono (g)	Poly (g)
21110	Fast Food, Sandwich, Hamburger (2 patty) plain	1 burger	176	543.8	29.9	42.9	0.0	27.9	12.1	2.3
21111	Fast Food, Sandwich, Hamburger (2 patty) w/condiments	1 burger	215	576.2	31.8	38.7	0.0	32.5	14.1	2.8
921929	Fast Food, Sandwich, Hamburger, Big Classic/Wendy	1 burger	277	570.6	27.0	46.0	1.0	33.0	13.0	8.0
921887	Fast Food, Sandwich, Hamburger, Big Mac/MCD	1 burger	215	559.0	25.2	42.5	1.0	32.5	20.9	1.5
921931	Fast Food, Sandwich, Hamburger, junior/Wendy	1 burger	111	259.7	14.0	30.0		9.0	0.0	0.0
21107	Fast Food, Sandwich, Hamburger, plain	1 burger	90	274.5	12.3	30.5	0.0	11.8	5.5	0.9
921930	Fast Food, Sandwich, Hamburger, single/Wendy	1 burger	126	340.2	24.0	38.0	1.0	17.0	9.0	1.0
921894	Fast Food, Sandwich, Hamburger/MCD	1 burger	102	260.1	12.2	30.6	0.5	9.5	5.1	0.8
921825	Fast Food, Sandwich, Hot Dog w/cheese/DQ	1 hot dog	113	330.0	15.0	21.0	0.5	21.0	8.0	2.0
921827	Fast Food, Sandwich, Hot Dog w/chili/DQ	1 hot dog	128	320.0	13.0	23.0	0.5	20.0	8.0	2.0
921844	Fast Food, Sandwich, Hot Dog/DQ	1 hot dog	99	280.2	11.0	21.0	0.5	16.0	7.0	2.0
921976	Fast Food, Sandwich, Jr Roast Beef/Arby	1 sandwich	74	218.3	12.0	22.0	0.5	8.0	3.0	2.0
921973	Fast Food, Sandwich, Roast Beef/Arby	1 sandwich	140	350.0	22.0	32.0	0.5	15.0	5.0	2.0
921972	Fast Food, Sandwich, Roast Beef/Hardee	1 sandwich	114	259.9	15.0	31.0	0.5	10.0	4.0	2.0
921806	Fast Food, Sandwich, Sausage McMuffin/MCD	1 sandwich	117	369.7	16.5	27.3	0.5	21.9	11.7	2.4
921978	Fast Food, Sandwich, Turkey Deluxe/Arby	1 sandwich	236	375.2	24.0	32.0	0.5	17.0	5.0	8.0
921890	Fast Food, Scrambled Eggs/MCD	1 serving	100	140.0	12.4	1.2	0.0	9.8	5.0	1.4
921988	Fast Food, Shake, Chocolate/Hardee	1 shake	341	460.4	11.0	85.0	0.0	8.0	2.0	0.0
921932	Fast Food, Shake, Frosty/Wendy	1 shake	243	401.0	8.0	59.0	0.0	14.0	3.0	2.0
921903	Fast Food, Shake, Strawberry/MCD	1 shake	239	320.3	10.7	67.0	0.0	1.3	0.6	0.1
921821	Fast Food, Shake, Vanilla/BK	1 shake	284	335.1	9.0	51.0	0.0	10.0	3.0	0.0
921904	Nutrient/Protein Supplement, Liquid Nutrition, Boost, vanilla	8 oz.	260	239.2	10.1	41.1	0.0	4.1	0.0	0.0
21059	Fast Food, Shrimp (shellfish) breaded, fried	6-8 shrimp	164	454.3	18.9	40.0	0.0	24.9	17.4	0.6
21123	Fast Food, Steak Sandwich	1 sandwich	204	459.0	30.3	52.0	0.0	14.1	5.3	3.3
21124	Fast Food, Submarine Sandwich, cold cuts	1 sub	228	456.0	21.8	51.0	0.0	18.6	8.2	2.3
21125	Fast Food, Submarine Sandwich, roast beef	1 sub	216	410.4	28.6	44.3	0.0	13.0	1.8	2.6
21126	Fast Food, Submarine Sandwich, tuna salad	1 sub	256	583.7	29.7	55.4	0.0	28.0	13.4	7.3
21082	Fast Food, Taco	1 small taco	171	369.4	20.7	26.7	0.0	20.6	6.6	1.0
921958	Fast Food, Taco/JB	1 taco	81	191.2	8.0	16.0	1.2	11.0	4.4	1.0
21085	Fast Food, Tostada w/beans & cheese	1 tostada	144	223.2	9.6	26.5	0.0	9.9	3.1	0.7
21086	Fast Food, Tostada w/beans, beef & cheese	1 tostada	225	333.0	16.1	29.7	0.0	16.9	3.5	0.6
4002	Fat, Animal, Lard, Pork	1 cup	205	1849.1	0.0	0.0	0.0	205.0	92.5	23.0
924073	Fish Cakes, fried	4.0 oz	120	206.4	17.6	11.2	0.0	9.6	0.0	0.0
924074	Fish Cakes, frozen	4.0 oz	119	253.5	11.6	27.3	0.0	10.8	0.0	0.0
15187	Fish, Bass, Freshwater, cooked w/dry heat	3.5 oz	100	146.0	24.2	0.0	0.0	4.7	1.8	1.4
15188	Fish, Bass, Striped, cooked w/dry heat	1 fillet	124	153.8	28.2	0.0	0.0	3.7	1.0	1.2
15189	Fish, Bluefish, cooked w/dry heat	1 fillet	117	186.0	30.1	0.0	0.0	6.4	2.7	1.6
15009	Fish, Carp, baked or broiled (dry heat)	1 fillet	170	275.4	38.9	0.0	0.0	12.2	5.1	3.1
15235	Fish, Catfish, Channel, Farmed, cooked w/dry heat	1 fillet	143	217.4	26.8	0.0	0.0	11.5	5.9	2.0
15233	Fish, Catfish, Channel, Wild, cooked w/dry heat	1 fillet	143	150.2	26.4	0.0	0.0	4.1	1.6	0.9
15012	Fish, Caviar, black/red, granular	1.0 oz	29	73.1	7.1	1.2	0.0	5.2	1.3	2.1
15016	Fish, Cod, Atlantic, baked/broiled (dry heat)	1 fillet	180	189.0	41.1	0.0	0.0	1.5	0.2	0.5
15018	Fish, Cod, Atlantic, dried & salted	1 piece (5.5" x 1.5" x 0.5")	80	232.0	50.3	0.0	0.0	1.9	0.3	0.6
15192	Fish, Cod, Pacific, cooked w/dry heat	3.0 oz	85	89.3	19.5	0.0	0.0	0.7	0.1	0.3
15027	Fish, Fish Sticks, frozen & reheated	1 piece (4" x 2" x 0.5")	57	155.0	8.9	13.5	0.0	7.0	2.9	1.8
15032	Fish, Grouper, baked or broiled (dry heat)	3.0 oz	85	100.3	21.1	0.0	0.0	1.1	0.2	0.3
15034	Fish, Haddock, baked or broiled (dry heat)	3.0 oz	85	95.2	20.6	0.0	0.0	0.8	0.1	0.3
15035	Fish, Haddock, smoked	1 cubic inch, boneless	17	19.7	4.3	0.0	0.0	0.2	0.0	0.1
15037	Fish, Halibut, Atlantic & Pacific, baked or broiled (dry heat)	3.0 oz	85	119.0	22.7	0.0	0.0	2.5	0.8	0.8
15196	Fish, Halibut, Greenland, cooked w/dry heat	3.0 oz	85	203.2	15.7	0.0	0.0	15.1	9.1	1.5
15040	Fish, Herring, Atlantic, baked or broiled (dry heat)	3.5 oz	100	203.0	23.0	0.0	0.0	11.6	4.8	2.7
15042	Fish, Herring, Atlantic, kippered	1.5 oz (1 piece 4⅜" x 1 ¾ " x ¼ ")	44	95.5	10.8	0.0	0.0	5.4	2.2	1.3
15041	Fish, Herring, Atlantic, pickled	0.5 oz (1 piece ¾ " x ⅞" x ½ ")	15	39.3	2.1	1.4	0.0	2.7	1.8	0.3
15121	Fish, Light Tuna, canned in H₂O, drained	3.5 oz	100	116.0	25.5	0.0	0.0	0.8	0.2	0.3
15183	Fish, Light Tuna, canned in oil w/o salt, drained	3.5 oz	100	198.0	29.1	0.0	0.0	8.2	2.9	2.9
15119	Fish, Light Tuna, canned in oil, drained	3.0 oz, 1 sm can	85	168.3	24.8	0.0	0.0	7.0	2.5	2.5
15047	Fish, Mackerel, Atlantic, baked or broiled (dry heat)	3.5 oz	100	262.0	23.9	0.0	0.0	17.8	7.0	4.3
15200	Fish, Mackerel, King, cooked w/dry heat	3.5 oz	100	134.0	26.0	0.0	0.0	2.6	1.0	0.6
15058	Fish, Ocean Perch, Atlantic, baked or broiled (dry heat)	3.5 oz	100	121.0	23.9	0.0	0.0	2.1	0.8	0.5
15061	Fish, Perch, baked or broiled (dry heat)	3.5 oz	100	117.0	24.9	0.0	0.0	1.2	0.2	0.5
15063	Fish, Pike, Northern, baked or broiled (dry heat)	3.5 oz	100	113.0	24.7	0.0	0.0	0.9	0.2	0.3
15204	Fish, Pike, Walleye, cooked w/dry heat	3.5 oz	100	119.0	24.5	0.0	0.0	1.6	0.4	0.6
15205	Fish, Pollock, Atlantic, cooked w/dry heat	3.5 oz	100	118.0	24.9	0.0	0.0	1.3	0.1	0.6
15067	Fish, Pollock, Walleye, baked or broiled	3.5 oz	100	113.0	23.5	0.0	0.0	1.1	0.2	0.5
15069	Fish, Pompano, Florida, baked or broiled (dry heat)	3.5 oz	100	211.0	23.7	0.0	0.0	12.1	3.3	1.5
915902	Fish, Roe, canned	1.0 oz	28	33.0	6.0	0.1	0.0	0.8	0.0	0.0
15232	Fish, Roughy, Orange, cooked w/dry heat	3.5 oz	100	89.0	18.9	0.0	0.0	0.9	0.6	0.0
15237	Fish, Salmon, Atlantic, Farmed, cooked w/dry heat	3.5 oz	100	206.0	22.1	0.0	0.0	12.4	4.4	4.4
15209	Fish, Salmon, Atlantic, Wild, cooked w/dryheat	3.5 oz	100	182.0	25.4	0.0	0.0	8.1	2.7	3.3

Sat (g)	Chol (mg)	Cal (mg)	Iron (mg)	Magn (mg)	Phos (mg)	Pota (mg)	Sodi (mg)	Zinc (mg)	Vit A (RE)	Vit C (mg)	Vit E (mg)	Thia (mg)	Ribo (mg)	Niac (mg)	Vit B-6 (mg)	Fol (µg)	Vit B-12 (µg)	Wat (g)
10.4	98.6	86.2	4.6	37.0	234.1	362.6	554.4	5.7	0.0	0.0	1.3	0.3	0.4	8.3	0.3	77.4	2.9	72.3
12.0	103.2	92.5	5.5	45.2	283.8	526.8	741.8	5.8	4.3	1.1	0.0	0.3	0.4	6.7	0.4	83.9	3.3	108.6
7.0	85.0	48.0	6.3	0.0	339.0	590.0	1075.0	8.4	25.6	0.0	0.0	0.2	0.4	9.0	0.5	29.0	0.0	0.0
10.1	103.0	256.0	4.0	0.0	314.0	249.0	950.0	4.7	70.4	2.0	0.0	0.5	0.4	6.8	0.3	21.0	1.8	0.0
0.0	34.0	0.0	0.0	0.0	0.0	220.0	545.0	0.0	0.0	0.0	0.0	0.0	0.0	0.0	0.0	0.0	0.0	0.0
4.1	35.1	63.0	2.4	18.9	102.6	144.9	387.0	2.0	0.0	0.0	0.5	0.3	0.3	3.7	0.1	53.1	0.9	33.8
7.0	65.0	32.0	4.5	0.0	118.0	275.0	475.0	2.0	18.8	0.0	0.0	0.2	0.2	5.0	0.1	0.5	0.0	0.0
3.6	37.0	122.0	2.3	0.0	126.0	142.0	500.0	2.1	30.4	2.0	0.0	0.3	0.2	3.8	0.1	17.0	0.8	0.0
8.0	55.0	150.0	1.4	0.0	200.0	140.0	990.0	1.9	20.0	0.0	0.0	0.1	0.2	3.0	0.1	25.0	1.2	0.0
8.0	55.0	80.0	1.8	0.0	150.0	175.0	985.0	1.8	30.0	0.0	0.0	0.1	0.3	4.0	0.2	30.0	1.2	0.0
6.0	45.0	80.0	1.4	21.0	80.0	130.0	830.0	1.4	0.0	0.0	0.0	0.1	0.1	3.0	0.1	20.0	0.9	0.0
3.0	20.0	40.0	1.8	0.0	60.0	197.0	345.0	1.2	0.0	0.0	0.0	0.2	0.3	4.0	0.1	7.0	0.0	0.0
7.0	39.0	80.0	3.6	0.0	0.0	422.0	590.0	0.0	17.0	1.0	0.0	0.2	0.4	7.6	0.2	14.0	0.0	0.0
4.0	34.0	105.0	4.0	0.0	0.0	260.0	730.0	0.0	108.4	3.0	0.0	0.9	0.2	3.7	0.0	0.0	0.0	0.0
7.8	64.0	235.0	2.3	0.0	353.0	231.0	820.0	1.3	48.0	0.0	0.0	0.6	0.3	4.8	0.1	12.0	0.0	0.0
4.0	39.0	80.0	2.7	0.0	250.0	346.0	850.0	2.2	60.0	4.8	0.0	0.2	0.4	12.0	0.5	20.0	0.0	0.0
3.3	399.0	57.0	2.1	0.0	264.0	135.0	290.0	1.7	103.6	0.0	0.0	0.1	0.3	0.1	0.2	65.0	0.9	0.0
5.0	45.0	480.0	1.0	0.0	429.0	520.0	340.0	1.6	58.4	0.0	0.0	0.2	0.8	0.4	0.1	0.0	1.1	0.0
5.0	50.0	45.0	0.9	0.0	238.0	585.0	220.0	0.9	71.0	0.0	0.0	0.2	0.6	0.5	0.1	17.0	0.0	0.0
0.6	10.0	327.0	0.1	0.0	289.0	487.0	170.0	1.0	61.2	0.0	0.0	0.1	0.5	0.3	0.1	11.0	1.6	0.0
6.0	33.0	295.0	0.0	32.0	284.0	508.0	213.0	1.0	0.0	0.0	0.0	0.1	0.6	0.0	0.0	0.0	0.0	0.0
0.5	4.9	299.0	3.6	100.0	249.6	400.4	130.0	4.4	249.6	59.8	29.9	0.4	0.4	5.0	0.7	140.4	2.1	199.9
5.4	200.1	83.6	3.0	39.4	344.4	183.7	1446.5	1.2	36.1	0.0	0.0	0.2	0.9	0.0	0.1	36.1	0.1	78.4
3.8	73.4	91.8	5.2	49.0	297.8	524.3	797.6	4.5	44.9	5.5	0.0	0.4	0.4	7.3	0.4	89.8	1.6	104.2
6.8	36.5	189.2	2.5	68.4	287.3	394.4	1650.7	2.6	79.8	12.3	0.0	1.0	0.8	5.5	0.1	86.6	1.1	131.8
7.1	73.4	41.0	2.8	67.0	192.2	330.5	844.6	4.4	49.7	5.6	0.0	0.4	0.4	6.0	0.3	71.3	1.8	127.4
5.3	48.6	74.2	2.6	79.4	220.2	335.4	1292.8	1.9	41.0	3.6	0.0	0.5	0.3	11.3	0.2	102.4	1.6	139.0
11.4	56.4	220.6	2.4	70.1	203.5	473.7	802.0	3.9	147.1	2.2	0.0	0.2	0.4	3.2	0.2	68.4	1.0	99.9
5.2	21.0	100.0	1.1	0.0	146.0	257.0	406.0	1.2	80.0	2.8	0.0	0.1	0.2	1.0	0.1	0.0	0.5	0.0
5.4	30.2	210.2	1.9	59.0	116.6	403.2	542.9	1.9	85.0	1.3	0.0	0.1	0.3	1.3	0.2	43.2	0.7	95.4
11.5	74.3	189.0	2.5	67.5	173.3	490.5	870.8	3.2	173.3	4.1	0.0	0.1	0.5	2.9	0.2	85.5	1.1	158.5
80.4	194.8	0.1	0.0	0.0	0.0	0.0	0.0	0.2	0.0	0.0	2.5	0.0	0.0	0.0	0.0	0.0	0.0	0.0
0.0	0.0	56.0	0.9	0.0	266.0	0.0	0.0	12.8	0.0	0.0	0.0	0.0	0.0	0.0	0.0	0.0	0.0	79.2
0.0	0.0	79.0	1.6	0.0	0.0	242.2	824.6	0.0	0.0	0.0	0.0	0.2	0.3	1.6	0.0	0.0	0.0	0.0
1.0	87.0	103.0	1.9	38.0	256.0	456.0	90.0	0.8	35.0	2.1	0.0	0.1	0.1	1.5	0.1	17.0	2.3	68.8
0.8	127.7	23.6	1.3	63.2	315.0	406.7	109.1	0.6	38.4	0.0	0.0	0.1	0.0	3.2	0.4	12.4	5.5	91.0
1.4	88.9	10.5	0.7	49.1	340.5	558.1	90.1	1.2	161.5	0.0	0.0	0.1	0.1	8.5	0.5	2.3	7.3	73.3
2.4	142.8	88.4	2.7	64.6	902.7	725.9	107.1	3.2	15.3	2.7	0.0	0.2	0.1	3.6	0.4	29.4	2.5	118.4
2.6	91.5	12.9	1.2	37.2	350.4	459.0	114.4	1.5	21.5	1.1	0.0	0.6	0.1	3.6	0.2	10.0	4.0	102.4
1.1	103.0	15.7	0.5	40.0	434.7	599.2	71.5	0.9	21.5	1.1	0.0	0.3	0.1	3.4	0.1	14.3	4.1	111.1
1.2	170.5	79.8	3.4	87.0	103.2	52.5	435.0	0.3	162.4	0.0	2.0	0.1	0.2	0.0	0.1	14.5	5.8	13.8
0.3	99.0	25.2	0.9	75.6	248.4	439.2	140.4	1.0	25.2	1.8	0.5	0.2	0.1	4.5	0.5	14.6	1.9	136.7
0.4	121.6	128.0	2.0	106.4	760.0	1166.4	5621.6	1.3	33.6	2.8	0.5	0.2	0.2	6.0	0.7	19.8	8.0	12.9
0.1	40.0	7.7	0.3	26.4	189.6	439.5	77.4	0.4	8.5	2.6	0.0	0.0	0.0	2.1	0.4	6.8	0.9	64.6
1.8	63.8	11.4	0.4	14.3	103.2	148.8	331.7	0.4	17.7	0.0	0.8	0.1	0.1	1.2	0.0	10.4	1.0	26.4
0.3	40.0	17.9	1.0	31.5	121.6	403.8	45.1	0.4	42.5	0.0	0.0	0.1	0.0	0.3	0.3	8.7	0.6	62.4
0.1	62.9	35.7	1.1	42.5	204.9	339.2	74.0	0.4	16.2	0.0	0.0	0.0	0.0	3.9	0.3	11.3	1.2	63.1
0.0	13.1	8.3	0.2	9.2	42.7	70.6	129.7	0.1	3.7	0.0	0.1	0.0	0.0	0.9	0.1	2.6	0.3	12.2
0.4	34.9	51.0	0.9	91.0	242.3	489.6	58.7	0.5	45.9	0.0	0.9	0.1	0.1	6.1	0.3	11.7	1.2	60.9
2.6	50.2	3.4	0.7	28.1	178.5	292.4	87.6	0.4	15.3	0.0	0.0	0.1	0.1	1.6	0.4	0.9	0.8	52.6
2.6	77.0	74.0	1.4	41.0	303.0	419.0	115.0	1.3	31.0	0.7	1.3	0.1	0.3	4.1	0.3	11.5	13.1	64.2
1.2	36.1	37.0	0.7	20.2	143.0	196.7	403.9	0.6	17.2	0.4	0.4	0.1	0.1	1.9	0.2	6.0	8.2	26.3
0.4	2.0	11.6	0.2	1.2	13.4	10.4	130.5	0.1	38.7	0.0	0.2	0.0	0.0	0.5	0.0	0.4	0.6	8.3
0.2	30.0	11.0	1.5	27.0	163.0	237.0	338.0	0.8	17.0	0.0	0.5	0.0	0.1	13.3	0.4	4.0	3.0	74.5
1.5	18.0	13.0	1.4	31.0	311.0	207.0	50.0	0.9	23.0	0.0	0.0	0.0	0.1	12.4	0.1	5.3	2.2	59.8
1.3	15.3	11.1	1.2	26.4	264.4	176.0	300.9	0.8	19.6	0.0	1.0	0.0	0.1	10.5	0.1	4.5	1.9	50.9
4.2	75.0	15.0	1.6	97.0	278.0	401.0	83.0	0.9	54.0	0.4	0.0	0.2	0.4	6.9	0.5	1.5	19.0	53.3
0.5	68.0	40.0	2.3	41.0	318.0	558.0	203.0	0.7	252.0	1.6	0.0	0.1	0.6	10.5	0.5	9.0	18.0	69.0
0.3	54.0	137.0	1.2	39.0	277.0	350.0	96.0	0.6	14.0	0.8	0.0	0.1	0.1	2.4	0.3	10.4	1.2	72.7
0.2	115.0	102.0	1.2	38.0	257.0	344.0	79.0	1.4	10.0	1.7	0.0	0.1	0.1	1.9	0.1	5.8	2.2	73.3
0.2	50.0	73.0	0.7	40.0	282.0	331.0	49.0	0.9	24.0	3.8	0.0	0.1	0.1	2.8	0.1	17.3	2.3	73.0
0.3	110.0	141.0	1.7	38.0	269.0	499.0	65.0	0.8	24.0	0.0	0.0	0.3	0.2	2.8	0.1	17.0	2.3	73.5
0.2	91.0	77.0	0.6	86.0	283.0	456.0	110.0	0.6	12.0	0.0	0.0	0.1	0.2	4.0	0.3	3.0	3.7	72.0
0.2	96.0	6.0	0.3	73.0	482.0	387.0	116.0	0.6	23.0	0.0	0.2	0.1	0.1	1.7	0.1	3.6	4.2	74.1
4.5	64.0	43.0	0.7	31.0	341.0	636.0	76.0	0.7	36.0	0.0	0.0	0.7	0.2	3.8	0.2	17.3	1.2	63.0
0.0	0.0	4.2	0.3	0.0	96.9	0.0	0.0	0.0	0.0	0.0	0.0	0.0	0.0	0.0	0.0	0.0	0.0	20.3
0.0	26.0	38.0	0.2	38.0	256.0	385.0	81.0	1.0	24.0	0.0	0.0	0.1	0.2	3.7	0.3	8.0	2.3	69.1
2.5	63.0	15.0	0.3	30.0	252.0	384.0	61.0	0.4	15.0	3.7	0.0	0.3	0.1	8.0	0.6	34.0	2.8	64.8
1.3	71.0	15.0	1.0	37.0	256.0	628.0	56.0	0.8	13.0	0.0	0.0	0.3	0.5	10.1	0.9	29.0	3.1	59.6

Code	Food Name	Unit/Amt	Wt (g)	Energy (Kcal)	Prot (g)	Carb (g)	Fiber (g)	Fat (g)	Mono (g)	Poly (g)
15210	Fish, Salmon, Chinook, cooked w/dry heat	3.5 oz	100	231.0	25.7	0.0	0.0	13.4	5.7	2.7
15077	Fish, Salmon, Chinook, smoked	3.5 oz	100	117.0	18.3	0.0	0.0	4.3	2.0	1.0
15179	Fish, Salmon, Chinook, smoked, lox, regular	1.0 oz	28	32.8	5.1	0.0	0.0	1.2	0.6	0.3
15239	Fish, Salmon, Coho, Farmed, cooked w/dry heat	3.5 oz	100	178.0	24.3	0.0	0.0	8.2	3.6	2.0
15247	Fish, Salmon, Coho, Wild, cooked w/dry heat	3.5 oz	100	139.0	23.5	0.0	0.0	4.3	1.6	1.3
15082	Fish, Salmon, Coho, Wild, cooked w/moist heat	3.5 oz	100	184.0	27.4	0.0	0.0	7.5	2.7	2.5
15084	Fish, Salmon, Pink, canned, solids & liquid	3.5 oz	100	139.0	19.8	0.0	0.0	6.1	1.8	2.0
15212	Fish, Salmon, Pink, cooked w/dry heat	3.5 oz	100	149.0	25.6	0.0	0.0	4.4	1.2	1.7
15088	Fish, Sardine, Atlantic, w/bone, canned in oil, drained	1 small fish (2.66 x 0.5" x 0.25")	12	25.0	3.0	0.0	0.0	1.4	0.5	0.6
15089	Fish, Sardine, Pacific, w/bone, canned in tom sauce, drained	1 sardine	38	67.6	6.2	0.0	0.0	4.6	2.1	0.9
15092	Fish, Sea Bass, baked or broiled (dry heat)	3.5 oz	100	124.0	23.6	0.0	0.0	2.6	0.5	1.0
15214	Fish, Sea Trout, cooked w/dry heat	3.5 oz	100	133.0	21.5	0.0	0.0	4.6	1.1	0.9
15215	Fish, Shad, American, cooked w/dry heat	3.5 oz	100	252.0	21.7	0.0	0.0	17.7	0.0	0.0
15096	Fish, Shark, battered, fried	4.0 oz	120	273.6	22.3	7.7	0.0	16.6	7.1	4.4
15102	Fish, Snapper, baked or broiled (dry heat)	3.5 oz	100	128.0	26.3	0.0	0.0	1.7	0.3	0.6
15218	Fish, Sunfish/Pumpkin Seed, cooked w/dry heat	3.5 oz	100	114.0	24.9	0.0	0.0	0.9	0.2	0.3
15109	Fish, Surimi	3.0 oz	85	84.2	12.9	5.8	0.0	0.8	0.1	0.4
15111	Fish, Swordfish, baked or broiled (dry heat)	3.5 oz	100	155.0	25.4	0.0	0.0	5.1	2.0	1.2
15219	Fish, Trout, cooked w/dry heat	3.5 oz	100	190.0	26.6	0.0	0.0	8.5	4.2	1.9
15241	Fish, Trout, Rainbow, Farmed, cooked w/dry heat	3.5 oz	100	169.0	24.3	0.0	0.0	7.2	2.1	2.3
15116	Fish, Trout, Rainbow, Wild, cooked w/dry heat	3.5 oz	100	150.0	22.9	0.0	0.0	5.8	1.7	1.8
924207	Fish, Tuna Noodle Casserole	6.0 oz	170	193.8	11.4	15.8	1.0	9.4	0.0	0.0
924208	Fish, Tuna Pot Pie, frozen/Banquet	7.0 oz	198	540.5	17.0	44.0	0.0	33.0	0.0	0.0
15128	Fish, Tuna Salad	3.0 oz	85	159.0	13.6	8.0	0.0	7.9	2.5	3.5
15118	Fish, Tuna, Bluefin, baked or broiled (dry heat)	3.0 oz	85	156.4	25.4	0.0	0.0	5.3	1.7	1.6
915905	Fish, Tuna, canned, low sodium	2.0 oz	58	70.2	15.0	0.0	0.0	1.0	0.0	0.8
15221	Fish, Tuna, Yellowfin, fresh, cooked w/dry heat	3.5 oz	100	139.0	30.0	0.0	0.0	1.2	0.2	0.4
15222	Fish, Turbot, European, cooked w/dry heat	3.5 oz	100	122.0	20.6	0.0	0.0	3.8	0.0	0.0
15126	Fish, White Tuna, canned in H20, drained	3.0 oz	85	108.8	20.1	0.0	0.0	2.5	0.7	0.9
15124	Fish, White Tuna, canned in oil, drained	3.0 oz	85	158.1	22.6	0.0	0.0	6.9	2.1	2.9
15223	Fish, Whitefish, cooked w/dry heat	3.0 oz	85	146.2	20.8	0.0	0.0	6.4	2.2	2.3
15133	Fish, Whiting, baked or broiled (dry heat)	1 fillet	72	83.5	16.9	0.0	0.0	1.2	0.3	0.4
15225	Fish, Yellowtail, cooked w/dry heat	3.5 oz	85	159.0	25.2	0.0	0.0	5.7	0.0	0.0
2050	Flavoring, Vanilla Extract	1 tsp	4.2	12.1	0.0	0.5	0.0	0.0	0.0	0.0
20003	Flour, Arrowroot	1 tbsp	8	28.6	0.0	7.1	0.3	0.0	0.0	0.0
20130	Flour, Barley Flour or Meal	1 tbsp	9.25	31.9	1.0	6.9	0.9	0.1	0.0	0.1
20131	Flour, Barley Malt Flour	1 tbsp	10.1	36.5	1.0	7.9	0.7	0.2	0.0	0.1
920904	Flour, Bisquick Mix	½ cup	57	240.0	4.0	37.0	0.0	8.0	5.0	1.0
20090	Flour, Brown Rice	1 cup	158	573.5	11.4	120.8	7.3	4.4	1.6	1.6
20011	Flour, Buckwheat, Whole Groat	1 cup	120	402.0	15.1	84.7	12.0	3.7	1.1	1.1
20017	Flour, Corn, Masa, enriched	1 cup	114	416.1	10.6	86.9	10.9	4.3	1.1	2.0
20316	Flour, Corn, White, Whole Grain	1 cup	117	422.4	8.1	89.9	11.2	4.5	1.2	2.1
20016	Flour, Corn, Yellow, Whole Grain	1 cup	117	422.4	8.1	89.9	15.7	4.5	1.2	2.1
924291	Flour, Potato	½ cup	90	315.9	7.2	71.9	0.0	0.7	0.0	0.3
20061	Flour, Rice, White	1 cup	163	596.6	9.7	130.6	3.9	2.3	0.7	0.6
920906	Flour, Rye&Wheat	1 cup	128	457.0	14.1	96.5	0.0	1.7	0.0	0.0
20063	Flour, Rye, Dark	1 cup	128	414.7	18.0	88.0	28.9	3.4	0.4	1.5
20065	Flour, Rye, Light	1 cup	128	469.8	10.7	102.7	18.7	1.7	0.2	0.7
20064	Flour, Rye, Medium	1 cup	128	453.1	12.0	99.2	18.7	2.3	0.3	1.0
20070	Flour, Triticale, Whole Grain	1 cup	128	432.6	16.9	93.6	18.7	2.3	0.2	1.0
20081	Flour, Wheat, White, All Purpose, bleached, enriched	1 cup	125	455.0	12.9	95.4	3.4	1.2	0.1	0.5
20082	Flour, Wheat, White, All Purpose, Selfrise, enriched	1 cup	125	442.5	12.4	92.8	3.4	1.2	0.1	0.5
20083	Flour, Wheat, White, Bread, enriched	1 cup	125	451.3	15.0	90.7	3.0	2.1	0.2	0.9
20084	Flour, Wheat, White, Cake, enriched	1 cup	125	452.5	10.3	97.5	2.1	1.1	0.1	0.5
20086	Flour, Wheat, White, Tortilla Mix, enriched	1 cup	125	506.3	12.1	83.9	0.0	13.3	5.7	1.9
20080	Flour, Whole Wheat, whole grain	1 cup	125	423.8	17.1	90.7	15.3	2.3	0.3	1.0
18268	French Toast, frozen	1 piece	59	125.7	4.4	18.9	0.7	3.6	1.2	0.7
18269	French Toast, homemade w/reduced fat (2%) milk	1 slice	65	148.9	5.0	16.3	0.0	7.0	2.9	1.7
918381	French Toast, homemade w/whole milk	1 slice	65	150.8	5.0	16.2	0.0	7.3	0.0	0.0
924287	Frozen Meal, Beef Chop Suey	12.0 oz	340	282.2	13.6	38.8	0.0	8.2	0.0	0.0
924062	Frozen Meal, Beef Chop Suey/Banquet	8.0 oz	227	104.4	9.8	9.8	0.0	3.0	0.0	0.0
924255	Frozen Meal, Beef Enchilada/Banquet	7.0 oz	198	269.3	10.0	28.0	0.0	13.0	0.0	0.0
22402	Frozen Meal, Beef Macaroni/Healthy Choice	1 serving	240	211.2	14.1	33.5	4.6	2.2	1.2	0.3
924026	Frozen Meal, Beef Oriental/LeMenuLite	10.0 oz	284	221.5	18.8	24.5	0.0	5.4	3.0	0.9
924080	Frozen Meal, Beef Pepper Steak, diet/Armour	11.25 oz	319	220.1	17.0	29.0	0.0	4.0	0.0	0.0
22578	Frozen Meal, Beef Pot Roast w/whipped potatoes/ Stoffer Lean Cuisine Homestyle	1 package	255	206.6	17.3	22.4	3.6	5.4	2.3	0.8
22616	Frozen Meal, Beef Sirloin Salisbury Steak w/red skinned pots & vege/ Budget Gourm	1 package	311	261.2	18.3	33.9	7.2	5.9	1.8	0.9

Sat (g)	Chol (mg)	Cal (mg)	Iron (mg)	Magn (mg)	Phos (mg)	Pota (mg)	Sodi (mg)	Zinc (mg)	Vit A (RE)	Vit C (mg)	Vit E (mg)	Thia (mg)	Ribo (mg)	Niac (mg)	Vit B-6 (mg)	Fol (µg)	Vit B-12 (µg)	Wat (g)
3.2	85.0	28.0	0.9	122.0	371.0	505.0	60.0	0.6	149.0	4.1	0.0	0.0	0.2	10.0	0.5	35.0	2.9	65.6
0.9	23.0	11.0	0.9	18.0	164.0	175.0	784.0	0.3	26.0	0.0	1.4	0.0	0.1	4.7	0.3	1.9	3.3	72.0
0.3	6.4	3.1	0.2	5.0	45.9	49.0	560.0	0.1	7.3	0.0	0.0	0.0	0.0	1.3	0.1	0.5	0.9	20.2
1.9	63.0	12.0	0.4	34.0	332.0	460.0	52.0	0.5	59.0	1.5	0.0	0.1	0.1	7.4	0.6	14.0	3.2	67.0
1.1	55.0	45.0	0.6	33.0	322.0	434.0	58.0	0.6	39.0	1.4	0.8	0.1	0.1	8.0	0.6	13.0	5.0	71.5
1.6	57.0	46.0	0.7	35.0	298.0	455.0	53.0	0.5	32.0	1.0	0.0	0.1	0.2	7.8	0.6	9.0	4.5	65.4
1.5	55.0	213.0	0.8	34.0	329.0	326.0	554.0	0.9	17.0	0.0	1.4	0.0	0.2	6.5	0.3	15.4	4.4	68.8
0.7	67.0	17.0	1.0	33.0	295.0	414.0	86.0	0.7	41.0	0.0	0.0	0.2	0.1	8.5	0.2	5.0	3.5	69.7
0.2	17.0	45.8	0.4	4.7	58.8	47.6	60.6	0.2	8.0	0.0	0.0	0.0	0.0	0.6	0.0	1.4	1.1	7.2
1.2	23.2	91.2	0.9	12.9	139.1	129.6	157.3	0.5	26.6	0.4	1.4	0.0	0.1	1.6	0.0	9.2	3.4	26.0
0.7	53.0	13.0	0.4	53.0	248.0	328.0	87.0	0.5	64.0	0.0	0.0	0.1	0.2	1.9	0.5	5.8	0.3	72.1
1.3	106.0	22.0	0.4	40.0	321.0	437.0	74.0	0.6	35.0	0.0	0.0	0.1	0.2	2.9	0.5	6.0	3.5	71.9
0.0	96.0	60.0	1.2	38.0	349.0	492.0	65.0	0.5	36.0	0.0	0.0	0.2	0.3	10.8	0.5	17.0	0.1	59.2
3.8	70.8	60.0	1.3	51.6	232.8	186.0	146.4	0.6	64.8	0.0	0.0	0.1	0.1	3.3	0.4	18.0	1.5	72.1
0.4	47.0	40.0	0.2	37.0	201.0	522.0	57.0	0.4	35.0	1.6	0.0	0.1	0.0	0.3	0.5	5.8	3.5	70.4
0.2	86.0	103.0	1.5	38.0	231.0	449.0	103.0	2.0	17.0	1.0	0.0	0.1	0.1	1.5	0.1	17.0	2.3	73.7
0.2	25.5	7.7	0.2	36.6	239.7	95.2	121.6	0.3	17.0	0.0	0.0	0.0	0.0	0.2	0.0	1.4	1.4	64.9
1.4	50.0	6.0	1.0	34.0	337.0	369.0	115.0	1.5	41.0	1.1	0.0	0.0	0.1	11.8	0.4	2.3	2.0	68.8
1.5	74.0	55.0	1.9	28.0	314.0	463.0	67.0	0.9	19.0	0.5	0.0	0.4	0.4	5.8	0.2	15.0	7.5	63.4
2.1	68.0	86.0	0.3	32.0	266.0	441.0	42.0	0.5	86.0	3.3	0.0	0.2	0.1	8.8	0.4	24.0	5.0	67.5
1.6	69.0	86.0	0.4	31.0	269.0	448.0	56.0	0.5	15.0	2.0	0.0	0.2	0.1	5.8	0.3	19.0	6.3	70.5
0.0	27.0	102.0	1.0	0.0	0.0	238.0	731.0	0.0	13.6	0.0	0.0	0.1	0.3	3.4	0.0	0.0	0.0	130.9
0.0	30.0	146.0	2.0	0.0	228.0	280.0	810.0	0.0	116.0	2.0	0.0	0.4	0.4	6.3	0.0	0.0	0.0	0.0
1.3	11.0	14.5	0.9	16.2	151.3	151.3	341.7	0.5	23.0	1.9	0.0	0.0	0.1	5.7	0.1	6.8	1.0	53.7
1.4	41.7	8.5	1.1	54.4	277.1	274.6	42.5	0.7	642.6	0.0	0.0	0.2	0.3	9.0	0.4	1.9	9.2	50.2
0.2	20.0	3.0	0.7	54.0	83.0	85.0	120.0	0.3	0.0	0.0	0.0	0.0	0.0	7.5	0.2	2.0	0.8	0.0
0.3	58.0	21.0	0.9	64.0	245.0	569.0	47.0	0.7	20.0	1.0	0.0	0.5	0.1	11.9	1.0	2.0	0.6	62.8
0.0	62.0	23.0	0.5	65.0	165.0	305.0	192.0	0.3	12.0	1.7	0.0	0.1	0.1	2.7	0.2	9.0	2.5	70.5
0.7	35.7	11.9	0.8	28.1	184.5	201.5	320.5	0.4	5.1	0.0	1.4	0.0	0.0	4.9	0.2	1.7	1.0	62.2
1.4	26.4	3.4	0.6	28.9	227.0	283.1	336.6	0.4	20.4	0.0	0.0	0.0	0.1	9.9	0.4	3.9	1.9	54.4
1.0	65.5	28.1	0.4	35.7	294.1	345.1	55.3	1.1	33.2	0.0	0.0	0.1	0.1	3.3	0.3	14.5	0.8	55.3
0.3	60.5	44.6	0.3	19.4	205.2	312.5	95.0	0.4	24.5	0.0	0.2	0.0	0.1	1.2	0.1	10.8	1.9	53.8
0.0	60.4	24.7	0.5	32.3	170.9	457.3	42.5	0.6	26.4	2.5	0.0	0.1	0.0	7.4	0.2	3.4	1.1	57.2
0.0	0.0	0.5	0.0	0.5	0.3	6.2	0.4	0.0	0.0	0.0	0.0	0.0	0.0	0.0	0.0	0.0	0.0	2.2
0.0	0.0	3.2	0.0	0.2	0.4	0.9	0.2	0.0	0.0	0.0	0.0	0.0	0.0	0.0	0.0	0.6	0.0	0.9
0.0	0.0	3.0	0.2	8.9	27.4	28.6	0.4	0.2	0.0	0.0	0.0	0.0	0.0	0.6	0.0	0.7	0.0	1.1
0.0	0.0	3.7	0.5	9.8	30.6	22.6	1.1	0.2	0.2	0.1	0.0	0.0	0.0	0.6	0.1	3.8	0.0	0.8
2.0	0.0	0.0	0.0	0.0	0.0	80.0	700.0	0.0	0.0	0.0	0.0	0.0	0.0	0.0	0.0	0.0	0.0	0.0
0.9	0.0	17.4	3.1	177.0	532.5	456.6	12.6	3.9	0.0	0.0	1.1	0.7	0.1	10.0	1.2	25.3	0.0	18.9
0.8	0.0	49.2	4.9	301.2	404.4	692.4	13.2	3.7	0.0	0.0	1.2	0.5	0.2	7.4	0.7	64.8	0.0	13.4
0.6	0.0	160.7	8.2	125.4	254.2	339.7	5.7	2.0	0.0	0.0	0.3	1.6	0.9	11.2	0.4	213.2	0.0	10.3
0.6	0.0	8.2	2.8	108.8	318.2	368.6	5.9	2.0	0.0	0.0	0.3	0.3	0.1	2.2	0.4	29.3	0.0	12.8
0.6	0.0	8.2	2.8	108.8	318.2	368.6	5.9	2.0	55.0	0.0	0.3	0.3	0.1	2.2	0.4	29.3	0.0	12.8
0.2	0.0	30.0	15.5	0.0	160.0	1429.0	31.0	0.0	0.0	17.0	0.0	0.4	0.1	3.1	0.0	0.0	0.0	6.8
0.6	0.0	16.3	0.6	57.1	159.7	123.9	0.0	1.3	0.0	0.0	0.2	0.2	0.0	4.2	0.7	6.5	0.0	19.4
0.0	0.0	27.4	4.6	0.0	224.0	190.9	2.3	0.0	0.0	0.0	0.0	0.6	0.3	5.0	0.0	0.0	0.0	14.7
0.4	0.0	71.7	8.3	317.4	809.0	934.4	1.3	7.2	0.0	0.0	3.3	0.4	0.3	5.5	0.6	76.8	0.0	14.2
0.2	0.0	26.9	2.3	89.6	248.3	298.2	2.6	2.2	0.0	0.0	0.7	0.4	0.1	1.0	0.3	28.2	0.0	11.2
0.3	0.0	30.7	2.7	96.0	265.0	435.2	3.8	2.5	0.0	0.0	1.7	0.4	0.1	2.2	0.3	24.3	0.0	12.6
0.4	0.0	44.8	3.3	195.8	410.9	596.5	2.6	3.4	0.0	0.0	2.4	0.5	0.2	3.7	0.5	94.7	0.0	12.8
0.2	0.0	18.8	5.8	27.5	135.0	133.8	2.5	0.9	0.0	0.0	0.1	1.0	0.6	7.4	0.1	192.5	0.0	14.9
0.2	0.0	422.5	5.8	23.8	743.8	155.0	1587.5	0.8	0.0	0.0	0.1	0.8	0.5	7.3	0.1	192.5	0.0	13.2
0.3	0.0	18.8	5.5	31.3	121.3	125.0	2.5	1.1	0.0	0.0	0.1	1.0	0.6	9.4	0.0	192.5	0.0	16.7
0.2	0.0	17.5	9.2	20.0	106.3	131.3	2.5	0.8	0.0	0.0	0.1	1.1	0.5	8.5	0.0	192.5	0.0	15.6
5.1	0.0	256.3	8.8	26.3	262.5	125.0	846.3	0.8	0.0	0.0	0.0	0.9	0.6	7.3	0.1	170.0	0.0	12.6
0.4	0.0	42.5	4.9	172.5	432.5	506.3	6.3	3.7	0.0	0.0	1.5	0.6	0.3	8.0	0.4	55.0	0.0	12.8
0.9	48.4	63.1	1.3	10.0	82.0	79.1	292.1	0.5	31.9	0.2	0.4	0.2	0.2	1.6	0.3	30.7	1.0	31.0
1.8	75.4	65.0	1.1	11.1	76.1	87.1	311.4	0.4	85.8	0.2	0.0	0.1	0.2	1.1	0.0	28.0	0.2	35.6
1.7	3.0	64.4	1.1	11.1	76.1	86.5	310.7	0.4	80.6	0.2	0.0	0.1	0.2	1.1	0.0	15.0	0.2	35.4
0.0	0.0	44.0	2.4	0.0	116.0	173.0	1802.0	0.0	68.0	4.0	0.0	0.1	0.1	3.0	0.0	0.0	0.0	0.0
1.5	0.0	32.0	2.1	0.0	68.0	136.0	1334.0	0.0	32.2	2.0	0.0	0.0	0.1	1.1	0.0	0.0	0.0	0.0
0.0	0.0	52.0	1.0	0.0	207.0	92.0	1477.0	0.0	35.8	0.0	0.0	0.0	0.2	1.9	0.0	0.0	0.0	0.0
0.7	14.4	45.6	2.7	36.0	134.4	364.8	444.0	1.2	50.4	58.1	1.5	0.3	0.2	3.1	0.2	105.6	0.1	187.7
1.5	39.0	39.0	3.4	0.0	0.0	362.0	560.0	0.0	289.8	9.0	0.0	0.1	0.5	3.4	0.0	0.0	0.0	0.0
0.0	35.0	50.0	2.0	0.0	139.0	320.0	970.0	0.0	105.4	15.0	0.0	0.2	0.3	1.6	0.0	0.0	0.0	0.0
1.3	38.3	0.0	0.0	0.0	0.0	0.0	494.7	0.0	0.0	0.0	0.0	0.0	0.0	0.0	0.0	0.0	0.0	206.8
2.0	43.5	0.0	3.0	0.0	0.0	0.0	494.5	0.0	0.0	51.0	0.0	0.0	0.0	0.0	0.0	0.0	0.0	249.7

Code	Food Name	Unit/Amt	Wt (g)	Energy (Kcal)	Prot (g)	Carb (g)	Fiber (g)	Fat (g)	Mono (g)	Poly (g)
924032	Frozen Meal, Beef Stew/Stouffer	5.0 oz	142	129.2	9.7	7.2	0.0	6.8	0.0	0.0
924229	Frozen Meal, Beef Stroganoff, diet/Armour	11.25 oz	319	248.8	18.0	33.0	0.0	6.0	0.0	0.0
924230	Frozen Meal, Beef Stroganoff/LeMenu	10.0 oz	284	383.4	26.5	23.8	0.0	20.3	0.0	0.0
924137	Frozen Meal, Beef Szechuan/LeanCuisine	9.2 oz	262	280.3	20.0	25.0	0.0	11.0	6.0	2.0
924231	Frozen Meal, Beef Teriyaki	9.0 oz	255	270.3	20.0	36.0	0.0	5.0	0.0	0.0
924025	Frozen Meal, Beef w/gravy/Banquet	4.0 oz	113	99.4	8.0	5.0	0.0	5.0	0.0	0.0
924268	Frozen Meal, Belgian Waffles&Berries/Swanson	3.5 oz	99	201.0	3.2	30.8	0.0	7.1	0.0	0.0
22679	Frozen Meal, Breakfast Burrito, Ham & Cheese Flavor	1 package	99	211.9	9.6	27.8	1.4	6.9	2.1	1.8
924031	Frozen Meal, Cannelloni/LeanCuisine	9.6 oz	273	270.3	19.0	25.0	0.0	10.0	5.0	1.0
924232	Frozen Meal, Cheese Cannelloni/Stouffer	5.5 oz	156	171.6	10.1	13.7	0.0	8.7	0.0	0.0
924292	Frozen Meal, Cheese Enchilada/Banquet	12.0 oz	340	550.8	22.0	71.0	0.0	19.0	0.0	0.0
924122	Frozen Meal, Cheese Lasagna/DiningLite	9.0 oz	225	261.0	14.0	36.0	0.0	6.0	0.0	0.0
924233	Frozen Meal, Cheese Tomato Cannelloni/LeanCuisine	9.1 oz	258	270.9	22.0	24.0	0.0	10.0	4.0	1.0
22577	Frozen Meal, Chicken & Vegetables w/vermicelli/Stouffer Lean Cuisine	1 package	297	252.5	18.7	32.1	5.0	5.6	2.1	1.4
22581	Frozen Meal, Chicken a l'Orange in Sauce w/broccoli & rice/ Stouffer's Lean Cuisi	1 package	255	267.8	24.5	38.5	0.0	1.8	0.5	0.4
924040	Frozen Meal, Chicken ala King&Rice/Swanson	9.0 oz	255	275.4	14.4	32.1	1.0	9.9	0.0	0.0
22610	Frozen Meal, Chicken Alfredo w/fettucini & vege/Stouffer's Lunch Express	1 package	272	372.6	19.0	32.6	3.8	18.5	6.3	2.4
924048	Frozen Meal, Chicken Cacciatore/LeanCuisine	10.9 oz	308	280.3	23.0	25.0	0.0	10.0	7.0	2.0
924234	Frozen Meal, Chicken Cannelloni, diet/LeMenu	10.3 oz	291	261.9	14.9	39.2	0.0	5.0	1.6	1.8
924254	Frozen Meal, Chicken Chow Mein/LeanCuisine	11.3 oz	319	248.8	14.0	36.0	0.0	5.0	3.0	1.0
22588	Frozen Meal, Chicken Enchilada Suprema w/green chili sauce, rice, corn&apple ras	1 package	320	297.6	13.0	46.0	4.2	6.7	2.6	1.0
924257	Frozen Meal, Chicken Enchilada/LeMenuLite	8.25 oz	234	269.1	19.1	33.2	0.0	6.6	2.7	1.9
924084	Frozen Meal, Chicken Fettucini/Armour	11.0 oz	312	259.0	17.0	28.0	0.0	9.0	0.0	0.0
924326	Frozen Meal, Chicken Fried Steak/Worthington	6.2 oz	176	580.8	28.0	25.0	1.0	41.0	0.0	0.0
924244	Frozen Meal, Chicken Parmesan/LeanCuisine	10.0 oz	283	249.0	25.0	19.0	0.0	8.0	4.0	2.0
924240	Frozen Meal, Chicken Piccata	11.0 oz	312	343.2	21.0	22.9	0.0	18.5	0.0	0.0
22906	Frozen Meal, Chicken Pot Pie, frozen entree	1 serving	217	483.9	13.0	42.7	1.7	29.1	12.5	4.5
22587	Frozen Meal, Chicken Teriyaki w/rice, mixed vege w/butter sauce& apple cherry com	1 package	312	268.3	17.1	37.1	2.8	5.6	2.2	0.5
924283	Frozen Meal, Chicken&Noodle/Armour	11.0 oz	312	230.9	19.0	23.0	0.0	7.0	0.0	0.0
924091	Frozen Meal, Chicken, Sweet&Sour Dinner/LeMenu	10.5 oz	298	381.4	18.8	41.0	0.0	15.7	0.0	0.0
924289	Frozen Meal, Corned Beef Hash	10.0 oz	284	372.0	19.9	42.6	0.0	13.3	0.0	0.0
924180	Frozen Meal, Egg Souffle w/broccoli&cheese/Stouffer	4.0 oz	113	151.4	8.4	7.7	0.0	9.6	0.0	0.0
22614	Frozen Meal, Escalloped Chicken & Noodles/Stouffer's	1 package	283	365.1	17.0	3.7	0.0	31.4	7.7	13.6
924294	Frozen Meal, Filet of Sole/LeMenu	10.0 oz	284	355.0	17.9	43.5	3.7	12.1	0.0	0.0
924216	Frozen Meal, Fried Chicken/Banquet	10.0 oz	284	400.4	15.0	45.0	0.0	22.0	0.0	0.0
924046	Frozen Meal, Glazed Chicken/LeanCuisine	8.5 oz	241	269.9	26.0	23.0	0.0	8.0	3.0	4.0
924261	Frozen Meal, Green Pepper Steak/Stouffer	3.0 oz	85	85.9	7.7	3.8	0.0	4.4	0.0	0.0
22673	Frozen Meal, Italian Sausage Lasagna/Budget Gourmet	1 package	298	455.9	20.6	39.9	3.0	23.8	9.8	2.0
924296	Frozen Meal, Lasagna	13.0 oz	369	391.1	13.0	54.0	0.0	14.0	0.0	0.0
22570	Frozen Meal, Lasagna w/meat & sauce/Stouffer	1 package	595	767.6	51.8	73.2	8.9	29.8	9.6	1.5
924117	Frozen Meal, Lasagna/LeanCuisine	10.3 oz	291	279.4	27.0	24.0	0.0	8.0	5.0	0.0
924267	Frozen Meal, Linguini w/clam sauce/LeanCuisine	9.6 oz	272	261.1	16.0	32.0	0.0	7.0	4.0	2.0
22576	Frozen Meal, Macaroni & Beef in Tomato Sauce/Stouffer Lean Cuisine	1 package	283	249.0	13.9	36.5	3.4	5.4	2.1	0.7
22680	Frozen Meal, Macaroni & Beef in Tomato Sauce/WW	1 package	269	282.5	15.6	44.7	6.7	4.6	1.8	0.6
924092	Frozen Meal, Macaroni&Cheese Dinner/Banquet	10.0 oz	284	420.3	14.0	46.0	0.0	20.0	0.0	0.0
924280	Frozen Meal, Manicotti w/tomato sauce/LeMenu	11.7 oz	333	392.9	20.0	44.3	0.0	15.2	0.0	0.0
22675	Frozen Meal, Meat Loaf w/tomato sauce, mashed pot & carrots in seasoned sauce/B	1 package	453	611.6	29.1	33.6	6.3	40.0	17.3	7.2
924114	Frozen Meal, Meatballs Italian Style/Stouffer	13.0 oz	369	483.4	24.5	60.4	0.2	15.9	0.0	0.0
924093	Frozen Meal, Meatloaf/LeMenu	10.0 oz	284	301.0	17.8	27.3	0.0	13.3	0.0	0.0
924302	Frozen Meal, Mexican Combo Dinner/Banquet	12.0 oz	340	520.2	20.0	72.0	0.0	17.0	0.0	0.0
924305	Frozen Meal, Noodles&Chicken/Banquet	10.0 oz	284	349.3	10.0	42.0	0.0	15.0	0.0	0.0
22571	Frozen Meal, Original Fried Chicken Meal w/mashed pots & corn in seasoned sauce/	1 package	228	469.7	21.5	35.1	2.1	27.0	15.4	2.4
924238	Frozen Meal, Pasta Primavera/Campbell	10.0 oz	284	14.2	22.2	39.9	0.0	0.0	0.0	0.0
924177	Frozen Meal, Pasta, Cheese Tortellini/Stouffer	4.5 oz	128	267.5	15.4	26.9	0.0	10.9	0.0	0.0
924308	Frozen Meal, Pasta, Ravioli Dinner/Swanson	16.0 oz	468	486.7	16.1	68.3	0.0	16.8	0.0	0.0
924193	Frozen Meal, Pasta, Spaghetti w/meat sauce/Banquet	8.0 oz	227	270.1	14.0	35.0	1.0	8.0	0.0	0.0
924191	Frozen Meal, Pasta, Spaghetti w/meat sauce/LeMenuLite	9.5 oz	269	285.1	12.6	44.6	0.0	6.1	3.6	1.3
924311	Frozen Meal, Pasta, Spaghetti&Meatballs/Swanson	12.5 oz	354	375.2	13.5	46.0	0.0	15.1	0.0	0.0
22569	Frozen Meal, Pepper, Stuffed w/Beef in Tomato Sauce/Stouffer	1 package	439	377.5	15.8	41.7	10.5	16.2	7.5	1.1
924090	Frozen Meal, Pork Ham/LeMenu	10.0 oz	284	286.8	18.3	31.0	0.0	10.1	0.0	0.0
22609	Frozen Meal, Rice & Chicken Stir-Fry w/vegetables/ Stouffer's Lean Cuisine Lunch	1 package	255	270.3	11.7	39.5	5.9	7.4	3.5	2.0
924156	Frozen Meal, Rigatoni Pasta/Stouffer	6.0 oz	170	180.2	11.7	17.0	0.0	7.1	0.0	0.0

Sat (g)	Chol (mg)	Cal (mg)	Iron (mg)	Magn (mg)	Phos (mg)	Pota (mg)	Sodi (mg)	Zinc (mg)	Vit A (RE)	Vit C (mg)	Vit E (mg)	Thia (mg)	Ribo (mg)	Niac (mg)	Vit B-6 (mg)	Fol (µg)	Vit B-12 (µg)	Wat (g)
0.0	28.0	14.0	1.3	0.0	0.0	213.0	540.0	0.0	213.0	3.0	0.0	0.1	0.1	1.4	0.0	0.0	0.0	116.4
0.0	55.0	56.0	2.0	0.0	196.0	320.0	510.0	0.0	580.8	43.0	0.0	0.3	0.2	1.6	0.0	0.0	0.0	0.0
0.0	0.0	107.0	4.3	0.0	0.0	469.0	867.0	0.0	220.6	1.0	0.0	0.1	0.3	5.1	0.0	0.0	0.0	0.0
3.0	95.0	40.0	1.8	0.0	0.0	320.0	720.0	0.0	250.0	12.0	0.0	0.1	0.3	4.0	0.0	0.0	0.0	0.0
0.0	45.0	29.0	2.0	0.0	152.0	370.0	850.0	0.0	146.4	2.0	0.0	0.2	0.2	3.4	0.0	0.0	0.0	0.0
0.0	40.0	10.0	2.0	0.0	0.0	81.0	426.0	0.0	5.8	0.0	0.0	0.0	0.1	1.2	0.0	0.0	0.0	0.0
0.0	0.0	45.0	1.1	0.0	0.0	165.0	235.0	0.0	3.8	3.0	0.0	0.1	0.1	0.7	0.0	0.0	0.0	0.0
2.0	192.1	0.0	3.2	0.0	0.0	0.0	404.9	0.0	0.0	0.0	0.0	0.0	0.0	0.0	0.0	0.0	0.0	53.3
4.0	45.0	200.0	1.4	0.0	0.0	400.0	940.0	0.0	400.0	0.0	0.0	0.2	0.3	2.0	0.0	0.0	0.0	0.0
0.0	20.0	218.0	0.6	0.0	0.0	218.0	608.0	0.0	156.0	17.0	0.0	0.1	0.2	0.9	0.0	0.0	0.0	121.7
0.0	0.0	281.0	3.0	0.0	388.0	420.0	2170.0	0.0	142.2	7.0	0.0	0.4	0.3	2.4	0.0	0.0	0.0	0.0
0.0	0.0	307.0	2.0	0.0	0.0	770.0	800.0	0.0	397.6	7.0	0.0	0.2	0.3	1.9	0.0	0.0	0.0	0.0
5.0	30.0	300.0	0.7	0.0	0.0	330.0	900.0	0.0	150.0	6.0	0.0	0.1	0.3	1.2	0.0	0.0	0.0	0.0
1.0	23.8	104.0	1.3	0.0	0.0	0.0	582.1	0.0	0.0	14.6	0.0	0.0	0.0	0.0	0.0	0.0	0.0	237.9
0.4	45.9	0.0	0.0	0.0	0.0	0.0	359.6	0.0	0.0	18.1	0.0	0.0	0.0	0.0	0.0	0.0	0.0	188.4
0.0	0.0	64.0	0.9	0.0	0.0	217.0	859.0	0.0	116.6	2.0	0.0	0.1	0.3	5.0	0.0	0.0	0.0	0.0
7.0	57.1	146.9	0.0	0.0	0.0	0.0	587.5	0.0	0.0	24.2	0.0	0.0	0.0	0.0	0.0	0.0	0.0	199.1
1.0	45.0	40.0	1.8	0.0	0.0	440.0	950.0	0.0	100.0	12.0	0.0	0.1	0.2	5.0	0.0	0.0	0.0	0.0
1.6	38.0	93.0	3.1	0.0	0.0	368.0	621.0	0.0	350.6	9.0	0.0	0.6	0.4	3.2	0.0	0.0	0.0	0.0
1.0	30.0	40.0	1.1	0.0	0.0	270.0	1030.0	0.0	20.0	15.0	0.0	0.1	0.2	4.0	0.0	0.0	0.0	0.0
3.1	38.4	134.4	0.8	0.0	236.8	384.0	563.2	0.0	0.0	18.2	0.0	0.0	0.0	0.0	0.0	0.0	0.0	251.5
2.0	33.0	215.0	1.8	0.0	0.0	624.0	537.0	0.0	68.8	11.0	0.0	0.1	0.4	3.2	0.0	0.0	0.0	0.0
0.0	50.0	146.0	2.0	0.0	300.0	400.0	660.0	0.0	329.8	61.0	0.0	0.2	0.2	3.8	0.0	0.0	0.0	0.0
0.0	95.0	20.0	4.1	0.0	198.0	390.0	1040.0	0.0	9.4	0.0	0.0	0.2	0.2	4.9	0.0	0.0	0.0	0.0
2.0	70.0	150.0	1.4	0.0	0.0	750.0	850.0	0.0	100.0	6.0	0.0	0.2	0.3	7.0	0.0	0.0	0.0	0.0
0.0	0.0	96.0	2.9	0.0	0.0	135.0	1148.0	0.0	178.6	6.0	0.0	0.2	0.1	8.0	0.0	0.0	0.0	0.0
9.7	41.2	32.6	2.1	23.9	119.4	256.1	857.2	1.0	342.9	1.5	3.8	0.3	0.4	4.1	0.2	52.1	0.2	130.0
3.0	43.7	37.4	1.1	0.0	224.6	424.3	602.2	0.0	0.0	12.2	0.0	0.0	0.0	0.0	0.0	0.0	0.0	249.6
0.0	50.0	87.0	2.0	0.0	213.0	540.0	660.0	0.0	895.6	57.0	0.0	0.2	0.2	4.7	0.0	0.0	0.0	0.0
0.0	0.0	80.0	2.1	0.0	0.0	400.0	1020.0	0.0	329.6	5.0	0.0	0.1	0.2	5.5	0.0	0.0	0.0	0.0
0.0	0.0	65.0	4.0	0.0	148.0	318.0	1752.0	0.0	70.4	13.0	0.0	0.2	0.1	3.1	0.0	0.0	0.0	0.0
0.0	141.0	130.0	0.9	0.0	0.0	158.0	509.0	0.0	65.6	9.0	0.0	0.1	0.3	0.5	0.0	0.0	0.0	84.8
6.6	76.4	116.0	1.1	0.0	0.0	0.0	1211.2	0.0	0.0	0.0	0.0	0.0	0.0	0.0	0.0	0.0	0.0	202.9
0.0	0.0	105.0	2.0	0.0	0.0	341.0	956.0	0.0	415.8	2.0	0.0	0.2	0.3	2.4	0.0	0.0	0.0	0.0
0.0	0.0	46.0	1.0	0.0	0.0	480.0	1100.0	0.0	112.8	8.0	0.0	0.1	0.1	4.9	0.0	0.0	0.0	0.0
1.0	60.0	20.0	0.7	0.0	0.0	390.0	710.0	0.0	20.0	2.0	0.0	0.1	0.1	8.0	0.0	0.0	0.0	0.0
0.0	19.0	14.0	0.9	0.0	0.0	170.0	527.0	0.0	27.2	7.0	0.0	0.0	0.1	1.5	0.0	0.0	0.0	67.2
8.2	47.7	315.9	2.7	0.0	0.0	0.0	902.9	0.0	0.0	0.0	0.0	0.0	0.0	0.0	0.0	0.0	0.0	209.5
0.0	0.0	0.0	0.0	0.0	0.0	0.0	825.0	0.0	0.0	0.0	0.0	0.0	0.0	0.0	0.0	0.0	0.0	0.0
13.0	113.1	636.7	0.0	0.0	0.0	0.0	2034.9	0.0	0.0	0.0	0.0	0.0	0.0	0.0	0.0	0.0	0.0	431.4
3.0	70.0	250.0	1.4	0.0	0.0	540.0	1000.0	0.0	400.0	5.0	0.0	0.9	0.4	4.0	0.0	0.0	0.0	0.0
1.0	30.0	20.0	1.8	0.0	0.0	100.0	800.0	0.0	0.0	0.0	0.0	0.1	0.1	1.2	0.0	0.0	0.0	0.0
1.6	22.6	0.0	2.2	0.0	0.0	0.0	563.2	0.0	0.0	157.3	0.0	0.0	0.0	0.0	0.0	0.0	0.0	224.7
1.6	13.5	0.0	5.7	0.0	0.0	0.0	492.3	0.0	0.0	27.4	0.0	0.0	0.0	0.0	0.0	0.0	0.0	201.5
0.0	30.0	272.0	3.0	0.0	0.0	340.0	450.0	0.0	1517.6	7.0	0.0	0.3	0.4	2.4	0.0	0.0	0.0	0.0
0.0	0.0	493.0	3.1	0.0	0.0	4.0	871.0	0.0	22.0	17.0	0.0	0.3	0.4	4.0	0.0	0.0	0.0	0.0
15.5	113.3	77.0	3.9	0.0	0.0	0.0	1943.4	0.0	0.0	7.7	0.0	0.0	0.0	0.0	0.0	0.0	0.0	343.4
0.0	0.0	148.0	5.7	0.0	0.0	645.0	935.0	0.0	335.8	16.0	0.0	0.3	0.4	4.9	0.0	0.0	0.0	0.0
0.0	0.0	97.0	4.0	0.0	0.0	626.0	860.0	0.0	934.4	5.0	0.0	0.2	0.3	4.3	0.0	0.0	0.0	0.0
0.0	0.0	194.0	3.0	0.0	418.0	420.0	1980.0	0.0	107.8	7.0	0.0	0.4	0.2	2.7	0.0	0.0	0.0	0.0
0.0	45.0	29.0	2.0	0.0	0.0	250.0	460.0	0.0	1378.0	2.0	0.0	0.2	0.2	3.8	0.0	0.0	0.0	0.0
9.3	88.9	38.8	1.4	0.0	0.0	0.0	1500.2	0.0	0.0	1.4	0.0	0.0	0.0	0.0	0.0	0.0	0.0	140.8
0.0	0.0	265.0	2.4	0.0	0.0	80.0	882.0	0.0	204.4	2.0	0.0	0.1	0.3	2.1	0.0	0.0	0.0	0.0
0.0	77.0	243.0	1.0	0.0	0.0	95.0	326.0	0.0	7.6	1.0	0.0	0.1	0.2	1.2	0.0	0.0	0.0	73.0
0.0	0.0	162.0	4.4	0.0	0.0	275.0	975.0	0.0	196.6	25.0	0.0	0.3	0.3	4.2	0.0	0.0	0.0	0.0
0.0	0.0	29.0	3.0	0.0	188.0	421.0	1250.0	0.0	179.6	14.0	0.0	0.1	0.1	3.2	0.0	0.0	0.0	0.0
1.2	14.0	45.0	3.9	0.0	0.0	494.0	406.0	0.0	146.4	32.0	0.0	0.2	0.3	3.0	0.0	0.0	0.0	0.0
0.0	0.0	113.0	3.1	0.0	177.0	411.0	1097.0	2.4	242.4	14.0	0.0	0.2	0.2	3.4	0.2	0.0	0.5	0.0
5.4	43.9	0.0	0.0	0.0	0.0	0.0	1154.6	0.0	0.0	173.0	0.0	0.0	0.0	0.0	0.0	0.0	0.0	360.9
0.0	0.0	67.0	2.2	0.0	0.0	426.0	1486.0	0.0	1479.4	31.0	0.0	0.6	0.3	4.5	0.0	0.0	0.0	0.0
0.9	25.5	0.0	0.0	0.0	0.0	0.0	632.4	0.0	0.0	23.7	0.0	0.0	0.0	0.0	0.0	0.0	0.0	193.8
0.0	22.0	170.0	1.7	0.0	0.0	357.0	510.0	0.0	85.0	9.0	0.0	0.1	0.2	2.2	0.0	0.0	0.0	130.9

Code	Food Name	Unit/Amt	Wt (g)	Energy (Kcal)	Prot (g)	Carb (g)	Fiber (g)	Fat (g)	Mono (g)	Poly (g)
22712	Frozen Meal, Roasted Chicken w/garlic sauce, pasta & vegetable medley/Tyson	1 package	255	214.2	16.9	21.5	3.6	6.7	2.3	2.1
22583	Frozen Meal, Salisbury Steak in gravy & macaroni & cheese/ Stouffer Homestyle	1 package	272	386.2	22.6	26.4	0.0	21.2	7.9	1.8
924157	Frozen Meal, Salisbury Steak/Banquet	5.0 oz	142	190.3	9.0	8.0	0.5	14.0	0.0	0.0
924204	Frozen Meal, Sliced Beef/Swanson	15.2 oz	432	453.6	37.8	50.0	0.0	11.3	0.0	0.0
22580	Frozen Meal, Spaghetti w/meat sauce/Stouffer's Lean Cuisine	1 package	326	313.0	14.3	50.5	5.5	5.9	2.3	1.3
924260	Frozen Meal, Stuffed Shells/LeMenuLite	10.0 oz	284	269.8	17.3	33.5	0.0	7.3	2.8	1.2
22573	Frozen Meal, Swedish Meatballs w/pasta/Stouffer's Lean Cuisine	1 package	258	276.1	21.7	31.2	2.6	7.2	2.3	1.0
924101	Frozen Meal, Swiss Steak/Swanson	10.0 oz	284	346.5	26.2	37.0	0.0	10.5	0.0	0.0
22683	Frozen Meal, Teriyaki Chicken Breast w/Oriental veges/ Budget Gourmet Light & Hea	1 package	311	317.2	18.7	52.2	4.0	3.7	0.9	1.6
924176	Frozen Meal, Turkey w/gravy	5.0 oz	142	95.1	8.4	6.6	0.1	3.7	1.4	0.7
924215	Frozen Meal, Turkey w/gravy/Banquet	5.0 pz	142	99.4	7.0	5.0	0.1	6.0	0.0	0.0
924175	Frozen Meal, Turkey&Dressing/Armour	11.5 oz	326	319.5	19.0	34.0	0.0	12.0	0.0	0.0
924103	Frozen Meal, Turkey/Banquet	10.5 oz	298	390.4	18.0	35.0	0.0	20.0	0.0	0.0
924304	Frozen Meal, Veal Marsala/LeMenuLite	10.0 oz	284	249.9	25.3	25.4	0.0	5.2	3.2	1.0
924314	Frozen Meal, Veal Parmigiana Dinner/Armour	11.25 oz	319	398.8	18.0	34.0	0.0	22.0	0.0	0.0
924061	Frozen Meal, Vegetable Chow Mein/LeanCuisine	¾ cup	128	34.6	2.0	6.0	2.0	0.0	0.0	0.0
924115	Frozen Meal, Vegetable Lasagna/LeMenuLite	10.5 oz	298	253.3	12.4	34.0	0.0	7.4	3.2	1.5
924121	Frozen Meal, Vegetarian Lasagna	7.8 oz	221	316.0	20.0	30.0	2.0	14.0	5.0	1.5
924301	Frozen Meal, Ziti w/meat sauce/Swanson	17.6 oz	489	557.5	28.4	58.4	0.0	23.5	0.0	0.0
914896	Fruit Beverage Mix, Fruit Punch Drink, dry, prep	8 fl oz	262	96.9	0.0	24.8	0.0	23.6	0.0	0.0
914847	Fruit Beverage Mix, Grape/Crystal Light	8 fl oz	238	2.4	0.1	0.3	0.0	0.0	0.0	0.0
914844	Fruit Beverage Mix, Kool-Aid	8 fl oz	240	98.4	0.0	25.1	0.0	0.0	0.0	0.0
14127	Fruit Beverage Mix, Kool-Aid, sugar free w/aspartame & Vit C, dry mix, cherry fl	⅛ envelope	1.2	3.5	0.1	1.0	0.0	0.0	0.0	0.0
14290	Fruit Beverage Mix, Lemonade w/aspartame, low kcal, dry, prep	1 fl oz	29.6	0.6	0.0	0.1	0.0	0.0	0.0	0.0
14288	Fruit Beverage Mix, Lemonade, dry, prep w/H$_2$O	1 cup H$_2$O & 2 tbsp mix	264	103.0	0.0	26.9	0.0	0.0	0.0	0.0
914845	Fruit Beverage Mix, Lemonade/CountryTime	8 fl oz	240	81.6	0.0	20.5	0.0	0.0	0.0	0.0
14408	Fruit Beverage Mix, Orange Flavor Drink, dry, prep w/H$_2$O	1 oz	31	14.3	0.0	3.7	0.0	0.0	0.0	0.0
914807	Fruit Beverage Mix, w/sugar/Kool-Aid	8 fl oz	240	81.6	0.0	21.0	0.0	0.0	0.0	0.0
914897	Fruit Beverage, Cherry Juice Drink	6 fl oz	182	96.5	0.2	23.6	0.0	0.1	0.0	0.1
14263	Fruit Beverage, Citrus Drink, frozen concentrate, prep w/H$_2$O	1 cup (8 fl oz)	245	112.7	0.7	28.2	0.0	0.0	0.0	0.0
14238	Fruit Beverage, Cranberry-Apple Drink, bottled	1 cup (8 fl oz)	245	164.2	0.2	41.9	0.2	0.0	0.0	0.0
14242	Fruit Beverage, Cranberry Cocktail, bottled	12 fl oz can	435	248.0	0.0	62.6	0.4	0.4	0.1	0.2
14431	Fruit Beverage, Cranberry Juice Cocktail, frozen concentrate, prep w/H$_2$O	1 cup (8 fl oz)	262	144.1	0.0	36.7	0.3	0.0	0.0	0.0
14267	Fruit Beverage, Fruit Punch, canned	1 cup	247	116.1	0.0	29.4	0.2	0.0	0.0	0.0
14269	Fruit Beverage, Fruit Punch, frozen concentrate, prep w/H$_2$O	1 cup	247	113.6	0.0	28.9	0.2	0.0	0.0	0.0
14282	Fruit Beverage, Grape Juice Drink, canned	6 fl oz glass	188	94.0	0.2	24.3	0.2	0.0	0.0	0.0
914848	Fruit Beverage, Grapefruit Juice Cocktail	6 fl oz	180	79.2	0.0	20.0	0.1	0.0	0.0	0.0
914842	Fruit Beverage, Hawaiian Punch	8 fl oz	247	121.0	0.0	29.0	0.0	0.0	0.0	0.0
14406	Fruit Beverage, Juice Drink, frozen concentrate, prep	1 fl oz	31	15.5	0.0	3.8	0.0	0.1	0.0	0.0
914898	Fruit Beverage, Lemonade, canned	6 fl oz	184	64.4	0.0	16.5	0.0	0.0	0.0	0.0
14543	Fruit Beverage, Lemonade, Pink, frozen conc, prep w/H$_2$O	6 fl oz	186	74.4	0.2	19.5	0.0	0.0	0.0	0.0
14293	Fruit Beverage, Lemonade, White, frozen, prep w/H$_2$O	6 fl oz	186	74.4	0.2	19.5	0.2	0.0	0.0	0.0
14303	Fruit Beverage, Limeade, frozen concentrate, prep w/H$_2$O	6 fl oz	186	76.3	0.0	20.5	0.2	0.0	0.0	0.0
914843	Fruit Beverage, low kcal/Hawaiian Punch	8 fl oz	247	34.6	0.1	8.0	0.0	0.0	0.0	0.0
14323	Fruit Beverage, Orange Drink, canned	6 fl oz	186	94.9	0.0	24.0	0.2	0.0	0.0	0.0
914900	Fruit Beverage, Orange-Pineapple Juice Drink	6 fl oz	180	93.6	0.6	23.0	1.0	0.0	0.0	0.0
14334	Fruit Beverage, Pineapple & Grapefruit Juice Drink, canned	6 fl oz	186	87.4	0.4	21.6	0.2	0.2	0.0	0.1
14341	Fruit Beverage, Pineapple & Orange Juice Drink, canned	6 fl oz	186	93.0	2.4	21.9	0.2	0.2	0.0	0.1
914808	Fruit Beverage, Sugar Free/Kool-Aid	8 fl oz	240	2.4	0.1	0.3	0.0	0.0	0.0	0.0
914903	Fruit Beverage, Wild Berry Juice Drink	6 fl oz	185	90.7	0.0	23.0	0.0	0.0	0.0	0.0
9101	Fruit Cocktail (peach,pineapple,pear,grape&cherry)canned in ex-heavy syrup	½ cup	130	114.4	0.5	29.8	1.4	0.1	0.0	0.0
9098	Fruit Cocktail (peach,pineapple,pear,grape&cherry)canned in extralite syrup	½ cup	122	54.9	0.5	14.2	1.3	0.1	0.0	0.0
914839	Fruit Juice, Apple Juice Works/Campbells	6 fl oz	180	97.2	0.3	23.7	0.0	0.1	0.0	0.0
9400	Fruit Juice, Apple, canned or bottled, unsweetened w/added Vit C	6 fl oz	180	84.6	0.1	21.0	0.2	0.2	0.0	0.1
9411	Fruit Juice, Apple, frozen concentrate, unsweetened w/added Vit C, prep	6 fl oz container	211	99.2	0.3	24.3	0.2	0.2	0.0	0.1
9403	Fruit Juice, Apricot Nectar, canned, w/added Vit C	6 fl oz container	211	118.2	0.8	30.4	1.3	0.2	0.1	0.0
914910	Fruit Juice, Cranberry Apple Juice	6 fl oz container	211	192.0	1.1	48.8	1.1	10.2	0.0	0.0
914907	Fruit Juice, Cranberry Apple Juice, low kcal	6 fl oz container	211	35.9	0.2	8.4	0.0	0.2	0.0	0.2
9137	Fruit Juice, Grape, frozen concentrate, sweetened w/added Vit C, prep	6 fl oz container	216	110.2	0.4	27.5	0.2	0.2	0.0	0.1
9124	Fruit Juice, Grapefruit, canned, sweetened	6 fl oz container	216	99.4	1.3	24.0	0.2	0.2	0.0	0.0
9123	Fruit Juice, Grapefruit, canned, unsweetened	6 fl oz container	216	82.1	1.1	19.4	0.2	0.2	0.0	0.0
9126	Fruit Juice, Grapefruit, frozen concentrate, unsweetened, prep	1 fl oz	30.9	12.7	0.2	3.0	0.0	0.0	0.0	0.0
9404	Fruit Juice, Grapefruit, Pink or Red, fresh	1 cup	247	96.3	1.2	22.7	0.0	0.2	0.0	0.1
9128	Fruit Juice, Grapefruit, white, fresh	juice from 1 fruit	196	76.4	1.0	18.0	0.2	0.2	0.0	0.0
9153	Fruit Juice, Lemon, canned or bottled	1 tbsp	15.2	3.2	0.1	1.0	0.1	0.0	0.0	0.0

Sat (g)	Chol (mg)	Cal (mg)	Iron (mg)	Magn (mg)	Phos (mg)	Pota (mg)	Sodi (mg)	Zinc (mg)	Vit A (RE)	Vit C (mg)	Vit E (mg)	Thia (mg)	Ribo (mg)	Niac (mg)	Vit B-6 (mg)	Fol (µg)	Vit B-12 (µg)	Wat (g)
1.3	28.1	0.0	1.6	0.0	0.0	0.0	466.7	0.0	0.0	0.0	0.0	0.0	0.0	0.0	0.0	0.0	0.0	207.5
8.0	62.6	195.8	2.3	0.0	0.0	0.0	1014.6	0.0	0.0	0.0	0.0	0.0	0.0	0.0	0.0	0.0	0.0	198.0
0.0	35.0	49.0	1.9	0.0	0.0	180.0	766.0	0.0	5.8	0.0	0.0	0.1	0.1	1.1	0.2	0.0	1.2	0.0
0.0	0.0	43.0	5.9	0.0	0.0	772.0	1003.0	0.0	105.2	7.0	0.0	0.2	0.4	7.7	0.0	0.0	0.0	0.0
1.4	13.0	0.0	2.1	0.0	0.0	0.0	609.6	0.0	0.0	34.9	0.0	0.0	0.0	0.0	0.0	0.0	0.0	252.3
3.3	20.0	241.0	2.7	0.0	0.0	315.0	686.0	0.0	268.2	34.0	0.0	0.1	0.1	2.0	0.0	0.0	0.0	0.0
2.4	46.4	0.0	2.1	0.0	0.0	0.0	562.4	0.0	0.0	0.0	0.0	0.0	0.0	0.0	0.0	0.0	0.0	195.6
0.0	0.0	49.0	4.4	0.0	0.0	483.0	701.0	0.0	112.6	11.0	0.0	0.2	0.2	4.6	0.0	0.0	0.0	0.0
0.6	24.9	0.0	0.0	0.0	0.0	0.0	674.9	0.0	0.0	44.5	0.0	0.0	0.0	0.0	0.0	0.0	0.0	233.9
1.2	45.0	20.0	1.3	12.0	114.0	0.0	786.0	1.0	11.8	0.0	0.0	0.0	0.2	2.6	0.1	0.0	0.0	120.8
0.0	45.0	19.0	0.7	0.0	0.0	83.0	586.0	0.0	1.6	0.0	0.0	0.0	0.1	1.7	0.0	0.0	0.0	0.0
0.0	50.0	95.0	2.0	0.0	206.0	520.0	1280.0	0.0	601.2	8.0	0.0	0.3	0.2	5.5	0.0	0.0	0.0	0.0
0.0	40.0	49.0	1.0	0.0	228.0	500.0	1110.0	0.0	109.2	6.0	0.0	0.1	0.2	5.8	0.0	0.0	0.0	0.0
1.0	112.0	33.0	1.8	0.0	0.0	492.0	728.0	0.0	243.2	3.0	0.0	0.2	0.5	7.4	0.0	0.0	0.0	0.0
0.0	55.0	164.0	3.0	0.0	169.0	520.0	1320.0	0.0	220.4	27.0	0.0	0.3	0.3	3.6	0.0	0.0	0.0	0.0
0.0	0.0	80.0	0.7	0.0	0.0	175.0	780.0	0.0	200.0	15.0	0.0	0.0	0.4	0.0	0.0	0.0	0.0	0.0
2.7	24.0	174.0	2.8	0.0	0.0	531.0	462.0	0.0	367.6	44.0	0.0	0.2	0.4	2.8	0.0	0.0	0.0	0.0
7.0	30.0	457.0	2.4	0.0	345.0	424.0	760.0	2.0	33.6	7.0	0.0	0.2	0.3	2.0	0.2	14.0	0.0	0.0
0.0	0.0	255.0	7.5	0.0	0.0	1027.0	1689.0	0.0	476.2	38.0	0.0	0.4	0.4	6.6	0.0	0.0	0.0	0.0
0.0	0.0	41.0	0.1	3.0	52.0	2.0	38.0	0.1	0.0	31.0	0.0	0.0	0.0	0.0	0.0	0.0	0.0	236.8
0.0	0.0	0.0	0.0	14.0	0.0	0.0	0.0	0.0	0.0	6.0	0.0	0.0	0.0	0.0	0.0	0.0	0.0	236.8
0.0	0.0	15.0	0.0	0.0	7.0	1.0	14.0	0.0	0.0	6.0	0.0	0.0	0.0	0.0	0.0	0.0	0.0	0.0
0.0	0.0	0.0	0.0	0.0	0.0	0.0	5.1	0.0	0.0	6.7	0.0	0.0	0.0	0.0	0.0	0.0	0.0	0.0
0.0	0.0	6.2	0.0	0.3	3.0	0.0	0.9	0.0	0.0	0.7	0.0	0.0	0.0	0.0	0.0	0.0	0.0	29.4
0.0	0.0	71.3	0.2	2.6	34.3	34.3	13.2	0.1	0.0	8.4	0.0	0.0	0.0	0.0	0.0	3.4	0.0	236.8
0.0	0.0	1.0	0.0	16.0	0.0	12.0	21.0	0.0	0.0	6.0	0.0	0.0	0.0	0.0	0.0	0.0	0.0	220.0
0.0	0.0	7.8	0.0	0.3	4.7	6.2	1.6	0.0	68.8	15.1	0.0	0.0	0.0	0.0	0.0	17.9	0.0	27.3
0.0	0.0	26.0	0.0	0.0	11.0	1.0	19.0	0.0	0.0	6.0	0.0	0.0	0.0	0.0	0.0	0.0	0.0	0.0
0.0	0.0	20.0	0.9	0.0	0.0	118.0	18.0	0.0	0.0	7.0	0.0	0.0	0.0	0.4	0.0	0.0	0.0	0.0
0.0	0.0	22.1	2.7	14.7	24.5	274.4	7.4	0.1	9.8	66.4	0.0	0.0	0.0	0.4	0.1	4.9	0.0	215.1
0.0	0.0	17.2	0.1	4.9	7.4	66.2	4.9	0.1	0.0	78.4	0.0	0.0	0.0	0.1	0.1	0.5	0.0	202.9
0.0	0.0	13.1	0.7	8.7	8.7	78.3	8.7	0.3	0.0	154.0	0.0	0.0	0.0	0.2	0.1	0.9	0.0	371.9
0.0	0.0	13.1	0.2	2.6	2.6	36.7	7.9	0.1	2.6	25.9	0.0	0.0	0.0	0.0	0.0	0.0	0.0	225.1
0.0	0.0	19.8	0.5	4.9	2.5	61.8	54.3	0.3	2.5	73.1	0.0	0.1	0.1	0.1	0.0	3.2	0.0	217.4
0.0	0.0	9.9	0.2	4.9	2.5	32.1	9.9	0.1	2.5	108.4	0.0	0.0	0.0	0.1	0.0	2.2	0.0	217.9
0.0	0.0	5.6	0.2	7.5	7.5	65.8	1.9	0.1	0.0	30.1	0.0	0.0	0.0	0.2	0.0	1.5	0.0	163.6
0.0	0.0	14.0	0.2	8.0	16.0	125.0	15.0	0.1	0.0	100.0	0.0	0.0	0.0	0.0	0.0	0.0	0.0	0.0
0.0	0.0	4.0	0.4	0.0	3.0	40.0	23.0	0.0	2.6	80.0	0.0	0.0	0.0	0.0	0.0	0.0	0.0	0.0
0.0	0.0	2.2	0.1	1.2	0.0	23.9	1.6	0.1	0.3	1.7	0.0	0.0	0.0	0.0	0.0	0.0	0.0	27.1
0.0	0.0	0.0	0.0	0.0	0.0	5.5	33.0	0.0	0.0	22.0	0.0	0.0	0.0	0.0	0.0	0.0	0.0	0.0
0.0	0.0	5.6	0.3	3.7	3.7	27.9	5.6	0.1	0.0	7.3	0.0	0.0	0.0	0.0	0.0	4.1	0.0	166.1
0.0	0.0	5.6	0.3	3.7	3.7	27.9	5.6	0.1	3.7	7.3	0.0	0.0	0.0	0.0	0.0	4.1	0.0	166.1
0.0	0.0	5.6	0.1	1.9	1.9	24.2	3.7	0.0	0.0	5.0	0.0	0.0	0.0	0.0	0.0	1.9	0.0	165.4
0.0	0.0	0.0	0.0	0.0	0.0	0.0	0.0	0.0	0.0	0.0	0.0	0.0	0.0	0.0	0.0	0.0	0.0	0.0
0.0	0.0	11.2	0.5	3.7	1.9	33.5	29.8	0.2	3.7	63.4	0.0	0.0	0.0	0.1	0.0	4.1	0.0	161.6
0.0	0.0	0.0	0.0	0.0	0.0	64.0	1.0	0.0	115.2	60.0	0.0	0.0	0.0	0.0	0.0	0.0	0.0	157.3
0.0	0.0	13.0	0.6	11.2	11.2	113.5	26.0	0.1	7.4	85.6	0.0	0.1	0.0	0.5	0.1	19.5	0.0	163.5
0.0	0.0	9.3	0.5	11.2	7.4	85.6	5.6	0.1	98.6	41.9	0.0	0.1	0.0	0.4	0.1	20.3	0.0	161.6
0.0	0.0	24.0	0.0	0.0	17.0	9.0	13.0	0.0	0.0	6.0	0.0	0.0	0.0	0.0	0.0	0.0	0.0	0.0
0.0	0.0	2.0	0.4	0.0	2.0	26.0	19.0	0.0	2.8	60.0	0.0	0.0	0.0	0.0	0.0	0.0	0.0	0.0
0.0	0.0	7.8	0.4	6.5	14.3	111.8	7.8	0.1	26.0	2.5	0.0	0.0	0.0	0.5	0.1	3.4	0.0	99.4
0.0	0.0	9.8	0.4	7.3	14.6	126.9	4.9	0.1	28.1	3.7	0.0	0.0	0.0	0.6	0.1	3.3	0.0	107.0
0.0	0.0	19.0	0.9	0.0	0.0	125.0	30.0	0.0	0.0	5.0	0.0	0.0	0.0	0.3	0.0	0.2	0.0	0.0
0.0	0.0	12.6	0.7	5.4	12.6	214.2	5.4	0.1	0.0	74.9	0.0	0.0	0.0	0.0	0.1	0.2	0.0	158.3
0.0	0.0	12.7	0.5	10.6	14.8	265.9	14.8	0.1	0.0	52.8	0.0	0.0	0.0	0.1	0.1	0.6	0.0	185.5
0.0	0.0	14.8	0.8	10.6	19.0	240.5	6.3	0.2	278.5	114.8	0.0	0.0	0.0	0.5	0.0	2.7	0.0	179.1
0.0	0.0	20.4	0.2	0.0	7.9	77.1	5.7	0.1	0.2	90.8	0.0	0.0	0.1	0.2	0.1	1.1	0.0	0.0
0.0	0.0	19.3	0.1	0.0	2.3	90.8	9.1	0.0	0.0	68.1	0.0	0.0	0.0	0.0	0.0	0.0	0.0	0.0
0.1	0.0	8.6	0.2	8.6	8.6	45.4	4.3	0.1	2.2	51.6	0.1	0.0	0.1	0.3	0.1	2.8	0.0	187.7
0.0	0.0	17.3	0.8	21.6	23.8	349.9	4.3	0.1	0.0	58.1	0.1	0.1	0.0	0.7	0.0	22.5	0.0	188.7
0.0	0.0	15.1	0.4	21.6	23.8	330.5	2.2	0.2	2.2	63.1	0.1	0.1	0.0	0.5	0.0	22.5	0.0	194.6
0.0	0.0	2.5	0.0	3.4	4.3	42.0	0.3	0.0	0.3	10.4	0.0	0.0	0.0	0.1	0.0	1.1	0.0	27.6
0.0	0.0	22.2	0.5	29.6	37.1	400.1	2.5	0.1	108.7	93.9	0.0	0.1	0.0	0.5	0.1	25.2	0.0	222.3
0.0	0.0	17.6	0.4	23.5	29.4	317.5	2.0	0.1	2.0	74.5	0.1	0.1	0.0	0.4	0.1	20.0	0.0	176.4
0.0	0.0	1.7	0.0	1.2	1.4	15.5	3.2	0.0	0.3	3.8	0.0	0.0	0.0	0.0	0.0	1.5	0.0	14.1

Code	Food Name	Unit/Amt	Wt (g)	Energy (Kcal)	Prot (g)	Carb (g)	Fiber (g)	Fat (g)	Mono (g)	Poly (g)
9152	Fruit Juice, Lemon, fresh	1 tbsp	15	3.8	0.1	1.3	0.1	0.0	0.0	0.0
9161	Fruit Juice, Lime, canned or bottled unsweetened	1 tbsp	15	3.2	0.0	1.0	0.1	0.0	0.0	0.0
9160	Fruit Juice, Lime, fresh	1 tbsp	15	4.1	0.1	1.4	0.1	0.0	0.0	0.0
9207	Fruit Juice, Orange, canned, unsweetened	1 fl oz	31.1	13.1	0.2	3.1	0.1	0.0	0.0	0.0
9206	Fruit Juice, Orange, fresh	juice from 1 fruit (2.6" diam)	86	38.7	0.6	8.9	0.2	0.2	0.0	0.0
9215	Fruit Juice, Orange, frozen concentrate, unsweetened, prep	1 fl oz	31.1	14.0	0.2	3.4	0.1	0.0	0.0	0.0
914889	Fruit Juice, Orange-Grapefruit Juice	1 cup	245	110.3	1.6	25.5	0.1	0.1	0.0	0.1
9229	Fruit Juice, Papaya Nectar, canned	6 fl oz	213	121.4	0.4	30.9	1.3	0.3	0.1	0.1
9232	Fruit Juice, Passion Fruit, Purple, fresh	6 fl oz	218	111.2	0.9	29.6	0.4	0.1	0.0	0.1
9407	Fruit Juice, Peach Nectar, canned, w/added Vit C	6 fl oz	213	115.0	0.6	29.6	1.3	0.0	0.0	0.0
9408	Fruit Juice, Pear Nectar, canned, w/added Vit C	6 fl oz	213	127.8	0.2	33.6	1.3	0.0	0.0	0.0
9409	Fruit Juice, Pineapple, canned, unsweetened w/added Vit C	6 fl oz	213	119.3	0.7	29.4	0.4	0.2	0.0	0.1
9294	Fruit Juice, Prune, canned	6 fl oz	213	151.2	1.3	37.2	2.1	0.1	0.0	0.0
9223	Fruit Juice, Tangerine, canned, sweetened	6 fl oz	213	106.5	1.1	25.6	0.4	0.4	0.0	0.1
9105	Fruit Salad (peach,pineapple,pear,apricot&cherry)canned in heavy syrup	½ cup	127	92.7	0.4	24.3	1.3	0.1	0.0	0.0
9103	Fruit Salad (peach,pineapple,pear,apricot&cherry)canned in juice	½ cup	124	62.0	0.6	16.2	1.2	0.0	0.0	0.0
9104	Fruit Salad (peach,pineapple,pear,apricot&cherry)canned in lite syrup	½ cup	126	73.1	0.4	19.1	1.3	0.1	0.0	0.0
9003	Fruit, Apple w/skin, raw	1 medium (2.75" dia) (3/lb)	138	81.4	0.3	21.0	3.7	0.5	0.0	0.1
9009	Fruit, Apple, dehydrated, sulfured	1 cup	60	207.6	0.8	56.1	7.4	0.3	0.0	0.1
9014	Fruit, Apple, frozen, unsweetened	1 cup slices	173	83.0	0.5	21.3	3.3	0.6	0.0	0.2
9004	Fruit, Apple, peeled, raw, medium	1 fruit (2.75" dia) (3/lb)	128	73.0	0.2	19.0	2.4	0.4	0.0	0.1
9007	Fruit, Apple, slices, sweetened, canned, drained	½ cup slices	102	68.3	0.2	17.0	1.7	0.5	0.0	0.1
9402	Fruit, Applesauce, canned, sweetened w/added Vit C	½ cup	127	96.5	0.2	25.3	1.5	0.2	0.0	0.1
9401	Fruit, Applesauce, canned, unsweetened w/added Vit C	½ cup	122	52.5	0.2	13.8	1.5	0.1	0.0	0.0
9024	Fruit, Apricot w/skin, canned in juice	½ cup of halves	123	59.0	0.8	15.2	2.0	0.0	0.0	0.0
9026	Fruit, Apricot w/skin, canned in lite syrup	½ cup of halves	123	77.5	0.7	20.3	2.0	0.1	0.0	0.0
9032	Fruit, Apricot, dried, sulfured	½ cup of halves	3.5	8.3	0.1	2.2	0.3	0.0	0.0	0.0
9035	Fruit, Apricot, frozen, sweetened	1 tbsp cup	121	118.6	0.8	30.4	2.7	0.1	0.1	0.0
9023	Fruit, Apricot, peeled, canned in H₂O	4 halves & 2 tbsp liquid	90	19.8	0.6	4.9	1.0	0.0	0.0	0.0
9028	Fruit, Apricot, peeled, canned in heavy syrup	4 halves & 2 tbsp liquid	90	74.7	0.5	19.3	1.4	0.1	0.0	0.0
9021	Fruit, Apricot, raw	1 apricot	35	16.8	0.5	3.9	0.8	0.1	0.1	0.0
9037	Fruit, Avocado, All Varieties, peeled, raw	1 fruit w/o pit	115	185.2	2.3	8.5	5.8	17.6	11.0	2.2
9040	Fruit, Banana, peeled, raw	1 small	100	92.9	1.0	23.7	2.4	0.5	0.0	0.1
9041	Fruit, Banana, dried or powder	1 tbsp	50	173.0	1.9	44.1	3.8	0.9	0.1	0.2
9048	Fruit, Blackberries, frozen, unsweetened	1 cup	255	163.2	3.0	40.0	12.8	1.1	0.1	0.6
9042	Fruit, Blackberries, raw	1 cup	144	74.9	1.0	18.4	7.6	0.6	0.1	0.3
9052	Fruit, Blueberries, canned in heavy syrup	½ cup	129	113.5	0.8	28.5	1.9	0.4	0.1	0.4
9054	Fruit, Blueberries, frozen, unsweetened	½ cup	142	72.4	0.6	17.3	3.8	0.9	0.1	0.4
9050	Fruit, Blueberries, raw	1 cup	145	81.2	1.0	20.5	3.9	0.6	0.1	0.2
9056	Fruit, Boysenberries, canned in heavy syrup	½ cup	142	125.0	1.4	31.7	3.7	0.2	0.0	0.1
9057	Fruit, Boysenberries, frozen, unsweetened	½ cup	142	71.0	1.6	17.3	5.5	0.4	0.0	0.2
9059	Fruit, Breadfruit, peeled, raw	¼ small fruit w/o seeds	96	98.9	1.0	26.0	4.7	0.2	0.0	0.1
9060	Fruit, Carambola (Starfruit) raw	1 small (3" long)	70	23.1	0.4	5.5	1.9	0.2	0.0	0.1
9061	Fruit, Carissa (Natal-plum) peeled, raw	1 fruit w/o seeds	20	12.4	0.1	2.7	0.0	0.3	0.0	0.0
9062	Fruit, Cherimoya, peeled, raw	1 fruit w/o seeds	547	514.2	7.1	131.3	13.1	2.2	0.0	0.0
9065	Fruit, Cherries, Sour, Red, canned in lite syrup	½ cup	126	94.5	0.9	24.3	1.0	0.1	0.0	0.0
9068	Fruit, Cherries, Sour, Red, frozen, unsweetened	½ cup	125	57.5	1.2	13.8	2.0	0.6	0.2	0.2
9063	Fruit, Cherries, Sour, Red, raw	1 cup w/pits	103	51.5	1.0	12.5	1.6	0.3	0.1	0.1
9064	Fruit, Cherries, Sour/Tart, Red, canned in H₂O	½ cup	122	43.9	0.9	10.9	1.3	0.1	0.0	0.0
9072	Fruit, Cherries, Sweet, canned in juice	½ cup w/o pits	125	67.5	1.1	17.3	1.9	0.0	0.0	0.0
9073	Fruit, Cherries, Sweet, canned in lite syrup	½ cup w/o pits	126	84.4	0.8	21.8	1.9	0.2	0.1	0.1
9076	Fruit, Cherries, Sweet, frozen, sweetened	10 oz package	142	126.4	1.6	31.8	3.0	0.2	0.1	0.1
9070	Fruit, Cherries, Sweet, raw	1 cup w/pits, edible part	117	84.2	1.4	19.4	2.7	1.1	0.3	0.3
9078	Fruit, Cranberries, raw	1 cup whole	95	46.6	0.4	12.0	4.0	0.2	0.0	0.1
9082	Fruit, Cranberry-Orange Relish, canned	½ cup	138	245.6	0.4	63.8	0.0	0.1	0.0	0.0
9081	Fruit, Cranberry Sauce, canned, sweetened	1 slice (0.5" thick, ~8 slices/can)	57	86.1	0.1	22.2	0.6	0.1	0.0	0.0
9083	Fruit, Currant, European, Black, raw	1 cup	112	70.6	1.6	17.2	0.0	0.5	0.1	0.2
9084	Fruit, Currant, Red or White, raw	1 cup	112	62.7	1.6	15.5	4.8	0.2	0.0	0.1
9087	Fruit, Dates, Domestic, Natural, dried	1 date	8.3	22.8	0.2	6.1	0.6	0.0	0.0	0.0
9091	Fruit, Figs, canned in lite syrup	1 fig w/liquid	28	19.3	0.1	5.0	0.5	0.0	0.0	0.0
9094	Fruit, Figs, Dried, raw	1 fig	19	48.5	0.6	12.4	2.3	0.2	0.0	0.1
9095	Fruit, Figs, Dried, stewed	½ cup	130	140.4	1.7	35.8	6.6	0.6	0.1	0.3
9089	Fruit, Figs, raw	1 small (1.5" dia)	40	29.6	0.3	7.7	1.3	0.1	0.0	0.1
9107	Fruit, Gooseberries, raw	½ cup	75	33.0	0.7	7.6	3.2	0.4	0.0	0.2
9120	Fruit, Grapefruit, canned in juice	½ cup	125	46.3	0.9	11.5	0.5	0.1	0.0	0.0
9121	Fruit, Grapefruit, canned in lite syrup	½ cup	158	94.8	0.9	24.4	0.6	0.2	0.0	0.0
9111	Fruit, Grapefruit, Red, White or Pink, peeled, raw	1.2 cup sections w/ juice	135	43.2	0.9	10.9	1.5	0.1	0.0	0.0
9131	Fruit, Grapes, American type (slip skin) raw	1 cup	92	61.6	0.6	15.8	0.9	0.3	0.0	0.1
9139	Fruit, Guava, Common, raw	½ cup	85	43.4	0.7	10.1	4.6	0.5	0.0	0.2

Sat (g)	Chol (mg)	Cal (mg)	Iron (mg)	Magn (mg)	Phos (mg)	Pota (mg)	Sodi (mg)	Zinc (mg)	Vit A (RE)	Vit C (mg)	Vit E (mg)	Thia (mg)	Ribo (mg)	Niac (mg)	Vit B-6 (mg)	Fol (µg)	Vit B-12 (µg)	Wat (g)
0.0	0.0	1.1	0.0	0.9	0.9	18.6	0.2	0.0	0.3	6.9	0.0	0.0	0.0	0.0	0.0	1.9	0.0	13.6
0.0	0.0	1.8	0.0	1.1	1.5	11.3	2.4	0.0	0.3	1.0	0.0	0.0	0.0	0.0	0.0	1.2	0.0	13.9
0.0	0.0	1.4	0.0	0.9	1.1	16.4	0.2	0.0	0.2	4.4	0.0	0.0	0.0	0.0	0.0	1.2	0.0	13.5
0.0	0.0	2.5	0.1	3.4	4.4	54.4	0.6	0.0	5.6	10.7	0.0	0.0	0.0	0.1	0.0	5.6	0.0	27.7
0.0	0.0	9.5	0.2	9.5	14.6	172.0	0.9	0.0	17.2	43.0	0.1	0.1	0.0	0.3	0.0	26.1	0.0	75.9
0.0	0.0	2.8	0.0	3.1	5.0	59.1	0.3	0.0	2.5	12.1	0.1	0.0	0.0	0.1	0.0	13.6	0.0	27.4
0.0	0.0	24.0	0.3	25.0	41.0	459.0	1.0	0.2	56.2	107.0	0.0	0.2	0.0	0.7	0.1	7.0	0.0	217.3
0.1	0.0	21.3	0.7	6.4	0.0	66.0	10.7	0.3	23.4	6.4	0.0	0.0	0.0	0.3	0.0	4.5	0.0	181.1
0.0	0.0	8.7	0.5	37.1	28.3	606.0	13.1	0.1	157.0	65.0	0.1	0.0	0.3	3.2	0.1	15.3	0.0	186.7
0.0	0.0	10.7	0.4	8.5	12.8	85.2	14.9	0.2	55.4	57.1	0.0	0.0	0.0	0.6	0.0	3.0	0.0	182.4
0.0	0.0	10.7	0.6	6.4	6.4	27.7	8.5	0.1	0.0	57.5	0.0	0.0	0.0	0.3	0.0	2.6	0.0	178.9
0.0	0.0	36.2	0.6	27.7	17.0	285.4	2.1	0.2	0.0	51.1	0.0	0.1	0.0	0.5	0.2	49.2	0.0	182.2
0.0	0.0	25.6	2.5	29.8	53.3	587.9	8.5	0.4	0.0	8.7	0.0	0.0	0.1	1.7	0.5	0.9	0.0	173.0
0.0	0.0	38.3	0.4	17.0	29.8	379.1	2.1	0.1	89.5	46.9	0.2	0.1	0.0	0.2	0.1	9.8	0.0	185.3
0.0	0.0	7.6	0.4	6.4	11.4	101.6	7.6	0.1	63.5	3.0	0.6	0.0	0.0	0.4	0.0	3.2	0.0	101.9
0.0	0.0	13.6	0.3	9.9	17.4	143.8	6.2	0.2	74.4	4.1	0.0	0.0	0.0	0.4	0.0	3.2	0.0	106.8
0.0	0.0	8.8	0.4	6.3	11.3	103.3	7.6	0.1	54.2	3.2	0.0	0.0	0.0	0.5	0.0	3.3	0.0	106.1
0.1	0.0	9.7	0.2	6.9	9.7	158.7	0.0	0.1	6.9	7.9	0.4	0.0	0.0	0.1	0.1	3.9	0.0	115.8
0.1	0.0	11.4	1.2	13.2	33.0	384.0	74.4	0.2	4.8	1.3	2.1	0.0	0.1	0.4	0.2	0.6	0.0	1.8
0.1	0.0	6.9	0.3	5.2	13.8	133.2	5.2	0.1	5.2	0.2	0.0	0.0	0.0	0.1	0.1	1.2	0.0	150.3
0.1	0.0	5.1	0.1	3.8	9.0	144.6	0.0	0.1	5.1	5.1	0.1	0.0	0.0	0.1	0.1	0.5	0.0	108.1
0.1	0.0	4.1	0.2	2.0	5.1	69.4	3.1	0.0	5.1	0.4	0.0	0.0	0.0	0.1	0.0	0.8	0.0	84.0
0.0	0.0	5.1	0.4	3.8	8.9	77.5	35.6	0.1	1.3	2.2	0.0	0.0	0.0	0.2	0.0	0.8	0.0	101.1
0.0	0.0	3.7	0.1	3.7	8.5	91.5	2.4	0.0	3.7	25.9	0.0	0.0	0.0	0.2	0.0	0.7	0.0	107.8
0.0	0.0	14.8	0.4	12.3	24.6	203.0	4.9	0.1	207.9	6.0	1.1	0.0	0.0	0.4	0.1	2.1	0.0	106.5
0.0	0.0	13.5	0.5	9.8	16.0	169.7	4.9	0.1	162.4	3.3	1.1	0.0	0.0	0.4	0.1	2.1	0.0	101.5
0.0	0.0	1.6	0.2	1.6	4.1	48.2	0.4	0.0	25.3	0.1	0.1	0.0	0.0	0.1	0.0	0.4	0.0	1.1
0.0	0.0	12.1	1.1	10.9	23.0	277.1	4.8	0.1	203.3	10.9	1.1	0.0	0.0	1.0	0.1	2.1	0.0	88.7
0.0	0.0	7.2	0.5	8.1	14.4	138.6	9.9	0.1	162.9	1.6	0.0	0.0	0.0	0.4	0.0	1.5	0.0	84.1
0.0	0.0	8.1	0.4	7.2	11.7	120.6	9.9	0.1	111.6	2.5	0.0	0.0	0.0	0.4	0.0	1.5	0.0	69.9
0.0	0.0	4.9	0.2	2.8	6.7	103.6	0.4	0.1	91.4	3.5	0.3	0.0	0.0	0.2	0.0	3.0	0.0	30.2
2.8	0.0	12.7	1.2	44.9	47.2	688.9	11.5	0.5	70.2	9.1	1.5	0.1	0.1	2.2	0.3	71.2	0.0	85.4
0.2	0.0	6.1	0.3	29.3	20.2	399.7	1.0	0.2	8.1	9.2	0.3	0.1	0.1	0.6	0.6	19.3	0.0	75.0
0.3	0.0	11.0	0.6	54.0	37.0	745.5	1.5	0.3	15.5	3.5	0.0	0.1	0.1	1.4	0.2	7.0	0.0	1.5
0.0	0.0	74.0	2.0	56.1	76.5	357.0	2.6	0.6	28.1	7.9	1.8	0.1	0.1	3.1	0.2	86.7	0.0	209.6
0.0	0.0	46.1	0.8	28.8	30.2	282.2	0.0	0.4	23.0	30.2	1.0	0.0	0.1	0.6	0.1	49.0	0.0	123.3
0.0	0.0	6.5	0.4	5.2	12.9	51.6	3.9	0.1	7.7	1.4	1.3	0.0	0.1	0.1	0.0	2.1	0.0	99.0
0.1	0.0	11.4	0.3	7.1	15.6	76.7	1.4	0.1	11.4	3.6	1.4	0.0	0.1	0.7	0.1	9.5	0.0	123.0
0.0	0.0	8.7	0.2	7.3	14.5	129.1	8.7	0.2	14.5	18.9	1.5	0.1	0.1	0.5	0.1	9.3	0.0	122.7
0.0	0.0	25.6	0.6	15.6	14.2	127.8	4.3	0.3	5.7	8.8	1.0	0.0	0.0	0.3	0.1	48.8	0.0	108.3
0.0	0.0	38.3	1.2	22.7	38.3	197.4	1.4	0.3	9.9	4.4	0.6	0.1	0.1	1.1	0.1	89.9	0.0	122.0
0.0	0.0	16.3	0.5	24.0	28.8	470.4	1.9	0.1	3.8	27.8	1.1	0.1	0.0	0.9	0.1	13.4	0.0	67.8
0.0	0.0	2.8	0.2	6.3	11.2	114.1	1.4	0.1	34.3	14.8	0.3	0.0	0.0	0.3	0.1	9.8	0.0	63.6
0.0	0.0	2.2	0.3	3.2	1.4	52.0	0.6	0.0	0.8	7.6	0.0	0.0	0.0	0.0	0.0	0.0	0.0	16.8
0.0	0.0	125.8	2.7	0.0	218.8	0.0	0.0	0.0	5.5	49.2	0.0	0.5	0.6	7.1	0.0	0.0	0.0	402.0
0.0	0.0	12.6	1.7	7.6	12.6	119.7	8.8	0.1	92.0	2.5	0.0	0.0	0.0	0.2	0.1	9.7	0.0	100.3
0.1	0.0	16.3	0.7	11.3	20.0	155.0	1.3	0.1	108.8	2.1	0.2	0.1	0.0	0.2	0.1	5.6	0.0	109.0
0.1	0.0	16.5	0.3	9.3	15.5	178.2	3.1	0.1	131.8	10.3	0.1	0.0	0.0	0.4	0.0	7.7	0.0	88.7
0.0	0.0	13.4	1.7	7.3	12.2	119.6	8.5	0.1	91.5	2.6	0.2	0.0	0.1	0.2	0.1	9.8	0.0	109.7
0.0	0.0	17.5	0.7	15.0	27.5	163.8	3.8	0.1	16.3	3.1	0.1	0.0	0.0	0.5	0.0	5.3	0.0	106.2
0.0	0.0	11.3	0.5	11.3	22.7	186.5	3.8	0.1	20.2	4.7	0.2	0.0	0.1	0.5	0.0	5.3	0.0	102.8
0.0	0.0	17.0	0.5	14.2	22.7	282.6	1.4	0.1	27.0	1.4	0.2	0.0	0.1	0.3	0.1	6.0	0.0	107.3
0.3	0.0	17.6	0.5	12.9	22.2	262.1	0.0	0.1	24.6	8.2	0.2	0.1	0.1	0.5	0.0	4.9	0.0	94.5
0.0	0.0	6.7	0.2	4.8	8.6	67.5	1.0	0.1	4.8	12.8	0.1	0.0	0.0	0.1	0.1	1.6	0.0	82.2
0.0	0.0	15.2	0.3	5.5	11.0	52.4	44.2	0.0	9.7	24.8	0.0	0.0	0.0	0.1	0.0	0.0	0.0	73.4
0.0	0.0	2.3	0.1	1.7	3.4	14.8	16.5	0.0	1.1	1.1	0.1	0.0	0.0	0.1	0.0	0.6	0.0	34.6
0.0	0.0	61.6	1.7	26.9	66.1	360.6	2.2	0.3	25.8	202.7	0.1	0.1	0.1	0.3	0.1	0.0	0.0	91.8
0.0	0.0	37.0	1.1	14.6	49.3	308.0	1.1	0.3	13.4	45.9	0.1	0.0	0.1	0.1	0.1	9.0	0.0	94.0
0.0	0.0	2.7	0.1	2.9	3.3	54.1	0.2	0.0	0.4	0.0	0.0	0.0	0.0	0.2	0.0	1.0	0.0	1.9
0.0	0.0	7.6	0.1	2.8	2.8	28.6	0.3	0.0	1.1	0.3	0.2	0.0	0.0	0.1	0.0	0.6	0.0	22.8
0.0	0.0	27.4	0.4	11.2	12.9	135.3	2.1	0.1	2.5	0.2	0.0	0.0	0.0	0.1	0.0	1.4	0.0	5.4
0.1	0.0	79.3	1.2	32.5	37.7	391.3	6.5	0.3	20.8	5.7	0.0	0.0	0.1	0.8	0.2	1.3	0.0	90.7
0.0	0.0	14.0	0.1	6.8	5.6	92.8	0.4	0.1	5.6	0.8	0.4	0.0	0.0	0.2	0.0	2.4	0.0	31.6
0.0	0.0	18.8	0.2	7.5	20.3	148.5	0.8	0.1	21.8	20.8	0.3	0.0	0.0	0.2	0.1	4.5	0.0	65.9
0.0	0.0	18.8	0.3	13.8	15.0	211.3	8.8	0.1	0.0	42.4	0.3	0.0	0.0	0.3	0.0	11.0	0.0	112.1
0.0	0.0	22.1	0.6	15.8	15.8	203.8	3.2	0.1	0.0	33.7	0.4	0.1	0.0	0.4	0.0	13.4	0.0	132.1
0.0	0.0	16.2	0.1	10.8	10.8	187.7	0.0	0.1	16.2	46.4	0.3	0.0	0.0	0.3	0.1	13.8	0.0	122.7
0.1	0.0	12.9	0.3	4.6	9.2	175.7	1.8	0.0	9.2	3.7	0.3	0.1	0.1	0.3	0.1	3.6	0.0	74.8
0.1	0.0	17.0	0.3	8.5	21.3	241.4	2.6	0.2	67.2	156.0	1.0	0.0	0.0	1.0	0.1	11.9	0.0	73.2

Code	Food Name	Unit/Amt	Wt (g)	Energy (Kcal)	Prot (g)	Carb (g)	Fiber (g)	Fat (g)	Mono (g)	Poly (g)
9148	Fruit, Kiwifruit (Chinese Gooseberry) peeled, raw	1 medium fruit	76	46.4	0.8	11.3	2.6	0.3	0.0	0.2
9149	Fruit, Kumquat, raw	1 fruit	19	12.0	0.2	3.1	1.3	0.0	0.0	0.0
9150	Fruit, Lemon, peeled, raw	1 medium fruit (2.1" dia)	58	16.8	0.6	5.4	1.6	0.2	0.0	0.1
9165	Fruit, Lychee (Litchi) shelled, dried	1 fruit	2.5	6.9	0.1	1.8	0.1	0.0	0.0	0.0
9176	Fruit, Mango, peeled, raw	1 fruit w/o seed	207	134.6	1.1	35.2	3.7	0.6	0.2	0.1
9185	Fruit, Melon Balls (cantaloupe & honeydew) frozen	1 cup thawed	173	57.1	1.5	13.7	1.2	0.4	0.0	0.2
9183	Fruit, Melon, Casaba, peeled, raw	1 cup cubes	170	44.2	1.5	10.5	1.4	0.2	0.0	0.1
9184	Fruit, Melon, Honeydew, peeled, wedges, raw	10 honeydew balls	138	48.3	0.6	12.7	0.8	0.1	0.0	0.1
9188	Fruit, Mixed (prune, apricot & pear) dried	3.5 w/o pits	100	243.0	2.5	64.1	7.8	0.5	0.2	0.1
9187	Fruit, Mixed, (peach, pear & pineapple) canned in heavy syrup	1 tbsp	15.9	11.4	0.1	3.0	0.2	0.0	0.0	0.0
9191	Fruit, Nectarine, raw	1 fruit w/o pit (2.5" diam)	136	66.6	1.3	16.0	2.2	0.6	0.2	0.3
9193	Fruit, Olives, Ripe, pitted, canned	1 tsp	2.8	3.2	0.0	0.2	0.1	0.3	0.2	0.0
90990	Fruit, Olives, Green	4 medium	13	14.9	0.0	0.0	0.4	2.0	1.2	0.1
9200	Fruit, Orange, All Varieties, peeled, raw	1 cup sections w/o membrane	180	84.6	1.7	21.2	4.3	0.2	0.0	0.0
9226	Fruit, Papayas, peeled, cubed/mashed, raw	1 cup cubes	140	54.6	0.9	13.7	2.5	0.2	0.1	0.0
9231	Fruit, Passion Fruit/Granadilla, Purple, peeled, raw	1 fruit	18	17.5	0.4	4.2	1.9	0.1	0.0	0.1
9241	Fruit, Peach, canned in heavy syrup	1 half w/liquid	98	72.5	0.4	19.5	1.3	0.1	0.0	0.0
9238	Fruit, Peach, canned in juice	1 half w/liquid	98	43.1	0.6	11.3	1.3	0.0	0.0	0.0
9240	Fruit, Peach, canned in lite syrup	1 half w/liquid	98	52.9	0.4	14.3	1.3	0.0	0.0	0.0
9246	Fruit, Peach, dried, sulfured	1 half	13	31.1	0.5	8.0	1.1	0.1	0.0	0.0
9250	Fruit, Peach, frozen, sweetened	10 slices	155	145.7	1.0	37.2	2.8	0.2	0.1	0.1
9236	Fruit, Peach, raw	1 large (2.75" dia) (2.5/lb)	157	67.5	1.1	17.4	3.1	0.1	0.1	0.1
9254	Fruit, Pear, canned in juice	½ cup halves	124	62.0	0.4	16.0	2.0	0.1	0.0	0.0
9256	Fruit, Pear, canned in lite syrup	½ cup halves	126	71.8	0.2	19.1	2.0	0.0	0.0	0.0
9259	Fruit, Pear, dried, sulfured	10 halves	175	458.5	3.3	122.0	13.1	1.1	0.2	0.3
9252	Fruit, Pear, raw	1 large pear (2/lb)	209	123.3	0.8	31.6	5.0	0.8	0.2	0.2
9265	Fruit, Persimmon, Native, raw	1 fruit w/o seeds	25	31.8	0.2	8.4	0.0	0.1	0.0	0.0
9268	Fruit, Pineapple, canned in juice	½ cup crushed, sliced of chunks	125	75.0	0.5	19.6	1.0	0.1	0.0	0.0
9269	Fruit, Pineapple, canned in lite syrup	½ cup crushed, sliced of chunks	126	65.5	0.5	16.9	1.0	0.2	0.0	0.1
9272	Fruit, Pineapple, frozen, chunks, sweetened	½ cup of chunks, frz sweetened	123	104.6	0.5	27.3	1.4	0.1	0.0	0.0
9266	Fruit, Pineapple, peeled, raw	1 fruit	472	231.3	1.8	58.5	5.7	2.0	0.2	0.7
9276	Fruit, Pitanga (Surinam Cherry) peeled, raw	1 fruit w/o seeds	7	2.3	0.1	0.5	0.0	0.0	0.0	0.0
9277	Fruit, Plantain, peeled, raw	1 medium fruit	179	218.4	2.3	57.1	4.1	0.7	0.1	0.1
9282	Fruit, Plum, Purple, canned in juice	½ cup w/o pits	126	73.1	0.6	19.1	1.3	0.0	0.0	0.0
9283	Fruit, Plum, Purple, canned in lite syrup	½ cup w/o pits	126	79.4	0.5	20.5	1.3	0.1	0.1	0.0
9279	Fruit, Plum, raw	1 fruit (2.1" diam) w/o pit	66	36.3	0.5	8.6	1.0	0.4	0.3	0.1
9286	Fruit, Pomegranates, peeled, raw	1 fruit: 3.35" dia	154	104.7	1.5	26.4	0.9	0.5	0.1	0.1
9287	Fruit, Prickly Pear, peeled, raw	1 fruit	103	42.2	0.8	9.9	3.7	0.5	0.1	0.2
9292	Fruit, Prune, dried, stewed w/o added sugar	1 tbsp w/o pits	15.5	16.6	0.2	4.4	1.0	0.0	0.0	0.0
9290	Fruit, Prunes, dehydrated, stewed	½ cup	140	158.2	1.7	41.6	0.0	0.3	0.2	0.1
9291	Fruit, Prunes, dried	1 prune	8.4	20.1	0.2	5.3	0.6	0.0	0.0	0.0
9295	Fruit, Pummelo, peeled, raw	1 fruit w/o seeds & membrane	609	231.4	4.6	58.6	6.1	0.2	0.0	0.0
9296	Fruit, Quinces, peeled, raw	1 fruit w/o seeds	92	52.4	0.4	14.1	1.7	0.1	0.0	0.0
9297	Fruit, Raisins, Golden, seedless	½ cup packed	83	250.7	2.8	66.0	3.3	0.4	0.0	0.1
9298	Fruit, Raisins, seedless	½ cup packed	83	249.0	2.7	65.7	3.3	0.4	0.0	0.1
9302	Fruit, Raspberries, raw	10 raspberries	19	9.3	0.2	2.2	1.3	0.1	0.0	0.1
9304	Fruit, Raspberries, Red, canned in heavy syrup	½ cup	128	116.5	1.1	29.9	4.2	0.2	0.0	0.1
9306	Fruit, Raspberries, Red, frozen, sweetened	10 oz package	284	292.5	2.0	74.3	12.5	0.5	0.0	0.3
9310	Fruit, Rhubarb, frozen, cooked w/sugar	½ cup	120	139.2	0.5	37.4	2.4	0.1	0.0	0.0
9307	Fruit, Rhubarb, raw	½ cup diced	61	12.8	0.5	2.8	1.1	0.1	0.0	0.1
9317	Fruit, Strawberries, canned in heavy syrup	½ cup	77	70.8	0.4	18.1	1.3	0.2	0.0	0.1
9320	Fruit, Strawberries, frozen, sliced, sweetened	1 cup thawed	255	244.8	1.4	66.1	4.8	0.3	0.0	0.2
9318	Fruit, Strawberries, unsweetened, frozen	1 cup	149	52.2	0.6	13.6	3.1	0.2	0.0	0.1
9322	Fruit, Tamarind, raw	1 fruit w/o pods & seeds:3x1"	2	4.8	0.1	1.3	0.1	0.0	0.0	0.0
9326	Fruit, Watermelon, balls, raw	1 cup balls	154	49.3	1.0	11.1	0.8	0.7	0.2	0.2
5308	Game, Cornish Game Hen w/skin, roasted	½ bird	129	335.4	28.7	0.0	0.0	23.5	10.3	4.6
5310	Game, Cornish Game Hens, no skin, roasted	½ bird	110	147.4	25.6	0.0	0.0	4.3	1.4	1.0
17167	Game, Elk, roasted	3.0 oz	85	124.1	25.7	0.0	0.0	1.6	0.4	0.3
17179	Game, Rabbit, Domestic, Composite, roasted	3.0 oz	85	167.5	24.7	0.0	0.0	6.8	1.8	1.3
17161	Game, Venison/Deer, roasted	3.0 oz	85	134.3	25.7	0.0	0.0	2.7	0.7	0.5
5150	Goose Liver Pate/Pate de Fois Gras, Smoked, canned	2 tbsp	28	129.4	3.2	1.3	0.0	12.3	7.2	0.2
5148	Goose, Domestic, meat & skin, roasted	3.5 oz	100	305.0	25.2	0.0	0.0	21.9	10.3	2.5
20001	Goose, Domestic, meat only, no skin, roasted	3.5 oz	100	238.0	29.0	0.0	0.0	12.7	4.3	1.5
20005	Grain, Barley	1 tbsp	11.5	40.7	1.4	8.5	2.0	0.3	0.0	0.1
20008	Grain, Barley, Pearled, ckd	1 tbsp	9.8	12.1	0.2	2.8	0.4	0.0	0.0	0.0
20009	Grain, Buckwheat Groats, roasted, ckd	1 tbsp	10.5	9.7	0.4	2.1	0.3	0.1	0.0	0.0
20012	Grain, Bulgar, ckd	1 tbsp	8.4	7.0	0.3	1.6	0.4	0.0	0.0	0.0
20014	Grain, Corn, White	1 tbsp	10.4	38.0	1.0	7.7	0.0	0.5	0.1	0.2
20029	Grain, Corn, Yellow	1 tbsp	10.4	38.0	1.0	7.7	0.0	0.5	0.1	0.2

Sat (g)	Chol (mg)	Cal (mg)	Iron (mg)	Magn (mg)	Phos (mg)	Pota (mg)	Sodi (mg)	Zinc (mg)	Vit A (RE)	Vit C (mg)	Vit E (mg)	Thia (mg)	Ribo (mg)	Niac (mg)	Vit B-6 (mg)	Fol (µg)	Vit B-12 (µg)	Wat (g)
0.0	0.0	19.8	0.3	22.8	30.4	252.3	3.8	0.1	13.7	74.5	0.9	0.0	0.0	0.4	0.1	28.9	0.0	63.1
0.0	0.0	8.4	0.1	2.5	3.6	37.1	1.1	0.0	5.7	7.1	0.0	0.0	0.0	0.1	0.0	3.0	0.0	15.5
0.0	0.0	15.1	0.3	4.6	9.3	80.0	1.2	0.0	1.7	30.7	0.1	0.0	0.0	0.1	0.0	6.1	0.0	51.6
0.0	0.0	0.8	0.0	1.1	4.5	27.8	0.1	0.0	0.0	4.6	0.0	0.0	0.0	0.1	0.0	0.3	0.0	0.6
0.1	0.0	20.7	0.3	18.6	22.8	322.9	4.1	0.1	805.2	57.3	2.3	0.1	0.1	1.2	0.3	29.0	0.0	169.1
0.1	0.0	17.3	0.5	24.2	20.8	484.4	53.6	0.3	306.2	10.7	0.3	0.3	0.0	1.1	0.2	44.5	0.0	156.1
0.0	0.0	8.5	0.7	13.6	11.9	357.0	20.4	0.3	5.1	27.2	0.3	0.1	0.0	0.7	0.2	28.9	0.0	156.4
0.0	0.0	8.3	0.1	9.7	13.8	374.0	13.8	0.1	5.5	34.2	0.2	0.1	0.0	0.8	0.1	8.3	0.0	123.7
0.0	0.0	38.0	2.7	39.0	77.0	796.0	18.0	0.5	244.0	3.8	0.0	0.0	0.2	1.9	0.2	3.9	0.0	31.2
0.0	0.0	0.2	0.1	0.8	1.6	13.4	0.6	0.0	3.0	11.0	0.0	0.0	0.0	0.1	0.0	0.5	0.0	12.8
0.1	0.0	6.8	0.2	10.9	21.8	288.3	0.0	0.1	100.6	7.3	1.2	0.0	0.1	1.3	0.0	5.0	0.0	117.3
0.0	0.0	2.5	0.1	0.1	0.1	0.2	24.4	0.0	1.1	0.0	0.1	0.0	0.0	0.0	0.0	0.0	0.0	2.2
0.2	0.0	8.0	0.2	0.0	2.0	7.0	312.0	0.1	8.0	6.0	0.0	0.0	0.0	0.0	0.0	0.4	0.0	0.0
0.0	0.0	72.0	0.2	18.0	25.2	325.8	0.0	0.1	37.8	95.8	0.4	0.2	0.1	0.5	0.1	54.5	0.0	156.2
0.1	0.0	33.6	0.1	14.0	7.0	359.4	4.2	0.1	39.2	86.5	1.6	0.0	0.0	0.5	0.0	53.2	0.0	124.4
0.0	0.0	2.2	0.3	5.2	12.2	62.6	5.0	0.0	12.6	5.4	0.2	0.0	0.0	0.3	0.0	2.5	0.0	13.1
0.0	0.0	2.9	0.3	4.9	10.8	90.2	5.9	0.1	32.3	2.7	0.9	0.0	0.0	0.6	0.0	3.1	0.0	77.7
0.0	0.0	5.9	0.3	6.9	16.7	125.4	3.9	0.1	37.2	3.5	1.5	0.0	0.0	0.6	0.0	3.3	0.0	85.7
0.0	0.0	2.9	0.4	4.9	10.8	95.1	4.9	0.1	34.3	2.4	0.9	0.0	0.0	0.6	0.0	3.2	0.0	83.0
0.0	0.0	3.6	0.5	5.5	15.5	129.5	0.9	0.1	28.1	0.6	0.0	0.0	0.0	0.6	0.0	0.0	0.0	4.1
0.0	0.0	4.7	0.6	7.8	17.1	201.5	9.3	0.1	43.4	146.0	1.4	0.0	0.1	1.0	0.0	5.0	0.0	115.8
0.0	0.0	7.9	0.2	11.0	18.8	309.3	0.0	0.2	84.8	10.4	1.1	0.0	0.1	1.6	0.0	5.3	0.0	137.6
0.0	0.0	11.2	0.4	8.7	14.9	119.0	5.0	0.1	1.2	2.0	0.6	0.0	0.0	0.2	0.0	1.5	0.0	107.2
0.0	0.0	6.3	0.4	5.0	8.8	83.2	6.3	0.1	0.0	0.9	0.6	0.0	0.0	0.2	0.0	1.5	0.0	106.4
0.1	0.0	59.5	3.7	57.8	103.3	932.8	10.5	0.7	0.0	12.3	0.0	0.0	0.3	2.4	0.1	0.0	0.0	46.7
0.0	0.0	23.0	0.5	12.5	23.0	261.3	0.0	0.3	4.2	8.4	1.0	0.0	0.1	0.2	0.0	15.3	0.0	175.2
0.0	0.0	6.8	0.6	0.0	6.5	77.5	0.3	0.0	0.0	16.5	0.0	0.0	0.0	0.0	0.0	0.0	0.0	16.1
0.0	0.0	17.5	0.4	17.5	7.5	152.5	1.3	0.1	5.0	11.9	0.1	0.1	0.0	0.4	0.1	6.0	0.0	104.4
0.0	0.0	17.6	0.5	20.2	8.8	132.3	1.3	0.2	1.3	9.5	0.1	0.1	0.0	0.4	0.1	5.9	0.0	108.0
0.0	0.0	11.1	0.5	12.3	4.9	123.0	2.5	0.1	3.7	9.8	0.1	0.1	0.0	0.4	0.1	13.0	0.0	94.8
0.2	0.0	33.0	1.7	66.1	33.0	533.4	4.7	0.4	9.4	72.7	0.5	0.4	0.2	2.0	0.4	50.0	0.0	408.3
0.0	0.0	0.6	0.0	0.8	0.8	7.2	0.2	0.0	10.5	1.8	0.0	0.0	0.0	0.0	0.0	0.0	0.0	6.4
0.3	0.0	5.4	1.1	66.2	60.9	893.2	7.2	0.3	202.3	32.9	0.5	0.1	0.1	1.2	0.5	39.4	0.0	116.9
0.0	0.0	12.6	0.4	10.1	18.9	194.0	1.3	0.1	127.3	3.5	0.9	0.0	0.1	0.6	0.0	3.3	0.0	105.9
0.0	0.0	11.3	1.1	6.3	16.4	117.2	25.2	0.1	32.8	0.5	0.9	0.0	0.0	0.4	0.0	3.3	0.0	104.6
0.0	0.0	2.6	0.1	4.6	6.6	113.5	0.0	0.1	21.1	6.3	0.4	0.0	0.1	0.3	0.1	1.5	0.0	56.2
0.1	0.0	4.6	0.5	4.6	12.3	398.9	4.6	0.2	0.0	9.4	0.8	0.0	0.0	0.5	0.2	9.2	0.0	124.7
0.1	0.0	57.7	0.3	87.6	24.7	226.6	5.2	0.1	5.2	14.4	0.0	0.0	0.1	0.5	0.1	6.2	0.0	90.2
0.0	0.0	3.6	0.2	3.1	5.4	51.8	0.3	0.0	4.8	0.4	0.0	0.0	0.0	0.1	0.0	0.0	0.0	10.8
0.0	0.0	33.6	1.6	29.4	51.8	494.2	2.8	0.4	72.8	0.0	0.0	0.1	0.0	1.4	0.3	0.3	0.0	95.2
0.0	0.0	4.3	0.2	3.8	6.6	62.6	0.3	0.1	16.7	0.3	0.1	0.0	0.0	0.2	0.0	0.3	0.0	2.7
0.0	0.0	24.4	0.7	36.5	103.5	1315.4	6.1	0.5	0.0	371.5	0.0	0.2	0.2	1.3	0.2	0.0	0.0	542.6
0.0	0.0	10.1	0.6	7.4	15.6	181.2	3.7	0.0	3.7	13.8	0.5	0.0	0.0	0.2	0.0	2.8	0.0	77.1
0.1	0.0	44.0	1.5	29.1	95.5	619.2	10.0	0.3	3.3	2.7	0.6	0.0	0.2	0.9	0.3	2.7	0.0	12.4
0.1	0.0	40.7	1.7	27.4	80.5	623.3	10.0	0.2	0.8	2.7	0.6	0.1	0.1	0.7	0.2	2.7	0.0	12.8
0.0	0.0	4.2	0.1	3.4	2.3	28.9	0.0	0.1	2.5	4.8	0.1	0.0	0.0	0.2	0.0	4.9	0.0	16.4
0.0	0.0	14.1	0.5	15.4	11.5	120.3	3.8	0.2	3.8	11.1	0.6	0.0	0.0	0.6	0.1	13.4	0.0	96.4
0.0	0.0	42.6	1.8	36.9	48.3	323.8	2.8	0.5	17.0	46.9	1.3	0.1	0.1	0.7	0.1	73.8	0.0	206.6
0.0	0.0	174.0	0.3	14.4	9.6	115.2	1.2	0.1	8.4	4.0	0.2	0.0	0.0	0.2	0.0	6.4	0.0	81.3
0.0	0.0	52.5	0.1	7.3	8.5	175.7	2.4	0.1	6.1	4.9	0.1	0.0	0.0	0.2	0.0	4.3	0.0	57.1
0.0	0.0	10.0	0.4	6.2	9.2	66.2	3.1	0.1	2.3	24.4	0.1	0.0	0.0	0.0	0.0	21.6	0.0	58.0
0.0	0.0	28.1	1.5	17.9	33.2	249.9	7.7	0.2	5.1	105.6	0.4	0.0	0.1	1.0	0.1	38.0	0.0	186.6
0.0	0.0	23.8	1.1	16.4	19.4	220.5	3.0	0.2	6.0	61.4	0.4	0.0	0.1	0.7	0.0	25.0	0.0	134.1
0.0	0.0	1.5	0.1	1.8	2.3	12.6	0.6	0.0	0.1	0.1	0.0	0.0	0.0	0.0	0.0	0.3	0.0	0.6
0.1	0.0	12.3	0.3	16.9	13.9	178.6	3.1	0.1	57.0	14.8	0.2	0.1	0.0	0.3	0.2	3.4	0.0	140.9
6.5	169.0	16.8	1.2	23.2	188.3	316.1	82.6	1.9	41.3	0.6	0.3	0.1	0.3	7.6	0.4	2.6	0.4	75.7
1.1	116.6	14.3	0.8	20.9	163.9	275.0	69.3	1.7	22.0	0.7	0.3	0.1	0.2	6.9	0.4	2.2	0.3	79.1
0.6	62.1	4.3	3.1	20.4	153.0	278.8	51.9	2.7	0.0	0.0	0.0	0.0	0.0	0.0	0.0	0.0	0.0	56.3
2.0	69.7	16.2	1.9	17.9	223.6	325.6	40.0	1.9	0.0	0.0	0.0	0.1	0.2	7.2	0.4	9.4	7.1	51.5
1.1	95.2	6.0	3.8	20.4	192.1	284.8	45.9	2.3	0.0	0.0	0.0	0.2	0.5	5.7	0.0	0.0	0.0	55.4
4.0	42.0	19.6	1.5	3.6	56.0	38.6	195.2	0.3	280.0	0.6	0.0	0.0	0.1	0.7	0.0	16.8	2.6	10.4
6.9	91.0	13.0	2.8	22.0	270.0	329.0	70.0	2.6	21.0	0.0	1.7	0.1	0.3	4.2	0.4	2.0	0.4	52.0
4.6	96.0	14.0	2.9	25.0	309.0	388.0	76.0	3.2	12.0	0.0	0.0	0.1	0.4	4.1	0.5	12.0	0.5	57.2
0.1	0.0	3.8	0.4	15.3	30.4	52.0	1.4	0.3	0.2	0.0	0.1	0.1	0.0	0.5	0.0	2.2	0.0	1.1
0.0	0.0	1.1	0.1	2.2	5.3	9.1	0.3	0.1	0.1	0.0	0.0	0.0	0.0	0.2	0.0	1.6	0.0	6.7
0.0	0.0	0.7	0.1	5.4	7.4	9.2	0.4	0.1	0.0	0.0	0.0	0.0	0.0	0.1	0.0	1.5	0.0	7.9
0.0	0.0	0.8	0.1	2.7	3.4	5.7	0.4	0.0	0.0	0.0	0.0	0.0	0.0	0.1	0.0	1.5	0.0	6.5
0.1	0.0	0.7	0.3	13.2	21.8	29.8	3.6	0.2	0.0	0.0	0.0	0.0	0.0	0.4	0.1	0.0	0.0	1.1
0.1	0.0	0.7	0.3	13.2	21.8	29.8	3.6	0.2	4.9	0.0	0.1	0.0	0.0	0.4	0.1	2.0	0.0	1.1

Code	Food Name	Unit/Amt	Wt (g)	Energy (Kcal)	Prot (g)	Carb (g)	Fiber (g)	Fat (g)	Mono (g)	Poly (g)
20030	Grain, Couscous, dry	1 tbsp	10.8	40.6	1.4	8.4	0.5	0.1	0.0	0.0
20330	Grain, Hominy, Yellow	1 cup	242	128.3	2.7	27.9	1.6	0.6	0.0	0.0
20031	Grain, Millet, ckd	1 tbsp	10.9	13.0	0.4	2.6	0.1	0.1	0.0	0.1
20035	Grain, Oats	1 tbsp	9.8	38.1	1.7	6.5	1.0	0.7	0.2	0.2
20036	Grain, Rice, Brown, Long grain, ckd	1 tbsp	12.2	13.5	0.3	2.8	0.2	0.1	0.0	0.0
20040	Grain, Rice, Brown, Medium grain, ckd	1 tbsp	12.2	13.7	0.3	2.9	0.2	0.1	0.0	0.0
20054	Grain, Rice, White, Glutinous, ckd	1 tbsp, cooked	10.9	10.6	0.2	2.3	0.1	0.0	0.0	0.0
20047	Grain, Rice, White, Long grain, enriched, ckd w/salt	1 tbsp	9.9	12.9	0.3	2.8	0.0	0.0	0.0	0.0
20048	Grain, Rice, White, Long grain, Precooked/Instant, enriched, ckd	1 tbsp	10.3	10.1	0.2	2.2	0.1	0.0	0.0	0.0
20044	Grain, Rice, White, Long grain, Regular, enriched, ckd	1 tbsp	9.9	12.9	0.3	2.8	0.0	0.0	0.0	0.0
20444	Grain, Rice, White, Long Grain, Regular, unenriched, ckd w/o salt	1 tbsp	9.8	12.7	0.3	2.8	0.0	0.0	0.0	0.0
20051	Grain, Rice, White, Long Grain, unenriched, ckd w/salt	1 tbsp	9.9	12.9	0.3	2.8	0.0	0.0	0.0	0.0
20050	Grain, Rice, White, Medium grain, ckd	1 tbsp	11.6	15.1	0.3	3.3	0.0	0.0	0.0	0.0
20450	Grain, Rice, White, Medium grain, unenriched, ckd	1 tbsp	11.6	15.1	0.3	3.3	0.0	0.0	0.0	0.0
20056	Grain, Rice, White, w/pasta, ckd	1 tbsp	12.6	15.4	0.3	2.7	0.3	0.4	0.1	0.1
20066	Grain, Rye	1 tbsp	10.6	35.5	1.6	7.4	1.5	0.3	0.0	0.1
20466	Grain, Semolina, enriched	1 tbsp	10.4	37.4	1.3	7.6	0.4	0.1	0.0	0.0
20068	Grain, Sorghum	1 tbsp	12	40.7	1.4	9.0	0.0	0.4	0.1	0.2
20069	Grain, Tapioca, Pearl, dry	1 tbsp	9.5	34.0	0.0	8.4	0.1	0.0	0.0	0.0
20076	Grain, Wheat Germ, crude	1 tbsp	9.6	34.6	2.2	5.0	1.3	0.9	0.1	0.6
20071	Grain, Wheat, Durum	1 tbsp	12	40.7	1.6	8.5	0.0	0.3	0.0	0.1
6115	Gravy, Au Jus, canned	1 cup	238.4	38.1	2.9	6.0	0.0	0.5	0.2	0.0
6116	Gravy, Au Jus, dry, made w/H_2O	1 cup (8 fl oz)	246	32.0	1.2	4.0	0.0	1.3	0.5	0.0
6561	Gravy, Beef, canned	1 cup	233	123.5	8.7	11.2	0.9	5.5	2.2	0.2
6118	Gravy, Brown Gravy, dry mix/Nestle Trio	1 tbsp	6	24.4	0.6	3.5	0.2	0.9	0.2	0.5
6119	Gravy, Brown, dry, made w/H_2O	1 cup (8 fl oz)	258	74.8	2.4	13.0	0.0	1.7	0.7	0.1
6120	Gravy, Chicken, canned	1 cup	238	188.0	4.6	12.9	1.0	13.6	6.1	3.6
6572	Gravy, Chicken, dry, made w/H_2O	1 cup (8 fl oz)	260	83.2	2.6	14.4	0.0	1.9	0.9	0.4
6746	Gravy, dry, made w/H_2O	¼ cup	66	21.8	0.8	3.6	0.0	0.5	0.2	0.1
6579	Gravy, Hearty Beef Gravy, glass jar/PepFarm	1 package	340	146.2	10.2	21.1	0.0	2.4	0.9	0.2
6122	Gravy, Mushroom, canned	¼ cup	60	30.0	0.8	3.3	0.2	1.6	0.7	0.6
6124	Gravy, Onion, dry, made w/H_2O	¼ cup	60	18.0	0.5	3.7	0.0	0.2	0.0	0.0
6563	Gravy, Pork, dry, made w/H_2O	¼ cup	60	18.0	0.4	3.1	0.2	0.4	0.2	0.0
6126	Gravy, Turkey, canned	1 tbsp	15	7.7	0.4	0.8	0.1	0.3	0.1	0.1
5151	Gravy, Turkey, dry, made w/H_2O	1 tbsp	15	5.0	0.2	0.9	0.1	0.1	0.0	0.0
22700	Hamburger Helper	1 serving	144	341.3	20.3	30.0	0.0	15.7	0.0	0.0
2023	Herb, Ginger Root, peeled, sliced, raw	5 slices (1″diam x 0.12″thick)	11	7.6	0.2	1.7	0.2	0.1	0.0	0.0
17170	Hopping John (rice&blackeyed peas)	⅓ cup	100	118.0	5.0	17.8	0.5	3.6	0.0	0.0
901932	Ice Cream Bar, Vanilla	1 bar	67	162.1	2.1	14.5	0.0	10.6	0.0	0.0
18272	Ice Cream Cone, Cake or Wafer	1 cone	4	16.7	0.3	3.2	0.1	0.3	0.1	0.1
901920	Ice Cream Cone, Sugar, Rolled	1 cone	10	40.2	0.8	8.4	0.2	0.4	0.1	0.1
19270	Ice Cream Sandwich	1 bar	62	166.8	3.1	26.1	0.1	6.2	0.0	0.3
901917	Ice Cream, Chocolate	1 individual container (3.5 fl oz)	58	125.3	2.2	16.4	0.7	6.4	1.9	0.2
901918	Ice Cream, Creamsicle	1 bar	67	103.2	1.2	17.6	0.0	3.1	0.0	0.0
19264	Ice Cream, Drumstick	1 stick	67	186.3	2.6	21.5	0.2	9.9	0.0	0.0
19090	Ice Cream, Eskimo Pie Vanilla Ice Cream Bar w/dark chocolate coating	1 bar	50	165.7	2.1	12.3	0.0	12.1	0.0	0.0
901919	Ice Cream, French Vanilla custard, soft serve	1 cup (8 fl oz)	172	369.8	7.1	38.2	0.0	22.4	6.0	0.8
19262	Ice Cream, Fudgsicle	1 bar	73	91.3	3.8	18.6	0.0	0.2	0.0	0.0
901922	Ice Cream, Klondike Vanilla Ice Cream Bar w/chocolate coating	1 bar (5 fl oz)	148	488.5	6.2	35.7	0.0	35.7	0.0	0.0
901923	Ice Cream, Light, Chocolate (ice milk)	2/3 cup	90	136.8	4.3	20.2	0.0	4.6	1.5	0.2
19088	Ice Cream, Light, Strawberry (ice milk)	2/3 cup	90	133.2	4.3	22.1	0.1	3.1	0.9	0.1
19096	Ice Cream, Light, Vanilla	1 cup (8 fl oz)	132	183.5	5.0	30.0	0.0	5.7	1.6	0.2
19260	Ice Cream, Light, Vanilla, soft serve	1 cup (8 fl oz)	176	221.8	8.6	38.4	0.0	4.6	1.3	0.2
19271	Ice Cream, Light, w/aspartame, no sugar, vanilla	1 tbsp	8.1	12.3	0.4	1.5	0.0	0.5	0.1	0.0
19095	Ice Cream, Strawberry	1 individual container (3.5 fl oz)	58	111.4	1.9	16.0	0.2	4.9	0.0	0.0
19089	Ice Cream, Vanilla	1 individual container (3.5 fl oz)	58	116.6	2.0	13.7	0.0	6.4	1.8	0.2
17003	Lamb, Domestic, Choice, Composite, lean (¼″ trim) ckd	3.0 oz	85	175.1	24.0	0.0	0.0	8.1	3.5	0.5
17001	Lamb, Domestic, Choice, Composite, lean (¼″ trim) raw	3.5 oz	100	134.0	20.3	0.0	0.0	5.3	2.1	0.5
17226	Lamb, Domestic, Choice, Composite, lean&fat (⅛″ trim) cooked	3.5 oz	100	271.0	25.5	0.0	0.0	18.0	7.6	1.3
18370	Leavening Agent, Baking Powder, Double Acting, Na Al sulfate	1 tsp	4.6	2.4	0.0	1.3	0.0	0.0	0.0	0.0
18373	Leavening Agent, Baking Soda	1 tbsp	13.8	0.0	0.0	0.0	0.0	0.0	0.0	0.0
18375	Leavening Agent, Cream of Tartar	1 tsp	3	7.7	0.0	1.8	0.0	0.0	0.0	0.0
18374	Leavening Agent, Yeast, Baker's, Active	1 package (0.25 oz)	7	20.7	2.7	2.7	1.5	0.3	0.2	0.0
7001	Lobster (shellfish) Egg Roll/LaChoy	1 medium	13	26.4	0.7	4.2	0.0	0.7	0.1	0.4
7274	Lunch Meat, Barbecue Loaf (Pork & Beef)	1.0 oz, 1 slice	28	48.4	4.4	1.8	0.0	2.5	1.2	0.2
7042	Lunch Meat, Beef Pastrami, cooked, smoked, chopped, pressed/Carl Buddig	2.5 oz, 1 pkg	71	100.1	13.9	0.7	0.0	4.6	0.0	0.2
7043	Lunch Meat, Beef, smoked, sliced/Carl Buddig	2.5 oz, 1 pkg	71	98.7	13.7	0.4	0.0	4.6	0.0	0.2
7008	Lunch Meat, Beef, thin slices	1.0 oz, 6 paper-thin slices	28	49.6	7.9	1.6	0.0	1.1	0.5	0.1
7202	Lunch Meat, Bologna (Beef & Pork)	1.0 oz, 1 slice	28	88.5	3.3	0.8	0.0	7.9	3.7	0.7

Sat (g)	Chol (mg)	Cal (mg)	Iron (mg)	Magn (mg)	Phos (mg)	Pota (mg)	Sodi (mg)	Zinc (mg)	Vit A (RE)	Vit C (mg)	Vit E (mg)	Thia (mg)	Ribo (mg)	Niac (mg)	Vit B-6 (mg)	Fol (µg)	Vit B-12 (µg)	Wat (g)
0.0	0.0	2.6	0.1	4.8	18.4	17.9	1.1	0.1	0.0	0.0	0.0	0.0	0.0	0.4	0.0	2.2	0.0	0.9
0.0	0.0	9.0	2.3	0.0	0.0	33.0	701.0	0.0	55.4	0.0	0.0	0.0	0.1	0.1	0.0	0.0	0.0	211.0
0.0	0.0	0.3	0.1	4.8	10.9	6.8	0.2	0.1	0.0	0.0	0.0	0.0	0.0	0.1	0.0	2.1	0.0	7.8
0.1	0.0	5.3	0.5	17.3	51.3	42.0	0.2	0.4	0.0	0.0	0.1	0.1	0.0	0.1	0.0	5.5	0.0	0.8
0.0	0.0	1.2	0.1	5.2	10.1	5.2	0.6	0.1	0.0	0.0	0.1	0.0	0.0	0.2	0.0	0.5	0.0	8.9
0.0	0.0	1.2	0.1	5.4	9.4	9.6	0.1	0.1	0.0	0.0	0.0	0.0	0.0	0.2	0.0	0.5	0.0	8.9
0.0	0.0	0.2	0.0	0.5	0.9	1.1	0.5	0.0	0.0	0.0	0.0	0.0	0.0	0.0	0.0	0.1	0.0	8.4
0.0	0.0	1.0	0.1	1.2	4.3	3.5	37.8	0.0	0.0	0.0	0.0	0.0	0.0	0.1	0.0	5.7	0.0	6.8
0.0	0.0	0.8	0.1	0.5	1.4	0.4	0.3	0.0	0.0	0.0	0.0	0.0	0.0	0.1	0.0	4.2	0.0	7.9
0.0	0.0	1.0	0.1	1.2	4.3	3.5	0.1	0.0	0.0	0.0	0.0	0.0	0.0	0.1	0.0	5.7	0.0	6.8
0.0	0.0	1.0	0.0	1.2	4.2	3.4	0.1	0.0	0.0	0.0	0.0	0.0	0.0	0.0	0.0	0.3	0.0	6.7
0.0	0.0	1.0	0.0	1.2	4.3	3.5	37.8	0.0	0.0	0.0	0.0	0.0	0.0	0.0	0.0	0.3	0.0	6.8
0.0	0.0	0.3	0.2	1.5	4.3	3.4	0.0	0.0	0.0	0.0	0.0	0.0	0.0	0.2	0.0	6.7	0.0	8.0
0.0	0.0	0.3	0.0	1.5	4.3	3.4	0.0	0.0	0.0	0.0	0.0	0.0	0.0	0.0	0.0	0.2	0.0	8.0
0.1	0.1	1.0	0.1	1.5	4.7	5.3	71.6	0.0	0.0	0.0	0.0	0.0	0.0	0.2	0.0	5.5	0.0	9.0
0.0	0.0	3.5	0.3	12.8	39.6	28.0	0.6	0.4	0.0	0.0	0.2	0.0	0.0	0.5	0.0	6.4	0.0	1.2
0.0	0.0	1.8	0.5	4.9	14.1	19.3	0.1	0.1	0.0	0.0	0.0	0.1	0.1	0.6	0.0	16.0	0.0	1.3
0.1	0.0	3.4	0.5	0.0	34.4	42.0	0.7	0.0	0.0	0.0	0.0	0.0	0.0	0.4	0.0	0.0	0.0	1.1
0.0	0.0	1.9	0.2	0.1	0.7	1.0	0.1	0.0	0.0	0.0	0.0	0.0	0.0	0.0	0.0	0.4	0.0	1.0
0.2	0.0	3.7	0.6	22.9	80.8	85.6	1.2	1.2	0.0	0.0	0.0	0.2	0.0	0.7	0.1	27.0	0.0	1.1
0.1	0.0	4.1	0.4	17.3	61.0	51.7	0.2	0.5	0.0	0.0	0.0	0.1	0.0	0.8	0.1	5.2	0.0	1.3
0.2	0.0	9.5	1.4	4.8	71.5	193.1	119.2	2.4	0.0	2.4	0.0	0.0	0.1	2.1	0.0	4.8	0.2	225.3
0.6	2.5	22.1	0.0	7.4	0.0	0.0	964.3	0.1	0.0	0.0	0.0	0.0	0.0	0.0	0.0	0.0	0.0	236.5
2.7	7.0	14.0	1.6	4.7	69.9	188.7	1304.8	2.3	0.0	0.0	0.1	0.1	0.1	1.5	0.0	4.7	0.2	203.8
0.3	0.0	2.2	0.1	0.5	7.3	0.8	261.8	0.0	0.0	0.0	0.0	0.0	0.0	0.0	0.0	1.6	0.0	0.3
0.8	2.6	67.1	0.2	10.3	43.9	56.8	1075.9	0.3	0.0	0.0	0.0	0.0	0.1	0.8	0.0	0.0	0.0	237.0
3.4	4.8	47.6	1.1	4.8	69.0	259.4	1373.3	1.9	264.2	0.0	0.4	0.0	0.1	1.1	0.0	4.8	0.2	203.1
0.5	2.6	39.0	0.3	10.4	46.8	62.4	1133.6	0.3	0.0	2.6	0.0	0.1	0.1	0.8	0.0	2.6	0.2	237.7
0.2	0.0	9.2	0.1	2.6	12.5	16.5	359.0	0.1	0.0	0.5	0.0	0.0	0.0	0.2	0.0	0.9	0.0	60.0
0.8	17.0	0.0	0.0	0.0	0.0	0.0	2145.4	0.0	0.0	0.0	0.0	0.0	0.0	0.0	0.0	0.0	0.0	300.6
0.2	0.0	4.2	0.4	1.2	9.0	63.6	342.0	0.4	0.0	0.0	0.0	0.0	0.0	0.4	0.0	7.2	0.0	53.4
0.1	0.0	16.8	0.0	0.6	0.0	0.0	232.8	0.1	0.0	0.0	0.0	0.0	0.0	0.0	0.0	0.0	0.0	54.7
0.2	0.6	7.2	0.1	2.4	10.2	13.2	287.4	0.1	0.0	0.4	0.0	0.0	0.0	0.2	0.0	0.7	0.0	55.2
0.1	0.3	0.6	0.1	0.3	4.4	16.4	86.6	0.1	0.0	0.0	0.0	0.0	0.0	0.2	0.0	0.3	0.0	13.3
0.0	0.2	2.9	0.0	0.6	2.9	3.8	86.0	0.0	0.0	0.1	0.0	0.0	0.0	0.1	0.0	0.2	0.0	13.6
0.0	0.0	0.0	0.0	0.0	0.0	436.0	1043.0	0.0	0.0	0.0	0.0	0.0	0.0	0.0	0.0	0.0	0.0	78.0
0.0	0.0	2.0	0.1	4.7	3.0	45.7	1.4	0.0	0.0	0.6	0.0	0.0	0.0	0.1	0.0	1.2	0.0	9.0
0.0	0.0	22.0	1.0	0.0	81.0	112.0	447.0	0.0	4.2	2.0	0.0	0.5	0.0	0.3	0.0	0.0	0.0	0.0
0.0	0.0	70.0	0.0	8.0	52.0	107.0	28.0	0.0	41.8	0.0	0.0	0.0	0.1	0.1	0.0	0.0	0.0	0.0
0.0	0.0	1.0	0.1	1.0	3.9	4.5	5.7	0.0	0.0	0.0	0.1	0.0	0.0	0.2	0.0	4.1	0.0	0.2
0.1	0.0	4.4	0.4	3.1	10.3	14.5	32.0	0.1	0.0	0.0	0.0	0.1	0.0	0.5	0.0	8.3	0.0	0.3
3.7	0.0	73.0	0.1	8.0	72.0	102.0	92.0	0.0	38.6	0.0	0.0	0.1	0.1	0.5	0.0	0.0	0.0	0.0
3.9	19.7	63.2	0.5	16.8	62.1	144.4	44.1	0.3	69.0	0.4	0.2	0.0	0.1	0.1	0.0	9.3	0.2	32.3
0.0	0.0	46.0	0.0	5.0	37.0	82.0	27.0	0.0	25.0	0.0	0.0	0.0	0.0	0.3	0.0	0.0	0.0	0.0
0.0	0.0	67.0	0.1	7.0	59.0	99.0	57.0	0.0	37.0	0.0	0.0	0.0	0.0	0.5	0.0	0.0	0.0	0.0
7.3	14.2	59.5	0.0	0.0	0.0	0.0	34.2	0.0	0.0	0.0	0.0	0.0	0.0	0.0	0.0	0.0	0.0	23.2
12.9	156.5	225.3	0.4	20.6	199.5	304.4	104.9	0.9	264.9	1.4	0.6	0.1	0.3	0.2	0.1	15.5	0.9	102.9
0.2	0.0	129.0	0.1	14.0	99.0	173.0	55.0	0.0	0.0	0.0	0.0	0.0	0.2	0.7	0.0	0.0	0.0	0.0
19.4	39.8	211.6	0.0	0.0	0.0	0.0	107.9	0.0	0.0	0.0	0.0	0.0	0.0	0.0	0.0	0.0	0.0	69.1
2.9	13.0	140.0	0.1	12.0	111.0	175.0	61.0	0.8	38.0	1.0	0.0	0.0	0.2	0.1	0.1	5.0	1.4	0.0
2.1	13.0	161.0	0.3	12.0	121.0	412.0	64.0	0.9	25.8	0.0	0.0	0.1	0.2	0.1	0.1	5.0	1.4	0.0
3.5	18.5	183.5	0.1	19.8	143.9	278.5	112.2	0.6	62.0	1.1	0.0	0.1	0.3	0.1	0.1	7.9	0.9	90.0
2.9	21.1	276.3	0.1	24.6	213.0	389.0	123.2	0.9	51.0	1.6	0.0	0.1	0.3	0.2	0.1	10.6	0.9	122.5
0.3	1.3	15.9	0.0	0.0	0.0	0.0	7.2	0.0	0.0	0.0	0.0	0.0	0.0	0.0	0.0	0.0	0.0	5.6
3.0	16.8	69.6	0.1	8.1	58.0	109.0	34.8	0.2	45.2	4.5	0.0	0.0	0.1	0.1	0.0	7.0	0.2	34.8
3.9	25.5	74.2	0.1	8.1	60.9	115.4	46.4	0.4	67.9	0.3	0.0	0.0	0.1	0.1	0.0	2.9	0.2	35.4
2.9	78.2	12.8	1.7	22.1	178.5	292.4	64.6	4.5	0.0	0.0	0.2	0.1	0.2	5.4	0.1	19.6	2.2	52.7
1.9	65.0	10.0	1.8	26.0	189.0	280.0	66.0	4.1	0.0	0.0	0.2	0.1	0.2	6.0	0.2	23.0	2.6	73.4
7.5	96.0	16.0	1.9	24.0	193.0	318.0	72.0	4.7	0.0	0.0	0.2	0.1	0.3	6.6	0.1	19.0	2.6	55.8
0.0	0.0	270.3	0.5	1.2	100.8	0.9	487.6	0.0	0.0	0.0	0.0	0.0	0.0	0.0	0.0	0.0	0.0	0.2
0.0	0.0	0.0	0.0	0.0	0.0	0.0	3775.7	0.0	0.0	0.0	0.0	0.0	0.0	0.0	0.0	0.0	0.0	0.1
0.0	0.0	0.2	0.1	0.1	0.2	495.0	1.6	0.0	0.0	0.0	0.0	0.0	0.0	0.0	0.0	0.0	0.0	0.1
0.0	0.0	4.5	1.2	6.9	90.3	140.0	3.5	0.4	0.0	0.0	0.0	0.2	0.4	2.8	0.1	163.8	0.0	0.5
0.1	0.0	3.9	0.2	0.0	0.0	24.6	52.7	0.0	1.8	1.1	0.0	0.0	0.0	0.3	0.0	0.0	0.0	0.0
0.9	10.4	15.4	0.3	4.8	37.0	92.1	373.5	0.7	2.0	0.0	0.0	0.1	0.1	0.6	0.1	2.5	0.5	18.1
2.1	46.2	12.1	1.7	0.0	0.0	259.2	749.8	0.0	0.0	0.0	0.0	0.1	0.2	2.9	0.0	0.0	0.0	49.6
1.8	47.6	9.9	1.6	0.0	0.0	238.6	1016.0	0.0	0.0	0.0	0.0	0.1	0.2	2.7	0.0	0.0	0.0	49.3
0.5	11.5	3.1	0.8	5.3	47.0	120.1	402.9	1.1	0.0	0.0	0.1	0.0	0.1	1.5	0.1	3.1	0.7	16.3
3.0	15.4	3.4	0.4	3.1	25.5	50.4	285.3	0.5	0.0	0.0	0.1	0.0	0.0	0.7	0.1	1.4	0.4	15.2

Code	Food Name	Unit/Amt	Wt (g)	Energy (Kcal)	Prot (g)	Carb (g)	Fiber (g)	Fat (g)	Mono (g)	Poly (g)
7007	Lunch Meat, Bologna (Beef light)/Oscar Mayer	1.0 oz, 2 slices	28	55.4	3.3	1.7	0.0	4.0	2.0	0.1
7201	Lunch Meat, Bologna (Beef)	1.0 oz, 1 slice	28	87.4	3.4	0.2	0.0	8.0	3.9	0.3
7010	Lunch Meat, Bologna (Chicken, Pork & Beef)/Oscar Mayer	1.0 oz, 1 slice	28	89.0	3.1	0.7	0.0	8.2	4.1	1.1
7011	Lunch Meat, Bologna (Pork)	1.0 oz, 1 slice	28	69.2	4.3	0.2	0.0	5.6	2.7	0.6
7206	Lunch Meat, Bologna (Turkey)	1.0 oz, 1 slice	28	55.7	3.8	0.3	0.0	4.3	1.3	1.2
7039	Lunch Meat, Bologna, fat free/Oscar Mayer	1.0 oz, 1 slice	28	22.1	3.5	1.7	0.0	0.2	0.1	0.0
7249	Lunch Meat, Braunschweiger Liver Sausage, sliced/Oscar Mayer	1.0 oz, 1 slice	28	94.1	3.9	0.6	0.1	8.5	4.3	1.0
7209	Lunch Meat, Chicken Breast Classic Baked/Grill, carving board/Louis Rich	1.0 oz, 1 slice	28	27.4	5.5	1.0	0.0	0.1	0.0	0.0
7250	Lunch Meat, Chicken Breast, honey glazed/Oscar Mayer	1.0 oz, 1 slice	28	30.5	5.5	1.2	0.0	0.4	0.2	0.1
7210	Lunch Meat, Chicken Breast, oven roasted deluxe/Louis Rich	1.0 oz, 1 slice	28	28.3	5.1	0.7	0.0	0.6	0.2	0.1
7053	Lunch Meat, Chicken Breast, oven roasted, fat free/Oscar Mayer	1.0 oz, 1 slice	28	23.8	5.1	0.5	0.0	0.2	0.0	0.0
7018	Lunch Meat, Chicken Roll, light meat	2.0 oz, 2 slices	57	90.6	11.1	1.4	0.0	4.2	1.7	0.9
7271	Lunch Meat, Chicken Spread, canned	1.5 oz.	43	82.6	6.6	2.3	0.0	5.0	2.1	1.1
7251	Lunch Meat, Chicken, light and dark meat, sliced, smoked/Carl Buddig	2.5 oz, 1 pkg	71	117.2	12.7	0.5	0.0	7.2	0.0	1.5
7021	Lunch Meat, Corned Beef, cooked, chopped, pressed/Carl Buddig	2.5 oz, 1 pkg	71	100.8	13.7	0.7	0.0	4.8	0.0	0.2
7252	Lunch Meat, Dutch Brand (Old Fashion) Loaf (Pork & Beef)	1.0 oz, 1 slice	28	67.2	3.8	1.6	0.0	5.0	2.3	0.5
7253	Lunch Meat, Franks (Turkey & Chicken Cheese)/Louis Rich	1.6 oz, 1 frank	45	90.5	5.7	2.3	0.0	6.5	2.8	1.3
7054	Lunch Meat, Franks (Turkey & Chicken)/Louis Rich	1.6 oz, 1 frank	45	84.6	5.0	2.4	0.0	6.1	2.5	1.4
7033	Lunch Meat, Ham & Cheese Loaf or Roll	1.0 oz, 1 slice	28	72.5	4.7	0.4	0.0	5.7	2.6	0.6
7211	Lunch Meat, Ham & Cheese Spread	3 tbsp	43	105.4	7.0	1.0	0.0	8.0	3.0	0.6
7031	Lunch Meat, Ham and Cheese Loaf/Oscar Mayer	1.0 oz, 1 slice	28	64.4	3.9	1.0	0.0	5.0	2.3	0.5
7212	Lunch Meat, Ham Salad Spread	1.0 oz, 1tbsp	28	60.5	2.4	3.0	0.0	4.3	2.0	0.8
7030	Lunch Meat, Ham, honey, water added/Oscar Mayer	1 slice	21	23.3	3.5	0.7	0.0	0.7	0.4	0.1
7028	Lunch Meat, Ham, minced	1 slice	21	55.2	3.4	0.4	0.0	4.3	2.0	0.5
7029	Lunch Meat, Ham, slices, extra lean (5% fat)	1 slice : 6.25 x 4 x 0.06"	28.35	37.1	5.5	0.3	0.0	1.4	0.7	0.1
7217	Lunch Meat, Ham, slices, regular (11% fat)	1 slice : 6.25 x 4 x 0.06"	28.35	51.6	5.0	0.9	0.0	3.0	1.4	0.3
7216	Lunch Meat, Ham, smoked, sliced/Carl Buddig	2.5 oz, 1 pkg	71	115.7	13.1	0.8	0.0	6.6	0.0	0.8
7214	Lunch Meat, Ham, water added, baked, 96% fat free/Oscar Mayer	2.25 oz	63	64.9	10.4	0.6	0.0	2.3	0.7	0.8
7035	Lunch Meat, Head Cheese/Oscar Mayer	1.0 oz, 1 slice	28	51.8	4.4	0.0	0.0	3.8	1.9	0.4
7219	Lunch Meat, Honey Loaf (Pork & Beef)	2 slices: 4 x 4 x 0.09"	57	73.0	9.0	3.0	0.0	2.5	1.1	0.3
7220	Lunch Meat, Jellied, Beef	1 slice (4 x 4 x 0.9" thick)	29	32.2	5.5	0.0	0.0	1.0	0.4	0.0
7055	Lunch Meat, Liver Cheese (Pork)	1.0 oz slice	28	85.1	4.3	0.6	0.0	7.2	3.4	1.0
7041	Lunch Meat, Liver Pate, canned	1.0 oz, 2 tbsp	28	89.3	4.0	0.4	0.0	7.8	3.5	0.9
7221	Lunch Meat, Liver Sausage (Liverwurst)	1 slice: 2.5"diam x 0.25"thick	18	58.7	2.5	0.4	0.0	5.1	2.4	0.5
7060	Lunch Meat, Luncheon Loaf, spiced/Oscar Mayer	1.0 oz, 1 slice	28	65.5	3.8	2.0	0.0	4.7	2.1	0.8
7223	Lunch Meat, Old Fashioned Loaf/Oscar Mayer	1.0 oz, 1 slice	28	64.7	3.7	2.2	0.0	4.6	2.2	0.7
7051	Lunch Meat, Olive Loaf (Chicken, Pork & Turkey)/Oscar Mayer	1.0 oz, 1 slice	28	73.6	2.8	1.9	0.0	6.1	3.1	0.7
13355	Lunch Meat, Olive Loaf (Pork)	1.0 oz, 1 slice	28	65.8	3.3	2.6	0.0	4.6	2.2	0.5
7052	Lunch Meat, Pastrami (Beef)	1.0 oz, 1 slice	28	97.7	4.8	0.9	0.0	8.2	4.1	0.3
7056	Lunch Meat, Pastrami (Turkey)	1.0 oz, 1 slice	28	39.5	5.1	0.5	0.0	1.7	0.6	0.4
7058	Lunch Meat, Peppered Loaf (Pork & Beef)	1.0 oz, 1 slice	28	41.4	4.8	1.3	0.0	1.8	0.8	0.1
7224	Lunch Meat, Pickle & Pimiento Loaf	1.0 oz, 1 slice	28	73.4	3.2	1.7	0.0	5.9	2.7	0.7
7045	Lunch Meat, Pork Sausage Links, cooked/Oscar Mayer	1 link	24	82.3	3.9	0.2	0.0	7.3	3.6	0.9
7067	Lunch Meat, Pork, canned	0.75 oz, 1 slice	21	70.1	2.6	0.4	0.0	6.4	3.0	0.7
7227	Lunch Meat, Salami Beef Cotto/Oscar Mayer	0.75 oz, 1 slice	21	43.3	3.0	0.4	0.0	3.3	1.5	0.2
7230	Lunch Meat, Salami Cotto (Beef, Pork & Chicken)/Oscar Mayer	0.75 oz, 1 slice	21	51.5	2.8	0.5	0.0	4.3	2.1	0.4
7073	Lunch Meat, Salami, hard/Oscar Mayer	0.33 oz, 1 slice	9	35.8	2.5	0.3	0.0	2.8	1.4	0.3
7231	Lunch Meat, Sandwich Spread (Pork & Beef)	1.0 oz, 2 tbsp	28	65.8	2.1	3.3	0.1	4.9	2.1	0.7
7232	Lunch Meat, Sandwich Spread (Pork, Chicken & Beef)/Oscar Mayer	1.0 oz, 2 tbsp	28	66.4	1.8	4.3	0.1	4.6	2.0	0.7
7233	Lunch Meat, Smokie Links Sausage/Oscar Mayer	1.5 oz, 1 link	43	129.9	5.3	0.7	0.0	11.7	5.7	1.2
7236	Lunch Meat, Smokies Sausage Little (Pork & Turkey)/Oscar Mayer	0.33 oz, 1 sm link	9	27.1	1.1	0.2	0.0	2.4	1.2	0.3
7237	Lunch Meat, Smokies Sausage Little Cheese (Pork & Turkey)/Oscar Mayer	0.33 oz, 1 sm link	9	28.4	1.2	0.2	0.0	2.5	1.2	0.3
7254	Lunch Meat, Summer Sausage Thuringer Cervalat/Oscar Mayer	1.0 oz, 1 slice	28	85.1	4.2	0.3	0.0	7.5	3.4	0.6
7255	Lunch Meat, Turkey Bacon/Louis Rich	0.5 oz, 1 slice	14	34.2	2.2	0.3	0.0	2.7	1.1	0.7
7256	Lunch Meat, Turkey Bologna/Louis Rich	1.0 oz, 1 slice	28	51.5	3.2	1.3	0.0	3.7	1.5	1.0
7259	Lunch Meat, Turkey Breast Meat	1.5 oz, 2 slices	42	46.2	9.5	0.0	0.0	0.7	0.2	0.1
7260	Lunch Meat, Turkey Breast, oven roasted, fat free/Louis Rich	1.0 oz, 1 slice	28	23.5	4.2	1.3	0.0	0.2	0.1	0.1
7239	Lunch Meat, Turkey Breast, smoked, carving board/Louis Rich	2, 1.0 oz slices	45	42.3	8.9	0.7	0.0	0.5	0.1	0.1
7080	Lunch Meat, Turkey Ham, 10% water added/Louis Rich	1.0 oz slice	28	31.6	5.1	0.3	0.0	1.1	0.3	0.2
7265	Lunch Meat, Turkey Ham, cured	2 slices	57	73.0	10.8	0.2	0.0	2.9	0.7	0.9
7081	Lunch Meat, Turkey Roll, light & dark meat	2.0 oz slice	56	83.4	10.2	1.2	0.0	3.9	1.3	1.0
7267	Lunch Meat, Turkey Roll, light meat	2.0 oz slice	56	82.3	10.5	0.3	0.0	4.0	1.4	1.0
7266	Lunch Meat, Turkey Salami Cotto/Louis Rich	1.0 oz, 1 slice	28	41.7	4.2	0.3	0.0	2.7	1.1	0.7
5300	Lunch Meat, Turkey Smoked Sausage/Louis Rich	2 oz, slice	56	89.6	8.1	2.2	0.0	5.4	2.0	1.5
7273	Lunch Meat, Turkey, honey roasted, fat free/Louis Rich	2.0 oz slice	56	57.1	10.8	2.5	0.0	0.4	0.1	0.1
7243	Lunch Meat, Wieners (Beef Franks) bun length/Oscar Mayer	1 frank	57	183.5	6.4	1.6	0.0	16.9	8.3	0.5
7241	Lunch Meat, Wieners (Beef Franks) light/Oscar Mayer	1 frank	57	110.0	6.1	2.3	0.0	8.5	4.3	0.6
7246	Lunch Meat, Wieners (Cheese Hot Dogs w/turkey)/Oscar Mayer	1 frank	45	143.1	5.4	1.3	0.0	12.9	5.9	1.7
7247	Lunch Meat, Wieners (Hot Dogs) fat free/Oscar Mayer	1 frank	50	36.5	6.3	2.2	0.0	0.3	0.1	0.1

Sat (g)	Chol (mg)	Cal (mg)	Iron (mg)	Magn (mg)	Phos (mg)	Pota (mg)	Sodi (mg)	Zinc (mg)	Vit A (RE)	Vit C (mg)	Vit E (mg)	Thia (mg)	Ribo (mg)	Niac (mg)	Vit B-6 (mg)	Fol (µg)	Vit B-12 (µg)	Wat (g)
1.6	12.6	3.6	0.3	3.9	49.8	43.7	313.9	0.5	0.0	0.0	0.0	0.0	0.0	0.0	0.0	0.0	0.0	18.2
3.4	16.2	3.4	0.5	3.4	24.6	44.0	274.7	0.6	0.0	0.0	0.1	0.0	0.0	0.7	0.0	1.4	0.4	15.5
2.9	28.8	19.3	0.5	5.9	55.7	43.1	289.2	0.4	0.0	0.0	0.0	0.0	0.0	0.0	0.0	0.0	0.0	15.0
1.9	16.5	3.1	0.2	3.9	38.9	78.7	331.5	0.6	0.0	0.0	0.1	0.1	0.0	1.1	0.1	1.4	0.3	17.0
1.4	27.7	23.5	0.4	3.9	36.7	55.7	245.8	0.5	0.0	0.0	0.1	0.0	0.0	1.0	0.1	2.0	0.1	18.2
0.1	7.0	4.2	0.3	6.2	43.1	43.7	273.6	0.3	0.0	0.0	0.0	0.0	0.0	0.0	0.0	0.0	0.0	21.8
3.1	49.0	2.5	2.7	3.9	55.7	56.6	324.0	1.0	0.0	2.5	0.0	0.1	0.4	2.6	0.1	13.2	5.3	14.1
0.0	14.6	2.2	0.4	9.0	79.0	81.5	319.8	0.2	0.0	0.0	0.0	0.0	0.0	0.0	0.0	0.0	0.0	20.4
0.1	15.1	2.8	0.3	10.1	80.9	92.1	388.1	0.2	0.0	0.0	0.0	0.0	0.0	0.0	0.0	0.0	0.0	19.7
0.2	13.7	2.0	0.3	6.7	74.5	74.2	332.6	0.2	0.0	0.0	0.0	0.0	0.0	0.0	0.0	0.0	0.0	20.6
0.0	12.3	3.4	0.4	10.1	71.7	88.5	347.8	0.2	0.0	0.0	0.0	0.0	0.0	0.0	0.0	0.0	0.0	21.2
1.2	28.5	24.5	0.6	10.8	89.5	130.0	332.9	0.4	13.7	0.0	0.2	0.0	0.1	3.0	0.1	1.1	0.1	39.1
1.5	22.4	53.8	1.0	5.2	38.3	45.6	166.0	0.5	10.8	0.0	0.0	0.0	0.0	1.2	0.1	1.3	0.1	28.5
1.8	37.6	88.0	1.1	0.0	0.0	181.8	677.3	0.0	0.0	0.0	0.0	0.0	0.2	4.8	0.0	0.0	0.0	48.4
2.0	46.2	12.1	1.7	0.0	0.0	249.9	952.8	0.0	0.0	0.0	0.0	0.1	0.2	3.0	0.0	0.0	0.0	49.1
1.8	13.2	23.5	0.3	5.9	45.4	105.3	350.0	0.5	0.0	0.0	0.1	0.1	0.1	0.7	0.1	0.6	0.4	16.6
2.3	42.3	109.4	0.9	9.9	91.8	71.1	481.5	0.8	0.0	0.0	0.0	0.0	0.0	0.0	0.0	0.0	0.0	28.8
1.7	41.4	59.0	1.0	10.4	66.2	72.0	511.2	0.8	0.0	0.0	0.0	0.0	0.0	0.0	0.0	0.0	0.0	30.1
2.1	16.0	16.2	0.3	4.5	70.8	82.3	376.0	0.6	6.4	0.0	0.1	0.2	0.1	1.0	0.1	0.8	0.2	16.2
3.7	26.2	93.3	0.3	7.7	212.9	69.7	514.7	1.0	39.1	0.0	0.0	0.1	0.1	0.9	0.1	1.3	0.3	25.4
1.8	18.5	18.8	0.2	5.3	75.6	74.2	350.8	0.5	0.0	0.0	0.0	0.2	0.1	1.0	0.1	0.8	0.2	17.0
1.4	10.4	2.2	0.2	2.8	33.6	42.0	255.4	0.3	0.0	0.0	0.5	0.1	0.0	0.6	0.0	0.3	0.2	17.5
0.2	9.5	2.1	0.3	6.5	54.4	59.0	262.1	0.4	0.0	0.0	0.0	0.0	0.0	0.0	0.0	0.0	0.0	15.3
1.5	14.7	2.1	0.2	3.4	33.0	65.3	261.5	0.4	0.0	0.0	0.0	0.1	0.0	0.9	0.1	0.2	0.2	12.0
0.5	13.3	2.0	0.2	4.8	61.8	99.2	405.1	0.5	0.0	0.0	0.1	0.3	0.1	1.4	0.1	1.1	0.2	20.0
1.0	16.2	2.0	0.3	5.4	70.0	94.1	373.4	0.6	0.0	0.0	0.1	0.2	0.1	1.5	0.1	0.9	0.2	18.3
2.2	39.1	11.4	1.4	0.0	0.0	241.4	980.5	0.0	0.0	0.0	0.0	0.5	0.2	3.7	0.0	0.0	0.0	47.6
0.5	30.2	6.3	0.8	19.5	146.8	168.8	764.8	1.1	0.0	0.0	0.0	0.0	0.0	0.0	0.0	0.0	0.0	47.1
1.2	25.5	5.9	0.5	3.1	17.6	8.1	300.4	0.3	0.0	0.0	0.0	0.0	0.0	0.3	0.0	0.3	0.3	18.9
0.8	19.4	9.7	0.8	9.7	81.5	195.5	752.4	1.4	0.0	0.0	0.1	0.3	0.1	1.8	0.2	4.6	0.6	40.2
0.4	9.9	2.9	1.0	5.2	40.3	116.6	383.4	1.0	0.0	0.0	0.0	0.0	0.1	1.4	0.1	2.0	1.5	21.6
2.5	48.7	2.2	3.0	3.4	58.0	63.3	343.0	1.0	1470.6	0.8	0.0	0.1	0.6	3.3	0.1	29.1	6.9	15.0
2.7	71.4	19.6	1.5	3.6	56.0	38.6	195.2	0.8	279.7	0.6	0.0	0.0	0.2	0.9	0.0	16.8	0.9	15.1
1.9	28.4	4.7	1.2	2.2	41.4	30.6	154.8	0.4	1494.0	0.0	0.0	0.0	0.2	0.8	0.0	5.4	2.4	9.4
1.5	18.8	30.5	0.4	6.7	54.6	75.6	343.3	0.5	0.0	0.0	0.0	0.0	0.0	0.0	0.0	0.0	0.0	16.4
1.6	17.1	31.6	0.4	6.4	58.2	82.3	331.5	0.5	0.0	0.0	0.0	0.0	0.0	0.0	0.0	0.0	0.0	16.5
2.0	19.9	31.1	0.5	7.6	37.0	52.1	369.0	0.3	0.0	0.0	0.0	0.0	0.0	0.0	0.0	0.0	0.0	16.1
1.6	10.6	30.5	0.2	5.3	35.6	83.2	415.5	0.4	5.6	0.0	0.1	0.1	0.1	0.5	0.1	0.6	0.4	16.3
2.9	26.0	2.5	0.5	5.0	42.0	63.8	343.6	1.2	0.0	0.0	0.1	0.0	0.1	1.4	0.1	2.0	0.5	13.1
0.5	15.1	2.5	0.5	3.9	56.0	72.8	292.6	0.6	0.0	0.0	0.1	0.0	0.1	1.0	0.1	1.4	0.1	19.8
0.6	12.9	15.1	0.3	5.6	47.6	110.3	426.4	0.9	0.0	0.0	0.1	0.1	0.1	0.9	0.1	0.6	0.5	18.9
2.2	10.4	26.6	0.3	5.0	39.2	95.2	388.9	0.4	2.0	0.0	0.1	0.1	0.1	0.6	0.1	1.4	0.3	16.0
2.6	18.5	3.8	0.4	4.3	37.9	57.1	200.6	0.6	0.0	0.0	0.0	0.0	0.0	0.0	0.0	0.0	0.0	11.9
2.3	13.0	1.3	0.2	2.1	17.2	45.2	270.7	0.3	0.0	0.0	0.2	0.1	0.1	0.7	0.0	1.3	0.2	10.8
1.4	17.4	1.5	0.6	3.6	47.0	43.5	274.9	0.4	0.0	0.0	0.0	0.0	0.0	0.0	0.0	0.0	0.0	13.5
1.8	16.8	15.8	0.6	6.1	51.9	45.6	230.0	0.4	0.0	0.0	0.0	0.0	0.0	0.0	0.0	0.0	0.0	12.7
1.0	8.6	1.1	0.2	1.9	16.2	32.0	169.4	0.3	0.0	0.0	0.0	0.1	0.0	0.5	0.0	0.3	0.2	3.0
1.7	10.6	3.4	0.2	2.2	16.5	30.8	283.6	0.3	2.5	0.0	0.5	0.0	0.0	0.5	0.0	0.6	0.3	16.9
1.6	12.6	7.6	0.2	3.4	19.3	33.0	229.9	0.2	0.0	0.0	0.0	0.0	0.0	0.0	0.0	0.0	0.0	16.6
4.0	27.1	4.3	0.5	7.3	103.2	77.4	433.0	0.9	0.0	0.0	0.0	0.0	0.0	0.0	0.0	0.0	0.0	23.9
0.8	5.8	1.0	0.1	1.5	19.1	15.6	92.0	0.2	0.0	0.0	0.0	0.0	0.0	0.0	0.0	0.0	0.0	5.0
1.0	6.0	6.0	0.1	1.9	22.3	13.7	93.2	0.2	0.0	0.0	0.0	0.0	0.0	0.0	0.0	0.0	0.0	4.8
3.0	23.5	2.5	0.6	4.2	36.4	63.8	400.4	0.6	0.0	0.0	0.0	0.1	0.1	1.2	0.1	1.4	1.1	14.9
0.7	12.5	5.6	0.2	2.7	27.9	29.1	184.2	0.4	0.0	0.0	0.0	0.0	0.0	0.0	0.0	0.0	0.0	8.3
1.1	19.0	34.7	0.5	6.2	54.9	42.6	269.9	0.5	0.0	0.0	0.0	0.0	0.0	0.0	0.0	0.0	0.0	19.0
0.2	17.2	2.9	0.2	8.4	96.2	116.8	601.0	0.5	0.0	0.0	0.0	0.0	0.0	3.5	0.2	1.7	0.8	30.2
0.1	9.0	3.1	0.3	7.6	65.0	57.4	333.8	0.2	0.0	0.0	0.0	0.0	0.0	0.0	0.0	0.0	0.0	21.4
0.1	19.4	6.8	0.7	14.0	143.1	140.4	540.5	0.4	0.0	0.0	0.0	0.0	0.0	0.0	0.0	0.0	0.0	33.4
0.3	18.8	1.4	0.4	6.2	82.3	81.2	315.6	0.7	0.0	0.0	0.0	0.0	0.0	0.0	0.0	0.0	0.0	20.5
1.0	31.9	5.7	1.6	9.1	108.9	185.3	567.7	1.7	0.0	0.0	0.4	0.0	0.1	2.0	0.1	3.4	0.1	40.7
1.1	30.8	17.9	0.8	10.1	94.1	151.2	328.2	1.1	0.0	0.0	0.2	0.1	0.2	2.7	0.2	2.8	0.1	39.3
1.1	24.1	22.4	0.7	9.0	102.5	140.6	273.8	0.9	0.0	0.0	0.1	0.0	0.1	3.9	0.2	2.2	0.1	40.1
0.8	21.6	8.7	0.5	5.9	76.2	61.6	285.0	0.7	0.0	0.0	0.0	0.0	0.0	0.0	0.0	0.0	0.0	20.0
1.5	35.8	14.6	0.8	11.8	114.2	112.6	515.2	1.2	0.0	0.0	0.0	0.0	0.0	0.0	0.0	0.0	0.0	38.7
0.1	22.4	8.4	0.6	15.7	154.6	146.7	660.8	0.6	0.0	0.0	0.0	0.0	0.0	0.0	0.0	0.0	0.0	40.3
7.1	32.5	7.4	0.9	8.6	59.9	90.1	575.7	1.3	0.0	0.0	0.0	0.0	0.0	0.0	0.0	0.0	0.0	30.6
3.6	27.9	12.0	0.9	10.3	93.5	228.6	615.0	1.2	0.0	0.0	0.0	0.0	0.0	0.0	0.0	0.0	0.0	38.1
4.5	33.3	73.8	0.7	11.3	96.8	59.0	514.4	0.8	0.0	0.0	0.0	0.0	0.0	0.0	0.0	0.0	0.0	23.8
0.1	14.5	7.5	0.5	10.5	81.0	235.5	487.0	0.6	0.0	0.0	0.0	0.0	0.0	0.0	0.0	0.0	0.0	39.4

Code	Food Name	Unit/Amt	Wt (g)	Energy (Kcal)	Prot (g)	Carb (g)	Fiber (g)	Fat (g)	Mono (g)	Poly (g)
7248	Lunch Meat, Wieners (Pork & Turkey)/Oscar Mayer	1 frank	45	144.9	5.0	1.3	0.0	13.3	6.2	1.9
924132	Macaroni&Beef/FrancoAm	7.5 oz	213	191.7	9.0	30.1	0.0	3.8	0.0	0.0
924274	Macaroni&Cheese Mix/Kraft	¾ cup	147	254.3	10.8	36.3	1.0	7.5	2.0	0.6
924275	Macaroni&Cheese, frozen	6.0 oz	170	195.5	11.0	21.8	1.0	7.1	0.0	0.0
924276	Macaroni&Cheese/FrancoAm	7.5 oz	213	166.1	6.5	23.1	1.0	5.4	0.0	0.0
20099	Macaroni, enriched, ckd	1 cup elbow shaped	140	197.4	6.7	39.7	1.8	0.9	0.1	0.4
20499	Macaroni, unenriched, ckd	1 cup	115	162.2	5.5	32.6	1.5	0.8	0.1	0.3
20105	Macaroni, Vegetable, enriched, ckd	1 cup elbow shaped	140	179.2	6.3	37.3	6.0	0.2	0.0	0.1
20107	Macaroni, Whole Wheat, ckd	1 cup	134	166.2	7.1	35.6	3.8	0.7	0.1	0.3
4585	Margarine (about 40% fat) Imitation	1 cup elbow shaped	140	483.3	0.7	0.6	0.0	54.3	22.0	19.3
4132	Margarine, blend: 60% corn oil & 40% butter	1 cup spiral shaped	105	753.9	0.9	0.7	0.0	84.7	34.4	16.7
4522	Margarine, Hard w/salt	1 tbsp	15	107.8	0.1	0.1	0.0	12.1	5.4	3.8
4067	Margarine, Hard, Corn, Corn-Hydrogenated	1 tbsp	15	107.8	0.1	0.1	0.0	12.1	5.8	3.6
4068	Margarine, Hard, Corn, Soybean-Hydrogenated & Cottonseed-Hydrogenated w/salt	1 tbsp	15	107.8	0.1	0.1	0.0	12.1	5.5	3.8
4071	Margarine, Hard, Corn, Soybean-Hydrogenated & Cottonseed-Hydrogenated, no salt	1 tbsp	15	107.1	0.1	0.1	0.0	12.0	5.5	3.8
4091	Margarine, Hard, Corn-Hydrogenated	1 tbsp	15	107.8	0.1	0.1	0.0	12.1	6.9	2.7
4131	Margarine, Hard, Lard-Hydrogenated	1 tbsp	15	110.0	0.1	0.1	0.0	12.1	5.7	1.1
4089	Margarine, Hard, no salt	1 tbsp	15	107.1	0.1	0.1	0.0	12.0	5.5	3.8
4079	Margarine, Hard, Safflower, Soybean-Hydrogenated	1 tbsp	15	107.8	0.1	0.1	0.0	12.1	4.8	4.7
4081	Margarine, Hard, Soybean, Soybean-Hydrogenated	1 tbsp	15	107.8	0.1	0.1	0.0	12.1	5.6	3.9
4076	Margarine, Hard, Soybean-Hydrogenated	1 tbsp	15	107.8	0.1	0.1	0.0	12.1	5.9	3.1
4082	Margarine, Hard, Soybean-Hydrogenated & Palm-Hydrogenated	1 tbsp	15	107.8	0.1	0.1	0.0	12.1	4.8	4.5
4521	Margarine, Hard, Soybean-Hydrogenated, Cottonseed	1 tbsp	15	107.8	0.1	0.1	0.0	12.1	6.1	3.0
4109	Margarine, Imitation (about 40% fat) Corn, Corn-Hydrogenated	1 tbsp	15	51.8	0.1	0.1	0.0	5.8	2.2	2.4
4112	Margarine, Imitation (about 40% fat) Soybean-Hydrogenated	1 tbsp	15	51.8	0.1	0.1	0.0	5.8	2.5	2.1
4130	Margarine, Liquid, Soybean-Hydrogenated, Soybean, Cottonseed	1 tbsp	15	108.2	0.3	0.0	0.0	12.1	4.2	5.4
4092	Margarine, Soft w/salt	1 tbsp	15	107.5	0.1	0.1	0.0	12.1	4.3	5.2
4129	Margarine, Soft, Corn, Corn-Hydrogenated	1 tbsp	15	107.5	0.1	0.1	0.0	12.1	4.7	4.7
4101	Margarine, Soft, no salt	1 tbsp	15	107.5	0.1	0.1	0.0	12.0	5.6	3.9
4094	Margarine, Soft, Safflower, Safflower-Hydrogenated	1 tbsp	15	107.5	0.1	0.1	0.0	12.1	3.5	6.7
4093	Margarine, Soft, Soybean, Soybean-Hydrogenated w/salt	1 tbsp	15	107.5	0.1	0.1	0.0	12.1	5.5	4.0
4103	Margarine, Soft, Soybean, Soybean-Hydrogenated, no salt	1 tbsp	15	107.5	0.1	0.1	0.0	12.0	5.5	4.0
4099	Margarine, Soft, Soybean, Soybean & Cottonseed-Hydrogenated	1 tbsp	15	107.5	0.1	0.1	0.0	12.1	4.6	4.5
4095	Margarine, Soft, Soybean-Hydrogenated & Safflower	1 tbsp	15	107.5	0.1	0.1	0.0	12.1	4.7	5.3
4523	Margarine, Soft, Soybean-Hydrogenated, Cottonseed	1 tbsp	15	107.5	0.1	0.1	0.0	12.1	4.7	4.4
4525	Margarine, Soft, Soybean-Hydrogenated, Palm-Hydrogenated & Palm	1 tbsp	15	107.5	0.1	0.1	0.0	12.1	3.8	5.2
4527	Margarine-Like Spread (about 60% fat) tub	1 tbsp	15	80.9	0.1	0.0	0.0	9.1	4.7	2.1
920900	Mayonnaise Dressing, low kcal	2 tbsp	30	42.9	0.0	4.3	0.0	4.3	1.3	2.1
20324	Meal, Corn, enriched, ckd	1 cup	170	85.0	2.1	18.4	2.1	0.2	0.1	0.1
20322	Meal, Corn, White w/wheat flour, Selfrise, enriched, bolted	1 cup	170	591.6	14.3	124.8	10.7	4.8	1.3	2.2
20325	Meal, Corn, White, Selfrise, enriched, bolted	1 cup	122	407.5	10.1	85.7	8.2	4.1	1.1	1.9
20024	Meal, Corn, White, Whole Grain	1 cup	122	441.6	9.9	93.8	8.9	4.4	1.2	2.0
20025	Meal, Corn, Yellow, Degermed, enriched	1 cup	138	505.1	11.7	107.2	10.2	2.3	0.6	1.0
20020	Meal, Corn, Yellow, Degermed, unenriched	1 cup	138	505.1	11.7	107.2	10.2	2.3	0.6	1.0
18236	Meal, Corn, Yellow, Whole Grain	1 cup	122	441.6	9.9	93.8	8.9	4.4	1.2	2.0
16106	Meal, Crackermeal	1 tbsp	1.2	4.6	0.1	1.0	0.0	0.0	0.0	0.0
902934	Meat Extender, Vegetarian, Meatless	1 cup	88	275.4	33.5	33.7	15.4	2.6	0.6	1.5
902935	Meat Tenderizer	1 tsp	5	2.0	0.0	0.0	0.0	0.0	0.0	0.0
924327	Meat&Shrimp (shellfish) Egg Roll/LaChoy	3 medium	37	79.9	3.0	11.0	0.0	3.0	1.2	1.2
14422	Meatloaf	3.5 oz	98	159.7	17.0	4.6	0.2	7.6	0.0	0.0
14423	Milk Beverage Mix, Chocolate Dairy Drink w/aspartame, low kcal, dry	½ cup H₂O, 3 icecubes, ¾ oz pkt	204	607.9	51.0	102.4	3.3	5.3	1.0	0.1
901916	Milk Beverage Mix, Dairy Drink w/aspartame, low kcal, dry, prep w/H₂O	½ cup	74	22.9	1.9	3.8	0.1	0.2	0.0	0.0
901900	Milk Dessert, frozen, Vanilla/Simple Pleasures	½ cup	89	115.7	5.9	21.1	0.0	0.7	0.1	0.0
19220	Milk Dessert, frozen, Vanilla/Simple Pleasures Lite	½ cup	74	71.8	4.6	15.0	1.0	0.4	0.1	0.1
19221	Milk Dessert, Rennin, Chocolate, dry mix prep w/reduced fat (2%) milk	½ cup	137	111.0	4.4	18.5	0.7	2.9	0.8	0.1
19225	Milk Dessert, Rennin, Chocolate, dry mix prep w/whole milk	½ cup	137	126.0	4.4	18.2	0.7	4.5	1.3	0.2
19223	Milk Dessert, Rennin, Vanilla, dry mix prep w/reduced fat (2%) milk	½ cup	137	104.1	4.2	16.9	0.0	2.5	0.7	0.1
919224	Milk Dessert, Rennin, Vanilla, dry mix prep w/whole milk	½ cup	137	119.2	4.1	16.7	0.0	4.2	1.2	0.2
901905	Milk Dessert, Rennin, Vanilla, homemade	½ cup	137	112.3	4.0	15.3	0.0	4.1	0.0	0.0
1110	Milk Drink, Vanilla Cream	12 fl oz	360	194.4	0.0	48.0	0.0	0.0	0.0	0.0
1111	Milk Shake, Thick, Chocolate	1 container (10.6 oz net wt)	300	355.8	9.2	63.5	0.9	8.1	2.3	0.3
1094	Milk Shake, Thick, Vanilla	1 container (11 oz net wt)	313	350.0	12.1	55.6	0.0	9.5	2.7	0.4
1088	Milk, Buttermilk, Dry	1 tbsp	6.5	25.1	2.2	3.2	0.0	0.4	0.1	0.0
1059	Milk, Buttermilk, Lowfat, Cultured	1 cup	245	99.0	8.1	11.7	0.0	2.2	0.6	0.1
1082	Milk, Human, Mature Breast	1 fl oz	30.8	21.4	0.3	2.1	0.0	1.3	0.5	0.2
1083	Milk, Lowfat, 1% fat w/added vitamin A	1 cup	244	102.1	8.0	11.7	0.0	2.6	0.7	0.1
1104	Milk, Lowfat, 1% fat w/NFDM & Vit A added	1 cup	245	104.4	8.5	12.2	0.0	2.4	0.7	0.1

Sat (g)	Chol (mg)	Cal (mg)	Iron (mg)	Magn (mg)	Phos (mg)	Pota (mg)	Sodi (mg)	Zinc (mg)	Vit A (RE)	Vit C (mg)	Vit E (mg)	Thia (mg)	Ribo (mg)	Niac (mg)	Vit B-6 (mg)	Fol (µg)	Vit B-12 (µg)	Wat (g)
4.3	32.4	27.0	0.5	7.7	61.7	72.9	434.7	0.8	0.0	0.0	0.0	0.0	0.0	0.0	0.0	0.0	0.0	24.0
0.0	0.0	43.0	2.2	0.0	113.0	333.0	792.0	0.0	192.6	7.0	0.0	0.2	0.2	3.2	0.0	0.0	0.0	0.0
4.2	18.0	123.0	1.9	29.0	345.0	94.0	652.0	1.3	77.6	0.0	0.0	0.3	0.2	1.7	0.0	12.0	0.2	90.3
0.0	17.0	269.0	0.7	0.0	197.0	73.0	358.0	0.0	17.6	4.0	0.0	0.2	0.2	0.9	0.0	0.0	0.0	0.0
0.0	0.0	95.0	1.5	0.0	117.0	114.0	934.0	1.4	173.4	0.0	0.0	0.2	0.2	2.1	0.0	0.0	0.0	0.0
0.1	0.0	9.8	2.0	25.2	75.6	43.4	1.4	0.7	0.0	0.0	0.0	0.3	0.1	2.3	0.0	98.0	0.0	92.4
0.1	0.0	8.1	0.6	20.7	62.1	35.7	1.2	0.6	0.0	0.0	0.0	0.0	0.0	0.5	0.0	8.1	0.0	75.9
0.0	0.0	15.4	0.7	26.6	70.0	43.4	8.4	0.6	7.0	0.0	0.1	0.2	0.1	1.5	0.0	91.0	0.0	95.7
0.1	0.0	20.1	1.4	40.2	119.3	59.0	4.0	1.1	0.0	0.0	0.1	0.1	0.1	0.9	0.1	6.7	0.0	90.0
10.8	0.0	24.9	0.0	2.2	19.2	35.4	1343.4	0.0	1118.6	0.1	3.3	0.0	0.0	0.0	0.0	1.0	0.1	81.3
29.9	92.4	29.4	0.1	2.1	24.2	37.8	941.9	0.0	839.0	0.1	8.0	0.0	0.0	0.0	0.0	2.1	0.1	16.6
2.4	0.0	4.5	0.0	0.4	3.4	6.4	141.5	0.0	119.9	0.0	1.9	0.0	0.0	0.0	0.0	0.2	0.0	2.4
2.1	0.0	4.5	0.0	0.4	3.4	6.4	141.5	0.0	119.9	0.0	2.2	0.0	0.0	0.0	0.0	0.2	0.0	2.4
2.3	0.0	4.5	0.0	0.4	3.4	6.4	141.5	0.0	119.9	0.0	0.0	0.0	0.0	0.0	0.0	0.2	0.0	2.4
2.3	0.0	2.6	0.0	0.2	2.0	3.7	0.3	0.0	119.9	0.0	1.7	0.0	0.0	0.0	0.0	0.1	0.0	2.8
2.0	0.0	4.5	0.0	0.4	3.4	6.4	141.5	0.0	119.9	0.0	0.0	0.0	0.0	0.0	0.0	0.2	0.0	2.4
4.7	7.7	0.0	0.0	0.0	0.0	6.4	141.5	0.0	0.0	0.0	0.0	0.0	0.0	0.0	0.0	0.0	0.0	2.4
2.3	0.0	2.6	0.0	0.2	2.0	3.7	0.3	0.0	119.9	0.0	1.9	0.0	0.0	0.0	0.0	0.1	0.0	2.8
2.1	0.0	4.5	0.0	0.4	3.4	6.4	141.5	0.0	119.9	0.0	0.0	0.0	0.0	0.0	0.0	0.2	0.0	2.4
2.0	0.0	4.5	0.0	0.4	3.4	6.4	141.5	0.0	119.9	0.0	0.0	0.0	0.0	0.0	0.0	0.2	0.0	2.4
2.5	0.0	4.5	0.0	0.4	3.4	6.4	141.5	0.0	119.9	0.0	1.6	0.0	0.0	0.0	0.0	0.2	0.0	2.4
2.3	0.0	4.5	0.0	0.4	3.4	6.4	141.5	0.0	119.9	0.0	0.0	0.0	0.0	0.0	0.0	0.2	0.0	2.4
2.4	0.0	4.5	0.0	0.4	3.4	6.4	141.5	0.0	119.9	0.0	0.0	0.0	0.0	0.0	0.0	0.2	0.0	2.4
1.0	0.0	2.7	0.0	0.2	2.1	3.8	143.9	0.0	119.9	0.0	0.0	0.0	0.0	0.0	0.0	0.1	0.0	8.7
1.0	0.0	2.7	0.0	0.2	2.1	3.8	143.9	0.0	119.9	0.0	0.0	0.0	0.0	0.0	0.0	0.1	0.0	8.7
2.0	0.0	9.9	0.0	0.9	7.6	14.1	117.1	0.0	119.9	0.1	0.8	0.0	0.0	0.0	0.0	0.4	0.0	2.4
2.1	0.0	4.0	0.0	0.3	3.0	5.7	161.8	0.0	119.9	0.0	1.8	0.0	0.0	0.0	0.0	0.2	0.0	2.4
2.1	0.0	4.0	0.0	0.3	3.0	5.7	161.8	0.0	119.9	0.0	0.0	0.0	0.0	0.0	0.0	0.2	0.0	2.4
2.1	0.0	4.0	0.0	0.3	3.0	5.7	4.1	0.0	119.9	0.0	1.3	0.0	0.0	0.0	0.0	0.2	0.0	2.7
1.4	0.0	4.0	0.0	0.3	3.0	5.7	161.8	0.0	119.9	0.0	0.0	0.0	0.0	0.0	0.0	0.2	0.0	2.4
2.0	0.0	4.0	0.0	0.3	3.0	5.7	161.8	0.0	119.9	0.0	0.0	0.0	0.0	0.0	0.0	0.2	0.0	2.4
2.0	0.0	4.0	0.0	0.3	3.0	5.7	4.1	0.0	119.9	0.0	0.0	0.0	0.0	0.0	0.0	0.2	0.0	2.7
2.4	0.0	4.0	0.0	0.3	3.0	5.7	161.8	0.0	119.9	0.0	0.0	0.0	0.0	0.0	0.0	0.2	0.0	2.4
1.6	0.0	4.0	0.0	0.3	3.0	5.7	161.8	0.0	119.9	0.0	0.0	0.0	0.0	0.0	0.0	0.2	0.0	2.4
2.5	0.0	4.0	0.0	0.3	3.0	5.7	161.8	0.0	119.9	0.0	0.0	0.0	0.0	0.0	0.0	0.2	0.0	2.4
2.6	0.0	4.0	0.0	0.3	3.0	5.7	161.8	0.0	119.9	0.0	0.0	0.0	0.0	0.0	0.0	0.2	0.0	2.4
1.9	0.0	3.1	0.0	0.3	2.4	4.5	149.1	0.0	119.9	0.0	1.4	0.0	0.0	0.0	0.0	0.1	0.0	5.6
0.9	4.3	6.4	0.0	0.0	8.6	2.1	40.7	0.0	17.1	0.0	0.0	0.0	0.0	0.0	0.0	0.0	0.0	0.0
0.0	0.0	1.4	1.0	70.8	24.1	26.9	0.0	0.2	19.8	0.0	0.0	0.1	0.1	0.9	0.0	4.3	0.0	0.0
0.7	0.0	508.3	8.4	91.8	1106.7	351.9	2242.3	2.4	0.0	0.0	0.0	1.2	0.7	8.8	0.7	312.8	0.0	17.6
0.6	0.0	440.4	7.0	104.9	980.9	311.1	1521.3	2.4	0.0	0.0	0.0	0.8	0.5	6.5	0.7	228.1	0.0	15.4
0.6	0.0	7.3	4.2	154.9	294.0	350.1	42.7	2.2	0.0	0.0	0.4	0.5	0.2	4.4	0.4	31.0	0.0	12.5
0.3	0.0	6.9	5.7	55.2	115.9	223.6	4.1	1.0	56.6	0.0	0.5	1.0	0.6	6.9	0.4	258.1	0.0	16.0
0.3	0.0	6.9	1.5	55.2	115.9	223.6	4.1	1.0	56.6	0.0	0.5	0.2	0.1	1.4	0.4	66.2	0.0	16.0
0.6	0.0	7.3	4.2	154.9	294.0	350.1	42.7	2.2	57.3	0.0	0.8	0.5	0.2	4.4	0.4	31.0	0.0	12.5
0.0	0.0	0.3	0.1	0.3	1.2	1.4	0.3	0.0	0.0	0.0	0.0	0.0	0.0	0.0	0.0	1.4	0.0	0.1
0.4	0.0	179.5	10.6	190.1	562.3	1673.8	8.8	1.9	2.6	0.0	0.0	0.6	0.8	19.4	1.2	174.2	5.3	6.6
0.0	0.0	11.0	0.1	2.0	0.0	2.0	1695.0	0.0	1.0	0.0	0.0	0.0	0.0	0.0	0.0	0.0	0.0	0.0
0.6	4.0	9.0	0.8	0.0	0.0	65.0	115.0	0.0	2.0	3.0	0.0	0.1	0.1	1.0	0.0	0.0	0.0	0.0
0.0	92.0	38.0	2.3	0.0	162.0	374.0	653.0	0.0	35.8	2.0	0.0	0.1	0.2	8.0	0.0	0.0	0.0	0.0
3.8	16.3	1795.2	15.7	428.4	1740.1	4569.6	1591.2	7.3	701.8	2.4	0.2	0.2	4.0	2.6	0.2	85.7	4.9	26.1
0.1	0.7	69.6	0.6	17.0	65.9	173.9	62.2	0.3	26.6	0.1	0.0	0.0	0.2	0.1	0.0	3.3	0.2	67.2
0.2	12.0	162.0	0.1	12.0	122.0	114.0	50.0	0.7	103.6	0.0	0.0	0.0	0.2	0.1	0.0	0.0	0.0	61.0
0.2	9.0	128.0	0.6	13.0	105.0	201.0	68.0	0.4	69.2	0.0	0.0	0.1	0.2	0.1	0.1	0.0	0.9	0.7
1.7	9.6	172.6	0.4	27.4	134.3	249.3	71.2	0.7	60.3	1.2	0.0	0.0	0.2	0.1	0.1	6.9	0.5	110.1
2.8	16.4	169.9	0.4	27.4	132.9	245.2	69.9	0.7	32.9	1.1	0.0	0.0	0.2	0.1	0.1	6.9	0.4	108.6
1.5	9.6	165.8	0.1	17.8	130.2	194.5	63.0	0.5	71.2	1.2	0.0	0.0	0.2	0.1	0.1	6.9	0.5	112.5
2.6	17.8	163.0	0.1	16.4	127.4	191.8	63.0	0.5	34.3	1.2	0.0	0.0	0.2	0.1	0.1	6.9	0.5	111.0
0.2	1.2	150.7	0.1	16.4	115.1	185.0	95.9	0.5	37.0	1.1	0.0	0.0	0.2	0.1	0.1	5.5	0.4	112.6
0.0	0.0	0.0	0.0	0.0	0.0	0.0	28.0	0.0	0.0	0.0	0.0	0.0	0.0	0.0	0.0	0.0	0.0	0.0
5.0	31.5	396.0	0.9	48.0	378.0	672.0	333.0	1.4	63.0	0.0	0.3	0.1	0.7	0.4	0.1	14.7	0.9	216.6
5.9	36.9	457.3	0.3	36.8	360.6	571.9	298.6	1.2	87.6	0.0	0.3	0.1	0.6	0.5	0.1	20.7	1.6	233.0
0.2	4.5	77.0	0.0	7.1	60.6	103.5	33.6	0.3	3.5	0.4	0.0	0.0	0.1	0.1	0.0	3.1	0.2	0.2
1.3	8.6	285.2	0.1	26.8	218.5	370.7	257.0	1.0	19.6	2.4	0.1	0.1	0.4	0.1	0.1	12.3	0.5	220.8
0.6	4.3	9.9	0.0	1.0	4.2	15.8	5.2	0.1	19.7	1.5	0.3	0.0	0.0	0.1	0.0	1.6	0.0	27.0
1.6	9.8	300.1	0.1	33.7	234.7	380.9	123.2	1.0	144.0	2.4	0.1	0.1	0.4	0.2	0.1	12.4	0.9	219.8
1.5	9.8	312.9	0.1	35.2	244.8	397.1	128.4	1.0	144.6	2.5	0.1	0.1	0.4	0.2	0.1	13.0	0.9	220.0

Code	Food Name	Unit/Amt	Wt (g)	Energy (Kcal)	Prot (g)	Carb (g)	Fiber (g)	Fat (g)	Mono (g)	Poly (g)
1084	Milk, Lowfat, 1% fat, Chocolate	1 cup	250	157.6	8.1	26.1	1.3	2.5	0.8	0.1
1154	Milk, Lowfat, 1% fat, protein fortified, Vit A added	1 cup	246	119.1	9.7	13.6	0.0	2.9	0.8	0.1
1093	Milk, Nonfat, Dry w/addedVit A	¼ cup	30	108.7	10.8	15.6	0.0	0.2	0.1	0.0
1092	Milk, Nonfat, Dry, Calcium Reduced	1.0 oz	28.35	100.3	10.1	14.7	0.0	0.1	0.0	0.0
1155	Milk, Nonfat, Dry, Instant w/added Vit A	1 cup	68	243.6	23.9	35.5	0.0	0.5	0.1	0.0
1091	Milk, Nonfat, Dry, Instant w/o Vit A added	1 cup	68	243.4	23.9	35.5	0.0	0.5	0.1	0.0
1097	Milk, Nonfat, Dry, Regular w/o Vit A added	1 tbsp	7.5	27.2	2.7	3.9	0.0	0.1	0.0	0.0
1085	Milk, Nonfat, Skim, Evaporated, canned	1 tbsp	16	12.5	1.2	1.8	0.0	0.0	0.0	0.0
1086	Milk, Nonfat/Fat Free, Skim w/added Vit A	1 cup	245	85.5	8.4	11.9	0.0	0.4	0.1	0.0
1151	Milk, Nonfat/Fat Free, Skim w/NFDM & Vit A added	1 cup	245	90.3	8.7	12.3	0.0	0.6	0.2	0.0
1087	Milk, Nonfat/Fat Free, Skim w/o added Vit A	1 cup	245	85.8	8.4	11.9	0.0	0.4	0.1	0.0
1079	Milk, Nonfat/Fat Free, Skim, protein fortified, Vit A added	1 cup	246	99.9	9.7	13.7	0.0	0.6	0.2	0.0
1080	Milk, Reduced Fat, 2% fat w/added vitamin A	1 cup	244	121.2	8.1	11.7	0.0	4.7	1.4	0.2
1152	Milk, Reduced Fat, 2% fat w/NFDM & Vit A added	1 cup	245	124.9	8.5	12.2	0.0	4.7	1.4	0.2
1103	Milk, Reduced Fat, 2% fat w/NFDM, w/o added Vit A	1 cup	245	136.0	9.7	13.5	0.0	4.9	0.2	0.0
1081	Milk, Reduced Fat, 2% fat, Chocolate	1.0 fl oz	31.2	22.3	1.0	3.2	0.2	0.6	0.2	0.0
16120	Milk, Reduced Fat, 2% fat, protein fortified, Vit A added	1 cup	246	136.6	9.7	13.5	0.0	4.9	1.4	0.2
1075	Milk, Soy, fluid	1 cup	240	79.2	6.6	4.3	3.1	4.6	0.8	2.0
1076	Milk, Substitute w/hydrogenated vege oils	1 cup	244	150.0	4.3	15.0	0.0	8.3	4.9	1.2
1095	Milk, Substitute w/lauric acid oil	1 cup	244	150.0	4.3	15.0	0.0	8.3	0.4	0.0
1077	Milk, Sweetened Condensed, canned	1.0 fl oz	38.2	122.5	3.0	20.8	0.0	3.3	0.9	0.1
1078	Milk, Whole, 3.25% fat	1 tbsp	15.2	9.3	0.5	0.7	0.0	0.5	0.1	0.0
1102	Milk, Whole, 3.7% fat	1 cup	244	156.6	8.0	11.3	0.0	8.9	2.6	0.3
1090	Milk, Whole, Chocolate	8.0 fl oz	266	221.7	8.4	27.5	2.1	9.0	2.6	0.3
1153	Milk, Whole, Dry	1 tbsp	8	39.7	2.1	3.1	0.0	2.1	0.6	0.1
1096	Milk, Whole, Evaporated, canned, w/added Vit A	1 fl oz	31.5	42.3	2.1	3.2	0.0	2.4	0.7	0.1
1106	Milk, Whole, Evaporated, canned, w/o Vit A added	1 tbsp	15.75	21.2	1.1	1.6	0.0	1.2	0.4	0.0
1108	Milk, Whole, Goat	1 fl oz	30.5	21.0	1.1	1.4	0.0	1.3	0.3	0.0
1089	Milk, Whole, Indian Buffalo	8.0 fl oz	244	235.8	9.2	12.6	0.0	16.8	4.4	0.4
1109	Milk, Whole, low sodium	1 cup	244	148.6	7.6	10.9	0.0	8.4	2.4	0.3
924033	Milk, Whole, Sheep	1 cup	244	263.1	14.6	13.1	0.0	17.1	4.2	0.8
18613	Muffin, Almond Poppyseed Mix, dry/Krusteaz	1 piece	2	8.4	0.1	1.5	0.0	0.2	0.0	0.0
18274	Muffin, Blueberry Mix/Martha White	1 small muffin	40	161.6	2.0	30.4	0.0	3.5	0.0	0.0
18275	Muffin, Blueberry, commercially prep	1 serving	40	110.8	2.2	19.2	1.0	2.6	0.8	1.0
18278	Muffin, Blueberry, dry mix, prep	1 muffin (2.25" dia x 1.75")	50	149.5	2.6	24.4	0.6	4.4	0.0	0.0
918391	Muffin, Blueberry, homemade w/reduced fat (2%) milk	1 muffin	57	162.5	3.7	23.2	0.0	6.2	1.5	3.1
18279	Muffin, Blueberry, homemade w/whole milk	1 muffin (2.75" dia x 2")	57	165.3	3.7	23.1	0.0	6.4	0.0	0.0
918280	Muffin, Corn, commercially prep	1 muffin (2.5" dia x 2.25")	57	173.9	3.4	29.0	1.9	4.8	1.2	1.8
918393	Muffin, Corn, homemade w/reduced fat (2%) milk	1 muffin (2.75" dia x 2")	57	180.1	4.0	25.2	0.0	7.0	1.7	3.5
18605	Muffin, Corn, homemade w/whole milk	1 muffin (2.75" dia x 2")	57	183.0	4.0	25.2	0.0	7.4	0.0	0.0
18273	Muffin, Oatbran	1 muffin (2.5" dia x 2.25")	57	153.9	4.0	27.5	2.6	4.2	1.0	2.4
918389	Muffin, Plain, homemade w/reduced fat (2%) milk	1 muffin	57	168.7	3.9	23.6	1.5	6.5	1.6	3.3
18639	Muffin, Plain, homemade w/whole milk	1 muffin (2.75" dia x 2")	57	171.6	3.9	23.6	1.5	6.8	0.0	0.0
18284	Muffin, Thomas' English Muffins, plain/Best Foods	1.0 oz	29	66.9	2.5	13.2	0.0	0.4	0.5	0.9
918287	Muffin, Wheat Bran, dry mix, prep	1 muffin (2.25" dia x 1.75")	50	138.0	3.3	23.3	2.1	4.6	0.0	0.0
918394	Muffin, Wheat Bran, homemade w/reduced fat (2%) milk	1 muffin (2.75" dia x 2")	57	161.3	4.0	23.9	0.0	7.0	0.0	0.0
18601	Muffin, Wheat Bran, homemade w/whole milk	1 muffin (2.75" dia x 2")	57	164.2	4.0	23.8	0.0	7.3	0.0	0.0
20134	Muffin, Wild Blueberry, dry mix/General Mills-Betty Crocker	1 serving	40	128.4	2.1	26.0	0.0	1.8	0.0	0.0
22702	Noodle Weenee/VanCamp	1 cup	220	244.2	9.3	32.9	0.0	8.5	0.0	0.0
16082	Noodles, Alfredo Egg Noodles in a Creamy Sauce, dry mix/Lipton	1 cup	93	388.6	14.4	58.0	0.0	11.0	3.6	1.2
20113	Noodles, Beans, Mung, Long Rice or Cellophane, dry	1 tbsp	8.8	30.9	0.0	7.6	0.0	0.0	0.0	0.0
20110	Noodles, Chinese, Chow Mein	1 tbsp	2.8	14.8	0.2	1.6	0.1	0.9	0.2	0.5
20310	Noodles, Egg, enriched, ckd w/salt	1 tbsp	10	13.3	0.5	2.5	0.1	0.1	0.0	0.0
20111	Noodles, Egg, Spinach, enriched, ckd	1 cup	160	211.2	8.1	38.8	3.7	2.5	0.8	0.6
20510	Noodles, Egg, unenriched, ckd w/o salt	1 cup	160	212.8	7.6	39.7	1.8	2.4	0.7	0.7
20409	Noodles, Egg, unenriched, ckd w/salt	1 cup	160	212.8	7.6	39.7	0.0	2.4	0.7	0.7
20114	Noodles, Japanese, Soba, ckd	1 cup	114	112.9	5.8	24.4	0.0	0.1	0.0	0.0
20116	Noodles, Japanese, Somen, ckd	1 cup	176	230.6	7.0	48.5	0.0	0.3	0.0	0.1
20133	Noodles, Ramen	1 cup	227	231.5	6.2	34.1	4.1	8.4	4.3	2.9
12195	Nut Butter, Almond Butter w/honey & cinnamon, w/salt	1 cup	250	1505.0	39.6	67.4	9.3	130.5	84.7	27.4
12088	Nut Butter, Almond Butter, Plain, w/salt	1 cup	250	1582.5	37.7	53.1	9.3	147.8	95.9	31.0
12060	Nut Butter, Cashew Butter, Plain, w/salt	1 tbsp	16	93.9	2.8	5.4	0.3	7.9	4.7	1.3
12168	Nut Flour, Acorn, full-fat	3.5 oz	100	501.0	7.5	54.7	0.0	30.2	19.1	5.8
12697	Nut Flour, Pecan	3.5 oz	100	329.0	31.9	50.7	0.0	1.4	0.7	0.3
12197	Nut Meal, Almond, partly defatted, w/salt	3.5 oz	100	408.0	39.5	28.9	0.0	18.3	11.9	3.8
16420	Nut Paste, Almond Paste	1 cup firmly packed	227	1039.7	20.4	108.5	10.9	63.0	40.9	13.2
16421	Nutrient/Protein Supplement, Soy Protein Conc prep w/acid wash	3.5 oz	100	332.0	58.1	31.2	5.5	0.5	0.1	0.2
16122	Nutrient/Protein Supplement, Soy Protein Conc, prep w/R-OH extraction	3.5 oz	100	332.0	58.1	31.2	5.5	0.5	0.1	0.2
16422	Nutrient/Protein Supplement, Soy Protein Isolate	3.5 oz	100	338.0	80.7	7.4	5.6	3.4	0.6	1.6

Sat (g)	Chol (mg)	Cal (mg)	Iron (mg)	Magn (mg)	Phos (mg)	Pota (mg)	Sodi (mg)	Zinc (mg)	Vit A (RE)	Vit C (mg)	Vit E (mg)	Thia (mg)	Ribo (mg)	Niac (mg)	Vit B-6 (mg)	Fol (µg)	Vit B-12 (µg)	Wat (g)
1.5	7.3	286.8	0.6	33.3	256.5	425.5	151.8	1.0	147.5	2.3	0.1	0.1	0.4	0.3	0.1	12.0	0.9	211.3
1.8	9.8	349.3	0.1	39.3	273.3	443.5	143.4	1.1	145.1	2.8	0.0	0.1	0.5	0.2	0.1	14.5	1.0	218.3
0.1	5.9	377.1	0.1	33.0	290.5	538.2	160.6	1.2	198.0	2.0	0.0	0.1	0.5	0.3	0.1	15.0	1.2	0.9
0.0	0.6	79.4	0.1	17.0	286.6	192.8	646.4	1.1	0.6	1.9	0.0	0.0	0.5	0.2	0.1	14.0	1.1	1.4
0.3	12.4	836.9	0.2	79.6	669.6	1159.7	373.1	3.0	482.8	3.8	0.0	0.3	1.2	0.6	0.2	33.9	2.7	2.7
0.3	12.2	837.1	0.2	79.6	669.8	1159.4	373.3	3.0	3.4	3.8	0.0	0.3	1.2	0.6	0.2	34.0	2.7	2.7
0.0	1.5	94.3	0.0	8.3	72.6	134.6	40.1	0.3	0.6	0.5	0.0	0.0	0.1	0.1	0.0	3.8	0.3	0.2
0.0	0.6	46.3	0.0	4.3	31.2	53.0	18.4	0.1	18.7	0.2	0.0	0.0	0.0	0.0	0.0	1.4	0.0	12.7
0.3	4.4	302.3	0.1	27.8	247.2	405.7	126.2	1.0	149.5	2.4	0.1	0.1	0.3	0.2	0.1	12.7	0.9	222.5
0.4	4.9	316.3	0.1	35.5	254.8	418.2	129.9	1.0	149.5	2.5	0.1	0.1	0.4	0.2	0.1	13.2	0.9	221.4
0.3	4.9	301.4	0.1	27.0	247.5	406.7	127.4	1.0	2.5	2.4	0.1	0.1	0.3	0.2	0.1	12.3	0.9	222.5
0.4	4.9	351.8	0.1	39.5	275.3	446.5	144.4	1.1	150.1	2.8	0.0	0.1	0.5	0.2	0.1	14.8	1.1	219.8
2.9	18.3	296.7	0.1	33.4	232.0	376.7	121.8	1.0	139.1	2.3	0.2	0.1	0.4	0.2	0.1	12.4	0.9	217.7
2.9	18.4	312.9	0.1	35.2	244.8	397.1	128.4	1.0	139.7	2.5	0.2	0.1	0.4	0.2	0.1	13.0	0.9	217.7
3.0	18.9	350.6	0.1	35.5	274.4	445.2	144.1	1.0	149.5	2.7	0.1	0.1	0.5	0.2	0.1	13.2	0.9	214.9
0.4	2.1	35.4	0.1	4.1	31.7	52.7	18.8	0.1	17.8	0.3	0.0	0.0	0.1	0.0	0.0	1.5	0.1	26.1
3.0	18.9	352.0	0.1	39.6	275.5	447.0	144.6	1.1	140.2	2.8	0.0	0.1	0.5	0.2	0.1	14.8	1.1	215.8
0.5	0.0	9.6	1.4	45.6	117.6	338.4	28.8	0.6	7.2	0.0	0.0	0.4	0.2	0.4	0.1	3.6	0.0	223.8
1.9	0.5	79.3	1.0	15.6	181.0	278.9	191.1	2.9	0.0	0.0	2.6	0.0	0.2	0.0	0.0	0.0	0.0	215.2
7.4	0.5	79.3	1.0	15.6	181.0	278.9	191.1	2.9	0.0	0.0	0.0	0.0	0.2	0.0	0.0	0.0	0.0	215.2
2.1	12.9	108.3	0.1	9.8	96.8	141.9	48.5	0.4	30.9	1.0	0.1	0.0	0.2	0.1	0.0	4.3	0.2	10.4
0.3	2.1	18.1	0.0	2.0	14.2	23.0	7.4	0.1	4.7	0.1	0.0	0.0	0.0	0.0	0.0	0.8	0.1	13.4
5.6	34.9	290.4	0.1	32.7	227.2	368.4	119.1	0.9	83.0	3.6	0.2	0.1	0.4	0.2	0.1	12.2	0.9	214.0
5.6	32.5	298.2	0.6	34.7	267.3	444.0	158.5	1.1	77.1	2.4	0.2	0.1	0.4	0.3	0.1	12.5	0.9	218.9
1.3	7.8	73.0	0.0	6.8	62.0	106.4	29.7	0.3	22.4	0.7	0.1	0.0	0.1	0.1	0.0	3.0	0.3	0.2
1.4	9.3	82.2	0.1	7.6	63.8	95.5	33.3	0.2	17.0	0.6	0.0	0.0	0.1	0.1	0.0	2.5	0.1	23.3
0.7	4.6	41.1	0.0	3.8	31.9	47.7	16.7	0.1	8.5	0.3	0.0	0.0	0.0	0.0	0.0	1.2	0.0	11.7
0.8	3.5	40.7	0.0	4.3	33.8	62.3	15.2	0.1	17.1	0.4	0.0	0.0	0.1	0.0	0.0	0.2	0.0	26.5
11.2	46.4	412.4	0.3	75.9	286.5	433.6	127.4	0.5	129.3	5.5	0.0	0.1	0.3	0.2	0.1	13.7	0.9	203.5
5.3	33.2	246.0	0.1	12.2	208.6	616.8	6.1	0.9	78.1	2.3	0.2	0.0	0.3	0.1	0.1	12.2	0.9	215.2
11.2	65.9	471.9	0.2	44.8	385.5	333.1	107.6	1.3	102.5	10.2	0.0	0.2	0.9	1.0	0.1	17.1	1.7	196.9
0.1	0.0	0.0	0.0	0.0	0.0	0.0	12.1	0.0	0.0	0.0	0.0	0.0	0.0	0.0	0.0	0.0	0.0	0.1
0.8	0.0	0.0	0.0	0.0	0.0	0.0	343.2	0.0	0.0	0.0	0.0	0.0	0.0	0.0	0.0	0.0	0.0	2.7
0.6	12.0	22.8	0.6	6.4	78.8	49.2	178.8	0.2	3.6	0.4	0.4	0.1	0.0	0.4	0.0	18.0	0.2	15.3
1.5	1.8	12.5	0.6	5.5	94.5	39.0	218.5	0.2	11.0	0.5	0.0	0.1	0.2	1.1	0.0	5.5	0.0	17.8
1.2	21.1	107.7	1.3	9.1	82.7	70.1	251.4	0.3	22.2	0.9	0.0	0.2	0.2	1.3	0.0	27.4	0.1	22.5
3.1	1.6	107.2	1.3	9.1	82.1	69.5	250.8	0.3	16.0	0.9	0.0	0.2	0.2	1.3	0.0	6.8	0.1	22.2
0.8	14.8	42.2	1.6	18.2	161.9	39.3	297.0	0.3	20.5	0.0	1.0	0.2	0.2	1.2	0.0	35.3	0.2	18.6
1.3	23.9	147.6	1.5	13.1	100.9	82.7	333.5	0.3	29.1	0.2	0.0	0.2	0.2	1.4	0.1	35.3	0.1	18.8
3.5	1.8	147.1	1.5	13.1	100.3	82.1	333.5	0.3	22.8	0.2	0.0	0.2	0.2	1.4	0.1	9.7	0.1	18.5
0.6	0.0	35.9	2.4	89.5	214.3	289.0	224.0	1.0	0.0	0.0	0.7	0.1	0.1	0.2	0.1	29.6	0.0	20.0
1.2	22.2	114.0	1.4	9.7	87.2	69.0	266.2	0.3	22.8	0.2	0.0	0.2	0.2	1.3	0.0	29.1	0.1	21.5
3.3	1.7	113.4	1.4	9.1	86.6	68.4	266.2	0.3	16.5	0.2	0.0	0.2	0.2	1.3	0.0	6.8	0.1	21.2
0.4	0.0	38.9	0.9	0.0	0.0	0.0	107.0	0.0	0.0	0.0	0.5	0.0	0.0	0.0	0.0	42.1	0.1	12.4
0.7	2.3	16.0	1.3	28.5	167.0	73.5	233.5	0.6	15.5	0.0	0.0	0.1	0.1	1.4	0.1	8.0	0.1	17.7
3.6	1.7	106.6	2.4	44.5	162.5	181.3	335.2	1.6	142.5	4.4	0.0	0.2	0.3	2.3	0.2	29.6	0.1	20.2
3.6	1.8	106.0	2.4	44.5	162.5	180.7	335.2	1.6	136.2	4.4	0.0	0.2	0.3	2.3	0.2	29.6	0.1	19.9
0.4	0.0	0.0	0.0	0.0	0.0	0.0	186.0	0.0	0.0	0.0	0.0	0.0	0.0	0.0	0.0	0.0	0.0	9.5
0.0	0.0	0.0	6.0	0.0	0.0	289.0	1245.0	0.0	134.4	0.0	0.0	0.1	0.2	2.1	0.0	0.0	0.0	187.2
4.3	104.2	118.1	2.8	0.0	0.0	0.0	1646.1	0.0	0.0	0.0	0.0	0.0	0.0	0.0	0.0	0.0	0.0	4.6
0.0	0.0	2.2	0.2	0.3	2.8	0.9	0.9	0.0	0.0	0.0	0.0	0.0	0.0	0.0	0.0	0.2	0.0	1.2
0.1	0.0	0.6	0.1	1.5	4.5	3.4	12.3	0.0	0.3	0.0	0.0	0.0	0.0	0.2	0.0	2.5	0.0	0.0
0.0	3.3	1.2	0.2	1.9	6.9	2.8	0.7	0.1	0.6	0.0	0.0	0.0	0.0	0.1	0.0	6.4	0.0	6.9
0.6	52.8	30.4	1.7	38.4	91.2	59.2	19.2	1.0	22.4	0.0	0.1	0.4	0.2	2.4	0.2	102.4	0.2	109.6
0.5	52.8	19.2	1.0	30.4	110.4	44.8	11.2	1.0	9.6	0.0	0.1	0.0	0.0	0.6	0.1	11.2	0.1	109.9
0.5	52.8	19.2	1.0	30.4	110.4	44.8	264.0	1.0	9.6	0.0	0.0	0.0	0.0	0.6	0.1	11.2	0.1	109.9
0.0	0.0	4.6	0.5	10.3	28.5	39.9	68.4	0.1	0.0	0.0	0.0	0.1	0.0	0.6	0.0	8.0	0.0	83.2
0.0	0.0	14.1	0.9	3.5	47.5	51.0	283.4	0.4	0.0	0.0	0.0	0.0	0.1	0.2	0.0	3.5	0.0	119.5
1.1	0.0	7.2	2.1	0.0	0.0	41.3	892.5	0.0	0.0	0.0	0.0	0.2	0.2	2.4	0.0	0.0	0.0	0.0
12.4	0.0	667.5	9.2	750.0	1295.0	1875.0	425.0	7.5	0.0	1.8	0.0	0.3	1.5	7.1	0.2	161.3	0.0	5.0
14.0	0.0	675.0	9.3	757.5	1307.5	1895.0	1125.0	7.6	0.0	1.8	50.7	0.3	1.5	7.2	0.2	163.0	0.0	2.5
1.6	0.0	6.9	0.8	41.3	73.1	87.4	98.2	0.8	0.0	0.0	0.0	0.2	0.0	0.3	0.0	10.9	0.0	0.5
3.9	0.0	43.0	1.2	110.0	103.0	712.0	0.0	0.6	5.0	0.0	0.0	0.1	0.2	2.4	0.7	113.5	0.0	6.0
0.1	0.0	32.0	2.0	120.0	274.0	334.0	1.0	5.1	12.0	1.8	0.0	0.8	0.1	0.8	0.2	36.7	0.0	10.7
1.7	0.0	424.0	8.5	288.0	914.0	1400.0	746.0	2.8	0.0	0.6	0.0	0.3	1.7	6.3	0.1	57.0	0.0	7.2
6.0	0.0	390.4	3.6	295.1	585.7	712.8	20.4	3.4	0.0	0.2	46.0	0.2	0.9	3.2	0.1	165.7	0.0	32.0
0.1	0.0	363.0	10.8	140.0	839.0	450.0	900.0	4.4	0.0	0.0	0.0	0.3	0.1	0.7	0.1	340.0	0.0	5.8
0.1	0.0	363.0	10.8	315.0	839.0	2202.0	3	4.4	0.0	0.0	0.0	0.3	0.1	0.7	0.1	340.0	0.0	5.8
0.4	0.0	178.0	14.5	39.0	776.0	81.0	1005.0	4.0	0.0	0.0	0.0	0.0	0.2	1.4	0.1	176.1	0.0	5.0

Code	Food Name	Unit/Amt	Wt (g)	Energy (Kcal)	Prot (g)	Carb (g)	Fiber (g)	Fat (g)	Mono (g)	Poly (g)
16423	Nutrient/Protein Supplement, Soy Protein Isolate, potassium type	3.5 oz	100	326.0	80.7	10.2	5.6	0.5	0.6	1.6
925044	Nutrient/Protein Supplement, Soy Protein Isolate, potassium type	3.5 oz	100	321.0	88.3	2.6	2.0	0.5	0.1	0.3
925074	Nutrient/Vitamin Supplement, 1-A-Day Essential	1 tablet	1	0.0	0.0	0.0	0.0	0.0	0.0	0.0
925042	Nutrient/Vitamin Supplement, 1-A-Day Maximum	1 tablet	1	0.0	0.0	0.0	0.0	0.0	0.0	0.0
925058	Nutrient/Vitamin Supplement, 1-A-Day plus Extra C	1 tablet	1	0.0	0.0	0.0	0.0	0.0	0.0	0.0
925033	Nutrient/Vitamin Supplement, Allbee C-800	1 tablet	1	0.0	0.0	0.0	0.0	0.0	0.0	0.0
925040	Nutrient/Vitamin Supplement, Bugs Bunny	1 tablet	1	0.0	0.0	0.0	0.0	0.0	0.0	0.0
925050	Nutrient/Vitamin Supplement, Bugs Bunny Extra C	1 tablet	1	0.0	0.0	0.0	0.0	0.0	0.0	0.0
925091	Nutrient/Vitamin Supplement, Bugs Bunny plus Iron	1 tablet	1	0.0	0.0	0.0	0.0	0.0	0.0	0.0
925045	Nutrient/Vitamin Supplement, Centrum Jr.	1 tablet	1	0.0	0.0	0.0	0.0	0.0	0.0	0.0
925088	Nutrient/Vitamin Supplement, Chew Vits	1 tablet	1	0.0	0.0	0.0	0.0	0.0	0.0	0.0
925046	Nutrient/Vitamin Supplement, Engran-HP	1 tablet	1	0.0	0.0	0.0	0.0	0.0	0.0	0.0
925098	Nutrient/Vitamin Supplement, FemIron	1 tablet	1	0.0	0.0	0.0	0.0	0.0	0.0	0.0
925034	Nutrient/Vitamin Supplement, Fero-Grad-500	1 tablet	1	0.0	0.0	0.0	0.0	0.0	0.0	0.0
925073	Nutrient/Vitamin Supplement, Flintstones	1 tablet	1	0.0	0.0	0.0	0.0	0.0	0.0	0.0
925041	Nutrient/Vitamin Supplement, Flintstones Complete	1 tablet	1	0.0	0.0	0.0	0.0	0.0	0.0	0.0
925023	Nutrient/Vitamin Supplement, Flintstones plus Iron	1 tablet	1	0.0	0.0	0.0	0.0	0.0	0.0	0.0
925024	Nutrient/Vitamin Supplement, Geritol Complete	1 tablet	1	0.0	0.0	0.0	0.0	0.0	0.0	0.0
925097	Nutrient/Vitamin Supplement, Geritol Tonic	15 ml	1	0.0	0.0	0.0	0.0	0.0	0.0	0.0
925093	Nutrient/Vitamin Supplement, Iron & Vitamin C	1 tablet	1	0.0	0.0	0.0	0.0	0.0	0.0	0.0
925055	Nutrient/Vitamin Supplement, Lifestage, Children	1 tablet	1	0.0	0.0	0.0	0.0	0.0	0.0	0.0
925059	Nutrient/Vitamin Supplement, Lifestage, Men	1 tablet	1	0.0	0.0	0.0	0.0	0.0	0.0	0.0
925025	Nutrient/Vitamin Supplement, Lifestage, Teen	1 tablet	1	0.0	0.0	0.0	0.0	0.0	0.0	0.0
925049	Nutrient/Vitamin Supplement, Lifestage, Women	1 tablet	1	0.0	0.0	0.0	0.0	0.0	0.0	0.0
925096	Nutrient/Vitamin Supplement, Minute Man plus Iron	1 tablet	1	0.0	0.0	0.0	0.0	0.0	0.0	0.0
925054	Nutrient/Vitamin Supplement, Mol-Iron with C	1 tablet	1	0.0	0.0	0.0	0.0	0.0	0.0	0.0
925089	Nutrient/Vitamin Supplement, Myadec	1 tablet	1	0.0	0.0	0.0	0.0	0.0	0.0	0.0
925035	Nutrient/Vitamin Supplement, Natalins	1 tablet	1	0.0	0.0	0.0	0.0	0.0	0.0	0.0
925052	Nutrient/Vitamin Supplement, Neovadrin child	1 tablet	1	0.0	0.0	0.0	0.0	0.0	0.0	0.0
925087	Nutrient/Vitamin Supplement, Neovadrin with Iron	1 tablet	1	0.0	0.0	0.0	0.0	0.0	0.0	0.0
925086	Nutrient/Vitamin Supplement, Os-Cal Forte	1 tablet	1	0.0	0.0	0.0	0.0	0.0	0.0	0.0
925047	Nutrient/Vitamin Supplement, Os-Cal Plus	1 tablet	1	0.0	0.0	0.0	0.0	0.0	0.0	0.0
925061	Nutrient/Vitamin Supplement, Pac-man plus Iron	1 tablet	1	0.0	0.0	0.0	0.0	0.0	0.0	0.0
925084	Nutrient/Vitamin Supplement, Poly-Vi-Flor	0.5 mg tab	1	0.0	0.0	0.0	0.0	0.0	0.0	0.0
925085	Nutrient/Vitamin Supplement, Poly-Vi-Flor 0.25mg drops	1 ml	1	0.0	0.0	0.0	0.0	0.0	0.0	0.0
925076	Nutrient/Vitamin Supplement, Poly-Vi-Flor 0.5 mg drops	1 ml	1	0.0	0.0	0.0	0.0	0.0	0.0	0.0
925077	Nutrient/Vitamin Supplement, Poly-Vi-Flor tablets	1 mg tab	1	0.0	0.0	0.0	0.0	0.0	0.0	0.0
925081	Nutrient/Vitamin Supplement, Poly-Vi-Flor w/iron	1 mg tab	1	0.0	0.0	0.0	0.0	0.0	0.0	0.0
925063	Nutrient/Vitamin Supplement, Poly-Vi-Sol w/iron & zinc	1 tablet	1	0.0	0.0	0.0	0.0	0.0	0.0	0.0
925095	Nutrient/Vitamin Supplement, Stresstab 600 Adv Formula	1 tablet	1	0.0	0.0	0.0	0.0	0.0	0.0	0.0
925094	Nutrient/Vitamin Supplement, Stresstabs 600 w/iron	1 tablet	1	0.0	0.0	0.0	0.0	0.0	0.0	0.0
925092	Nutrient/Vitamin Supplement, Stresstabs 600 w/zinc	1 tablet	1	0.0	0.0	0.0	0.0	0.0	0.0	0.0
925030	Nutrient/Vitamin Supplement, Theragran-M	1 tablet	1	0.0	0.0	0.0	0.0	0.0	0.0	0.0
925100	Nutrient/Vitamin Supplement, Theragran	1 tablet	1	0.0	0.0	0.0	0.0	0.0	0.0	0.0
925082	Nutrient/Vitamin Supplement, Theragran Stress Formula	1 tablet	1	0.0	0.0	0.0	0.0	0.0	0.0	0.0
925065	Nutrient/Vitamin Supplement, Tri-Vi-Flor	1 tablet	1	0.0	0.0	0.0	0.0	0.0	0.0	0.0
925031	Nutrient/Vitamin Supplement, Tri-Vi-Sol w/iron drops	1 dose	1	0.0	0.0	0.0	0.0	0.0	0.0	0.0
925032	Nutrient/Vitamin Supplement, Unicap	1 tablet	1	0.0	0.0	0.0	0.0	0.0	0.0	0.0
925057	Nutrient/Vitamin Supplement, Unicap Jr	1 tablet	1	0.0	0.0	0.0	0.0	0.0	0.0	0.0
925048	Nutrient/Vitamin Supplement, Unicap M	1 tablet	1	0.0	0.0	0.0	0.0	0.0	0.0	0.0
925070	Nutrient/Vitamin Supplement, Unicap plus Iron	1 tablet	1	0.0	0.0	0.0	0.0	0.0	0.0	0.0
925056	Nutrient/Vitamin Supplement, Unicap Senior	1 tablet	1	0.0	0.0	0.0	0.0	0.0	0.0	0.0
925039	Nutrient/Vitamin Supplement, Unicap T	1 tablet	1	0.0	0.0	0.0	0.0	0.0	0.0	0.0
925043	Nutrient/Vitamin Supplement, Z-Bec	1 tablet	1	0.0	0.0	0.0	0.0	0.0	0.0	0.0
12059	Nutrient/Vitamin Supplement, Zymacap	1 capsule	1	0.0	0.0	0.0	0.0	0.0	0.0	0.0
12072	Nuts, Acorns, raw	1.0 oz	28	108.4	1.7	11.4	0.0	6.7	4.2	1.3
12061	Nuts, Almonds, dried, blanched	1 tbsp	9.1	53.3	1.9	1.7	0.6	4.8	3.1	1.0
12066	Nuts, Almonds, oil roast, blanched w/salt	1 whole kernel	1	6.1	0.2	0.2	0.1	0.6	0.4	0.1
12563	Nuts, Almonds, toasted, unblanched	1.0 oz	28	164.9	5.7	6.4	3.1	14.2	9.2	3.0
12565	Nuts, Almonds, unblanched, dry roasted w/salt	1 kernel	1	5.9	0.2	0.2	0.1	0.5	0.3	0.1
12078	Nuts, Beechnuts, dried	1.0 oz	28	161.3	1.7	9.4	0.0	14.0	6.1	5.6
12084	Nuts, Brazilnuts, dried, unblanched	1.0 oz, 6-8 kernals	28	183.7	4.0	3.6	1.5	18.5	6.4	6.8
12585	Nuts, Butternuts, dried	1 cup	120	734.4	29.9	14.5	5.6	68.4	12.5	51.3
12085	Nuts, Cashews, dry roasted w/salt	1 nut	2	11.5	0.3	0.7	0.1	0.9	0.5	0.2
912903	Nuts, Cashews, dry roasted, w/o salt	1 cup, halves and whole	137	786.4	21.0	44.8	4.1	63.5	37.4	10.7
12586	Nuts, Cashews, honey roasted	1.0 oz	28	150.1	4.0	7.0	2.0	13.0	7.0	3.0
12086	Nuts, Cashews, oil roasted w/salt	1 nut	2	11.5	0.3	0.6	0.1	1.0	0.6	0.2
12095	Nuts, Cashews, oil roasted, w/o salt	1.0 oz, 18 kernals	28	161.3	4.5	8.0	1.1	13.5	8.0	2.3
12203	Nuts, Chestnuts, European, roasted	1 kernel	8	19.6	0.3	4.2	0.4	0.2	0.1	0.1

Sat (g)	Chol (mg)	Cal (mg)	Iron (mg)	Magn (mg)	Phos (mg)	Pota (mg)	Sodi (mg)	Zinc (mg)	Vit A (RE)	Vit C (mg)	Vit E (mg)	Thia (mg)	Ribo (mg)	Niac (mg)	Vit B-6 (mg)	Fol (µg)	Vit B-12 (µg)	Wat (g)
0.4	0.0	178.0	14.5	39.0	776.0	1590.0	50.0	4.0	0.0	0.0	0.0	0.2	0.1	1.4	0.1	176.1	0.0	5.0
0.1	0.0	178.0	14.5	39.0	776.0	1590.0	50.0	4.0	0.0	0.0	0.0	0.2	0.1	1.4	0.1	176.1	0.0	5.0
0.0	0.0	0.0	0.0	0.0	0.0	0.0	0.0	0.0	1000.0	60.0	0.0	1.5	1.7	20.0	2.0	0.4	6.0	0.0
0.0	0.0	0.0	18.0	0.0	0.0	0.0	0.0	15.0	1000.0	60.0	0.0	1.5	1.7	20.0	2.0	0.4	6.0	0.0
0.0	0.0	0.0	0.0	0.0	0.0	0.0	0.0	0.0	1000.0	300.0	0.0	1.5	1.7	20.0	2.0	0.4	6.0	0.0
0.0	0.0	0.0	0.0	0.0	0.0	0.0	0.0	0.0	0.0	800.0	0.0	15.0	17.0	100.0	25.0	0.0	12.0	0.0
0.0	0.0	0.0	0.0	0.0	0.0	0.0	0.0	0.0	500.0	60.0	0.0	1.0	1.2	13.5	1.0	0.3	4.5	0.0
0.0	0.0	0.0	0.0	0.0	0.0	0.0	0.0	0.0	500.0	250.0	0.0	1.0	1.2	13.5	1.0	0.3	4.5	0.0
0.0	0.0	0.0	15.0	0.0	0.0	0.0	0.0	0.0	500.0	60.0	0.0	1.0	1.2	13.5	1.0	0.3	4.5	0.0
0.0	0.0	0.0	18.0	0.0	0.0	0.0	0.0	0.0	1000.0	300.0	0.0	1.5	1.7	20.0	2.0	0.4	6.0	0.0
0.0	0.0	0.0	0.0	0.0	0.0	0.0	0.0	0.0	500.0	60.0	0.0	1.0	1.2	13.5	1.0	0.3	4.5	0.0
0.0	0.0	325.0	9.0	0.0	0.0	0.0	0.0	0.0	800.0	30.0	0.0	0.9	1.0	10.0	1.3	0.4	4.0	0.0
0.0	0.0	0.0	20.0	0.0	0.0	0.0	0.0	0.0	1000.0	60.0	0.0	1.5	1.7	20.0	2.0	0.4	6.0	0.0
0.0	0.0	0.0	105.0	0.0	0.0	0.0	0.0	0.0	0.0	500.0	0.0	0.0	0.0	0.0	0.0	0.0	0.0	0.0
0.0	0.0	0.0	0.0	0.0	0.0	0.0	0.0	0.0	500.0	60.0	0.0	1.0	1.2	13.5	1.0	0.3	4.5	0.0
0.0	0.0	0.0	18.0	0.0	0.0	0.0	0.0	15.0	1000.0	60.0	0.0	1.5	1.7	20.0	2.0	0.4	6.0	0.0
0.0	0.0	0.0	15.0	0.0	0.0	0.0	0.0	0.0	500.0	60.0	0.0	1.0	1.2	13.5	1.0	0.3	4.5	0.0
0.0	0.0	0.0	50.0	0.0	0.0	0.0	0.0	0.0	1000.0	60.0	0.0	1.5	1.7	20.0	2.0	0.4	6.0	0.0
0.0	0.0	0.0	50.0	0.0	0.0	0.0	0.0	0.0	0.0	0.0	0.0	2.5	2.5	50.0	0.5	0.4	0.8	0.0
0.0	0.0	0.0	50.0	0.0	0.0	0.0	0.0	0.0	0.0	25.0	0.0	0.0	0.0	0.0	0.0	0.0	0.0	0.0
0.0	0.0	0.0	4.5	0.0	0.0	0.0	0.0	0.0	500.0	30.0	0.0	0.8	0.9	10.0	1.0	0.2	3.0	0.0
0.0	0.0	0.0	18.0	0.0	0.0	0.0	0.0	22.5	2000.0	500.0	0.0	20.0	10.0	100.0	10.0	0.4	25.0	0.0
0.0	0.0	0.0	18.0	0.0	0.0	0.0	0.0	0.0	1000.0	100.0	0.0	15.0	10.0	50.0	7.5	0.4	12.5	0.0
0.0	0.0	0.0	27.0	0.0	0.0	0.0	0.0	0.0	1000.0	100.0	0.0	3.0	3.4	40.0	4.0	0.4	12.0	0.0
0.0	0.0	0.0	18.0	0.0	0.0	0.0	0.0	0.0	1000.0	60.0	0.0	1.5	1.7	20.0	2.0	0.4	6.0	0.0
0.0	0.0	0.0	39.0	0.0	0.0	0.0	0.0	0.0	0.0	75.0	0.0	0.0	0.0	0.0	0.0	0.0	0.0	0.0
0.0	0.0	0.0	20.0	0.0	0.0	0.0	0.0	20.0	2000.0	250.0	0.0	10.0	10.0	100.0	5.0	0.4	6.0	0.0
0.0	0.0	200.0	45.0	0.0	0.0	0.0	0.0	0.0	1600.0	90.0	0.0	1.7	2.0	20.0	4.0	0.8	8.0	0.0
0.0	0.0	0.0	0.0	0.0	0.0	0.0	0.0	0.0	500.0	60.0	0.0	1.0	1.2	13.5	1.0	0.3	4.5	0.0
0.0	0.0	0.0	15.0	0.0	0.0	0.0	0.0	0.0	500.0	60.0	0.0	1.0	1.2	13.5	1.0	0.3	4.5	0.0
0.0	0.0	250.0	5.0	0.0	0.0	0.0	0.0	0.5	333.6	50.0	0.0	1.7	1.7	15.0	2.0	0.0	1.6	0.0
0.0	0.0	250.0	16.6	0.0	0.0	0.0	0.0	0.8	333.2	33.0	0.0	0.5	0.7	3.3	0.5	0.0	0.0	0.0
0.0	0.0	0.0	18.0	0.0	0.0	0.0	0.0	0.0	1000.0	60.0	0.0	1.5	1.7	20.0	2.0	0.4	6.0	0.0
0.0	0.0	0.0	0.0	0.0	0.0	0.0	0.0	10.0	500.0	60.0	0.0	1.0	1.2	13.5	1.0	0.3	4.5	0.0
0.0	0.0	0.0	0.0	0.0	0.0	0.0	0.0	0.0	300.0	35.0	0.0	0.5	0.6	8.0	0.4	0.0	2.0	0.0
0.0	0.0	0.0	0.0	0.0	0.0	0.0	0.0	0.0	300.0	35.0	0.0	0.5	0.6	8.0	0.4	0.0	2.0	0.0
0.0	0.0	0.0	0.0	0.0	0.0	0.0	0.0	0.0	500.0	60.0	0.0	1.0	1.2	13.5	1.0	0.3	4.5	0.0
0.0	0.0	0.0	12.0	0.0	0.0	0.0	0.0	10.0	500.0	60.0	0.0	1.0	1.2	13.5	1.0	0.3	4.5	0.0
0.0	0.0	0.0	12.0	0.0	0.0	0.0	0.0	0.0	500.0	60.0	0.0	1.1	1.2	13.5	1.1	0.3	4.5	0.0
0.0	0.0	0.0	0.0	0.0	0.0	0.0	0.0	0.0	0.0	600.0	0.0	15.0	15.0	100.0	5.0	0.4	12.0	0.0
0.0	0.0	0.0	27.0	0.0	0.0	0.0	0.0	0.0	0.0	600.0	0.0	15.0	15.0	100.0	5.0	0.4	12.0	0.0
0.0	0.0	0.0	0.0	0.0	0.0	0.0	0.0	23.9	0.0	600.0	0.0	20.0	10.0	50.0	5.0	0.4	12.0	0.0
0.0	0.0	40.0	27.0	0.0	0.0	0.0	0.0	15.0	1100.0	120.0	0.0	3.0	3.4	30.0	3.0	0.4	9.0	0.0
0.0	0.0	0.0	0.0	0.0	0.0	0.0	0.0	0.0	1100.0	120.0	0.0	3.0	3.4	30.0	3.0	0.4	9.0	0.0
0.0	0.0	0.0	27.0	0.0	0.0	0.0	0.0	0.0	0.0	600.0	0.0	15.0	15.0	100.0	5.0	0.4	12.0	0.0
0.0	0.0	0.0	0.0	0.0	0.0	0.0	0.0	0.0	500.0	60.0	0.0	0.0	0.0	0.0	0.0	0.0	0.0	0.0
0.0	0.0	0.0	10.0	0.0	0.0	0.0	0.0	0.0	300.0	35.0	0.0	0.0	0.0	0.0	0.0	0.0	0.0	0.0
0.0	0.0	0.0	0.0	0.0	0.0	0.0	0.0	0.0	1000.0	60.0	0.0	1.5	1.7	20.0	2.0	0.4	6.0	0.0
0.0	0.0	0.0	0.0	0.0	0.0	0.0	0.0	0.0	1000.0	60.0	0.0	1.5	1.7	20.0	2.0	0.4	6.0	0.0
0.0	0.0	0.0	18.0	0.0	0.0	0.0	0.0	15.0	1000.0	600.0	0.0	15.0	10.0	100.0	5.0	0.4	12.0	0.0
0.0	0.0	0.0	18.0	0.0	0.0	0.0	0.0	0.0	1000.0	60.0	0.0	1.5	1.7	20.0	2.0	0.4	6.0	0.0
0.0	0.0	0.0	10.0	0.0	0.0	0.0	0.0	15.0	1000.0	60.0	0.0	1.2	1.7	14.0	2.0	0.4	6.0	0.0
0.0	0.0	0.0	18.0	0.0	0.0	0.0	0.0	15.0	1000.0	500.0	0.0	10.0	10.0	100.0	6.0	0.4	18.0	0.0
0.0	0.0	0.0	0.0	0.0	0.0	0.0	0.0	22.5	0.0	600.0	0.0	15.0	10.2	100.0	10.0	25.0	6.0	0.0
0.0	0.0	0.0	0.0	0.0	0.0	0.0	0.0	0.0	1000.0	90.0	0.0	2.3	2.6	30.0	3.0	0.4	9.0	0.0
0.9	0.0	11.5	0.2	17.4	22.1	150.9	0.0	0.1	1.1	0.0	0.0	0.0	0.0	0.5	0.1	24.4	0.0	7.8
0.5	0.0	22.5	0.3	26.0	48.4	68.3	0.9	0.3	0.0	0.1	1.8	0.0	0.1	0.3	0.0	3.5	0.0	0.5
0.1	0.0	1.9	0.1	2.9	5.8	6.9	7.8	0.0	0.0	0.0	0.1	0.0	0.0	0.0	0.0	0.6	0.0	0.5
1.3	0.0	79.2	1.4	85.4	154.0	216.4	3.1	1.4	0.0	0.2	4.5	0.0	0.2	0.8	0.0	17.9	0.0	0.7
0.0	0.0	2.8	0.0	3.0	5.5	7.7	7.8	0.0	0.0	0.0	0.1	0.0	0.0	0.0	0.0	0.6	0.0	0.0
1.6	0.0	0.3	0.7	0.0	0.0	284.8	10.6	0.1	0.0	4.3	0.0	0.1	0.1	0.2	0.2	31.6	0.0	1.8
4.5	0.0	49.3	1.0	63.0	168.0	168.0	0.6	1.3	0.0	0.2	2.1	0.3	0.0	0.5	0.1	1.1	0.0	0.9
1.6	0.0	63.6	4.8	284.4	535.2	505.2	1.2	3.8	14.4	3.8	4.2	0.5	0.2	1.3	0.7	79.4	0.0	4.0
0.2	0.0	0.9	0.1	5.2	9.8	11.3	12.8	0.1	0.0	0.0	0.0	0.0	0.0	0.0	0.0	1.4	0.0	0.0
12.5	0.0	61.7	8.2	356.2	671.3	774.1	21.9	7.7	0.0	0.0	0.8	0.3	0.3	1.9	0.4	94.8	0.0	2.3
3.0	0.0	12.0	1.2	0.0	120.0	135.0	90.0	1.4	0.0	0.0	0.0	0.1	0.1	0.4	0.1	20.0	0.0	0.0
0.2	0.0	0.8	0.1	5.1	8.5	10.6	12.5	0.1	0.0	0.0	0.0	0.0	0.0	0.0	0.0	1.4	0.0	0.1
2.7	0.0	11.5	1.1	71.4	119.3	148.4	4.8	1.3	0.0	0.0	0.4	0.1	0.0	0.5	0.1	19.0	0.0	1.1
0.0	0.0	2.3	0.1	2.6	8.6	47.4	0.2	0.0	0.2	2.1	0.1	0.0	0.0	0.0	0.0	5.6	0.0	3.2

Code	Food Name	Unit/Amt	Wt (g)	Energy (Kcal)	Prot (g)	Carb (g)	Fiber (g)	Fat (g)	Mono (g)	Poly (g)
12118	Nuts, Coconut Meat, raw	1 cup shredded or grated	80	283.2	2.7	12.2	7.2	26.8	1.1	0.3
12176	Nuts, Coconut Milk, canned (liquid expressed from grated meat&water)	1 tbsp	15	29.6	0.3	0.4	0.0	3.2	0.1	0.0
12177	Nuts, Coconut Water (liquid from coconuts)	1 tbsp	15	2.9	0.1	0.6	0.2	0.0	0.0	0.0
12114	Nuts, Coconut, Creamed, dried, creamed	1.0 oz	28	191.5	1.5	6.0	0.0	19.3	0.8	0.2
12109	Nuts, Coconut, dried, toasted	1.0 oz	28	165.8	1.5	12.4	0.0	13.2	0.6	0.1
12108	Nuts, Coconut, Sweetened, shredded, dried	7 oz pkg	199	997.0	5.7	94.9	9.0	70.6	3.0	0.8
12121	Nuts, Coconut, Unsweetened, dried	1.0 oz	28	184.8	1.9	6.8	4.6	18.1	0.8	0.2
12120	Nuts, Filberts/Hazelnuts, dried, blanched	1.0 oz	28	188.2	3.6	4.5	1.8	18.8	14.8	1.8
12633	Nuts, Macadamia, dried	1 kernel	2	14.0	0.2	0.3	0.2	1.5	1.2	0.0
12138	Nuts, Mixed (no peanuts) oil roasted w/salt	1.0 oz	28	172.2	4.3	6.2	1.5	15.7	9.3	3.2
12135	Nuts, Mixed w/o peanuts, oil roasted, w/o salt	1.0 oz	28	172.2	4.3	6.2	1.5	15.7	9.3	3.2
12635	Nuts, Mixed w/peanuts, dry roast, w/o salt	1.0 oz	28	166.3	4.8	7.1	2.5	14.4	8.8	3.0
12137	Nuts, Mixed w/peanuts, dry roasted w/salt	1.0 oz	28	166.3	4.8	7.1	2.5	14.4	8.8	3.0
12637	Nuts, Mixed w/peanuts, oil roast, w/o salt	1 tbsp	8.9	54.9	1.5	1.9	0.9	5.0	2.8	1.2
12142	Nuts, Mixed w/peanuts, oil roasted w/salt	1 nut	1	6.2	0.2	0.2	0.1	0.6	0.3	0.1
12143	Nuts, Pecans, dried	2 halves	3	20.0	0.2	0.5	0.2	2.0	1.3	0.5
12643	Nuts, Pecans, dry roasted w/o salt	1.0 oz	28	184.5	2.2	6.3	2.6	18.1	11.3	4.5
12144	Nuts, Pecans, dry roasted w/salt	1.0 oz	28	184.5	2.2	6.3	2.6	18.1	11.3	4.5
12644	Nuts, Pecans, oil roasted w/o salt	2 halves	4	27.4	0.3	0.6	0.3	2.8	1.8	0.7
12145	Nuts, Pecans, oil roasted w/salt	2 halves	4	27.4	0.3	0.6	0.3	2.8	1.8	0.7
12149	Nuts, Pine Nut, Pignolias, dried	1 cup	136	769.8	32.6	19.3	6.1	69.0	25.9	29.0
12152	Nuts, Pistachios, dried	2 kernels	1	5.8	0.2	0.2	0.1	0.5	0.3	0.1
12652	Nuts, Pistachios, dry roasted w/o salt	1.0 oz	28	169.7	4.2	7.7	3.0	14.8	10.0	2.2
12154	Nuts, Pistachios, dry roasted w/salt	1.0 oz	28	169.7	4.2	7.7	3.0	14.8	10.0	2.2
12155	Nuts, Walnut, Black, dried	1 tbsp	7.8	47.3	1.9	0.9	0.4	4.4	1.0	2.9
4590	Oil, Fish, Cod Liver	1 cup	218	1966.4	0.0	0.0	0.0	218.0	101.8	49.1
4501	Oil, Vegetable, Canola	1 tbsp	13.6	120.2	0.0	0.0	0.0	13.6	8.0	4.0
4047	Oil, Vegetable, Cocoa Butter	1 tbsp	13.6	120.2	0.0	0.0	0.0	13.6	4.5	0.4
904902	Oil, Vegetable, Coconut	1 tbsp	13.6	117.2	0.0	0.0	0.0	13.6	0.8	0.2
4541	Oil, Vegetable, Crisco	1 tbsp	13.6	120.5	0.0	0.0	0.0	13.6	4.8	7.1
4532	Oil, Vegetable, Grapeseed	1 tbsp	13.6	120.2	0.0	0.0	0.0	13.6	2.2	9.5
4055	Oil, Vegetable, Oat	1 tbsp	13.6	120.2	0.0	0.0	0.0	13.6	4.8	5.6
4513	Oil, Vegetable, Palm	1 tbsp	13.6	120.2	0.0	0.0	0.0	13.6	5.0	1.3
4514	Oil, Vegetable, Palm Kernel	1 tbsp	13.6	117.2	0.0	0.0	0.0	13.6	1.6	0.2
4037	Oil, Vegetable, Poppyseed	1 tbsp	13.6	120.2	0.0	0.0	0.0	13.6	2.7	8.5
4536	Oil, Vegetable, Rice Bran	1 tbsp	13.6	120.2	0.0	0.0	0.0	13.6	5.3	4.8
4060	Oil, Vegetable, Soybean Lecithin	1 tbsp	13.6	103.8	0.0	0.0	0.0	13.6	1.5	6.2
4506	Oil, Vegetable, Sunflower, linoleic <60%	1 tbsp	13.6	120.2	0.0	0.0	0.0	13.6	6.2	5.5
4584	Oil, Vegetable, Sunflower, linoleic >60%	1 tbsp	13.6	120.2	0.0	0.0	0.0	13.6	2.7	8.9
4545	Oil, Vegetable, Sunflower, oleic >70%	1 tbsp	13.6	120.2	0.0	0.0	0.0	13.6	11.4	0.5
4516	Oil, Vegetable, Sunflower-Hydrogenated, linoleic	1 tbsp	13.6	120.2	0.0	0.0	0.0	13.6	6.3	5.0
4528	Oil, Vegetable, Ucuhuba Butter	1 tbsp	13.6	120.2	0.0	0.0	0.0	13.6	0.9	0.4
4502	Oil, Vegetable/Salad/Cooking, Corn	1 tbsp	13.6	120.2	0.0	0.0	0.0	13.6	3.3	8.0
4053	Oil, Vegetable/Salad/Cooking, Cottonseed	1 tbsp	13.6	120.2	0.0	0.0	0.0	13.6	2.4	7.1
4042	Oil, Vegetable/Salad/Cooking, Olive	1 tbsp	13.5	119.3	0.0	0.0	0.0	13.5	9.9	1.1
4510	Oil, Vegetable/Salad/Cooking, Peanut	1 tbsp	13.5	119.3	0.0	0.0	0.0	13.5	6.2	4.3
4511	Oil, Vegetable/Salad/Cooking, Safflower, linoleic >70%	1 tbsp	13.6	120.2	0.0	0.0	0.0	13.6	1.6	10.1
4058	Oil, Vegetable/Salad/Cooking, Safflower, oleic >70%	1 tbsp	13.6	120.2	0.0	0.0	0.0	13.6	10.2	1.9
4044	Oil, Vegetable/Salad/Cooking, Sesame	1 tbsp	13.6	120.2	0.0	0.0	0.0	13.6	5.4	5.7
4034	Oil, Vegetable/Salad/Cooking, Soybean	1 tbsp	13.6	120.2	0.0	0.0	0.0	13.6	3.2	7.9
4543	Oil, Vegetable/Salad/Cooking, Soybean, hydrogenated	1 tbsp	13.6	120.2	0.0	0.0	0.0	13.6	5.8	5.1
18294	Pancake/Waffle, Buttermilk, Eggo/Kellogg	1 serving (2 waffles)	78	181.7	4.7	29.7	0.9	5.2	2.3	1.7
18295	Pancakes, Blueberry, homemade	1 pancake (4" dia)	38	84.4	2.3	11.0	0.0	3.5	0.9	1.6
18611	Pancakes, Buckwheat, incomplete dry mix, prep	1 pancake (4" dia)	30	62.4	2.4	8.5	0.7	2.3	0.0	0.0
918298	Pancakes, Buttermilk, homemade	1 pancake (4" dia)	38	86.3	2.6	10.9	0.0	3.5	0.9	1.7
18297	Pancakes, dry mix, prep, special dietary	1 pancake (4" dia)	38	75.6	1.9	16.0	0.0	0.3	0.0	0.0
918292	Pancakes, Plain, homemade	1.0 oz	28	63.6	1.8	7.9	0.0	2.7	0.7	1.2
18289	Pancakes, Plain, incomplete dry mix, prep	1 pancake (4" dia)	38	82.8	3.0	11.0	0.7	2.9	0.0	0.0
18288	Pancakes, Plain/Buttermilk, complete dry mix, prep	1 pancake (4" dia)	38	73.7	2.0	13.9	0.5	1.0	0.0	0.0
18291	Pancakes, Plain/Buttermilk, frozen	1 pancake (4" dia)	36	82.4	1.9	15.7	0.6	1.2	0.4	0.3
20097	Pancakes, Whole Wheat, incomplete dry mix, prep	1 pancake (4" dia)	38	79.0	3.2	11.2	1.1	2.5	0.0	0.0
22907	Pasta w/egg, homemade, ckd	2.0 oz, ckd	57	74.1	3.0	13.4	0.0	1.0	0.3	0.3
20098	Pasta w/meatballs in tomato sauce, canned entree	1 can	425	437.8	18.4	52.2	11.5	17.3	7.1	1.0
22522	Pasta w/o egg, homemade, ckd	2.0 oz	57	70.7	2.5	14.3	0.0	0.6	0.1	0.3
22515	Pasta w/sliced franks in tomato sauce, canned entree	1 can	418	434.7	15.5	49.7	3.8	19.2	7.9	2.5
924169	Pasta, Beef Ravioli w/meat sauce, canned	1 can, 7.8 oz serving	213	268.4	9.8	34.8	0.0	10.1	0.0	0.0
924206	Pasta, Beefaroni, Macaroni w/beef in tomato sauce, canned entree/ Chef Boyardee	1 package	212	184.4	8.2	31.1	3.0	2.9	1.3	0.3
20092	Pasta, Cheese Ravioli/Contadina	4.5 oz	128	369.9	18.0	39.0	0.0	15.0	5.0	0.0

Sat (g)	Chol (mg)	Cal (mg)	Iron (mg)	Magn (mg)	Phos (mg)	Pota (mg)	Sodi (mg)	Zinc (mg)	Vit A (RE)	Vit C (mg)	Vit E (mg)	Thia (mg)	Ribo (mg)	Niac (mg)	Vit B-6 (mg)	Fol (µg)	Vit B-12 (µg)	Wat (g)
23.8	0.0	11.2	1.9	25.6	90.4	284.8	16.0	0.9	0.0	2.6	0.6	0.1	0.0	0.4	0.0	21.1	0.0	37.6
2.8	0.0	2.7	0.5	6.9	14.4	33.0	2.0	0.1	0.0	0.2	0.0	0.0	0.0	0.1	0.0	2.0	0.0	10.9
0.0	0.0	3.6	0.0	3.8	3.0	37.5	15.8	0.0	0.0	0.4	0.0	0.0	0.0	0.0	0.0	0.4	0.0	14.2
17.2	0.0	7.3	0.9	25.8	58.5	154.3	10.4	0.6	0.0	0.4	0.0	0.0	0.0	0.2	0.1	2.5	0.0	0.5
11.7	0.0	7.6	0.9	25.8	59.1	155.1	10.4	0.6	0.0	0.4	0.0	0.0	0.0	0.2	0.1	2.6	0.0	0.3
62.6	0.0	29.9	3.8	99.5	212.9	670.6	521.4	3.6	0.0	1.4	2.7	0.1	0.0	0.9	0.5	16.1	0.0	25.0
16.0	0.0	7.3	0.9	25.2	57.7	152.0	10.4	0.6	0.0	0.4	0.4	0.0	0.0	0.2	0.1	2.5	0.0	0.8
1.4	0.0	54.6	0.9	82.9	90.4	129.4	0.8	0.7	2.0	0.3	7.2	0.1	0.0	0.3	0.2	20.9	0.0	0.5
0.2	0.0	1.4	0.0	2.3	2.7	7.4	0.1	0.0	0.0	0.0	0.0	0.0	0.0	0.0	0.0	0.3	0.0	0.1
2.5	0.0	29.7	0.7	70.3	125.7	152.3	196.0	1.3	0.6	0.1	1.7	0.1	0.1	0.5	0.1	15.8	0.0	0.9
2.5	0.0	29.7	0.7	70.3	125.7	152.3	3.1	1.3	0.6	0.1	1.7	0.1	0.1	0.5	0.1	15.8	0.0	0.9
1.9	0.0	19.6	1.0	63.0	121.8	167.2	3.4	1.1	0.3	0.1	1.7	0.1	0.1	1.3	0.1	14.1	0.0	0.5
1.9	0.0	19.6	1.0	63.0	121.8	167.2	187.3	1.1	0.3	0.1	1.7	0.1	0.1	1.3	0.1	14.1	0.0	0.5
0.8	0.0	9.6	0.3	20.9	41.3	51.7	1.0	0.5	0.2	0.0	0.5	0.0	0.0	0.5	0.0	7.4	0.0	0.2
0.1	0.0	1.1	0.0	2.4	4.6	5.8	6.5	0.1	0.0	0.0	0.1	0.0	0.0	0.1	0.0	0.8	0.0	0.0
0.2	0.0	1.1	0.1	3.8	8.7	11.8	0.0	0.2	0.4	0.1	0.1	0.0	0.0	0.0	0.0	1.2	0.0	0.1
1.4	0.0	9.8	0.6	37.2	85.1	103.6	0.3	1.6	3.6	0.6	0.9	0.1	0.0	0.3	0.1	11.4	0.0	0.3
1.4	0.0	9.8	0.6	37.2	85.1	103.6	218.4	1.6	3.6	0.6	0.0	0.1	0.0	0.3	0.1	11.4	0.0	0.3
0.2	0.0	1.4	0.1	5.2	11.8	14.4	0.0	0.2	0.5	0.1	0.0	0.0	0.0	0.0	0.0	1.6	0.0	0.2
0.2	0.0	1.4	0.1	5.2	11.8	14.4	30.2	0.2	0.5	0.1	0.0	0.0	0.0	0.0	0.0	1.6	0.0	0.2
10.6	0.0	35.4	12.5	316.9	690.9	814.6	5.4	5.8	4.1	2.6	4.8	1.1	0.3	4.9	0.1	77.9	0.0	9.1
0.1	0.0	1.4	0.1	1.6	5.0	10.9	0.1	0.0	0.2	0.1	0.1	0.0	0.0	0.0	0.0	0.6	0.0	0.0
1.9	0.0	19.6	0.9	36.4	133.3	271.6	1.7	0.4	6.7	2.0	1.5	0.1	0.1	0.4	0.1	16.5	0.0	0.6
1.9	0.0	19.6	0.9	36.4	133.3	271.6	218.4	0.4	6.7	2.0	1.8	0.1	0.1	0.4	0.1	16.5	0.0	0.6
0.3	0.0	4.5	0.2	15.8	36.2	40.9	0.1	0.3	2.3	0.2	0.2	0.0	0.0	0.1	0.0	5.1	0.0	0.3
49.3	1242.6	0.0	0.0	0.0	0.0	0.0	0.0	0.0	65406.5	0.0	0.0	0.0	0.0	0.0	0.0	0.0	0.0	0.0
1.0	0.0	0.0	0.0	0.0	0.0	0.0	0.0	0.0	0.0	0.0	2.8	0.0	0.0	0.0	0.0	0.0	0.0	0.0
8.1	0.0	0.0	0.0	0.0	0.0	0.0	0.0	0.0	0.0	0.0	0.0	0.0	0.0	0.0	0.0	0.0	0.0	0.0
11.8	0.0	0.0	0.0	0.0	0.0	0.0	0.0	0.0	0.0	0.0	0.0	0.0	0.0	0.0	0.0	0.0	0.0	0.0
1.7	0.0	0.0	0.0	0.0	0.0	0.0	0.0	0.0	0.0	0.0	0.0	0.0	0.0	0.0	0.0	0.0	0.0	0.0
1.3	0.0	0.0	0.0	0.0	0.0	0.0	0.0	0.0	0.0	0.0	0.0	0.0	0.0	0.0	0.0	0.0	0.0	0.0
2.7	0.0	0.0	0.0	0.0	0.0	0.0	0.0	0.0	0.0	0.0	2.0	0.0	0.0	0.0	0.0	0.0	0.0	0.0
6.7	0.0	0.0	0.0	0.0	0.0	0.0	0.0	0.0	0.0	0.0	3.0	0.0	0.0	0.0	0.0	0.0	0.0	0.0
11.1	0.0	0.0	0.0	0.0	0.0	0.0	0.0	0.0	0.0	0.0	0.5	0.0	0.0	0.0	0.0	0.0	0.0	0.0
1.8	0.0	0.0	0.0	0.0	0.0	0.0	0.0	0.0	0.0	0.0	0.0	0.0	0.0	0.0	0.0	0.0	0.0	0.0
2.7	0.0	0.0	0.0	0.0	0.0	0.0	0.0	0.0	0.0	0.0	0.0	0.0	0.0	0.0	0.0	0.0	0.0	0.0
2.0	0.0	0.0	0.0	0.0	0.0	0.0	0.0	0.0	0.0	0.0	0.7	0.0	0.0	0.0	0.0	0.0	0.0	0.0
0.8	0.0	0.0	0.0	0.0	0.0	0.0	0.0	0.0	0.0	0.0	0.0	0.0	0.0	0.0	0.0	0.0	0.0	0.0
1.9	0.0	0.0	0.0	0.0	0.0	0.0	0.0	0.0	0.0	0.0	6.9	0.0	0.0	0.0	0.0	0.0	0.0	0.0
2.0	0.0	0.0	0.0	0.0	0.0	0.0	0.0	0.0	0.0	0.0	0.0	0.0	0.0	0.0	0.0	0.0	0.0	0.0
1.8	0.0	0.0	0.0	0.0	0.0	0.0	0.0	0.0	0.0	0.0	6.9	0.0	0.0	0.0	0.0	0.0	0.0	0.0
11.6	0.0	0.0	0.0	0.0	0.0	0.0	0.0	0.0	0.0	0.0	0.0	0.0	0.0	0.0	0.0	0.0	0.0	0.0
1.7	0.0	0.0	0.0	0.0	0.0	0.0	0.0	0.0	0.0	0.0	2.9	0.0	0.0	0.0	0.0	0.0	0.0	0.0
3.5	0.0	0.0	0.0	0.0	0.0	0.0	0.0	0.0	0.0	0.0	5.2	0.0	0.0	0.0	0.0	0.0	0.0	0.0
1.8	0.0	0.0	0.1	0.0	0.2	0.0	0.0	0.0	0.0	0.0	1.7	0.0	0.0	0.0	0.0	0.0	0.0	0.0
2.3	0.0	0.0	0.0	0.0	0.0	0.0	0.0	0.0	0.0	0.0	1.7	0.0	0.0	0.0	0.0	0.0	0.0	0.0
1.2	0.0	0.0	0.0	0.0	0.0	0.0	0.0	0.0	0.0	0.0	5.9	0.0	0.0	0.0	0.0	0.0	0.0	0.0
0.8	0.0	0.0	0.0	0.0	0.0	0.0	0.0	0.0	0.0	0.0	4.7	0.0	0.0	0.0	0.0	0.0	0.0	0.0
1.9	0.0	0.0	0.0	0.0	0.0	0.0	0.0	0.0	0.0	0.0	0.6	0.0	0.0	0.0	0.0	0.0	0.0	0.0
2.0	0.0	0.0	0.0	0.0	0.0	0.0	0.0	0.0	0.0	0.0	2.5	0.0	0.0	0.0	0.0	0.0	0.0	0.0
2.0	0.0	0.0	0.0	0.0	0.0	0.0	0.0	0.0	0.0	0.0	2.5	0.0	0.0	0.0	0.0	0.0	0.0	0.0
1.1	8.6	27.3	2.4	14.0	266.0	80.3	413.4	0.5	0.0	1.1	0.0	0.2	0.2	2.7	0.3	40.6	0.8	36.8
0.8	21.3	78.3	0.7	6.1	57.4	52.4	156.6	0.2	19.4	0.8	0.0	0.1	0.1	0.6	0.0	13.7	0.1	20.2
0.8	0.6	76.8	0.6	16.8	122.1	69.9	159.9	0.4	20.1	0.2	0.0	0.1	0.1	0.4	0.0	5.1	0.1	16.1
0.7	22.0	59.7	0.6	5.7	52.8	55.1	198.4	0.2	11.4	0.2	0.0	0.1	0.1	0.6	0.0	14.4	0.1	20.0
0.1	0.1	22.0	0.7	10.3	129.2	146.7	99.6	0.3	3.8	0.0	0.0	0.1	0.0	0.6	0.0	1.9	0.0	18.6
0.6	16.5	61.3	0.5	4.5	44.5	37.0	122.9	0.2	15.1	0.1	0.0	0.1	0.1	0.4	0.0	10.6	0.1	14.8
1.1	0.8	81.7	0.5	8.4	118.9	75.6	191.9	0.3	27.4	0.2	0.0	0.1	0.1	0.5	0.0	4.2	0.1	20.1
0.3	0.3	47.9	0.6	7.6	126.9	66.5	238.6	0.1	3.4	0.1	0.0	0.1	0.1	0.7	0.0	3.4	0.1	20.1
0.3	3.2	22.3	1.3	5.0	133.9	26.3	183.2	0.2	10.4	0.1	0.1	0.1	0.2	1.4	0.0	18.0	0.1	16.3
0.9	0.7	95.0	1.2	17.5	141.7	106.0	217.4	0.4	24.3	0.2	0.0	0.1	0.2	0.9	0.0	8.0	0.1	20.1
0.2	23.4	5.7	0.7	8.0	29.6	12.0	47.3	0.3	9.7	0.0	0.0	0.1	0.1	0.7	0.0	24.5	0.1	39.2
6.8	34.0	46.8	4.0	59.5	195.5	701.3	1776.5	3.1	157.3	12.8	2.1	0.3	0.3	5.6	0.3	89.3	1.0	330.8
0.1	0.0	3.4	0.6	8.0	22.8	10.8	42.2	0.2	0.0	0.0	0.0	0.1	0.1	0.8	0.0	24.5	0.0	39.3
6.1	37.6	0.0	3.8	0.0	0.0	0.0	2014.8	0.0	0.0	0.0	0.0	0.0	0.0	0.0	0.0	0.0	0.0	326.9
0.0	0.0	51.0	2.2	0.0	0.0	371.0	814.0	0.0	196.0	7.0	0.0	0.2	0.2	3.3	0.0	0.0	0.0	0.0
1.2	17.0	17.0	1.5	0.0	0.0	0.0	799.2	0.0	0.0	0.4	0.0	0.0	0.0	0.0	0.0	0.0	0.0	167.0
10.0	110.0	340.0	1.4	34.0	320.0	120.0	540.0	1.1	103.0	0.0	0.0	0.2	0.3	1.2	0.1	13.0	0.5	0.0

Code	Food Name	Unit/Amt	Wt (g)	Energy (Kcal)	Prot (g)	Carb (g)	Fiber (g)	Fat (g)	Mono (g)	Poly (g)
20094	Pasta, Fettucini Alfredo	2.0 oz dry, @ 1 cup cooked	29	30.7	1.3	46.0	0.0	0.9	0.0	0.0
20093	Pasta, Fresh-refrigerated, Plain, ckd	2.0 oz dry, @ 1 cup cooked	57	74.7	2.9	14.2	0.0	0.6	0.1	0.2
20095	Pasta, Fresh-refrigerated, Spinach, ckd	2.0 oz	57	74.1	2.9	14.3	0.0	0.5	0.2	0.1
924170	Pasta, Mini beef Ravioli in tomato & meat sauce, canned entree/Chef Boyardee	1 package	425	403.8	14.8	68.5	5.5	8.0	3.4	0.3
924270	Pasta, Ravioli, frozen	1.0 oz	28	59.9	2.0	7.0	0.0	2.0	0.0	0.0
924014	Pasta, Spaghetti w/meat sauce	1 cup	248	332.3	18.6	38.7	0.0	11.7	0.0	0.0
924126	Pasta, Spaghetti w/tomato sauce&cheese	1 cup	250	260.0	9.0	37.0	2.0	9.0	3.6	1.2
924189	Pasta, Spaghetti&Meatballs	1 cup	248	329.8	19.0	39.0	1.0	12.0	4.4	2.2
20121	Pasta, Spaghetti, canned	1 cup	250	190.0	6.0	39.0	2.0	2.0	0.4	0.5
20321	Pasta, Spaghetti, enriched, ckd w/o salt	1 cup	140	197.4	6.7	39.7	2.4	0.9	0.1	0.4
20120	Pasta, Spaghetti, enriched, ckd w/salt	1 cup	140	197.4	6.7	39.7	2.4	0.9	0.1	0.4
20126	Pasta, Spaghetti, Spinach, ckd	1 cup	140	182.0	6.4	36.6	0.0	0.9	0.1	0.4
20521	Pasta, Spaghetti, unenriched, ckd w/o salt	1 cup	140	197.4	6.7	39.7	2.4	0.9	0.1	0.4
20420	Pasta, Spaghetti, unenriched, ckd w/salt	1 cup	140	197.4	6.7	39.7	0.0	0.9	0.1	0.4
20124	Pasta, Spaghetti, Whole Wheat, ckd	1 cup	140	173.6	7.5	37.2	6.3	0.8	0.1	0.3
924172	Pasta, Spaghettios&Franks/FrancoAm	8.0 oz	227	227.0	8.3	28.3	1.1	9.1	0.0	0.0
924194	Pasta, Spaghettios&Meatballs/FrancoAm	8.0 oz	227	222.5	9.9	27.3	0.9	8.2	0.0	0.0
22520	Pasta, Spinach Tortellini/Contadina	8.0 oz	227	656.0	31.9	97.5	0.0	14.2	5.3	1.8
18640	Pasta, Whole Wheat Macaroni and Cheese Dinner, dry mix/Hodgson Mill	8.0 oz	227	852.4	32.0	157.1	17.3	10.7	0.0	0.0
18635	Pastry, Chocolate Eclairs, frozen/WW	1 eclair, frozen	59	140.5	2.4	23.5	0.9	4.1	0.0	0.0
18238	Pastry, Cinnamon Rolls w/icing, refrigerated dough/Pillsbury	1 serving	44	150.2	2.4	23.9	0.0	5.0	0.0	0.0
18237	Pastry, Cream Puff/Eclair Shell, homemade w/custard	1 miniature cream puff	23	59.3	1.5	5.3	0.1	3.6	1.5	1.0
18240	Pastry, Cream Puff/Eclair Shell, homemade	1 cream puff shell	66	238.9	5.9	15.0	0.5	17.1	7.3	4.9
18241	Pastry, Croissant, Butter	1 mini croissant	29	117.7	2.4	13.3	0.8	6.1	1.6	0.3
918816	Pastry, Croissant, Cheese	1 small croissant	42	173.9	3.9	19.7	1.1	8.8	2.7	1.0
18244	Pastry, Danish, Cheese	1 pastry	71	265.5	5.7	26.4	0.7	15.5	8.0	1.8
18431	Pastry, Danish, Fruit (Apple/Cinn/Raisin/Lemon/Raspberry/Strawberry)enrich	1 large (7" dia)	142	526.8	7.7	67.9	2.7	26.3	14.2	3.4
18435	Pastry, Danish, Nut (Almond/Raisin Nut/Cinnamon Nut)	1 piece (⅛ of 15 oz ring)	53	227.9	3.8	24.2	1.1	13.4	7.3	2.3
18338	Pastry, Eclair/Cream Puff, homemade, custard filled w/chocolate icing	1 eclair (5" x 2" x 1.75")	100	262.0	6.4	24.2	0.6	15.7	6.5	3.9
18337	Pastry, Phyllo Dough	1.0 oz	28	83.7	2.0	14.7	0.5	1.7	0.9	0.3
18354	Pastry, Puff, frozen, baked	1 shell	40	223.2	3.0	18.3	0.6	15.4	3.5	8.9
18368	Pastry, Strudel, Apple	1 piece	71	194.5	2.3	29.2	1.6	8.0	2.3	3.8
16398	Peanut Butter, chunky w/salt	2 tbsp	32	188.5	7.7	6.9	2.1	16.0	7.5	4.5
16099	Peanut Butter, smooth w/salt	2 tbsp	32	189.8	8.1	6.2	1.9	16.3	7.8	4.4
16100	Peanut Flour, defatted	1 cup	60	196.2	31.3	20.8	9.5	0.3	0.1	0.1
912902	Peanut Flour, low fat	1 cup	60	256.8	20.3	18.8	9.5	13.1	6.5	4.2
16090	Peanuts, All Types, dry roasted w/o salt	1 peanut	1	5.9	0.2	0.2	0.1	0.5	0.2	0.2
16389	Peanuts, All Types, dry roasted w/salt	1.0 oz	28	163.8	6.6	6.0	2.2	13.9	6.9	4.4
16089	Peanuts, All Types, oil roasted w/o salt	1 nut	1	5.8	0.3	0.2	0.1	0.5	0.2	0.2
16087	Peanuts, All Types, oil roasted w/salt	1 peanut	0.9	5.2	0.2	0.2	0.1	0.4	0.2	0.1
912901	Peanuts, All Types, raw	1.0 oz	28	158.8	7.2	4.5	2.4	13.8	6.8	4.4
16392	Peanuts, honey roasted	1.0 oz	28	150.1	7.0	4.0	3.0	13.0	7.0	4.0
16394	Peanuts, Spanish, raw	¼ cup (@ 1 handful)	37	210.9	9.7	5.9	3.5	18.4	8.3	6.4
16158	Peas, Chickpea/Garbanzo, Falafel, homemade	1 (2.25" diam) patty	17	56.6	2.3	5.4	0.0	3.0	1.7	0.7
16357	Peas, Chickpea/Garbanzo, Hummus, commercial	½ cup	125	207.5	9.9	17.9	7.5	12.0	0.0	0.0
16056	Peas, Chickpea/Garbanzo/Bengal gram, mature seeds, canned	½ cup	120	142.8	5.9	27.1	5.3	1.4	0.3	0.6
16063	Peas, Cowpea, Catjang, mature seeds, raw	½ cup	65	223.0	15.5	38.8	7.0	1.3	0.1	0.6
16363	Peas, Cowpea, Common (blackeyed,crowder,southern) mature seed, boiled w/o salt	½ cup	66	76.6	5.1	13.7	4.3	0.3	0.0	0.1
16101	Peas, Pigeon (red gram) mature seeds, boiled w/salt	½ cup	84	101.6	5.7	19.5	5.6	0.3	0.0	0.2
16086	Peas, Split, mature seed, boiled w/salt	½ cup	93	109.7	7.8	19.6	7.7	0.4	0.1	0.2
18398	Pie Crust, Chocolate Cookie	⅛ crust	20	96.0	1.2	13.4	0.0	4.2	3.4	0.2
18618	Pie Crust, Chocolate Wafer, baked	1 piece (⅛ of 9" dia)	27	139.3	1.4	15.0	0.0	8.6	0.0	0.0
18332	Pie Crust, Cookie Type Nilla Wafer, ready to use/Nabisco	1.0 oz	28	143.7	1.0	17.7	0.3	7.6	5.2	0.4
18335	Pie Crust, dry mix, prep, baked	1 piece (⅛ of 9" dia)	20	100.2	1.3	10.1	0.4	6.1	0.0	0.0
18334	Pie Crust, frozen, baked	1 piece (⅛ of 9" dia)	16	82.2	0.7	7.9	0.2	5.2	2.5	0.6
18336	Pie Crust, Graham Cracker/Cookie Type, baked	1 piece (⅛ of 9" dia)	30	148.2	1.3	19.6	0.5	7.5	3.4	2.1
18402	Pie Crust, homemade, baked	1 piece (⅛ of 9" dia)	23	121.2	1.5	10.9	0.4	8.0	3.5	2.1
19312	Pie Crust, Vanilla Wafer, baked	1 piece (⅛ of 9" dia)	22	119.0	0.8	11.3	0.0	8.1	0.0	0.0
19314	Pie Filling, Apple, canned	⅛ can	74	74.7	0.1	19.4	0.7	0.1	0.0	0.0
918888	Pie Filling, Cherry, canned	⅛ can	74	85.1	0.4	21.7	0.4	0.1	0.0	0.0
18628	Pie, Apple Snack Pie/Hostess	1 pie	128	390.4	5.0	45.0	0.0	20.0	0.0	0.0
18443	Pie, Apple Turnover, frozen, ready to bake/PepFarm	1 serving	89	284.1	3.7	31.2	1.6	16.0	0.0	0.0
18302	Pie, Apple, frozen/Banquet	1 serving	112	292.3	2.9	41.4	1.0	13.2	6.1	1.4
918871	Pie, Apple, homemade	1 oz	28.35	75.1	0.7	10.5	0.0	3.5	1.5	0.9
18304	Pie, Banana Cream, frozen	⅙ pie	66	180.2	2.0	21.0	2.0	10.0	0.0	0.0
18303	Pie, Banana Cream, homemade	1 piece (⅛ of 9" dia)	144	387.4	6.3	47.4	1.0	19.6	8.2	4.7
918872	Pie, Banana Cream, no bake mix	1 piece (⅛ of 9" dia)	92	230.9	3.1	29.1	0.6	11.9	4.2	0.7
918873	Pie, Banana Custard	⅛ pie	114	251.9	5.1	35.0	1.0	10.6	0.0	0.0

Sat (g)	Chol (mg)	Cal (mg)	Iron (mg)	Magn (mg)	Phos (mg)	Pota (mg)	Sodi (mg)	Zinc (mg)	Vit A (RE)	Vit C (mg)	Vit E (mg)	Thia (mg)	Ribo (mg)	Niac (mg)	Vit B-6 (mg)	Fol (µg)	Vit B-12 (µg)	Wat (g)
0.0	5.7	13.2	0.3	0.0	18.9	8.9	47.3	0.0	0.0	0.0	0.0	0.0	0.0	0.2	0.0	0.0	0.0	0.0
0.1	18.8	3.4	0.6	10.3	35.9	13.7	3.4	0.3	3.4	0.0	0.0	0.1	0.1	0.6	0.0	36.5	0.1	39.1
0.1	18.8	10.3	0.6	13.7	32.5	21.1	3.4	0.4	8.0	0.0	0.0	0.1	0.1	0.6	0.1	36.5	0.1	39.1
3.0	29.8	38.3	4.1	0.0	0.0	0.0	2018.8	0.0	0.0	0.0	0.4	0.0	0.0	0.0	0.0	0.0	0.0	327.5
0.0	0.0	12.0	0.7	0.0	34.0	40.0	80.0	0.0	0.0	0.0	0.0	0.1	0.1	0.8	0.0	0.0	0.0	0.0
3.3	0.0	124.0	3.7	0.0	236.0	665.0	1009.0	0.0	318.0	22.0	0.0	0.3	0.3	4.0	0.0	0.0	0.0	173.8
3.0	8.0	80.0	2.3	0.0	135.0	408.0	955.0	1.3	216.0	13.0	0.0	0.3	0.2	2.3	0.2	8.0	0.0	0.0
3.9	89.0	124.0	3.7	0.0	236.0	665.0	1009.0	2.5	318.0	22.0	0.0	0.3	0.3	4.0	0.2	10.0	0.0	0.0
0.4	3.0	40.0	2.8	0.0	88.0	303.0	955.0	1.1	186.0	10.0	0.0	0.4	0.3	4.5	0.1	6.0	0.0	0.0
0.1	0.0	9.8		25.2	75.6	43.4	1.4	0.7	0.0	0.0	0.1	0.3	0.1	2.3	0.0	98.0	0.0	92.4
0.1	0.0	9.8	2.0	25.2	75.6	43.4	140.0	0.7	0.0	0.0	0.0	0.3	0.1	2.3	0.0	98.0	0.0	92.4
0.1	0.0	42.0	1.5	86.8	151.2	81.2	19.6	1.5	21.0	0.0	0.0	0.1	0.1	2.1	0.1	16.8	0.0	95.4
0.1	0.0	9.8	0.7	25.2	75.6	43.4	1.4	0.7	0.0	0.0	0.1	0.0	0.0	0.6	0.0	9.8	0.0	92.4
0.1	0.0	9.8	0.7	25.2	75.6	43.4	140.0	0.7	0.0	0.0	0.0	0.0	0.0	0.6	0.0	9.8	0.0	92.4
0.1	0.0	21.0	1.5	42.0	124.6	61.6	4.2	1.1	0.0	0.0	0.1	0.2	0.1	1.0	0.1	7.0	0.0	94.0
0.0	0.0	34.8	2.4	0.0	118.4	325.8	1074.2	1.7	111.0	4.3	0.0	0.2	0.2	3.5	0.1	0.0	0.5	0.0
0.0	0.0	32.0	2.4	0.0	137.7	342.7	1024.8	2.2	112.8	4.4	0.0	0.2	0.2	3.3	0.1	0.0	0.8	0.0
7.1	115.3	540.9	6.4	16.0	532.0	478.8	1064.1	0.6	94.0	0.0	0.0	1.3	1.0	11.4	0.0	12.4	0.3	0.0
3.1	17.9	258.8	5.9	0.0	0.0	0.0	1387.0	0.0	0.0	0.0	0.0	0.0	0.0	0.0	0.0	0.0	0.0	19.3
0.7	30.1	0.0	0.0	0.0	0.0	0.0	185.9	0.0	0.0	0.0	0.0	0.0	0.0	0.0	0.0	0.0	0.0	28.3
1.2	0.0	0.0	0.0	0.0	0.0	0.0	334.4	0.0	0.0	0.0	0.0	0.0	0.0	0.0	0.0	0.0	0.0	11.7
0.8	30.8	15.2	0.3	2.8	25.1	26.5	78.4	0.1	45.8	0.1	0.5	0.0	0.1	0.2	0.0	6.4	0.1	12.3
3.7	129.4	23.8	1.3	7.9	78.5	64.0	367.6	0.5	203.3	0.0	2.5	0.1	0.2	1.0	0.0	31.7	0.3	26.7
3.4	19.4	10.7	0.6	4.6	30.5	34.2	215.8	0.2	53.9	0.1	0.1	0.1	0.1	0.6	0.0	18.0	0.1	6.7
4.5	23.9	22.3	0.9	10.1	54.6	55.4	233.1	0.4	82.7	0.1	0.4	0.2	0.1	0.9	0.0	31.1	0.1	8.8
4.8	11.4	24.9	1.1	10.7	76.7	69.6	319.5	0.5	32.0	0.1	1.8	0.1	0.2	1.4	0.0	42.6	0.1	22.3
6.9	161.9	65.3	2.5	21.3	126.4	117.9	502.7	0.8	31.2	5.5	3.5	0.4	0.3	2.8	0.1	46.9	0.1	38.5
3.1	24.4	49.8	1.0	17.0	58.3	50.4	192.4	0.5	7.4	0.9	1.9	0.1	0.1	1.2	0.1	44.0	0.1	10.8
4.1	127.0	63.0	1.2	15.0	107.0	117.0	337.0	0.6	191.0	0.3	2.1	0.1	0.3	0.8	0.1	28.0	0.3	52.4
0.4	0.0	3.1	0.9	4.2	21.0	20.7	135.2	0.1	0.0	0.0	0.3	0.2	0.1	1.1	0.0	20.7	0.0	9.1
2.2	0.0	4.0	1.0	6.4	24.0	24.8	101.2	0.2	0.0	0.0	1.0	0.1	0.1	1.5	0.0	18.8	0.0	3.0
1.5	4.3	10.7	0.3	6.4	23.4	105.8	191.0	0.1	6.4	1.2	2.2	0.0	0.0	0.2	0.0	9.9	0.2	30.9
3.1	0.0	13.1	0.6	50.9	101.4	239.0	155.5	0.9	0.0	0.0	0.0	0.0	0.0	4.4	0.1	29.4	0.0	0.4
3.3	0.0	12.2	0.6	50.9	118.1	214.1	149.4	0.9	0.0	0.0	3.2	0.0	0.4	4.3	0.0	23.7	0.0	0.4
0.0	0.0	84.0	1.3	222.0	456.0	774.0	108.0	3.1	0.0	0.0	0.0	0.4	0.3	16.2	0.3	148.9	0.0	4.7
1.8	0.0	78.0	2.8	28.8	304.8	814.8	0.6	3.6	0.0	0.0	0.0	0.3	0.1	6.9	0.2	80.0	0.0	4.7
0.1	0.0	0.5	0.0	1.8	3.6	6.6	0.1	0.0	0.0	0.0	0.1	0.0	0.0	0.1	0.0	1.5	0.0	0.0
1.9	0.0	15.1	0.6	49.3	100.2	184.2	227.6	0.9	0.0	0.0	2.1	0.1	0.0	3.8	0.1	40.7	0.0	0.4
0.1	0.0	0.9	0.0	1.9	5.2	6.8	0.1	0.1	0.0	0.0	0.1	0.0	0.0	0.1	0.0	1.3	0.0	0.0
0.1	0.0	0.8	0.0	1.7	4.7	6.1	3.9	0.1	0.0	0.0	0.1	0.0	0.0	0.1	0.0	1.1	0.0	0.0
1.9	0.0	25.8	1.3	47.0	105.3	197.4	5.0	0.9	0.0	0.0	2.6	0.2	0.0	3.4	0.1	67.1	0.0	1.8
2.0	0.0	15.0	0.6	0.0	100.0	160.0	110.0	0.9	0.0	0.0	0.0	0.1	0.0	3.8	0.1	41.0	0.0	0.0
2.8	0.0	39.2	1.4	69.6	143.6	275.3	8.1	0.8	0.0	0.0	0.0	0.2	0.0	5.9	0.1	88.8	0.0	2.4
0.4	0.0	9.2	0.6	13.9	32.6	99.5	50.0	0.3	0.2	0.3	0.0	0.0	0.0	0.2	0.0	15.8	0.0	5.9
0.0	0.0	47.5	3.1	88.8	220.0	285.0	473.8	2.3	3.8	0.0	0.0	0.2	0.1	0.7	0.3	103.8	0.0	83.2
0.1	0.0	38.4	1.6	34.8	108.0	206.4	358.8	1.3	2.4	4.6	0.0	0.0	0.0	0.2	0.6	80.2	0.0	83.6
0.4	0.0	55.3	6.5	216.5	284.7	893.8	37.7	4.0	2.0	1.0	0.0	0.4	0.1	1.8	0.2	415.4	0.0	7.2
0.1	0.0	15.8	1.7	35.0	103.0	183.5	2.6	0.9	1.3	0.3	0.2	0.1	0.0	0.3	0.1	137.2	0.0	46.2
0.1	0.0	36.1	0.9	38.6	100.0	322.6	202.4	0.8	0.0	0.0	0.0	0.1	0.0	0.7	0.0	93.1	0.0	57.6
0.1	0.0	13.0	1.2	33.5	92.1	336.7	221.3	0.9	0.9	0.4	0.0	0.2	0.1	0.8	0.0	60.4	0.0	64.6
0.6	0.0	5.0	0.6	0.0	0.0	62.0	107.0	0.0	0.0	0.0	0.0	0.1	0.2	0.6	0.0	0.0	0.0	0.0
2.1	4.1	8.4	0.8	11.1	28.9	46.2	185.2	0.2	60.2	0.0	0.0	0.0	0.1	0.6	0.0	0.0	0.0	1.5
1.4	2.8	11.5	0.5	2.2	23.2	19.3	62.7	0.1	0.0	0.0	0.0	0.0	0.1	0.7	0.0	8.4	0.0	0.9
0.8	3.5	12.0	0.4	3.0	16.8	12.4	145.8	0.1	0.0	0.0	0.0	0.1	0.0	0.5	0.0	2.4	0.0	2.1
1.7	0.0	3.4	0.4	2.9	9.4	17.6	103.5	0.1	0.0	0.0	0.8	0.0	0.1	0.4	0.0	6.2	0.0	1.8
1.6	0.0	6.3	0.7	5.4	19.5	26.4	171.3	0.1	60.6	0.0	1.2	0.0	0.1	0.6	0.0	7.2	0.0	1.3
2.0	0.0	2.3	0.7	3.2	15.4	15.4	124.7	0.1	0.0	0.0	0.0	0.1	0.1	0.8	0.0	15.4	0.0	2.3
2.4	3.5	9.5	0.4	2.4	17.4	17.8	115.7	0.1	64.0	0.0	0.0	0.0	0.1	0.5	0.0	1.5	0.0	1.5
0.0	0.0	3.0	0.2	1.5	5.2	33.3	32.6	0.0	0.7	0.0	0.0	0.0	0.0	0.0	0.0	0.0	0.0	54.3
0.0	0.0	8.1	0.2	5.2	11.1	77.7	6.7	0.0	15.5	2.7	0.0	0.0	0.0	0.1	0.0	3.0	0.0	51.6
0.0	18.0	26.0	1.4	0.0	0.0	0.0	540.0	0.0	0.0	1.0	0.0	0.1	0.1	1.6	0.0	0.0	0.0	37.3
4.0	0.0	0.0	1.2	0.0	0.0	0.0	176.2	0.0	0.0	0.0	0.0	0.0	0.0	0.0	0.0	0.0	0.0	54.3
5.7	8.7	10.1	0.3	0.0	0.0	0.0	360.6	0.0	0.0	0.0	0.0	0.0	0.0	0.0	0.0	0.0	0.0	54.3
0.9	0.0	2.0	0.3	2.0	7.9	22.4	59.8	0.1	3.4	0.5	0.0	0.0	0.0	0.3	0.0	6.8	0.0	13.4
0.0	0.0	32.0	1.0	0.0	100.0	120.0	150.0	0.0	1.4	1.0	0.0	0.0	0.1	2.0	0.3	15.0	0.0	0.0
5.4	73.4	108.0	1.5	23.0	132.5	237.6	345.6	0.7	100.8	2.3	2.1	0.2	0.3	1.5	0.2	38.9	0.4	69.0
6.4	26.7	67.2	0.4	11.0	153.6	104.0	266.8	0.3	92.0	0.5	0.0	0.1	0.1	0.7	0.0	19.3	0.2	46.8
3.4	0.0	75.0	0.6	0.0	93.0	231.0	221.0	0.0	58.0	1.0	0.0	0.0	0.1	0.3	0.0	0.0	0.0	60.2

Code	Food Name	Unit/Amt	Wt (g)	Energy (Kcal)	Prot (g)	Carb (g)	Fiber (g)	Fat (g)	Mono (g)	Poly (g)
918889	Pie, Blackberry	⅛ pie	118	286.7	3.1	40.6	5.0	13.0	0.0	0.0
18305	Pie, Blueberry Snack Pie/Hostess	1 pie	128	390.4	3.0	49.0	0.0	20.0	0.0	0.0
18306	Pie, Blueberry, commercially prep	1 piece (⅛ of 9″ dia)	125	290.0	2.3	43.6	1.3	12.5	5.3	4.4
918307	Pie, Blueberry, homemade	1 piece (⅛ of 9″ dia)	147	360.2	4.0	49.2	0.0	17.5	7.5	4.5
918890	Pie, Butterscotch Pudding, homemade	1 piece (⅛ of 9″ dia)	127	354.3	6.0	42.3	0.0	18.2	0.0	0.0
18308	Pie, Cherry Snack Pie/Hostess	1 pie	128	390.4	5.0	55.0	0.0	20.0	0.0	0.0
18444	Pie, Cherry, commercially prep	1 piece (⅛ of 9″ dia)	125	325.0	2.5	49.8	1.0	13.8	7.3	2.6
18309	Pie, Cherry, fried	1.0 oz	28	88.5	0.8	11.9	0.7	4.5	2.1	1.5
918874	Pie, Cherry, homemade	1.0 oz	29	78.3	0.8	11.2	0.0	3.5	1.5	0.9
18310	Pie, Chocolate Cream, frozen/Banquet	⅙ pie	66	190.1	2.0	24.0	1.0	10.0	0.0	0.0
918311	Pie, Chocolate Creme, commercially prep	1 piece (⅙ of 8″ pie)	113	343.5	2.9	38.0	2.3	21.9	12.6	2.7
18312	Pie, Chocolate Creme, homemade	1 piece (⅛ of 9″ dia)	142	400.4	6.8	44.3	0.0	22.9	0.0	0.0
918875	Pie, Chocolate Mousse, no bake mix	1 piece (⅛ of 9″ dia)	95	247.0	3.3	28.1	0.0	14.6	4.8	0.8
18313	Pie, Coconut Cream, frozen	1 piece (⅙ of 8″ pie)	100	288.0	3.0	33.3	0.0	16.7	0.0	0.0
918315	Pie, Coconut Creme, commercially prep	1 piece (⅛ of 7″ pie)	48	143.0	1.0	17.9	0.6	8.0	3.5	0.7
18314	Pie, Coconut Creme, homemade	1 piece (⅛ of 9″ dia)	133	396.3	6.4	45.5	0.0	21.3	0.0	0.0
918318	Pie, Egg Custard, commercially prep	1 piece (⅙ of 8″ pie)	105	220.5	5.8	21.8	1.7	12.2	5.0	3.9
18319	Pie, Egg Custard, homemade	1 piece (⅛ of 9″ dia)	127	261.6	6.5	34.0	0.0	11.3	0.0	0.0
918876	Pie, Fruit Pie, fried	1 fried pie (5 x 3.75″)	128	404.5	3.8	54.5	3.3	20.6	9.5	6.9
918877	Pie, Lemon Chiffon	1 piece (⅙ of 8″ pie)	81	254.3	5.7	35.5	1.0	10.2	0.0	0.0
18320	Pie, Lemon Cream, frozen/Banquet	1 piece (⅙ of 8″ pie)	66	170.3	2.0	23.0	1.0	9.0	0.0	0.0
18321	Pie, Lemon Meringue, commercially prep	1 piece (⅙ of 8″ pie)	113	302.8	1.7	53.3	1.4	9.8	3.0	4.1
18445	Pie, Lemon Meringue, homemade	1 piece (⅛ of 9″ dia)	127	362.0	4.8	49.7	0.0	16.4	7.1	4.2
18322	Pie, Lemon, fried	1 fried pie (5 x 3.75″)	128	404.5	3.8	54.5	3.3	20.6	9.5	6.9
918878	Pie, Mince, homemade	1 piece (⅛ of 9″ dia)	165	476.9	4.3	79.2	4.3	17.8	7.7	4.7
18323	Pie, Mincemeat, frozen/Banquet	1 piece (⅙ of 8″ pie)	94	260.4	3.0	38.0	0.0	11.0	0.0	0.0
918891	Pie, Peach	1.0 oz	28.5	63.6	0.5	9.4	0.2	2.9	1.2	1.1
918892	Pie, Peach Snack Pie/Hostess	1 pie	128	399.4	4.0	53.0	0.0	20.0	0.0	0.0
18324	Pie, Pecan Snack Pie/LittleDeb	1 pie	52	201.8	1.8	33.1	1.0	6.9	4.0	1.2
18325	Pie, Pecan, commercially prep	1 piece (⅙ of 8″ pie)	113	452.0	4.5	64.6	4.0	20.9	12.1	3.6
918879	Pie, Pecan, homemade	1 piece (⅛ of 9″ dia)	122	502.6	6.0	63.7	0.0	27.1	13.6	7.0
918880	Pie, Pineapple	1 piece (⅛ of 9″ dia)	118	298.5	2.6	45.0	0.6	12.6	0.0	0.0
918881	Pie, Pineapple Chiffon	1 piece (⅛ of 9″ dia)	81	233.3	5.3	31.7	0.3	9.8	0.0	0.0
18326	Pie, Pineapple Custard	1 piece (⅛ of 9″ dia)	114	250.8	4.6	36.6	0.5	9.9	0.0	0.0
18327	Pie, Pumpkin, commercially prep	1 piece (⅙ of 8″ pie)	180	378.0	7.0	49.1	4.9	17.1	7.3	5.7
918882	Pie, Pumpkin, homemade	1 piece (⅛ of 9″ dia)	114	232.6	5.1	30.1	0.0	10.6	4.2	2.1
918883	Pie, Raisin	1 piece (⅛ of 9″ dia)	118	318.6	3.1	50.7	0.8	12.6	0.0	0.0
918885	Pie, Rhubarb	1 piece (⅛ of 9″ dia)	118	298.5	3.0	45.1	2.0	12.6	0.0	0.0
18328	Pie, Strawberry	1 piece (⅛ of 9″ dia)	93	184.1	1.8	28.7	1.8	7.3	0.0	0.0
22531	Pie, Vanilla Creme, homemade	1 piece (⅛ of 9″ dia)	93	258.5	4.5	30.3	0.6	13.4	5.6	3.2
22533	Pizza Rolls Pizza Snacks, Hamburger, frozen/Totinos	1 serving (⅓ pkg)	85	231.2	9.4	26.4	0.0	9.8	0.0	0.0
22532	Pizza Rolls Pizza Snacks, Pepperoni, frozen/Totinos	1 serving	141	384.9	14.4	39.5	2.3	18.9	9.2	2.2
924142	Pizza Rolls Pizza Snacks, Sausage, frozen/Totinos	1 serving	141	351.1	14.1	40.2	2.8	14.9	7.2	2.2
924146	Pizza, Cheese Meat Vegetable	⅛ of alarge pizza	79	184.1	13.0	21.3	0.0	5.4	2.5	0.9
924141	Pizza, Cheese, frozen/Celeste	¼ of a medium pizza	126	317.5	14.2	27.8	2.2	16.6	3.0	1.0
22545	Pizza, Cheese, homemade	1 slice	65	152.8	7.8	18.4	1.0	5.4	0.0	0.0
924262	Pizza, Combination, Sausage & Pepperoni, frozen/Jeno's Crisp'n Tasty	1 package	198	491.0	16.8	51.7	2.8	24.2	11.9	3.1
22548	Pizza, Combo, frozen/Totino	⅙ pizza	91	234.8	11.3	20.0	0.0	12.2	0.0	0.0
22554	Pizza, Deep Dish Sausage, frozen/Tony's D'Primo	1 package	569	1576.1	50.1	163.9	0.0	80.2	29.3	17.0
22542	Pizza, Deluxe French Bread w/Sausage, Pepperoni & Mushroom, frozen/Stouffer	1 package	350	857.5	32.2	88.9	7.0	41.3	17.4	5.0
924148	Pizza, Deluxe w/Sausage, Green & Red Pepper & Mushrooms, frozen/Celeste	1 package	666	1538.5	66.6	132.5	0.0	82.6	30.4	9.7
924133	Pizza, Deluxe, frozen/Celeste	¼ pizza	158	377.6	15.5	29.3	3.1	22.1	7.0	2.0
22553	Pizza, French Bread Pizza/Pillsbury	5.7 oz	161	389.6	18.5	43.0	0.0	15.8	0.0	0.0
924149	Pizza, French Bread w/sausage & pepperoni, frozen/Stouffers	1 package	354	895.6	35.4	87.1	5.0	45.0	18.5	5.6
924264	Pizza, Ground Beef/Totino	3.5 oz	100	240.0	10.5	24.4	0.0	11.0	0.0	0.0
22560	Pizza, Mexican, frozen/Totino	½ pizza	145	381.4	13.1	35.5	0.0	20.3	0.0	0.0
22555	Pizza, Original Pepperoni, frozen, 12″/Tombstone	1 serving	113	311.9	14.5	28.3	0.0	15.7	5.3	2.0
22557	Pizza, Original Pepperoni, frozen, 9″/Tombstone	1 serving	152	413.4	17.8	38.6	0.0	20.8	7.1	2.4
22559	Pizza, Original Sausage & Mushroom, frozen/Tombstone	1 serving	132	306.2	14.4	31.2	0.0	13.7	4.4	2.1
22566	Pizza, Original Sausage & Pepperoni, frozen/Tombstone	1 serving	125	327.5	14.4	30.6	2.1	16.4	5.6	2.3
22562	Pizza, Pepperoni	⅛ pizza	71	181.1	10.1	19.9	0.0	7.0	3.1	1.2
22903	Pizza, Pepperoni w/Italian Pastry Crust, frozen/Tony's	1 seving	140	411.6	15.1	36.8	0.0	22.7	9.2	2.6
924151	Pizza, Pepperoni, frozen	1 seving	138	378.1	15.3	34.2	2.2	20.0	8.0	2.3
22546	Pizza, Pepperoni, frozen/Jack's Original	1 serving	122	323.3	15.0	29.5	0.0	16.1	5.2	2.1
22551	Pizza, Pepperoni/Pillsbury	½ pizza	120	302.4	13.4	29.0	2.0	14.4	0.0	0.0
22563	Pizza, Premium Deep Dish Singles, Pepperoni, frozen/Red Baron	1 serving	168	480.5	16.0	47.9	0.0	25.0	10.8	2.8
22543	Pizza, Sausage & pepperoni, frozen	1 serving	146	385.4	15.8	36.2	2.3	19.7	7.8	2.6
924158	Pizza, Sausage & Pepperoni, frozen/Jack's Great Combination	1 serving	137	348.0	17.4	30.1	0.0	17.5	6.1	2.3
924155	Pizza, Sausage Mushroom, frozen/Celentano	8.5 oz	241	592.9	23.9	51.3	4.5	32.3	10.0	3.0

Sat (g)	Chol (mg)	Cal (mg)	Iron (mg)	Magn (mg)	Phos (mg)	Pota (mg)	Sodi (mg)	Zinc (mg)	Vit A (RE)	Vit C (mg)	Vit E (mg)	Thia (mg)	Ribo (mg)	Niac (mg)	Vit B-6 (mg)	Fol (µg)	Vit B-12 (µg)	Wat (g)
3.2	0.0	22.0	0.6	0.0	31.0	118.0	316.0	0.0	22.0	5.0	0.0	0.0	0.0	0.4	0.0	0.0	0.0	60.2
0.0	18.0	28.0	1.5	0.0	0.0	0.0	450.0	0.0	0.0	2.0	0.0	0.2	0.1	1.8	0.0	0.0	0.0	0.0
2.1	0.0	10.0	0.4	6.3	28.8	62.5	406.3	0.2	42.5	3.4	2.5	0.0	0.0	0.0	0.0	27.5	0.0	65.6
4.3	0.0	10.3	1.8	11.8	44.1	73.5	272.0	0.3	5.9	1.0	0.0	0.2	0.2	1.8	0.0	33.8	0.0	75.3
4.3	7.6	128.3	1.6	21.6	134.6	221.0	335.3	0.7	106.7	0.6	0.0	0.2	0.3	1.3	0.1	14.0	0.4	58.8
0.0	18.0	29.0	1.4	0.0	0.0	0.0	530.0	0.0	0.0	2.0	0.0	0.2	0.1	1.6	0.0	0.0	0.0	0.0
3.2	0.0	15.0	0.6	10.0	36.3	101.3	307.5	0.2	67.5	1.1	1.9	0.0	0.0	0.3	0.1	27.5	0.0	57.8
0.7	0.0	6.2	0.3	2.8	12.0	18.2	104.7	0.1	4.8	0.4	0.0	0.0	0.0	0.4	0.0	5.0	0.0	10.5
0.9	0.0	2.9	0.5	2.6	8.7	22.3	55.4	0.1	13.9	0.3	0.0	0.0	0.0	0.4	0.0	7.8	0.0	13.3
0.0	0.0	38.0	1.0	0.0	0.0	86.0	110.0	0.0	1.4	0.0	0.0	0.0	0.1	0.2	0.0	0.0	0.0	0.0
5.6	5.7	40.7	1.2	23.7	76.8	143.5	153.7	0.3	0.0	3.1	0.0	0.1	0.0	0.8	0.0	14.7	0.0	49.2
4.8	9.4	115.0	1.8	36.9	156.2	208.7	347.9	0.9	103.7	0.7	0.0	0.2	0.3	1.5	0.1	14.2	0.4	66.2
7.8	33.3	73.2	1.0	30.4	219.5	270.8	437.0	0.6	96.0	0.5	0.0	0.0	0.1	0.6	0.0	24.7	0.2	47.2
0.0	0.0	45.5	1.5	0.0	0.0	116.7	181.8	0.0	0.3	0.0	0.0	0.0	0.1	0.3	0.0	0.0	0.0	0.0
3.3	0.0	13.9	0.4	9.6	40.8	31.2	122.4	0.2	0.0	0.0	0.9	0.0	0.0	0.1	0.0	3.4	0.1	20.7
4.5	8.0	113.1	1.5	21.3	139.7	183.5	356.4	0.8	105.1	0.7	0.0	0.2	0.3	1.3	0.1	14.6	0.4	58.1
2.5	34.7	84.0	0.6	11.6	117.6	111.3	252.0	0.5	70.4	0.6	2.0	0.0	0.2	0.3	0.1	21.0	0.5	63.9
2.4	4.6	106.7	1.0	16.5	124.5	158.8	256.5	0.6	81.3	0.5	0.0	0.1	0.3	0.8	0.1	12.7	0.3	73.9
3.1	0.0	28.2	1.6	12.8	55.0	83.2	478.7	0.3	3.8	1.7	3.8	0.2	0.1	1.8	0.0	23.0	0.1	48.1
2.7	0.0	19.0	0.7	0.0	67.0	66.0	211.0	0.0	28.0	2.0	0.0	0.0	0.1	0.2	0.0	0.0	0.0	28.8
0.0	0.0	30.0	1.0	0.0	0.0	70.0	120.0	0.0	0.4	2.0	0.0	0.0	0.0	0.2	0.0	0.0	0.0	0.0
2.0	50.9	63.3	0.7	17.0	118.7	100.6	165.0	0.6	58.8	3.6	2.5	0.1	0.2	0.7	0.0	14.7	0.2	47.1
4.0	67.3	15.2	1.3	7.6	53.3	82.6	307.3	0.4	55.9	4.2	0.0	0.1	0.2	1.2	0.0	31.8	0.2	55.0
3.1	0.0	28.2	1.6	12.8	55.0	83.2	478.7	0.3	3.8	0.0	0.0	0.2	0.1	1.8	0.0	23.0	0.1	48.1
4.4	0.0	36.3	2.5	23.1	69.3	335.0	419.1	0.4	3.3	9.7	3.1	0.2	0.2	2.0	0.1	38.0	0.0	61.7
0.0	0.0	19.0	1.0	0.0	45.0	110.0	370.0	0.0	0.4	1.0	0.0	0.0	0.0	0.3	0.0	0.0	0.0	0.0
0.4	0.0	2.3	0.1	1.7	6.3	35.6	77.0	0.0	6.3	0.3	0.6	0.0	0.0	0.1	0.0	6.8	0.0	15.5
0.0	18.0	37.0	2.0	0.0	0.0	0.0	445.0	0.0	0.0	1.0	0.0	0.2	0.2	2.3	0.0	0.0	0.0	0.0
1.6	1.0	8.0	0.6	0.0	50.0	50.0	184.0	0.5	0.0	0.0	0.0	0.1	0.1	0.5	0.0	5.0	0.0	9.8
4.0	36.2	19.2	1.2	20.3	87.0	83.6	479.1	0.6	53.1	1.2	2.1	0.1	0.1	0.3	0.0	30.5	0.1	21.8
4.9	106.1	39.0	1.8	31.7	114.7	162.3	319.6	1.2	108.6	0.2	0.0	0.2	0.2	1.0	0.1	31.7	0.2	23.8
3.1	0.0	15.0	0.6	0.0	25.0	85.0	320.0	0.0	4.0	1.0	0.0	0.0	0.0	0.5	0.0	0.0	0.0	56.6
2.6	0.0	19.0	0.7	0.0	62.0	79.0	207.0	0.0	56.0	1.0	0.0	0.1	0.3	0.0	0.0	0.0	0.0	33.3
3.0	0.0	27.0	0.5	0.0	74.0	111.0	212.0	0.0	42.0	1.0	0.0	0.1	0.1	0.5	0.0	0.0	0.0	61.9
3.2	36.0	108.0	1.4	27.0	127.8	277.2	507.6	0.8	669.6	1.8	3.1	0.1	0.3	0.3	0.1	36.0	0.5	104.6
3.6	47.9	107.2	1.4	21.7	111.7	212.0	256.5	0.5	891.5	1.9	0.0	0.1	0.2	0.9	0.1	23.9	0.1	66.7
3.1	0.0	21.0	1.1	0.0	47.0	227.0	336.0	0.0	2.0	1.0	0.0	0.0	0.0	0.4	0.0	0.0	0.0	50.2
3.1	0.0	76.0	0.8	0.0	31.0	188.0	319.0	0.0	12.0	4.0	0.0	0.0	0.0	0.4	0.0	0.0	0.0	55.9
1.8	0.0	15.0	0.7	0.0	23.0	112.0	180.0	0.0	8.0	23.0	0.0	0.0	0.0	0.4	0.0	0.0	0.0	54.3
3.7	57.7	83.7	0.9	12.1	96.7	117.2	241.8	0.5	79.1	0.5	1.3	0.1	0.2	0.9	0.0	24.2	0.3	43.7
0.0	0.0	0.0	0.0	0.0	0.0	0.0	417.4	0.0	0.0	0.0	0.0	0.0	0.0	0.0	0.0	0.0	0.0	37.7
5.0	31.0	102.9	0.0	0.0	0.0	0.0	865.7	0.0	0.0	0.0	0.0	0.0	0.0	0.0	0.0	0.0	0.0	65.3
3.5	24.0	101.5	0.0	0.0	0.0	0.0	631.7	0.0	0.0	0.0	0.0	0.0	0.0	0.0	0.0	0.0	0.0	69.2
1.5	21.0	101.0	1.5	18.0	131.0	178.0	382.0	1.1	101.0	2.0	0.0	0.2	0.2	2.0	0.1	27.0	0.4	37.7
7.0	20.0	204.0	1.0	30.0	266.0	268.0	770.0	3.0	155.8	0.0	0.0	0.1	0.4	1.1	0.1	14.0	1.0	62.1
2.1	0.0	144.0	0.7	0.0	127.0	85.0	456.0	3.0	82.0	5.0	0.0	0.0	0.1	0.7	0.2	100.0	2.0	31.4
5.7	25.7	166.3	0.0	0.0	0.0	0.0	1239.5	0.0	0.0	0.0	0.0	0.0	0.0	0.0	0.0	0.0	0.0	101.0
0.0	0.0	177.0	1.5	0.0	196.0	177.0	539.0	0.0	65.8	3.0	0.0	0.3	0.2	2.0	0.0	0.0	0.0	46.4
23.2	62.6	574.7	11.7	0.0	0.0	0.0	3351.4	0.0	0.0	0.0	0.0	0.0	0.0	0.0	0.0	0.0	0.0	261.7
12.7	66.5	462.0	5.4	0.0	0.0	0.0	1680.0	0.0	0.0	59.9	0.0	0.0	0.0	0.0	0.0	0.0	0.0	181.0
32.4	146.5	1118.9	0.0	0.0	0.0	0.0	3050.3	0.0	0.0	0.0	0.0	0.0	0.0	0.0	0.0	0.0	0.0	369.6
7.0	20.0	267.0	1.9	38.0	357.0	352.0	903.0	3.0	190.0	0.0	0.0	0.2	0.5	2.7	0.2	57.0	2.0	86.3
0.0	0.0	309.0	2.2	0.0	250.0	274.0	708.0	0.0	33.4	1.0	0.0	0.4	0.2	2.7	0.0	0.0	0.0	79.5
14.3	74.3	308.0	6.0	0.0	0.0	0.0	1720.4	0.0	0.0	0.0	0.0	0.0	0.0	0.0	0.0	0.0	0.0	179.5
0.0	0.0	134.0	1.7	0.0	190.0	178.0	712.0	0.0	53.2	3.0	0.0	0.1	0.2	2.4	0.0	0.0	0.0	51.2
0.0	0.0	213.0	3.3	0.0	296.0	270.0	973.0	0.0	84.2	10.0	0.0	0.4	0.3	3.3	0.0	0.0	0.0	64.2
6.0	31.6	202.3	0.0	0.0	0.0	0.0	551.4	0.0	0.0	0.0	0.0	0.0	0.0	0.0	0.0	0.0	0.0	52.1
7.8	41.0	272.1	0.0	0.0	0.0	0.0	869.4	0.0	0.0	0.0	0.0	0.0	0.0	0.0	0.0	0.0	0.0	71.0
5.1	26.4	200.6	0.0	0.0	0.0	0.0	718.1	0.0	0.0	0.0	0.0	0.0	0.0	0.0	0.0	0.0	0.0	69.7
6.1	31.3	178.8	0.0	0.0	0.0	0.0	790.0	0.0	0.0	0.0	0.0	0.0	0.0	0.0	0.0	0.0	0.0	60.8
2.2	14.0	65.0	0.9	8.0	75.0	153.0	267.0	0.5	54.0	2.0	0.0	0.1	0.2	3.1	0.0	53.0	0.2	33.0
7.7	32.2	218.4	2.8	0.0	0.0	0.0	845.6	0.0	0.0	0.0	0.0	0.0	0.0	0.0	0.0	0.0	0.0	61.7
6.7	31.7	0.0	2.5	23.5	209.8	209.8	830.8	1.7	62.1	1.7	1.6	0.4	0.3	3.4	0.1	51.1	0.1	65.1
6.2	40.3	220.8	0.0	0.0	0.0	0.0	612.4	0.0	0.0	0.0	0.0	0.0	0.0	0.0	0.0	0.0	0.0	58.4
0.0	0.0	194.0	1.6	0.0	184.0	205.0	790.0	4.0	87.8	9.0	0.0	0.2	0.2	2.3	0.0	0.0	0.0	60.2
8.2	28.6	152.9	3.5	0.0	0.0	0.0	888.7	0.0	0.0	0.0	0.0	0.0	0.0	0.0	0.0	0.0	0.0	75.6
6.3	30.7	191.3	2.8	26.3	207.3	255.5	854.1	1.6	62.8	3.2	1.4	0.4	0.3	3.6	0.1	51.1	0.4	71.0
6.6	43.8	224.7	0.0	0.0	0.0	0.0	708.3	0.0	0.0	0.0	0.0	0.0	0.0	0.0	0.0	0.0	0.0	68.8
11.0	20.0	362.0	2.4	60.0	504.0	459.0	1179.0	5.0	240.0	0.0	0.0	0.3	0.9	3.9	0.3	82.0	2.0	127.7

Code	Food Name	Unit/Amt	Wt (g)	Energy (Kcal)	Prot (g)	Carb (g)	Fiber (g)	Fat (g)	Mono (g)	Poly (g)
924153	Pizza, Sausage, frozen/LeanCuisine	6 oz	170	329.8	21.0	40.0	0.0	10.0	6.0	1.0
924139	Pizza, Sausage, homemade	1 slice	67	156.8	5.2	19.8	1.0	6.2	0.0	0.0
924140	Pizza, Sicilian Cheese, frozen	¼ pizza	140	329.0	15.4	42.5	1.5	10.6	0.0	0.0
924145	Pizza, Sicilian Deluxe	¼ pizza	182	425.9	18.6	43.8	1.5	19.5	0.0	0.0
22550	Pizza, Sicilian Sausage	¼ pizza	168	399.8	18.2	44.5	1.2	16.5	0.0	0.0
22598	Pizza, Supreme Italian Pastry Crust w/sausage, pepperoni, mushroom, green&red pe	1 serving	155	399.9	15.8	39.1	0.0	20.0	7.9	2.8
22564	Pizza, Supreme, Sausage, Mushrooms, Pepperoni, frozen/Red Baron	1 serving	136	344.1	13.6	31.8	0.0	18.1	7.2	2.5
924263	Pizza, Taco/Mexican Sausage & Tangy Taco Sauce on a Corn Crust, frozen/Tony's	1 serving	154	437.4	14.3	42.8	0.0	23.3	8.9	3.5
18339	Pizza, Vegetable, frozen/Totino	½ pizza	152	304.0	10.6	36.0	0.0	13.4	0.0	0.0
18447	Popover, dry mix, prep	1 popover	33	66.7	2.6	10.4	0.0	1.5	0.0	0.0
918395	Popover, homemade w/reduced fat (2%) milk	1 popover	40	87.6	3.5	11.2	0.4	3.0	0.0	0.0
10131	Pork Back Rib, Fresh, lean&fat, roasted	3.5 oz	100	370.0	24.3	0.0	0.0	29.6	13.5	2.3
10130	Pork Bacon, Canadian, Cured, grilled	3.5 oz	100	185.0	24.2	1.4	0.0	8.4	4.0	0.8
10123	Pork Bacon, Cured, broiled, pan-fried, or roasted	3.5 oz	100	576.0	30.5	0.6	0.0	49.2	23.7	5.8
10041	Pork Centerloin/Chop, Fresh, lean&fat w/bone, broiled	3.5 oz	100	240.0	28.7	0.0	0.0	13.1	5.9	1.0
10039	Pork Centerloin/Roast, Fresh, lean w/bone, roasted	3.5 oz	100	199.0	27.6	0.0	0.0	9.0	4.0	0.7
10098	Pork Centerloin/Roast, Fresh, lean&fat w/bone, roasted	3.5 oz	100	234.0	26.3	0.0	0.0	13.5	5.9	1.2
10093	Pork Chow Mein, canned/LaChoy	¾ cup	120	45.6	5.0	4.0	2.0	1.0	0.5	0.2
10137	Pork Ham, Cured, boneless, extra lean (4% fat) canned, roasted	3.5 oz	100	136.0	21.2	0.5	0.0	4.9	2.5	0.4
10140	Pork Ham, Cured, boneless, regular fat (11% fat) roasted	3.5 oz	100	178.0	22.6	0.0	0.0	9.0	4.4	1.4
10151	Pork Ham, Smoked	3.5 oz	100	122.0	18.9	0.0	0.0	4.7	2.6	0.4
10032	Pork Loin, Blade/Chops, Fresh, lean&fat w/bone, broiled	3.5 oz	100	320.0	22.5	0.0	0.0	24.9	10.7	2.3
10048	Pork Loin, Blade/Roasts, Fresh, lean&fat w/bone, roasted	3.5 oz	100	323.0	23.7	0.0	0.0	24.6	10.6	2.2
10045	Pork Loin, Center Rib Chop, Fresh, lean w/bone, broiled	3.5 oz	100	219.0	30.8	0.0	0.0	9.7	4.5	0.6
10200	Pork Loin, Center Rib Chop, Fresh, lean&fat, boneless, pan-fried	4.0 oz	119	266.6	32.9	0.0	0.0	14.0	6.3	1.8
10203	Pork Loin, Center Rib Roast, Fresh, lean&fat, boneless, roasted	3.5 oz	100	252.0	27.0	0.0	0.0	15.2	6.7	1.3
10215	Pork Sirloin Chop, Fresh, lean&fat, boneless, broiled	3.5 oz	100	208.0	30.5	0.0	0.0	8.6	3.8	0.7
10213	Pork Sirloin Chop, Fresh, lean, boneless, broiled	3.5 oz	100	193.0	31.1	0.0	0.0	6.7	2.9	0.5
10056	Pork Sirloin Roast, Fresh, lean&fat, boneless, roasted	3.5 oz	100	207.0	28.5	0.0	0.0	9.4	4.1	0.9
10053	Pork Sirloin, Chop, Fresh, lean w/bone, broiled	3.5 oz	100	213.0	28.5	0.0	0.0	10.1	4.5	0.9
10059	Pork Sirloin, Fresh, lean, boneless, roasted	3.5 oz	100	198.0	28.9	0.0	0.0	8.3	3.6	0.7
10218	Pork Tenderloin, Fresh, lean&fat, broiled	3.5 oz	100	201.0	29.9	0.0	0.0	8.1	3.3	0.7
10223	Pork Tenderloin, Fresh, lean&fat, roasted	3.5 oz	100	173.0	27.8	0.0	0.0	6.1	2.5	0.5
51612	Pork, Bacon Bits	¼ oz	7	21.0	2.6	0.2	0.0	1.1	0.6	0.2
10219	Pork, Ground, Fresh, ckd	3.5 oz	100	297.0	25.7	0.0	0.0	20.8	9.3	1.9
10088	Pork, Spareribs, Fresh, lean&fat, braised	3.5 oz	100	397.0	29.1	0.0	0.0	30.3	13.5	2.7
924165	Pork, Sweet&Sour, canned/LaChoy	¾ cup	128	249.6	6.0	48.0	3.0	4.0	2.4	0.2
19318	Pudding Pop, Chocolate/Vanilla swirl	1 pop	47	78.0	1.9	13.0	0.0	1.9	0.1	0.0
919167	Pudding, Banana, RTE	1.0 oz	28.35	36.0	0.7	6.0	0.0	1.0	0.4	0.4
901924	Pudding, Bread Pudding, homemade	½ cup	126	211.7	6.6	31.0	1.3	7.4	0.0	0.0
901927	Pudding, Chocolate, RTE	4.0 oz (1 snack-sized can)	113	150.3	3.1	25.8	1.1	4.5	1.9	1.6
19191	Pudding, Chocolate, sugar free	½ cup	133	91.8	4.5	13.0	0.0	2.7	1.0	0.1
901928	Pudding, Flan (Caramel Custard) dry mix prep w/whole milk	1 cup	266	300.6	8.0	50.8	0.3	8.2	2.3	0.3
19330	Pudding, Indian	⅔ cup	158	161.2	5.4	22.6	0.0	5.6	0.0	0.0
919182	Pudding, Lemon, RTE	1 oz	28.35	35.4	0.0	7.1	0.0	0.9	0.4	0.3
901929	Pudding, Mousse, Chocolate, homemade	½ cup	202	446.4	8.7	33.1	1.2	32.9	0.0	0.0
19194	Pudding, Pistachio	½ cup	147	170.5	4.2	28.2	0.0	4.8	1.9	0.3
19198	Pudding, Rice, RTE	1 oz	28.35	46.2	0.6	6.2	0.0	2.1	0.9	0.8
919210	Pudding, Tapioca, RTE	1 can (5 oz)	142	169.0	2.8	27.5	0.1	5.3	2.2	1.9
901930	Pudding, Vanilla, RTE	1 cup (8 oz)	226	293.8	5.2	49.5	0.2	8.1	3.5	3.0
14342	Pudding, Vanilla, sugar free	½ cup	131	82.5	4.2	11.0	0.0	2.4	0.8	0.1
924152	Rice Beverage, Rice Dream, canned/Imagine Foods	1 cup	245	120.1	0.4	24.8	0.0	2.0	1.3	0.3
924042	Rice, Chicken Fried Rice/Chun King	8 fl oz	227	261.1	14.0	41.0	0.0	4.0	0.0	0.0
924197	Rice, Pork Fried Rice/Chun King	8 fl oz	227	270.1	10.0	44.0	0.0	6.0	0.0	0.0
918814	Rice, Spanish	1 cup	245	213.2	4.4	40.7	1.6	4.2	0.0	0.0
918815	Roll, Brown & Serve	1 roll	28	80.1	2.0	13.0	0.5	2.0	0.0	0.0
18344	Roll, Buttermilk	1 roll	28	80.1	2.0	13.0	0.5	2.0	0.0	0.0
918343	Roll, Dinner, Egg	1 roll, (2.5" dia)	35	107.5	3.3	18.2	1.3	2.2	1.0	0.4
18396	Roll, Dinner, Oat Bran	1 roll	33	77.9	3.1	13.3	1.4	1.5	0.5	0.5
18347	Roll, Dinner, Rye	1 large (3.5" - 4" dia)	43	123.0	4.4	22.8	2.1	1.5	0.5	0.3
18342	Roll, Dinner, Wheat	1 roll (3 oz)	85	232.1	7.3	39.1	3.2	5.4	2.6	0.9
18351	Roll, French	1 roll	38	105.3	3.3	19.1	1.2	1.6	0.7	0.3
18350	Roll, Hamburger/HotDog, Mixed Grain	1 roll	43	113.1	4.1	19.2	1.6	2.6	0.8	0.4
18352	Roll, Hamburger/HotDog, Plain	1 roll	43	123.0	3.7	21.6	1.2	2.2	0.4	1.1
18353	Roll, Hamburger/HotDog, Whole Wheat	1 frankfurter roll	43	114.4	3.7	22.0	3.2	2.0	0.5	0.9
918817	Roll, Hard/Kaiser	1 roll (3.5" dia)	57	167.0	5.6	30.0	1.3	2.5	0.6	1.0
4023	Salad Dressing, 1000 Island, regular, w/salt	2.0 tbsp	30	113.2	0.3	4.6	0.0	10.7	2.5	5.9

Sat (g)	Chol (mg)	Cal (mg)	Iron (mg)	Magn (mg)	Phos (mg)	Pota (mg)	Sodi (mg)	Zinc (mg)	Vit A (RE)	Vit C (mg)	Vit E (mg)	Thia (mg)	Ribo (mg)	Niac (mg)	Vit B-6 (mg)	Fol (µg)	Vit B-12 (µg)	Wat (g)
3.0	30.0	300.0	3.6	0.0	0.0	390.0	1040.0	0.0	60.0	6.0	0.0	0.5	0.4	5.0	0.0	0.0	0.0	0.0
1.8	0.0	11.0	0.8	0.0	62.0	113.0	488.0	3.0	76.0	6.0	0.0	0.1	0.1	1.0	0.2	100.0	2.0	33.9
0.0	0.0	269.0	2.1	0.0	0.0	0.0	0.0	0.0	123.6	6.0	0.0	0.4	0.3	2.0	0.0	0.0	0.0	69.2
0.0	0.0	267.0	2.0	0.0	375.0	400.0	1000.0	4.0	200.0	6.0	0.0	0.3	0.7	3.0	0.2	65.0	2.5	96.8
0.0	0.0	267.0	1.6	0.0	300.0	300.0	1000.0	3.0	213.2	2.0	0.0	0.3	0.5	2.1	0.2	90.0	1.0	85.6
6.9	27.9	212.4	2.9	0.0	0.0	0.0	771.9	0.0	0.0	0.0	0.0	0.0	0.0	0.0	0.0	0.0	0.0	76.6
6.1	23.1	223.0	2.3	0.0	0.0	0.0	738.5	0.0	0.0	0.0	0.0	0.0	0.0	0.0	0.0	0.0	0.0	69.2
7.7	27.7	187.9	2.5	0.0	0.0	0.0	756.1	0.0	0.0	0.0	0.0	0.0	0.0	0.0	0.0	0.0	0.0	70.4
0.0	0.0	210.0	2.6	0.0	284.0	205.0	909.0	0.0	104.6	13.0	0.0	0.3	0.3	2.9	0.0	0.0	0.0	88.5
0.2	0.6	9.2	0.6	4.6	29.7	25.1	143.2	0.2	16.5	0.0	0.0	0.1	0.1	0.4	0.0	5.6	0.1	18.0
1.0	0.9	37.6	0.8	7.2	56.4	65.2	82.0	0.3	34.0	0.2	0.4	0.1	0.1	0.7	0.0	7.2	0.1	21.8
11.0	118.0	45.0	1.4	21.0	195.0	315.0	101.0	3.4	3.0	0.3	0.0	0.4	0.2	3.6	0.3	3.0	0.6	45.4
2.8	58.0	10.0	0.8	21.0	296.0	390.0	1546.0	1.7	0.0	0.0	0.3	0.8	0.2	6.9	0.5	4.0	0.8	61.7
17.4	85.0	12.0	1.6	24.0	336.0	486.0	1596.0	3.3	0.0	0.0	0.5	0.7	0.3	7.3	0.3	5.0	1.8	12.9
4.8	82.0	33.0	0.8	25.0	232.0	358.0	58.0	2.3	3.0	0.4	0.0	1.1	0.3	5.2	0.4	6.0	0.7	57.6
3.3	79.0	25.0	1.0	22.0	219.0	362.0	66.0	2.1	2.0	1.0	0.0	0.9	0.3	5.5	0.4	4.0	0.6	63.0
5.1	80.0	27.0	1.0	20.0	215.0	352.0	63.0	2.0	2.0	0.9	0.0	0.9	0.3	5.2	0.4	4.0	0.6	59.8
0.3	50.0	80.0	0.7	0.0	0.0	280.0	820.0	0.0	150.0	10.0	0.0	0.0	0.0	0.4	0.0	0.0	0.0	0.0
1.6	30.0	6.0	0.9	21.0	209.0	348.0	1135.0	2.2	0.0	0.0	0.3	1.0	0.2	4.9	0.5	5.0	0.7	69.5
3.1	59.0	8.0	1.3	22.0	281.0	409.0	1500.0	2.5	0.0	0.0	0.3	0.7	0.3	6.2	0.3	3.0	0.7	64.5
1.5	38.8	6.1	1.0	17.3	228.6	371.4	1280.6	2.0	0.0	27.6	0.0	0.9	0.5	5.4	0.5	6.1	0.8	75.0
9.3	86.0	29.0	0.9	22.0	212.0	344.0	70.0	3.4	2.0	0.7	0.0	0.7	0.3	4.1	0.4	4.0	0.8	51.8
9.2	93.0	34.0	1.1	20.0	210.0	326.0	30.0	3.3	3.0	0.2	0.0	0.5	0.3	4.2	0.4	4.0	0.7	51.2
3.5	81.0	31.0	0.8	28.0	245.0	420.0	65.0	2.4	2.0	0.3	0.3	1.1	0.3	6.2	0.5	3.0	0.8	57.0
5.1	83.3	6.0	0.9	32.1	282.0	540.3	61.9	2.5	2.4	0.4	0.3	0.9	0.4	6.1	0.5	9.5	0.7	72.4
5.4	81.0	6.0	0.9	22.0	214.0	346.0	48.0	2.6	3.0	0.4	0.0	0.6	0.3	5.0	0.4	8.0	0.6	57.3
2.9	91.0	18.0	1.2	27.0	243.0	372.0	56.0	2.6	2.0	0.4	0.3	1.0	0.4	4.7	0.5	6.0	0.8	60.1
2.2	92.0	18.0	1.2	27.0	246.0	377.0	56.0	2.7	2.0	0.4	0.3	1.0	0.4	4.8	0.5	6.0	0.8	61.4
3.4	86.0	16.0	1.2	26.0	252.0	402.0	56.0	2.5	2.0	1.0	0.3	0.9	0.4	5.1	0.5	5.0	0.8	60.5
3.6	85.0	13.0	1.1	31.0	257.0	401.0	72.0	2.7	2.0	1.0	0.3	1.0	0.4	4.8	0.6	5.0	0.8	60.5
3.0	86.0	17.0	1.2	27.0	254.0	405.0	56.0	2.5	2.0	1.0	0.3	0.9	0.4	5.1	0.5	5.0	0.8	61.3
2.9	94.0	5.0	1.4	35.0	290.0	444.0	64.0	2.9	2.0	1.0	0.0	1.0	0.4	5.1	0.5	6.0	1.0	61.1
2.1	79.0	6.0	1.5	27.0	257.0	433.0	55.0	2.6	2.0	0.4	0.3	0.9	0.4	4.7	0.4	6.0	0.6	65.4
0.3	6.0	1.0	0.1	2.0	40.0	38.0	181.0	0.3	0.0	1.0	0.0	0.0	0.0	0.7	0.0	1.0	0.2	2.6
7.7	94.0	22.0	1.3	24.0	226.0	362.0	73.0	3.2	2.0	0.7	0.3	0.7	0.2	4.2	0.4	6.0	0.5	52.8
11.1	121.0	47.0	1.9	24.0	261.0	320.0	93.0	4.6	3.0	0.0	0.3	0.4	0.4	5.5	0.4	4.0	1.1	40.4
1.4	18.0	20.0	1.4	0.0	0.0	215.0	1540.0	0.0	125.0	4.0	0.0	0.1	0.1	1.2	0.0	0.0	0.0	0.0
1.8	1.0	71.0	0.2	7.0	51.0	70.0	66.0	0.1	13.4	0.0	0.0	0.0	0.1	0.1	0.0	2.0	0.1	30.4
0.2	0.0	24.1	0.0	2.3	19.6	31.2	55.6	0.1	8.5	0.1	0.0	0.0	0.0	0.0	0.0	0.6	0.1	20.4
1.2	2.7	143.6	1.4	23.9	137.3	282.2	291.1	0.7	81.9	1.0	0.0	0.1	0.3	0.8	0.1	16.4	0.3	79.3
0.8	3.4	101.7	0.6	23.7	90.4	203.4	145.8	0.5	12.4	2.0	0.1	0.0	0.2	0.4	0.0	3.4	0.0	78.3
1.6	9.0	152.0	0.3	25.0	289.0	256.0	381.0	0.6	50.2	1.0	0.0	0.1	0.2	0.1	0.1	6.0	0.4	1.6
5.1	31.9	300.6	0.2	31.9	228.8	383.0	130.3	0.9	69.2	1.9	0.0	0.1	0.4	0.2	0.1	10.6	0.7	197.4
0.0	0.0	221.0	1.4	0.0	151.0	0.0	0.0	0.0	79.0	0.0	0.0	0.1	0.3	0.4	0.0	0.0	0.0	0.0
0.1	0.0	0.6	0.0	0.3	1.4	0.3	39.7	0.0	0.0	0.0	0.0	0.0	0.0	0.0	0.0	0.0	0.0	20.3
1.7	10.3	202.0	1.3	44.4	258.6	296.9	86.9	1.4	323.2	1.2	0.0	0.1	0.4	0.3	0.1	32.3	0.9	125.4
2.6	17.0	149.0	0.1	19.0	307.0	194.0	408.0	0.5	30.8	1.0	0.0	0.0	0.2	0.1	0.0	7.0	0.4	107.8
0.3	0.3	14.7	0.1	2.3	19.3	17.0	24.1	0.1	9.9	0.1	0.4	0.0	0.0	0.0	0.0	0.9	0.1	19.2
0.9	1.4	119.3	0.3	11.4	112.2	137.7	225.8	0.4	0.0	1.0	0.1	0.0	0.1	0.4	0.0	4.3	0.3	105.4
1.3	15.8	198.9	0.3	18.1	153.7	255.4	305.1	0.6	13.6	0.0	0.3	0.0	0.3	0.6	0.0	0.0	0.2	160.9
1.5	9.0	152.0	0.1	18.0	117.0	189.0	199.0	0.5	50.0	1.0	0.0	0.0	0.2	0.1	0.0	6.0	0.5	109.5
0.2	0.0	19.6	0.2	9.8	34.3	68.6	85.8	0.2	0.0	1.2	1.8	0.1	0.0	1.9	0.0	90.7	0.0	217.5
0.0	0.0	38.0	2.0	0.0	128.0	190.0	1460.0	0.0	136.0	7.0	0.0	0.7	0.2	1.5	0.0	0.0	0.0	0.0
0.0	0.0	26.0	1.0	0.0	129.0	180.0	1210.0	0.0	170.0	4.0	0.0	0.3	0.2	1.5	0.0	0.0	0.0	0.0
0.0	0.0	34.0	1.5	0.0	96.0	566.0	774.0	0.0	324.0	37.0	0.0	0.1	0.1	1.7	0.0	0.0	0.0	192.3
0.0	5.0	14.0	0.6	0.0	25.0	28.0	140.0	0.0	0.0	1.0	0.0	0.1	0.1	0.6	0.0	0.0	0.0	0.0
0.0	5.0	0.0	0.0	0.0	0.0	0.0	140.0	0.0	0.0	0.0	0.0	0.0	0.0	0.0	0.0	0.0	0.0	0.0
0.6	17.5	20.7	1.2	8.8	35.4	36.4	190.8	0.4	2.8	0.0	0.3	0.2	0.2	1.2	0.0	36.8	0.1	10.6
0.2	0.0	28.1	1.4	10.9	38.0	39.9	136.3	0.3	0.0	0.0	0.2	0.1	0.1	1.6	0.0	31.4	0.0	14.5
0.3	0.0	12.9	1.2	23.2	68.4	77.4	383.6	0.4	0.4	0.0	0.2	0.2	0.1	1.7	0.0	37.0	0.0	12.9
1.3	0.0	149.6	3.0	30.6	88.4	97.8	289.0	0.8	0.0	0.0	0.8	0.4	0.2	3.5	0.1	43.4	0.0	31.5
0.4	0.0	34.6	1.0	7.6	31.9	43.3	231.4	0.3	0.0	0.0	0.2	0.2	0.1	1.7	0.0	36.1	0.0	13.2
0.4	0.0	40.9	1.7	18.9	52.5	68.8	196.9	0.5	0.0	0.0	0.2	0.2	0.1	1.9	0.0	40.9	0.0	16.3
0.5	0.0	59.8	1.4	8.6	37.8	60.6	240.8	0.3	0.0	0.0	0.7	0.2	0.1	1.7	0.0	40.9	0.0	14.6
0.4	0.0	45.6	1.0	36.6	96.3	117.0	205.5	0.9	0.0	0.0	0.6	0.1	0.1	1.6	0.1	13.3	0.0	14.2
0.3	0.0	54.2	1.9	15.4	57.0	61.6	310.1	0.5	0.0	0.0	0.2	0.3	0.2	2.4	0.0	54.2	0.0	17.7
1.8	7.8	3.3	0.2	0.6	5.1	33.9	210.0	0.0	28.8	0.0	0.3	0.0	0.0	0.0	0.0	1.9	0.1	13.8

Code	Food Name	Unit/Amt	Wt (g)	Energy (Kcal)	Prot (g)	Carb (g)	Fiber (g)	Fat (g)	Mono (g)	Poly (g)
902921	Salad Dressing, 1000 Island, w/salt, low kcal (10kcal/tsp)	2.0 tbsp	30	47.6	0.2	4.9	0.4	3.2	0.7	1.9
4539	Salad Dressing, Blue Cheese, low kcal	2.0 tbsp	30	80.1	0.6	3.0	0.0	7.4	1.8	3.8
4140	Salad Dressing, Blue/Roquefort Cheese, regular w/salt	2.0 tbsp	30	151.2	1.4	2.2	0.0	15.7	3.7	8.3
4120	Salad Dressing, French, low fat, w/salt, diet (5kcal/tsp)	2.0 tbsp	30	40.3	0.1	6.5	0.0	1.7	0.4	1.0
4141	Salad Dressing, French, regular w/salt	2.0 tbsp	30	128.9	0.2	5.3	0.0	12.3	2.4	6.5
4114	Salad Dressing, Italian, no salt, diet (2kcal/tsp)	2.0 tbsp	30	31.6	0.0	1.5	0.0	2.9	0.6	1.8
4143	Salad Dressing, Italian, regular w/salt	2.0 tbsp	30	140.2	0.2	3.1	0.0	14.5	3.4	8.4
4145	Salad Dressing, Mayonnaise, Safflower & Soybean Oil, w/salt	2.0 tbsp	30	215.0	0.3	0.8	0.0	23.8	3.9	16.5
18625	Salad Dressing, Mayonnaise-type, regular, w/salt	2.0 tbsp	30	116.9	0.3	7.2	0.0	10.0	2.7	5.4
4022	Salad Dressing, Russian w/salt	2.0 tbsp	30	148.2	0.5	3.1	0.0	15.2	3.5	8.8
4030	Salad Dressing, Russian, w/salt, low kcal	2.0 tbsp	30	42.4	0.2	8.3	0.1	1.2	0.3	0.7
4016	Salad Dressing, Sandwich Spread w/chopped pickle, regular	2.0 tbsp	30	116.7	0.3	6.7	0.1	10.2	2.2	6.0
902932	Salad Dressing, Sesame Seed	2.0 tbsp	30	132.9	0.9	2.6	0.3	13.6	3.6	7.5
902933	Salad Dressing, Sweet & Sour	2.0 tbsp	30	57.9	0.4	13.8	0.2	0.6	0.0	0.0
4135	Salad Dressing, Vinaigrette	2.0 tbsp	30	99.9	0.0	8.0	0.0	7.6	3.2	2.8
902910	Salad Dressing, Vinegar & Oil, homemade	2.0 tbsp	30	134.6	0.0	0.8	0.0	15.0	4.4	7.2
902909	Salt Substitute, lite/Morton	1 tsp	6	0.0	0.0	0.0	0.0	0.0	0.0	0.0
22539	Salt Substitute/Morton	1 tsp	6	0.0	0.0	0.1	0.0	0.0	0.0	0.0
2047	Salt, Table (Sodium Chloride)	1 tsp	6	0.0	0.0	0.0	0.0	0.0	0.0	0.0
22535	Sandwich, Hot Pockets, Beef & Cheddar Stuffed, frozen	1 package	142	403.3	16.3	39.2	0.0	20.2	6.7	1.2
22537	Sandwich, Hot Pockets, Croissant Pocket w/chicken, broccoli, & cheddar, frozen	1 package	256	601.6	22.8	77.8	2.8	22.0	8.8	3.3
22002	Sandwich, Lean Pockets, Glazed Chicken Supreme Stuffed, frozen	1 package	255	464.1	19.6	68.1	0.0	12.5	4.9	1.9
22540	Sandwich, Pizza Burger	1 burger	92	243.8	18.2	2.3	0.5	18.0	0.0	0.0
6931	Sandwich, Sausage Biscuits, breakfast sandwich, frozen/Jimmy Dean	1 package	96	384.6	9.5	23.1	1.4	28.2	0.0	0.0
6932	Sauce, Pasta, Spaghetti/Marinara, RTE	½ cup	125	71.3	1.8	10.3	2.0	2.6	1.1	0.9
906961	Sauce, 100% Natural Spaghetti Sauce, Traditional, jar/Prego	½ cup	125	130.9	2.1	20.0	3.9	4.9	0.0	0.0
6721	Sauce, Alfredo	1 tbsp	16	42.6	1.6	0.4	0.0	3.8	0.0	0.0
6921	Sauce, Barbecue, RTE	1 tbsp	18	13.5	0.3	2.3	0.2	0.3	0.1	0.1
6140	Sauce, Bearnaise, dry, made w/milk & butter	1 cup (8 fl oz)	250	687.5	8.2	17.2	0.0	67.0	19.6	3.0
906978	Sauce, Cheddar Cheese Sauce/LaVictoria	1 tbsp	16.29	26.2	0.3	1.5	0.0	2.1	1.0	0.5
6713	Sauce, Cheese	2.0 oz	56	59.9	2.3	3.5	0.0	4.1	0.0	0.0
6139	Sauce, Chili	1 tbsp	15	17.0	0.2	3.8	0.0	0.0	0.0	0.0
6923	Sauce, Chunky Chili Dip, Salsa, canned/LaVictoria	1 tbsp	15	4.7	0.1	1.0	0.1	0.0	0.0	0.0
6135	Sauce, Con Queso Sauce, RTE/Nestle Que Bueno	1 cup	252	335.2	15.4	14.3	0.0	24.1	6.8	3.0
6903	Sauce, Coney Island Style Hot Dog Sauce, RTE/Nestle Chef-Mate	¼ cup	62	75.6	2.2	5.6	1.4	4.9	1.5	2.1
6104	Sauce, Creole Sauce, RTE/Nestle Chef-Mate	¼ cup	62	24.8	0.9	3.7	0.8	0.7	0.2	0.3
6901	Sauce, Curry, dry, made w/milk	¼ cup	68	67.3	2.7	6.4	0.0	3.7	1.3	0.7
6152	Sauce, Deluxe Marinara Sauce, RTE/Contadina	¼ cup	64	37.1	0.8	4.4	0.8	1.8	0.9	0.5
6153	Sauce, Deluxe Pizza Sauce, RTE/Contadina	¼ cup	63	34.0	1.4	5.5	1.3	0.7	0.3	0.1
6179	Sauce, Enchilada Sauce/LaVictoria	1 tbsp	15.08	5.0	0.0	0.7	0.1	0.2	0.0	0.0
6273	Sauce, Green Chile Salsa, mild/LaVictoria	1 tbsp	15.23	3.8	0.2	0.7	0.1	0.0	0.0	0.0
6259	Sauce, Green Taco Sauce, medium/LaVictoria	1 tbsp	15.09	4.5	0.1	0.9	0.1	0.1	0.0	0.0
906965	Sauce, Hoisin, RTE	1 tbsp	16	35.2	0.5	7.1	0.4	0.5	0.2	0.3
6155	Sauce, Hollandaise	¼ cup	50	264.0	3.1	6.7	0.0	25.6	8.8	1.1
6181	Sauce, Hot Dog Chili Sauce, RTE/Nestle Chef-Mate	2.25 oz , ¼ cup	63	69.3	2.7	9.2	1.7	2.4	1.0	0.2
6922	Sauce, Italian Sauce, RTE/Nestle Chef-Mate	2.25 oz , ¼ cup	63	61.7	1.1	11.6	0.9	1.2	0.8	0.2
6905	Sauce, Jalapeno Cheese Sauce, RTE/Nestle Que Bueno	1 package	3005	3876.5	95.9	369.6	0.0	224.2	81.3	35.8
906970	Sauce, Lemon Sauce, RTE/Nestle Chef-Mate	1 package	2126	2848.8	4.7	678.6	0.0	12.5	3.6	6.0
906960	Sauce, Marinara/Contadina	7.5 oz	213	100.1	4.0	12.0	0.0	4.0	0.0	0.0
906966	Sauce, Medium White	1 cup	250	395.0	10.0	24.0	0.5	30.0	11.9	7.2
6136	Sauce, Mole Poblano, dry mix	1 tbsp	16.5	94.2	1.2	6.9	1.7	6.9	0.0	0.0
6714	Sauce, Mushroom, dry, made w/milk	1 cup (8 fl oz)	267	227.0	11.3	23.8	0.0	10.3	3.3	1.1
6910	Sauce, Nacho Cheese Sauce, mild, RTE/Nestle Que Bueno	1 cup	252	476.3	18.1	10.1	2.0	40.5	12.4	8.5
6168	Sauce, Oyster, RTE	1 tbsp	4	2.0	0.1	0.4	0.0	0.0	0.0	0.0
6169	Sauce, Pepper or Hot, RTE	¼ tsp	1.2	0.1	0.0	0.0	0.0	0.0	0.0	0.0
924173	Sauce, Pepperoni Pizza/Contadina	¼ cup	60	40.2	1.0	5.0	0.0	2.2	1.1	0.7
6157	Sauce, Pesto	1 oz	28	155.1	2.8	3.0	0.7	14.6	0.0	0.0
906968	Sauce, Picante Sauce, RTE/Que Bueno Nestle	1 serving	30	10.2	0.4	2.0	0.0	0.1	0.0	0.0
6151	Sauce, Pizza/Contadina	¼ cup	60	30.0	1.0	5.0	0.0	1.0	0.0	0.0
6153	Sauce, Plum, RTE	1 tbsp	19	35.0	0.2	8.1	0.1	0.2	0.0	0.1
6274	Sauce, Red Clam (Shellfish)	4 oz	112	80.6	3.6	9.3	1.0	3.2	0.0	0.0
6907	Sauce, Salsa, RTE	1 packet	8.9	2.5	0.1	0.6	0.1	0.0	0.0	0.0
906969	Sauce, Sofrito, homemade	1 tbsp	14.9	35.3	1.9	0.8	0.3	2.7	0.0	0.0
6148	Sauce, Sour Cream	¼ cup	52	123.8	2.8	1.9	0.0	11.9	4.6	1.2
906134	Sauce, Sour Cream, dry, made w/milk	1 cup (8 fl oz)	314	508.7	19.1	45.3	3.5	30.2	9.9	2.8
924192	Sauce, Soy Sauce, RTE	1 tbsp	18	9.5	0.9	1.5	0.0	0.0	0.0	0.0
924195	Sauce, Spaghetti Sauce w/meat	4 oz	113	70.1	2.0	12.0	2.0	2.0	0.8	0.9
6904	Sauce, Spaghetti Sauce w/mushrooms	4 oz	113	107.4	1.6	14.5	0.6	4.7	0.0	0.0
924162	Sauce, Spaghetti w/mushrooms, dry	2 tsp	10	30.4	1.0	4.9	0.0	0.9	0.3	0.0

Sat (g)	Chol (mg)	Cal (mg)	Iron (mg)	Magn (mg)	Phos (mg)	Pota (mg)	Sodi (mg)	Zinc (mg)	Vit A (RE)	Vit C (mg)	Vit E (mg)	Thia (mg)	Ribo (mg)	Niac (mg)	Vit B-6 (mg)	Fol (µg)	Vit B-12 (µg)	Wat (g)
0.5	4.5	3.3	0.2	0.2	5.1	33.9	300.0	0.0	28.8	0.0	0.4	0.0	0.0	0.0	0.0	1.7	0.1	20.8
1.6	2.0	0.0	0.0	0.0	0.0	0.0	394.0	0.0	0.0	0.0	0.0	0.0	0.0	0.0	0.0	0.0	0.0	0.0
3.0	5.1	24.3	0.1	0.0	22.2	11.1	328.2	0.1	19.8	0.6	2.8	0.0	0.0	0.0	0.0	2.4	0.1	9.7
0.2	0.0	3.3	0.1	0.0	4.2	23.7	236.1	0.1	39.0	0.0	0.4	0.0	0.0	0.0	0.0	0.0	0.0	20.8
2.9	0.0	3.3	0.1	0.0	4.2	23.7	411.0	0.0	39.0	0.0	2.5	0.0	0.0	0.0	0.0	1.3	0.0	11.4
0.4	1.8	0.6	0.1	0.0	1.5	4.5	9.0	0.0	0.0	0.0	0.0	0.0	0.0	0.0	0.0	0.0	0.0	25.1
2.1	0.0	3.0	0.1	0.2	1.5	4.5	236.1	0.0	7.2	0.0	3.1	0.0	0.0	0.0	0.0	1.5	0.0	11.5
2.6	17.7	5.4	0.2	0.3	8.4	10.2	170.5	0.0	25.2	0.0	0.0	0.0	0.0	0.0	0.2	2.3	0.1	4.6
1.5	7.8	4.2	0.1	0.6	7.8	2.7	213.2	0.1	25.2	0.0	1.2	0.0	0.0	0.0	0.0	1.9	0.1	12.0
2.2	5.4	5.7	0.2	0.5	11.1	47.1	260.4	0.1	62.1	1.8	3.1	0.0	0.0	0.2	0.0	3.1	0.1	10.4
0.2	1.8	5.7	0.2	0.1	11.1	47.1	260.4	0.0	4.8	1.8	0.2	0.0	0.0	0.0	0.0	1.0	0.0	19.5
1.5	22.8	4.2	0.1	0.6	7.8	10.5	300.0	0.2	25.2	0.0	2.1	0.0	0.0	0.0	0.0	1.8	0.1	12.2
1.9	0.0	5.7	0.2	0.0	11.1	47.1	300.0	0.0	62.1	0.0	0.0	0.0	0.0	0.0	0.0	0.0	0.0	11.8
0.0	0.0	2.0	0.0	0.0	2.0	28.0	136.0	0.0	0.0	0.0	0.0	0.0	0.0	0.0	0.0	0.0	0.0	0.0
1.2	0.0	0.0	0.0	0.0	0.0	0.0	432.0	0.0	0.0	0.0	0.0	0.0	0.0	0.0	0.0	0.0	0.0	0.0
2.7	0.0	0.0	0.0	0.0	0.0	2.3	0.2	0.0	0.0	0.0	2.6	0.0	0.0	0.0	0.0	0.0	0.0	14.2
0.0	0.0	0.0	0.0	4.0	0.0	1500.0	1100.0	0.0	0.0	0.0	0.0	0.0	0.0	0.0	0.0	0.0	0.0	0.0
0.0	0.0	30.0	0.0	0.0	28.0	2800.0	0.0	0.0	0.0	0.0	0.0	0.0	0.0	0.0	0.0	0.0	0.0	0.0
0.0	0.0	1.4	0.0	0.1	0.0	0.5	2325.5	0.0	0.0	0.0	0.0	0.0	0.0	0.0	0.0	0.0	0.0	0.0
8.8	52.5	336.5	2.9	0.0	0.0	0.0	906.0	0.0	0.0	0.0	0.0	0.0	0.0	0.0	0.0	0.0	0.0	62.5
6.7	74.2	0.0	7.6	0.0	0.0	0.0	1303.0	0.0	0.0	12.5	0.0	0.0	0.0	0.0	0.0	0.0	0.0	128.0
3.8	45.9	242.3	0.0	0.0	0.0	0.0	1119.5	0.0	0.0	0.0	0.0	0.0	0.0	0.0	0.0	0.0	0.0	150.2
0.0	62.0	109.0	2.3	16.0	205.0	263.0	615.0	3.3	72.6	4.0	0.0	0.1	0.2	6.5	0.0	0.0	0.0	51.0
8.6	31.4	75.5	1.6	0.0	0.0	0.0	881.3	0.0	0.0	0.0	0.0	0.0	0.0	0.0	0.0	0.0	0.0	32.2
0.4	0.0	27.5	0.9	21.3	40.0	368.8	515.0	0.2	47.5	10.0	1.6	0.1	0.1	1.3	0.1	12.5	0.0	108.6
1.1	0.0	0.0	0.0	0.0	0.0	0.0	537.5	0.0	0.0	13.0	0.0	0.0	0.0	0.0	0.0	0.0	0.0	96.0
0.0	0.0	28.9	0.2	0.0	0.0	4.6	104.4	0.0	4.2	0.1	0.0	0.0	0.0	0.0	0.0	0.0	0.0	0.0
0.0	0.0	3.4	0.2	3.2	3.6	31.3	146.7	0.0	15.7	1.3	0.2	0.0	0.0	0.2	0.0	0.7	0.0	14.6
41.0	185.0	225.0	0.3	25.0	182.5	292.5	1240.0	0.8	742.5	1.8	0.0	0.1	0.3	0.3	0.1	10.0	0.5	153.1
0.6	0.5	15.0	0.1	0.0	0.0	0.0	158.2	0.0	0.0	0.0	0.0	0.0	0.0	0.0	0.0	0.0	0.0	11.9
0.0	0.0	63.0	0.2	0.0	0.0	23.0	288.0	3.5	32.2	0.0	0.0	0.0	0.1	0.0	0.0	0.0	0.0	0.0
0.0	0.0	3.0	0.1	0.0	8.0	56.0	191.0	0.0	42.0	2.0	0.0	0.0	0.2	0.0	0.0	9.0	0.0	0.0
0.0	0.0	2.1	0.0	0.0	0.0	0.0	74.0	0.0	0.0	1.6	0.0	0.0	0.0	0.0	0.0	0.0	0.0	13.6
11.7	63.0	471.2	0.0	15.1	206.6	65.5	2220.1	1.3	148.7	0.0	1.3	0.0	0.2	0.2	0.0	7.6	0.2	190.8
0.9	1.9	19.8	1.1	11.8	29.1	197.8	383.2	0.3	63.2	0.1	1.1	0.0	0.0	0.8	0.1	8.1	0.0	47.9
0.1	0.0	34.7	0.3	8.7	17.4	187.2	339.1	0.1	23.6	0.0	0.6	0.0	0.0	0.5	0.1	8.7	0.0	55.3
1.5	8.8	121.0	0.3	11.6	70.0	123.8	318.9	0.3	10.2	0.7	0.0	0.0	0.1	0.1	0.0	4.1	0.3	53.9
0.3	0.0	12.2	0.4	7.7	16.6	132.5	240.0	0.1	22.4	4.5	0.0	0.0	0.0	0.4	0.1	5.8	0.0	56.1
0.3	1.9	34.0	0.6	13.2	31.5	223.0	116.6	0.2	42.2	7.1	1.6	0.0	0.0	0.9	0.1	6.3	0.0	54.6
0.0	0.0	1.8	0.0	0.0	0.0	0.0	99.2	0.0	0.0	0.7	0.0	0.0	0.0	0.0	0.0	0.0	0.0	13.9
0.0	0.0	2.3	0.1	0.0	0.0	0.0	87.4	0.0	0.0	2.0	0.0	0.0	0.0	0.0	0.0	0.0	0.0	14.0
0.0	0.0	1.2	0.0	0.0	0.0	0.0	95.7	0.0	0.0	0.7	0.0	0.0	0.0	0.0	0.0	0.0	0.0	13.7
0.1	0.5	5.1	0.2	3.8	6.1	19.0	258.4	0.1	0.2	0.1	0.0	0.0	0.0	0.2	0.0	3.7	0.0	7.1
15.7	71.0	23.0	0.9	0.0	78.0	0.0	425.0	0.0	205.0	0.0	0.0	0.0	0.0	0.0	0.0	0.0	0.0	58.5
1.0	4.4	19.5	1.0	12.6	39.7	149.3	398.8	0.5	42.2	0.1	0.3	0.0	0.0	0.7	0.1	22.1	0.1	47.2
0.2	0.0	34.7	0.4	20.2	43.5	383.0	308.7	0.3	24.6	4.2	1.2	0.1	0.0	1.1	0.2	16.4	0.0	47.8
86.2	300.5	2554.3	5.7	180.3	2464.1	781.3	27255.4	16.2	811.4	24.0	15.7	0.1	2.0	2.0	0.4	90.2	2.7	2230.3
1.5	0.0	85.0	8.1	42.5	85.0	425.2	170.1	0.9	0.0	182.8	0.9	0.1	0.1	0.7	0.2	21.3	0.0	1427.6
0.0	0.0	73.0	2.6	0.0	0.0	810.0	700.0	0.0	413.2	20.0	0.0	0.2	0.4	2.2	0.0	0.0	0.0	0.0
9.1	32.0	292.0	0.9	0.0	238.0	381.0	888.0	0.5	238.0	2.0	0.0	0.2	0.4	0.8	0.1	12.0	0.0	0.0
0.0	0.0	49.8	0.9	21.0	41.9	99.3	192.1	0.4	0.0	0.0	0.0	0.0	0.1	0.4	0.1	12.2	0.0	0.7
5.4	34.7	293.7	0.5	37.4	165.5	494.0	1535.3	1.3	93.5	1.9	0.0	0.2	0.8	4.8	0.2	40.1	0.8	215.7
16.9	80.6	471.2	0.8	25.2	420.8	80.6	1968.1	2.6	126.0	0.3	1.0	0.0	0.3	0.1	0.0	12.6	0.4	177.5
0.0	0.0	1.3	0.0	0.2	0.9	2.2	109.3	0.0	0.3	0.0	0.0	0.0	0.0	0.1	0.0	0.6	0.0	3.2
0.0	0.0	0.1	0.0	0.1	0.1	1.7	31.7	0.0	0.4	0.9	0.0	0.0	0.0	0.0	0.0	0.1	0.0	1.1
0.4	0.0	13.0	0.7	8.0	16.0	260.0	390.0	0.0	131.8	13.0	0.0	0.0	0.1	0.0	0.0	0.0	0.0	48.2
0.0	0.0	98.0	0.3	0.0	0.0	27.0	244.0	0.0	98.8	0.0	0.0	0.1	0.2	0.0	0.0	0.0	0.0	0.0
0.0	0.0	12.6	0.2	4.5	8.4	80.4	252.0	0.1	8.4	0.6	0.4	0.0	0.0	0.3	0.0	3.0	0.0	26.8
0.0	0.0	13.0	0.7	8.0	14.0	220.0	330.0	0.0	133.8	14.0	0.0	0.0	0.6	0.0	0.0	0.0	0.0	50.0
0.0	0.0	2.3	0.3	2.3	4.2	49.2	102.2	0.0	0.8	0.1	0.0	0.0	0.0	0.2	0.0	1.1	0.0	10.2
0.0	0.0	32.0	1.2	0.0	0.0	274.0	556.0	0.0	128.2	9.0	0.0	0.1	0.1	0.9	0.0	0.0	0.0	0.0
0.0	0.0	2.7	0.1	1.2	2.3	19.0	38.6	0.0	5.3	1.2	0.1	0.0	0.0	0.1	0.0	1.4	0.0	8.1
0.0	0.0	3.0	0.1	3.7	20.7	59.7	170.6	0.2	0.0	3.0	0.0	0.0	0.0	0.4	0.1	6.4	0.0	8.9
6.1	1966.0	23.0	0.3	3.0	75.0	13.0	7.0	0.5	82.0	0.0	0.0	0.0	0.1	0.0	0.0	23.0	0.6	11.9
16.1	91.1	546.4	0.6	44.0	310.9	731.6	1004.8	1.4	144.4	2.5	0.0	0.1	0.7	0.6	0.1	15.7	0.9	215.5
0.0	0.0	3.1	0.4	6.1	19.8	32.4	1028.7	0.1	0.0	0.0	0.0	0.0	0.0	0.6	0.0	2.8	0.0	12.8
0.3	2.0	18.0	1.8	0.0	51.0	650.0	570.0	0.0	156.0	18.0	0.0	0.1	0.1	1.8	0.0	0.0	0.0	0.0
0.0	0.0	21.0	1.1	0.0	30.0	428.0	499.0	0.0	129.8	12.0	0.0	0.1	0.1	1.3	0.0	0.0	0.0	0.0
0.6	2.8	39.9	0.2	3.6	28.6	41.1	942.0	0.2	4.9	0.2	0.0	0.0	0.0	0.2	0.0	2.8	0.0	0.3

Code	Food Name	Unit/Amt	Wt (g)	Energy (Kcal)	Prot (g)	Carb (g)	Fiber (g)	Fat (g)	Mono (g)	Poly (g)
6107	Sauce, Spaghetti&Meat/FrancoAm	7.5 oz	212	212.0	8.5	26.2	1.0	8.1	0.0	0.0
906972	Sauce, Steak	1 tbsp	15	18.0	0.0	2.5	0.1	0.0	0.0	0.0
6109	Sauce, Steak & Mushrooms	1 fl oz	30	9.0	0.3	1.9	0.2	0.1	0.1	0.0
6716	Sauce, Stroganoff, dry, made w/H₂O	1 cup (8 fl oz)	296	272.3	11.7	33.9	0.0	10.7	3.0	0.4
6110	Sauce, Sweet & Sour	¼ cup	59	54.9	0.2	13.6	0.0	0.0	0.0	0.0
906975	Sauce, Szechuan, RTE/Nestle Chef-Mate	1 tbsp	16	20.8	0.2	2.9	0.0	0.9	0.3	0.4
906974	Sauce, Tabasco	1 tsp	5	0.8	0.1	0.1	0.0	0.0	0.0	0.0
6111	Sauce, Tartar	1 tbsp	14	70.0	0.2	0.1	0.1	8.1	2.4	4.5
6129	Sauce, Teriyaki, RTE	1 tbsp	18	15.1	1.1	2.9	0.0	0.0	0.0	0.0
906977	Sauce, Thick White	¼ cup	66	130.7	2.6	7.3	0.3	10.3	3.8	1.3
924111	Sauce, Thin White	¼ cup	61	73.8	2.4	4.6	0.1	5.2	1.9	0.7
6113	Sauce, White Clam (Shellfish)	4.0 oz	112	121.0	4.5	4.2	0.5	9.6	0.0	0.0
7006	Sausage, Blood	1slice: 5 x 4.6 x 0.06"	25	94.5	3.7	0.3	0.0	8.6	4.0	0.9
7014	Sausage, Bratwurst (Pork) ckd	1 link (4/12 oz)	85	255.9	12.0	1.8	0.0	22.0	10.4	2.3
7022	Sausage, Frankfurter (weiner) (Beef & Pork)	1 frank:0.85"diam x 5"long-8/lb	57	182.4	6.4	1.5	0.0	16.6	7.8	1.6
7024	Sausage, Frankfurter (weiner) (Beef)	1 frank:0.75"diam x 5"long-10/lb	45	141.8	5.4	0.8	0.0	12.8	6.1	0.6
7025	Sausage, Frankfurter (weiner) (Chicken)	1 frank	45	115.7	5.8	3.1	0.0	8.8	3.8	1.8
7016	Sausage, Frankfurter (weiner) (Turkey)	1 frank	45	101.7	6.4	0.7	0.0	8.0	2.5	2.3
7089	Sausage, Italian (Pork & Beef)	1 slice: 4"diam x 0.12"thick	23	59.8	3.5	0.4	0.0	4.8	2.3	0.5
7038	Sausage, Kielbasa (Kolbassy) (Pork, Beef & NFD Milk)	1slice: 6 x 3.75 x 0.06"	26	80.6	3.4	0.6	0.0	7.1	3.4	0.8
7091	Sausage, Mortadella (Beef & Pork)	1 slice (15/8 oz)	15	46.7	2.5	0.5	0.0	3.8	1.7	0.5
7059	Sausage, Pepperoni (Pork & Beef)	1 sausage @ 9.0 oz.	251	1247.5	52.6	7.1	0.0	110.4	53.0	11.0
7064	Sausage, Pork, bulk/links/patties, frozen, raw/USDA Commodity	3.5 oz	100	231.0	15.0	0.0	0.0	18.6	8.1	2.2
7068	Sausage, Salami (Cotto) (Beef & Pork) ckd	1 slice: 4"diam x 0.12"thick (10/8 oz)	23	57.5	3.2	0.5	0.0	4.6	2.1	0.5
7072	Sausage, Salami, (Turkey) ckd	2 slices	57	111.7	9.3	0.3	0.0	7.9	2.6	2.0
7074	Sausage, Smoked Link (Pork & Beef)	2.4 oz	68	228.5	9.1	1.0	0.0	20.6	9.6	2.2
7077	Sausage, Smoked Link (Pork)	2.4 oz	68	264.5	15.1	1.4	0.0	21.6	10.0	2.6
7076	Sausage, Smoked Link (Pork, Beef & NFD Milk)	2.4 oz	68	212.8	9.0	1.3	0.0	18.8	8.6	2.1
7083	Sausage, Vegetarian, Meatless	2.4 oz	68	174.1	12.6	6.7	1.9	12.3	3.1	6.3
924160	Sausage, Vienna, canned (Beef & Pork)	1 sm sausage	16	44.6	1.6	0.3	0.0	4.0	2.0	0.3
12037	Seeds, Sunflower Kernels, dried	1 cup w/hulls (edible part)	46	262.2	10.5	8.6	4.8	22.8	4.4	15.1
12537	Seeds, Sunflower Kernels, dry roast w/o salt	1.0 oz	28.35	165.0	5.5	6.8	3.1	14.1	2.7	9.3
12538	Seeds, Sunflower Kernels, oil roast w/o salt	1.0 oz	28.35	174.4	6.1	4.2	1.9	16.3	3.1	10.8
15155	Shellfish, Abalone, fried	3.0 oz	85	160.7	16.7	9.4	0.0	5.8	2.3	1.4
15158	Shellfish, Clams, boiled/steamed (moist heat)	3.0 oz	85	125.8	21.7	4.4	0.0	1.7	0.1	0.5
15162	Shellfish, Clams, breaded & fried	3.0 oz	85	171.7	12.1	8.8	0.0	9.5	3.9	2.4
15160	Shellfish, Clams, canned with liquid	3.0 oz	85	1.7	0.3	0.1	0.0	0.0	0.0	0.0
15157	Shellfish, Clams, canned, drained	3.0 oz	85	125.8	21.7	4.4	0.0	1.7	0.1	0.5
15138	Shellfish, Crab, Alaskan King, boiled/steamed	3.0 oz	85	82.5	16.4	0.0	0.0	1.3	0.2	0.5
15136	Shellfish, Crab, Alaskan King, imitation surimi	3.0 oz	85	86.7	10.2	8.7	0.0	1.1	0.2	0.6
15139	Shellfish, Crab, Blue, Crab Cakes	1 cake	60	93.0	12.1	0.3	0.0	4.5	1.7	1.4
15143	Shellfish, Crab, Dungeness, cooked w/moist heat	3.0 oz	85	93.5	19.0	0.8	0.0	1.1	0.2	0.3
15147	Shellfish, Lobster, Northern, boiled/steamed (moist heat)	3.0 oz	85	83.3	17.4	1.1	0.0	0.5	0.1	0.1
15154	Shellfish, Lobster, Spiny, cooked w/moist heat	3.0 oz	85	121.6	22.4	2.7	0.0	1.6	0.3	0.6
15164	Shellfish, Mussel, Blue, boiled/steamed	3.0 oz	85	146.2	20.2	6.3	0.0	3.8	0.9	1.0
15246	Shellfish, Oyster, Eastern, breaded & fried	3.0 oz	85	167.5	7.5	9.9	0.0	10.7	4.0	2.8
15245	Shellfish, Oyster, Eastern, Farmed, cooked w/dry heat	6 medium oysters	59	46.6	4.1	4.3	0.0	1.3	0.1	0.4
15244	Shellfish, Oyster, Eastern, Farmed, raw	6 medium oysters	84	49.6	4.4	4.6	0.0	1.3	0.1	0.5
15174	Shellfish, Scallops, breaded, fried	2 large scallops	31	66.7	5.6	3.1	0.0	3.4	1.4	0.9
15172	Shellfish, Scallops, imitation surimi	3.0 oz	85	84.2	10.9	9.0	0.0	0.3	0.1	0.2
924252	Shellfish, Shrimp Chow Mein, frozen	1 cup	227	72.6	5.9	10.9	0.0	0.7	0.0	0.0
15151	Shellfish, Shrimp Egg Roll/LaChoy	3 medium	37	75.1	2.0	12.0	0.0	2.4	0.5	1.5
15150	Shellfish, Shrimp, boiled/steamed (moist heat)	1 large shrimp	6	5.9	1.3	0.0	0.0	0.1	0.0	0.0
15152	Shellfish, Shrimp, breaded & fried	1 large shrimp	7	16.9	1.5	0.8	0.0	0.9	0.3	0.4
15153	Shellfish, Shrimp, canned	1 cup	128	153.6	29.5	1.3	0.0	2.5	0.4	1.0
15149	Shellfish, Shrimp, Imitation Surimi	3.0 oz	85	85.9	10.5	7.8	0.0	1.2	0.2	0.6
4550	Sherbet, Orange	1 sherbert bar	66	91.1	0.7	20.1	0.0	1.3	0.3	0.1
4546	Shortening, Animal & Vegetable Fat, Lard & Vege Oil	1 cup	205	1845.0	0.0	0.0	0.0	205.0	91.0	22.3
4556	Shortening, Vegetable Fat, Crisco	1 tbsp	12	106.0	0.0	0.0	0.0	12.0	5.3	3.6
19002	Snack, Banana Chips	1.0 oz	28.35	147.1	0.7	16.6	2.2	9.5	0.6	0.2
919972	Snack, Beef Jerky	1.0 oz	28.35	116.2	9.4	3.1	0.5	7.3	3.2	0.3
18501	Snack, Bugles	1.0 oz	28	150.1	2.0	18.0	0.0	8.0	0.0	0.0
19419	Snack, Chex Party Mix	1.0 oz (⅔ cup)	28	119.0	3.1	18.2	1.6	4.8	0.0	0.0
19800	Snack, Corn Cakes	1 cake	9	34.8	0.7	7.5	0.2	0.2	0.1	0.1
919973	Snack, Corn Chips, BBQ flavor	1.0 oz	28.35	148.3	2.0	15.9	1.5	9.3	2.7	4.6
19003	Snack, Corn Chips, light/Fritos	1.0 oz	28	155.1	1.9	15.9	0.8	9.7	0.0	0.0
19803	Snack, Corn Chips, Plain	1.0 oz	28.35	152.8	1.9	16.1	1.4	9.5	2.7	4.7
19401	Snack, Corn Cones, Plain	1.0 oz	28.35	144.6	1.6	17.8	0.3	7.6	0.5	0.2

Sat (g)	Chol (mg)	Cal (mg)	Iron (mg)	Magn (mg)	Phos (mg)	Pota (mg)	Sodi (mg)	Zinc (mg)	Vit A (RE)	Vit C (mg)	Vit E (mg)	Thia (mg)	Ribo (mg)	Niac (mg)	Vit B-6 (mg)	Fol (µg)	Vit B-12 (µg)	Wat (g)
0.0	0.0	28.0	2.2	0.0	138.0	391.0	1101.0	0.0	185.6	5.0	0.0	0.2	0.2	3.5	0.0	0.0	0.0	0.0
0.0	0.0	6.0	0.4	0.0	1.0	64.0	149.0	0.0	10.2	11.0	0.0	0.0	0.1	0.0	0.0	0.0	0.0	0.0
0.0	0.0	2.0	0.2	0.0	5.0	10.0	157.0	0.0	0.8	2.0	0.0	0.0	0.0	0.1	0.0	0.0	0.0	0.0
6.8	38.5	521.0	1.3	38.5	301.9	671.9	1829.3	1.1	127.3	1.5	0.0	0.9	0.8	0.8	0.1	8.9	0.6	231.4
0.0	0.0	8.0	0.3	0.0	0.0	12.0	146.0	0.0	0.0	0.0	0.0	0.0	0.0	0.0	0.0	0.0	0.0	44.7
0.1	0.0	1.8	0.1	1.6	5.9	12.8	218.1	0.0	9.9	0.3	0.1	0.0	0.0	0.1	0.0	0.6	0.1	11.3
0.0	0.0	0.0	0.0	0.0	0.0	3.0	22.0	0.0	0.0	0.0	0.0	0.0	0.0	0.0	0.0	0.0	0.0	0.0
1.2	5.0	2.0	0.0	0.0	4.0	1.0	190.0	0.0	30.0	0.0	0.0	0.0	0.0	0.0	0.0	0.0	0.0	5.2
0.0	0.0	4.5	0.3	11.0	27.7	40.5	689.9	0.0	0.0	0.0	0.0	0.0	0.0	0.2	0.0	3.6	0.0	12.2
5.2	24.0	71.0	0.2	0.0	0.0	0.0	263.0	0.0	75.2	0.0	0.0	0.0	0.1	0.2	0.0	0.0	0.0	44.8
2.6	18.0	73.0	0.1	0.0	59.0	89.0	214.0	0.3	42.6	0.0	0.0	0.0	0.1	0.1	0.0	0.0	0.0	48.0
0.0	0.0	28.0	1.3	0.0	0.0	139.0	639.0	0.0	22.4	2.0	0.0	0.0	0.0	0.4	0.0	0.0	0.0	0.0
3.3	30.0	1.5	1.6	2.0	5.5	9.5	170.0	0.3	0.0	0.0	0.1	0.0	0.0	0.3	0.0	1.3	0.3	11.8
7.9	51.0	37.4	1.1	12.8	126.7	180.2	473.5	2.0	0.0	0.0	0.9	0.2	0.4	2.7	0.2	1.7	0.8	47.7
6.1	28.5	6.3	0.7	5.7	49.0	95.2	638.4	1.0	0.0	0.0	0.1	0.1	0.1	1.5	0.1	2.3	0.7	30.7
5.4	27.5	9.0	0.6	1.4	39.2	74.7	461.7	1.0	0.0		0.1	0.0	0.0	1.1	0.1	1.8	0.7	24.6
2.5	45.5	42.8	0.9	4.5	48.2	37.8	616.5	0.5	17.1	0.0	0.1	0.0	0.1	1.4	0.1	1.8	0.1	25.9
2.7	48.2	47.7	0.8	6.3	60.3	80.6	641.7	1.4	0.0	0.0	0.3	0.0	0.1	1.9	0.1	3.6	0.1	28.3
1.8	14.7	3.0	0.3	3.2	28.1	56.4	271.9	0.6	0.0	0.0	0.0	0.0	0.0	0.8	0.0	0.7	0.5	13.5
2.6	17.4	11.4	0.4	4.2	38.5	70.5	279.8	0.5	0.0	0.0	0.1	0.1	0.1	0.7	0.0	1.3	0.4	14.0
1.4	8.4	2.7	0.2	1.7	14.6	24.5	186.9	0.3	0.0	0.0	0.0	0.0	0.0	0.4	0.0	0.5	0.2	7.8
40.5	198.3	25.1	3.5	40.2	298.7	871.0	5120.4	6.3	0.0	0.0	0.6	0.8	0.6	12.4	0.6	10.0	6.3	67.9
5.0	73.0	9.0	1.0	17.0	162.0	231.0	507.0	2.4	8.0	0.0	0.6	0.7	0.2	2.6	0.2	3.0	0.8	64.9
1.9	15.0	3.0	0.6	3.5	26.5	45.5	245.0	0.5	0.0	0.0	0.1	0.1	0.1	0.8	0.0	0.5	0.8	13.9
2.3	46.7	11.4	0.9	8.6	60.4	139.1	572.3	1.0	0.0	0.0	0.3	0.0	0.1	2.0	0.1	2.3	0.1	37.5
7.2	48.3	6.8	1.0	8.2	72.8	128.5	642.6	1.4	0.0	0.0	0.1	0.2	0.1	2.2	0.1	1.4	1.0	35.5
7.7	46.2	20.4	0.8	12.9	110.2	228.5	1020.0	1.9	0.0	1.4	0.2	0.5	0.2	3.1	0.2	3.4	1.1	26.7
6.6	44.2	27.9	1.0	10.9	93.2	194.5	797.6	1.3	0.0	0.0	0.0	0.1	0.1	1.9	0.1	1.4	1.1	36.7
2.0	0.0	42.8	2.5	24.5	153.0	157.1	603.8	1.0	43.5	0.0	1.4	1.6	0.3	7.6	0.6	17.7	0.0	34.3
1.5	8.3	1.6	0.1	1.1	7.8	16.2	152.5	0.3	0.0	0.0	0.0	0.0	0.0	0.3	0.0	0.6	0.2	9.6
2.4	0.0	53.4	3.1	162.8	324.3	316.9	1.4	2.3	2.3	0.6	23.1	1.1	0.1	2.1	0.4	104.6	0.0	2.5
1.5	0.0	19.8	1.1	36.6	327.4	241.0	0.9	1.5	0.0	0.4	14.3	0.0	0.1	2.0	0.2	67.3	0.0	0.3
1.7	0.0	15.9	1.9	36.0	322.9	136.9	0.9	1.5	1.4	0.4	14.3	0.1	0.1	1.2	0.2	66.3	0.0	0.7
1.4	79.9	31.5	3.2	47.6	184.5	241.4	502.4	0.8	1.7	1.5	0.0	0.2	0.1	1.6	0.1	11.9	0.6	51.1
0.2	57.0	78.2	23.8	15.3	287.3	533.8	95.2	2.3	145.4	18.8	0.0	0.1	0.4	2.9	0.1	24.5	84.1	54.1
2.3	51.9	53.6	11.8	11.9	159.8	277.1	309.4	1.2	76.5	8.5	0.0	0.1	0.2	1.8	0.1	30.6	34.2	52.3
0.0	2.6	11.1	0.3	9.4	96.9	126.7	182.8	0.1	7.7	0.9	0.9	0.0	0.0	0.2	0.0	1.7	4.3	83.0
0.2	57.0	78.2	23.8	15.3	287.3	533.8	95.2	2.3	145.4	18.8	0.9	0.1	0.4	2.9	0.1	24.5	84.1	54.1
0.1	45.1	50.2	0.6	53.6	238.0	222.7	911.2	6.5	7.7	6.5	0.0	0.0	0.0	1.1	0.2	43.4	9.8	65.9
0.2	17.0	11.1	0.3	36.6	239.7	76.5	714.9	0.3	17.0	0.0	0.1	0.0	0.0	0.2	0.0	1.4	1.4	62.6
0.9	90.0	63.0	0.6	19.8	127.8	194.4	198.0	2.5	48.6	1.7	0.0	0.1	0.0	1.7	0.1	31.8	3.6	42.6
0.1	64.6	50.2	0.4	49.3	148.8	346.8	321.3	4.6	26.4	3.1	0.0	0.0	0.2	3.1	0.1	35.7	8.8	62.3
0.1	61.2	51.9	0.3	29.8	157.3	299.2	323.0	2.5	22.1	0.0	0.9	0.0	0.1	0.9	0.1	9.4	2.6	64.6
0.3	76.5	53.6	1.2	43.4	194.7	176.8	193.0	6.2	5.1	1.8	0.0	0.0	0.0	4.2	0.1	0.9	3.4	56.7
0.7	47.6	28.1	5.7	31.5	242.3	227.8	313.7	2.3	77.4	11.6	0.0	0.3	0.4	2.6	0.1	64.3	20.4	52.0
2.7	68.9	52.7	5.9	49.3	135.2	207.4	354.5	74.1	76.5	3.2	0.0	0.1	0.2	1.4	0.1	26.4	13.3	55.0
0.4	22.4	33.0	4.6	19.5	67.9	89.7	96.2	26.6	11.2	3.5	0.0	0.1	0.0	1.1	0.0	14.2	14.3	48.4
0.4	21.0	37.0	4.9	27.7	78.1	104.2	149.5	31.9	6.7	3.9	0.0	0.1	0.1	1.1	0.1	15.1	13.6	72.4
0.8	18.9	13.0	0.3	18.3	73.2	103.2	143.8	0.3	6.8	0.7	0.0	0.0	0.0	0.5	0.0	11.5	0.4	18.1
0.1	18.7	6.8	0.3	36.6	239.7	87.6	675.8	0.3	17.0	0.0	0.0	0.0	0.0	0.3	0.0	1.4	1.4	62.7
0.0	0.0	0.0	0.0	0.0	0.0	0.0	985.0	0.0	0.0	0.0	0.0	0.0	0.0	0.0	0.0	0.0	0.0	0.0
0.4	4.0	11.0	0.8	0.0	0.0	65.0	120.0	0.0	5.0	4.0	0.0	0.1	0.1	0.8	0.0	0.0	0.0	0.0
0.0	11.7	2.3	0.2	2.0	8.2	10.9	13.4	0.1	4.0	0.1	0.0	0.0	0.0	0.2	0.0	0.2	0.1	4.6
0.1	12.4	4.7	0.1	2.8	15.3	15.8	24.1	0.1	3.9	0.1	0.0	0.0	0.0	0.2	0.0	0.6	0.1	3.7
0.5	221.4	75.5	3.5	52.5	298.2	268.8	216.3	1.6	23.0	2.9	1.2	0.0	0.0	3.5	0.1	2.3	1.4	92.9
0.2	30.6	16.2	0.5	36.6	239.7	75.7	599.3	0.3	17.0	0.0	0.0	0.0	0.0	0.1	0.0	1.4	1.4	63.7
0.8	4.0	35.6	0.1	5.3	26.4	63.4	30.4	0.3	9.2	2.0	0.1	0.0	0.1	0.0	0.0	3.3	0.1	43.6
82.6	114.8	0.0	0.0	0.0	0.0	0.0	0.0	0.0	0.0	0.0	0.0	2.5	0.0	0.0	0.0	0.0	0.0	0.0
3.1	0.0	0.0	0.0	0.0	0.0	0.0	0.0	0.0	0.0	0.0	0.0	0.0	0.0	0.0	0.0	0.0	0.0	0.0
8.2	0.0	5.1	0.4	21.5	15.9	152.0	1.7	0.2	2.3	1.8	1.5	0.0	0.0	0.2	0.1	4.0	0.0	1.2
3.1	13.6	5.7	1.5	14.5	115.4	169.2	627.4	2.3	0.0	0.0	0.1	0.0	0.0	0.5	0.1	38.0	0.3	6.6
0.0	0.0	2.0	0.2	0.0	13.0	20.0	290.0	0.0	0.0	0.0	0.0	0.0	0.0	0.3	0.0	0.0	0.0	0.0
1.5	0.0	9.8	6.9	17.6	52.4	75.3	284.8	0.6	3.9	13.3	0.0	0.4	0.1	4.7	0.4	0.0	3.5	1.0
0.0	0.0	1.7	0.1	10.3	14.1	14.1	43.9	0.2	2.2	0.0	0.0	0.0	0.0	0.5	0.0	1.7	0.0	0.4
1.3	0.0	37.1	0.4	21.8	58.7	66.9	216.3	0.3	17.3	0.5	0.0	0.0	0.1	0.5	0.1	11.1	0.0	0.3
0.0	0.0	25.0	0.3	21.0	52.0	48.0	194.0	0.3	7.4	0.0	0.0	0.0	0.0	0.4	0.1	0.0	0.0	0.2
1.3	0.0	36.0	0.4	21.5	52.4	40.3	178.6	0.4	2.6	0.0	0.4	0.0	0.0	0.3	0.1	5.7	0.0	0.3
6.4	0.0	0.9	0.7	3.1	12.5	23.0	289.7	0.1	9.1	0.0	0.0	0.1	0.1	0.4	0.0	0.9	0.0	0.6

Code	Food Name	Unit/Amt	Wt (g)	Energy (Kcal)	Prot (g)	Carb (g)	Fiber (g)	Fat (g)	Mono (g)	Poly (g)
19402	Snack, Corn Nuts, BBQ flavor	1.0 oz	28.35	123.6	2.6	20.3	2.4	4.1	2.1	0.9
19008	Snack, Corn Nuts, Plain	1.0 oz	28.35	124.5	2.4	20.8	2.0	4.0	2.1	0.9
19016	Snack, Doo Dads Party Mix, Original flavor	1 tbsp	3.5	16.0	0.4	2.3	0.2	0.6	0.0	0.0
19015	Snack, Granola Bar, Hard, peanut butter	1.0 oz	28.35	136.9	2.8	17.7	0.8	6.7	2.0	3.4
19017	Snack, Granola Bar, Hard, Plain	1.0 oz bar	28.35	133.5	2.9	18.3	1.5	5.6	1.2	3.4
19405	Snack, Granola Bar, Hard, w/chocolate chips	1.0 oz	28.35	124.2	2.1	20.4	1.2	4.6	0.7	0.4
19024	Snack, Granola Bar, Soft, chocolate chip, graham & marshmallow	1.0 oz bar	28.35	121.1	1.7	20.1	1.1	4.4	0.8	0.7
19406	Snack, Granola Bar, Soft, Chocolate Chip, milk chocolate cover	1.0 oz bar	28.35	132.1	1.6	18.1	1.0	7.1	2.2	0.5
19027	Snack, Granola Bar, Soft, Peanut Butter	1.0 oz bar	28.35	120.8	3.0	18.3	1.2	4.5	1.9	1.2
19022	Snack, Granola Bar, Soft, Plain	1.0 oz bar	28.35	125.6	2.1	19.1	1.3	4.9	1.1	1.5
19404	Snack, Granola Bar, Soft, Raisin	1.0 oz bar	28.35	127.0	2.2	18.8	1.2	5.0	0.8	0.9
19440	Snack, Granola Bar, Soft, w/chocolate chips	1.0 oz bar	28.35	119.1	2.1	19.6	1.4	4.7	1.0	0.6
19439	Snack, Kudos Whole Grain Bars, chocolate chip/M&M Mars	4.0 oz bar	100	437.0	5.8	67.7	3.6	16.4	5.2	0.9
19407	Snack, Low Fat Granola Bar, Crunchy Almond/Brown Sugar/Kellogg's	4.0 oz bar	100	390.0	8.0	78.0	6.2	7.4	1.8	4.5
19441	Snack, Meat-Based Sticks, smoked	1.0 oz	28.35	155.9	6.1	1.5	0.0	14.1	5.8	1.3
19031	Snack, Nutri-Grain Cereal Bars, fruit/Kellogg's	4.0 oz bar	100	368.0	4.4	72.9	2.1	7.5	5.0	0.9
19034	Snack, Popcorn Cakes	1 cake	10	38.4	1.0	8.0	0.3	0.3	0.1	0.1
19806	Snack, Popcorn, air-popped	1 tbsp	0.5	1.9	0.1	0.4	0.1	0.0	0.0	0.0
19039	Snack, Popcorn, caramel coated w/peanuts	1.0 oz (⅔ cup)	28.35	113.4	1.8	22.9	1.1	2.2	0.8	0.9
19040	Snack, Popcorn, caramel coated, no peanuts	1.0 oz	28.35	122.2	1.1	22.4	1.5	3.6	0.8	1.3
19807	Snack, Popcorn, Cheese flavor	1 tbsp	0.7	3.7	0.1	0.4	0.1	0.2	0.1	0.1
19035	Snack, Popcorn, oil-popped, white corn	1.0 oz	28.35	141.8	2.6	16.2	2.8	8.0	2.3	3.8
19408	Snack, Popcorn, prep in microwave	3 cups	40	210.0	3.0	20.4	1.0	13.2	8.3	3.2
19412	Snack, Pork Skins, Plain	1.0 oz	28.35	154.5	17.4	0.0	0.0	8.9	4.2	1.0
19042	Snack, Potato Chips w/o salt	1.0 oz	28.35	157.9	2.1	14.5	1.0	10.6	2.0	5.7
919975	Snack, Potato Chips, BBQ flavor	1.0 oz	28.35	139.2	2.2	15.0	1.2	9.2	1.9	4.6
19809	Snack, Potato Chips, light	1.0 oz	28.35	133.5	2.0	19.0	1.7	5.9	1.4	3.1
19411	Snack, Potato Chips, Plain, no salt	1.0 oz	28.35	152.0	2.0	15.0	1.4	9.8	2.8	3.5
19043	Snack, Potato Chips, Plain, salted	1.0 oz	28.35	152.0	2.0	15.0	1.3	9.8	2.8	3.5
919985	Snack, Potato Chips, sour cream & onion	1.0 oz	28.35	150.5	2.3	14.6	1.5	9.6	1.7	4.9
19047	Snack, Pretzel, Hard, Plain, no salt	1.0 oz	28.35	108.0	2.6	22.5	0.8	1.0	0.4	0.3
19813	Snack, Pretzel, Hard, Plain, salted	1.0 oz	28.35	108.0	2.6	22.5	0.9	1.0	0.4	0.3
19050	Snack, Pretzels, Hard, chocolate coated	1.0 oz	28.35	129.8	2.1	20.1	0.0	4.7	1.5	0.6
919978	Snack, Pretzels, Hard, whole wheat	1.0 oz, (2 sm pretzels)	28	101.4	3.1	22.7	2.2	0.7	0.3	0.2
19052	Snack, Rice Cake	1 cake	5	21.0	0.5	4.6	0.4	0.0	0.0	0.0
19818	Snack, Rice Cake, brown rice & multigrain	1 cake	9	34.8	0.8	7.2	0.3	0.3	0.1	0.1
19816	Snack, Rice Cake, brown rice, Plain	1 cake	9	34.8	0.7	7.3	0.4	0.3	0.1	0.1
19524	Snack, Sesame Stick, wheat based, no salt	1.0 oz	28.35	153.4	3.1	13.2	0.0	10.4	3.1	4.9
19857	Snack, Taro Chips	1.0 oz	28.35	141.2	0.7	19.3	2.0	7.1	1.3	3.7
19424	Snack, Tortilla Chips, Nacho flavor	1.0 oz	28.35	141.2	2.2	17.7	1.5	7.3	4.3	1.0
19056	Snack, Tortilla Chips, Nacho, light	1.0 oz	28.35	126.2	2.5	20.3	1.4	4.3	2.5	0.6
19058	Snack, Tortilla Chips, Plain	1.0 oz	28.35	142.0	2.0	17.8	1.8	7.4	4.4	1.0
19063	Snack, Tortilla Chips, Ranch flavor	1.0 oz	28.35	138.9	2.2	18.3	1.1	6.7	4.0	0.9
19059	Snack, Tortilla Chips, Taco flavor	1.0 oz	28.35	136.1	2.2	17.9	1.5	6.9	4.1	1.0
19062	Snack, Trail Mix, regular	1.0 oz	28.35	131.0	3.9	12.7	0.0	8.3	3.6	2.7
6201	Soup, Asparagus, canned, made w/H₂O	1 cup (8 fl oz)	244	85.4	2.3	10.7	0.5	4.1	1.0	1.9
6009	Soup, Beans w/ham, chunky, RTE, canned	1 cup (8 fl oz)	243	230.9	12.6	27.1	11.2	8.5	3.8	0.9
6748	Soup, Beef Noodle, condensed, canned	1 cup (8 fl oz)	251	168.2	9.7	18.0	1.5	6.2	2.5	1.0
6008	Soup, Beef Broth or Bouillon, dry, made w/H₂O	1 packet (6 fl oz)	183	14.6	1.0	1.4	0.0	0.5	0.2	0.0
6147	Soup, Beef Mushroom, canned, made w/H₂O	1 cup (8 fl oz)	244	73.2	5.8	6.3	0.2	3.0	1.2	0.1
6743	Soup, Beef Vegetable, canned, RTE/Progresso Healthy Classics	1 cup	250	160.0	10.5	25.6	6.0	1.6	0.6	0.2
6722	Soup, Beef, chunky, RTE, canned	1 cup (8 fl oz)	240	170.4	11.7	19.6	1.4	5.1	2.1	0.2
6724	Soup, Beefy Mushroom, dry mix/Lipton Recipe Secrets	1 serving	11	32.8	0.9	6.6	0.1	0.4	0.0	0.0
6402	Soup, Beefy Onion, dry mix/Lipton Recipe Secrets	1 serving	8	25.1	0.5	4.7	0.4	0.6	0.0	0.0
6002	Soup, Black Bean, canned, made w/H₂O	1 cup (8 fl oz)	247	116.1	5.6	19.8	4.4	1.5	0.5	0.5
906161	Soup, Broccoli & Cheese, dry mix/Lipton Soup Secrets	1 serving	16	66.9	1.8	8.9	0.7	2.9	0.0	0.0
6411	Soup, Cauliflower, dry, made w/H₂O	1 cup (8 fl oz)	256.1	69.1	2.9	10.7	0.0	1.7	0.7	0.6
6011	Soup, Cheese, canned, made w/milk	1 cup (8 fl oz)	251	230.9	9.5	16.2	1.0	14.6	4.1	0.5
6413	Soup, Chicken Broth or Bouillon, dry, made w/H₂O	1 cup (8 fl oz)	244	22.0	1.3	1.4	0.0	1.1	0.4	0.4
6017	Soup, Chicken Gumbo, canned, made w/H₂O	1 cup (8 fl oz)	244	56.1	2.6	8.4	2.0	1.4	0.7	0.3
6549	Soup, Chicken Mushroom Chowder, chunky, RTE		0.0	0.0	0.0	0.0	0.0	0.0	0.0	0.0
6727	Soup, Chicken Noodle, chunky, canned, RTE	1 cup (8 fl oz)	240	175.2	12.7	17.0	3.8	6.0	2.7	1.5
6022	Soup, Chicken Rice, canned, made w/H₂O	1 cup (8 fl oz)	241	60.3	3.5	7.2	0.7	1.9	0.9	0.4
6025	Soup, Chicken Vegetable, chunky, RTE, canned	1 cup (8 fl oz)	240	165.6	12.3	18.9	0.0	4.8	2.2	1.0
6012	Soup, Chicken w/dumplings, canned, made w/H₂O	1 cup (8 fl oz)	241	96.4	5.6	6.0	0.5	5.5	2.5	1.3
6034	Soup, Consomme w/gelatin, dry, made w/H₂O	1 cup (8 fl oz)	250	17.5	2.2	2.1	0.0	0.0	0.0	0.0
6001	Soup, Crab, RTE, canned	1 cup (8 fl oz)	244	75.6	5.5	10.3	0.7	1.5	0.7	0.4
6410	Soup, Cream of Broccoli, canned, RTE/Progresso Healthy Classics	1 cup (8 fl oz)	356	128.2	3.5	19.4	3.6	4.1	1.3	0.8
6210	Soup, Cream of Celery, canned, made w/H₂O	1 cup (8 fl oz)	244	90.3	1.7	8.8	0.7	5.6	1.3	2.5

Sat (g)	Chol (mg)	Cal (mg)	Iron (mg)	Magn (mg)	Phos (mg)	Pota (mg)	Sodi (mg)	Zinc (mg)	Vit A (RE)	Vit C (mg)	Vit E (mg)	Thia (mg)	Ribo (mg)	Niac (mg)	Vit B-6 (mg)	Fol (µg)	Vit B-12 (µg)	Wat (g)
0.7	0.0	4.8	0.5	30.9	80.2	81.1	276.7	0.5	9.6	0.1	0.0	0.1	0.0	0.4	0.1	0.0	0.0	0.5
0.7	0.0	2.6	0.5	32.0	78.0	78.8	155.6	0.5	0.0	0.0	0.3	0.0	0.0	0.5	0.1	0.0	0.0	0.4
0.1	0.0	2.6	0.1	2.1	10.4	9.7	44.5	0.1	1.5	0.0	0.0	0.0	0.0	0.2	0.0	1.4	0.0	0.1
0.9	0.0	11.6	0.7	15.6	39.4	82.5	80.2	0.4	0.6	0.1	0.0	0.1	0.0	0.6	0.0	5.1	0.0	0.7
0.7	0.0	17.3	0.8	27.5	78.5	95.3	83.3	0.6	4.3	0.3	0.0	0.1	0.0	0.4	0.0	6.5	0.0	1.1
3.2	0.0	21.8	0.9	20.4	57.8	71.2	97.5	0.5	1.1	0.0	0.0	0.1	0.0	0.2	0.0	3.7	0.0	0.7
2.6	0.3	25.2	0.7	20.1	57.3	78.0	89.6	0.4	1.4	0.0	0.0	0.0	0.0	0.3	0.0	6.0	0.0	1.7
4.0	1.4	29.2	0.7	18.7	56.4	88.7	56.7	0.4	2.0	0.0	0.0	0.0	0.1	0.2	0.0	7.4	0.2	1.0
1.0	0.3	25.8	0.6	24.4	70.9	82.5	116.0	0.5	0.6	0.0	0.0	0.1	0.0	0.9	0.0	9.1	0.1	2.1
2.1	0.3	29.8	0.7	21.0	65.2	92.1	78.8	0.4	0.0	0.0	0.0	0.0	0.1	0.1	0.0	6.8	0.1	1.8
2.7	0.3	28.6	0.7	20.4	62.4	102.6	79.9	0.4	0.0	0.0	0.0	0.1	0.0	0.3	0.0	6.0	0.1	1.8
2.9	0.3	26.4	0.7	22.1	65.2	96.4	77.1	0.4	1.4	0.0	0.0	0.1	0.0	0.3	0.0	6.2	0.0	1.5
9.5	136.0	783.0	9.2	70.0	207.0	279.0	280.0	1.4	1253.0	46.6	10.8	0.2	0.2	1.5	0.1	13.0	0.1	4.9
1.1	0.0	35.0	8.6	87.0	248.0	249.0	291.0	2.2	713.0	0.0	0.0	0.7	0.8	9.5	1.0	0.0	0.0	5.0
5.9	37.7	19.3	1.0	6.0	51.0	72.9	419.6	0.7	47.9	1.9	0.0	0.0	0.1	1.3	0.1	0.0	0.3	5.4
1.5	0.0	41.0	4.9	27.0	103.0	197.0	297.0	4.1	614.0	0.0	0.0	1.0	1.1	13.5	1.4	108.0	0.0	14.5
0.0	0.0	0.9	0.2	15.9	27.7	32.7	28.8	0.4	0.7	0.0	0.0	0.0	0.0	0.6	0.0	1.8	0.0	0.5
0.0	0.0	0.1	0.0	0.7	1.5	1.5	0.0	0.0	0.1	0.0	0.0	0.0	0.0	0.0	0.0	0.1	0.0	0.1
0.3	0.0	18.7	1.1	22.7	36.0	100.6	83.6	0.4	1.7	0.0	0.4	0.0	0.0	0.6	0.1	4.5	0.0	0.9
1.0	1.4	12.2	0.5	9.9	23.5	30.9	58.4	0.2	2.8	0.0	0.3	0.0	0.0	0.6	0.0	0.6	0.0	0.8
0.0	0.1	0.8	0.0	0.6	2.5	1.8	6.2	0.0	0.3	0.0	0.0	0.0	0.0	0.0	0.0	0.1	0.0	0.0
1.4	0.0	2.8	0.8	30.6	70.9	63.8	250.6	0.7	0.6	0.1	0.0	0.0	0.0	0.4	0.1	4.8	0.0	0.8
1.7	0.0	8.0	0.7	0.0	73.0	96.0	415.0	0.0	10.8	3.0	0.0	0.1	0.3	0.7	0.0	0.0	0.0	0.0
3.2	26.9	8.5	0.2	3.1	24.1	36.0	521.1	0.2	11.1	0.1	0.2	0.0	0.1	0.4	0.0	0.0	0.2	0.5
2.9	0.0	6.1	0.4	19.2	50.6	384.8	4.1	0.2	1.6	12.1	0.0	0.1	0.0	1.1	0.2	13.2	0.0	0.5
2.3	0.0	14.2	0.5	21.3	52.7	357.5	212.6	0.3	6.2	9.6	1.4	0.1	0.1	1.3	0.2	23.5	0.0	0.5
1.2	0.0	6.0	0.4	25.2	54.7	494.4	139.5	0.0	0.0	7.3	0.8	0.1	0.1	2.0	0.2	7.7	0.0	0.3
3.1	0.0	6.8	0.5	19.0	46.8	361.5	2.3	0.3	0.0	8.8	1.4	0.0	0.1	1.1	0.2	12.8	0.0	0.5
3.1	0.0	6.8	0.5	19.0	46.8	361.5	168.4	0.3	0.0	8.8	1.4	0.0	0.1	1.1	0.2	12.8	0.0	0.5
2.5	2.0	20.4	0.5	21.0	49.9	377.3	177.2	0.3	6.0	10.6	0.0	0.1	0.1	1.1	0.2	17.6	0.3	0.5
0.2	0.0	10.2	1.2	9.9	32.0	41.4	81.9	0.2	0.0	0.0	0.1	0.1	0.2	1.5	0.0	23.5	0.0	0.9
0.2	0.0	10.2	1.2	9.9	32.0	41.4	486.2	0.2	0.0	0.0	0.1	0.1	0.2	1.5	0.0	48.5	0.0	0.9
2.2	0.0	21.0	0.6	11.6	41.1	63.8	161.3	0.3	0.6	0.1	0.0	0.0	0.1	0.2	0.0	2.6	0.0	0.7
0.2	0.0	7.8	0.8	8.4	35.0	120.4	56.8	0.2	0.0	0.0	0.3	0.1	0.1	1.8	0.1	15.1	0.0	1.1
0.0	0.0	0.0	0.1	0.0	0.0	25.0	16.0	0.0	2.8	0.0	0.0	0.0	0.0	0.6	0.0	0.0	0.0	0.0
0.1	0.0	1.9	0.2	12.3	33.3	26.5	22.7	0.2	0.0	0.0	0.0	0.0	0.0	0.6	0.0	1.8	0.0	0.6
0.1	0.0	1.0	0.1	11.8	32.4	26.1	29.3	0.3	0.5	0.0	0.1	0.0	0.0	0.7	0.0	1.9	0.0	0.5
1.8	0.0	48.2	0.2	12.8	39.1	50.2	8.2	0.3	2.6	0.0	0.0	0.0	0.0	0.4	0.0	6.2	0.0	0.6
1.8	0.0	17.0	0.3	23.8	37.1	214.0	97.0	0.1	0.0	1.4	1.4	0.0	0.0	0.1	0.1	5.7	0.0	0.6
1.4	0.9	41.7	0.4	23.2	69.2	61.2	200.7	0.3	11.6	0.5	0.0	0.1	0.1	0.4	0.0	4.0	0.0	0.5
0.8	0.9	45.1	0.5	27.5	90.2	77.1	284.4	0.0	11.9	0.1	0.0	0.1	0.1	0.1	0.1	7.4	0.0	0.4
1.4	0.0	43.7	0.4	24.9	58.1	55.8	149.7	0.4	5.7	0.0	0.4	0.0	0.1	0.4	0.1	2.8	0.0	0.5
1.3	0.3	40.0	0.4	25.2	67.8	69.2	173.5	0.4	7.7	0.3	0.0	0.0	0.1	0.4	0.1	4.8	0.0	0.5
1.3	1.4	43.9	0.6	24.9	67.8	61.5	223.1	0.4	25.8	0.3	0.0	0.1	0.1	0.6	0.1	6.0	0.0	0.5
1.6	0.0	22.1	0.9	44.8	97.8	194.2	64.9	0.9	0.6	0.4	0.0	0.1	0.1	1.3	0.1	20.1	0.0	2.6
1.0	4.9	29.3	0.8	4.9	39.0	173.2	980.9	0.9	43.9	2.7	0.7	0.1	0.1	0.8	0.0	22.0	0.0	224.0
3.3	21.9	77.8	3.2	46.2	143.4	425.3	972.0	1.1	396.1	4.4	0.0	0.1	0.1	1.7	0.1	29.2	0.1	191.1
2.3	10.0	30.1	2.2	12.6	92.9	198.3	1905.1	3.1	125.5	0.8	0.0	0.1	0.1	2.1	0.1	37.7	0.4	211.9
0.3	0.0	7.3	0.0	5.5	18.3	27.5	1021.1	0.1	0.0	0.0	0.0	0.0	0.0	0.3	0.0	0.0	0.0	177.0
1.5	7.3	4.9	0.9	9.8	34.2	153.7	941.8	1.5	0.0	4.6	0.0	0.0	0.1	1.0	0.0	9.8	0.2	225.9
0.6	15.0	15.0	1.9	32.5	102.5	627.5	420.0	1.3	215.0	4.8	0.5	0.1	0.1	2.9	0.3	25.0	0.3	212.5
2.5	14.4	31.2	2.3	4.8	120.0	336.0	866.4	2.6	261.6	7.0	0.2	0.1	0.2	2.7	0.1	13.4	0.6	200.0
0.1	0.2	10.8	0.1	0.0	0.0	0.0	645.2	0.0	0.0	0.2	0.0	0.0	0.0	0.1	0.0	0.0	0.0	0.4
0.1	0.0	11.2	0.1	0.0	0.0	0.0	606.6	0.0	0.0	0.0	0.0	0.0	0.0	0.1	0.0	0.0	0.0	0.3
0.4	0.0	44.5	2.1	42.0	106.2	274.2	1198.0	1.4	49.4	0.7	0.1	0.1	0.1	0.5	0.1	24.7	0.0	215.6
0.8	2.9	46.4	0.2	0.0	0.0	0.0	545.3	0.0		3.0	0.0	0.0	0.0	0.1	0.0	3.7	0.0	0.6
0.3	0.0	10.2	0.5	2.6	51.2	105.0	842.6	0.3	0.0	2.6	0.0	0.1	0.1	0.5	0.0	2.6	0.2	238.0
9.1	47.7	288.7	0.8	20.1	251.0	341.4	1019.1	0.7	148.1	1.3	0.3	0.1	0.3	0.5	0.1	10.0	0.4	206.9
0.3	0.0	14.6	0.1	4.9	12.2	24.4	1483.5	0.0	12.2	0.0	0.0	0.0	0.0	0.2	0.0	2.4	0.0	236.2
0.3	4.9	24.4	0.9	4.9	24.4	75.6	954.0	0.4	14.6	4.9	0.0	0.0	0.0	0.7	0.1	4.9	0.0	229.0
0.0	0.0	0.0	0.0	0.0	0.0	0.0	0.0	0.0	0.0	0.0	0.0	0.0	0.0	0.0	0.0	0.0	0.0	
1.4	19.2	24.0	1.4	9.6	72.0	108.0	849.6	1.0	122.4	0.0	0.8	0.1	0.2	4.3	0.0	38.4	0.3	201.6
0.5	7.2	16.9	0.7	0.0	21.7	101.2	814.6	0.3	65.1	0.2	0.1	0.0	0.0	1.1	0.0	1.0	0.1	226.1
1.4	16.8	26.4	1.5	9.6	105.6	367.2	1068.0	2.2	600.0	5.5	0.0	0.0	0.2	3.3	0.1	12.0	0.2	200.3
1.3	33.7	14.5	0.6	4.8	60.3	115.7	860.4	0.4	53.0	0.0	0.1	0.0	0.1	1.8	0.0	2.4	0.2	221.2
0.0	0.0	7.5	0.1	7.5	40.0	57.5	3312.5	0.0	0.0	0.0	0.0	0.0	0.0	0.6	0.0	4.0	0.1	237.4
0.4	9.8	65.9	1.2	14.6	87.8	327.0	1234.6	1.5	51.2	0.0	0.0	0.2	0.1	1.3	0.1	14.6	0.2	223.3
1.0	7.1	60.5	1.8	21.4	57.0	235.0	843.7	0.4	46.3	8.5	0.6	0.0	0.1	0.5	0.1	42.7	0.0	327.5
1.4	14.6	39.0	0.6	7.3	36.6	122.0	949.2	0.2	31.7	0.2	0.9	0.0	0.0	0.3	0.0	2.4	0.2	225.1

Code	Food Name	Unit/Amt	Wt (g)	Energy (Kcal)	Prot (g)	Carb (g)	Fiber (g)	Fat (g)	Mono (g)	Poly (g)
6216	Soup, Cream of Chicken, canned, made w/H_2O	1 cup (8 fl oz)	240	115.2	3.4	9.1	0.2	7.2	3.2	1.5
6243	Soup, Cream of Mushroom, canned, made w/H_2O	1 cup (8 fl oz)	244	129.3	2.3	9.3	0.5	9.0	1.7	4.2
6246	Soup, Cream of Onion, canned, made w/H_2O	1 cup (8 fl oz)	244	107.4	2.8	12.7	1.0	5.3	2.1	1.5
6253	Soup, Cream of Potato, canned, made w/H_2O	1 cup (8 fl oz)	244	73.2	1.8	11.5	0.5	2.4	0.6	0.4
6256	Soup, Cream of Shrimp, canned, made w/H_2O	1 cup (8 fl oz)	244	90.3	2.8	8.2	0.2	5.2	1.5	0.2
6582	Soup, Cream of Vegetable, dry, made w/H_2O	1 cup (8 fl oz)	260	106.6	1.9	12.3	0.5	5.7	2.5	1.5
6035	Soup, Cup Noodles, Ramen, chicken flavor, dry/Nissin	1 individual container	64	296.2	5.6	36.8	0.0	14.1	0.0	0.0
6283	Soup, Gazpacho, RTE, canned	1 cup (8 fl oz)	244	46.4	7.1	4.4	0.5	0.2	0.0	0.1
6249	Soup, Green Pea, canned, made w/H_2O	1 cup (8 fl oz)	250	165.0	8.6	26.5	2.8	2.9	1.0	0.4
6287	Soup, Hearty Chicken Noodle, dry mix/Lipton Cup-a-Soup	1 envelope	16	61.4	2.6	10.2	0.3	1.2	0.0	0.0
6204	Soup, Lentil Ham, RTE, canned	1 cup (8 fl oz)	248	138.9	9.3	20.2	0.0	2.8	1.3	0.3
6027	Soup, Manhattan Clam Chowder, canned, made w/H_2O	1 cup (8 fl oz)	244	78.1	2.2	12.2	1.5	2.2	0.4	1.3
6039	Soup, Minestrone, canned, RTE/Progresso Healthy Classics	1 cup (8 fl oz)	241	122.9	4.8	20.3	1.2	2.5	0.9	1.0
6430	Soup, Nacho Cheese	1 cup (8 fl oz)	251	105.4	3.8	6.4	0.0	7.2	0.0	0.0
6230	Soup, New England Clam Chowder, canned, made w/H_2O	1 cup (8 fl oz)	244	95.2	4.8	12.4	1.5	2.9	1.2	1.1
6302	Soup, Noodle w/real Chicken Broth, dry mix/Lipton Soup Secrets	1 tbsp	16	62.1	2.1	9.2	0.3	1.9	0.0	0.0
6045	Soup, Onion, canned, made w/H_2O	1 cup (8 fl oz)	241	57.8	3.8	8.2	1.0	1.7	0.7	0.7
6730	Soup, Split Pea w/ham, canned, made w/H_2O	1 cup (8 fl oz)	253	189.8	10.3	28.0	2.3	4.4	1.8	0.6
6192	Soup, Split Pea w/ham, chunky, RTE, canned	1 cup (8 fl oz)	240	184.8	11.1	26.8	4.1	4.0	1.6	0.6
6099	Soup, Tomato Rice, made w/H_2O	1 cup (8 fl oz)	247	118.6	2.1	21.9	1.5	2.7	0.6	1.4
6559	Soup, Tomato Vegetable, dry, made w/H_2O	1 cup (8 fl oz)	253	55.7	2.0	10.2	0.5	0.9	0.3	0.1
6359	Soup, Tomato, canned, made w/H_2O	1 cup (8 fl oz)	244	85.4	2.0	16.6	0.5	1.9	0.4	1.0
6159	Soup, Tomato, canned, made w/milk	1 cup (8 fl oz)	248	161.2	6.1	22.3	2.7	6.0	1.6	1.1
6065	Soup, Turkey Noodle, canned, made w/H_2O	1 cup (8 fl oz)	251	70.3	4.0	8.9	0.8	2.1	0.8	0.5
6066	Soup, Turkey Vegetable, canned, made w/H_2O	1 cup (8 fl oz)	240	72.0	3.1	8.6	0.5	3.0	1.3	0.7
6471	Soup, Turkey, chunky, RTE, canned	1 cup (8 fl oz)	236	134.5	10.2	14.1	0.0	4.4	1.8	1.1
6301	Soup, Vegetable, chunky, RTE, canned	1 cup (8 fl oz)	240	122.4	3.5	19.0	1.2	3.7	1.6	1.4
6068	Soup, Vegetarian Vegetable, canned, made w/H_2O	1 cup (8 fl oz)	241	72.3	2.1	12.0	0.5	1.9	0.8	0.7
22693	Stew, Beef Stew, canned entree	1 cup	232	218.1	11.5	15.7	3.5	12.5	5.5	0.5
924055	Stew, Beef&Vegetable	1 cup	245	220.5	16.0	15.0	2.0	11.0	4.5	0.5
906162	Stew, Chicken Vegetable/Bounty	7.5 oz	213	166.1	10.5	15.1	0.0	7.0	0.0	0.0
924190	Stew, Ratatouille, homemade	½ cup	107	132.7	1.2	5.9	0.0	12.3	9.0	1.1
19337	Stuffing, Brownberry Sage and Onion Stuffing Mix, dry mix/Best Foods	½ cup	67	255.3	8.9	47.2	3.6	3.4	0.0	0.0
919908	Sugar Substitute, Aspartame/Nutrasweet/Equal	1 tsp	3.5	12.3	0.1	3.0	0.0	0.0	0.0	0.0
924174	Sugar Substitute, Equal	1 package	1	4.0	0.0	1.0	0.0	0.0	0.0	0.0
18356	Sweet Roll, Cheese	1 oz	28.4	102.2	2.0	12.4	0.3	5.2	2.6	0.6
18357	Sweet Roll, Cinnamon-Raisin, commercially prep	1 large	83	308.8	5.1	42.2	2.0	13.6	4.0	6.2
919959	Sweet, All-Fruit Strawberry Spread/Polaner	1 tbsp	18	41.5	0.1	10.3	0.0	0.0	0.0	0.0
919904	Sweet, Baking Chocolate/Bakers	1 oz	28	141.1	3.1	9.0	0.5	14.6	5.5	0.4
919916	Sweet, Chewing Gum	1 stick	3	10.2	0.0	2.9	0.0	0.0	0.0	0.0
919902	Sweet, Chewing Gum, Sugarless	1 piece	3	8.0	0.0	2.0	0.0	0.0	0.0	0.0
19166	Sweet, Cocoa, dry powder, unsweetened	1 tbsp	5.4	12.4	1.1	2.9	1.8	0.7	0.2	0.0
19240	Sweet, Frosting, Chocolate creamy, RTE, no added phosphorus & Vit A	1/12 package	38	150.9	0.4	24.0	0.2	6.7	3.4	0.8
19375	Sweet, Frosting, Cream Cheese flavor, RTE	1/12 package	38	156.9	0.0	25.3	0.0	6.6	3.4	0.9
19714	Sweet, Frosting, Glaze, homemade	1/12 recipe	27	96.9	0.2	19.8	0.0	2.1	0.9	0.6
919377	Sweet, Frosting, Sour Cream flavor, RTE	1/12 package	38	156.6	0.0	25.7	0.0	6.5	3.4	0.9
19715	Sweet, Frosting, Vanilla, Creamy, RTE	1/12 package	38	159.2	0.0	26.4	0.0	6.4	3.3	0.9
19712	Sweet, Frosting, White, fluffy, dry mix prep w/H_2O	1/12 package	26	63.4	0.4	16.3	0.0	0.0	0.0	0.0
19172	Sweet, Fruit Butter, Apple	1 tbsp	17	29.4	0.1	7.3	0.3	0.0	0.0	0.0
19703	Sweet, Gelatin, dry mix, low kcal w/aspartame, prep w/H_2O	1 cup	234	16.4	2.6	1.6	0.0	0.0	0.0	0.0
19296	Sweet, Gelatin, dry, prep w/H_2O	1 cup	270	159.3	3.2	37.8	0.0	0.0	0.0	0.0
19283	Sweet, Honey, strained/extracted	1 tbsp	21	63.8	0.1	17.3	0.0	0.0	0.0	0.0
19717	Sweet, Ice Popsicle	1 double stick	128	92.2	0.0	24.2	0.0	0.0	0.0	0.0
19280	Sweet, Ices/Sorbet, pineapple-coconut	1 tbsp	12.4	14.0	0.0	3.0	0.1	0.3	0.0	0.0
918860	Sweet, Ices/Sorbet/Water, fruit, low kcal w/aspartame	1 bar	51	12.2	0.3	3.2	0.0	0.1	0.0	0.0
919905	Sweet, Italian Ice, restaurant-prep	1.0 fl oz	29	15.4	0.0	3.9	0.0	0.0	0.0	0.0
19297	Sweet, Jam, low kcal	1 tbsp	6	18.0	0.0	5.1	0.5	0.0	0.0	0.0
19719	Sweet, Jams & Preserves	1 tbsp	20	48.4	0.1	12.9	0.2	0.0	0.0	0.0
919907	Sweet, Jellies	1 tbsp	19	51.5	0.1	13.5	0.2	0.0	0.0	0.0
919906	Sweet, Jelly, low kcal	1.0 oz	28	4.2	0.0	1.0	0.5	0.0	0.0	0.0
19303	Sweet, Maraschino Cherry	1.0 oz	28	96.0	0.1	24.6	0.3	0.1	0.0	0.1
19304	Sweet, Marmalade, orange	1 tbsp	20	49.2	0.1	13.3	0.0	0.0	0.0	0.0
19305	Sweet, Molasses	1 tbsp	20	53.2	0.0	13.8	0.0	0.0	0.0	0.0
19251	Sweet, Pectin, unsweetened, dry mix	¼ package	12	39.0	0.0	10.8	1.0	0.0	0.0	0.0
19334	Sweet, Solo Poppy Seed Filling/Sokol	1 tbsp	18	59.7	0.9	10.5	0.0	1.6	0.2	1.0
19335	Sweet, Sugar, brown	1 tsp, packed	4.6	17.3	0.0	4.5	0.0	0.0	0.0	0.0
19340	Sweet, Sugar, granulated, white	1 tsp	4.2	16.3	0.0	4.2	0.0	0.0	0.0	0.0
19336	Sweet, Sugar, Maple	1 piece (1 oz/1.75 x 1.25 x 0.5")	28	99.1	0.0	25.5	0.0	0.1	0.0	0.0
19113	Sweet, Sugar, powdered/confectioner's, white	1 tsp	2.5	9.7	0.0	2.5	0.0	0.0	0.0	0.0

Sat (g)	Chol (mg)	Cal (mg)	Iron (mg)	Magn (mg)	Phos (mg)	Pota (mg)	Sodi (mg)	Zinc (mg)	Vit A (RE)	Vit C (mg)	Vit E (mg)	Thia (mg)	Ribo (mg)	Niac (mg)	Vit B-6 (mg)	Fol (µg)	Vit B-12 (µg)	Wat (g)
2.0	9.6	33.6	0.6	2.4	36.0	86.4	969.6	0.6	55.2	0.2	0.2	0.0	0.1	0.8	0.0	1.7	0.1	217.5
2.4	2.4	46.4	0.5	4.9	48.8	100.0	880.8	0.6	0.0	1.0	1.2	0.0	0.1	0.7	0.0	4.9	0.0	220.4
1.5	14.6	34.2	0.6	4.9	36.6	119.6	927.2	0.1	29.3	1.2	0.0	0.1	0.1	0.5	0.0	6.8	0.0	220.8
1.2	4.9	19.5	0.5	2.4	46.4	136.6	1000.4	0.6	29.3	0.0	0.0	0.0	0.0	0.5	0.0	2.9	0.0	225.7
3.2	17.1	17.1	0.5	9.8	31.7	58.6	976.0	0.8	14.6	0.0	0.8	0.0	0.0	0.4	0.0	3.7	0.6	225.0
1.4	0.0	31.2	0.5	10.4	54.6	96.2	1170.0	0.3	2.6	3.9	1.2	1.2	0.1	0.5	0.0	7.8	0.1	237.1
6.3	0.0	0.0	2.2	0.0	0.0	0.0	1433.6	0.0	0.0	0.0	0.0	0.0	0.0	0.0	0.0	0.0	0.0	3.8
0.0	0.0	24.4	1.0	7.3	36.6	224.5	739.3	0.2	261.1	7.1	0.5	0.0	0.0	0.9	0.1	9.8	0.0	228.8
1.4	0.0	27.5	2.0	40.0	125.0	190.0	917.5	1.7	20.0	1.8	0.1	0.1	0.1	1.2	0.1	1.8	0.0	208.7
0.4	14.2	5.9	0.5	0.0	0.0	0.0	591.4	0.0	0.0	0.1	0.1	0.1	0.1	1.3	0.0	17.0	0.0	0.6
1.1	7.4	42.2	2.7	22.3	183.5	357.1	1319.4	0.7	34.7	4.2	0.0	0.2	0.1	1.4	0.2	49.6	0.3	212.7
0.4	2.4	26.8	1.6	12.2	41.5	187.9	578.3	1.0	97.6	3.9	0.7	0.0	0.0	0.8	0.1	9.8	4.1	224.2
0.4	0.0	38.6	1.7	31.3	86.8	306.1	470.0	0.7	135.0	0.7	0.7	0.1	0.1	1.0	0.1	60.3	0.0	208.9
0.0	0.0	78.0	0.6	0.0	0.0	56.0	754.0	0.0	270.8	5.0	0.0	0.1	0.1	0.3	0.0	0.0	0.0	0.0
0.4	4.9	43.9	1.5	7.3	53.7	146.4	915.0	0.8	0.0	2.0	0.1	0.0	0.0	1.0	0.1	3.7	8.0	220.9
0.6	14.4	3.4	0.5	0.0	0.0	0.0	723.8	0.0	0.0	0.1	0.0	0.2	0.1	1.0	0.0	19.8	0.0	0.6
0.3	0.0	26.5	0.7	2.4	12.1	67.5	1053.2	0.6	0.0	1.2	0.3	0.0	0.0	0.6	0.0	15.2	0.0	224.3
1.8	7.6	22.8	2.3	48.1	212.5	399.7	1006.9	1.3	45.5	1.5	0.0	0.1	0.1	1.5	0.1	2.5	0.3	206.9
1.6	7.2	33.6	2.1	38.4	177.6	304.8	964.8	3.1	487.2	7.0	0.1	0.1	0.1	2.5	0.2	4.6	0.2	194.3
0.5	2.5	22.2	0.8	4.9	34.6	331.0	815.1	0.5	76.6	14.8	0.8	0.1	0.0	1.1	0.1	13.6	0.0	217.6
0.4	0.0	7.6	0.6	20.2	30.4	103.7	1146.1	0.2	20.2	6.1	0.8	0.1	0.0	0.8	0.1	10.1	0.0	236.6
0.4	0.0	12.2	1.8	7.3	34.2	263.5	695.4	0.2	68.3	66.4	2.5	0.1	0.1	1.4	0.1	14.6	0.0	220.5
2.9	17.4	158.7	1.8	22.3	148.8	448.9	744.0	0.3	109.1	67.7	2.6	0.1	0.2	1.5	0.2	20.8	0.4	209.8
0.6	5.0	12.6	1.0	5.0	50.2	77.8	838.3	0.6	30.1	0.3	0.1	0.1	0.1	1.4	0.0	20.1	0.2	233.4
0.9	2.4	16.8	0.8	4.8	40.8	175.2	902.4	0.6	242.4	0.0	0.1	0.0	0.0	1.0	0.0	4.8	0.2	222.9
1.2	9.4	49.6	1.9	23.6	103.8	361.1	922.8	2.1	715.1	6.4	0.0	0.0	0.1	3.6	0.3	11.1	2.1	203.8
0.6	0.0	55.2	1.6	7.2	72.0	396.0	1010.4	3.1	588.0	6.0	0.6	0.1	0.1	1.2	0.2	16.6	0.0	210.2
0.3	0.0	21.7	1.1	7.2	33.7	209.7	821.8	0.5	301.3	1.4	0.8	0.1	0.0	0.9	0.1	10.6	0.0	222.5
5.2	37.1	27.8	1.6	32.5	127.6	403.7	946.6	1.9	494.2	10.2	0.2	0.2	0.1	2.9	0.3	25.5	0.9	189.1
4.4	71.0	29.0	2.9	0.0	184.0	613.0	292.0	5.3	1138.0	17.0	0.0	0.1	0.2	4.7	0.3	37.0	0.0	0.0
0.0	0.0	29.0	1.2	0.0	109.0	315.0	1055.0	0.0	1463.4	5.0	0.0	0.0	0.1	3.4	0.0	0.0	0.0	0.0
1.7	0.0	27.8	0.6	16.1	31.0	242.9	164.8	0.2	40.7	20.7	0.0	0.1	0.0	0.6	0.1	17.1	0.0	86.6
0.6	0.0	0.0	2.6	0.0	0.0	0.0	1125.6	0.0	0.0	0.0	0.0	0.0	0.0	0.0	0.0	0.0	0.0	4.2
0.0	0.0	0.0	0.0	0.0	0.0	0.1	0.1	0.0	0.0	0.0	0.0	0.0	0.0	0.0	0.0	0.0	0.0	0.4
0.0	0.0	0.0	0.0	0.0	0.0	0.0	0.0	0.0	0.0	0.0	0.0	0.0	0.0	0.0	0.0	0.0	0.0	0.0
1.7	21.6	33.5	0.2	5.4	27.8	38.9	101.4	0.2	21.9	0.1	0.0	0.0	0.0	0.2	0.0	12.2	0.1	8.3
2.6	54.8	59.8	1.3	14.1	63.1	92.1	317.9	0.5	53.1	1.7	3.6	0.3	0.2	2.0	0.1	43.2	0.1	20.6
0.0	0.0	0.0	0.0	0.0	0.0	0.0	3.6	0.0	0.0	0.0	0.0	0.0	0.0	0.0	0.0	0.0	0.0	7.5
8.7	0.0	23.0	2.0	86.0	113.0	245.0	1.0	1.0	3.4	0.0	0.0	0.0	0.1	0.4	0.0	3.0	0.0	0.4
0.0	0.0	0.0	0.0	0.0	0.0	0.1	0.2	0.0	0.0	0.0	0.0	0.0	0.0	0.0	0.0	0.0	0.0	0.1
0.0	0.0	5.0	0.0	0.0	0.0	0.0	0.0	0.0	0.0	0.0	0.0	0.0	0.0	0.0	0.0	0.0	0.0	0.0
0.4	0.0	6.9	0.7	26.9	39.6	82.3	1.1	0.4	0.1	0.0	0.0	0.0	0.0	0.1	0.0	1.7	0.0	0.2
2.1	0.0	3.0	0.5	8.0	22.4	74.5	69.5	0.1	0.0	0.0	0.0	0.0	0.0	0.0	0.0	0.0	0.0	6.5
1.9	0.0	1.1	0.1	0.8	1.1	13.3	90.1	0.0	44.1	0.0	0.0	0.0	0.0	0.0	0.0	0.0	0.0	5.7
0.5	0.5	5.9	0.0	0.8	4.9	8.1	25.4	0.0	21.9	0.1	0.2	0.0	0.0	0.0	0.0	0.3	0.0	4.8
1.9	0.0	0.8	0.0	0.8	1.5	73.7	77.5	0.0	46.4	0.0	0.0	0.0	0.0	0.3	0.0	0.4	0.0	5.4
1.9	0.0	1.1	0.0	0.4	14.8	14.1	34.2	0.0	85.9	0.0	1.8	0.0	0.0	0.0	0.0	0.0	0.0	5.0
0.0	0.0	1.0	0.0	0.5	1.3	20.0	40.6	0.0	0.0	0.0	0.0	0.0	0.0	0.2	0.0	0.5	0.0	9.2
0.0	0.0	2.4	0.1	0.9	1.7	15.5	0.7	0.0	2.0	0.1	0.0	0.0	0.0	0.0	0.0	0.2	0.0	9.6
0.0	0.0	4.7	0.0	2.3	63.2	0.0	112.3	0.1	0.0	0.0	0.2	0.0	0.0	0.0	0.0	0.0	0.0	229.3
0.0	0.0	5.4	0.1	2.7	59.4	2.7	113.4	0.1	0.0	0.0	0.0	0.0	0.0	0.0	0.0	0.0	0.0	228.4
0.0	0.0	1.3	0.1	0.4	0.8	10.9	0.8	0.0	0.0	0.1	0.0	0.0	0.0	0.0	0.0	0.4	0.0	3.6
0.0	0.0	0.0	0.0	1.3	0.0	5.1	15.4	0.0	0.0	0.0	0.0	0.0	0.0	0.0	0.0	0.0	0.0	102.4
0.3	0.0	0.0	0.4	0.6	1.1	2.1	4.3	0.0	0.0	1.6	0.0	0.0	0.0	0.0	0.0	0.1	0.0	9.1
0.0	0.0	1.0	0.1	1.0	0.0	13.3	2.6	0.0	0.0	0.0	0.0	0.0	0.0	0.1	0.0	0.0	0.0	47.5
0.0	0.0	0.3	0.0	0.0	0.0	1.7	1.2	0.0	0.0	0.1	0.0	0.0	0.0	0.2	0.0	1.5	0.0	25.1
0.0	0.0	1.0	0.0	0.0	8.0	9.0	7.0	0.0	0.0	0.0	0.0	0.0	0.0	0.0	0.0	1.0	0.0	3.8
0.0	0.0	4.0	0.1	0.8	2.2	15.4	8.0	0.0	0.2	1.8	0.0	0.0	0.0	0.0	0.0	6.6	0.0	6.9
0.0	0.0	1.5	0.0	1.1	1.0	12.2	6.8	0.0	0.4	0.2	0.0	0.0	0.0	0.0	0.0	0.2	0.0	5.4
0.0	0.0	1.0	0.0	0.0	8.0	20.0	4.0	0.0	0.0	0.0	0.0	0.0	0.0	0.0	0.0	5.0	0.0	
0.0	0.0	0.0	0.0	0.0	0.0	0.0	0.0	0.0	0.0	0.0	0.0	0.0	0.0	0.0	0.0	0.0	0.0	3.4
0.0	0.0	7.6	0.0	0.4	1.2	7.4	11.2	0.0	1.0	1.0	0.0	0.0	0.0	0.0	0.0	7.2	0.0	6.6
0.0	0.0	41.0	0.9	48.4	6.2	292.8	7.4	0.1	0.0	0.0	0.0	0.0	0.0	0.2	0.1	0.0	0.0	5.2
0.0	0.0	0.8	0.3	0.1	0.2	0.8	24.0	0.1	0.0	0.0	0.0	0.0	0.0	0.0	0.0	0.1	0.0	1.0
0.2	0.0	58.0	0.0	0.0	0.0	0.0	13.3	0.0	0.0	0.0	0.0	0.0	0.0	0.0	0.0	0.0	0.0	4.8
0.0	0.0	3.9	0.1	1.3	1.0	15.9	1.8	0.0	0.0	0.0	0.0	0.0	0.0	0.0	0.0	0.0	0.0	0.1
0.0	0.0	0.0	0.0	0.0	0.1	0.1	0.0	0.0	0.0	0.0	0.0	0.0	0.0	0.0	0.0	0.0	0.0	0.0
0.0	0.0	25.2	0.5	5.3	0.8	76.7	3.1	1.7	0.6	0.0	0.0	0.0	0.0	0.0	0.0	0.0	0.0	2.2
0.0	0.0	0.0	0.0	0.0	0.1	0.1	0.0	0.0	0.0	0.0	0.0	0.0	0.0	0.0	0.0	0.0	0.0	0.0

Code	Food Name	Unit/Amt	Wt (g)	Energy (Kcal)	Prot (g)	Carb (g)	Fiber (g)	Fat (g)	Mono (g)	Poly (g)
19349	Sweet, Syrup, Chocolate, fudge-type	1 tbsp	17	59.5	0.8	10.7	0.5	1.5	0.7	0.0
19351	Sweet, Syrup, Corn, dark	1 tbsp	20	56.4	0.0	15.3	0.0	0.0	0.0	0.0
19362	Sweet, Syrup, Corn, light	1 tbsp	20	56.4	0.0	15.3	0.0	0.0	0.0	0.0
19129	Sweet, Syrup, Maple	1 tbsp	20	52.4	0.0	13.4	0.0	0.0	0.0	0.0
19360	Sweet, Syrup, pancake	1 tbsp	20	57.4	0.0	15.1	0.0	0.0	0.0	0.0
19355	Sweet, Syrup, pancake, reduced-kcal	¼ cup	60	98.4	0.0	26.6	0.0	0.0	0.0	0.0
19365	Sweet, Topping, Butterscotch or Caramel	tbsp	20.5	51.7	0.3	13.5	0.2	0.0	0.0	0.0
19367	Sweet, Topping, Marshmallow Cream	1.0 oz	28	90.2	0.2	22.1	0.0	0.1	0.0	0.0
19137	Sweet, Topping, Pineapple	2 tbsp	42	106.3	0.0	27.9	0.4	0.0	0.0	0.0
919984	Sweet, Topping, strawberry	1 tbsp	21	53.3	0.0	13.9	0.2	0.0	0.0	0.0
924200	Syrups, Chocolate, Genuine Chocolate Flavor,lite/Hershey	1 tbsp	17.5	25.0	0.3	5.8	0.4	0.1	0.0	0.0
924201	Taco	6.0 oz	171	369.4	20.7	26.7	2.0	20.6	6.6	1.0
18386	Toaster Muffin, Blueberry	1 toaster muffin	33	103.3	1.5	17.6	0.6	3.1	0.7	1.8
918387	Toaster Muffin, Corn	1 toaster muffin	33	114.2	1.7	19.1	0.5	3.7	0.9	2.1
18493	Toaster Pastry, Pop Tart, Brown Sugar Cinnamon/Kellogg	1 pastry	50	219.0	2.7	32.2	0.8	9.2	3.6	4.6
18480	Toaster Pastry, Pop Tart, Cherry, low fat/Kellogg	1 pastry	52	191.9	2.3	39.8	0.6	2.9	1.6	0.7
18477	Toaster Pastry, Pop Tart, Frosted Apple Cinnamon, low fat/Kellogg	1 pastry	52	191.4	2.2	40.0	0.6	2.9	1.5	0.8
18479	Toaster Pastry, Pop Tart, Frosted Brown Sugar Cinnamon, low fat/Kellogg	1 pastry	50	188.0	2.4	39.2	0.6	2.8	1.5	0.7
18481	Toaster Pastry, Pop Tart, Frosted Brown Sugar Cinnamon/Kellogg	1 pastry	50	211.0	2.5	34.2	0.7	7.4	3.9	2.4
18489	Toaster Pastry, Pop Tart, Frosted Strawberry, low fat/Kellogg	1 pastry	52	190.8	2.1	40.3	0.6	3.0	1.4	1.0
18490	Toaster Pastry, Pop Tart, Frosted Strawberry/Kellogg	1 pastry	52	202.8	2.3	37.6	0.5	5.0	2.9	0.7
11693	Toaster Pastry/Pop Tart, Fruit (Apple/Blueberry/Cherry/Strawberry)	1 Pop Tart	52	204.4	2.4	37.0	1.1	5.3	2.2	2.0
18363	Tomato, crushed, canned	½ cup	50	16.0	0.8	3.6	1.0	0.1	0.0	0.1
18449	Tortilla, Corn, ready-to-cook	1 medium tortilla (6" dia)	26	57.7	1.5	12.1	1.4	0.7	0.2	0.3
18616	Tortilla, Flour, ready-to-cook	1 12" diameter	75	243.8	6.5	41.7	2.5	5.3	2.8	0.8
18360	Tortilla, Flour, w/o added calcium, ready to cook	1 8 " diameter	50	162.5	4.4	27.8	1.7	3.6	1.9	0.5
18448	Tortilla, Taco Shell, baked	1 large (6.5" dia)	21	98.3	1.5	13.1	1.6	4.7	1.9	1.8
5600	Tuna Helper	1 serving	184	301.8	14.4	29.4	0.0	14.0	0.0	0.0
924187	Turkey Patty, breaded, fried	1 patty	94	266.0	13.2	14.8	0.5	16.9	7.0	4.4
5296	Turkey Pot Pie, frozen/Swanson	7.0 oz	198	380.2	10.9	36.1	0.0	21.4	0.0	0.0
5295	Turkey Roast, Light & Dark Meat, no bone, frozen, seasoned, ckd	3.5 oz	100	155.0	21.3	3.1	0.0	5.8	1.2	1.7
5189	Turkey w/gravy, frozen	1 pkg (5.0 oz)	142	95.1	8.3	6.5	0.0	3.7	1.4	0.7
5293	Turkey, Breaded Turkey Nuggets w/USDA commodity meat, cooked/ Pierre product #193	3.5 oz	100	347.0	18.2	10.2	0.3	25.8	7.5	11.3
924210	Turkey, Breast w/skin, roasted	3.5 oz	100	189.0	28.7	0.0	0.0	7.4	2.5	1.8
5187	Turkey, Dark Meat w/skin, roasted	3.5 oz	100	221.0	27.5	0.0	0.0	11.5	3.7	3.1
51619	Turkey, Dark Meat, no skin, roasted	3.5 oz	100	187.0	28.6	0.0	0.0	7.2	1.6	2.2
5211	Turkey, Fryer/Roaster, Dark Meat w/skin, roasted	3.5 oz	100	182.0	27.7	0.0	0.0	7.1	2.3	1.9
5221	Turkey, Fryer/Roaster, Dark Meat, no skin, roasted	3.5 oz	100	162.0	28.8	0.0	0.0	4.3	1.0	1.3
5209	Turkey, Fryer/Roaster, Light Meat w/skin, roasted	3.5 oz	100	164.0	28.8	0.0	0.0	4.6	1.7	1.1
5201	Turkey, Fryer/Roaster, Light Meat, no skin, roasted	3.5 oz	100	140.0	30.2	0.0	0.0	1.2	0.2	0.3
51617	Turkey, Fryer/Roaster, Wing, no skin, roasted	3.5 oz	100	163.0	30.9	0.0	0.0	3.4	0.6	0.9
5305	Turkey, Ground, cooked	3.5 oz	100	235.0	27.4	0.0	0.0	13.2	4.9	3.2
5285	Turkey, Leg w/skin, roasted	3.5 oz	100	208.0	27.9	0.0	0.0	9.8	2.9	2.7
5181	Turkey, Light & Dark Meat, diced, seasoned	3.5 oz	100	138.0	18.7	1.0	0.0	6.0	2.0	1.5
5185	Turkey, Light Meat w/skin, roasted	3.5 oz	100	197.0	28.6	0.0	0.0	8.3	2.8	2.0
5165	Turkey, Light Meat, no skin, roasted	3.5 oz	100	157.0	29.9	0.0	0.0	3.2	0.6	0.9
5294	Turkey, Smoked	3.5 oz	100	118.0	19.6	0.7	0.0	3.9	1.4	1.1
5245	Turkey, Wing w/skin, roasted	3.5 oz	100	229.0	27.4	0.0	0.0	12.4	4.7	2.9
17089	Veal, Breast, Whole, boneless, lean, braised	3.5 oz	100	218.0	30.3	0.0	0.0	9.8	4.5	0.8
17138	Veal, Sirloin, lean&fat, roasted	6.0 oz	170	343.4	42.7	0.0	0.0	17.8	6.9	1.2
11886	Vege Juice, Carrot, canned	6.0 oz	184	73.6	1.7	17.1	1.5	0.3	0.0	0.1
11001	Vege Juice, Tomato, canned w/o salt	6.0 oz	184	31.3	1.4	7.8	1.5	0.1	0.0	0.0
11004	Vege, Alfalfa Seeds, sprouted, raw	1 cup	33	9.6	1.3	1.2	0.8	0.2	0.0	0.1
11009	Vege, Artichokes (Globe or French) boiled, drained, no salt	1 medium	300	150.0	10.4	33.5	16.2	0.5	0.0	0.2
11705	Vege, Arugula/Roquette, raw	1 cup	20	5.0	0.5	0.7	0.3	0.1	0.0	0.1
11015	Vege, Asparagus, boiled, drained	½ cup	90	21.6	2.3	3.8	1.4	0.3	0.0	0.1
11707	Vege, Asparagus, canned, drained	½ cup	90	17.1	1.9	2.2	1.4	0.6	0.0	0.3
11011	Vege, Asparagus, frozen, boiled, drained, no salt	4 spears	60	16.8	1.8	2.9	1.0	0.3	0.0	0.1
11028	Vege, Bamboo Shoots, canned, drained	½ cup	60	7.2	0.9	1.2	0.6	0.1	0.0	0.1
11045	Vege, Bean Sprouts, Mung, mature seeds, sprouted, stir fried	½ cup	30	3.6	0.4	0.6	0.2	0.0	0.0	0.0
11046	Vege, Bean Sprouts, Navy, mature seeds, sprouted, raw	1 cup	120	93.6	8.5	18.0	0.0	1.0	0.1	0.6
11052	Vege, Beans, Snap, Green, raw	1 cup	125	35.0	1.9	8.1	3.8	0.2	0.0	0.1
11722	Vege, Beans, Snap, Yellow, raw	1 cup	135	37.8	2.0	8.7	4.1	0.2	0.0	0.1
11081	Vege, Beets, boiled, drained	½ cup	85	37.4	1.4	8.5	1.7	0.2	0.0	0.1
11090	Vege, Broccoli florets, raw	1 cup	88	63.4	4.9	10.3	3.7	0.5	0.0	0.3
22600	Vege, Broccoli in Cheese Flavored Sauce, frozen/GreenGiant	½ cup	142	39.8	4.2	7.4	0.0	0.5	0.0	0.2
11095	Vege, Broccoli Spears, frozen, boiled, drained, no salt	½ cup	78	21.8	2.4	4.2	2.3	0.1	0.0	0.0
11093	Vege, Broccoli, chopped, frozen, boiled, drained, no salt	½ cup	84	23.5	2.6	4.5	2.5	0.1	0.0	0.0

Sat (g)	Chol (mg)	Cal (mg)	Iron (mg)	Magn (mg)	Phos (mg)	Pota (mg)	Sodi (mg)	Zinc (mg)	Vit A (RE)	Vit C (mg)	Vit E (mg)	Thia (mg)	Ribo (mg)	Niac (mg)	Vit B-6 (mg)	Fol (µg)	Vit B-12 (µg)	Wat (g)
0.7	0.3	13.8	0.2	8.7	23.0	61.5	58.8	0.1	0.7	0.0	0.5	0.0	0.0	0.1	0.0	0.7	0.0	3.7
0.0	0.0	3.6	0.1	1.6	2.2	8.8	31.0	0.0	0.0	0.0	0.0	0.0	0.0	0.0	0.0	0.0	0.0	4.6
0.0	0.0	0.6	0.0	0.4	0.4	0.8	24.2	0.0	0.0	0.0	0.0	0.0	0.0	0.0	0.0	0.0	0.0	4.6
0.0	0.0	13.4	0.2	2.8	0.4	40.8	1.8	0.8	0.0	0.0	0.0	0.0	0.0	0.0	0.0	0.0	0.0	6.4
0.0	0.0	0.2	0.0	0.4	1.8	0.4	16.6	0.0	0.0	0.0	0.0	0.0	0.0	0.0	0.0	0.0	0.0	4.8
0.0	0.0	0.6	0.0	0.0	25.8	1.8	120.0	0.0	0.0	0.0	0.0	0.0	0.0	0.0	0.0	0.0	0.0	32.9
0.0	0.2	10.9	0.0	1.4	9.6	17.2	71.5	0.0	5.5	0.1	0.0	0.0	0.0	0.0	0.0	0.4	0.0	6.6
0.0	0.0	0.8	0.1	0.6	2.2	1.4	13.7	0.0	0.0	0.0	0.0	0.0	0.0	0.0	0.0	0.3	0.0	5.5
0.0	0.0	9.2	0.2	0.8	3.4	133.1	26.5	0.2	0.8	24.6	0.0	0.0	0.0	0.0	0.0	1.3	0.0	13.9
0.0	0.0	5.0	0.2	0.8	2.7	15.3	4.4	0.1	0.4	5.2	0.0	0.0	0.0	0.1	0.0	0.4	0.0	6.9
0.0	0.0	1.9	0.0	2.6	4.0	13.5	24.0	0.0	0.0	0.0	0.0	0.0	0.0	0.0	0.0	0.2	0.0	11.3
11.4	57.0	221.0	2.4	71.0	203.0	473.0	802.0	3.9	147.0	2.0	0.0	0.2	0.1	3.2	0.2	23.0	1.0	99.9
0.5	2.0	4.3	0.2	4.0	19.5	27.4	157.7	0.1	22.1	0.0	0.6	0.1	0.1	0.7	0.0	18.2	0.0	10.2
0.6	4.3	6.3	0.5	4.6	49.8	30.4	141.9	0.1	6.6	0.0	0.0	0.1	0.1	0.8	0.0	18.8	0.0	7.8
1.0	0.0	15.5	1.8	8.0	31.5	67.5	214.0	0.6	0.0	0.0	0.0	0.2	0.2	2.0	0.2	40.0	0.0	5.3
0.6	0.0	5.7	1.8	4.7	22.4	29.6	221.5	0.2	0.0	0.0	0.0	0.2	0.2	2.0	0.2	52.0	0.0	6.5
0.6	0.0	5.7	1.8	4.7	21.3	28.1	205.9	0.2	0.0	0.0	0.0	0.2	0.2	2.0	0.2	52.0	0.0	6.5
0.6	0.0	7.0	1.8	5.0	22.5	30.5	209.5	0.2	0.0	0.0	0.0	0.2	0.2	2.0	0.2	50.0	0.0	5.3
1.1	0.0	14.5	1.8	7.5	46.5	55.5	184.5	1.2	0.0	0.0	0.0	0.2	0.2	2.0	0.2	40.0	0.0	5.3
0.6	0.0	5.2	1.8	4.2	20.3	25.5	201.2	0.2	0.0	0.0	0.0	0.2	0.2	2.0	0.2	52.0	0.0	6.5
1.4	0.0	11.4	1.8	5.2	26.5	44.2	169.0	0.2	0.0	0.0	0.0	0.2	0.2	2.0	0.2	52.0	0.0	6.5
0.8	0.0	13.5	1.8	9.4	57.7	58.2	217.9	0.3	1.6	0.3	1.2	0.2	0.2	2.0	0.2	33.8	0.0	6.4
0.0	0.0	17.0	0.7	10.0	16.0	146.5	66.0	0.1	35.0	4.6	0.3	0.0	0.0	0.6	0.1	6.5	0.0	44.7
0.1	0.0	45.5	0.4	16.9	81.6	40.0	41.9	0.2	0.0	0.0	0.0	0.0	0.0	0.4	0.1	29.6	0.0	11.5
1.3	0.0	93.8	2.5	19.5	93.0	98.3	358.5	0.5	0.0	0.0	0.7	0.4	0.2	2.7	0.0	92.3	0.0	20.1
0.9	0.0	19.5	1.7	13.0	62.0	65.5	239.0	0.4	0.0	0.0	0.5	0.3	0.1	1.8	0.0	61.5	0.0	13.4
0.7	0.0	33.6	0.5	22.1	52.1	37.6	77.1	0.3	0.0	0.0	0.8	0.0	0.0	0.3	0.1	22.1	0.0	1.3
0.0	0.0	0.0	0.0	0.0	0.0	239.0	916.0	0.0	0.0	0.0	0.0	0.0	0.0	0.0	0.0	0.0	0.0	126.2
4.4	58.3	13.2	2.1	14.1	253.8	258.5	752.0	1.4	10.3	0.0	2.2	0.1	0.2	2.2	0.2	26.3	0.2	46.7
0.0	0.0	29.0	2.4	0.0	0.0	138.0	719.0	0.0	393.4	2.0	0.0	0.3	0.2	3.1	0.0	0.0	0.0	0.0
1.9	53.0	5.0	1.6	22.0	244.0	298.0	680.0	2.5	0.0	0.0	0.4	0.0	0.2	6.3	0.3	5.0	1.5	67.8
1.2	25.6	19.9	1.3	11.4	115.0	86.6	786.7	1.0	18.5	0.0	0.0	0.0	0.2	2.6	0.1	5.7	0.3	120.8
5.1	57.0	28.0	1.9	15.0	205.0	178.0	567.0	1.9	0.0	0.0	2.8	0.2	0.2	4.3	0.2	22.0	0.2	44.2
2.1	74.0	21.0	1.4	27.0	210.0	288.0	63.0	2.0	0.0	0.0	0.0	0.1	0.1	6.4	0.5	6.0	0.4	63.2
3.5	89.0	33.0	2.3	23.0	196.0	274.0	76.0	4.2	0.0	0.0	0.6	0.1	0.2	3.5	0.3	9.0	0.4	60.2
2.4	85.0	32.0	2.3	24.0	204.0	290.0	79.0	4.5	0.0	0.0	0.6	0.1	0.2	3.6	0.4	9.0	0.4	63.1
2.1	117.0	27.0	2.3	23.0	190.0	237.0	76.0	3.8	0.0	0.0	0.0	0.0	0.2	3.4	0.3	9.0	0.4	64.8
1.5	112.0	26.0	2.4	24.0	196.0	246.0	79.0	4.1	0.0	0.0	0.0	0.1	0.2	3.5	0.4	10.0	0.4	66.4
1.3	95.0	18.0	1.6	26.0	205.0	262.0	57.0	2.1	0.0	0.0	0.0	0.0	0.1	6.3	0.5	6.0	0.4	66.5
0.4	86.0	15.0	1.6	28.0	216.0	277.0	56.0	2.1	0.0	0.0	0.0	0.0	0.1	6.9	0.6	6.0	0.4	68.6
1.1	102.0	26.0	1.8	22.0	174.0	204.0	78.0	3.8	0.0	0.0	0.1	0.0	0.2	4.1	0.6	7.0	0.4	65.6
3.4	102.0	25.0	1.9	24.0	196.0	270.0	107.0	2.9	0.0	0.0	0.3	0.1	0.2	4.8	0.4	7.0	0.3	59.4
3.1	85.0	32.0	2.3	23.0	199.0	280.0	77.0	4.3	0.0	0.0	0.6	0.1	0.2	3.6	0.3	9.0	0.4	61.2
1.8	55.0	1.0	1.8	17.0	240.0	310.0	850.0	2.0	0.0	0.0	0.0	0.0	0.1	4.8	0.3	5.0	0.2	71.7
2.3	76.0	21.0	1.4	26.0	208.0	285.0	63.0	2.0	0.0	0.0	0.1	0.1	0.1	6.3	0.5	6.0	0.4	62.8
1.0	69.0	19.0	1.4	28.0	219.0	305.0	64.0	2.0	0.0	0.0	0.1	0.1	0.1	6.8	0.5	6.0	0.4	66.3
1.4	42.9	7.1	0.5	92.9	260.7	271.4	996.4	1.9	0.0	0.0	0.0	0.0	0.1	3.6	0.4	0.0	0.7	256.8
3.4	81.0	24.0	1.5	25.0	197.0	266.0	61.0	2.1	0.0	0.0	0.2	0.1	0.1	5.7	0.4	6.0	0.4	59.5
3.7	116.0	9.0	0.8	22.0	208.0	289.0	68.0	4.2	0.0	0.0	0.4	0.1	0.3	9.0	0.3	15.0	1.5	59.7
7.7	173.4	22.1	1.6	44.2	379.1	596.7	141.1	5.7	0.0	0.0	0.7	0.1	0.6	15.1	0.5	25.5	2.4	106.5
0.0	0.0	44.2	0.8	25.8	77.3	537.3	53.4	0.3	2014.8	15.6	0.0	0.2	0.1	0.7	0.4	7.0	0.0	163.5
0.0	0.0	16.6	1.1	20.2	35.0	404.8	18.4	0.3	103.0	33.7	1.7	0.1	0.1	1.2	0.2	36.6	0.0	172.8
0.0	0.0	10.6	0.3	8.9	23.1	26.1	2.0	0.0	5.3	2.7	0.0	0.0	0.0	0.2	0.0	11.9	0.0	30.1
0.1	0.0	135.0	3.9	180.0	258.0	1062.0	285.0	1.5	54.0	30.0	0.6	0.2	0.2	3.0	0.3	153.0	0.0	251.9
0.0	0.0	32.0	0.3	9.4	10.4	73.8	5.4	0.1	47.4	3.0	0.1	0.0	0.0	0.1	0.0	19.4	0.0	18.3
0.1	0.0	18.0	0.7	9.0	48.6	144.0	9.9	0.4	48.6	9.7	0.3	0.1	0.1	1.0	0.1	131.4	0.0	83.0
0.1	0.0	14.4	1.6	9.0	38.7	154.8	258.3	0.4	47.7	16.6	0.4	0.1	0.1	0.9	0.1	86.0	0.0	84.6
0.1	0.0	13.8	0.4	7.8	33.0	130.8	2.4	0.3	49.2	14.6	0.8	0.0	0.1	0.6	0.0	80.8	0.0	54.7
0.0	0.0	7.2	0.1	1.8	12.0	319.8	2.4	0.3	0.0	0.0	0.0	0.0	0.0	0.2	0.1	1.4	0.0	57.6
0.0	0.0	4.2	0.1	2.7	9.6	8.1	42.0	0.1	0.6	0.1	0.0	0.0	0.0	0.1	0.0	2.9	0.0	28.8
0.1	0.0	19.2	2.5	133.2	123.6	380.4	16.8	1.2	0.0	20.8	0.0	0.5	0.3	1.5	0.2	127.6	0.0	91.2
0.1	0.0	61.3	1.1	30.0	38.8	157.5	11.3	0.6	50.0	5.1	0.2	0.0	0.1	0.5	0.1	28.8	0.0	114.3
0.1	0.0	66.2	1.2	32.4	41.9	170.1	12.2	0.6	14.9	5.5	0.2	0.0	0.1	0.5	0.1	31.1	0.0	123.4
0.0	0.0	13.6	0.7	19.6	32.3	259.3	242.3	0.3	3.4	3.1	0.0	0.0	0.0	0.3	0.1	68.0	0.0	74.0
0.1	0.0	19.4	1.7	33.4	83.6	220.0	44.0	0.5	30.8	29.0	0.0	0.1	0.1	1.3	0.0	84.7	0.0	71.3
0.1	0.0	68.2	1.2	35.5	93.7	461.5	38.3	0.6	426.0	132.3	2.4	0.1	0.2	0.9	0.2	100.8	0.0	128.8
0.0	0.0	39.8	0.5	15.6	42.9	140.4	202.8	0.2	147.4	31.3	1.3	0.0	0.1	0.4	0.1	23.4	0.0	70.8
0.0	0.0	42.8	0.5	16.8	46.2	151.2	218.4	0.3	158.8	33.7	1.4	0.0	0.1	0.4	0.1	47.4	0.0	76.2

Code	Food Name	Unit/Amt	Wt (g)	Energy (Kcal)	Prot (g)	Carb (g)	Fiber (g)	Fat (g)	Mono (g)	Poly (g)
11099	Vege, Brussels Sprouts, boiled, drained, no salt	½ cup, 4 sprouts	78	32.0	2.0	6.8	2.0	0.4	0.0	0.2
11110	Vege, Cabbage, boiled, drained, no salt	½ cup	60	13.2	0.6	2.7	1.7	0.3	0.0	0.1
11749	Vege, Cabbage, Common (Danish/Domestic/Pointed) Fresh Harvest, raw	1 cup	70	15.4	0.7	3.1	1.6	0.3	0.0	0.1
11970	Vege, Cabbage, Napa, cooked	½ cup	35	8.4	0.4	1.9	0.8	0.1	0.0	0.0
11960	Vege, Carrots, Baby, raw	1 cup, or 6 baby carrots	140	28.0	1.0	6.8	2.2	0.1	0.0	0.1
11128	Vege, Carrots, canned, drained	½ cup	73	32.9	0.8	7.7	2.4	0.1	0.0	0.1
11131	Vege, Carrots, frozen, boiled, drained, no salt	½ cup	73	26.3	0.9	6.0	2.6	0.1	0.0	0.0
11136	Vege, Cauliflower, boiled, drained, no salt	½ cup	62	14.3	1.1	2.5	1.7	0.3	0.0	0.1
11138	Vege, Cauliflower, frozen, boiled, drained, no salt	½ cup	62	11.8	1.0	2.3	1.7	0.1	0.0	0.1
11967	Vege, Cauliflower, green, cooked, no salt	½ cup	90	28.8	2.7	5.7	3.0	0.3	0.0	0.1
11965	Vege, Cauliflower, Green, head, raw	1 cup	100	32.0	3.0	6.3	3.3	0.3	0.0	0.1
11142	Vege, Celeriac, boiled, drained, no salt	½ cup	100	27.0	1.0	5.9	0.0	0.2	0.0	0.1
11143	Vege, Celery, raw	½ cup or 2 stalks	80	14.4	0.7	3.2	1.3	0.1	0.0	0.1
11148	Vege, Chard, Swiss, boiled, drained, no salt	½ cup	88	17.6	1.7	3.6	1.8	0.1	0.0	0.0
11162	Vege, Collards, boiled, drained, no salt	½ cup	74	19.2	1.6	3.6	2.1	0.3	0.0	0.1
11656	Vege, Corn Pudding, homemade	1 cup	250	232.5	7.8	55.8	7.0	1.9	0.5	0.9
11190	Vege, Corn Salad, raw	⅔ cup (#6 scoop)	167	182.0	7.3	21.3	0.0	8.9	2.9	1.1
11774	Vege, Corn, Yellow, kernels, frozen, boiled w/salt, drained	½ cup	82	52.5	1.6	12.6	1.4	0.4	0.1	0.2
11771	Vege, Corn, Yellow, Sweet, canned, solids & liquid, no added salt	½ cup	123	88.6	2.1	22.3	1.5	0.5	0.2	0.2
11174	Vege, Corn, Yellow, Sweet, cream style, regular pack, canned	½ cup	105	83.0	2.5	20.4	2.1	0.5	0.2	0.2
11179	Vege, Corn, Yellow, Sweet, kernels, frozen, boiled, drained, no salt	½ cup	84	73.9	2.5	17.5	2.0	0.6	0.2	0.3
11172	Vege, Corn, Yellow, Sweet, whole kernel, canned, drained	½ cup	84	67.2	2.3	16.4	2.0	0.4	0.1	0.2
11192	Vege, Cowpeas (Blackeyes), immature seeds, boiled, drained, no salt	½ cup	84	81.5	2.7	17.1	4.2	0.3	0.0	0.1
11205	Vege, Cucumber, raw	1 cup	40	4.8	0.2	1.0	0.3	0.1	0.0	0.0
11210	Vege, Eggplant (Brinjal) boiled, drained, no salt	½ cup, 1″ cubes	99	27.7	0.8	6.6	2.5	0.2	0.0	0.1
11213	Vege, Endive (Escarole) raw	1 tbsp, 1″ pieces	5.1	1.3	0.1	0.3	0.1	0.0	0.0	0.0
11957	Vege, Fennel Bulb, raw	1 cup	100	150.0	4.6	31.7	0.0	1.8	0.0	0.0
11950	Vege, Fungi, Mushroom, Enoki, raw	1 cup	28	79.5	2.6	20.4	19.6	0.2	0.0	0.0
11987	Vege, Fungi, Mushroom, Oyster, raw	1 medium: 3.35″ long	3	1.0	0.1	0.2	0.1	0.0	0.0	0.0
11269	Vege, Fungi, Mushroom, Shiitake, ckd, no salt	½ cup, 4 mushrooms	72	39.6	1.1	10.3	1.5	0.2	0.0	0.0
11261	Vege, Fungi, Mushrooms, boiled, drained, no salt	1 mushroom	12	3.2	0.3	0.6	0.3	0.1	0.0	0.0
11260	Vege, Fungi, Mushrooms, slices, raw	10 slices	40	9.6	0.7	2.0	1.0	0.1	0.0	0.0
924135	Vege, Green Pepper, Stuffed, homemade	1 pepper	185	172.1	10.4	32.0	20.4	3.9	0.1	2.0
11961	Vege, Hearts of Palm, canned	½ cup	72	122.4	9.4	12.1	0.4	4.0	0.0	0.0
11971	Vege, Herb, Cilantro, raw	1 tbsp, chopped	8.1	2.3	0.2	0.4	0.2	0.1	0.0	0.0
11234	Vege, Kale, boiled, drained, no salt	½ cup	65	18.2	1.2	3.7	1.3	0.3	0.0	0.1
11242	Vege, Kohlrabi, boiled, drained, no salt	½ cup	85	24.7	1.5	5.7	0.9	0.1	0.0	0.0
11245	Vege, Lambsquarters, boiled, drained, no salt	1 tbsp, chopped	11.3	3.6	0.4	0.6	0.2	0.1	0.0	0.0
11246	Vege, Leeks (bulb & lower leaf-portion) raw	1 leek	124	38.4	1.0	9.4	1.2	0.2	0.0	0.1
11972	Vege, Lemon Grass (citronella), raw	1 leek	124	38.4	1.0	9.4	1.2	0.2	0.0	0.1
11250	Vege, Lettuce, Butterhead (Boston/Bibb) leaves, raw	3.5 grams	100	101.0	8.8	21.3	0.0	0.5	0.1	0.2
11251	Vege, Lettuce, Cos/Romaine, raw	1 small leaf	5	0.7	0.1	0.1	0.1	0.0	0.0	0.0
11252	Vege, Lettuce, Iceberg, head, raw	1 inner leaf	10	1.4	0.2	0.2	0.2	0.0	0.0	0.0
11253	Vege, Lettuce, Looseleaf, raw	1 small head	324	38.9	3.3	6.8	4.5	0.6	0.0	0.3
11796	Vege, Lotus Root, boiled w/salt, drained	1 cup, shredded	56	10.1	0.7	2.0	1.1	0.2	0.0	0.1
11974	Vege, Mushrooms, sauteed	1 tbsp, cubes	9.1	7.5	0.2	1.8	0.0	0.0	0.0	0.0
11805	Vege, Onions, boiled w/salt, chopped, drained	1 ring	10	40.7	0.5	3.8	0.1	2.7	1.1	0.5
11282	Vege, Onions, chopped, raw	1 tbsp, chopped	15	4.2	0.1	1.0	0.3	0.0	0.0	0.0
11291	Vege, Onions, Spring (tops & bulb) chopped, raw	1 tbsp	5	17.5	0.4	4.2	0.5	0.0	0.0	0.0
11298	Vege, Parsnip, peeled, raw	1 cup, slices	76	61.6	1.0	14.8	3.0	0.2	0.1	0.0
11318	Vege, Peas & Carrots, canned, regular pack, solids & liquid	½ cup	174	92.2	5.6	17.0	5.6	0.5	0.0	0.2
11323	Vege, Peas & Carrots, frozen, boiled, drained, no salt	½ cup	80	38.4	2.5	8.1	2.5	0.3	0.0	0.2
11301	Vege, Peas w/edible pod-Snow/Sugar, boiled, drained, no salt	½ cup	80	33.6	2.6	5.6	2.2	0.2	0.0	0.1
11305	Vege, Peas, Green, boiled, drained, no salt	½ cup	80	67.2	4.3	12.5	4.4	0.2	0.0	0.1
11308	Vege, Peas, Green, canned, regular pack, drained	½ cup	85	58.7	3.8	10.7	3.5	0.3	0.0	0.1
11980	Vege, Pepper, Chili, Green, canned	½ cup	62	16.7	1.0	3.3	2.1	0.3	0.0	0.2
11670	Vege, Pepper, Hot Chili, raw	½ cup	70	14.7	0.5	3.2	1.2	0.2	0.0	0.1
11632	Vege, Pepper, Jalapeno, canned, solids & liquid	1 pepper	27	7.8	0.2	1.8	0.0	0.1	0.0	0.1
11979	Vege, Pepper, Jalapeno, raw	½ cup chopped	85	23.0	0.8	4.0	2.2	0.8	0.0	0.4
11333	Vege, Pepper, Sweet, Green, chopped/sliced, raw	3.5 oz	100	18.0	1.0	3.9	0.9	0.2	0.0	0.1
11821	Vege, Pepper, Sweet, Red, raw	3.5 oz	100	18.0	1.0	3.9	0.0	0.2	0.0	0.1
11951	Vege, Pepper, Sweet, Yellow, raw	1 tbsp	9.3	2.5	0.1	0.6	0.2	0.0	0.0	0.0
11973	Vege, Pickles, Bread & Butter	10 strips	52	14.0	0.5	3.3	0.5	0.1	0.0	0.0
11937	Vege, Pickles, Cucumber, Dill	2 slices	15	13.2	1.2	2.6	0.0	0.1	0.0	0.1
11941	Vege, Pickles, Cucumber, Sour, slices/spears	1 large (4″ long)	135	14.9	0.4	3.0	1.6	0.3	0.0	0.1
11940	Vege, Pickles, Cucumber, Sweet, Gherkins	1 large Gherkin (3″ long)	35	3.9	0.1	0.8	0.4	0.1	0.0	0.0
11970	Vege, Pickles, Fresh Pack	1 medium	35	41.0	0.1	11.1	0.4	0.1	0.0	0.0
11975	Vege, Pickles, Kosher	2 slices	15	1.8	0.2	0.3	0.0	0.0	0.0	0.0
11976	Vege, Pickles, Sweet & Sour	1.0 oz	28	6.7	0.6	1.2	0.8	0.1	0.1	0.0

Sat (g)	Chol (mg)	Cal (mg)	Iron (mg)	Magn (mg)	Phos (mg)	Pota (mg)	Sodi (mg)	Zinc (mg)	Vit A (RE)	Vit C (mg)	Vit E (mg)	Thia (mg)	Ribo (mg)	Niac (mg)	Vit B-6 (mg)	Fol (μg)	Vit B-12 (μg)	Wat (g)
0.1	0.0	28.1	0.9	15.6	43.7	247.3	200.5	0.3	56.2	48.4	0.0	0.1	0.1	0.5	0.1	46.8	0.0	68.1
0.0	0.0	18.6	0.1	4.8	9.0	58.2	153.0	0.1	7.8	12.1	0.0	0.0	0.0	0.2	0.1	12.0	0.0	56.2
0.0	0.0	21.7	0.1	5.6	10.5	67.9	5.6	0.1	9.1	14.1	0.1	0.0	0.0	0.2	0.1	14.0	0.0	65.5
0.0	0.0	16.5	0.2	5.3	8.1	86.1	6.3	0.1	4.6	14.7	0.0	0.0	0.0	0.1	0.0	19.8	0.0	32.4
0.0	0.0	98.0	1.0	58.8	32.2	560.0	238.0	0.2	16.8	2.8	0.0	0.0	0.0	0.4	0.1	39.6	0.0	131.6
0.0	0.0	22.6	0.5	9.5	21.9	165.7	48.2	0.2	1792.2	1.7	0.3	0.0	0.0	0.4	0.2	10.1	0.0	63.8
0.0	0.0	20.4	0.3	7.3	19.0	115.3	215.4	0.2	1292.1	2.0	0.0	0.0	0.0	0.3	0.1	7.9	0.0	65.6
0.0	0.0	9.9	0.2	5.6	19.8	88.0	150.0	0.1	1.2	27.5	0.0	0.0	0.0	0.3	0.1	27.3	0.0	57.7
0.0	0.0	10.5	0.3	5.6	14.9	86.2	157.5	0.1	1.2	19.4	0.0	0.0	0.0	0.2	0.1	25.4	0.0	58.3
0.0	0.0	28.8	0.6	17.1	51.3	250.2	233.1	0.6	12.6	65.3	0.0	0.1	0.1	0.6	0.2	36.9	0.0	80.5
0.0	0.0	32.0	0.7	19.0	57.0	278.0	23.0	0.6	14.0	72.6	0.0	0.1	0.1	0.7	0.2	41.0	0.0	89.5
0.0	0.0	26.0	0.4	12.0	66.0	173.0	297.0	0.2	0.0	3.6	0.0	0.0	0.0	0.4	0.1	3.4	0.0	92.3
0.0	0.0	33.6	0.3	9.6	20.0	227.2	72.8	0.1	10.4	4.9	0.3	0.0	0.0	0.3	0.1	17.6	0.0	75.3
0.0	0.0	51.0	2.0	75.7	29.0	483.1	365.2	0.3	276.3	15.8	0.0	0.0	0.1	0.3	0.1	7.6	0.0	81.5
0.0	0.0	88.1	0.3	12.6	19.2	192.4	186.5	0.3	231.6	13.5	0.7	0.0	0.1	0.4	0.1	68.8	0.0	68.0
0.3	0.0	7.5	1.5	72.5	187.5	627.5	10.0	1.6	52.5	12.0	0.0	0.4	0.2	3.8	0.6	76.3	0.0	183.0
4.2	167.0	66.8	0.9	25.1	95.2	268.9	91.9	0.8	60.1	4.7	0.0	0.7	0.2	1.6	0.2	42.3	0.2	127.5
0.1	0.0	3.3	0.3	13.1	41.8	134.5	174.7	0.3	0.0	4.5	0.0	0.0	0.1	0.8	0.0	31.2	0.0	66.7
0.1	0.0	3.7	0.5	20.9	62.7	164.8	3.7	0.7	12.3	5.7	0.1	0.0	0.1	1.2	0.1	55.1	0.0	96.8
0.1	0.0	5.3	0.4	24.2	67.2	195.3	285.6	0.5	25.2	8.5	0.1	0.0	0.1	1.2	0.1	51.8	0.0	80.4
0.1	0.0	3.4	0.4	15.1	58.0	176.4	2.5	0.3	10.9	5.4	0.0	0.1	0.1	1.4	0.1	30.0	0.0	62.9
0.1	0.0	3.4	0.3	16.0	47.9	123.5	4.2	0.3	18.5	2.6	0.1	0.1	0.1	1.1	0.1	26.0	0.0	64.5
0.1	0.0	107.5	0.9	43.7	42.8	351.1	201.6	0.9	66.4	1.8	0.0	0.1	0.1	1.2	0.1	106.7	0.0	63.4
0.0	0.0	5.6	0.1	4.8	8.4	59.2	0.8	0.1	2.8	1.1	0.0	0.0	0.0	0.0	0.0	5.6	0.0	38.6
0.0	0.0	5.9	0.3	12.9	21.8	245.5	236.6	0.1	5.9	1.3	0.0	0.1	0.0	0.6	0.1	14.3	0.0	90.9
0.0	0.0	0.4	0.0	0.7	1.1	11.1	0.2	0.0	0.4	0.1	0.0	0.0	0.0	0.0	0.0	1.0	0.0	4.7
0.0	0.0	110.0	1.2	32.0	165.0	340.0	12.0	1.2	0.0	13.0	0.0	0.1	0.1	0.3	0.2	24.3	0.0	60.0
0.0	0.0	44.5	1.6	23.2	51.5	211.1	9.8	0.4	0.0	0.0	0.0	0.0	0.2	1.8	0.0	10.6	0.0	4.1
0.0	0.0	0.0	0.0	0.5	3.4	11.4	0.1	0.0	0.0	0.4	0.0	0.0	0.0	0.1	0.0	0.9	0.0	2.7
0.0	0.0	2.2	0.3	10.1	20.9	84.2	172.8	1.0	0.0	0.2	0.0	0.0	0.0	1.1	0.1	15.0	0.0	60.1
0.0	0.0	0.7	0.2	1.4	10.4	42.7	28.6	0.1	0.0	0.5	0.0	0.0	0.0	0.5	0.0	2.2	0.0	10.9
0.0	0.0	4.4	0.3	6.0	26.4	51.6	170.0	0.3	0.0	0.0	0.0	0.0	0.0	0.6	0.0	4.9	0.0	36.4
0.6	0.0	671.6	4.9	175.8	168.4	503.2	16.7	1.2	4993.2	20.5	3.7	0.1	0.7	4.4	0.7	153.6	0.0	135.6
1.9	0.0	30.4	1.5	0.0	87.2	185.6	226.1	0.0	40.5	28.8	0.0	0.1	0.3	1.8	0.0	0.0	0.0	45.4
0.0	0.0	4.7	0.3	3.1	5.3	14.3	34.5	0.1	0.0	0.6	0.0	0.0	0.0	0.0	0.0	3.2	0.0	7.3
0.0	0.0	46.8	0.6	11.7	18.2	148.2	168.4	0.2	481.0	26.7	0.0	0.0	0.0	0.3	0.1	8.6	0.0	59.3
0.0	0.0	21.3	0.3	16.2	38.3	289.0	218.5	0.3	3.4	45.9	0.0	0.0	0.0	0.3	0.1	10.3	0.0	76.8
0.0	0.0	29.2	0.1	2.6	5.1	32.5	29.9	0.0	109.6	4.2	0.0	0.0	0.0	0.1	0.0	1.5	0.0	10.0
0.0	0.0	37.2	1.4	17.4	21.1	107.9	12.4	0.1	6.2	5.2	0.0	0.0	0.0	0.2	0.1	30.1	0.0	112.6
0.0	0.0	37.2	1.4	17.4	21.1	107.9	305.0	0.1	6.2	5.2	0.0	0.0	0.0	0.2	0.1	30.1	0.0	112.6
0.1	0.0	14.0	3.1	35.0	153.0	284.0	10.0	1.6	4.0	12.6	0.0	0.2	0.1	1.2	0.2	67.0	0.0	68.7
0.0	0.0	1.6	0.0	0.7	1.2	12.9	0.3	0.0	4.9	0.4	0.0	0.0	0.0	0.0	0.0	3.7	0.0	4.8
0.0	0.0	3.6	0.1	0.6	4.5	29.0	0.8	0.0	26.0	2.4	0.0	0.0	0.0	0.1	0.0	13.6	0.0	9.5
0.1	0.0	61.6	1.6	29.2	64.8	511.9	29.2	0.7	106.9	12.6	0.9	0.1	0.1	0.6	0.1	181.4	0.0	310.7
0.0	0.0	38.1	0.8	6.2	14.0	147.8	5.0	0.2	106.4	10.1	0.2	0.0	0.0	0.2	0.0	27.9	0.0	52.6
0.0	0.0	0.7	0.0	0.9	3.6	45.0	1.1	0.0	0.0	0.0	0.0	0.0	0.0	0.0	0.0	1.1	0.0	7.0
0.9	0.0	3.1	0.2	1.9	8.1	12.9	37.5	0.0	2.3	0.1	0.0	0.0	0.0	0.4	0.0	6.6	0.0	2.9
0.0	0.0	2.4	0.0	0.9	2.9	16.2	1.8	0.0	0.5	0.4	0.0	0.0	0.0	0.0	0.0	2.0	0.0	13.8
0.0	0.0	12.9	0.1	4.6	15.2	81.1	1.1	0.1	0.0	3.8	0.1	0.0	0.0	0.0	0.1	8.3	0.0	0.2
0.0	0.0	28.1	0.4	22.0	52.4	278.9	7.6	0.2	0.0	9.9	0.8	0.1	0.0	0.6	0.1	44.2	0.0	59.1
0.1	0.0	31.3	1.8	29.6	92.2	174.0	15.7	1.2	66.1	17.1	0.7	0.2	0.1	1.5	0.1	49.6	0.0	149.5
0.1	0.0	18.4	0.8	12.8	39.2	126.4	243.2	0.4	620.8	6.5	0.0	0.2	0.1	0.9	0.1	20.8	0.0	68.6
0.0	0.0	33.6	1.6	20.8	44.0	192.0	192.0	0.3	10.4	38.3	0.0	0.1	0.1	0.4	0.1	23.3	0.0	71.1
0.0	0.0	21.6	1.2	31.2	93.6	216.8	191.2	1.0	48.0	11.4	0.0	0.2	0.1	1.6	0.2	50.6	0.0	62.3
0.1	0.0	17.0	0.8	14.5	57.0	147.1	1.7	0.6	65.5	8.2	0.3	0.1	0.1	0.6	0.1	37.7	0.0	69.4
0.0	0.0	8.7	0.3	10.5	19.8	158.7	8.1	0.2	21.1	51.3	0.4	0.1	0.0	0.8	0.2	18.0	0.0	56.9
0.0	0.0	25.2	0.9	2.8	7.7	79.1	277.9	0.1	9.1	23.9	0.0	0.0	0.0	0.4	0.1	37.8	0.0	65.3
0.0	0.0	3.2	0.1	4.3	7.8	54.5	0.3	0.1	3.8	25.1	0.0	0.0	0.0	0.3	0.1	14.3	0.0	24.7
0.1	0.0	19.6	1.6	12.8	15.3	164.1	1420.4	0.3	144.5	8.5	0.6	0.0	0.0	0.3	0.2	11.9	0.0	75.6
0.0	0.0	8.0	0.5	7.0	13.0	72.0	4.0	0.1	29.0	41.2	0.0	0.1	0.0	1.1	0.1	9.9	0.0	94.7
0.0	0.0	8.0	0.5	7.0	13.0	72.0	4.0	0.1	334.0	41.2	0.0	0.1	0.0	1.1	0.1	9.9	0.0	94.7
0.0	0.0	0.8	0.0	0.9	1.8	16.5	0.2	0.0	53.0	17.7	0.1	0.0	0.0	0.0	0.0	2.0	0.0	8.6
0.0	0.0	5.7	0.2	6.2	12.5	110.2	1.0	0.1	12.5	95.4	0.0	0.0	0.0	0.5	0.1	13.5	0.0	47.9
0.0	0.0	5.6	0.2	5.0	19.4	49.8	3.8	0.2	5.0	0.6	0.0	0.0	0.0	0.3	0.0	22.2	0.0	10.9
0.1	0.0	0.0	0.5	5.4	18.9	31.1	24.3	0.0	20.3	1.4	0.1	0.0	0.0	0.0	0.0	1.0	0.0	127.0
0.0	0.0	0.0	0.1	1.4	4.9	8.1	422.8	0.0	5.3	0.4	0.1	0.0	0.0	0.0	0.0	0.2	0.0	32.9
0.0	0.0	1.4	0.2	1.4	4.2	11.2	6.3	0.0	4.6	0.4	0.1	0.0	0.0	0.1	0.0	0.4	0.0	22.8
0.0	0.0	4.4	0.1	1.2	2.9	13.1	1.7	0.6	1.4	0.5	0.0	0.0	0.0	0.1	0.0	6.5	0.0	14.4
0.0	0.0	18.8	0.5	7.3	15.1	142.8	15.1	0.0	171.6	9.9	0.6	0.0	0.1	0.4	0.0	17.4	0.0	25.7

Code	Food Name	Unit/Amt	Wt (g)	Energy (Kcal)	Prot (g)	Carb (g)	Fiber (g)	Fat (g)	Mono (g)	Poly (g)
11383	Vege, Potato Mashed, granules w/milk, prep w/water & margarine	½ cup	100	358.0	10.9	77.7	0.0	1.1	0.2	0.3
11672	Vege, Potato Pancakes, homemade	½ cup	105	83.0	2.1	13.8	1.9	2.3	0.7	0.7
11414	Vege, Potato Salad, homemade	1 cup	128	284.2	4.3	39.0	4.1	13.7	5.6	1.0
11410	Vege, Potato Wedges, frozen, USDA Commodity	1 cup	250	357.5	6.7	27.9	3.3	20.5	6.2	9.3
11385	Vege, Potato, Au Gratin, mix, prep w/H₂O, whole milk & butter	⅙ of 5.5 oz package	26	81.6	2.3	19.3	1.1	1.0	0.3	0.0
11376	Vege, Potato, canned, drained	1 potato (2.5"diam)	135	116.1	2.3	27.0	2.7	0.1	0.0	0.1
11675	Vege, Potato, Flesh & Skin cooked in microwave, no salt	½ cup of whole potatoes	150	66.0	1.8	14.8	2.1	0.2	0.0	0.1
11674	Vege, Potato, Flesh & Skin, baked, no salt	1 potato: 2.33 x 4.75"	202	220.2	4.6	51.0	4.8	0.2	0.0	0.1
11363	Vege, Potato, Flesh only, baked, no salt	1 potato: 2.33 x 4.75"	156	145.1	3.1	33.6	2.3	0.2	0.0	0.1
11365	Vege, Potato, Flesh only, boiled in skin, no salt	1 potato (2.5"diam)	136	118.3	2.5	27.4	2.7	0.1	0.0	0.1
11367	Vege, Potato, Flesh only, boiled w/o skin, no salt	1 potato (2.5"diam)	136	118.3	2.5	27.4	2.4	0.1	0.0	0.1
911405	Vege, Potato, French Fries, frozen, fried in oil & lard	10 strips	65	101.4	1.6	15.8	2.0	3.8	2.4	0.4
11403	Vege, Potato, French Fries, frozen, oven heated, no salt	10 strips	50	157.5	2.0	19.8	1.6	8.3	4.0	0.5
11391	Vege, Potato, Hashed Brown, plain, frozen, cooked	4.0 oz	115	94.3	2.4	20.4	1.6	0.7	0.0	0.3
11930	Vege, Potato, Mashed, dried flakes w/o milk, prep w/whole milk & margarine	½ cup	105	118.7	2.0	15.8	2.4	5.9	1.7	0.3
11371	Vege, Potato, Mashed, homemade w/milk & margarine	½ cup	105	113.4	2.2	15.1	2.3	5.2	2.1	1.4
11396	Vege, Potato, O'Brien, frozen	½ cup	105	111.3	2.0	17.5	2.1	4.4	1.2	0.2
11387	Vege, Potato, Scalloped, mix, prep w/H₂O, whole milk & butter	⅙ of 5.5 oz package	26	93.1	2.0	19.2	2.2	1.2	0.0	0.5
11364	Vege, Potato, Skin only, baked, no salt	skin from 1 potato: 2.33 x 4.75"	58	114.8	2.5	26.7	4.6	0.1	0.0	0.0
11401	Vege, Potato, whole, frozen, boiled, drained, no salt	3.5 oz	100	65.0	2.0	14.5	1.4	0.1	0.0	0.1
11426	Vege, Pumpkin Pie Mix, canned	½ cup	39	7.4	1.2	0.9	0.0	0.2	0.0	0.0
11424	Vege, Pumpkin, canned, no salt	½ cup	122	41.5	1.3	9.9	3.5	0.3	0.0	0.0
11952	Vege, Radicchio, raw	1 cup	43	6.9	0.6	1.5	0.0	0.1	0.0	0.0
11676	Vege, Radish Sprouts, raw	1 cup, shredded	40	9.2	0.6	1.8	0.4	0.1	0.0	0.0
11430	Vege, Radish, Oriental (Daikon) raw	1 cup	116	314.4	9.2	73.5	0.0	0.8	0.1	0.4
11439	Vege, Sauerkraut, canned, solids & liquid	1 cup, slices	133	109.1	4.4	24.7	4.4	0.3	0.0	0.0
11677	Vege, Shallots, peeled, raw	¼ cup	3.6	12.5	0.4	2.9	0.0	0.0	0.0	0.0
11452	Vege, Soybean Sprouts, mature seeds, sprouted, raw	3.5 oz	100	72.0	2.5	16.8	0.0	0.1	0.0	0.0
11853	Vege, Soybeans, Green, boiled w/salt, drained	½ cup	47	38.1	4.0	3.1	0.4	2.1	0.5	1.2
11461	Vege, Spinach, canned, drained	½ cup	60	13.8	1.8	2.3	1.4	0.2	0.0	0.1
11463	Vege, Spinach, chopped or leaf, frozen	½ cup	117	22.2	2.5	3.4	2.6	0.4	0.0	0.2
11457	Vege, Spinach, raw	10 oz package	220	61.6	6.9	11.7	6.6	0.5	0.0	0.2
11484	Vege, Squash, Acorn, boiled, drained, no salt	1 cup	30	6.6	0.9	1.1	0.8	0.1	0.0	0.0
11486	Vege, Squash, Butternut, baked, no salt	1 cup	30	12.0	0.3	3.1	0.0	0.0	0.0	0.0
11493	Vege, Squash, Spaghetti, boiled or baked, drained, no salt	1 cup, cubes	205	55.4	1.4	13.2	2.9	0.5	0.0	0.3
11642	Vege, Squash, Summer, All Varieties, boiled, drained, no salt	½ cup	77	15.4	0.7	3.3	1.1	0.2	0.0	0.1
11641	Vege, Squash, Summer, All Varieties, slices, raw	½ cup	90	18.0	0.8	3.9	1.3	0.3	0.0	0.1
11644	Vege, Squash, Winter, All Varieties, baked, no salt	½ cup	190	74.1	1.7	16.6	5.3	1.2	0.1	0.5
11872	Vege, Succotash (corn & lima beans) frozen, boiled w/salt, drained	1 large: 3.12 x 0.6"	16	18.4	0.8	3.9	0.0	0.1	0.0	0.1
11508	Vege, Sweet Potato, baked in skin, no salt	½ cup	96	98.9	1.7	23.3	2.9	0.1	0.0	0.0
11659	Vege, Sweet Potato, Candied, homemade	½ cup	164	172.2	2.7	39.8	3.0	0.5	0.0	0.2
11647	Vege, Sweet Potato, canned w/syrup, drained	½ cup	164	224.7	1.4	45.7	3.9	5.3	1.0	0.2
11954	Vege, Tomatillos, raw	1 can (No. 3 vacuum/404 x 307)	638	280.7	26.5	43.7	0.0	4.3	0.4	1.8
11540	Vege, Tomato Juice, canned, w/salt	½ cup, sliced	68	21.8	0.7	4.0	1.3	0.7	0.1	0.3
11887	Vege, Tomato Paste, canned w/salt	½ cup, chopped	67	11.4	0.5	2.8	0.3	0.0	0.0	0.0
11888	Vege, Tomato Puree, canned w/salt	½ cup	131	395.6	16.9	97.8	21.6	0.6	0.1	0.2
11549	Vege, Tomato Sauce, canned	½ cup	123	39.4	1.6	8.7	1.7	0.5	0.1	0.2
11533	Vege, Tomato, Red, canned, stewed	1 slice or wedge	20	3.2	0.2	0.6	0.2	0.0	0.0	0.0
11531	Vege, Tomato, Red, canned, whole	1 tomato	111	31.1	1.1	7.5	1.1	0.1	0.0	0.1
11883	Vege, Tomato, Red, Cherry, ripe, raw, Jun-Oct	½ cup	123	23.4	1.1	5.4	1.2	0.2	0.0	0.1
11660	Vege, Tomato, Red, ripe, stewed	1 tbsp	15	4.1	0.2	0.9	0.2	0.1	0.0	0.0
11885	Vege, Tomato, Red, ripe, whole, canned, no added salt	1 medium	123	97.2	2.4	16.1	2.1	3.3	1.3	1.1
11529	Vege, Tomato, Red, ripe, whole, raw	yield from recipe	604	114.8	5.6	26.4	6.0	0.8	0.1	0.3
11537	Vege, Tomato, Red, w/green chilies, canned	½ cup	123	25.8	1.0	5.7	1.4	0.4	0.1	0.2
11955	Vege, Tomato, Sun-dried	½ cup	123	32.0	1.0	7.8	0.0	0.2	0.0	0.1
11956	Vege, Tomato, Sun-dried, oil packed, drained	1 cup	261	673.4	36.8	145.5	32.1	7.8	1.3	2.9
11565	Vege, Turnip, boiled, drained, no salt	1 piece	3	0.6	0.0	0.1	0.1	0.0	0.0	0.0
11590	Vege, Waterchestnut, Chinese, canned, solids & liquid	10 oz package, mashed	284	309.6	13.6	66.9	21.9	1.8	0.0	0.0
11578	Vegetable Juice Cocktail, canned	3.5 oz	100	48.0	0.6	11.0	0.2	0.2	0.0	0.0
11159	Vegetable Salad, Coleslaw, homemade	1 cup	241	48.2	1.7	10.2	1.7	0.1	0.0	0.1
11581	Vegetables, Mixed, canned, drained solids	½ cup	60	41.4	0.8	7.4	0.9	1.6	0.4	0.8
924281	Vegetarian Manicotti	10 oz package	275	162.3	7.9	36.0	12.1	0.4	0.0	0.2
22246	Vegetarian, Beef Stew, canned entree/Nestle Chef-Mate	1 serving	71	190.3	14.0	21.0	0.0	5.3	1.7	1.3
22121	Vegetarian, Better'n Burgers/Vegan Burgers, frozen/Worthington, Morningstar	1 patty	38	28.9	2.3	2.9	0.5	0.9	0.4	0.0
22126	Vegetarian, Big Franks, meatless, frozen/Worthingfoods, Loma Linda	1 patty	85	91.0	13.9	7.5	4.3	0.5	0.3	0.2
22122	Vegetarian, Breakfast Patties/Worthington, Morningstar	1 patty	38	88.2	9.0	1.1	1.1	5.3	1.1	2.7
22363	Vegetarian, Breakfast Stuff-Its, egg & cheese pockets, frozen/SunnyFresh	1 patty	38	79.4	9.9	3.7	2.0	2.8	0.7	1.3
22120	Vegetarian, Burger Crumbles/Worthington, Morningstar	1 serving	64	147.2	6.8	14.7	1.0	7.6	0.9	0.6
924269	Vegetarian, Chili Mac/Worthington	1 cup	110	231.0	22.2	6.6	5.1	12.9	4.6	4.9

Sat (g)	Chol (mg)	Cal (mg)	Iron (mg)	Magn (mg)	Phos (mg)	Pota (mg)	Sodi (mg)	Zinc (mg)	Vit A (RE)	Vit C (mg)	Vit E (mg)	Thia (mg)	Ribo (mg)	Niac (mg)	Vit B-6 (mg)	Fol (µg)	Vit B-12 (µg)	Wat (g)
0.5	2.0	142.0	3.5	74.0	237.0	1848.0	82.0	1.2	9.0	16.0	0.0	0.2	0.3	4.2	0.9	29.9	0.0	6.3
0.7	2.1	32.6	0.6	16.8	46.2	351.8	245.7	0.3	13.7	3.2	0.0	0.0	0.1	0.8	0.2	7.5	0.0	85.5
6.5	0.0	38.4	2.0	24.3	61.4	486.4	954.9	0.4	2.6	8.8	0.1	0.3	0.1	2.8	0.3	21.1	0.0	67.7
3.6	170.0	47.5	1.6	37.5	130.0	635.0	1322.5	0.8	82.5	25.0	0.0	0.2	0.2	2.2	0.4	16.8	0.0	190.0
0.6	0.0	80.9	0.4	16.6	105.0	257.4	544.7	0.2	18.7	4.0	0.0	0.0	0.1	1.1	0.0	10.5	0.0	1.3
0.0	0.0	10.8	0.4	27.0	54.0	442.8	325.4	0.4	0.0	10.0	0.1	0.1	0.0	1.8	0.4	12.0	0.0	104.6
0.0	0.0	58.5	1.1	21.0	33.0	307.5	325.5	0.6	0.0	11.4	0.1	0.1	0.0	1.3	0.2	6.8	0.0	131.7
0.1	0.0	20.2	2.7	54.5	115.1	844.4	492.9	0.6	0.0	26.1	0.0	0.2	0.1	3.3	0.7	22.2	0.0	143.8
0.0	0.0	7.8	0.5	39.0	78.0	610.0	376.0	0.5	0.0	20.0	0.0	0.2	0.0	2.2	0.5	14.2	0.0	117.7
0.0	0.0	6.8	0.4	29.9	59.8	515.4	326.4	0.4	0.0	17.7	0.1	0.1	0.0	2.0	0.4	13.6	0.0	104.7
0.0	0.0	6.8	0.4	29.9	59.8	515.4	5.4	0.4	0.0	17.7	0.1	0.1	0.0	2.0	0.4	13.6	0.0	104.7
0.6	0.0	3.9	0.6	11.1	41.6	211.9	15.0	0.2	0.0	6.4	0.1	0.1	0.0	1.1	0.2	7.8	0.0	43.3
3.4	6.5	9.5	0.4	17.0	46.5	366.0	108.0	0.2	0.0	5.2	0.0	0.1	0.0	1.6	0.1	14.5	0.0	19.0
0.2	0.0	11.5	1.1	12.7	54.1	327.8	25.3	0.2	0.0	9.4	0.0	0.1	0.0	1.9	0.1	4.8	0.0	90.7
3.6	14.7	51.5	0.2	18.9	58.8	244.7	348.6	0.2	22.1	10.2	0.7	0.1	0.1	0.7	0.0	7.8	0.1	80.1
1.3	3.2	36.8	0.2	20.0	63.0	152.3	276.2	0.3	21.0	6.3	0.0	0.1	0.0	0.8	0.0	7.4	0.0	81.4
2.9	12.6	27.3	0.3	18.9	48.3	303.5	309.8	0.3	21.0	6.4	0.0	0.1	0.0	1.1	0.2	8.3	0.0	80.1
0.3	1.3	16.1	0.5	15.3	51.2	235.3	410.3	0.2	0.0	4.3	0.1	0.0	0.0	1.2	0.0	8.2	0.0	1.6
0.0	0.0	19.7	4.1	24.9	58.6	332.3	149.1	0.3	0.0	7.8	0.0	0.1	0.1	1.8	0.4	12.5	0.0	27.4
0.0	0.0	7.0	0.8	11.0	26.0	287.0	256.0	0.3	0.0	9.4	0.0	0.1	0.0	1.3	0.2	8.4	0.0	82.8
0.1	0.0	15.2	0.9	14.8	40.6	170.0	4.3	0.1	75.7	4.3	0.0	0.0	0.0	0.4	0.1	14.1	0.0	36.2
0.2	0.0	31.7	1.7	28.1	42.7	251.3	294.0	0.2	2691.3	5.1	0.0	0.0	0.1	0.4	0.1	15.0	0.0	109.8
0.0	0.0	28.0	0.9	29.2	18.9	212.4	19.4	0.1	56.8	9.0	0.0	0.0	0.0	0.2	0.0	4.9	0.0	40.4
0.0	0.0	7.6	0.2	5.2	16.0	120.8	8.8	0.2	1.2	3.2	0.9	0.0	0.0	0.1	0.0	24.0	0.0	37.3
0.3	0.0	729.6	7.8	197.2	236.6	4053.0	322.5	2.5	0.0	0.0	0.0	0.3	0.8	3.9	0.7	341.9	0.0	22.8
0.0	0.0	79.8	0.9	30.6	99.8	505.4	26.6	0.5	0.0	10.6	0.0	0.1	0.3	0.7	0.4	35.0	0.0	102.4
0.0	0.0	6.6	0.2	3.7	10.7	59.4	2.1	0.1	202.0	1.4	0.0	0.0	0.0	0.0	0.1	4.2	0.0	0.1
0.0	0.0	37.0	1.2	21.0	60.0	334.0	12.0	0.4	119.0	8.0	0.0	0.1	0.0	0.2	0.3	34.2	0.0	79.8
0.3	0.0	27.7	0.6	28.2	63.5	166.9	4.7	0.5	0.5	3.9	0.0	0.1	0.0	0.5	0.0	37.6	0.0	37.3
0.0	0.0	81.6	2.1	52.2	33.6	279.6	42.0	0.5	491.4	5.9	0.6	0.1	0.1	0.3	0.1	87.5	0.0	54.7
0.1	0.0	97.1	1.8	65.5	37.4	269.1	87.8	0.5	752.3	15.8	1.1	0.0	0.1	0.3	0.1	67.9	0.0	109.1
0.1	0.0	321.2	3.3	151.8	105.6	655.6	708.4	1.5	1711.6	27.1	0.0	0.1	0.4	0.9	0.3	236.5	0.0	198.0
0.0	0.0	29.7	0.8	23.7	14.7	167.4	23.7	0.2	201.6	8.4	0.6	0.0	0.1	0.2	0.1	58.3	0.0	27.5
0.0	0.0	12.3	0.2	8.7	8.1	85.2	72.0	0.0	210.0	4.5	0.0	0.0	0.0	0.3	0.0	5.8	0.0	26.3
0.1	0.0	43.1	0.7	22.6	0.0	239.9	520.7	0.4	22.6	7.2	0.0	0.1	0.0	1.7	0.2	16.4	0.0	189.2
0.0	0.0	20.8	0.3	18.5	30.0	147.8	182.5	0.3	22.3	4.2	0.0	0.0	0.0	0.4	0.1	15.5	0.0	72.1
0.1	0.0	24.3	0.3	21.6	35.1	172.8	0.9	0.4	26.1	5.0	0.1	0.0	0.0	0.5	0.1	18.1	0.0	84.3
0.2	0.0	26.6	0.6	15.2	38.0	830.3	450.3	0.5	676.4	18.2	0.0	0.2	0.0	1.3	0.1	53.2	0.0	169.1
0.0	0.0	2.7	0.2	8.5	18.7	65.6	40.5	0.1	4.6	1.3	0.0	0.0	0.0	0.2	0.0	5.2	0.0	10.9
0.0	0.0	26.9	0.4	19.2	52.8	334.1	236.2	0.3	2094.7	23.6	0.3	0.1	0.1	0.6	0.2	21.7	0.0	69.9
0.1	0.0	34.4	0.9	16.4	44.3	301.8	21.3	0.4	2796.2	28.0	0.5	0.1	0.2	1.0	0.4	18.2	0.0	119.5
2.2	13.1	42.6	1.9	18.0	42.6	310.0	114.8	0.2	687.2	11.0	0.0	0.0	0.1	0.6	0.1	18.7	0.0	109.8
0.9	0.0	950.6	10.0	325.4	427.5	3974.7	1850.2	0.6	1122.9	242.4	0.0	0.3	1.3	3.1	0.7	45.9	0.0	551.6
0.1	0.0	4.8	0.4	13.6	26.5	182.2	0.7	0.1	7.5	8.0	0.3	0.0	0.0	1.3	0.0	4.8	0.0	62.3
0.0	0.0	6.0	0.4	7.4	12.7	147.4	241.9	0.1	37.5	12.3	0.6	0.0	0.0	0.5	0.1	13.3	0.0	62.9
0.1	0.0	217.5	6.0	233.2	386.5	2524.4	175.5	2.2	2259.8	152.9	0.7	1.2	1.0	12.0	0.6	157.1	0.0	4.0
0.1	0.0	12.3	0.8	24.6	51.7	458.8	18.5	0.2	98.4	26.4	0.0	0.1	0.1	1.5	0.2	11.6	0.0	109.6
0.0	0.0	1.0	0.1	1.6	5.8	42.4	8.4	0.0	30.0	3.2	0.0	0.0	0.0	0.1	0.0	5.8	0.0	19.0
0.0	0.0	36.6	0.8	13.3	22.2	264.2	245.3	0.2	59.9	12.7	0.4	0.1	0.0	0.8	0.0	6.0	0.0	101.0
0.0	0.0	36.9	0.7	14.8	23.4	271.8	182.0	0.2	73.8	17.5	0.4	0.1	0.0	0.9	0.1	9.6	0.0	115.2
0.0	0.0	0.9	0.1	2.1	4.7	41.9	1.7	0.0	11.1	3.4	0.1	0.0	0.0	0.1	0.0	2.0	0.0	13.8
0.6	0.0	32.0	1.3	18.5	46.7	303.8	559.7	0.2	82.4	22.4	1.6	0.1	0.1	1.4	0.1	13.5	0.0	99.2
0.1	0.0	181.2	3.3	72.5	114.8	1371.1	60.4	1.0	362.4	85.8	2.3	0.3	0.2	4.4	0.5	47.1	0.0	565.6
0.1	0.0	6.2	0.6	13.5	29.5	273.1	11.1	0.1	76.3	23.5	0.5	0.1	0.1	0.8	0.1	18.5	0.0	115.3
0.0	0.0	32.0	0.6	13.5	28.3	308.7	266.9	0.2	71.3	18.2	0.0	0.1	0.0	0.8	0.1	12.4	0.0	112.9
1.1	0.0	287.1	23.7	506.3	929.2	8944.5	5468.0	5.2	227.1	102.3	0.0	1.4	1.3	23.6	0.9	177.5	0.0	38.0
0.0	0.0	0.7	0.0	0.2	0.6	4.1	8.6	0.0	0.0	0.3	0.0	0.0	0.0	0.0	0.0	0.3	0.0	2.8
0.0	0.0	363.5	2.9	196.0	227.2	1613.1	48.3	4.6	14.2	119.0	0.0	0.4	0.3	2.1	0.8	51.1	0.0	196.3
0.0	0.0	12.0	0.6	22.0	78.0	90.0	362.0	1.1		4.1	0.0	0.0	0.0	0.2	0.1	15.9	30.6	87.4
0.0	0.0	31.8	1.5	0.0	67.5	508.5	732.3	0.5	611.2	49.0	0.0	0.1	0.1	1.6	0.5	0.0	0.0	0.0
0.2	4.8	27.0	0.4	6.0	19.2	108.6	13.8	0.1	49.2	19.6	0.0	0.0	0.0	0.2	0.1	15.9	0.0	48.9
0.1	0.0	68.8	2.3	60.5	140.3	464.8	96.3	1.3	1177.0	8.8	1.0	0.2	0.3	2.3	0.2	52.3	0.0	228.9
1.3	128.5	39.8	0.7	3.6	88.8	68.2	283.3	0.3	0.0	0.0	0.2	0.0	0.2	0.1	0.0	0.0	0.4	29.2
0.3	4.9	9.5	0.2	5.3	23.9	58.5	179.0	0.4	46.7	0.4	0.1	0.0	0.0	0.5	0.0	0.0	0.1	31.4
0.1	0.0	86.7	2.9	16.2	181.1	433.5	382.5	0.7	0.0	0.0	0.0	0.3	0.6	4.1	0.2	245.7	0.0	60.6
0.6	0.0	7.6	0.7	0.0	63.1	45.2	166.8	0.9	0.0	0.0	0.0	0.2	0.5	4.3	0.5	0.0	2.2	21.9
0.5	0.8	18.2	1.9	1.1	106.4	101.8	259.2	0.4	0.0	0.0	0.3	5.4	0.1	1.8	0.2	0.0	1.5	20.4
3.1	93.4	62.7	0.9	2.6	38.4	30.7	233.0	0.2	65.3	0.0	0.1	0.1	0.2	1.5	0.0	0.0	0.2	34.4
3.3	0.0	79.2	6.4	2.2	173.8	178.2	476.3	1.6	0.0	0.0	0.7	9.9	0.4	3.0	0.5	0.0	4.4	66.3

Code	Food Name	Unit/Amt	Wt (g)	Energy (Kcal)	Prot (g)	Carb (g)	Fiber (g)	Fat (g)	Mono (g)	Poly (g)
22215	Vegetarian, Chili w/beans, canned entree/Nestle Chef-Mate	1 cup	220	316.8	11.5	22.9	0.0	19.9	0.0	0.0
924060	Vegetarian, Chili w/beans/Worthington	1 cup	253	412.4	17.7	29.0	11.1	25.0	10.7	1.4
22216	Vegetarian, Chili w/o beans, canned entree/Nestle Chef-Mate	1 cup	220	323.4	14.1	20.6	6.0	20.6	0.0	0.0
22217	Vegetarian, Corned Beef Hash, canned entree/Nestle Chef-Mate	1 cup	250	430.0	18.6	17.6	3.0	31.6	13.6	1.8
22119	Vegetarian, Deli Franks/Worthington, Morningstar	1 cup	253	485.8	24.2	29.1	6.1	30.3	14.7	1.1
22118	Vegetarian, Garden Patties, frozen/Worthington, Morningstar	1 patty	67	166.2	15.5	5.5	4.1	9.2	2.9	4.9
22125	Vegetarian, Harvest Burger, Original Flavor, vege protein patty, original flavor	1 patty	90	160.2	15.1	13.7	5.4	5.1	1.4	2.9
22223	Vegetarian, Macaroni And Cheese, canned entree/Nestle Chef-Mate	1 patty	90	137.3	18.0	7.0	5.7	4.1	0.0	0.0
22127	Vegetarian, Natural Touch Garden Vege Patty, frozen/Worthington	1 cup	253	283.4	10.8	35.4	3.3	11.0	3.0	0.5
22128	Vegetarian, Natural Touch Vegan Burgers, frozen/Worthington	1 cup	252	448.6	42.2	38.4	15.1	14.2	4.0	8.1
22360	Vegetarian, Sandwich, Egg & Cheese Biscuit, pre-ckd, frozen/SunnyFresh	1 patty	85	91.0	13.9	7.5	4.3	0.5	0.3	0.2
22361	Vegetarian, Sandwich, Egg, Ham & Cheese Biscuit, pre-ckd, frozen/SunnyFresh	1 serving	99	223.7	9.9	24.6	0.0	8.9	1.1	3.7
22224	Vegetarian, Sausage N' Shells, canned entree/Nestle Chef-Mate	½ cup	121	244.4	12.3	25.3	0.1	9.8	1.2	3.8
22123	Vegetarian, Spicy Black Bean Burger/Worthington, Morningstar	1 patty	78	117.8	4.6	5.8	0.3	8.5	3.8	1.1
22218	Vegetarian, Spicy Chili With Beans, canned entree/Nestle Chef-Mate	1 cup	253	371.9	38.2	49.3	15.4	2.5	0.8	1.1
924030	Vegetarian, Stew, Beef Vegetable/Worthington	1 cup	253	422.5	16.9	32.8	4.3	24.7	10.7	1.1
18367	Waffle, Plain, homemade	1 lg	75	217.5	4.6	26.4	1.1	10.3	0.0	0.0
18365	Waffle, Plain/Buttermilk, frozen, ready-to-heat	1 sm	34	98.9	2.7	11.2	0.0	4.8	1.2	2.3
1072	Whipped Dessert Topping, Nondairy, pressurized can	2 tbsp	7	13.2	0.3	1.2	0.0	0.9	0.1	0.0
1073	Whipped Dessert Topping, Nondairy, semi solid, frozen	1 tbsp	4	10.5	0.0	0.6	0.0	0.9	0.1	0.0
901913	Whipped Topping, Nondairy/Cool Whip	2 tbsp	9	28.6	0.1	2.1	0.0	2.3	0.1	0.0
19393	Yogurt, Frozen, Chocolate, soft serve	½ cup	72	129.6	2.9	14.4	0.0	5.8	1.4	0.0
19293	Yogurt, Frozen, Vanilla, soft serve	½ cup	72	115.2	2.9	17.9	1.6	4.3	1.3	0.2
1121	Yogurt, Lowfat w/fruit, 10g protein/8 oz	8.0 oz	227	360.9	9.1	54.9	0.0	12.7	3.6	0.5
1117	Yogurt, Lowfat, Plain, 12g protein/8 oz	8.0 oz	227	225.3	9.0	42.3	0.0	2.6	0.7	0.1
1119	Yogurt, Lowfat, Vanilla, 11g protein/8 oz	8.0 oz	227	143.7	11.9	16.0	0.0	3.5	1.0	0.1
901906	Yogurt, Lowfat, Yoplait	6 oz.	170	145.3	8.4	23.5	0.0	2.1	0.6	0.1
1118	Yogurt, Nonfat, Skim, 13g protein/8 oz	8.0 oz	227	276.9	10.4	52.6	2.7	4.3	1.3	0.8
901909	Yogurt, Whole Milk w/fruit	8.0 oz	227	120.3	13.0	18.0	0.0	0.0	0.0	0.0
1116	Yogurt, Whole Milk, Plain, 8g protein/8 oz	8.0 oz	227	256.5	9.6	42.6	0.0	7.9	2.6	0.2
				0.0	0.0	0.0	0.0	0.0	0.0	0.0

Sat (g)	Chol (mg)	Cal (mg)	Iron (mg)	Magn (mg)	Phos (mg)	Pota (mg)	Sodi (mg)	Zinc (mg)	Vit A (RE)	Vit C (mg)	Vit E (mg)	Thia (mg)	Ribo (mg)	Niac (mg)	Vit B-6 (mg)	Fol (µg)	Vit B-12 (µg)	Wat (g)
0.0	0.0	28.0	1.9	28.0	136.0	337.0	854.0	2.0	490.0	4.0	0.0	0.1	0.5	3.5	0.1	40.0	2.0	154.2
10.9	55.7	88.6	4.8	45.5	167.0	511.1	1171.4	3.9	301.1	0.8	1.2	0.1	0.2	3.5	0.2	0.0	1.4	175.8
0.0	0.0	55.0	2.4	53.0	236.0	593.0	926.0	2.0	738.0	4.0	0.0	0.1	0.8	2.5	0.2	30.0	0.0	151.5
14.4	85.0	67.5	4.5	45.0	162.5	530.0	1587.5	4.5	302.5	1.8	1.6	0.1	0.3	4.8	0.3	0.0	1.8	176.4
13.4	88.6	45.5	3.0	38.0	240.4	536.4	1593.9	7.5	0.0	1.5	0.3	0.2	0.3	6.3	0.6	0.0	2.5	163.9
1.3	0.7	25.5	0.9	5.4	63.0	74.4	641.2	0.6	0.0	0.0	1.9	0.2	0.0	0.0	0.0	0.0	0.0	34.6
0.7	0.9	64.8	1.6	39.6	166.5	241.2	513.0	0.8	102.6	0.0	1.3	8.7	0.1	0.0	0.0	38.7	0.0	53.9
1.0	0.0	101.7	3.9	0.0	0.0	0.0	411.3	0.0	0.0	0.0	0.0	0.0	0.0	0.0	0.0	0.0	0.0	58.5
6.2	27.8	202.4	1.9	32.9	250.5	151.8	1343.4	1.6	55.7	0.0	0.2	0.3	0.3	2.5	0.1	0.0	0.2	191.3
2.0	2.5	181.4	4.6	110.9	466.2	675.4	1436.4	2.2	287.3	0.0	3.7	24.3	0.4	0.0	0.0	0.0	0.0	150.9
0.1	0.0	86.7	2.9	16.2	181.1	433.5	382.5	0.7	0.0	0.0	0.0	0.3	0.6	4.1	0.2	245.7	0.0	60.6
2.4	110.9	101.0	2.2	3.0	49.5	39.6	563.3	0.3	57.4	0.0	2.0	0.2	0.3	2.0	0.0	0.0	0.3	53.0
2.6	115.0	106.5	2.5	3.6	54.5	47.2	728.4	0.3	59.3	0.1	2.4	0.2	0.3	2.0	0.0	0.0	0.3	70.2
2.7	16.4	12.5	1.0	6.4	64.7	293.3	304.2	0.7	42.1	0.0	1.4	0.2	0.1	2.0	0.2	0.0	0.4	57.9
0.6	2.5	182.2	6.0	141.7	485.8	872.9	1619.2	3.0	45.5	0.0	1.2	26.1	0.5	0.0	0.7	0.0	0.2	152.9
10.7	55.7	83.5	5.4	53.1	177.1	647.7	1485.1	2.8	210.0	1.3	2.1	0.1	0.1	3.0	0.3	0.0	0.9	172.9
5.2	2.7	93.0	1.2	15.0	252.0	134.3	458.3	0.4	19.5	0.2	0.0	0.2	0.2	1.2	0.1	9.0	0.2	31.9
1.0	23.5	86.7	0.8	6.5	64.6	54.1	173.7	0.2	22.1	0.1	0.0	0.1	0.1	0.7	0.0	15.6	0.1	14.3
0.7	0.7	6.3	0.0	0.7	6.0	10.5	4.6	0.0	3.4	0.0	0.0	0.0	0.0	0.0	0.0	0.3	0.0	4.7
0.8	0.0	0.2	0.0	0.0	0.7	0.8	2.5	0.0	1.9	0.0	0.0	0.0	0.0	0.0	0.0	0.0	0.0	2.4
2.0	0.0	0.6	0.0	0.2	0.7	1.6	2.3	0.0	7.7	0.0	0.0	0.0	0.0	0.0	0.0	0.0	0.0	4.5
4.3	14.4	72.0	0.0	14.4	57.6	100.8	57.6	0.3	28.8	0.0	0.0	0.0	0.1	0.0	0.0	0.0	0.1	47.5
2.6	3.6	105.8	0.9	19.4	100.1	187.9	70.6	0.4	31.0	0.2	0.1	0.0	0.2	0.2	0.1	7.9	0.2	45.9
7.8	4.5	324.6	0.7	31.8	292.8	479.0	197.5	1.0	129.4	1.8	0.1	0.1	0.5	0.7	0.2	13.6	0.7	148.2
1.7	10.2	313.9	0.1	30.1	246.7	402.0	120.8	1.5	27.2	1.4	0.1	0.1	0.4	0.2	0.1	19.3	1.0	170.9
2.3	13.8	414.5	0.2	39.6	325.7	530.7	159.4	2.0	36.3	1.8	0.1	0.1	0.5	0.3	0.1	25.4	1.3	193.1
1.4	8.3	291.2	0.1	27.9	228.8	372.8	111.9	1.4	22.1	1.3	0.1	0.1	0.3	0.2	0.1	17.9	0.9	134.3
2.1	13.4	0.0	0.0	0.0	0.0	475.4	121.5	0.0	0.0	0.0	0.0	0.0	0.0	0.0	0.0	0.0	0.0	0.0
0.0	5.0	0.0	0.0	0.0	0.0	590.0	160.0	0.0	0.0	0.0	0.0	0.0	0.0	0.0	0.0	0.0	0.0	0.0
5.1	30.9	292.0	0.1	0.0	229.1	374.1	111.9	1.4	59.5	1.1	0.0	0.1	0.3	0.2	0.1	18.1	0.9	0.0
0.0	0.0	0.0	0.0	0.0	0.0	0.0	0.0	0.0	0.0	0.0	0.0	0.0	0.0	0.0	0.0	0.0	0.0	

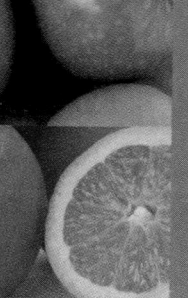

Appendix B

Dietary Advice for Canadians

Excellent World Wide Web resources for Canadians are Health Canada (hc-sc.gc.ca), Dietitians of Canada (www.dietitians.ca), and the National Institute of Nutrition (www.nin.ca).

The following chart (Table B.1) includes information on macronutrients from the Recommended Nutrient Intakes (RNIs) listed in *The Report of the Scientific Review Committee,* last published in 1990. Previous RNIs for micronutrients have been replaced by the Dietary Reference Intakes (DRIs) set by the Food and Nutrition Board of the National Academy of Sciences that apply to Canadian and U.S. citizens. These are listed on the inside cover. Both Canadian and American scientists worked on the various DRI committees, coming up with a set of harmonized Dietary Reference Intakes for both countries. The remaining DRIs for macronutrients are still under development, so these older RNIs for energy, protein, and omega-3 and omega-6 fatty acids, listed on the next page, remain as the current standard for Canadians.

Summary of the Nutrition Recommendations for Canadians

1. *The Canadian diet should provide energy consistent with the maintenance of body weight within the recommended range.* Physical activity should be appropriate to circumstances and capabilities. Although the importance of maintaining some activity throughout life can be stressed, it is not possible to specify a level of physical activity for the whole population. As a general guideline, it is desirable that adults, for as long as possible, maintain an activity level that permits an energy intake of at least 1800 kcal while keeping weight within the recommended range.
2. *The Canadian diet should include essential nutrients in amounts recommended in this report.* Although it is important that the diet provide the recommended amounts of nutrients, it should be understood that no evidence was found that intakes in excess of the RNI confer any health benefit. There is no general need for supplements, except for vitamin D for infants and folate during pregnancy. Vitamin D supplementation might be required for older persons not exposed to the sun and iron for pregnant women with low iron stores.
3. *The Canadian diet should include no more than 30% of energy as fat (33 grams per 1000 kcal) and no more than 10% as saturated fat (11 grams per 1000 kcal).* Dietary cholesterol, though not as influential in affecting blood cholesterol, is not without importance. A reduction in cholesterol intake normally will accompany a reduction in total fat and saturated fat. The recommendation to reduce total fat intake does not apply to children under the age of 2 years.
4. *The Canadian diet should provide 55% of energy as carbohydrate (138 grams per 1000 kcal) from a variety of sources.* Sources should be selected that provide complex carbohydrates, a variety of dietary fiber, and beta-carotene.
5. *The sodium content of the Canadian diet should be reduced.* The present food supply provides sodium in an amount greatly exceeding requirements. Although insufficient evidence exists to support a precise recommendation, potential benefit would be expected from a reduction in current sodium intake.
6. *The Canadian diet should include no more than 5% of total energy as alcohol, or two drinks daily, whichever is less.* The harmful influence of alcohol on blood pressure provides a more urgent reason for moderation. During pregnancy, it is prudent to abstain from alcoholic beverages because a safe intake is not known with certainty.

Table B.1 Summary of Examples of Recommended Macronutrient Intakes Based on Energy Expressed As Daily Rates

Age	Gender	Energy (kcal)	Protein (grams)	ω-3 PUFA* (grams)	ω-6 PUFA (grams)
Months					
0–4	Both	600	12[†]	0.50	3.0
5–12	Both	900	12	0.50	3.0
Years					
1	Both	1100	13	0.60	4.0
2–3	Both	1300	16	0.70	4.0
4–6	Both	1800	19	1.00	6.0
7–9	M	2200	26	1.20	7.0
	F	1900	26	1.00	6.0
10–12	M	2500	34	1.40	8.0
	F	2200	36	1.20	7.0
13–15	M	2800	49	1.50	9.0
	F	2200	46	1.20	7.0
16–18	M	3200	58	1.80	11.0
	F	2100	47	1.20	7.0
19–24	M	3000	61	1.60	10.0
	F	2100	50	1.20	7.0
25–49	M	2700	64	1.50	9.0
	F	1900	51	1.10	7.0
50–74	M	2300	63	1.30	8.0
	F	1800	54	1.10[‡]	7.0[‡]
75+	M	2000	59	1.10	7.0
	F[SS]	1700	55	1.10[‡]	7.0[‡]
Pregnancy (additional)					
1st trimester		100	5	0.05	0.3
2nd trimester		300	20	0.16	0.9
3rd trimester		300	24	0.16	0.9
Lactation		450	20	0.25	1.5

*PUFA, polyunsaturated fatty acids

[†]Protein is assumed to be from breast milk and must be adjusted for infant formula.

[‡]Level below which intake should not fall

[SS]Assumes moderate physical activity

From Scientific Review Committee: *Nutrition recommendations*. Ottawa, Canada, 1990. Health and Welfare.

7. *The Canadian diet should contain no more caffeine than the equivalent of four regular cups of coffee per day.* This is a prudent measure in view of the increased risk for cardiovascular disease associated with high intakes of caffeine.
8. *Community water supplies containing less fluoride than 1 milligram per liter should be fluoridated to that level.* Fluoridation of community water supplies has proven to be a safe, effective, and economical method of improving dental health.

In essence, suggested actions toward healthful eating as listed in Canada's Guidelines for Healthy Eating include the following:

- Enjoy a variety of foods.
- Emphasize cereals, breads, other grain products, vegetables, and fruits.
- Choose low-fat dairy products, lean meats, and foods prepared with little or no fat.
- Achieve and maintain a healthful body weight by enjoying regular physical activity and healthful eating.
- Limit salt, alcohol, and caffeine.

The *Canadian Food Guide* is a guide to help Canadians make wise food choices (Fig. B-1). The rainbow side of the Food Guide places foods into four groups: grain products;

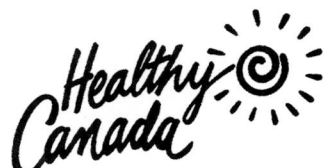

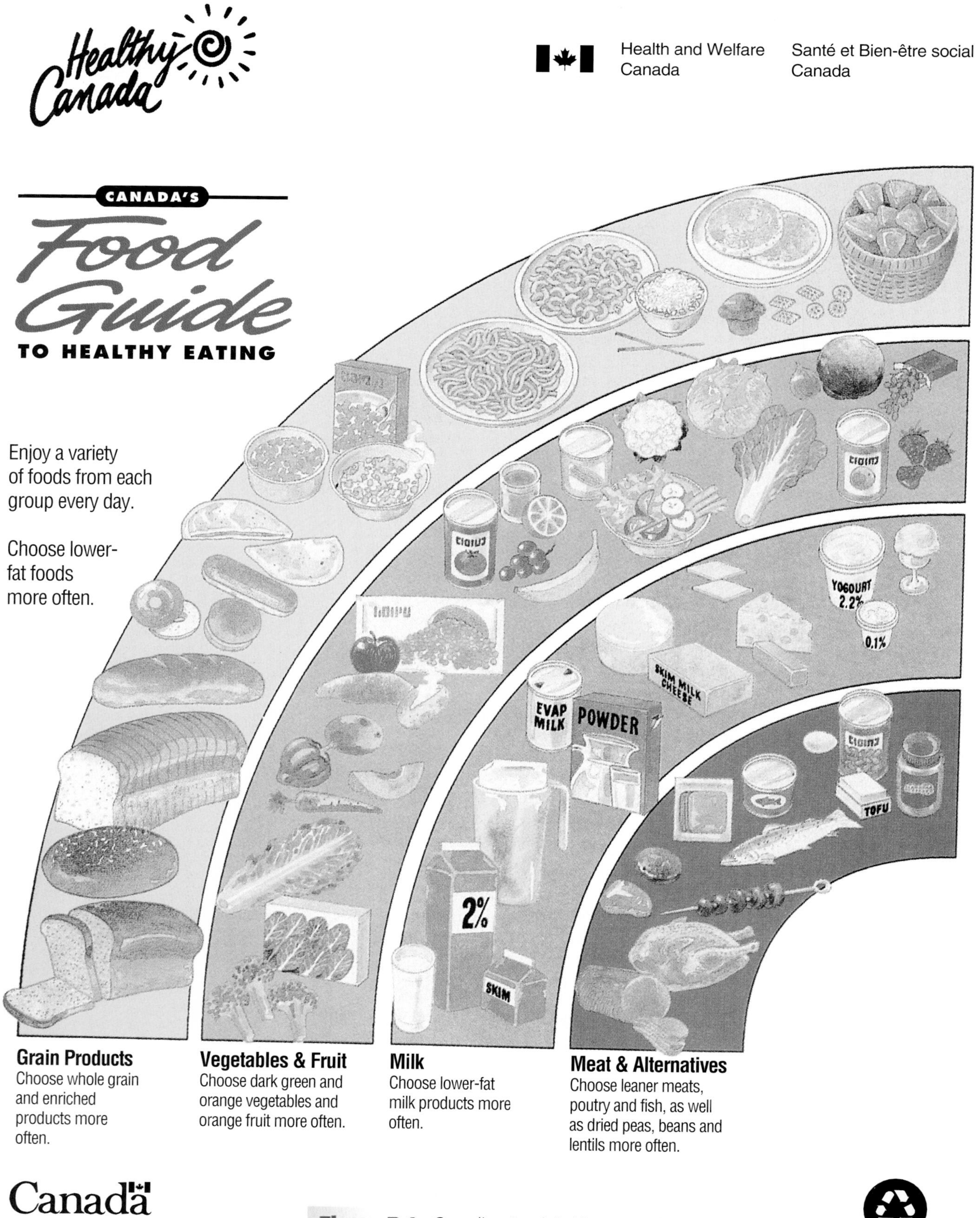
Healthy Canada
Health and Welfare Canada
Santé et Bien-être social Canada
CANADA'S
Food Guide
TO HEALTHY EATING
Enjoy a variety of foods from each group every day.
Choose lower-fat foods more often.
YOGOURT 2.2%
0.1%
SKIM MILK CHEESE
EVAP MILK
POWDER
2%
SKIM
TOFU
Grain Products
Choose whole grain and enriched products more often.
Vegetables & Fruit
Choose dark green and orange vegetables and orange fruit more often.
Milk
Choose lower-fat milk products more often.
Meat & Alternatives
Choose leaner meats, poutry and fish, as well as dried peas, beans and lentils more often.
Canada

Figure B.1 Canadian Food Guide to Healthy Eating

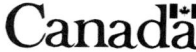

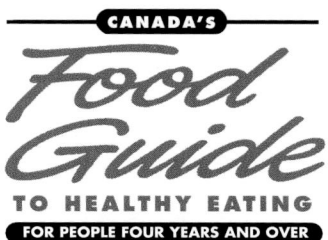

CANADA'S

Food Guide

TO HEALTHY EATING

FOR PEOPLE FOUR YEARS AND OVER

Different People Need Different Amounts of Food

The amount of food you need every day from the four food groups and other foods depends on your age, body size, activity level, whether you are male or female and if you are pregnant or breastfeeding. That's why the Food Guide gives a lower and higher number of servings for each food group. For example, young children can choose the lower number of servings, while male teenagers can go to the higher number. Most other people can choose servings somewhere in between.

Grain Products

5–12

SERVINGS PER DAY

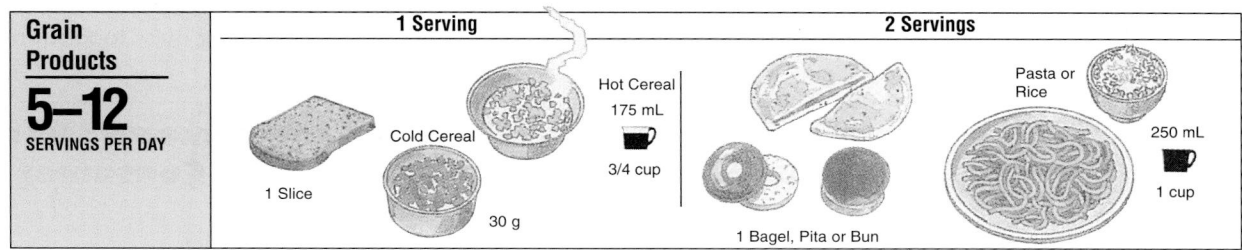

Vegetables & Fruit

5–10

SERVINGS PER DAY

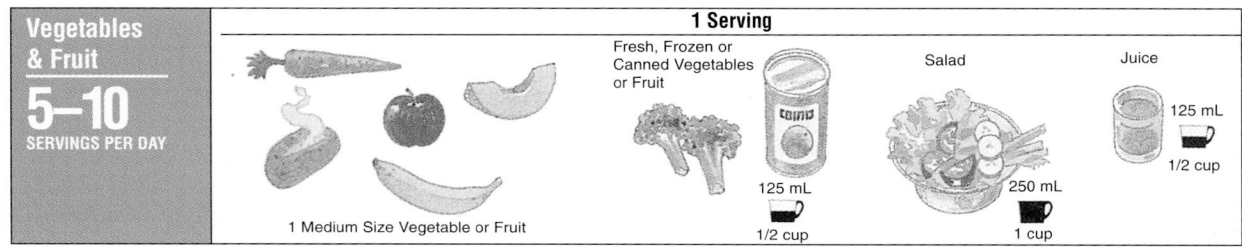

Milk Products

SERVINGS PER DAY

Children 4–9 years: 2-3
Youth 10–16 years: 3–4
Adults: 2-4
Pregnant & Breast-feeding
Women: 3-4

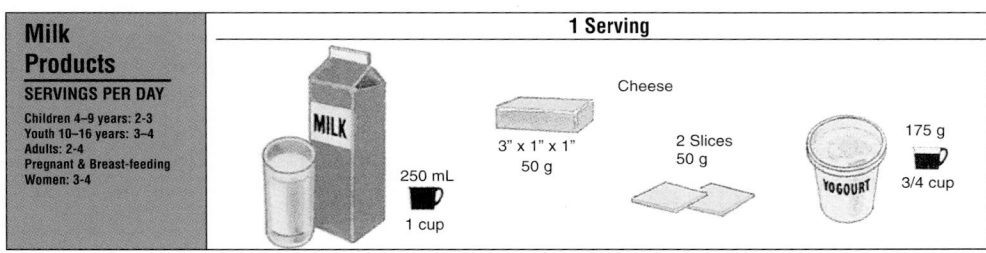

Other Foods

Taste and enjoyment can also come from other foods and beverages that are not part of the 4 food groups. Some of these foods are higher in fat or Calories, so use these foods in moderation.

Meat & Alternatives

2–3

SERVINGS PER DAY

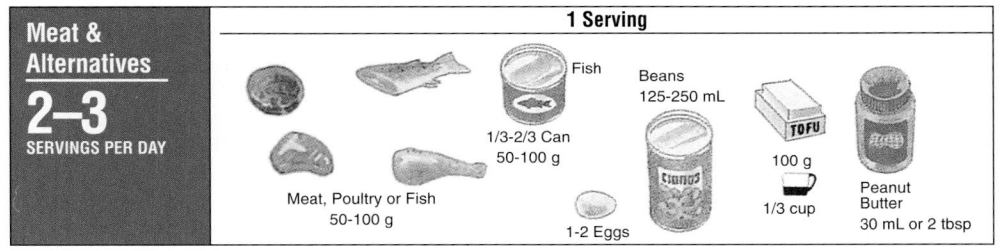

Enjoy eating well, being active, and feeling good about yourself. That's VITALITé®

© Minister of Supply and Services Canada 1992   Cat. No. H39-252 / 1992E   No changes permitted. Reprint permission not required.
ISBN 0-662-19648-1

Figure B.1 Concluded

vegetables and fruit; milk products; and meat and meat alternatives. The rainbow includes information about the types of foods to choose from each food group for healthy eating.

The bar side of the Food Guide helps Canadians decide how much they need from each group every day. The guide gives a range for the number of servings for each food group, since different people need different amounts of food. The Food Guide also shows serving sizes for different foods.

The bar side of the Food Guide also tells how other foods that are not part of the four food groups can have a role in healthy eating. Since some of these "other foods" are higher in fat or calories, the Food Guide recommends using these foods in moderation.

Canada's Basic Labeling Requirements: Under the Food and Drugs Act and the Consumer Packaging and Labeling Act

In general, prepackaged products must show the following basic label information:

1. THE COMMON NAME. This is either the name by which the food is generally known (e.g., orange drink, vanilla cookies, chocolate candies) or the name prescribed by a regulation (e.g., orange juice from concentrate, 60% whole-wheat bread, milk chocolate, mayonnaise). When a prescribed common name is used, the product must conform to the compositional standard set forth in the regulations. The common name is to be shown on the principal display panel (i.e., main panel) in English and French in a minimum type height of 1.6 millimeters, based on the lower case letter *o*.

2. A Metric Net Quality declaration by volume (e.g., milliliters, liters), weight (e.g., grams, kilograms) or by count, as applicable. The net quantity declaration is to be shown on the principal display panel in English and French. The following symbols are considered to be bilingual:

   grams—g
   kilograms—k
   milliliters—ml or mL
   liters—l or L

A minimum type height of 1.6 millimeters, based on the lowercase letter *o*, is required for all information in the net declaration, except for the numbers, which are to be shown in boldface type of not less than the following height:

a. 1/16 inch (1.6 millimeters), where the principal display surface of the container is not more than 5 square inches (32 square centimeters)

b. 1/8 inch (3.2 millimeters), where the principal display surface of the container is more than 5 square inches (32 square centimeters) but not more than 40 square inches (258 square centimeters)

c. 1/4 inch (6.4 millimeters), where the principal display surface of the container is more than 40 square inches (258 square centimeters) but not more than 100 square inches (645 square centimeters)

d. 3/8 inch (9.5 millimeters), where the principal display surface of the container is more than 100 square inches (645 square centimeters) but not more than 400 square inches (25.8 square decimeters) and

e. 1/2 inch (12.7 millimeters), where the principal display surface of the container is more than 400 square inches (25.8 square decimeters)

Additional nonmetric declarations (e.g., fluid ounces, pounds) are not required but may be shown grouped with the metric statement provided they are not false or misleading.

3. A LIST OF INGREDIENTS and their components (i.e., ingredients of ingredients) in descending order of proportion by weight. Spices, seasonings, and herbs except salt, natural and artificial flavors, flavor enhancers, food additives, and vitamin and mineral nutrients may be shown at the end of the list in any order. Some components are completely exempt from a component declaration, whereas others are exempt depending on the amount used. Components of natural or artificial flavoring preparations, seasonings, and spice or herb mixtures are:

a. flavor enhancers
b. salt
c. food additives that affect the finished product
d. Food additives listed in Table X of Division 16 of the Food and Drug Regulations must be shown in the ingredient list as if they were an ingredient of the finished food.

An ingredient or component must be shown in the list of ingredients by its common name. The list of ingredients is to be shown in English and French on any label panel except the bottom. It is required to be displayed clearly and prominently and be readily discernible. A minimum type height of 1.6 millimeter based on the lowercase letter *o* will usually satisfy this requirement.

4. THE NAME AND ADDRESS declaration of the responsible company. The company name must be the legal registered company name. The address should be complete enough for postal purposes and include the name of the country, if other than Canada or USA. This information is to be shown in either English or French on any label panel except the bottom, in a minimum type height of 1.6 millimeter based on the lowercase letter *o*. If only a Canadian company name and address are shown on an imported product that has been wholly manufactured outside of Canada, the Canadian declaration must be preceded by the appropriate terms "imported by/importÈ par" or "imported from/importÈ pour." Alternatively, the country of origin may be declared adjacent to the Canadian company name and address.
5. When a food has a DURABLE LIFE of 90 days or less, a "best before" date and storage instructions if they differ from normal room storage conditions must be declared. Additional information is available upon request.
6. When artificial flavors are used whether alone or with natural flavoring agents and a vignette on the label indicates a natural flavor source (e.g., picture of an apple), information that the added flavoring ingredient is imitation, artificial, or simulated must appear on or adjacent to the vignette in French and English in at least the same type height as required for the numbers in the net quantity.
7. Standard container sizes are specified for wine, glucose and refined sugar syrups, peanut butter, cookies, and biscuits. Specific information is available upon request.

Health Canada, a Canadian government agency, has proposed a new policy on nutrition labeling that would result in important changes to food labels. The proposal is that nutrition labeling will be mandatory on most foods (with some exceptions) and will be consistent in look, easy to find, legible, and readable. Nutrition labels will provide core information on calories, fat, saturated fat, trans fat, cholesterol, sodium, carbohydrate, fiber, sugar, protein, vitamin A, vitamin C, calcium, and iron. These changes will make nutrition information easier to find, more complete, and available on more foods and will allow Canadians to use this basic knowledge to make healthy food choices. The labels should appear on foods sold in Canada over the next few years.

HOW TO READ A CURRENT CANADIAN NUTRITION INFORMATION LABEL

Nutrition information is expressed per **suggested serving**. The serving size will vary according to food type and brand. Consider this fact when comparing foods.

Gives the calorie content (Cal)

Indicates the quantity of naturally occurring and added sugars as well as dietary fibre

Indicates the level of sodium from salt and all other sources

Vitamins and minerals are expressed as a percentage of the highest recommended amount

millilitres:
5 mL = 1 teaspoon

kilojoules:
metric unit of energy
1 Cal = 4.18kJ

grams: 28 g = 1 ounce

LASAGNA
Nutrition Information
per 275 g serving
(1 cup/250 mL)

Energy	275	Cal
	1140	kJ
Protein	19	g
Fat	7	g
Polyunsaturates	0.8	g
Monounsaturates	1.9	g
Saturates	2.5	g
Cholesterol	46	mg
Carbohydrate	34	g
Starch	29	g
Sugars	5	g
Dietary Fibre	0.2	g
Sodium	850	mg
Potassium	675	mg

Percentage of Recommended Daily Intake

Thiamine	20%
Riboflavin	19%
Niacin	18%
Calcium	12%
Iron	28%

Proposed New Canadian Label

Nutrition Facts
Per 1 cup (264g)

Amount	% Daily Value
Calories 260	
Fat 13g	**20**%
Saturated Fat 3g + Trans Fat 2g	**25**%
Cholesterol 30mg	
Sodium 660mg	**28**%
Carbohydrate 31g	**10**%
Fibre 0g	**0**%
Sugars 5g	
Protein 5g	

Vitamin A 4%	Vitamin C 2%
Calcium 15%	Iron 4%

Appendix C

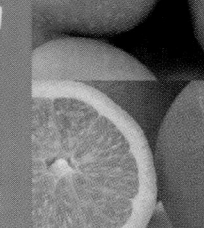

The Exchange System: A Helpful Menu-Planning Tool

The Exchange System

The **Exchange System** is a valuable tool for roughly estimating the energy, protein, carbohydrate, and fat content of a food or meal. This tool organizes many details of the nutrient composition of foods into a manageable framework. By using the Exchange System, you can plan daily menus to fall roughly within specific percentages of macronutrients without having to look up or memorize the nutrient values of numerous foods, so the time you spend now becoming familiar with the Exchange System will pay dividends in the future.

In the Exchange System, individual foods are placed into three broad groups: carbohydrate, meat and meat substitutes, and fat. Within these groups are lists that contain foods of similar macronutrient composition: various types of milk; fruit; vegetables; starch; other carbohydrates; meat and meat substitutes; and fat. These lists are designed so that, when the proper serving size is observed, each food on a list provides about the same amount of carbohydrate, protein, fat, and energy. This equality allows the exchange of foods on each list, hence the term *Exchange System*.

The Exchange System was originally developed for planning diabetic diets. Diabetes is easier to control if the person's diet has about the same composition day after day. If a certain number of **exchanges** from each of the various lists is eaten each day, that regularity is easier to achieve. However, because the Exchange System provides a quick way to estimate the energy, carbohydrate, protein, and fat content in any food or meal, it is a valuable menu-planning tool.

Becoming Familiar with the Exchange System

To use the Exchange System, you must know which foods are on each list and the serving sizes for each food.

Table C.1 gives the serving sizes for foods on each exchange list, as well as the carbohydrate, protein, fat, and energy content per exchange. Note that the meat and milk lists are divided into subclasses, which vary in fat content and, hence, in the amount of energy they provide. Foods on the meat and fat lists contain essentially no carbohydrate; those on the fruit and fat lists lack appreciable amounts of protein; and those on the vegetable, fruit, and other carbohydrates lists contain essentially no fat. You need to study Table C.1 and Figure C.1 to become familiar with the exchange lists, the sizes of the exchanges (that is, serving sizes) on each list, and the amounts of carbohydrate, protein, fat, and energy per exchange.

Before you can turn a group of exchanges into a daily meal plan, you must be aware of which foods are on each exchange list (Figure C.1). The entire U.S. Exchange System is presented in Appendix D, which you should consult frequently while exploring the system to discover its various peculiarities. For example, the starch list includes not only bread, dry cereal, cooked cereal, rice, and pasta, but also baked beans, corn on the cob, and potatoes. These foods are not identical to those composing the bread, cereal, rice, and pasta group in the Food Guide Pyramid. The Exchange System is not concerned with the origin of a food, whether animal or vegetable. It is primarily concerned with the macronutrients carbohydrate, protein, and fat in each food on a specific list. For example, the carbohydrate composition of potatoes resembles that of bread more than that of broccoli, although potatoes are vegetables. In addition, several foods on the

Exchange System *A system for classifying foods into numerous lists based on the foods' macronutrient composition and establishing serving sizes, so that one serving of each food on a list contains the same amount of carbohydrate, protein, fat, and energy content.*

exchange *The serving size of a food on a specific exchange list.*

Table C.1 Nutrient Composition of Exchange System Lists (1995 Edition)

Groups/Lists	Household Measures*	Carbohydrate (grams)	Protein (grams)	Fat (grams)	Energy (kcal)
Carbohydrate Group					
Starch	1 slice, ¾ cup raw, or ½ cup cooked	15	3	1 or less†	80
Fruit	1 small/medium piece	15	—	—	60
Milk	1 cup				
Nonfat/very low-fat		12	8	0–3†	90
Low-fat		12	8	5	120
Whole		12	8	8	150
Other carbohydrates	Varies	15	Varies	Varies	Varies
Vegetables	1 cup raw or ½ cup cooked	5	2	—	25
Meat and Meat Substitutes Group	1 ounce				
Very lean		—	7	0–1	35
Lean		—	7	3	55
Medium-fat		—	7	5	75
High-fat		—	7	8	100
Fat Group	1 teaspoon	—	—	5	45

*Just an estimate; see exchange lists for actual amounts.
†Calculated as 1 gram for purposes of energy contribution.

meat and meat substitutes list are not meats. The list of other carbohydrates includes jam, angel food cake, fat-free frozen yogurt, and foods such as frosted cake that count as both other carbohydrate exchanges and fat exchanges. Bacon appears in the fat list, rather than the high-fat meat category.

Free foods (essentially calorie-free) include bouillon, diet soda, coffee, tea, dill pickles, and vinegar, as well as herbs and spices. Most vegetables, such as cabbage, celery, mushrooms, lettuce, and zucchini, also can be considered free foods; their minimal energy contribution need not count in the calculations when they are eaten in moderation (1 to 2 servings per meal or snack).

▪ Using the Exchange System to Develop Daily Menus

Now let's use the Exchange System to plan a 1-day menu. Let's target an energy content of 2000 kcal, with 55% derived from carbohydrates (1100 kcal), 15% from protein (300 kcal), and 30% from fat (600 kcal). This can be translated into 2 low-fat milk exchanges, 3 vegetable exchanges, 5 fruit exchanges, 11 starch exchanges, 4 lean meat exchanges, and 6 fat exchanges (Table C.2). Note that this is only one of many possible combinations; the Exchange System offers great flexibility.

Table C.3 arbitrarily separates these exchanges into breakfast, lunch, dinner, and a snack. Breakfast includes 1 low-fat milk exchange, 2 fruit exchanges, 2 starch exchanges, and 1 fat exchange. This total corresponds to ¾ cup of a ready-to-eat breakfast cereal, 1 cup of reduced-fat milk, 1 slice of bread with 1 teaspoon margarine, and 1 cup of orange juice.

Lunch consists of 2 fat exchanges, 4 starch exchanges, 1 vegetable exchange, 1 low-fat milk exchange, and 2 fruit exchanges. This translates into one slice of bacon with 1 teaspoon mayonnaise on two slices of bread, with tomato—in other words, a bacon

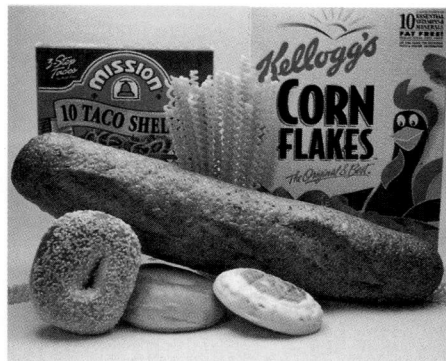

Starch exchange choices

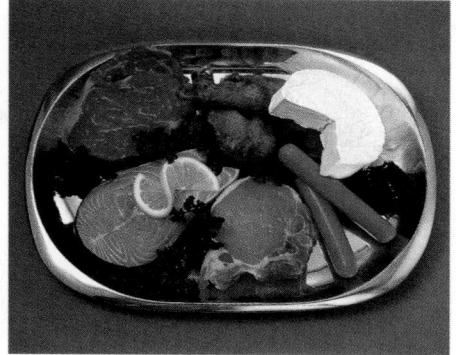

Meat and meat substitutes exchange choices

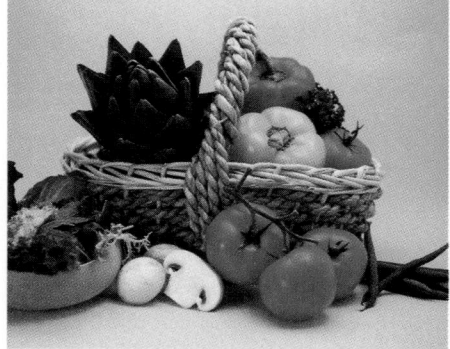

Vegetable exchange choices

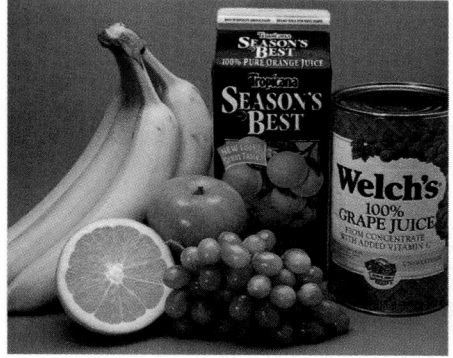

Fruit exchange choices

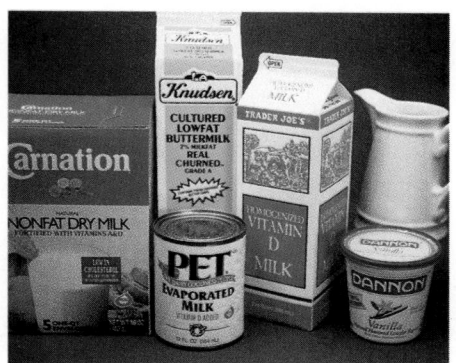

Milk exchange choices

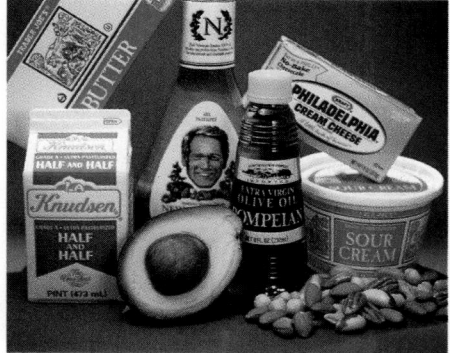

Fat exchange choices

Figure C.1   Foods Arranged According to the Exchange System Lists.

Table C.2 Possible Exchange Patterns That Yield 55% of Energy As Carbohydrate, 30% As Fat, and 15% As Protein for Energy Intakes Greater Than 2000 kcal

Exchange List	kcal/Day						
	1200*	1600*	2000	2400	2800	3200	3600
Milk (low fat)	2	2	2	2	2	2	2
Vegetable	3	3	3	4	4	4	4
Fruit	3	4	5	6	8	9	9
Starch	5	8	11	13	15	18	21
Meat (lean)	4	4	4	5	6	7	8
Fat	2	4	6	8	10	11	13

This is just one set of options. More meat could be included if less milk were used, for example.
*Energy intakes of 1200 and 1600 kcal contain 20% of energy as protein and 50% energy as carbohydrate to allow for greater flexibility in diet planning.

and tomato sandwich. You can also add lettuce to the sandwich. This can be considered a free vegetable choice. Add to this meal a 9-inch banana (1 exchange = 1 small banana), 1 cup of reduced fat milk, and 6 graham crackers (2½ inches by 2½ inches). Later add a snack of ¾ ounce of pretzels for another starch exchange.

Dinner consists of 4 lean meat exchanges, 1 fruit exchange, 2 vegetable exchanges, 1 fat exchange, and 2 starch exchanges. This total corresponds to a 4-ounce broiled steak (meat only, no bone), 1 medium baked potato (1 exchange = 1 small baked potato) with 1 teaspoon of margarine, 1 cup of broccoli, and 1 kiwi fruit. Coffee (if desired) is not counted, since it contains no appreciable energy.

Table C.3 Sample 1-Day 2000 kcal Menu Based on the Exchange System Plan*

Breakfast

1 low-fat milk exchange	1 cup reduced-fat milk (some on cereal)
2 fruit exchanges	1 cup orange juice
2 starch exchanges	¾ cup ready-to-eat breakfast cereal, 1 piece whole-wheat toast
1 fat exchange	1 teaspoon soft margarine on toast

Lunch

4 starch exchanges	2 slices whole-wheat bread, 6 graham crackers (2½ inches by 2½ inches)
2 fat exchanges	1 slice bacon, 1 teaspoon mayonnaise
1 vegetable exchange	1 sliced tomato
2 fruit exchanges	1 banana (9 inches)
1 low-fat milk exchange	1 cup reduced-fat milk

Snack

1 starch exchange	¾ ounce pretzels

Dinner

4 lean meat exchanges	4 ounces lean steak (well trimmed)
2 starch exchanges	1 medium baked potato
1 fat exchange	1 teaspoon soft margarine
2 vegetable exchanges	1 cup cooked broccoli
1 fruit exchange	1 kiwi fruit
	Coffee (if desired)

Snack

2 starch exchanges	1 bagel
2 fat exchanges	2 tablespoons regular cream cheese

*The target plan was a 2000 kcal energy intake, with 55% from carbohydrate, 15% from protein, and 30% from fat. Computer analysis indicates that this menu yielded 2040 kcal, with 53% from carbohydrate, 16% from protein, and 31% from fat—in close agreement with the targeted goals.

Finally, we have a snack containing 2 starch exchanges and 2 fat exchanges. This translates into 1 bagel with 2 tablespoons of regular cream cheese.

This 1-day menu is only one of many that are possible with the exchange lists. Apple juice could replace the orange juice; two apples could be exchanged for the banana. The choices are endless. Notice that an exchange diet is much easier to plan if you use individual foods, as was done here; however, the Exchange System tables list some combination foods to help you (see Appendix D). Using combination foods, such as pizza or lasagna, however, makes it more difficult to calculate the number of exchanges in a serving. For instance, lasagna typically has meat exchanges, vegetable exchanges, and starch exchanges. With experience, you will be able to tackle such complex foods (Fig. C.2). For now, using individual foods makes learning the Exchange System much easier. Finally, you might want to prove to yourself that the food choices listed in Table C.3 really meet the exchange plan. This demonstration will give you practice turning exchanges into actual food servings.

Exchange List	Total Exchanges to Be Consumed Daily	Exchanges Consumed at Each Meal		
		Breakfast	Lunch	Dinner
MILK				
VEGETABLE				
FRUIT				
STARCH				
MEAT AND SUBSTITUTES				
FAT				

Figure C.2   Record the Exchange System pattern you have chosen in the left-hand column. Then distribute the exchanges throughout the day, noting the food to be used and the serving size.

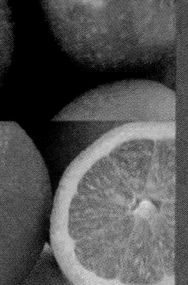

Appendix D

Exchange System Lists

Milk Exchange List

Skim and Very Low-Fat Milk

(12 grams carbohydrate, 8 grams protein, 0–3 grams fat, 90 kcal)

1 cup	skim or nonfat milk (½% and 1%)
⅓ cup	powdered (nonfat dry, before adding liquid)
½ cup	canned, evaporated skim milk
1 cup	buttermilk made from nonfat or low-fat milk
¾ cup	yogurt made from nonfat milk (plain, unflavored)
1 cup	nonfat or low-fat fruit-flavored yogurt sweetened with aspartame or nonnutritive sweetener

Low-Fat Milk

(12 grams carbohydrate, 8 grams protein, 5 grams fat, 120 kcal)

1 cup	2% milk
¾ cup	plain low-fat yogurt (added milk solids)
1 cup	sweet acidophilus milk

Whole Milk

(12 grams carbohydrate, 8 grams protein, 8 grams fat, 150 kcal)

1 cup	whole milk
½ cup	evaporated whole milk
1 cup	goat's milk
1 cup	kefir

Vegetable Exchange List

(5 grams carbohydrate, 2 grams protein, 0 grams fat, 25 kcal)
1 vegetable exchange equals:

½ cup cooked vegetables or vegetable juice
1 cup raw vegetables

artichoke	cucumber	peppers (all varieties)
artichoke hearts	eggplant	radishes
asparagus	green onions or scallions	salad greens
beans (green, wax, Italian)	greens (e.g., collard)	sauerkraut
bean sprouts	kohlrabi	spinach
beets	leeks	squash (summer)
broccoli	mixed vegetables (without corn, peas, or pasta)	tomato (fresh, canned, sauce)
brussels sprouts		tomato/vegetable juice
cabbage	mushrooms	turnips
carrots	okra	water chestnuts
cauliflower	onions	watercress
celery	pea pods	zucchini

Fruit Exchange List

Fruit

(15 grams carbohydrate, 0 grams protein, 0 grams fat, 60 kcal)
1 fruit exchange equals:

1	apple (small)	1	banana (small)	½ cup	cherries, canned
4 rings	apple, dried	¾ cup	blackberries	3	dates
½ cup	applesauce (unsweetened)	¾ cup	blueberries	2	figs, fresh (3½ ounces)
		⅓ melon	cantaloupe (small)	1½	figs, dried
4	apricots, fresh	1 cup cubes	cantaloupe	½ cup	fruit cocktail
8 halves	apricots, dried	12	cherries (3 ounces)	½	grapefruit

The Exchange Lists are the basis of a meal planning system designed by a committee of the American Diabetes Association and The American Dietetic Association. While designed primarily for people with diabetes and others who must follow special diets, the Exchange Lists are based on principles of good nutrition that apply to everyone. Copyright © 1995 by the American Diabetes Association and The American Dietetic Association.

¾ cup	grapefruit sections	½ cup	pear, canned	**Fruit Juice**
17	grapes (small)	¾ cup	pineapple, fresh	½ cup	apple juice/cider
1 slice	honeydew melon (or 1 cup cubes)	½ cup	pineapple, canned	⅓ cup	cranberry juice cocktail
1	kiwi	2	plums (small)	1 cup	cranberry juice cocktail, reduced-calorie
¾ cup	mandarin orange sections	½ cup	plums, canned	⅓ cup	fruit juice blends, 100% juice
½	mango (or ½ cup cubes)	3	prunes, dried	⅓ cup	grape juice
1	nectarine (small)	2 tablespoons	raisins	½ cup	grapefruit juice
1	orange (small)	1 cup	raspberries	½ cup	orange juice
½	papaya (or 1 cup cubes)	1¼ cup	strawberries (raw, whole)	½ cup	pineapple juice
1	peach, fresh (medium)	2	tangerines	⅓ cup	prune juice
½ cup	peaches, canned	1 slice	watermelon (or 1¼ cups cubes)		
½	pear, fresh				

▌ Starch Exchange List

(15 grams carbohydrate, 3 grams protein, 0–1 gram fat, 80 kcal)
1 starch exchange equals:

Bread

½ (1 ounce)	bagel
2 slices (1½ ounces)	bread, reduced-calorie
1 slice (1 ounce)	bread, white, whole-wheat, pumpernickel, or rye
2 (⅔ ounces)	bread sticks, crisp, 4 inches long × 3½ inches
½	English muffin
½ (1 ounce)	hot dog or hamburger bun
½	pita, 6 inches across
1 slice (1 ounce)	raisin bread, unfrosted
1 (1 ounce)	roll, plain (small)
1	tortilla, corn, 6 inches across
1	tortilla, flour, 7–8 inches across
1	waffle, 4½ inches square, reduced-fat

Cereals and Grains

½ cup	bran cereal
½ cup	bulgur
½ cup	cereal
¾ cup	cereal, unsweetened, ready-to-eat
3 tablespoons	cornmeal (dry)
⅓ cup	couscous
3 tablespoons	flour (dry)
¼ cup	granola, low-fat
¼ cup	Grape-Nuts
½ cup	grits
½ cup	kasha
¼ cup	millet
¼ cup	muesli
½ cup	oats
½ cup	pasta
1½ cups	puffed cereal
½ cup	rice milk
⅓ cup	rice, white or brown
½ cup	Shredded Wheat
½ cup	sugar-frosted cereal
3 tablespoons	wheat germ

Starchy Vegetables

⅓ cup	baked beans
½ cup	corn
1 (5 ounces)	corn on the cob (medium)
1 cup	mixed vegetables with corn, peas, or pasta
½ cup	peas, green
½ cup	plantain
1 (3 ounces)	potato, baked or boiled (small)
½ cup	potato, mashed
1 cup	squash, winter (acorn, butternut)
½ cup	yam, sweet potato, plain

Crackers and Snacks

8	animal crackers
3	graham crackers, 2½-inch square
¾ ounce	matzoh
4 slices	melba toast
24	oyster crackers
3 cups	popcorn (popped, no fat added or low-fat microwave)
¾ ounce	pretzels
2	rice cakes, 4 inches across
6	saltine-type crackers
15–20 (¾ ounce)	snack chips, fat-free (tortilla, potato)
2–5 (¾ ounce)	whole-wheat crackers, no fat added

Dried Beans, Peas, and Lentils

(counts as 1 starch exchange plus 1 very lean meat exchange)

½ cup	beans and peas (garbanzo, pinto, kidney, white, split, black-eyed)
⅔ cup	lima beans
½ cup	lentils
3 tablespoons	miso

Starchy Foods Prepared with Fat
(counts as 1 starch exchange plus 1 fat exchange)

1	biscuit, 2½ inches across
½ cup	chow mein noodles
1 (2 ounces)	corn bread, 2-inch cube
6	crackers, round butter type
1 cup	croutons
16–25 (3 ounces)	French-fried potatoes
¼ cup	granola
1 (1½ ounces)	muffin (small)
2	pancakes, 4 inches across
3 cups	popcorn, microwave
3	sandwich crackers, cheese or peanut butter filling
⅓ cup	stuffing, bread (prepared)
2	taco shells, 6 inches across
1	waffle, 4½-inch square
4–6 (1 ounce)	whole-wheat crackers, fat added

■ Other Carbohydrates Exchange List

One exchange equals 15 grams carbohydrate, or 1 starch, or 1 fruit, or 1 milk.

Exchanges per Serving

¹⁄₁₂th cake	angel food cake, unfrosted	2 carbohydrates
2-inch square	brownie, unfrosted (small)	1 carbohydrate, 1 fat
2-inch square	cake, unfrosted	1 carbohydrate, 1 fat
2-inch square	cake, frosted	2 carbohydrates, 1 fat
2	cookies, fat-free (small)	1 carbohydrate
2	cookies or sandwich cookies with creme filling (small)	1 carbohydrate, 1 fat
¼ cup	cranberry sauce, jellied	1½ carbohydrates
1	cupcake, frosted (small)	2 carbohydrates, 1 fat
1 (1½ ounces)	doughnut, plain cake (medium)	1½ carbohydrates, 2 fats
3¾ inches across (2 ounces)	doughnuts, glazed	2 carbohydrates, 2 fats
1 bar (3 ounces)	fruit juice bars, frozen, 100% juice	1 carbohydrate
1 roll (¾ ounce)	fruit snacks, chewy (puréed fruit concentrate)	1 carbohydrate
1 tablespoon	honey	1 carbohydrate
1 tablespoon	sugar	1 carbohydrate
1 tablespoon	fruit spread, 100% fruit	1 carbohydrate
½ cup	gelatin, regular	1 carbohydrate
3	gingersnaps	1 carbohydrate
1 bar	granola bar	1 carbohydrate, 1 fat
1 bar	granola bar, fat-free	2 carbohydrates
⅓ cup	hummus	1 carbohydrate, 1 fat
½ cup	ice cream	1 carbohydrate, 2 fats
½ cup	ice cream, light	1 carbohydrate, 1 fat
½ cup	ice cream, fat-free, no sugar added	1 carbohydrate
1 tablespoon	jam or jelly, regular	1 carbohydrate
1 cup	milk, chocolate, whole	2 carbohydrates, 1 fat
⅙ pie	pie, fruit, 2 crusts	3 carbohydrates, 2 fats
⅛ pie	pie, pumpkin or custard	1 carbohydrate, 2 fats
12–18 (1 ounce)	potato chips	1 carbohydrate, 2 fats
½ cup	pudding, regular (made with low-fat milk)	2 carbohydrates
½ cup	pudding, sugar-free (made with low-fat milk)	1 carbohydrate
¼ cup	salad dressing, fat-free	1 carbohydrate
½ cup	sherbet, sorbet	2 carbohydrates
½ cup	spaghetti or pasta sauce, canned	1 carbohydrate, 1 fat
1 (2½ ounces)	sweet roll or Danish	2½ carbohydrates, 2 fats
2 tablespoons	syrup, light	1 carbohydrate
1 tablespoon	syrup, regular	1 carbohydrate
6–12 (1 ounce)	tortilla chips	1 carbohydrate, 2 fats
5	vanilla wafers	1 carbohydrate, 1 fat
⅓ cup	yogurt, frozen, low-fat or fat-free	1 carbohydrate, 0–1 fat
½ cup	yogurt, frozen, fat-free, no sugar added	1 carbohydrate
1 cup	yogurt, low-fat, with fruit	3 carbohydrates, 0–1 fat

■ Meat and Meat Substitutes Exchange List

Very Lean Meat and Substitutes List

(0 grams carbohydrate, 7 grams protein, 0–1 gram fat, and 35 kcal)
One very lean meat exchange equals:

	Poultry		**Cheese with 1 gram or less fat per ounce**
1 ounce	chicken or turkey (white meat, no skin), Cornish hen (no skin)	¼ cup	nonfat or low-fat cottage cheese
		1 ounce	fat-free cheese
	Fish		**Other**
1 ounce	fresh or frozen cod, flounder, haddock, halibut, trout; tuna, fresh or canned in water	1 ounce	processed sandwich meats with 1 gram or less fat per ounce, such as deli thin, shaved meats, chipped beef, turkey, ham
	Shellfish	2	egg whites
1 ounce	clams, crab, lobster, scallops, shrimp, imitation shellfish	¼ cup	egg substitute, plain
		1 ounce	hot dogs with 1 gram or less fat per ounce
		1 ounce	kidney (high in cholesterol)
	Game	1 ounce	sausage with 1 gram or less fat per ounce
1 ounce	duck or pheasant (no skin), venison, buffalo, ostrich		

Counts as one very lean meat and one starch exchange:
½ cup   dried beans, peas, lentils (cooked)

Lean Meat and Substitutes List

(0 grams carbohydrate, 7 grams protein, 3 grams fat, and 55 kcal)
One lean meat exchange equals:

	Beef		**Fish**
1 ounce	USDA Select or Choice grades of lean beef trimmed of fat, such as round, sirloin, and flank steak; tenderloin; roast (rib, chuck, rump); steak (T-bone, porterhouse, cubed), ground round	1 ounce	herring (uncreamed or smoked)
		6	oysters (medium)
		1 ounce	salmon (fresh or canned), catfish
		2	sardines (canned, medium)
		1 ounce	tuna (canned in oil, drained)
	Pork		**Game**
1 ounce	lean pork, such as fresh ham; canned, cured, or boiled ham; Canadian bacon; tenderloin, center loin chop	1 ounce	goose (no skin), rabbit
			Cheese
	Lamb	¼ cup	4.5%–fat cottage cheese
1 ounce	roast, chop, leg	2 tablespoons	grated Parmesan
		1 ounce	cheeses with 3 grams or less fat per ounce
	Veal		**Other**
1 ounce	lean chop, roast	1½ ounce	hot dogs with 3 grams or less fat per ounce
	Poultry	1 ounce	processed sandwich meat with 3 grams or less fat per ounce, such as turkey pastrami or kielbasa
1 ounce	chicken, turkey (dark meat, no skin), chicken white meat (with skin), domestic duck or goose (well drained of fat, no skin)	1 ounce	liver, heart (high in cholesterol)

Medium-Fat Meat and Substitutes List

(0 grams carbohydrate, 7 grams protein, 5 grams fat, and 75 kcal)
One medium-fat meat exchange equals:

	Beef		**Pork**
1 ounce	most beef products (ground beef, meatloaf, corned beef, short ribs, prime grades of meat trimmed of fat, such as prime rib)	1 ounce	top loin, chop, Boston butt, cutlet
			Lamb
		1 ounce	rib roast, ground

	Veal		**Cheese (with 5 grams or less fat per ounce)**
1 ounce	cutlet (ground or cubed, unbreaded)	1 ounce	feta
		1 ounce	mozzarella
	Poultry	¼ cup (2 ounces)	ricotta
1 ounce	chicken dark meat (with skin), ground turkey or ground chicken, fried chicken (with skin)		**Other**
		1	egg (high in cholesterol, limit to 3 per week)
	Fish	1 ounce	sausage with 5 grams or less fat per ounce
1 ounce	any fried fish product	1 cup	soy milk
		¼ cup	tempeh
		4 ounces or ½ cup	tofu

High-Fat Meat and Substitutes List

(0 grams carbohydrate, 7 grams protein, 8 grams fat, and 100 kcal)
One high-fat meat exchange equals:

	Pork	1 ounce	sausage, such as bratwurst, Italian, knockwurst, Polish, smoked
1 ounce	spareribs, ground pork, pork sausage	1 (10 per pound)	hot dog (turkey or chicken)
	Cheese	3 slices (20 slices per pound)	bacon
1 ounce	all regular cheeses, such as American, cheddar, Monterey Jack, Swiss		
	Other	Counts as one high-fat meat plus one fat exchange:	
1 ounce	processed sandwich meats with 8 grams or less fat per ounce, such as bologna, pimento loaf, salami	1 (10 per pound)	hot dog (beef, pork, or combination)
		2 tablespoons	peanut butter (contains unsaturated fat)

■ Fat Exchange List

Monosaturated Fats List

(5 grams fat and 45 kcal)
One exchange equals:

⅛ (1 ounce)	avocado (medium)	6 nuts	almonds, cashews
1 teaspoon	oil (canola, olive, peanut)	6 nuts	mixed (50% peanuts)
	olives:	10 nuts	peanuts
8	ripe, black (large)	4 halves	pecans
10	green, stuffed (large)	2 teaspoons	peanut butter, smooth or crunchy
		1 tablespoon	sesame seeds
		2 teaspoons	tahini paste

Polyunsaturated Fats List

(5 grams fat and 45 kcal)
One exchange equals:

	margarine:	1 teaspoon	oil (corn, safflower, soybean)
1 teaspoon	stick, tub, or squeeze		salad dressing:
1 tablespoon	lower-fat (30 to 50% vegetable oil)	1 tablespoon	regular
	mayonnaise:	2 tablespoons	reduced-fat
1 teaspoon	regular		Miracle Whip Salad Dressing®:
1 tablespoon	reduced-fat	2 teaspoons	regular
4 halves	nuts, walnuts, English	1 tablespoon	reduced-fat
		1 tablespoon	seeds: pumpkin, sunflower

Saturated Fats List

(5 grams fat and 45 kcal)
One exchange equals:

1 slice (20 slices per pound)	bacon, cooked	2 tablespoons	chitterlings, boiled (½ ounce)
1 teaspoon	bacon, grease	2 tablespoons	coconut, sweetened, shredded
	butter:	2 tablespoons	cream, half and half
1 teaspoon	stick		
2 teaspoons	whipped		
1 tablespoon	reduced-fat		

	cream cheese:		sour cream:
1 tablespoon (½ ounce)	regular	2 tablespoons	regular
2 tablespoons (1 ounce)	reduced-fat	3 tablespoons	reduced-fat
1 teaspoon	fatback, salt pork,* shortening, or lard		

■ Free Foods List

A *free food* is any food or drink that contains less than 20 kcal or less than 5 grams of carbohydrate per serving. Foods with a serving size listed should be limited to three servings per day. Foods listed without a serving size can be eaten as often as you like.

Fat-Free or Reduced-Fat Foods

1 tablespoon	cream cheese, fat-free	1 teaspoon	Miracle Whip®, reduced-fat nonstick
1 tablespoon	creamers, nondairy, liquid		cooking spray
2 teaspoons	creamers, nondairy, powdered	1 tablespoon	salad dressing, fat-free
1 tablespoon	mayonnaise, fat-free	2 tablespoons	salad dressing, fat-free, Italian
1 teaspoon	mayonnaise, reduced-fat	¼ cup	salsa
4 tablespoons	margarine, fat-free	1 tablespoon	sour cream, fat-free, reduced-fat
1 teaspoon	margarine, reduced-fat	2 tablespoons	whipped topping, regular or light
1 tablespoon	Miracle Whip®, nonfat		

Sugar-Free or Low-Sugar Foods

1 candy	candy, hard, sugar-free	2 teaspoons	jam or jelly, low-sugar, or light sugar
	gelatin dessert, sugar-free		substitutes†
	gelatin, unflavored	2 tablespoons	syrup, sugar-free
	gum, sugar-free		

Drinks

	bouillon, broth, consommé		coffee
	bouillon or broth, low-sodium		diet soft drinks, sugar-free
	carbonated or mineral water		drink mixes, sugar-free
	club soda		tea
1 tablespoon	cocoa powder, unsweetened		tonic water, sugar-free

Condiments

1 tablespoon	catsup	1½	pickles, dill (large)
	horseradish		soy sauce, regular or light
	lemon juice	1 tablespoon	taco sauce
	lime juice		vinegar
	mustard		

Seasonings

flavoring extracts	spices
garlic	Tabasco® or hot pepper sauce
herbs, fresh or dried	wine, used in cooking
pimento	worcestershire sauce

*Use a piece 1 in × 1 in × ¼ in if you plan to eat the fatback cooked with vegetables. Use a piece 2 in × 1 in × ½ in when eating only the vegetables with the fatback removed.

†Sugar substitutes, alternatives, or replacements that are approved by the Food and Drug Administration (FDA) are safe to use. Common brand names include.
  Equal® (aspartame)
  Sprinkle Sweet® (saccharin)
  Sweet One® (acesulfame-K)
  Sweet-10® (saccharin)
  Sugar Twin® (saccharin)
  Sweet 'n Low® (saccharin)
  Splenda® (sucralose)

amount and type.
• For breads
  — Indicate whether whole wheat, rye, white, and so on.

■ Combination Foods List

1 cup (8 ounces)	Entrées	Exchanges per Serving
	tuna noodle casserole, lasagna, spaghetti ~~with meatballs, chili with beans~~	2 carbohydrates, 2 medium-fat meats

III. Complete the following table as you summarize your dietary intake.

Percentage of kcal from Protein, Fat, Carbohydrate, and Alcohol

Intake

Protein (P): ____ grams/day × 4 kcal/gram = (P) ____ kcal/day
Fat (F): ____ grams/day × 9 kcal/gram = (F) ____ kcal/day
Carbohydrate (C): ____ grams/day × 4 kcal/gram = (C) ____ kcal/day
Alcohol (A): (A) ____ kcal/day*
Total kcal (T)/day = (T) ____ kcal/day

Percentage of kcal from protein:

$$\frac{(P)}{(T)} \times 100 = \underline{\quad}\% \text{ of total kcal}$$

Percentage of kcal from fat:

$$\frac{(F)}{(T)} \times 100 = \underline{\quad}\% \text{ of total kcal}$$

Percentage of kcal from carbohydrate:

$$\frac{(C)}{(T)} \times 100 = \underline{\quad}\% \text{ of total kcal}$$

Percentage of kcal from alcohol:

$$\frac{(A)}{(T)} \times 100 = \underline{\quad}\% \text{ of total kcal}$$

NOTE: The four percentages can total 99, 100, or 101, depending on the way in which figures were rounded off earlier.

*To calculate how many kcal in a beverage are from alcohol, look up the beverage in Appendix A. Determine how many kcal are from carbohydrate (multiply carbohydrate grams times 4), fat (fat grams times 9), and protein (protein grams times 4). The remaining kcal are from alcohol.

IV. Use the following table to again record your food intake for one day, placing each food item in the correct category of the Food Guide Pyramid, with the correct number of servings (see Table 2.6 in Chapter 2). Note that a food such as toast with margarine contributes to two categories—namely, to the bread, cereal, rice, and pasta group and to the fats, oils, and sweets group. You can expect that many food choices will contribute to more than one group. Indicate the number of servings from the Food Guide Pyramid that each food yields.

Indicate the Number of Servings from the Food Guide Pyramid That Each Food Yields

Food or Beverage	Amount Eaten	Milk, Yogurt, and Cheese	Meat, Poultry, Fish, Dry Beans, Eggs, and Nuts	Fruits	Vegetables	Bread, Cereal, Rice, and Pasta	Fats, Oils, and Sweets
Group totals							
Recommended servings							In moderation
Shortages in numbers of servings							

V. Evaluation. Are there weaknesses suggested in your nutrient intake that correspond to missing servings in the Food Guide Pyramid? Consider replacing the missing servings to improve your nutrient intake.

VI. For the same day you keep your food record, also keep a 24-hour record of your activities. Include sleeping, sitting, and walking, as well as the obvious forms of exercise. Calculate your energy expenditure for these activities using Table 10.5 in Chapter 10 or the software available with this book. Try to substitute a similar activity if your particular activity is not listed. Calculate the total kcal you used for the day (total for column 3). Following is an example of an activity record. A blank form follows for your use. Ask your professor whether you are to turn in the form or the activity printout from the software.

Weight (kilograms)*: 70 kilograms

		Energy Cost		
Activity	Time (Minutes): Convert to Hours	Column I kcal/kilograms/hr (from Table 10.5)	Column 2 (Column 1 × Time)	Column 3 (Column 2 × Weight in kilograms)
Brisk walking	(60 min) 1 hr	4.4	(× 1) = 4.4	(× 70) = 308

*pounds/2.2

Weight (kilograms)*:

		Energy Cost		
Activity	Time (Minutes): Convert to Hours	Column I kcal/kilograms/hr (from Table 10.5)	Column 2 (Column 1 × Time)	Column 3 (Column 2 × Weight in kilograms)

Total kcal used (from adding all of column 3)

*pounds/2.2

Important Chemical Structures in Nutrition

Amino Acids

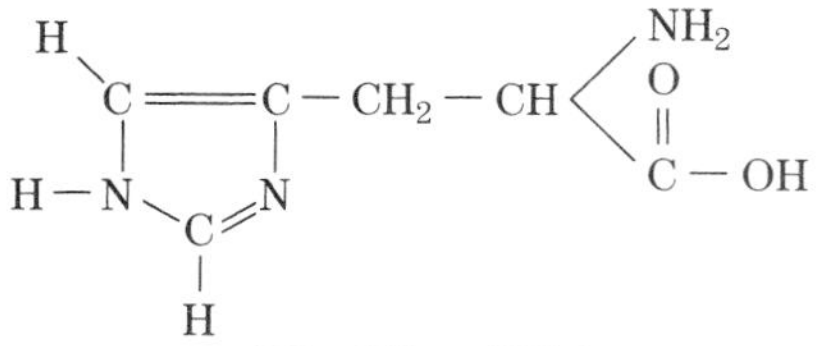

Histidine (His)
(essential)

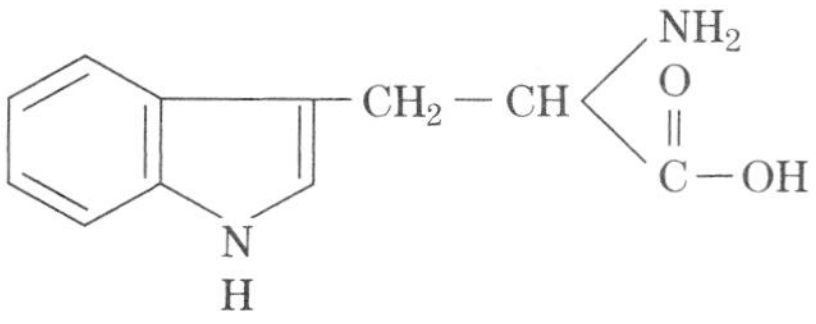

Tryptophan (Trp)
(essential)

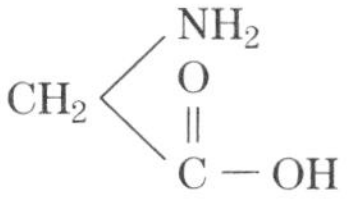

Glycine (Gly)

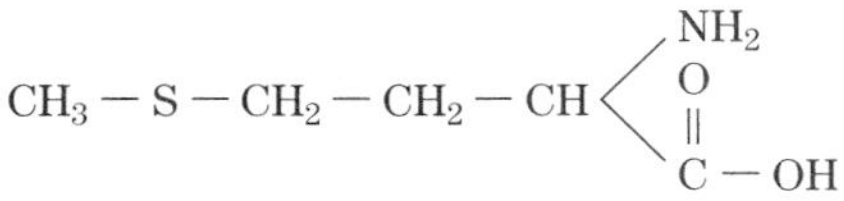

Methionine (Met)
(essential)

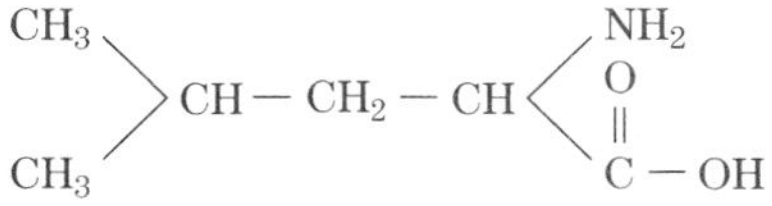

Leucine (Leu)
(essential)

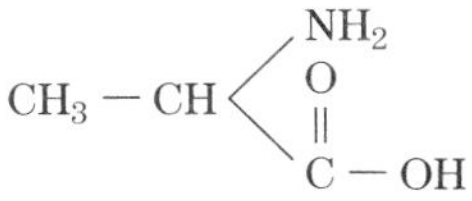

Alanine (Ala)

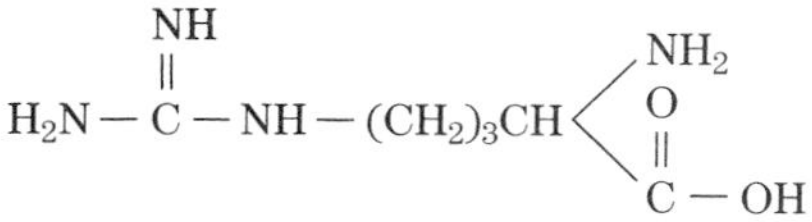

Arginine (Arg)
(essential in infancy)

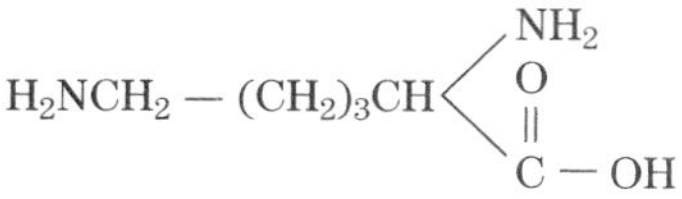

Lysine (Lys)
(essential)

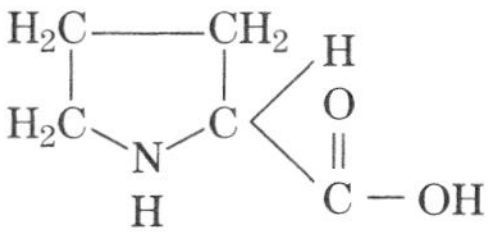

Proline (Pro)

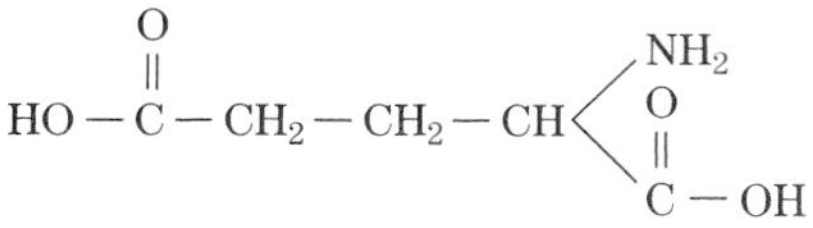

Glutamic Acid (Glu)

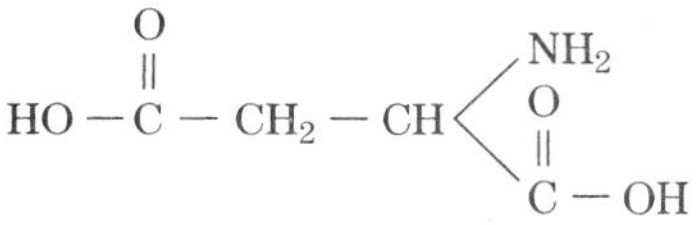

Aspartic Acid (Asp)

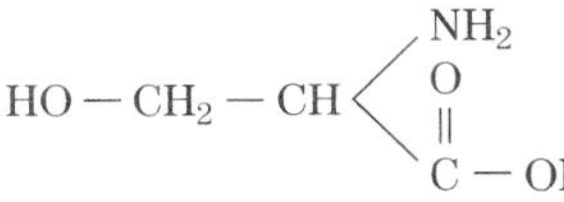

Serine (Ser)

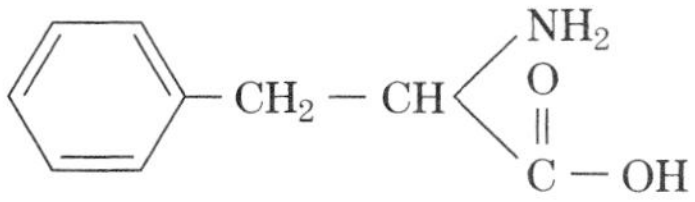

Phenylalanine (Phe)
(essential)

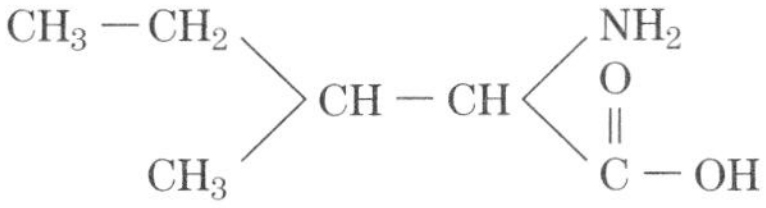

Isoleucine (Ile)
(essential)

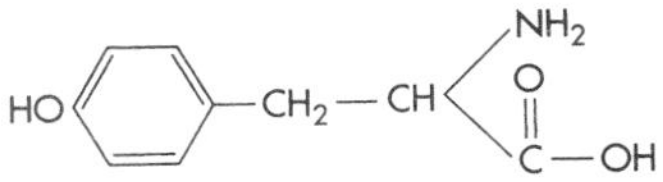

Tyrosine (Tyr)

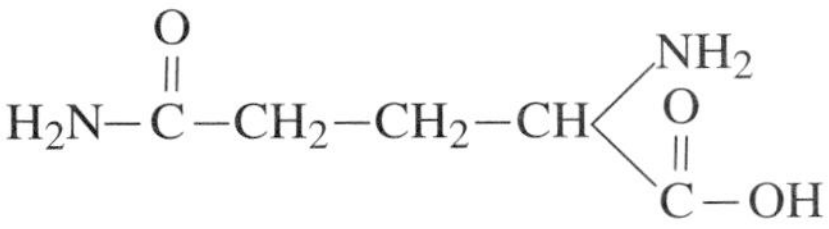

Glutamine (Gln)

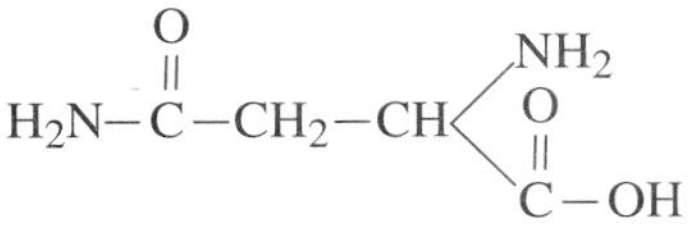

Asparagine (Asn)

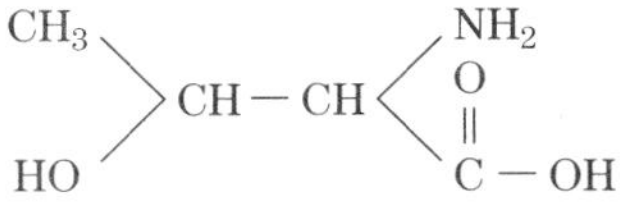

Threonine (Thr)
(essential)

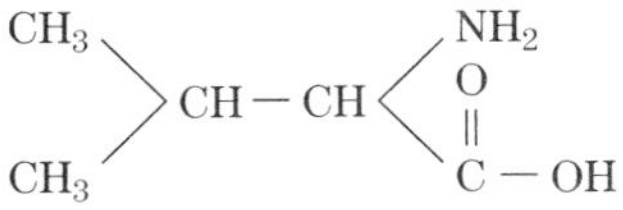

Valine (Val)
(essential)

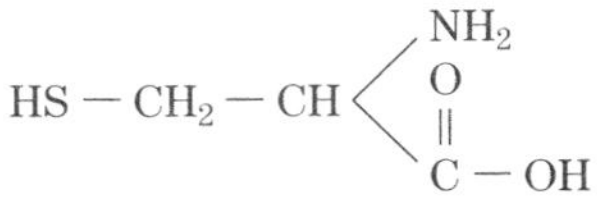

Cysteine (Cys)

Vitamins

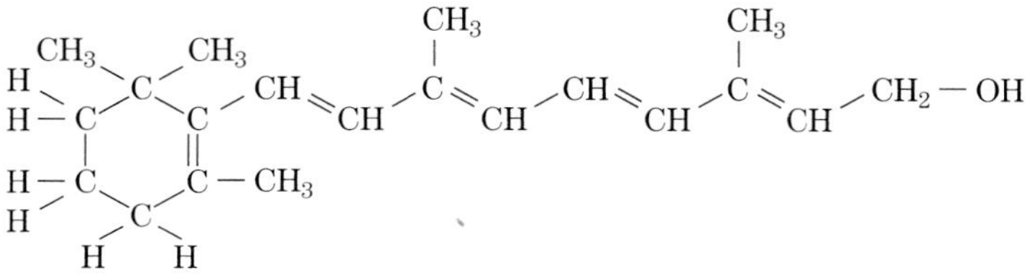

Vitamin A: retinol

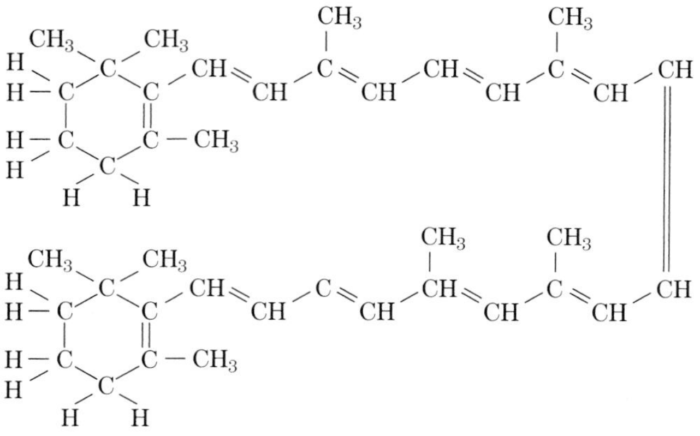

Beta-carotene

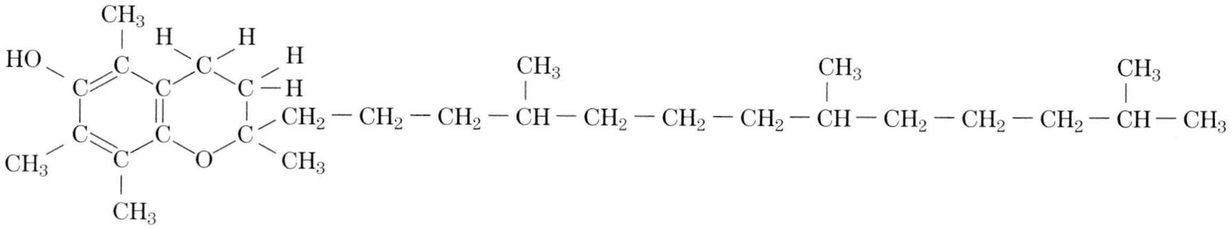

Vitamin E

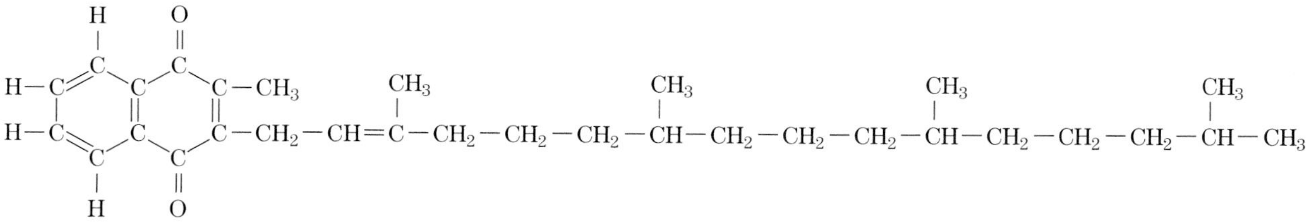

Vitamin K

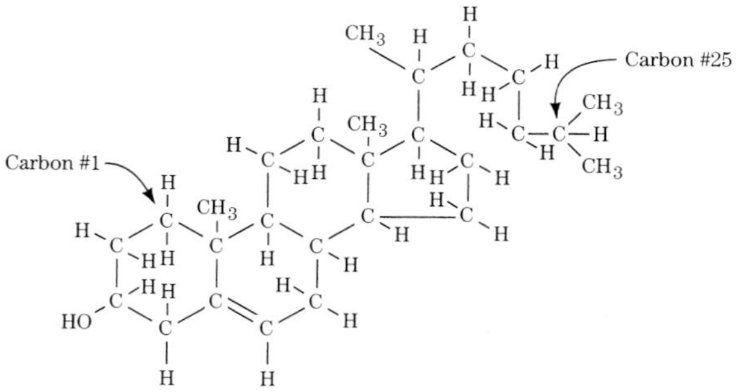

7-dehydrocholesterol

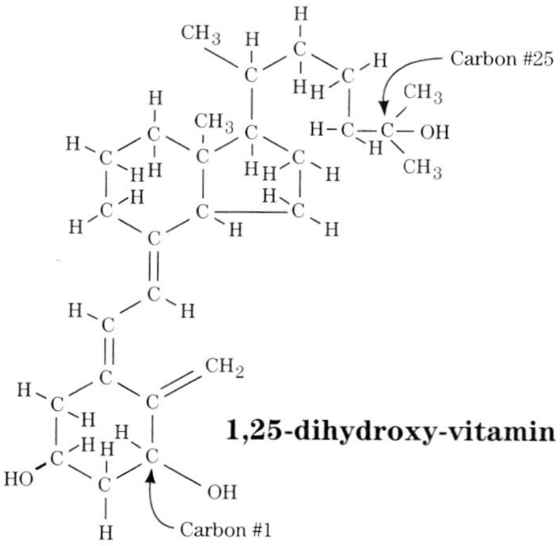

1,25-dihydroxy-vitamin D₃ (calcitriol)

Active vitamin D (calcitriol) and its precursor 7-dehydrocholesterol

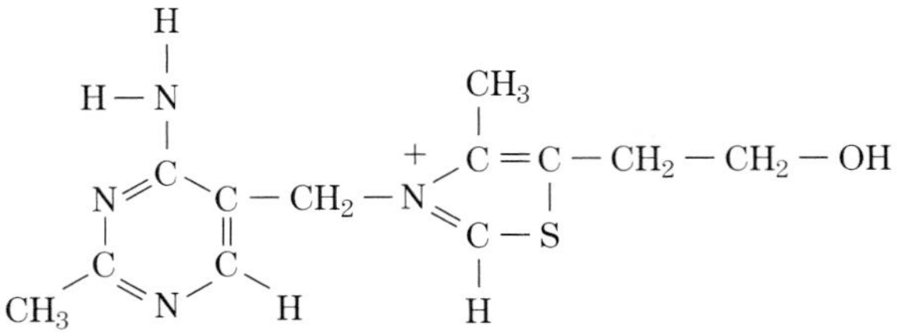

Thiamin

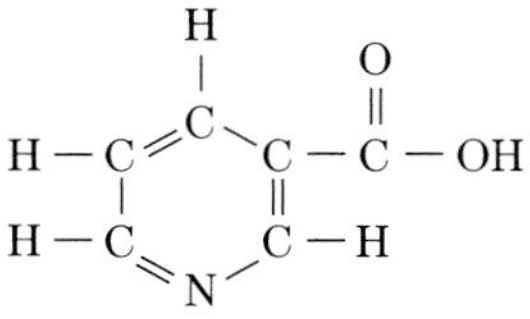

Niacin (nicotinic acid and nicotinamide)

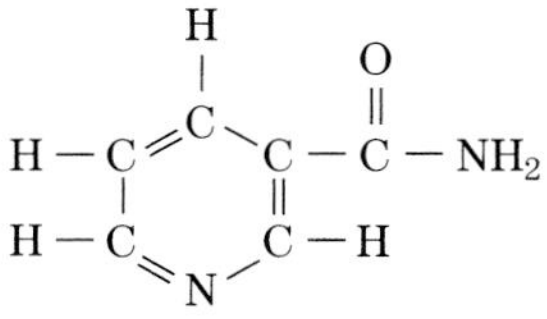

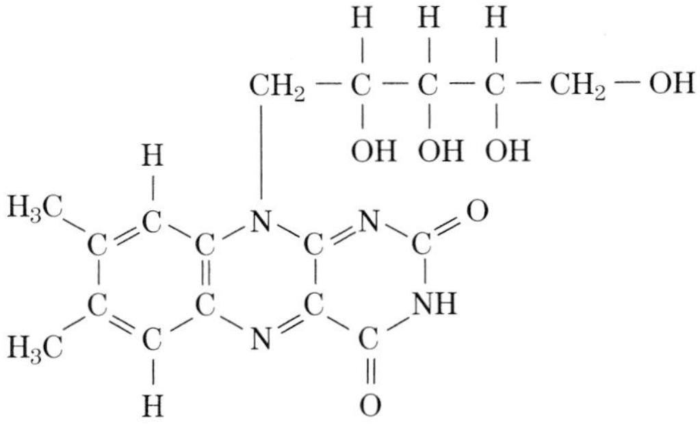

Nicotinic acid   Nicotinamide

Riboflavin

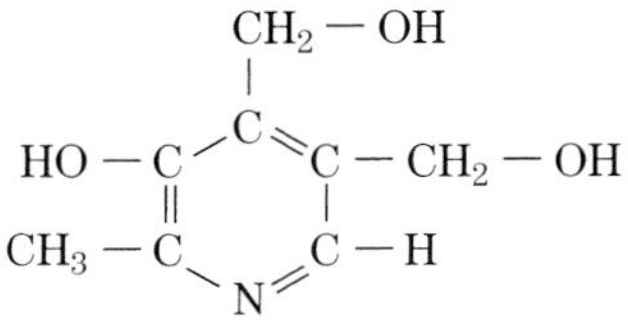

Pyridoxine 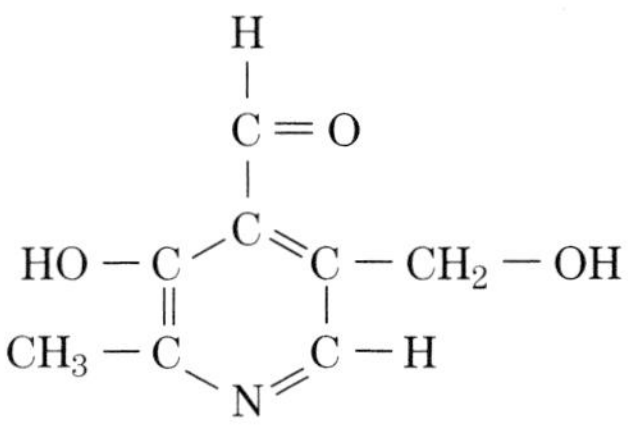   Pyridoxal 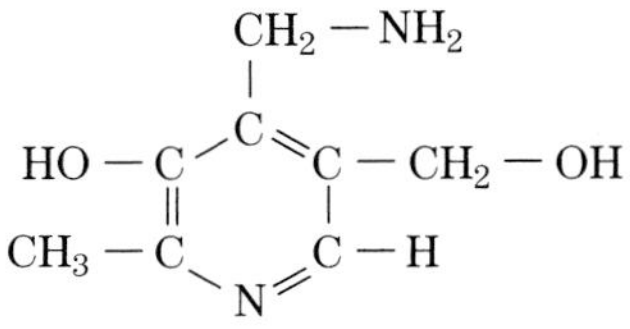   Pyridoxamine

Vitamin B-6 (a general name for three compounds— pyridoxine, pyridoxal, and pyridoxamine).

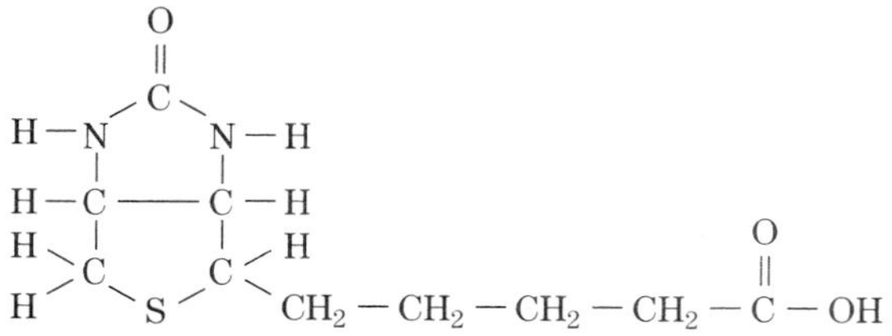

Biotin

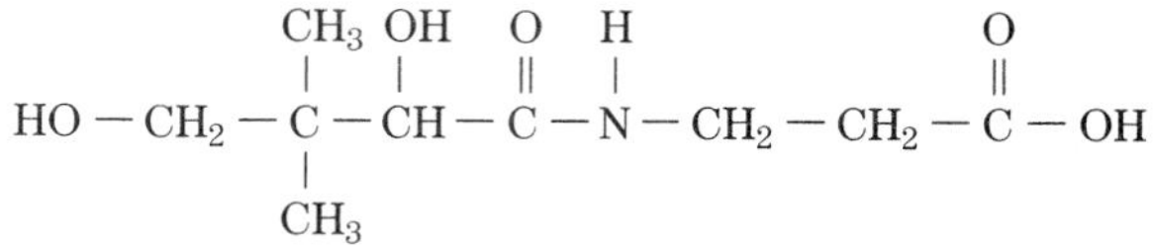

Pantothenic acid

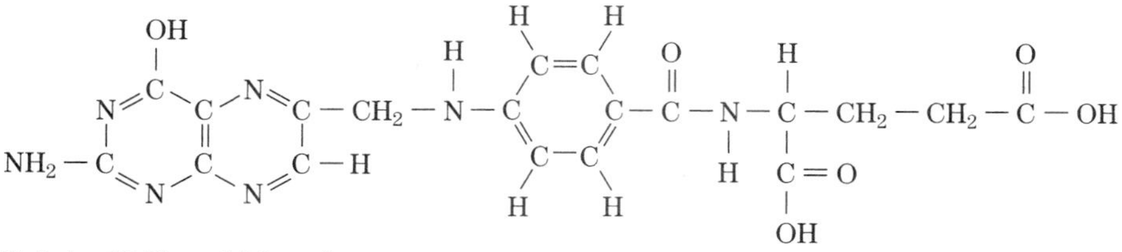

Folate (folic acid form)

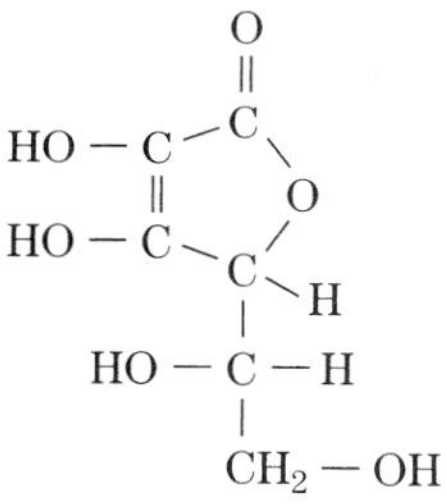

Vitamin C (ascorbic acid)

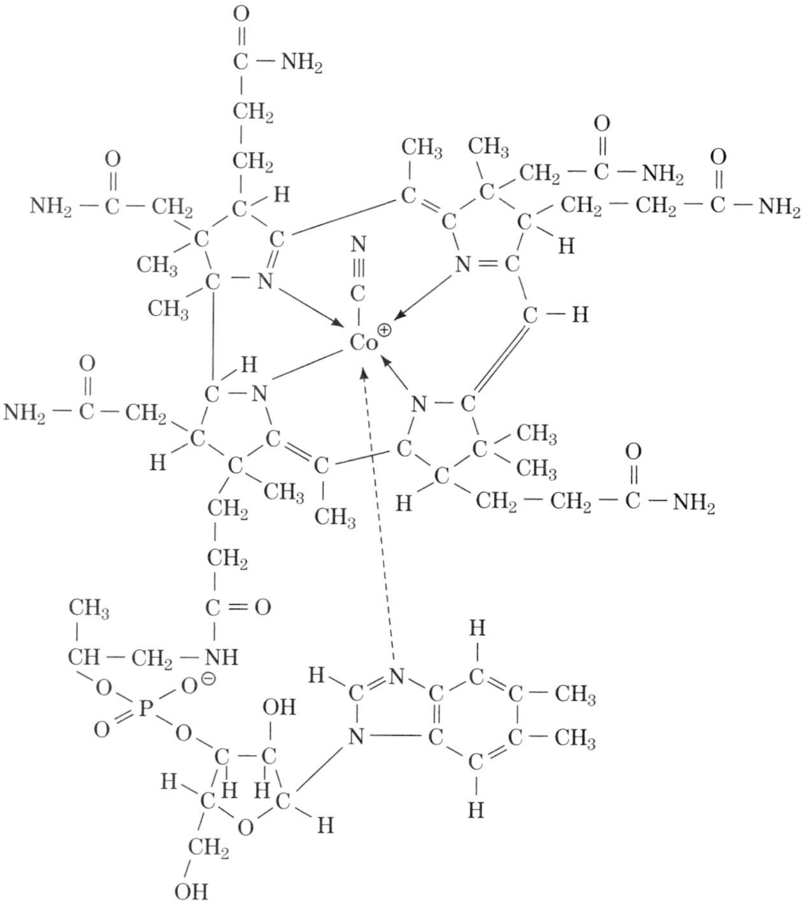

Vitamin B-12 (cyanocobalamin) The arrows in this diagram indicate that the spare electrons on the nitrogens attract them to the cobalt atom.

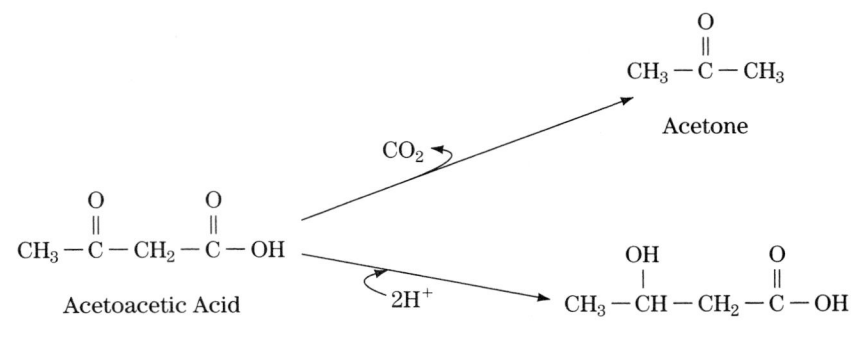

Ketone Bodies

Acetone

Acetoacetic Acid

β-Hydroxybutyric Acid

Point of cleavage to yield
ADP and energy release

Triphosphate

Adenine

Ribose
(a sugar)

**Adenosine Triphosphate
(ATP)**

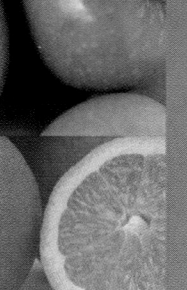

Appendix G

The 1983 Metropolitan Life Insurance Company Height-Weight Table and Determination of Frame Size

1983 Metropolitan Life Insurance Company Height-Weight Table*†

Women						Men					
Height		Frame				Height		Frame			
Ft.	In.	Small	Medium	Large		Ft.	In.	Small	Medium	Large	
4	10	102–111	109–121	118–131		5	2	128–134	131–141	138–150	
4	11	103–113	111–123	120–134		5	3	130–136	133–143	140–153	
5	0	104–115	113–126	122–137		5	4	132–138	135–145	142–156	
5	1	106–118	115–129	125–140		5	5	134–140	137–148	144–160	
5	2	108–121	118–132	128–143		5	6	136–142	139–151	146–164	
5	3	111–124	121–135	131–147		5	7	138–145	142–154	149–168	
5	4	114–127	124–138	134–151		5	8	140–148	145–157	152–172	
5	5	117–130	127–141	137–155		5	9	142–151	148–160	155–176	
5	6	120–133	130–144	140–159		5	10	144–154	151–163	158–180	
5	7	123–136	133–147	143–163		5	11	146–157	154–166	161–184	
5	8	126–139	136–150	146–167		6	0	149–160	157–170	164–188	
5	9	129–142	139–153	149–170		6	1	152–164	160–174	168–192	
5	10	132–145	142–156	152–173		6	2	155–168	164–178	172–197	
5	11	135–148	145–159	155–176		6	3	158–172	167–182	176–202	
6	0	138–151	148–162	158–179		6	4	162–176	171–187	181–207	

Permission granted courtesy of Metropolitan Life Insurance Company, *Statistical Bulletin*.

*Based on a weight-height mortality study conducted by the Society of Actuaries and the Association of Life Insurance Medical Directors of America, Metropolitan Life Insurance Medical Directors of America, Metropolitan Life Insurance Company, revised 1983.

†Weights at ages 25 to 59 based on lowest mortality. Height includes 1-inch heel. Weight for women includes 3 pounds for indoor clothing. Weight for men includes 5 pounds for indoor clothing.

■ Using the Metropolitan Life Insurance Table to Estimate Healthy Weight

The Metropolitan Life Insurance Table is one method for estimating healthy weight. The table lists for any height the weight that is associated with a maximum life span. The table does not tell the healthiest weight for a living person; it simply lists the weight associated with longevity.

There are many criticisms of this table. These stem from the inclusion of some people and the exclusion of others. For example, only policyholders of life insurance are included. In addition, smokers are included, but anyone over the age of 60 is excluded. Weight is only measured at the time of purchase of insurance, and there is no follow-up. All of these factors contribute to the fact that this table is to be used only as a rough screening tool; not meeting the exact recommendations should not be cause for alarm.

To diagnose overweight or obesity using the table, calculate the percentage of the Metropolitan Life Insurance Table weight. Use the midpoint of a weight range for a specific height.

$$\frac{(\text{Current weight} - \text{weight from table})}{\text{Weight from table}} \times 100$$

Example:

$$\frac{140 - 120}{120} \times 100 = 17\% \text{ over standard}$$

Overweight can be defined as weighing at least 10% more than the weight listed on the table. Obesity weighs in at 20% more than that listed on the table. Moreover, this measure of obesity comes in degrees. Whereas mild obesity carries little health risk, severe obesity raises overall health risk twelvefold.

Degrees of Obesity

% Over Healthy Body Weight	Form of Obesity
20–40%	Mild
41–99%	Moderate
100%+	Severe

■ Determining Frame Size

Method 1

Height is recorded without shoes.

Wrist circumference is measured just beyond the bony (styloid) process at the wrist joint on the right arm, using a tape measure.

The following formula is used:

$$r = \frac{\text{Height (centimeters)}}{\text{Wrist circumference (centimeters)}}$$

Frame size can be determined as follows:[†]

Males	Females
$r > 10.4$ small	$r > 11$ small
$r = 9.6–10.4$ medium	$r = 10.1–11$ medium
$r < 9.6$ large	$r < 10.1$ large

Method 2

The patient's right arm is extended forward, perpendicular to the body, with the arm bent so the angle at the elbow forms 90 degrees, with the fingers pointing up and the palm turned away from the body. The greatest breadth across the elbow joint is measured with a sliding caliper along the axis of the upper arm, on the two prominent bones on either side of the elbow. This is recorded as the elbow breadth. The following tables give elbow breadth measurements for medium-framed men and women of various heights. Measurements lower than those listed indicate a small frame size; higher measurements indicate a large frame size.[‡]

Men		Women	
Height in 1″ Heels	Elbow Breadth	Height in 1″ Heels	Elbow Breadth
5′2″–5′3″	2½–2⅞″	4′10″–4′11″	2¼–2½″
5′4″–5′7″	2⅝–2⅞″	5′0″–5′3″	2¼–2½″
5′8″–5′11″	2¾–3″	5′4″–5′7″	2⅜–2⅝″
6′0″–6′3″	2¾–3⅛″	5′8″–5′11″	2⅜–2⅝″
6′4″ and over	2⅞–3¼″	6′0″ and over	2½–2¾″

[†]From Grant JP: *Handbook of total parenteral nutrition.* Philadelphia: WB Saunders, 1980.
[‡]From Metropolitan Life Insurance Co., 1983.

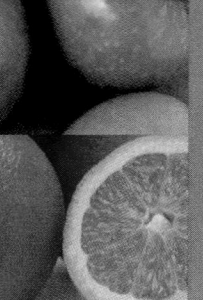

Appendix H

Caffeine Content of Foods

Beverages	Milligrams
Carbonated Beverages*	
Cherry Coke, Coca-Cola—12 fl oz (370 g)	46
Cherry cola, Slice—12 fl oz (360 g)	48
Cherry RC—12 fl oz (360 g)	12
Coca-Cola—12 fl oz (370 g)	46
Coca-Cola Classic—12 fl oz (369 g)	46
Cola, RC—12 fl oz (360 g)	18
Mello Yello—12 fl oz (372 g)	52
Mr. Pibb—12 fl oz (369 g)	40
Mountain Dew—12 fl oz (360 g)	54
Dr. Pepper-type soda—12 fl oz (368 g)	41
Pepsi Cola—12 fl oz (360 g)	38
Carbonated Beverages, Low-Calorie*	
Diet Cherry Coke, Coca-Cola—12 fl oz (354 g)	46
Diet cherry cola, Slice—12 fl oz (360 g)	41
Diet Coke, Coca-Cola—12 fl oz (354 g)	46
Diet cola, aspartame-sweetened—12 fl oz (355 g)	50
Diet Pepsi—12 fl oz (360 g)	36
Diet RC—12 fl oz (360 g)	48
Coffee	
Brewed—6 fl oz (177 g)	103
Instant powder—1 tsp (1.8 g)	57
Decaffeinated—1 rounded tsp (1.8 g)	2
With chicory—1 tsp (1.8 g)	37
Prepared from instant powder—6 fl oz & 1 tsp powder (179 g)	57
Amaretto, General Foods—6 fl oz & 11.5 g powder (189 g)	60
Amaretto, sugar-free, General Foods—6 fl oz water & 7.7 g powder (185 g)	60
Decaffeinated—6 fl oz water & 1 tsp powder (179 g)	2
Francais, General Foods—6 fl oz water & 11.5 g powder (189 g)	53
Francais, sugar-free, General Foods—6 fl oz water & 7.7 g powder (185 g)	59
Irish creme, General Foods—6 fl oz water & 12.8 g powder (190 g)	53
Irish creme, sugar free, General Foods—6 fl oz water & 7.1 g powder (185 g)	48
Irish mocha mint, General Foods—6 fl oz water & 11.5 g powder (189 g)	27
Irish mocha mint, sugar-free, General Foods—6 fl oz water & 6.4 g powder (189 g)	25
Orange cappuccino, General Foods—6 fl oz water & 14 g powder (191 g)	73
Orange cappuccino, sugar-free, General Foods—6 fl oz water & 6.7 g powder (184 g)	71
Suisse mocha, General Foods—6 fl oz water & 11.5 g powder (189 g)	41
Suisse mocha, sugar-free, General Foods—6 fl oz water & 6.4 g powder (184 g)	40
Vienna, General Foods—6 fl oz water & 14 g powder (191 g)	56
Vienna, sugar-free, General Foods—6 fl oz water & 6.7 g powder (184 g)	55
with chicory—6 fl oz water & 1 tsp powder (179 g)	38
Tea, Hot/Iced	
Brewed 3 min—6 fl oz water (178 g)	36
Instant powder—1 tsp (0.7 g)	31
With lemon flavor—1 rounded tsp (1.4 g)	25
With sugar & lemon flavor—3 tsp (23 g)	29
With sodium saccharin & lemon flavor—2 tsp (1.6 g)	36
Prepared from instant powder	
1 tsp powder in 8 fl oz water (237 g)	31
Crystal Light—8 fl oz (238 g)	11
With lemon flavor—1 tsp powder in 8 fl oz water (238 g)	26

With sugar & lemon flavor—3 tsp powder in 8 fl oz water (259 g)	29
With sodium, saccharin & lemon flavor—2 tsp powder in 8 fl oz water (238 g)	36
Candy	
Chocolate	
German sweet, Bakers—1 oz square (28 g)	8
Semi-sweet, Bakers—1 oz square (28 g)	13
Chocolate chips	
Bakers—1/4 cup (43 g)	12
German sweet, Bakers—1/4 cup (43 g)	15
Semi-sweet, Bakers—1/4 cup (43 g)	14
Desserts	
Frozen Desserts	
Pudding pops, Jell-O	
Chocolate—1 pop (47 g)	2
Chocolate caramel swirl—1 pop (47 g)	1
Chocolate fudge—1 pop (47 g)	3
Chocolate vanilla swirl—1 pop (47 g)	2
Chocolate with chocolate coating—1 pop (49 g)	3
Double chocolate swirl pop (47 g)	2
Milk chocolate—1 pop (47 g)	2
Pies	
Chocolate mousse, from mix, Jell-O—1/8 pie (95 g)	6
Puddings, from Instant Mix	
Chocolate	
Jell-O—1/2 cup (150 g)	5
Sugar-free, D-Zerta—1/2 cup (130 g)	4
Sugar-free, Jell-O—1/2 cup (133 g)	4
Chocolate fudge	
Jell-O—1/2 cup (150 g)	8
Chocolate fudge mousse, Jell-O—1/2 cup (86 g)	12
Chocolate mousse, Jell-O—1/2 cup (86 g)	9
Chocolate tapioca, Jell-O—1/2 cup (147 g)	8
Milk chocolate, Jell-O—1/2 cup (150 g)	5
Milk Beverages	
Chocolate flavor mix in whole milk—2–3 tsp powder in 8 fl oz milk (266 g)	8
Chocolate malted milk flavor powder	
In whole milk—3 tsp powder in 8 fl oz milk (265 g)	8
With added nutrients in whole milk—4–5 tsp powder in 8 fl oz milk (265 g)	5
Chocolate syrup in whole milk—2 tbsp syrup in 8 fl oz milk (282 g)	6
Cocoa/hot chocolate, prepared with water from mix —3–4 tsp powder in 6 fl oz water (206 g)	4
Milk Beverage Mixes	
Chocolate flavor mix, powder—2–3 tsp (22 g)	8
Chocolate malted milk flavor mix, powder—3/4 oz (3 tsp) (21 g)	8
Chocolate malted milk flavor mix with added nutrients, powder—3/4 oz (4–5 tsp) (21 g)	6
Chocolate syrup—2 tbsp (1 fl oz) (38 g)	5
Cocoa mix powder—1 oz pkt (3–4 tsp) (28 g)	5
Miscellaneous	
Baking chocolate, unsweetened, Bakers—1 oz (28 g)	25

Abbreviations: g for grams

*Caffeine-free carbonated beverages and most noncarbonated beverages contain no caffeine.
Data from Pennington JAT, *Bowes and Church's food values of portions commonly consumed,* ed. 17, 1998, JB Lippincott. Reprinted with permission.

Consider the following reliable sources of food and nutrition information:

Journals That Regularly Cover Nutrition Topics

American Family Physician*
American Journal of Clinical Nutrition
American Journal of Epidemiology
American Journal of Medicine
American Journal of Nursing
American Journal of Obstetrics and
  Gynecology
American Journal of Physiology
American Journal of Public Health
American Scientist
Annals of Internal Medicine
Annual Reviews of Medicine
Annual Reviews of Nutrition
Archives of Disease in Childhood
Archives of Internal Medicine
British Journal of Nutrition
BMJ (British Medical Journal)
Cancer
Cancer Research
Circulation
Diabetes
Diabetes Care

Disease-a-Month
FASEB Journal
FDA Consumer*
Food Chemical Toxicology
Food Engineering
Gastroenterology
Geriatrics
Gut
Human Nutrition: Applied Nutrition
Human Nutrition: Clinical Nutrition
Journal of the American College of
  Nutrition*
Journal of The American Dietetic
  Association*
Journal of the American Geriatric Society
JAMA (Journal of the American Medical
  Association)
Journal of Applied Physiology
Journal of Canadian Dietetic Association*
Journal of Clinical Investigation
Journal of Food Service
Journal of Food Technology

JNCI (Journal of the National Cancer
  Institute)
Journal of Nutrition
Journal of Nutritional Education*
Journal of Nutrition for the Elderly
Journal of Nutrition Research
Journal of Pediatrics
Lancet
Mayo Clinic Proceedings
Medicine and Science in Sports and Exercise
Nature
The New England Journal of Medicine
Nutrition
Nutrition Reviews
Nutrition Today*
Pediatrics
The Physician and Sports Medicine
Postgraduate Medicine*
Proceedings of the Nutrition Society
Science
Science News*
Scientific American*

The majority of these journals are available in college and university libraries or in a specialty library on campus, such as one designated for health services or home economics. As indicated, a few journals will be filed under their abbreviations, rather than the first word in their full name. A reference librarian can help you locate any of these sources. The asterisked (*) journals are ones you may find especially interesting and useful because of the number of nutrition articles presented each month or the less technical nature of the presentation.

Magazines for the Consumer That Cover Nutrition Topics

American Health for Women
Better Homes and Gardens

Good Housekeeping
Health

Parents
Self

Textbooks and Other Sources for Advanced Study of Nutrition Topics

Brody T: Nutritional biochemistry. 2nd ed. San Diego: Academic Press, 1999.
Groff JL, Gropper SS: Advanced human nutrition and metabolism. St Paul, MN: West, 2000.
International Life Sciences Institute: Present knowledge in nutrition. 8th ed. Washington DC: The Nutrition Foundation, 2001.
Mahan LK, Escott-Stump S: Krause's food, nutrition, and diet therapy. 10th ed. Philadelphia: WB Saunders, 2000.
Murray RK and others: Harper's biochemistry. 25th ed. Norwalk, CT: Appleton & Lange, 2000.
Schils ME, Olson JA, Shike M, Ross AC: Modern nutrition in health and disease. 9th ed. Philadelphia: Lea & Febiger, 1999.
Stipanuk MH: Biochemical and physiological aspects of human nutrition. Philadephia: WB Saunders, 2000.

Newsletters That Cover Nutrition Issues on a Regular Basis

American Institute for Cancer Research
(AICR) Washington, DC 20069
www.icr.ac.uk/

CNI Nutrition Week
Community Nutrition Institute
910 17th St. N.W., Suite 413
Washington, DC 20006
www.unidial.com

Dairy Council Digest
National Dairy Council
10255 West Higgins Road, Suite 900
Rosemont, IL 60018
(inexpensive)
www.national/dairycouncil.com

Dietetic Currents
Ross Laboratories
Director of Professional Services
625 Cleveland Ave.
Columbus, OH 43216
(free)
www.ross.com

Egg Nutrition Center
1819 H St. N.W., No. 510
Washington, DC 20009
(free)
www.enc-online.org/

Environmental Nutrition
52 Riverside Dr.
New York, NY 10024
www.eatright.org

Food and Nutrition News
National Cattlemen's Beef Association
444 Michigan Ave.
Chicago, IL 60611
(free)
www.beef.org

Harvard Medical School Health Letter
Department of Continuing Education
25 Shattuck St.
Boston, MA 02115
www.hms.harvard.edu/news/index.html

Mayo Clinic Health Letter
P.O. Box 53889
Boulder, CO 80322-3889
mayohealth.org

National Council Against Health Fraud
Newsletter (NCAHF)
P.O. Box 1276
Loma Linda, CA 92354
www.ncahf.org/

Nutrition Action Healthletter
1875 Connecticut Ave.
Washington, DC 20009-5728
www.cspinet.org

Nutrition Forum
George Stickley Co.
210 Washington Square
Philadelphia, PA 19106
www.quackwatch.com

Nutrition & the M.D.
Raven Press
1185 Avenue of the Americas
New York, NY 10036
www.lww.com

Nutrition Research Newsletter
P.O. Box 700
Pallisades, NY 10964
www.biz-lib.com/ZTINR.html

Soy Connection
United Soybean Board
16305 Swingley Ridge Drive
Suite 110
Chesterfield, MO 63017
(free)
smartsoy.ag.uiuc.edu/usb/speced.html/

Tufts University Diet & Nutrition Letter
P.O. Box 10948
Des Moines, IA 50940
www.healthletter.tufts.edu/

University of California at Berkeley
Wellness Letter
P.O. Box 420148
Palm Coast, FL 32142
magazines.enews.com/magazines/vcbw

Professional Organizations with a Commitment to Nutrition Issues

American Academy of Pediatrics
P.O. Box 1034
Evanston, IL 60204
www.aap.org

American Cancer Society
90 Park Ave.
New York, NY 10016
www.cancer.org

American College of Sports Medicine
P.O. Box 1440
Indianapolis, IN 46204
www.acsm.org/

American Dental Association
211 E. Chicago Ave.
Chicago, IL 60611
www.ada.org

American Diabetes Association
2 Park Ave.
New York, NY 10016
www.diabetes.org

American Dietetic Association
216 W. Jackson Blvd.
Suite 800
Chicago, IL 60606
www.eatright.org

American Geriatrics Society
770 Lexington Ave.
Suite 400
New York, NY 10021
www.americangeriatrics.org

American Heart Association
7272 Greenville Ave.
Dallas, TX 75231
www.americanheart.org

American Home Economics Association
2010 Massachusetts Ave. N.W.
Washington, DC 20036
www.orst.edu

American Society for Nutritional Sciences
9650 Rockville Pike
Bethesda, MD 20014
www.faseb.org/asns

American Medical Association
Nutrition Information Section
535 N. Dearborn St.
Chicago, IL 60610
www.ama-assn org/

American Public Health Association
1015 Fifteenth St. N.W.
Washington, DC 20005
www.apha.org

American Society for Clinical Nutrition
9650 Rockville Pike
Bethesda, MD 20014
www.faseb.org/ajcn

The Canadian Diabetes Association
15 Toronto St.
Suite 1001
Toronto, Ontario M5C 2E3 Canada
www.diabetes.ca

The Canadian Dietetic Association
480 University Ave.
Suite 601
Toronto, Ontario M5G 1V2 Canada
www.dietitians.ca

The Canadian Society for Nutritional Sciences
Department of Foods and Nutrition
University of Manitoba
Winnipeg, Manitoba, R3T 2N2 Canada
www.hc-sc.gc.ca

Food and Nutrition Board
National Research Council
National Academy of Sciences
2101 Constitution Ave. N.W.
Washington, DC 20418
www.nas.edu/fnb/

Institute of Food Technologies
221 N. LaSalle St.
Chicago, IL 60601
www.ift.org

National Council on the Aging
1828 L St. N.W.
Washington, DC 20036
www.ncoa.org

National Institute of Nutrition
1335 Carling Ave.
Suite 210
Ottawa, Ontario K1Z OL2 Canada
www.nines.com

National Osteoporosis Foundation
1150 Seventeenth St. N.W., Suite 500
Washington, DC 20036
www.nof.org

Society for Nutrition Education
2001 Killebrew Dr., Suite 340
Minneapolis, MN 55425
www.sne.org

Professional or Lay Organizations Concerned with Nutrition Issues

Bread for the World Institute
1100 Wayne Ave.
Silver Springs, MD 20910
www.bread.org

California Council Against Health Fraud, Inc.
P.O. Box 1276
Loma Linda, CA 92354
www.ncahf.org

Children's Foundation
1420 New York Ave. N.W.
Suite 800
Washington, DC 20005
www.childrenfoundation.com

Food Research and Action Center (FRAC)
1875 Connecticut Ave. N.W. #540
Washington, DC 20009
www.iglou.com/why/resource/1100.htm

Institute for Food and Development Policy
1885 Mission St.
San Francisco, CA 94103
www.foodfirst.org

La Leche League International, Inc.
9616 Minneapolis Ave.
Franklin Park, IL 60131
www.lalecheleague.org

March of Dimes Birth Defects Foundation
(National Headquarters)
1275 Mamaroneck Ave.
White Plains, NY 10605
www.modimes.org

Overeaters Anonymous (OA)
2190 190th St.
Torrance, CA 90504
www.overeatersanonymous.org

Oxfam America
115 Broadway
Boston, MA 02116
www.oxfamamerica.org

Local Resources for Advice on Nutrition Issues

Cooperative extension agents in county extension offices
Dietitians (contact the state or local Dietetics Association)
Nutrition faculty affiliated with departments of food and nutrition, home economics, and dietetics
Registered dietitians (RDs or in Canada also RDNs) in city, county, or state agencies

Government Agencies Concerned with Nutrition Issues or That Distribute Nutrition Information

United States
The Consumer Information Center
Department 609K
Pueblo, CO 81009
www.pueblo.gsa.gov

Food and Drug Administration (FDA)
5600 Fishers Lane
Rockville, MD 20852
www.fda.gov

*Food and Nutrition Information and
   Education Resources Center*
National Library of Congress
Beltsville, MD 20705
www.nal.usda.gov

Human Nutrition Research Division
Agricultural Research Center
Beltsville, MD 20705
www.usda.gov

National Center for Health Statistics
3700 East-West
Hyattsville, MD 20782
www.cdc.gov/nchswww

National Heart, Lung, and Blood Institute
9000 Rockville Pike, Building 31, Room 4A21
Bethesda, MD 20892
www.nhlbi.gov

National Institute on Aging
Information Office
Building 31, Room 5C35
Bethesda, MD 20205
www.nih.gov/nia/

Office of Cancer Communications
National Cancer Institute
Building 31, Room 10A18
90 Rockville Pike
Bethesda, MD 20205
www.nci.nih.gov

USDA, Agricultural Research Service
6505 Belcrest Rd., Room 344
Hyattsville, MD 20782
www.usda.gov

USDA, Food Safety & Inspection Service
Room 1180 South, 14th and Independence
Ave. S.W.
Washington, DC 20250
www.usda.gov

U.S. Government Printing Office
The Superintendent of Documents
Washington, DC 20402
www.printgovt.org

Canada
Canadian Food Inspection Agency
59 Camelot Dr.
Nepean, Ontario K1A OY9
www.cfia-acia.agr.ca

Health and Welfare Canada
Canadian Government Publishing Center
Minister of Supply and Services
Ottawa, Ontario K1A 0S9
www.hc-sc-gc.ca

Home Economics Directorate
880 Portage Ave.
Second Floor
Winnipeg, Manitoba R3G 0P1
www.mbnet.mb.ca

Nutrition Programs
446 Jeanne Mance Building
Tunney's Pasture
Ottawa, Ontario K1A 1B4
www.hc-sc.gc.ca

Nutrition Services
P.O. Box 488
Halifax, Nova Scotia B3J 3R8
www.fns.usda.gov

United Nations
Food and Agriculture Organization (FAO)
North American Regional Office
1001 22nd St. N.W.
Washington, DC 20437
or
Via della Terma di Caracella
0100 Rome, Italy
www.fao.org

World Health Organization (WHO)
1211 Geneva 27
Switzerland
www.who.org

Trade Organizations and Companies That Distribute Nutrition Information

American Institute of Baking
P.O. Box 1148
Manhattan, KS 66502
www.aibonline.org

American Meat Institute
P.O. Box 3556
Washington, DC 20007
www.meatami.org

Beech-Nut Nutrition Corporation
Booth 1414
Checkerboard Square
St. Louis, MO 63164
www.beech-nut.com/index.htm

Best Foods
Consumer Service Department
Division of CPC International
International Plaza
Englewood Cliffs, NJ 07632
www.bestfoods.com

Campbell Soup Co.
Food Service Products Division
Campbell Plaza
Camden, NJ 08103
www.campbellsoups.com

Continental Baking Company
Checkerboard Square
St. Louis, MO 63164
www.scisoc.org

The Dannon Company, Inc.
120 White Plains Rd.
Tarrytown, NY 10591-5536
www.dannon.com

Del Monte Foods
One Market Plaza
San Francisco, CA 94105
www.delmonte-international.com

General Mills
P.O. Box 1113
Minneapolis, MN 55440
www.generalmills.com

Gerber Products Co.
445 State St.
Fremont, MI 49413
www.gerber.com/home1.html

H.J. Heinz
Consumer Relations
P.O. Box 57
Pittsburgh, PA 15230
www.heinzbaby.com

Idaho Potato Commission
P.O. Box 1968
Boise, ID 83701
www.idahopotatoes.com

Kellogg Company
Department of Home Economics Services
Battle Creek, MI 49016
www.kellog.com

Kraft General Foods
Three Lakes Dr.
Northfield, IL 60093
www.kraftfoods.com

Mead Johnson Nutritionals
2404 Pennsylvania Ave.
Evansville, IN 47721
www.meadjohnson.com

National Dairy Council
10255 W. Higgins Rd.
Rosemont, IL 60018-4233
www.natdairycoun.org

The NutraSweet Kelco Company
1751 Lake Cook Rd.
Deerfield, IL 60015
www.nutrasweetkelco.com/
default.htm

Pillsbury Company
1177 Pillsbury Building
608 Second Ave. S.
Minneapolis, MN 55402
www.pillsbury.com

Ross Laboratories
Director of Professional Services
625 Cleveland Ave.
Columbus, OH 43216
www.ross.com

Sunkist Growers, Inc.
14130 Riverside Dr.
Sherman Oaks, CA 91423
www.sunkist.com/index.html

Vitamin Nutrition Information Service
(VNIS)
Hoffmann-LaRoche
340 Kingsland Ave.
Nutley, NJ 07110
www.rocheusa.com

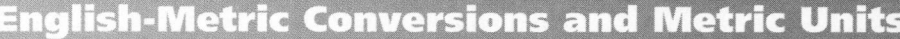

English-Metric Conversions

Length

English (USA)	= Metric
inch (in)	= 2.54 cm, 25.4 mm
foot (ft)	= 0.30 m, 30.48 cm
yard (yd)	= 0.91 m, 91.4 cm
mile (statute) (5280 ft)	= 1.61 km, 1609 m
mile (nautical) (6077 ft, 1.15 statute mi)	= 1.85 km, 1850 m

Metric	= English (USA)
millimeter (mm)	= 0.039 in (thickness of a dime)
centimeter (cm)	= 0.39 in
meter (m)	= 3.28 ft, 39.37 in
kilometer (km)	= 0.62 mi, 1091 yd, 3273 ft

Weight

English (USA)	= Metric
grain	= 64.80 mg
ounce (oz)	= 28.35 g
pound (lb)	= 453.60 g, 0.45 kg
ton (short—2000 lb)	= 0.91 metric ton (907 kg)

Metric	= English (USA)
milligram (mg)	= 0.002 grain (0.000035 oz)
gram (g)	= 0.04 oz (1/28 of an oz)
kilogram (kg)	= 35.27 oz, 2.20 lb
metric ton (1000 kg)	= 1.10 tons

Volume

English (USA)	= Metric
cubic inch	= 16.39 cc
cubic foot	= 0.03 m³
cubic yard	= 0.765 m³
ounce	= 0.03 liter (30 ml)*
pint (pt)	= 0.47 liter
quart (qt)	= 0.95 liter
gallon (gal)	= 3.79 liters

Metric	= English (USA)
milliliter (ml)	= 0.03 oz
liter (L)	= 2.12 pt
liter	= 1.06 qt
liter	= 0.27 gal

1 liter ÷ 1000 = 1 milliliter or 1 cubic centimeter (10^{-3} liter)
1 liter ÷ 1,000,000 = 1 microliter (10^{-6} liter)
*Note: 1 ml = 1 cc

Fahrenheit-Celsius Temperature Conversion Scale

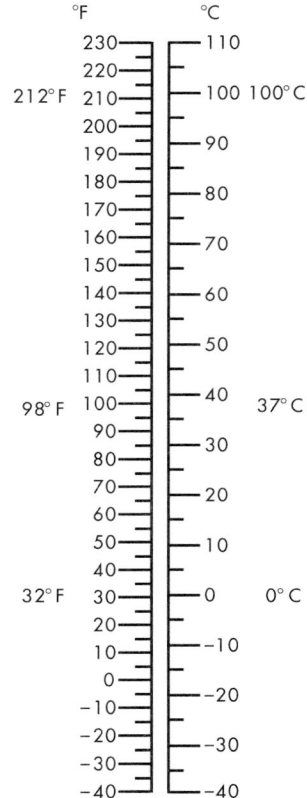

To convert temperature scales:
Fahrenheit to Celsius °C = (°F − 32) × 5/9
Celsius to Fahrenheit °F = 9/5 (°C) + 32

Additional Metric and Other Units Commonly Used in Nutrition

Unit/Abbreviation	Other Equivalent Measure
milligram/mg	1/1000 of a gram
microgram/μg	1/1,000,000 of a gram
deciliter/dl	1/10 of a liter (about ½ cup)
milliliter/ml	1/1000 of a liter (5 ml is about 1 tsp)
International Unit/IU	Crude measure of vitamin activity generally based on growth rate seen in animals

Overall, it is important to know what meter, gram, and liter represent, as well as the prefixes micro (1/1,000,000), milli (1/1000), centi (1/100), and kilo (1000).

Answers

Chapter 1

1. Supplements purchased in a store can provide vitamins and minerals. However, that is all they provide. Foods, on the other hand, supply not only vitamins and minerals but also carbohydrates, proteins, fats, and dietary fiber. These provide energy, as well as bulk for a healthy digestive system. The phytochemicals present are another bonus (see Chapter 2 for details). In addition, it is easy to overdose on certain vitamins and minerals when supplements are used.

2. A diet consisting primarily of foods derived from animal sources contains mostly proteins and fats, with a high percentage of fats as saturated fats. Saturated fats lead to a rise in blood cholesterol in many people. High blood cholesterol is linked to increased risk of cardiovascular disease. A diet high in fat is also related to increased risk of colon and prostate cancer in men.

   Fruits and vegetables are rich in dietary fiber, which helps decrease blood cholesterol and increases the rate of flow in the gastrointestinal tract. Fruits and vegetables, for the most part, contain low amounts of fat, if any, and are low in calories, thus helping maintain healthy body weight.

   Early humans lived only 30 years or so. Today our life expectancy is more than double that. History can give us clues to improve our diets, but only actual studies—such as double-blind research—can establish the actual advantages of any diet. Subjects could be placed on one of the two diets and followed for a number of years. Tests such as blood pressure, blood cholesterol, and body weight would show how the diets affect overall health.

Chapter 2

1. Increasing one's fruit and vegetable intake can be easy; it just takes planning.

   - Search for quick-service (fast food) restaurants with a salad bar.
   - Buy a variety of fruits and vegetables at the grocery store.
   - Include a fruit and/or vegetable at every meal.
   - Carry snacks, such as an apple, a banana, or carrots, with you so that, when you get hungry, you can avoid grabbing a candy bar.
   - Buy canned fruits and vegetables. These are convenient, and, because they are canned immediately after harvest, they retain their vitamins and minerals.
   - Keep a bowl of fresh vegetables in the refrigerator handy for snacks.
   - Drink fruit and vegetable juices (preferably 100% varieties).

2. Since the typical North American diet consists of many foods high in saturated fat and low in dietary fiber, Athe should assess her diet with respect to these components. She should list all of the foods she eats, preferably for a whole week, and estimate how much saturated fat and dietary fiber she consumes. She could use Appendix A in this textbook or the accompanying software. She then should change her eating habits to obtain recommended amounts of saturated fat and dietary fiber. Most likely, Athe will need to decrease saturated fat intake as well as increase dietary fiber.

Chapter 3

1. The small intestine is the most important absorption site in the digestive system because of its large surface area. Since much of the young girl's small intestine was removed, many of the nutrients she consumes are escaping absorption. It is likely that only a highly refined diet or intravenous total parenteral nutrition therapy will succeed in keeping her adequately nourished.

2. Unfortunately for Wesley, he is at high risk for developing alcoholism. He should carefully consider the consequences of alcohol use. Wesley may choose to avoid alcohol completely or consume it in moderation only. It may be helpful for him to recognize the signs of alcohol abuse to prevent any problems before they begin.

Chapter 4

1. Diverticulosis is a condition in which tiny pouches form in the wall of the colon. When foods are eaten that are not fully chewed and digested, such as hulls and nuts, undigested pieces may become trapped in the pouches. Bacteria then metabolize these particles into acids and gases, which irritate the diverticula, causing them to swell; this condition is called *diverticulitis*. The acids and gases in the swollen pouches cause cramping and abdominal pain.

2. Foods that remain in the mouth, usually caught between the teeth, are a source of food that bacteria can metabolize. As a byproduct of this metabolism, bacteria produce acids, which can decay tooth enamel, causing caries. Chewing sugar-free gum after meals decreases the risk of caries because chewing stimulates the secretion of saliva, which helps dislodge foods that remain in the mouth. Sugar-free gums also contain sugar substitutes, which bacteria can't metabolize. In addition, saliva is more alkaline than the acids produced by bacterial metabolism. This helps neutralize the acids.

Chapter 5

1. The general term *fats* refers to lipids in foods without reference to their structure. Only dietary fats with a high proportion of saturated fatty acids (or trans fatty acids) have been associated with an increased risk of cardiovascular disease. In the body, fat (primarily in the form of triglycerides) has many beneficial functions. Triglycerides form the main energy stores in the body and can release fatty acids, which serve as fuel for many cells, such as those in muscles at rest and during light activity. Stored fat insulates the body and protects vital organs. Absorption of fat-soluble vitamins from the intestine is aided by their association with dietary fats. In addition, the two essential fatty acids, linoleic acid and alpha-linolenic acid, are not synthesized by

the body and must be in the diet to maintain health. Thus, some fat is needed in the diet; moderation of intake, not elimination, is the goal.

2. The amount of cholesterol carried in HDL (high-density lipoprotein) also indicates the risk of cardiovascular disease. If one's HDL is greater than 60 mg/dl, the risk of cardiovascular disease is low. If it's less than 40 mg/dl, the risk is high. The ratio of total serum cholesterol to HDL-cholesterol is also a good indicator of one's risk. If the ratio exceeds 4 to 1, the risk is high. Since Juan's total cholesterol was 210 mg/dl and HDL cholesterol was 65 mg/dl, the ratio was 3.2 to 1 (210 mg/dl ÷ 65 mg/dl), which means he has a low risk for developing cardiovascular disease. LDL-cholesterol, which is 125 mg/dl, is also not elevated (LDL = total cholesterol − HDL − (triglycerides ÷ 5); 210 mg/dl − 65 mg/dl − [100 mg/dl ÷ 5] = 125 mg/dl).

Chapter 6

1. PKU is the abbreviation for the disease *phenylketonuria*. The liver of a person with phenylketonuria cannot readily convert phenylalanine, an essential amino acid, to tyrosine, a nonessential amino acid. Insufficient enzyme action causes this defect.

   The inability to metabolize excess phenylalanine to tyrosine leads to the formation of abnormal products that arise from alternative metabolic pathways; these products can cause mental retardation. Thus, it is vital to determine which infants have PKU, since the amount of phenylalanine in their diets must be monitored. However, because it is an essential amino acid, some phenylalanine must be consumed. Since phenylalanine cannot be sufficiently metabolized to tyrosine, the latter must be considered an essential amino acid for people with PKU.

2. Protein synthesis is a complex process by which a specific sequence and number of amino acids determine the ultimate structure of a protein. If a given amino acid is not present during protein synthesis, production will stop. In other words, protein synthesis is an all-or-none process: All of the amino acids necessary to make the protein must be available, or the protein will not be made at all. A mixed diet of plant products will likely contain enough of all nine essential amino acids, so the all-or-none principle won't typically be an issue in diet planning, even in vegetarianism.

Chapter 7

1. Many risks and diseases correlate with behaviors often combined with alcohol abuse. Unplanned sexual activity can lead to the contraction of STDs and other diseases, feelings of guilt, unplanned pregnancy, and toxicity to a fetus. If property is damaged, others can be harmed, and the persons responsible must deal with the legal and financial consequences. Both cigarettes and excessive alcohol use can cause cancer. When alcohol is used, the liver and other gastrointestinal tract organs can be harmed. The addition of smoking can compound poor health by increasing the risk of oral cancer.

2. Typical signs of alcohol abuse in teenagers are withdrawal from family activities, poor (failing) school performance, and increased colds and other general ills. José may also be making references to suicide.

Chapter 8

1. People with alcoholism usually have unbalanced diets, which can impair absorption of vitamins and minerals from the GI tract. An associated problem is poor metabolism. The B-vitamins are essential for metabolism of carbohydrates, proteins, and fats. Alcohol consumption decreases the absorption of many B-vitamins, such as thiamin, riboflavin, niacin, and folate. All of these vitamins are important in maintaining proper metabolic and nervous system function.

2. Humans must obtain vitamin C from foods because the body cannot synthesize it. A major function of this vitamin is to promote the formation of collagen, an important protein found in connective tissue. Collagen is an integral component of bone, skin, and blood vessels. Thus, a low intake of vitamin C will impair wound healing. Deficiency can also lead to scurvy, whose symptoms include bleeding gums and pinpoint hemorrhages on the skin.

   Vitamin C is an antioxidant. It works with vitamin E against free radicals and helps "reactivate" vitamin E so that it can continue to function. Vitamin C also deters certain forms of cancer, enhances iron absorption and aids in the synthesis of norepinephrine, a neurotransmitter.

   Finally, vitamin C is essential for activity within the immune system. Maintaining appropriate vitamin C intake gives the body the building blocks it needs to fight off infections. However, vitamin C does not *cure* the common cold.

Chapter 9

1. Almost all foods contain sodium. Most of the sodium in our diets is added during food processing, during cooking, and at mealtimes. The American Heart Association recommends that people generally limit sodium intake, and those at increased risk for cardiovascular disease should limit their sodium intake to no more than 2.4 grams per day. Still, sodium is essential to maintenance of normal fluid balance throughout the body and to normal nerve impulse conduction. If sodium intake is inadequate, neuromuscular symptoms will appear, including muscle weakness, headache, irritability, and confusion.

2. The mineral selenium is a cofactor for an enzyme that participates in a system that metabolizes peroxides into less toxic alcohol derivatives and water. Peroxides tend to become free radicals, which in turn can attack and break down cell membranes, causing cell damage. Selenium is considered to be important in protecting heart cells and other cells against oxidative damage. In addition, because it reduces the amount of free-radical damage to cells, selenium may be important in protecting against cancer, such as prostate cancer.

Chapter 10

1. Energy intake must equal energy output for body weight to remain the same. Weight increases when energy intake is more than output. Since basal metabolism decreases by 2% for every decade over 30 years of age, either energy intake or energy output must be modified to maintain the same weight.

   Energy balance can be attained in this case by increasing physical activity, a facet of life that tends to decrease with aging. Taking up a sport, jogging, or even parking the car farther away from a building to increase walking distance are all good strategies. People tend to become less active and therefore expend less energy without reducing food intake as they age. By increasing physical activity, energy balance and desirable weight can be maintained.

2. Although Hal has seen a steady decrease in his weight for the duration of his diet thus far, his body has built-in mechanisms that tend to fight weight loss. One of those factors is his basal metabolism. This tends to decrease to conserve energy as the number of calories in the diet decreases. Also, fat uptake into adipose cells from the blood is more efficient after the dieting has stopped.

Thus, the body resists weight loss by physiological means; however, it may finally surrender to persistent dieting, and Hal will continue to lose weight as long as he continues to diet.

Chapter 11

1. Marty has enhanced his cardiovascular fitness, a laudable goal. In addition, after a period of training, muscle cells worked on a regular basis will make more mitochondria. Since mitochondria are the sites of aerobic metabolism, this means that more ATP can be generated. ATP is a necessary component for muscle action.

2. Many wrestlers and other athletes lose weight quickly by losing large amounts of water, usually by sweating. By doing so, an athlete can compete in a lower weight class and thus gain an advantage over an opponent. However, losing weight this way can significantly impede performance. Over time, repeated dehydration episodes can lead to serious complications, such as kidney failure. Athletes also risk developing heat stress during the event.

The loss of water before a competition is the quick method of losing weight. But, if an athlete is serious about his or her sport, a gradual change in diet to create the best possible weight/muscle composition should be the goal.

Chapter 12

1. Signs that indicate an eating disorder include the following:

   a. Refusal to eat much food
   b. Obsession with being and looking thin
   c. Obsession with counting calories
   d. Not wanting to eat with others (e.g., refusing to go to a restaurant)
   e. Continually criticizing one's looks and comparing oneself to others, especially slender people
   f. Being convinced that one is overly fat when one is not

2. One of the most important topics Tom should discuss is proper nutrition. Using the concepts of adequacy, balance, and moderation, he can teach students about their diets. He could also present case studies of real people who have anorexia nervosa and bulimia nervosa, so that his students can see firsthand the outcome of these diseases. Tom should also focus on increasing awareness of the challenges facing these young adults. The prepuberty and teenage years are a time of self-evaluation and criticism. It is important for Tom to help his students feel good from within by emphasizing the importance of self-worth, regardless of one's physical appearance. Finally, Tom can teach his students how to cope with difficult situations by showing them how to alleviate stress in positive and constructive ways.

Chapter 13

1. Many changes occur in a woman during pregnancy. Her uterus and breasts grow, and her total blood volume increases. The placenta develops, the heart and kidneys work harder, stores of body fat increase, and, toward the latter part of the pregnancy, mammary glands prepare to produce milk. The nutrients needed to support these changes are:

   a. Increased energy, about 300 more kcal per day is necessary, especially during the second and third trimesters. This amount should allow adequate weight gain (25 to 35 pounds for a woman who begins pregnancy at a normal (healthy) weight).
   b. Protein needs are also increased by about 10 grams per day for women over 24 years of age and about 15 grams per day for women under 24. She likely eats this much protein already. This amount should support adequate growth.
   c. Carbohydrate intake should be at least 100 grams per day to prevent ketosis.
   d. Vitamin D should be increased to 10 micrograms per day by either increasing sunlight exposure or increasing vitamin D–fortified milk consumption. This amount will support fetal bone growth.
   e. Folate intake should increase to 600 micrograms per day to support red blood cell formation and DNA synthesis.
   f. Iron intake should increase to about 27 milligrams per day. This will support hemoglobin synthesis.
   g. Calcium is needed to promote mineralization of fetal bones and teeth. Calcium intake should meet 1000 milligrams per day.
   h. Zinc is important for growth and development. Intake should increase to 11 milligrams per day to support this.

   These nutrients should be obtained mostly from foods. However, a general multivitamin and mineral or prenatal supplement can aid in supplying these nutrients to the pregnant woman, especially in circumstances that may prevent her from adequately consuming sufficient nutrients from foods.

2. As the pregnancy advances, the uterus continues to grow to accommodate the growing fetus. As it does, it presses against the stomach as well as the intestines. Also, hormones produced in increased amounts during pregnancy relax muscles. This explains why heartburn may occur; the lower esophageal sphincter relaxes somewhat, allowing some foods and acid to regurgitate back into the esophagus—hence the heartburn. It is recommended that smaller quantities of foods be ingested and that the woman not recline after eating. High amounts of fats also decrease the rate of stomach emptying; therefore, decreasing the amounts of fats in the diet should also help. Since hormones relax muscles, the rate of peristalsis may also decrease and constipation may develop. It would be wise to gradually increase the amount of dietary fiber in Sandy's diet to improve her digestive system's peristaltic activity.

Chapter 14

1. Human milk is low in iron. Although it provides many essential nutrients to the baby, it doesn't meet all of a baby's needs after about 6 months, since iron stores are depleted by this time. This iron deficiency leads to a form of *anemia*. To prevent iron-deficiency anemia in infants, it is wise to begin feeding them iron-fortified cereal by about 6 months of age. In addition, to prevent anemia, some pediatricians recommend giving iron supplements to breastfed infants beginning shortly after birth.

2. Typical breakfast foods include cereal, eggs, toast, and pancakes, but any food can be a breakfast, lunch, or dinner food as long as it is nutrient dense. If Tim doesn't like the traditional breakfast foods but enjoys a sandwich, macaroni and cheese, or yogurt, his parents can offer them. These nutritious foods are no more beneficial at lunchtime than they are at 7 A.M.

The depletion of carbohydrate stores that occurs during the night can cause children to be lethargic and inattentive in the morning. Eating early in the morning replenishes carbohydrate stores. Many experts believe that the nutrients consumed stimulate attention in children, allowing them to perform better in school.

Chapter 15

1. Science has established a considerable link between nutrition (diet) and health. For example, very-low-fat diets have been shown to reverse atherosclerosis, and weight loss can improve type 2 diabetes in some people by reducing body fat. Although body cells will age no matter what health practices are followed, chronic disease can be

decreased through diet and lifestyle. A consistently healthful diet and a regimen of regular physical activity have proven effective in maintaining a healthful body: Muscles are firmer, bone fractures are less likely, and the person looks and feels better. The secret to enjoying "youth" throughout life is to establish a healthful physical, mental, and social framework.

2. The 1994 DSHEA Law allows companies to market herbal products in the United States without prior approval by FDA as long as they make vague structure/function claims. Jamila has to rely on the truthfulness of the manufacturer of the herbal product concerning any possible health benefits from use. Ideally, Jamila should make sure that any use of herbal products follow three specific guidelines:

   a. Follow label directions carefully and start with a low dose.
   b. Increase the dose gradually as needed, watching for potential side effects. These potential side effects should be listed on the label.
   c. Avoid products that contain mixtures of herbal substances. Many of these products have been especially linked to health problems with use.

Chapter 16

1. Bacteria thrive at room temperature, especially between 41°F and 140°F. Bacteria cause food-borne illness by releasing toxins. Cooling by refrigeration slows down bacterial growth, but it does not stop it or destroy toxins already produced. Foods left at room temperature for 2 hours, or even 1 hour in hot weather, provide microbes with the opportunity to grow. Refrigeration after that time is too late. Diana is correct in wanting to discard the food.

2. Bacteria and other microbes in foods cause more than 96% of all food-related illness. Only a small minority of people are susceptible to the health effects of food additives, such as sulfites. USDA states that most foodborne illnesses arise from poor food-handling practices by consumers. Thus, Joseph is at more risk from how he stores and prepares food rather than the food additives in the snack cakes he eats on occasion.

Chapter 17

1. Undernourished children (and adults) often show apathy, muscular weakness, and decreased physical activity and work capability. Since undernutrition decreases resistance to disease, undernourished children are likely to have more frequent infections and to recover more slowly from illness than are well-fed children.

2. Where extreme food shortages exist, there is no choice but to supply hungry people with food—they are starving and dying. However, reliance on outside help is not a long-range solution. Rather, developing countries need to develop their economies and infrastructures, so that people are able to produce or buy sufficient amounts of nutritious food to meet their needs. Appropriate development includes many aspects: education, control of population growth (if indicated), availability of machinery and other agricultural tools, and nonfarm employment opportunities. Small farms and businesses should be encouraged. As the overall economy expands, more people will be able to afford nutritious food. Agricultural production should focus on basic food crops to be consumed by a country's own citizens, rather than primarily on cash crops for export.

absorption The process by which substances are taken up from the GI tract and enter the bloodstream or the lymph. p. 88

absorptive cells A class of cells, also called *enterocytes*, that line the villi. These villi are fingerlike projections in the small intestine that participate in nutrient absorption. p. 93

acesulfame K (ay-SUL-fame) An alternative sweetener that yields no energy to the body; it is 200 times sweeter than sucrose. p. 121

acquired immunodeficiency syndrome (AIDS) A disorder in which a virus (human immunodeficiency virus [HIV]) infects specific types of immune system cells. This leaves the person with reduced immune function and, in turn, defenseless against numerous infectious agents; typically contributes to the person's death. p. 588

active absorption transport Absorption using a carrier and expending energy. In this way, the absorptive cell absorbs nutrients, such as glucose, when a high concentration of the nutrient is already present in the absorptive cells. p. 93

acute alcohol intoxication A temporary deterioration in mental function, accompanied by muscular incoordination and partial paralysis as a result of drinking alcoholic beverages too rapidly. p. 237

adenosine diphosphate (ADP) (ah-DEN-o-scene di-FOS-fate) A breakdown product of ATP. ADP is synthesized into ATP using energy from foodstuffs and a phosphate group (abbreviated Pi). p. 390

adenosine triphosphate (ATP) (ah-DEN-o-scene tri-FOS-fate) The main energy currency for cells. ATP energy is used to promote ion pumping, enzyme activity, and muscular contraction. p. 390

adequate intake (AI) Recommendations for nutrient intake when not enough information is available to establish an RDA. AIs are based on observed or experimentally determined estimates of the average nutrient intake that appears to maintain a defined nutritional state (e.g., bone health) in a specific population. Used when no RDA can be set. p. 50

adipose tissue (ad-i-POSE) A group of fat-storing cells. p. 85

aerobic (air-ROW-bic) Requiring oxygen. p. 76

alcohol Ethyl alcohol (CH_3CH_2OH). p. 10

alcohol abuse Severe alcohol-related problems, such as a person's inability to fulfill major obligations, use in hazardous situations (e.g.,

when driving), related legal problems, or use despite social and interpersonal difficulties. p. 229

alcohol dehydrogenase (dee-high-DRO-jen-ase) The enzyme used in alcohol (ethanol) metabolism; the major enzyme used in the liver when alcohol is in low concentration. p. 222

alcohol dependence Repeated alcohol-related difficulties, such as a person's inability to control use, spending a great deal of time associated with alcohol use, continued use of alcohol despite physical or psychological consequences, persistent desire or unsuccessful efforts to cut down or control alcohol use, and withdrawal symptoms. Tolerance is also seen. p. 229

aldosterone (al-DOS-ter-own) A hormone produced by the adrenal glands that acts on the kidneys to cause sodium reabsorption and, in turn, water conservation. p. 295

allergen A foreign protein, or antigen, that induces excess production of certain immune system antibodies; subsequent exposure to the same protein leads to allergic symptoms. Whereas all allergens are antigens, not all antigens are allergens. p. 509

allergy A hypersensitive immune response that occurs when antibodies produced by the body react with a protein foreign to the body (antigen). p. 481

alpha-linolenic acid (AL-fah-lin-oh-LE-nik) An essential omega-3 fatty acid with 18 carbons and 3 double bonds (C18:3, omega-3). p. 149

alpha-tocopherol (to-ca-FUR-all) The most potent form of vitamin E in terms of antioxidant function in humans. p. 254

amino acid (ah-MEE-noh) The building block for proteins containing a central carbon atom with a nitrogen atom and other atoms attached. p. 9

amniotic fluid (am-nee-OTT-ik) Fluid contained in a sac within the uterus. This fluid surrounds and protects the fetus during development. p. 293

amphetamine (am-FET-ah-mean) A group of medications that stimulate the central nervous system, among other effects. Abuse is linked to physical and psychological dependence. p. 368

amylase (AM-uh-lace) Starch-digesting enzyme from the salivary glands or pancreas. p. 122

amylopectin (AM-uh-low-pek-tin) A digestible branched-chain type of starch composed of multiple glucose units. p. 113

amylose (AM-uh-los) A digestible straight-chain type of starch made of multiple glucose units. p. 113

anaerobic (AN-ah-ROW-bic) Not requiring oxygen. p. 76

analog (AN-a-log) A chemical compound that differs slightly from another, usually natural, compound. Analogs generally contain extra or altered chemical groups and may have similar or opposite metabolic effects compared with the native compound. p. 248

anal sphincters A group of two sphincters (inner and outer) that help control expulsion of feces from the body. p. 97

anaphylactic shock (an-ah-fih-LAK-tic) A severe allergic response that results in lowered blood pressure and respiratory and gastrointestinal distress. This can be fatal. p. 509

android obesity (AN-droyd) The type of obesity in which fat is stored primarily in the abdominal area; defined as a waist circumference greater than 40 inches (102 centimeters) in men and greater than 35 inches (89 centimeters) in women; closely associated with a high risk for cardiovascular disease, hypertension, and type 2 diabetes. p. 352

anemia (ah-NEM-ee-a) Generally refers to a decreased oxygen-carrying capacity of the blood. This can be caused by many factors, such as iron deficiency or blood loss. p. 4

animal model Study of disease in animals that duplicates human disease. This can be used to understand more about human disease. p. 26

anorexia nervosa (an-oh-REX-ee-uh ner-VOH-sah) An eating disorder involving a psychological loss or denial of appetite and self-starvation, related in part to a distorted body image and to various social pressures commonly associated with puberty. p. 162

anthropometry (an-throw-PO-meh-tree) Pertaining to the measurement of body weight and the lengths, circumferences, and thicknesses of parts of the body. p. 40

antibody (AN-tih-bod-ee) Blood protein that inactivates foreign proteins found in the body. This helps prevent and control infections. p. 88

antidiuretic hormone (ADH) (an-tie-dye-u-RET-ik) A hormone secreted by the pituitary gland that acts on the kidney to cause a decrease in water excretion. It is also called arginine vasopressin (AVP). p. 295

antigen (AN-ti-jen) Any substance that induces a state of sensitivity and/or resistance to microbes or toxic substances after a lag period; substance that stimulates a specific aspect of the immune system. p. 88

antioxidant (an-tie-OX-ih-dant) Generally a compound that stops the damaging effects of reactive substances seeking an electron (i.e., oxidizing agent). This prevents the breakdown of substances in food or the body, particularly lipids. Antioxidants are especially important in preventing the breakdown of polyunsaturated lipids in the membranes of cells. An antioxidant is able to donate electrons to electron-seeking compounds. This in turn reduces electron capture and, thus, breakdown of unsaturated fatty acids and other cell components by oxidizing agents. Vitamin E is one antioxidant that cells use for protection. Some compounds have antioxidant capabilities (i.e., stop oxidation) but are not electron donors per se. p. 158

anus (A-nus) Last portion of the GI tract; serves as an outlet for that organ. p. 97

appetite The primarily psychological (external) influences that encourage us to find and eat food, often in the absence of obvious hunger. p. 16

arachidonic acid (ar-a-kih-DON-ik) An omega-6 fatty acid with 20 carbon atoms and 4 carbon-carbon double bonds (C20:4, omega-6). p. 149

arithmetic ratio A group of numbers wherein the difference between each number is the same. p. 581

aromatherapy The use of the vapors of essential oils extracted from flowers, leaves, stalks, fruits, and roots for therapeutic purposes. p. 534

artery A blood vessel that carries blood away from the heart. p. 82

aseptic processing (ah-SEP-tik) A method by which food and containers are simultaneously sterilized; it allows manufacturers to produce boxes of milk that can be stored at room temperature. Variations of this process are also known as *ultrahigh temperature (UHT)* packaging. p. 546

aspartame (AH-spar-tame) An alternative sweetener made of two amino acids and methanol; it is about 200 times sweeter than sucrose. p. 121

atherosclerosis (ath-e-roh-scle-ROH-sis) A buildup of fatty material (plaque) in the arteries, including those surrounding the heart. p. 180

atom Smallest combining unit of an element. p. 6

bacteria Single-cell microorganisms, some of which produce poisonous substances that cause illness in humans. They contain only one chromosome and lack many of the organelles found in human cells. Some can live without oxygen and survive harsh conditions by means of spore formation. p. 541

baryophobia (bear-ee-oh-FO-bee-ah) A disorder of young children and young adults characterized by stunted growth. It results from parental underfeeding in an attempt to prevent development of obesity and cardiovascular disease. p. 432

basal metabolism The minimal energy the body requires to support itself in a fasting state when resting and awake in a warm, quiet environment. It amounts to roughly 1 kcal per kilogram per hour for men and 0.9 kcal per kilogram per hour for women; these values are often referred to as basal metabolic rate (BMR). p. 344

benign Noncancerous; tumors that do not spread. p. 282

beriberi (BEAR-ee-BEAR-ee) The thiamin deficiency disorder characterized by muscle weakness, loss of appetite, nerve degeneration, and sometimes edema. p. 263

BHA Butylated hydroxyanisol, a synthetic antioxidant added to food. 167

BHT Butylated hydroxytoluene, a synthetic antioxidant added to food. 167

bile A liver secretion that is stored in the gallbladder and released through the common bile duct into the duodenum. It is essential for the absorption of fat. 97

bile acids Emulsifiers synthesized by the liver and released by the gallbladder during digestion. p. 155

binge-eating disorder An eating disorder characterized by recurrent binge eating and feelings of loss of control over eating. Binge episodes can be triggered by frustration, anger, depression, anxiety, permission to eat forbidden foods, and excessive hunger. p. 418

bioavailability The degree to which the amount of an ingested nutrient is absorbed and is available to the body. p. 297

biochemical lesion An indication of reduced biochemical function (e.g., low concentrations of nutrient by-products or enzyme activities in the blood or urine) resulting from a nutritional deficiency. p. 41

bioelectrical impedance A method to estimate total body fat that uses a low-energy electrical current. The more fat storage a person has, the more impedance (resistance) to electrical flow will be exhibited. p. 350

biotechnology A collection of processes that involve the use of advanced scientific techniques to alter and, ideally, improve characteristics of animals, plants, and other forms of life. p. 595

bisphosphonates (bis-FOS-foh-nates) Compounds primarily composed of carbon and phosphorus that bind to bone mineral and in turn reduce bone breakdown. p. 338

blood doping A technique by which an athlete's red blood cell count is increased. Blood is taken from the athlete, and the red blood cells are concentrated and then later reinjected into the athlete. Alternately, a hormone may be injected to increase red blood cell sythesis (erythropoetin [Epogen]). p. 412

body mass index (BMI) Weight (in kilograms) divided by height (in meters) squared. A normal value is 18.5 to 24.9. A value of 25 or greater indicates a risk for body weight-related health disorders. 1 BMI unit equals 6–7 pounds. p. 348

bomb calorimeter (kal-oh-RIM-eh-ter) An instrument used to determine the energy content of a food. p. 343

bond A sharing of electrons, charges, or attractions linking two atoms. p. 10

bone mass Total mineral substance (such as calcium or phosphorus) in a cross section of bone, generally expressed as grams per centimeter of length. p. 336

bone mineral density Total mineral content of bone at a specific bone site divided by the width of the bone at that site, generally expressed as grams per cubic centimeter. p. 336

brown adipose tissue (ADD-ih-pose) A specialized form of adipose tissue that produces large amounts of heat by metabolizing energy-yielding nutrients without synthesizing much useful energy for the body. The unused energy is released as heat. p. 346

buffers Compounds that cause a solution to resist changes in acid-base balance. p. 203

bulimia nervosa (boo-LEEM-ee-uh) An eating disorder in which large quantities of food are eaten at one time (binge eating) and then purged from the body by vomiting, or misuse of laxatives, diuretics, or enemas. Alternate means to counteract the caloric excess are fasting and excessive exercise. p. 418

cancer A condition characterized by uncontrolled growth of abnormal body cells. p. 78

cancer initiation The step in the process of cancer development that begins with alterations in DNA, the genetic material in a cell. This may cause the cell to no longer respond to normal physiological controls. p. 284

cancer progression The final stage in the cancer process, during which the cancer cells proliferate, forming a mass large enough to significantly affect body functions. p. 285

cancer promotion The stage in the cancer process when cell division increases, in turn decreasing the time available for repair enzymes to act on altered DNA, and encouraging cells with altered DNA to develop and grow. Anything that increases the rate of cell division decreases the chance that the repair enzymes will find the altered part of the DNA in time to do their work. p. 285

capillary (KAP-ill-air-ee) Microscopic blood vessel that connects the smallest arteries and veins; site of nutrient, oxygen, and waste exchange between body cells and the blood. p. 82

carbohydrate (kar-bow-HIGH-drate) A compound containing carbon, hydrogen, and oxygen atoms; most are known as *sugars, starches,* and *dietary fibers.* p. 6

carbohydrate loading A process in which a very high carbohydrate intake is consumed for 6 days before an athletic event while tapering exercise duration in an attempt to increase muscle glycogen stores. p. 398

carbon skeleton Amino acid after the amino group has been removed. p. 204

carcinogenic Describes a compound with the potential to cause cancer. p. 133

cardiac muscle Muscle that makes up the walls of the heart. Produces rhythmical involuntary contractions. p. 81

cardiovascular disease A disease characterized by the deposition of fatty material in the blood vessels that serve the heart, often called hardening of the arteries. These deposits restrict blood flow through the heart, which in turn can lead to heart damage and death. Also termed *coronary heart disease* (CHD), as the vessels of the heart are the primary site of disease. The term cardiovascular disease (CVD) is typically used, since in addition to the heart, the arteries that serve the rest of the body can experience the same deterioration. p. 78

cardiovascular system The body system consisting of the heart, blood vessels, and blood. This system transports nutrients, waste products, gases, and hormones throughout the body and plays an important role in immune responses and regulation of body temperature. p. 81

cariogenic (CARE-ee-oh-jen-ik) Literally "caries producing"; a substance often carbohydrate-rich (such as caramel), that promotes dental caries. p. 133

carnitine (CAR-nih-teen) A compound used to shuttle fatty acids from the cytoplasm of the cell into mitochondria. p. 278

carotenoids (kah-ROT-en-oyds) Pigment materials in fruits and vegetables that range in color from yellow to orange to red; 3 yield vitamin A activity in humans and thus are called provitamin A. Many have antioxidant properties as well. One example is beta-carotene. p. 158

cartilage Connective tissue, usually part of the skeleton, that is composed of cells in a flexible network. p. 81

case-control study Individuals who have the condition in question, such as lung cancer, are compared with individuals who do not have the condition. p. 26

cash crop A crop grown specifically for export, so that goods from other countries can be purchased. Cultivation of cash crops diverts agricultural resources necessary to feed a country's own citizens. Examples are coffee, tea, cocoa, and bananas. p. 585

cell A minute structure; the living basis of plant and animal organization. In animals it is bounded by a cell membrane. Cells contain both genetic material and systems for synthesizing energy-yielding compounds. Cells have the ability to take up compounds from and excrete compounds into their surroundings. p. 10

cell-mediated immunity A process in which white blood cells come in actual contact with the invading cells in order to destroy them. p. 88

cell nucleus Organelle bound by its own double membrane and containing chromosomes, the genetic information for cell protein synthesis and cell replication. p. 76

cellulose (SELL-you-los) A straight-chain polysaccharide of glucose molecules that is undigestible because of the presence of beta bonds; part of insoluble fiber. p. 115

Celsius A centigrade measure of temperature. For conversion: (degrees in Fahrenheit − 32) × 5/9 = °C; (degrees in Celsius × 9/5) + 32 = °F. p. 11

central nervous system (CNS) The brain and spinal cord portions of the nervous system. p. 84

cerebrovascular accident (CVA) (se-REE-bro-VAS-cue-lar) Death of part of the brain tissue due typically to a blood clot; also called *stroke*. p. 179

chain-breaking Breaking the link between two or more actions that encourage overeating such as snacking while watching television. p. 363

chelation (key-LAY-shun) The use of medicinal compounds, such as ethylenediaminetetraacetic acid (EDTA), to bind metals and other constituents in the blood. p. 534

chemical reaction An interaction between two chemicals that changes both participants. p. 9

cholecystokinin (CCK) (ko-la-sis-toe-KY-nin) A hormone that stimulates enzyme release from the pancreas, bile release from the gallbladder, and hunger regulation. p. 18

cholesterol (ko-LES-te-rol) A waxy lipid found in all body cells. It has a structure containing multiple chemical rings that is found only in foods that contain animal products. p. 42

chromosome A single large DNA molecule and its associated proteins containing many genes; it stores and transmits genetic information. p. 76

chronic (KRON-ik) Long-standing, developing over time. When referring to disease, this term indicates that the disease progress, once developed, is slow and tends to remain; a good example is cardiovascular disease. p. 4

chylomicron (kye-lo-MY-kron) Lipoprotein made of dietary fats that are surrounded by a shell of cholesterol, phospholipids, and protein. Chylomicrons are formed in the absorptive cells (enterocytes) in the small intestine after fat absorption and travel through the lymphatic system to the bloodstream. p. 156

chyme (KIME) A mixture of stomach secretions and partially digested food. p. 91

cirrhosis (see-ROH-sis) A loss of functioning liver cells, which are replaced by nonfunctioning connective tissue. Any substance that poisons liver cells can lead to cirrhosis. The most common cause is chronic, excessive alcohol intake. p. 222

cis isomer (sis EYE-so-mer) An isomer form seen in compounds with double bonds, such as fatty acids, in which the hydrogens on both ends of the double bond lie on the same side of the plane of that bond. p. 166

clinical symptoms Generally, a change in health status noted by the individual (such as stomach pain) or noticed by a clinician during physical examination (the latter is technically called a clinical sign). p. 41

Clostridium botulinum (klo-STRID-ee-um BOT-you-LY-num) A bacterium that can cause a fatal type of foodborne illness. p. 489

coenzyme A compound that combines with an inactive protein to form a catalytically active protein. In this manner, coenzymes aid in enzyme function. p. 241

cognitive behavior therapy Psychological therapy in which the person's assumptions about dieting, body weight, and related issues are challenged. New ways of thinking are explored and then practiced by the person. In this way, the person can learn new ways to control disordered eating behaviors and related life stress. p. 426

cognitive restructuring Changing one's frame of mind regarding eating—for example, instead of using a difficult day as an excuse to overeat, substituting other pleasures for rewards, such as a relaxing walk with a friend. p. 363

colic (KOL-ik) Periodic, inconsolable crying in a healthy young infant associated with sharp abdominal pain. p. 491

colostrum (ko-LAHS-trum) The first fluid secreted by the breast during late pregnancy and the first few days after birth. This thick fluid is rich in immune factors and protein. p. 463

complement A series of blood proteins that participate in a complex reaction cascade following stimulation by an antigen-antibody complex or the surface of a bacterial cell. Various activated complement proteins can enhance phagocytosis, contribute to inflammation, and destroy bacteria. p. 88

complementary proteins Two food protein sources that make up for each other's inadequate supply of specific essential amino acids; together they yield a sufficient amount of all nine and so provide high-quality (complete) protein for the diet. p. 192

complete proteins Proteins that contain ample amounts of all nine essential amino acids. p. 191

compound A group of different types of atoms bonded together in definite proportion (see also molecule). Not all chemical compounds exist as molecules. Some compounds are made up of ions attracted to each other, such as Na^+Cl^- (table salt). p. 10

connective tissue Protein tissue that holds different structures in the body together. Some structures are made up of connective tissue—notably, tendons and cartilage. Connective tissue also forms part of bone and the nonmuscular structures of arteries and veins. p. 77

constipation A condition in which bowel movements are infrequent. p. 106

contingency management Forming a plan of action to respond to a situation in which overeating is likely, such as when snacks are within arm's reach at a party. p. 363

control group Participants in an experiment who are not given the treatment being tested. p. 26

cortical bone (KORT-ih-kal) Tightly packed bone; also called compact or dense bone. p. 336

cortisol (KORT-ih-sol) A hormone made by the adrenal glands that, among other functions, stimulates the production of glucose from amino acids and increases the desire to eat. p. 17

creatinine (cree-A-tin-in) Nitrogenous waste product of the compound creatine found in muscles. p. 99

cretinism (KREET-in-ism) The stunting of body growth and poor mental development in the offspring that results from inadequate maternal intake of iodide during pregnancy. p. 243

cryptosporidiosis (krip-toe-spore-id-ee-O-sis) An intestinal disease, characterized by diarrhea, that originates from a protozoan parasite of the genus *Cryptosporidium*. p. 296

cystic fibrosis (SIS-tik figh-BRO-sis) A disease that often leads to overproduction of mucus. Mucus can invade the pancreas, decreasing enzyme output. The lack of lipase enzyme output then contributes to severe fat malabsorption. p. 94

cytoplasm (SITE-o-plas-um) The semifluid part of the cell between the cell membrane and the nucleus; it also does not include membrane-bound organelles. The cytoplasm contains many enzymes and structural proteins. p. 76

Daily Values A set of standard nutrient-intake values developed by FDA and used as a reference for expressing nutrient content on nutrition labels. p. 50

Delaney Clause A clause to the 1958 Food Additives Amendment of the Pure Food and Drug Act in the United States that prevents the intentional (direct) addition to foods of a compound that has been shown to cause cancer in laboratory animals or humans. p. 552

dementia (de-MEN-sha) General persistent loss or decrease in mental function. p. 265

denature (dee-NAY-ture) Alteration of a protein's three-dimensional structure, usually because of treatment by heat, enzymes, acid or alkaline solutions, or agitation. p. 196

dental caries (KARE-ees) Erosions in the surface of a tooth caused by acids made by bacteria as they metabolize sugars. p. 120

deoxyribonucleic acid (DNA) The site of hereditary information in cells; DNA directs the synthesis of cell proteins. p. 76

DEXA bone scan Method to measure bone density that uses small amounts of x-ray radiation. The ability of a bone to block the path of the radiation is used as a measure of bone density at that bone site. DEXA stands for dual energy x-ray absorptiometry. p. 338

diabetes (DYE-uh-BEET-eez) A disease characterized by high blood glucose, resulting from either insufficient or no release of the hormone insulin by the pancreas or the general inability of insulin to act on certain body cells, such as muscle cells. The two major forms are type 1 (requires daily insulin therapy) and type 2 (may or may not require insulin therapy). p. 78

diastolic blood pressure (dye-ah-STOL-ik) The pressure in the arterial blood vessels when the heart is between beats. p. 181

dietary fiber Substances in plant foods that are not digested by the processes that take place in the stomach or small intestine. These add bulk to feces. p. 8

Dietary Guidelines for Americans General goals for nutrient intake and diet composition set by USDA and the Department of Health and Human Services (DHHS). p. 49

Dietary Reference Intakes (DRIs) The overarching frameworks for nutrient recommendations made by the Food and Nutrition Board, a part of the National Academy of Science. p. 50

dietitian See *Registered Dietitian*. p. 30

digestion The process by which large ingested molecules are mechanically and chemically broken down to produce smaller forms that can be absorbed across the wall of the GI tract. p. 88

digestive system The body system consisting of the gastrointestinal tract and accessory structures such as the liver, gallbladder, and pancreas. This system performs the mechanical and chemical processes of digestion, absorption of nutrients, and elimination of wastes. p. 88

direct calorimetry (kal-oh-RIM-eh-tree) A method of determining a body's energy use by measuring heat that emanates from the body, usually using an insulated chamber. p. 347

disaccharides (dye-SACK-uh-rides) Class of sugars formed by the chemical bonding of two monosaccharides. p. 113

disordered eating Mild and short-term changes in eating patterns that occur in relation to a stressful event, an illness, or desire to modify one's diet for a variety of health and personal appearance reasons. p. 418

distillation (dis-te-LAY-shun) A physical method used to separate liquids based on their boiling points. p. 220

diuretic (dye-u-RET-ik) A substance that, when ingested, increases the flow of urine. p. 303

diverticula (DYE-ver-TIK-you-luh) Pouches that protrude through the exterior wall of the large intestine. p. 115

diverticulitis (DYE-ver-tik-you-LITE-us) An inflammation of the diverticula caused by acids produced by bacterial metabolism inside the diverticula. p. 115

diverticulosis (DYE-ver-tik-you-LOW-sus) The condition of having many diverticula in the large intestine. p. 115

docosahexaenoic acid (DHA) (DOE-co-sa-hex-ee-no-ik) An omega-3 fatty acid with 22 carbons and 6 carbon-carbon double bonds (C22:6, omega-3). It is present in large amounts in fatty fish and is synthesized in the body from alpha-linolenic acid. DHA is especially present in the retina of the eye. p. 159

dopamine (DOE-pah-mean) A type of neurotransmitter in the central nervous system that leads to feelings of euphoria, among other functions; it is also used to form norepinephrine, another neurotransmitter molecule. p. 85

double-blind study An experiment in which the participants and researchers are unaware of the participant's assignment (test or placebo) or the outcome of the study until it is completed. An independent third party holds the code and the data until the study is completed. p. 26

early childhood caries Tooth decay that results from formula or juice (and even human milk) bathing the teeth as the child sleeps with a bottle in his or her mouth. The upper teeth are mostly

affected, as the lower teeth are protected by the tongue; formerly called *nursing bottle syndrome*. p. 488

eating disorder Severe alterations in eating patterns linked to physiological changes. The alterations are associated with food restricting, binge eating, purging, and fluctuations in weight. They also involve a number of emotional and cognitive changes that affect the way a person perceives and experiences his or her body. p. 418

ecosystem A "community" in nature that includes plants, animals, and the environment. p. 585

ectomorph (EK-toe-morf) A body type associated with very long, thin bones and very long, thin fingers. p. 354

edema (uh-DEE-muh) The buildup of excess fluid in extracellular spaces. p. 202

eicosapentaenoic acid (EPA) (eye-KOH-sah-pen-tah-ee-NO-ik) An omega-3 fatty acid with 20 carbons and 5 carbon-carbon double bonds (C20:5, omega-3). It is present in large amounts in fatty fish and is synthesized in the body from alpha-linolenic acid. p. 159

electrolytes (ih-LEK-tro-lites) Compounds that separate into ions in water and, in turn, are able to conduct an electrical current. These include sodium, chloride, and potassium. p. 291

elements Substances that cannot be separated into simpler substances by chemical processes. Common elements in nutrition include carbon, oxygen, hydrogen, nitrogen, calcium, phosphorus, and iron. p. 7

elimination diet A restrictive diet that systematically tests foods that may cause an allergic response by first eliminating them for 1 to 2 weeks and then adding them back, one at a time. p. 510

embryo (EM-bree-oh) In humans, the developing in utero offspring from about the beginning of the third to the end of the eighth week after conception. p. 446

emulsifier (ee-MULL-sih-fire) A compound that can suspend fat in water by isolating individual fat droplets using a shell of water molecules or other substances to prevent the fat from coalescing. p. 155

endocrine gland (EN-doh-krin) A hormone-producing gland. p. 85

endocrine system (EN-doh-krin) The body system consisting of the various glands and the hormones these glands secrete. This system has major regulatory functions in the body, such as in reproduction and cell metabolism. p. 85

endometrium (en-doh-ME-tree-um) The membrane that lines the inside of the uterus. It increases in thickness during the menstrual cycle until ovulation occurs. The surface layers are shed during menstruation if conception does not take place. p. 285

endomorph (EN-dough-morf) A body type characterized by short, stubby bones, a short trunk, and short fingers. p. 354

endoplasmic reticulum (ER) (en-doh-PLAZ-mik re-TIK-u-lum) An organelle in the cytoplasm composed of a network of canals running through the cystoplasm. Rough ER contains ribosomes. Smooth ER does not contain ribosomes. p. 76

endorphins (en-DOR-fins) Natural body tranquilizers that may be involved in the feeding response. p. 17

energy balance A state in which energy intake, in the form of food and/or alcohol, matches the energy expended, primarily through basal metabolism and physical activity. p. 341

energy density A state determined by comparing the energy (kcal) content of a food to its weight of the food. An energy-dense food is high in calories but weighs very little (e.g., many fried foods), whereas a food low in energy density has few calories but weighs a lot, such as an orange. p. 36

enriched A term generally meaning that the vitamins thiamin, niacin, riboflavin, and folate and the mineral iron have been added to a grain product to improve nutritional quality. p. 59

enterocytes (en-TER-oh-sites) Epithelial cells, which are highly specialized for digestion and absorption, that line the intestinal villi. p. 93

enterohepatic circulation (EN-ter-oh-heh-PAT-ik) Recycling of compounds between the small intestine and the liver over and over again, as happens with certain bile constituents. p. 97

enzyme (EN-zime) A compound that speeds the rate of a chemical process but is not altered by the process. Almost all enzymes are proteins. p. 8, 74

epidemiology (ep-uh-dee-me-OLL-uh-gee) The study of how disease patterns vary between different population groups, such as the cases of stomach cancer in Japan compared with that in Germany. p. 25

epiglottis (ep-ih-GLOT-iss) Flap that folds down over the trachea during swallowing. p. 91

epinephrine (ep-ih-NEF-rin) A hormone also known as adrenaline; it is released by the adrenal gland (located on each kidney) and various nerve endings in the body. It acts to increase glycogen breakdown in the liver, among other functions. p. 127

epithelial cells (ep-ih-THEE-lee-ul) The surface cells that line the outside of the body and all external passages within it. p. 247

epithelial tissue The covering in internal and external surfaces of the body, including the lining of vessels and other small cavities. It consists of epithelial cells joined by a small amount of cementing material. p. 77

equilibrium (ee-kwih-LIB-ree-um) In nutrition, a state in which nutrient intake equals nutrient losses. Thus, the body maintains a stable condition. p. 204

ergogenic (ur-go-JEN-ic) Work-producing. An ergogenic acid is a mechanical, nutritional, psychological, pharmacological, or physiological substance or treatment that is intended to directly improve exercise performance. p. 411

erythrocyte (eh-RITH-row-site) Mature red blood cell that has no nucleus and a life span of about 120 days; it contains hemoglobin, which transports oxygen and carbon dioxide. p. 269

erythropoietin (eh-REE-throw-POY-eh-tin) A hormone secreted mostly by the kidneys that enhances red blood cell synthesis and stimulates red blood cell release from bone marrow. p. 99

esophagus (eh-SOF-ah-gus) A tube in the GI tract that connects the pharynx with the stomach. p. 91

essential fatty acids Fatty acids that must be supplied by the diet to maintain health. Currently only linoleic acid and alpha-linolenic acid are classified as essential fatty acids. p. 149

essential (indispensable) amino acids Amino acids that cannot be synthesized by humans in sufficient amounts and therefore must be included in the diet; there are nine essential amino acids. These are also called indispensable amino acids. p. 190

essential nutrient In nutritional terms, a substance that, when left out of a diet, leads to signs of poor health. The body either can't produce this nutrient or can't produce it fast enough to meet its needs. Then, if added back to a diet before permanent damage occurs, the affected aspects of health are restored. p. 3

exchange system A system for classifying foods into numerous lists based on their macronutrient composition and establishing serving sizes, so that one serving of each food on a list contains the same amount of carbohydrate, protein, fat, and energy content. p. 60

experiment A test made to examine the validity of a hypothesis. p. 24

extracellular fluid Fluid present outside the cells; represents one-third of all body fluid. p. 291

extracellular space The space outside cells. p. 202

facilitated diffusion The carrier-mediated transport of molecules through the cell membrane along the direction of their concentration gradients. It does not require the expenditure of energy. p. 95

famine An extreme shortage of food that leads to massive starvation in a population; often associated with crop failures, war, and political strife. p. 572

fasting hypoglycemia (HIGH-po-gligh-SEE-me-ah) Low blood glucose that follows after about a day of fasting. p. 142

fat-soluble vitamins Vitamins that dissolve in such substances as ether and benzene, but not readily in water. These vitamins are A, D, E, and K. p. 241

fatty acid Major part of most lipids; composed of a chain of carbons flanked by hydrogen with an

$$acid\ group\ (-\overset{O}{\overset{\|}{C}}-OH)$$

at one end and a methyl group ($-CH_3$) at the other. p. 8

feces (FEE-seas) Substances discharged from the bowel during defecation, consisting of the undigested residue of food, dead GI tract cells, mucus, bacteria, and other waste material. Another term for feces is stool. p. 97

female athlete triad A condition characterized by disordered eating, lack of menstrual periods, and osteoporosis. p. 432

fermentation The conversion, without the use of oxygen, of carbohydrates to alcohols, acids, and carbon dioxide. p. 113

fetal alcohol effect (FAE) Hyperactivity, attention deficit disorder, poor judgment, sleep disorders, and delayed learning as a result of being prenatally exposed to alcohol. p. 472

fetal alcohol syndrome (FAS) (FEET-al) A group of irreversible physical and mental abnormalities in the infant that result from the mother's consuming alcohol during pregnancy. p. 472

fetus (FEET-us) The developing life form from about the beginning of the ninth week after conception until birth. p. 250

folk medicine A medical treatment based on the beliefs, traditions, or customs of a particular society or ethnic/cultural group. p. 533

foodborne illness Sickness caused by the ingestion of food containing toxic substances produced by microorganisms. p. 541

food intolerance An adverse reaction to food that does not involve an allergic reaction. p. 509

food sensitivity A mild reaction to a substance in a food that might be expressed as slight itching or redness of the skin. p. 509

fortified A term generally meaning that vitamins, minerals, or both have been added to a food product in excess of what was originally found in the product. p. 59

fraternal twins Offspring that develop from two separate ova and sperm and therefore have separate genetic identities, although they develop simultaneously in the mother. p. 355

free radicals Short-lived form of compounds that exist with an unpaired electron, causing it to seek an electron from another compound. Free radicals can be very destructive to electron-dense components, such as the DNA and cell membranes. p. 227

fructose (FROOK-tose) A monosaccharide with six carbons that form a five-membered ring or six-membered ring with oxygen in the ring; found in fruits and honey. p. 112

fruitarian (froot-AIR-ee-un) A person who eats primarily fruits, nuts, honey, and vegetable oils. p. 214

functional foods Foods that provide health benefits beyond those supplied by the traditional nutrients they contain. For example, a tomato contains the phytochemical lycopene, so it can be called a functional food. p. 35

fungi Simple parasitic life forms, including molds, mildews, yeasts, and mushrooms. They live on dead or decaying organic matter. Fungi can grow as single cells, like yeast, or as multicellular colonies, as seen with molds. p. 541

galactose (gah-LAK-tos) A six-carbon monosaccharide that forms a six-membered ring with oxygen in the ring; closely related to glucose. p. 113

galactosemia (gah-LAK-toh-SEE-mee-ah) A rare genetic disease characterized by the buildup of the single sugar galactose in the bloodstream, resulting from the inability of the liver to metabolize it. If present at birth and left untreated, this disease causes severe mental and growth retardation in the infant. p. 203

gallbladder The organ attached to the underside of the liver and in which bile is stored and secreted. p. 97

gastrin (GAS-trin) A hormone that stimulates enzyme and acid secretion in the stomach. p. 86

gastroesophageal reflux disease (GERD) (gas-troh-eh-SOF-ah-jee-al) Disease that results from stomach acid backing up into the esophagus. The acid irritates the lining of the esophagus, causing pain. p. 106

gastrointestinal (GI) tract The main sites in the body used for digestion and absorption of nutrients. It consists of the mouth, esophagus, stomach, small intestine, large intestine, rectum, and anus. p. 17

gastroplasty (GAS-troh-plas-tee) Surgery performed on the stomach to limit its volume to approximately 30 milliliters. p. 369

generally recognized as safe (GRAS) A list of food additives that in 1958 were considered safe for consumption. Manufacturers were allowed to continue to use these additives, without special clearance, when needed for food products. FDA bears responsibility for proving they are not safe but can remove unsafe products from the list. p. 551

genes (JEANs) The hereditary material on chromosomes. Genes provide the blueprint for the production of cell proteins. The nucleus of the cell contains about 30,000 genes. p. 10, 76

genetic engineering Alteration of genetic material in plants or animals with the intent of improving growth, disease resistance, or other characteristics. p. 595

genetically modified organism (GMO) Any organism created by genetic engineering. p. 596

geometric ratio A group of numbers wherein the division of each number by the one to the left of it yields the same answer. p. 581

gestation (jes-TAY-shun) The period of intrauterine development of offspring, from conception to birth; in humans, gestation lasts for about 37 to 41 weeks after the woman's last menstrual period. p. 448

gestational diabetes (jes-TAY-shun-al) Elevated blood glucose that develops during pregnancy and returns to normal after birth; one cause is placental production of hormones that interfere with the regulation of blood glucose by insulin. p. 460

glucagon (GLOO-kuh-gon) A hormone made by the pancreas that stimulates the breakdown of glycogen in the liver into glucose; this increases blood glucose. Glucagon also performs other functions. p. 125

glucose (GLOO-kos) A six-carbon monosaccharide that forms a six-membered ring with oxygen in the ring; found as such in blood, and in table sugar bound to fructose; also known as *dextrose*, it is one of the simple sugars. p. 7, 112

glycemic index (GI) (gli-SEA-mik) The blood glucose response of a given food, compared to a standard (typically, glucose or white bread). Glycemic index of a food is influenced by starch structure, fiber content, food processing, physical structure, and macronutrients in the meal, such as fat. p. 134

glycerol (GLIS-er-ol) A three-carbon alcohol used to form triglycerides. p. 145

glycogen (GLI-ko-jen) A carbohydrate made of multiple units of glucose with a highly branched structure; sometimes known as *animal starch*. It is the storage form of glucose in humans and is synthesized (and stored) in the liver and muscles. p. 111

goiter (GOY-ter) An enlargement of the thyroid gland that can be caused by a lack of iodide in the diet. p. 324

Golgi complex (GOAL-jee) The cell organelle near the nucleus that processes newly synthesized protein for secretion or distribution to other organelles. p. 77

gout Joint inflammation caused by accumulation of a body compound called uric acid. Obesity is a risk factor for developing gout. p. 351

green revolution Increases in crop yields accompanying the introduction of new agricultural technologies in less developed countries, beginning in the 1960s. The key technologies were high-yielding, disease-resistant strains of rice, wheat, and corn; greater use of fertilizer and water; and improved cultivation practices. p. 585

growth hormone A pituitary hormone that stimulates body growth and release of fat from storage; it also has other effects. p. 412

gums Dietary fiber containing chains of galactose, glucuronic acid, and other monosaccharides; characteristically found in exudates from plant stems. p. 115

H₂ blockers Medications, such as cimetidine (Tagamet), that block the stimulation of stomach acid production caused by histamine. p. 105

heart attack Rapid fall in heart function caused by reduced blood flow through the heart's blood vessels. Often part of the heart dies in the process. It is technically called a *myocardial infarction*. p. 42

heartburn A pain emanating from the esophagus, caused by stomach acid backing up into the esophagus and irritating the esophageal tissue. p. 105

heart disease See *cardiovascular disease.*

heat cramps Heat cramps are a frequent complication of heat exhaustion. They usually occur in individuals exercising for several hours in a hot climate who have experienced large sweat losses and have consumed a large volume of water. The cramps occur in skeletal muscles and consist of contractions for 1 to 3 minutes at a time. p. 401

heat exhaustion The first stage of heat-related illness that occurs because of depletion of blood volume from fluid loss by the body. This increases body temperature and can lead to headache,

dizziness, muscle weakness, and visual disturbances, among other effects. p. 401

heatstroke Heatstroke can occur when internal body temperature reaches 105°F. Sweating generally ceases if left untreated, and blood circulation is greatly reduced. Nervous system damage may ensue and death is likely. Often in individuals who suffer heatstroke the skin is hot and dry. p. 401

hematocrit (hee-MAT-oh-krit) The percentage of total blood volume made up of red blood cells. p. 317

heme iron (HEEM) Iron provided from animal tissues as hemoglobin and myoglobin. Approximately 40% of the iron in meat is heme iron; it is readily absorbed. p. 315

hemicellulose (hem-ih-SELL-you-los) A dietary fiber containing xylose, galactose, glucose, and other monosaccharides bonded together. p. 115

hemochromatosis (heem-oh-krom-ah-TOE-sis) A disorder of iron metabolism characterized by increased iron absorption and deposition in the liver and heart tissue. This eventually poisons the cells in those organs. p. 320

hemoglobin (HEEM-oh-glow-bin) The iron-containing part of the red blood cell that carries oxygen to the cells and some carbon dioxide away from the cells. It is also responsible for the red color of blood. p. 315

hemolysis (hee-MOL-ih-sis) Destruction of red blood cells caused by the breakdown of the red blood cell membranes. This causes the cell contents to leak into the fluid portion (plasma) of the blood. p. 254

hemorrhage (hem-OR-ij) An escape of blood from blood vessels. p. 255

hemorrhagic stroke (hem-oh-RAJ-ik) Damage to part of the brain resulting from rupture of a blood vessel and subsequent bleeding within or over the internal surface of the brain. p. 160

hemorrhoid (HEM-or-oid) A pronounced swelling in a large vein, particularly veins found in the anal region. p. 107

herbicide (ERB-ih-side) A compound that reduces the growth and reproduction of plants. p. 563

high-density lipoprotein (HDL) The lipoprotein that picks up cholesterol from dying cells and other sources and transfers it to the other lipoproteins in the bloodstream, as well as directly to the liver. A low blood HDL value increases the risk for cardiovascular disease. p. 128

high-fructose corn syrup A corn syrup that has been manufactured to contain between 40% and 90% fructose. p. 112

high-quality (complete) proteins Dietary proteins that contain ample amounts of all nine essential amino acids. p. 191

homocysteine (homo-CYS-ti-ene) An amino acid not used in protein synthesis, but instead arises during metabolism of the amino acid methionine. Homocysteine is likely toxic to many cells, such as those that line blood vessels. p. 158

hormone A compound secreted into the bloodstream by one type of cell that acts to control the function of another type of cell. For example, certain cells in the pancreas produce insulin, which in turn acts on muscle and other types of cells. Protein forms, such as insulin or leptin, must be injected if used as therapy since they would be digested and broken down if taken orally. p. 17

hospice units (HAHS-pis) A facility offering care that emphasizes comfort and dignity in death. p. 527

human immunodeficiency virus (HIV) The virus that leads to acquired immune deficiency syndrome (AIDS). p. 588

hunger The primarily physiological (internal) drive to find and eat food, mostly regulated by innate cues to eating. p. 16

hydrogen peroxide Chemically, H_2O_2. p. 77

hydrogenation (high-dro-jen-AY-shun) Addition of hydrogen to a carbon-carbon double bond, producing a single bond. Because hydrogenation of unsaturated fatty acids in a vegetable oil increases its hardness, this process is used to convert liquid oils into more solid fats, which are used in making margarine and shortening. Trans fatty acids are a by-product of hydrogenation of vegetable oils. p. 164

hyperglycemia (HIGH-per-gligh-SEE-me-uh) High blood glucose, above 125 milligrams per 100 milliliters (dl) of blood. p. 127

hypertension (high-per-TEN-shun) A condition in which blood pressure remains persistently elevated. Obesity, inactivity, excess alcohol intake, and excess salt intake all can contribute to the problem. p. 78

hypoglycemia (HIGH-po-gligh-SEE-me-uh) Low blood glucose, below 40 to 50 milligrams per 100 milliliters (dl) of blood. p. 127

hypothalamus (high-po-THALL-uh-mus) A region at the base of the brain that contains cells that play a role in the regulation of hunger, respiration, body temperature, and other body functions. p. 17

hypothesis (high-POTH-eh-sis) An "educated guess" by a scientist to explain a phenomenon. p. 24

identical twins Two offspring that develop from a single ovum and sperm and, consequently, have the same genetic makeup. p. 354

ileocecal sphincter (ill-ee-oh-SEE-kal SFINK-ter) Ring of smooth muscle between the end of the small intestine and the large intestine. p. 95

immune system The body system consisting of white blood cells, lymph glands and vessels, and various other body tissues. The immune system provides defense against foreign invaders, primarily due to the action of various types of white blood cells. p. 86

immunoglobulins (em-you-no-GLOB-you-lins) Proteins found in the blood that bind to specific antigens, also called antibodies. The five major classes of immunoglobins play different roles in antibody-related immunity. p. 87

incidence The number of new cases of a disease in a defined population over a specific period of time, such as 1 year. p. 26

incidental food additives Additives that appear in food products indirectly, from environmental contamination of food ingredients or during the manufacturing process. p. 551

incomplete (lower-quality) protein Food protein that lacks ample amount of one or more of the essential amino acids needed to support human protein needs. p. 191

indirect calorimetry (kal-oh-RIM-eh-tree) A method to measure the energy use by the body by measuring oxygen uptake. Formulas are then used to convert this gas exchange value into energy use. p. 347

infancy Earliest stage of childhood—from birth to 1 year of age. p. 478

infectious disease (in-FEK-shus) Any disease caused by an invasion of the body by microorganisms, such as bacteria, fungi, or viruses. p. 26

infrastructure (IN-fra-struck-sure) The basic framework of a system or organization. For society, this includes roads, bridges, telephones, and other basic technologies. p. 581

inorganic (in-or-GAN-ik) Any substance lacking carbon atoms bonded to hydrogen atoms in the chemical structure. p. 9

insoluble fibers Fibers that mostly do not dissolve in water and are not metabolized by bacteria in the large intestine. These include cellulose, some hemicelluloses, and lignins. p. 115

insulin (IN-su-lynn) A hormone produced by the beta cells of the pancreas. Among other processes, insulin increases the synthesis of glycogen in the liver and the movement of glucose from the bloodstream into body cells. p. 126

integumentary system (in-teg-you-MEN-tah-ree) The body system consisting of the skin, hair, glands, and nails; the largest organ in the body. p. 81

intentional food additive Additives knowingly (directly) incorporated into food products by manufacturers. p. 551

interferons (in-ter-FEAR-ons) A group of proteins released by virus-infected cells that bind to other cells, stimulating synthesis of antiviral proteins, which in turn inhibit viral multiplication. p. 88

international unit (IU) A crude measure of vitamin activity, often based on the growth rate of animals. Today these units have generally been replaced by precise measurement of actual quantities in milligrams or micrograms. p. 249

intracellular fluid Fluid contained within a cell; represents about two-thirds of all body fluid. p. 291

intrinsic factor (in-TRIN-zik) A substance present in gastric juice that enhances vitamin B-12 absorption. p. 272

in utero (in-YOU-ter-oh) "In the uterus," or during pregnancy.

ion (EYE-on) An atom with an unequal number of electrons and protons. Negative ions have more electrons than protons; positive ions have more protons than electrons. p. 10

irradiation (ir-RAY-dee-AY-shun) A process in which radiation energy is applied to foods, creating compounds (free radicals) within the food that destroy cell membranes, break down DNA, link proteins together, limit enzyme activity, and alter a variety of other proteins and cell functions that would otherwise lead to food spoilage. This process does not make the food radioactive. p. 546

ischemic stroke (ih-SKI-mik) A stroke caused by the absence of blood flow to a part of the brain. p. 224

isomers (EYE-so-mers) Different chemical structures for compounds that share the same chemical formula. p. 254

ketone bodies (KEE-tone) Incomplete breakdown products of fat, containing three or four carbons. p. 125

ketosis (kee-TOE-sis) The condition of having a high concentration of ketone bodies and related breakdown products in the bloodstream and tissues. p. 125

kidney nephrons (NEF-rons) Units of kidney cells that filter wastes from the bloodstream and deposit them in the urine. p. 519

kilocalorie (kill-oh-KAL-oh-ree) (kcal) The heat energy needed to raise the temperature of 1000 grams (1 L) of water 1 degree Celsius; also written as Calories, with a capital C. p. 5

kwashiorkor (kwash-ee-OR-core) A disease occurring primarily in young children who have an existing disease and who consume a marginal amount of energy and minimal amounts of protein in relation to needs. The child suffers from infections and exhibits edema, poor growth, weakness, and an increased susceptibility to further illness. p. 208

lactase An enzyme made by cells of the intestinal wall; this enzyme digests lactose into glucose and galactose. p. 123

lacteal (LACK-tee-al) A small lymphatic duct associated with a villus of the small intestine. p. 83

lactic acid (LAK-tik) A three-carbon acid formed during anaerobic cell metabolism; a partial breakdown product of glucose; also called *lactate*. p. 391

lactobacillus bifidus **factor (lak-toe-bah-SIL-us BIFF-id-us)** A protective factor secreted in the colostrum that encourages growth of beneficial bacteria in the newborn's intestines. p. 463

lactoovovegetarian (lak-toe-o-vo-vej-eh-TEAR-ree-an) A person who consumes only plant products, dairy products, and eggs. p. 214

lactose (LAK-tose) Glucose bonded to another sugar galactose. p. 113

lactose intolerance A condition where noticeable symptoms such as abdominal gas and bloating appear as a result of severe lactose maldigestion. p. 135

lactose maldigestion (primary and secondary) Primary lactose maldigestion occurs when lactase production declines for no apparent reason.

Secondary lactose maldigestion occurs when a specific cause, such as long-standing diarrhea, results in a decline in lactase production. Severe cases resulting in profound clinical symptoms are also called *lactose intolerance.* p. 135

lacto-vegetarian (lak-toe-vej-eh-TEAR-ree-an) A person who consumes only plant products and dairy products. p. 214

lanugo (lah-NEW-go) Downlike hair that appears after a person has lost much body fat through semistarvation. The hair stands erect and traps air, acting as insulation for the body to compensate for the relative lack of body fat, which usually functions as insulation. p. 162

laxative A medication or other substance that stimulates evacuation of the intestinal tract. p. 106

lean body mass The part of the human body that is free of all but essential body fat; calculated as body weight minus fat storage weight. This includes organs such as the brain, muscles, and liver, as well as blood and other body fluids. p. 345

lecithin (LESS-uh-thin) A group of phospholipids containing two fatty acids, a phosphate group, and a choline molecule. Lecithins are a group of compounds, since they can differ based on the types of fatty acids found on each lecithin molecule. p. 149

leptin (LEP-tin) A hormone made by adipose tissue in proportion to total fat mass in the body that influences long-term regulation of fat mass. Leptin also influences reproductive functions, as well as other body processes, such as release of the hormone insulin. p. 18

"let-down reflex" A reflex stimulated by infant suckling that causes the release (ejection) of milk from milk ducts in the mother's breasts, also called *milk ejection reflex.* p. 462

life expectancy The average length of life for a given group of people born in a certain year, such as this year. p. 518

life span The potential oldest age to which a person can reach. p. 518

lignins (LIG-nins) Insoluble fiber made up of a multiringed alcohol (noncarbohydrate) structure. p. 115

limiting amino acid The essential amino acid in the lowest concentration in a food or diet relative to body needs. p. 192

linoleic acid (lin-oh-LEE-ik) An essential omega-6 fatty acid with 18 carbon and 2 double bonds (C18:2, omega-6). p. 149

lipase (LYE-pase) Fat-digesting enzyme; lipase is produced by the stomach, salivary glands, and the pancreas. p. 154

lipid (LIP-id) A compound composed of much carbon and hydrogen, little oxygen, and sometimes other elements. Lipids dissolve in ether or benzene, but not water, and include fats, oils, and cholesterol. p. 6

lipoprotein (ly-poh-PRO-teen) A compound found in the bloodstream containing a core of lipids with a shell composed of protein, phospholipid, and cholesterol. p. 156

liter (LEE-ter) (L) A measure of volume in the metric system. One liter equals 0.96 quarts. p. 13

liver Largest organ in the body, located in the abdominal cavity below the diaphragm; performs many vital functions that maintain balance in blood composition. p. 97

lobules (LOB-you-els) Saclike structures in the breast that store milk. p. 462

long-chain fatty acids Fatty acids that contain 12 or more carbons. p. 148

low birth weight (LBW) Referring to any infant weighing less than 5.5 pounds (2.5 kilograms) at birth; most commonly results from preterm birth. p. 449

low-density lipoprotein (LDL) The lipoprotein in the blood containing primarily cholesterol; elevated LDL-cholesterol is strongly linked to cardiovascular disease risk. p. 134

lower-body obesity The type of obesity, also called *gynoid,* in which fat storage is primarily located in the buttocks and thigh area. p. 352

lower esophageal sphincter (en-sof-ah-GEE-al SFINK-ter) A circular muscle that constricts the opening of the esophagus to the stomach. p. 91

lower-quality (incomplete) proteins Dietary proteins that are low in or lack one or more essential amino acids. p. 191

lumen (LOO-men) The inside cavity of a tube, such as the GI tract or a blood vessel. p. 93

lymph (limf) A clear, plasmalike fluid that flows through lymph vessels. p. 84

lymphatic system (lim-FAT-ick) System of vessels that can accept fluid surrounding cells and large particles, such as products of fat absorption. This lymph fluid eventually passes into the bloodstream via the lymphatic system. p. 82

lysosome (LYE-so-som) A cellular organelle that contains digestive enzymes for use inside the cell for turnover of cell parts. p. 77

lysozyme (LYE-so-zime) A set of enzyme substances produced by a variety of cells; it can destroy bacteria by rupturing cell membranes. p. 87

macrocytic anemia (mack-ro-SIT-ik ah-NEM-ee-a) Anemia characterized by the presence of abnormally large red blood cells. A typical cause is folate or vitamin B-12 deficiency. p. 269

macular degeneration A painless condition leading to disruption of the central part of the retina and, in turn, blurred vision. p. 247

major mineral A mineral vital to health that is required in the diet in amounts greater than 100 milligrams per day. p. 9

malignant (ma-LIG-nant) Essentially, to do anything malicious. In reference to a tumor, the property of spreading locally and to distant sites. p. 282

malnutrition Failing health that results from long-standing dietary practices that do not coincide with nutritional needs. p. 39

maltase (MALL-tase) An enzyme made by cells of the intestinal wall; this enzyme digests maltose to two glucose molecules. p. 123

maltose (MALL-tos) Glucose bonded to glucose. p. 113

marasmus (ma-RAZ-mus) A disease that results from consuming a minimal amount of protein and energy; one of the diseases classed as protein-energy malnutrition. Victims have little or no fat stores, little muscle mass, and poor strength. Death from infection is common. p. 208

meconium (me-KO-nee-um) The first thick, mucuslike stool passed by the infant after birth. p. 463

medium-chain fatty acid A fatty acid that contains 6 to 10 carbons. p. 148

megadose Generally an intake of a nutrient in excess of 10 times human need. p. 30

megaloblast (MEG-ah-low-blast) A large, nucleated, immature red blood cell that results from the inability of a precursor cell to divide when it normally should. p. 269

menarche (men-AR-kee) The onset of menstruation. Menarche usually occurs around age 13, 2 or 3 years after the first signs of puberty start to appear. p. 451

menopause (MEN-oh-paws) The cessation of menses in women, usually beginning at about 50 years of age. p. 159

mesomorph (MEZ-oh-morf) A body type associated with average bone size, trunk size, and finger length. p. 354

metabolism (meh-TAB-oh-lizm) Chemical processes in the body that provide energy in useful forms and sustain vital activities. p. 10

metastasize (ma-TAS-tah-size) The spreading of disease from one part of the body to another, even to parts of the body that are remote from the site of original tumor. Cancer cells can spread via blood vessels, the lymphatic system, or direct growth of the tumor. p. 282

meter A measure of length in the metric system. One meter equals 39.4 inches. p. 13

microvilli (my-kro-VIL-eye) Microscopic, hairlike projections of cell membranes of certain epithelial cells. p. 94

minerals Elements used in the body to promote chemical reactions and to form body structures. p. 6

miscarriage Termination of pregnancy that occurs before the fetus can survive; typically called *spontaneous abortion.* p. 447

mitochondria (my-toe-KON-dree-ah) The main sites of energy production in a cell. They also contain the pathway for oxidizing fat for fuel, among other metabolic pathways. p. 76

monoglyceride (mon-oh-GLIS-er-ide) A breakdown product of a triglyceride consisting of one fatty acid bonded to a glycerol backbone. A diglyceride contains 2 fatty acids bonded to glycerol. p. 149

monosaccharide (mon-oh-SACK-uh-ride) A simple sugar, such as glucose, that is not broken down further during digestion. p. 112

monounsaturated fatty acid (mon-oh-un-SAT-ur-ated) A fatty acid containing one carbon-carbon double bond. p. 147

motility Generally, the ability to move spontaneously. It also refers to movement of food through the GI tract. p. 88

mottling (MOT-ling) The discoloration or marking of the surface of teeth from fluorosis. p. 326

mucilages (MYOU-sih-laj) Dietary fiber consisting of chains of galactose, mannose, and other monosaccharides; characteristically found in seaweed. p. 115

mucosa (MYOO-co-sa) Mucous membrane consisting of cells and supporting connective tissue. In the digestive tract, there is also a layer of smooth muscle supporting the mucosa. Mucosa lines cavities that open to the outside of the body, such as the stomach and intestine, and generally contains glands that secrete mucus. p. 87

mucous membranes (MYOO-cuss) Also called mucosae, these line passageways open to the exterior environment. p. 87

mucus (MYOO-cuss) A thick fluid secreted by glands throughout the body. It contains a compound that has both carbohydrate and protein parts. It acts as a lubricant and means of protection for cells. p. 90

muscle tissue A type of tissue adapted to contract. p. 77

mutation (myoo-TAY-shun) A change in the chemistry of a gene that remains in subsequent divisions of the cell in which it occurred. p. 284

mycotoxin (MY-ko-tok-sin) A group of toxic compounds produced by molds, such as aflatoxin B-1 found on moldy grains. p. 242

myelin sheath (MY-eh-lyn) A combined lipid and protein (lipoprotein) that covers nerve fibers. p. 85

myocardial infarction (MY-oh-CARD-ee-ahl in-FARK-shun) Death of part of the heart muscle. p. 179

myoglobin (my-oh-GLOW-bin) The iron-containing protein that controls the rate of diffusion of oxygen (O_2) from red blood cells into the muscle cells. p. 315

negative protein balance The state in which protein losses from the body exceed intake, as in cases of starvation. p. 205

negative energy balance The state in which energy intake is less than energy expended, resulting in weight loss. p. 341

neoplasm (KNEE-oh-plaz-em) New and abnormal growth of tissues, which may be benign or cancerous. p. 282

nervous system The body system consisting of the brain, spinal cord, nerves, and sensory receptors. This system detects sensations and controls physiological and intellectual functions and movement. p. 84

neural tube defect A defect in the formation of the neural tube occurring during early fetal development. These are seen in about 2500 infants per year in the United States. This type of defect results in various nervous system disorders, such as spina bifida. Folate deficiency in the pregnant woman increases the risk of the fetus's developing this disorder. p. 270

neuron (NYOUR-on) The structural and functional unit of the nervous system. Consists of cell body, dendrites, and axon. p. 84

neuropeptide Y (nyoo-row-PEP-tide) A chemical substance made in the hypothalamus that stimulates food intake. The hormone leptin inhibits neuropeptide Y production. p. 18

neurotransmitter (nyoo-row-TRANS-mit-er) A compound made by a nerve cell that allows for communication between it and other cells. p. 85

night blindness A vitamin A deficiency condition in which the retina in the eye cannot adjust to low amounts of light. p. 246

nitrate (NI-trait) A nitrogen-containing compound used to cure meats. Its use contributes a pink color to meats and confers some resistance to bacterial growth. p. 554

nitrosamine (ni-TROH-sa-mean) A carcinogen formed from nitrates and breakdown products of amino acids; can lead to stomach cancer. p. 287

nonessential (dispensable) amino acids Amino acids that can be synthesized by a healthy body in sufficient amounts; there are 11 nonessential amino acids. These are also termed dispensable amino acids. p. 190

nonexercise activity thermogenesis (NEAT) Adaptive energy expended via increased heat production, such as when one is fidgeting. p. 346

nonheme iron (non-HEEM) Iron provided from plant sources and animal tissues other than hemoglobin and myoglobin. Nonheme iron is less efficiently absorbed than heme iron, as absorption is also more closely dependent on body needs. p. 315

nonspecific immunity Defenses that stop the invasion of pathogens. Requires no previous encounter with a pathogen. p. 87

norepinephrine (nor-ep-ih-NEF-rin) A neurotransmitter from nerve endings and a hormone from the adrenal gland. It is involved in hunger regulation, blood glucose regulation, and other body processes. p. 85

nucleolus (NEW-klee-o-lus) Center for production of ribosomes within the cell nucleus. p. 75

nutrient density The ratio calculated by dividing a food's contribution to the needs for a nutrient by its contribution to energy needs. When its contribution to nutrient needs exceeds its energy contribution, the food is considered to have a favorable nutrient density. p. 35

nutrients Chemical substances in food that contribute to health, many of which are essential parts of a diet. Nutrients nourish us by providing energy, materials for building body parts, and factors to regulate necessary chemical processes in the body. p. 3

nutrition The Council on Food and Nutrition of the American Medical Association defines nutrition as "the science of food; the nutrients and the substances therein; their action, interaction, and balance in relation to health and disease; and the process by which the organism (i.e., body)

ingests, digests, absorbs, transports, utilizes, and excretes food substances." p. 3

nutritional state The nutritional health of a person as determined by anthropometric measures (height, weight, circumferences, and so on), biochemical measures of nutrients or their by-products in blood and urine, a clinical (physical) examination, a dietary analysis, and a review of economic status; also called nutritional status. p. 39

obesity (oh-BEES-ih-tee) A condition characterized by excess body fat, typically defined in clinical settings as body mass index (BMI) of 30 or more. p. 78

oleic acid (oh-LAY-ik) An omega-9 fatty acid with 18 carbons and one double bond (C18:1, omega-9). p. 149

omega-3 (ω-3) fatty acid Unsaturated fatty acid with the first double bond on the third carbon atom from the methyl end ($-CH_3$). p. 149

omega-6 (ω-6) fatty acid Unsaturated fatty acid with the first double bond on the sixth carbon atom from the methyl end ($-CH_3$). p. 149

organ A group of tissues designed to perform a specific function—for example, the heart. It contains muscle tissue, nerve tissue, and so on. p. 73

organelles (OAR-gan-ells) A compartment, particle, or filament that performs specialized functions within a cell. p. 74

organic Any substance that contains carbon atoms bonded to hydrogen atoms in the chemical structure. p. 9

organism A living thing. The human body is an organism consisting of many organs, which act in a coordinated manner to support life. p. 74

osmosis (oz-MO-sis) The passage of a solvent such as water through a semipermeable membrane from a less concentrated solution to a more concentrated compartment. p. 292

osteomalacia (OS-tee-oh-mal-AY-shuh) Softening of the bones that occurs in adults as the result of bone decalcification linked to inadequate vitamin D status. p. 251

osteoporosis (os-tee-oh-po-ROH-sis) Decreased bone mass wherein no outward causes can be found. This bone loss is related to the effects of aging, poor diet, and hormonal effects of menopause in women. p. 78

overnutrition A state in which nutritional intake greatly exceeds the body's needs. p. 39

ovum (OH-vum) The egg cell from which a fetus eventually develops if the egg is fertilized by a sperm cell. p. 446

oxalic acid (oxalate) An organic acid found in spinach, rhubarb, and other leafy green vegetables that can depress the absorption of certain minerals present in the food, such as calcium. p. 297

oxidation (ox-ih-DAY-shun) Loss of an electron by an atom or a molecule; in metabolism, often associated with a gain of oxygen or loss of hydrogen. Oxidation (loss of an electron) and reduction (gain of an electron) take place simultaneously in metabolism, because an electron that is lost by one atom is accepted by another. p. 158

oxidize (OX-ih-dize) In the most basic sense, this means a chemical substance has either lost an electron or gained an oxygen. This change typically alters the shape and/or function of the substance. An oxidizing agent then is a substance capable of capturing an electron from another source. That source is then "oxidized" when it loses the electron. p. 158

oxytocin (ok-si-TO-sin) A hormone secreted by the posterior part of the pituitary gland. It causes contraction of the musclelike cells surrounding the ducts of the breasts and the smooth muscle of the uterus. p. 462

pancreas (pan-KREE-us) Endocrine organ, located near the stomach, that secretes digestive enzymes into the small intestine and produces hormones, notably insulin. p. 97

parasite An organism that lives in or on another organism and derives nourishment from it. p. 541

parathyroid hormone (PTH) A hormone made by the parathyroid glands that increases synthesis of the vitamin D hormone and aids calcium release from bone and calcium uptake by the kidneys, among other functions. p. 251

passive absorption (transport) Absorption that uses no energy. It requires permeability for the substance through the wall of the small intestine and a concentration gradient higher in the lumen of the intestine than in the absorptive cell. The higher concentration of the substance in the lumen of the intestine in comparison with that in the absorptive cells promotes the absorption of the nutrient. p. 93

pasteurizing (PAS-tur-i-zing) Heating food products rapidly to kill pathogenic microorganisms. p. 541

pectins (PEK-tin) Dietary fiber containing chains of galacturonic acid and other monosaccharides; characteristically found between plant cell walls. p. 115

peer-reviewed journal A journal that publishes research only after two or three scientists who were not part of the study agree it was well conducted and the results are fairly represented. Thus, the research has been approved by peers of the research team. p. 28

pellagra (peh-LAHG-rah) A disease characterized by inflammation of the skin, diarrhea, and eventual mental incapacity; results from an insufficient amount of the vitamin niacin in the diet. p. 24

pepsin (PEP-sin) A protein-digesting enzyme produced by the stomach. p. 200

peptide A few amino acids chemically bonded together; often two to four. p. 193

peptide bond A chemical bond formed between amino acids in a protein.

$$\overset{O}{\underset{\parallel}{}}$$

The acid group $-C-OH_2$ from one amino acid reacts with the amino group ($-NH_2$) of another amino acid to form the

$$\overset{O}{\underset{\parallel}{}}$$

peptide bond $-C-NH-$. Water (H_2O) is a by-product of the reaction. p. 193

percentile Classification of a measurement of a unit into divisions of 100 units. p. 479

peripheral nervous system (PNS) (peh-RIF-er-al) The nerves of the nervous system that lie outside the brain and spinal cord. p. 84

peristalsis (per-ih-STALL-sis) A coordinated muscular contraction that is used to propel food down the gastrointestinal tract. p. 91

pernicious anemia The anemia that results from the inability to absorb sufficient vitamin B-12; it is associated with nerve degeneration, which can result in eventual paralysis and death. p. 273

peroxisome (per-OK-si-som) Cell organelle that destroys toxic products within the cell. p. 77

pesticide A general term for an agent that can destroy bacteria, fungi, insects, rodents, or other pests. p. 563

pH A measure of relative acidity or alkalinity of a solution. The pH scale is 0–14. A ph below 7 is acidic; a pH above 7 is alkaline. p. 99

phagocytic cells (fag-oh-SIT-ick) Cells that engulf substances; these cells include neutrophils and macrophages. p. 88

phagocytosis (FAG-oh-sigh-TOW-sis) A form of active absorption in which the absorptive cell forms an indentation, and particles or fluids entering the indentation are then engulfed by the cell. p. 88

pharynx (FAIR-ingks) The organ of the digestive tract and respiratory tract located at the back of the oral and nasal cavities. p. 91

phenylalanine (fen-ihl-AL-ah-neen) An essential (indispensable) amino acid. p. 7

phenylketonuria (PKU) (fen-ihl-kee-toh-NEW-ree-ah) A disease caused by a defect in the ability of the liver to metabolize the amino acid phenylalanine into the amino acid tyrosine. Toxic by-products of phenylalanine can then build up in the body and lead to mental retardation. p. 121

phosphocreatine (PCr) (fos-fo-CREE-a-tin) A high-energy compound that can be used to re-form ATP. It is used primarily during bursts of activity, such as lifting and jumping. p. 390

phospholipid Any of a class of fat-related substances that contain phosphorus, fatty acids, and a nitrogen-containing component. The phospholipids are an essential part of every cell. p. 74

photosynthesis (foto-SIN-tha-sis) The process by which plants use solar energy from the sun to produce energy-yielding compounds, such as glucose. p. 111

phylloquinone (fil-oh-KWIN-own) A form of vitamin K that comes from plants; also called *vitamin K₁*. p. 245

physiological anemia The normal increase in blood volume in pregnancy that dilutes the concentration of red blood cells, resulting in anemia; also called *hemodilution*. p. 460

phytic acid (phytate) (FY-tick, FY-tate) A constituent of plant fibers that binds positive ions to its multiple phosphate groups. p. 298

phytobezoar (fy-tow-BEE-zor) A pellet of fiber characteristically found in the stomach. p. 129

phytochemical A chemical found in plants. Some phytochemicals may contribute to a reduced risk of cancer or cardiovascular disease in people who consume them regularly. p. 34

pica (PIE-kah) The practice of eating nonfood items, such as dirt, laundry starch, or clay. p. 453

pinocytosis (pee-no-sigh-TOE-sis) Formation of a vesicle that brings molecules into a cell; also called cell drinking. p. 94

placebo (plah-SEE-bo) A fake medicine used to disguise the roles of participants in an experiment; if fake surgery is performed, that is called a *sham operation*. p. 27

placenta (plah-SEN-tah) An organ that forms in pregnant women. Through this organ, oxygen and nutrients from the mother's blood are transferred to the fetus and fetal wastes are removed. The placenta also releases hormones that maintain the pregnant state. p. 446

plaque (PLACK) A cholesterol-rich substance deposited in the blood vessels; it contains various white blood cells, smooth muscle cells, various proteins, cholesterol and other lipids, and eventually calcium. p. 158

plasma The fluid, extracellular portion of the blood that results when blood is centrifuged but is not allowed to clot beforehand. This includes the blood serum plus all blood-clotting factors. p. 82

polypeptide (POL-ee-PEP-tide) A group of amino acids bonded together; from a few to a thousand or more. p. 193

polysaccharide (POL-ee-SACK-uh-ride) Large carbohydrates containing from hundreds to 3000 or more glucose units; also known as *complex carbohydrates*. p. 113

polyunsaturated fatty acid A fatty acid containing two or more carbon-carbon double bonds. p. 148

pool The amount of a nutrient found within the body that can be easily mobilized when needed. p. 202

portal system A process that utilizes a vein to convey blood from capillaries in the intestines and portions of the stomach to the liver. p. 82

portal vein A large vein that distributes blood from the intestine to the liver through capillaries. p. 82

positive protein balance A state in which protein intake exceeds related losses. This causes a net gain of protein in the body, such as when tissue protein is gained during growth. p. 205

positive energy balance State in which energy intake is greater than energy expended, generally resulting in weight gain. p. 341

prebiotic A substance that stimulates bacterial growth in the large intestines. p. 97

preeclampsia (pre-ee-KLAMP-see-ah) Part of the disease pregnancy-induced hypertension. This serious disorder can include high blood pressure, kidney failure, convulsions, and even death of the mother and fetus. Mild cases are known as preeclampsia: more severe cases are called eclampsia or, more correctly, toxemia. p. 460

pregnancy-induced hypertension A serious disorder that can include high blood pressure, kidney failure, convulsions, and even death of the mother and fetus. Although its exact cause is not known, meeting nutrient needs and obtaining prenatal care may prevent or limit its severity. Mild cases are known as *preeclampsia; more severe cases are called *eclampsia* (or more correctly *toxemia*). p. 460

premenstrual syndrome A disorder (also referred to as *PMS*) found in some women a few days before the onset of menses and characterized by depression, anxiety, headache, bloating, and mood swings. Severe cases are currently termed *premenstrual dysphoric disorder (PDD)*. p. 268

preservatives Compounds that extend the shelf life of foods by inhibiting microbial growth or minimizing the destructive effect of oxygen and metals. p. 553

preterm An infant born before 37 weeks of gestation; also referred to as *premature*. p. 449

primary disease A disease process that is not simply caused by another disease process. p. 135

probiotic (PRO-bye-ah-tic) A product that contains specific types of bacteria. Use is intended to colonize the large intestine with the specific bacteria in the product. An example is yogurt. p. 97

prognosis (prog-NO-sis) A forecast of the course and end of a disease. p. 510

prolactin (pro-LACK-tin) A hormone secreted by the mother that stimulates the synthesis of milk. p. 462

prostate gland (PROS-tait) A solid, chestnut-shaped organ surrounding the first part of the urethra in the male. The prostate gland is situated immediately under the bladder and in front of the rectum. The prostate gland secretes substances into the semen as the fluid passes through ducts leading from the seminal vesicles into the urethra. p. 79

protein Food and body components made of amino acids; proteins contain carbon, hydrogen, oxygen, nitrogen, and sometimes other atoms, in a specific configuration. Proteins contain the form of nitrogen most easily used by the human body. p. 6

protein-energy malnutrition (PEM) A condition resulting from regularly consuming insufficient amounts of energy and protein. The deficiency eventually results in body wasting of primarily lean tissue and an increased susceptibility to infection. p. 208

psyllium (SIL-ee-um) A mostly soluble type of dietary fiber found in the seeds of the plantain plant. p. 115

pulmonary circulation (pulmonary circuit) The system of blood vessels from the right side of the heart to the lungs and back to the left side of the heart. p. 82

pyloric sphincter (pi-LOR-ik SFINK-ter) Ring of smooth muscle between the stomach and the small intestine. p. 92

pyruvic acid A three-carbon compound formed during glucose metabolism; also called *pyruvate*. p. 391

radiation Literally, energy that is emitted from a center in all directions. Various forms of radiation energy include X rays and ultraviolet rays from the sun. p. 284

rancid (RAN-sid) Containing products of decomposed fatty acids; they yield unpleasant flavors and odors. p. 160

reactive hypoglycemia (HIGH-po-gligh-SEE-mee-uh) Low blood glucose that may follow a meal high in simple sugars, with corresponding symptoms of irritability, headache, nervousness, sweating, and confusion; actually called *postprandial hypoglycemia*. p. 142

receptive framework for learning The process by which a person opens up to learning more about a problem; it usually involves seeking more information about the issue from books and people. In the case of seeking behavior changes, it involves examining background experience to evaluate whether a behavior change is feasible. p. 374

receptor (ri-SEP-ter) A site in a cell at which compounds (such as hormones) bind. Cells that contain receptors for a specific compound are partially controlled by that compound. p. 86

recombinant DNA (re-KOM-bih-nant) A molecule composed of the DNA of two different species spliced together, such as a combination of bacterial and human DNA used to produce unique bacteria that now can synthesize human proteins. p. 595

Recommended Dietary Allowances (RDAs) Recommended intakes of nutrients that meet the needs of nearly all (97% to 98%) healthy individuals of similar age and gender. These are established by the Food and Nutrition Board of the National Academy of Sciences. p. 50

rectum Terminal portion of the large intestine. p. 97

Registered Dietitian (RD) (dye-eh-TISH-shun) A person who has completed a baccalaureate degree program approved by The American Dietetic Association, performed at least 900 hours of supervised professional practice, and passed a registration examination. p. 30

relapse prevention A series of strategies used to help prevent and cope with weight-control lapses, such as recognizing high-risk situations and deciding beforehand on appropriate responses. p. 366

reserve capacity The extent to which an organ can preserve essentially normal function despite decreasing cell number or cell activity. p. 519

respiratory system The body system consisting of the lungs and various associated organs such as the nose and various conducting tubes. This system transports oxygen from outside air to the lungs, and allows carbon dioxide to be expelled from the body. Oxygen and carbon dioxide are exchanged with the blood in the lungs. p. 81

retinoids (RET-ih-noyds) A collective term for the biologically active forms of vitamin A, including retinol, retinal, and retinoic acid. p. 246

riboneucleic acid (RNA) (RI-bow-new-CLAY-ik) Single-stranded nucleic acid involved in the transcription of genetic information and translation of that information into protein structure. p. 76

ribose (RIGH-bos) A five-carbon sugar found in genetic material—specifically, RNA. p. 414

ribosomes (RI-bow-soms) Cytoplasmic particles that mediate the linking together of amino acids to form proteins; attached to endoplasmic reticulum as bound ribosomes, or suspended in cytoplasm as free ribosomes. p. 76

rickets (RIK-its) A disease characterized by soft, unmineralized bones caused by limited calcium deposition. This deficiency disease arises in infants and children with a poor vitamin D status. p. 251

risk factor A term used frequently when discussing diseases and factors contributing to their development. A risk factor is an aspect of our lives—such as heredity, lifestyle choices (e.g., smoking), or nutritional habits—that make us more likely to develop a disease. p. 4

rough endoplasmic reticulum Portion of the endoplasmic reticulum that contains ribosomes. This is the site of protein synthesis in a cell. p. 76

saccharin (SACK-ah-rin) An alternate sweetener that yields no energy to the body; it is 300 times sweeter than sucrose. p. 121

saliva (sah-LIGH-vah) A watery fluid, produced by the salivary glands in the mouth, that contains lubricants, enzymes, and other substances. p. 90

salivary amylase (SAL-ih-var-ee AM-ih-lace) Starch-digesting enzyme produced by salivary glands. p. 90

salt Generally refers to a compound of sodium and chloride in a 40:60 ratio. p. 14

satiety (suh-TIE-uh-tee) State in which there is no longer a desire to eat; a feeling of satisfaction. p. 17

saturated fatty acid A fatty acid containing no carbon-carbon double bonds. p. 147

scurvy (SKER-vee) The deficiency disease that results after a few weeks to months of consuming a diet that lacks vitamin C; pinpoint sites of bleeding on the skin are an early sign. p. 25

secretory vesicles (see-KRE-tor-ee VES-ih-kels) Membrane-bound vesicles produced by the Golgi apparatus; contains protein and other compounds to be secreted by the cell. p. 77

segmentation Contractions of the circular muscles in the intestines that lead to a dividing and mixing of the intestinal contents. This action aids digestion and absorption of nutrients. p. 92

self-monitoring A process of tracking a behavior and conditions affecting that behavior; actions are usually recorded in a diary, along with location, time, and state of mind. This can be a tool to help people understand more about their eating habits. p. 363

semiessential amino acids Amino acids that, when consumed, spare the need to use an essential amino acid for their synthesis. Tyrosine in the diet, for example, spares the need to use phenylalanine for tyrosine synthesis. p. 190

sequesterants (see-KWES-ter-ants) Compounds that bind free metal ions. By so doing, they reduce the ability of ions to cause rancidity in foods containing fat. p. 553

serotonin (ser-oh-TONE-in) A neurotransmitter synthesized from the amino acid tryptophan that appears to decrease the desire to eat carbohydrates and to induce sleep. p. 18

serum (SEER-um) The portion of the blood fluid remaining after (1) the blood is allowed to clot and (2) the red and white blood cells and other solid matter are removed by centrifugation. p. 181

set point Often refers to the close regulation of body weight. It is not known what cells control this set point or how it actually functions in weight regulation. There is evidence, however, that mechanisms exist that help regulate weight. p. 355

sexually transmitted disease (STD) A contagious disease usually acquired by sexual intercourse or genital contact. Common examples include AIDS, gonorrhea, and syphilis. Also called *venereal disease*. p. 228

short-chain fatty acids Fatty acids that contain fewer than eight carbon atoms. p. 148

sickle cell disease (sickle cell anemia) An anemia that results from a malformation of the red blood cell because of an incorrect primary structure in part of its hemoglobin protein chains. The disease can lead to episodes of severe bone and joint pain, abdominal pain, headache, convulsions, paralysis, and even death. p. 195

simple sugar Term used to describe the group of typical sugars in our diets: glucose, fructose, and sucrose. p. 131

skeletal muscle Muscle responsible for voluntary body movements. p. 81

slough (SLUF) To shed or cast off. p. 194

small-for-gestational age (SGA) (jes-TAY-shun-al) Referring to infants who weigh less than the expected weight for their length of gestation. This corresponds to less than 5.5 pounds (2.5 kilograms) in a full-term newborn. A preterm infant who is also SGA will most likely develop some medical complications. p. 449

smooth endoplasmic reticulum Portion of the endoplasmic reticulum that does not contain ribosomes. This is the site of lipid synthesis in a cell. p. 76

smooth muscle Muscle under involuntary control; found in GI tract, artery walls, respiratory passages, urinary tract, and reproductive tract. p. 81

sodium bicarbonate (SO-dee-um bi-KAR-bow-nait) An alkaline substance made basically of sodium and carbon dioxide ($NaHCO_3$). p. 412

soluble fibers (SOL-you-bull) Fibers that either dissolve or swell in water and are metabolized (fermented) by bacteria in the large intestine. These include pectins, gums, and mucilages. p. 115

solvent A substance that other substances dissolve in. p. 9

sorbitol (SOR-bih-tol) An alcohol derivative of glucose. p. 120

specific immunity Function of white blood cells directed at specific antigens. p. 87

sphincter (SFINK-ter) A muscular valve that controls flow of foodstuff in the GI tract. p. 97

spontaneous abortion Any cessation of pregnancy and expulsion of the embryo or nonviable fetus as the result of natural causes, such as a genetic defect or developmental problem; also called *miscarriage*. p. 447

spores Dormant reproductive cells capable of forming into adult organisms without the help of another cell. Various fungi and bacteria form spores. p. 541

sports anemia (ah-NEE-me-ah) A decrease in the blood's ability to carry oxygen, found in athletes, which may be caused by iron loss through perspiration and feces or increased blood volume. p. 400

starch A carbohydrate made of multiple units of glucose attached together in a form the body can digest; also known as *complex carbohydrate*. p. 122

sterol (STARE-ol) A compound containing a multiring (steroid) structure and a hydroxyl group (–OH). p. 145

stimulus control Altering the environment to minimize the stimuli for eating—for example, removing foods from sight and storing them in kitchen cabinets. p. 363

stress fracture A fracture that occurs from repeated jarring of a bone. Common sites include bones of the foot. p. 400

stroke The loss of body function that results from a blood clot or other change in the brain that affects blood flow. This in turn causes the death of brain tissue. Also called a *cerebrovascular accident*. p. 179

subclinical Not seen on a clinical (physical) examination. p. 39

subclinical Disease or disorder that is present but not severe enough to produce symptoms that can be detected or diagnosed. p. 39

sucralose (SOO-kra-los) An alternative sweetener that has chlorines in place of three hydroxyl (–OH) groups on sucrose. It is 600 times sweeter than sucrose. p. 121

sucrase An enzyme made by cells of the intestinal wall; this enzyme digests sucrose to glucose and galactose. p. 123

sucrose (SOO-kros) Fructose bonded to another sugar glucose; table sugar. p. 112

sugar Simple carbohydrate form with a chemical composition $(CH_2O)_n$. Most sugars form ringed structures when in solution. p. 111

symptom A change in health status noted by the person with the problem, such as a stomach pain. p. 40

synapse (SIN-aps) The space between the axon of one neuron and the dendrite of another neuron. p. 85

Syndrome X A condition in which the person has insulin resistance, hypertension, increased blood triglycerides, and decreased HDL-cholesterol. This condition is usually accompanied by obesity, lack of physical activity, and a diet high in refined carbohydrates. Also called *metabolic syndrome*. p. 128

system A collection of organs that work together to perform an overall function. p. 81

systemic circulation (system circuit) The part of the circulatory system concerned with the flow of blood from the left ventricle to the body and back to the right atrium. p. 82

systolic blood pressure (sis-TOL-lik) The pressure in the arterial blood vessels associated with the pumping of blood from the heart. p. 181

telomerase (teh-LO-mer-ace) Enzyme that maintains length and completeness of chromosomes. p. 284

tetany (TET-ah-nee) A state marked by sharp contraction of muscles with failure to relax afterward; usually caused by abnormal calcium metabolism. p. 308

theory An explanation for a phenomenon that has numerous lines of evidence to support it. p. 24

thermic effect of food (TEF) The increase in metabolism that occurs during the digestion, absorption, and metabolism of energy-yielding nutrients. This represents 5% to 10% of energy consumed. p. 345

thrifty metabolism A metabolism that characteristically conserves more energy than normal, such that it increases risk of weight gain and obesity. p. 355

thyroid hormone Hormone produced by the thyroid gland that increases the rate of overall metabolism in the body. p. 86

tissue (TISH-you) Collection of cells adapted to perform a specific function. p. 73

tocopherols (tuh-KOFF-er-alls) A group of four structurally similar compounds that have vitamin E activity. The alpha form is the most potent form. p. 254

tocotrienols (toe-co-TRY-en-ols) A group of four compounds with the same basic chemical structure as the tocopherols but containing slightly altered side chains. They exhibit much less vitamin E activity than the corresponding tocopherols. p. 254

tolerable upper intake level (UL) Maximum chronic daily intake of a nutrient that is unlikely to cause adverse health effects in almost all people in a population. This number applies to a chronic daily use. p. 50

total parenteral nutrition The intravenous provision of all necessary nutrients, including the most basic forms of protein, carbohydrates, lipids, vitamins, minerals, and electrolytes. p. 161

toxic Poisonous; caused by a poison. p. 542

toxicity The capacity of a substance to produce injury or illness at some dosage. p. 542

toxin Poisonous compounds produced by an organism that can cause disease. p. 542

trabecular bone (trah-BEK-you-lar) Bone tissue with a lattice-like structure; also called *spongy* or *cancellous* bone. p. 336

trace mineral A mineral vital to health that is required in the diet in amounts less than 100 milligrams per day. p. 9

***trans* fatty acids** A form of an unsaturated fatty acid, usually a monounsaturated one when found in food, in which the hydrogens on both carbons forming that double bond lie on opposite sides of that bond. Stick margarine, shortenings, and deep-fat fried foods in general are rich sources. p. 139

triglyceride (try-GLISS-uh-ride) The major form of lipid in the body and in food. It is composed of three fatty acids bonded to glycerol, an alcohol. p. 8

trimesters Three 13- to 14-week periods into which the normal pregnancy of about 37 to 41 weeks is divided somewhat arbitrarily for purposes of discussion and analysis. Development of the embryo and fetus, however, is continuous throughout pregnancy, with no specific physiological markers demarcating the transition from one trimester to the next. p. 446

trypsin (TRIP-sin) A protein-digesting enzyme secreted by the pancreas to act in the small intestine. p. 201

tumor Mass of cells; may be cancerous (malignant) or noncancerous (benign). p. 282

type 1 diabetes A form of diabetes that is prone to ketosis and requires insulin therapy. p. 139

type 2 diabetes A form of diabetes in which ketosis is not commonly seen. Insulin therapy can be used but often is not required. This form of the disease is often associated with obesity. p. 139

ulcer (UL-sir) Erosion of the tissue lining, usually in the stomach (gastric ulcer) or the upper small intestine (duodenal ulcer). These are generally referred to as *peptic ulcers*. p. 24

umami (you-MA-mee) A brothy, meaty, savory flavor in some foods. Monosodium glutamate enhances this flavor when added to foods. p. 90

undernutrition Failing health that results from a longstanding dietary intake that does not meet nutritional needs. p. 39

underwater weighing A method of estimating total body fat by weighing the individual on a standard scale and then weighing him or her again submerged in water. The difference between the two weights is used to estimate total body fat. p. 350

underweight A body mass index below 18.5. The cutoff is less precise than for obesity because this condition has been studied less. p. 369

unsaturated fatty acid A fatty acid with one or more carbon-carbon double bonds in its chemical structure. p. 8

upper-body obesity The type of obesity, also called android, in which fat is stored primarily in the abdominal area; defined as a waist circumference greater than 40 inches in men and greater than 35 inches in women; closely associated with a high risk of cardiovascular disease, hypertension, and type 2 diabetes. p. 352

urea (yoo-REE-ah) Nitrogenous waste product of protein metabolism; major source of nitrogen in the urine, chemically $NH_2-\overset{\overset{O}{\|}}{C}-NH_2$. p. 82

ureter (YOUR-ih-ter) Tube that transports urine from the kidney to the urinary bladder. p. 99

urethra (yoo-REE-thra) Tube that transports urine from the urinary bladder to the outside of the body. p. 99

urinary system The body system consisting of the kidneys, urinary bladder, and the ducts that carry urine. This system removes waste products from the circulatory system and regulates blood acid-base balance, overall chemical balance, and water balance in the body. p. 99

vegan (VEE-gun) A person who eats only plant foods. p. 168

vegetarian A person who avoids eating animal products to a varying degree, ranging from consuming no animal products to simply not consuming four-footed animal products. p. 214

vein A blood vessel that conveys blood to the heart. p. 82

very-low-calorie diet (VLCD) Known also as *protein-sparing modified fast (PSMF)*, this diet allows a person 400 to 800 kcal per day, often in liquid form. Of this, 120 to 480 kcals are carbohydrate; the rest is mostly high-quality protein. p. 368

very-low-density lipoprotein (VLDL) The lipoprotein created in the liver that carries both the cholesterol and lipids taken up by the liver, as well as newly synthesized by the liver. p. 157

villi (VIL-eye) Fingerlike protrusions into the small intestine that participate in digestion and absorption of foodstuff. p. 93

virus (VI-rus) The smallest known type of infectious agent, many of which cause disease in humans. Viruses do not metabolize, grow, or move by themselves. They reproduce by the aid of a living cellular host. Viruses are essentially a piece of genetic material surrounded by a coat of protein. p. 541

vitamins Compounds needed in very small amounts in the diet to help regulate and support chemical reactions in the body. p. 6, 241

water The universal solvent of life; chemically, H_2O. The body is composed of about 60% water. Water (fluid) needs are about 8 cups per day; needs are greater if one exercises heavily. p. 6

water-soluble vitamins Vitamins that dissolve in water. These vitamins are the B-vitamins and vitamin C. p. 241

white blood cells One of the formed elements of the circulating blood system; also called *leukocytes*. Five types of leukocytes are lymphocytes, monocytes, neutrophils, basophils, and eosinophils. White blood cells are able to squeeze through intracellular spaces and migrate. Leukocytes phagocytize bacteria, fungi, and viruses, as well as detoxify proteins that may result from allergic reactions, cellular injury, and other immune system cells. p. 88

whole grains Grains containing the entire seed of the plant, including the bran, germ, and endosperm (starchy interior). Examples are whole wheat and brown rice. p. 115

xerophthalmia (zer-op-THAL-mee-uh) A condition marked by dryness of the cornea and eye membranes that results from vitamin A deficiency and can lead to blindness. The specific cause is a lack of mucus production by the eye, which then leaves it more vulnerable to surface dirt and bacterial infections. p. 246

xylitol (ZIGH-lih-tol) An alcohol derivative of a five-carbon monosaccharide, called xylose. p. 120

zygote (ZIGH-goat) The fertilized ovum; the cell resulting from union of an egg cell (ovum) and sperm until it divides. p. 446

Credits

Chapter 1

Opener: © Vol. 79/PhotoDisc; p. 5 (top): © Vol. 30/CORBIS; p. 5 (bottom): © James Mulligan; 1.1 (top): Courtesy of Wheat Foods Council; 1.1 (mid): Courtesy of National Sunflower Association; 1.1 (bottom): Courtesy of the National Fisheries Institute; p. 9: © CORBIS website; p. 10: © Ken Halfman/Photographics; 1.2 (left & right): © PhotoDisc website; p. 14: © Greg Kidd and Joanne Scott; p. 15: © The Ohio State University Communications Photo Service; p. 16: © PhotoDisc website; 1.4: © Vol. 115/CORBIS; p. 19: © Gordon Wardlaw; p. 20: © The Ohio State University Communications Photo Service; p. 26: USDA; p. 28: © The Ohio State University Communications Photo Service

Chapter 2

Opener: © Vol. 67/Photodisc; p. 34: Courtesy of U.S. Rice Federation; p. 35: Reproduction with permission. © Culinary Hearts Kitchen, 1982; p. 36: © Quaker® Oats; p. 38: © Vol. 67/PhotoDisc; 2.2a: © Vol. 76/CORBIS; 2.2b: © Vol. 29/PhotoDisc; 2.2c: © PhotoDisc website; 2.2d: © Vol. 102/CORBIS; 2.2e: © Vol. 81/CORBIS; 2.4 (golf ball): © Vol. 127/CORBIS; 2.4 (tennis ball): © Object Series 25/PhotoDisc; 2.4 (yoyo): © CORBIS website; 2.4 (mouse): © Vol. 127/CORBIS; 2.4 (baseball): © Object Series 25/PhotoDisc; 2.4 (fist): © Object Series 02/PhotoDisc; p. 48: © Object Series 49/Photo Disc; p. 54: © The Ohio State University Communications Photo Service, Jodi Miller; p. 55 (top): © Vol. 25/PhotoDisc; p. 55 (bottom): © Mark Kempf; p. 58: © Greg Kidd and Joanne Scott; p. 64 © Joanne Scott; p. 66: Courtesy of Gordon Wardlaw; p. 67: Courtesy of National Cattlemen's Beef Association; p. 68: © William Wardlaw

Chapter 3

Opener: © Vol. 38/PhotoDisc; p. 76: © Digital Art/CORBIS; p. 80: © Vol. 40/CORBIS; p. 81: © PhotoDisc; p. 91: Courtesy of National Cattlemen's Beef Association; p. 95: © Science Photo Library/Photo Researchers; p. 99: © PhotoDisc; p. 105: © Gordon Wardlaw

Chapter 4

Opener: © Vol. 43/CORBIS; p. 112: © Object Series 49/PhotoDisc; p. 114: © Greg Kidd and Joanne Scott; p. 118: Courtesy of The Sugar Association, Inc., Washington, D.C.; p. 120: USDA Rice Federation; p. 122: © PhotoDisc website; p. 127: © The Ohio State University Communications Photo Service; p. 130: Courtesy of Wheat Foods Council; p. 131: © The Ohio State University Communications Photo Service, Jodi Miller; p. 135: © Vol. 49/PhotoDisc; p. 140: © William Wardlaw; p. 141: © Vol. 70/PhotoDisc

Chapter 5

Opener: © Vol. 67/PhotoDisc; p. 147: © Greg Kidd and Joanne Scott; p. 151: © Object Series 49/PhotoDisc; p. 160: Courtesy of National Fisheries Institute; p. 152: © Vol. 48/PhotoDisc; p. 161: © Gordon Wardlaw; p. 155: © Vol. 18/PhotoDisc; p. 164: © Vol. 20/PhotoDisc; p. 165: © Saffola Quality Foods, Inc.; p. 166: © CORBIS website; p. 169: © William Wardlaw; p. 171: © Mark Kempf; p. 182: © American Egg Board; p. 183: Courtesy of Avocado Commission

Chapter 6

Opener: © Vol. 192/CORBIS; p. 189: Courtesy of Florida Tomato Committee; p. 192: © Vol. 20/Photodisc; p. 193: © PhotoDisc; 6.3 (left & right): © Bill Longcore/SPL/Photo Researchers; p. 196: Courtesy of Walnut Marketing Board; p. 197: © Greg Kidd & Joanne Scott; p. 198: Beano® is a registered trademark of AkPharma Inc.; p. 206: © Greg Kidd and Joanne Scott; p. 207: © The Ohio State University Communications Photo Service; p. 210: © PhotoDisc website; p. 216: © Gordon Wardlaw

Chapter 7

Opener: © PhotoDisc website; p. 219: © Greg Kidd and Joanne Scott; p. 220 (top): © Vol. 7/PhotoDisc; p. 220 (bottom): © CORBIS website; p. 222: © CORBIS website; p. 224 (top): © Vol. 20/PhotoDisc; p. 224 (bottom): © Vol. 48/PhotoDisc; p. 227: © James Mulligan; p. 228: © Vol. 94/CORBIS; p. 229: © CORBIS website; p. 233: © PhotoDisc website; p. 237: © Vol. 178/CORBIS; p. 238: © CORBIS website

Chapter 8

Opener: © Vol. 130/CORBIS; 8.2a-e and g: © *A Colour Atlas and Text of Nutritional Disorders* by Dr. Donald D. McLaren/Mosby-Woolfe Europe, Ltd.; 8.2f: © BioPhoto Associates/SPL/Photo Researchers; p. 244 and 250: © Object Series 49/PhotoDisc; p. 252: © Vol. 130/CORBIS; p. 253: © Greg Kidd and Joanne Scott; p. 257: © The Ohio State University Communications Photo Service, Jodi Miller; p. 258: © Vol. 67/PhotoDisc; p. 264: Courtesy of National Pork Producers Council; p. 266 (top): © Vol. 43/CORBIS; p. 266 (bottom): © American Egg Board; p. 267: © Vol. 130/CORBIS; p. 271: CORBIS website; p. 274: © Vol. 30/CORBIS; p. 276 (top): © The Ohio State University Communications Photo Service, Jodi Miller; p. 276 (bottom): Courtesy of California Strawberry Commission; p. 277: © CORBIS website; p. 285 (top & bottom): © Object Series 49/PhotoDisc

Chapter 9

Opener: © Vol. 172/CORBIS; p. 293: © PhotoDisc; p. 296: © Gordon Wardlaw; p. 301: © Vol. 83/CORBIS; p. 298: © The Ohio State University Communications Photo Service, Malcolm W. Emmons; p. 302: © Vol. 83/CORBIS; p. 304: © PhotoDisc; p. 308: USDA; p. 310: © William Wardlaw; p. 312: Courtesy of National Dairy Council®; p. 314: © CORBIS website; p. 315: Courtesy of Florida Tomato Committee; p. 318: Courtesy of National Cattlemen's Beef Association; p. 321: © The Ohio State University Communications Photo Service; p. 324: © Vol. 130/CORBIS; p. 325: Courtesy of Fishery Products International, Danvers, MA; p. 326: © Gordon Wardlaw; p. 327: © CORBIS website; p. 328: Photo courtesy of Almond Board of California; p. 335: © Vol. 40/PhotoDisc; p. 338: © Vol. 46/PhotoDisc

Chapter 10

Opener: © Vol. 67/PhotoDisc; p. 343: © Vol. 130/CORBIS; p. 345: © PhotoDisc website; 10.3: © Medical Graphics, Inc.; 10.5: © Diana Linsley/Linsley Photographics; 10.6: © Gordon Wardlaw; p. 353: © CORBIS website; p. 354: © Signature Series 79/PhotoDisc; p. 357: © The Ohio State University Communications Photo Service, Jodi Miller; p. 359: © The Ohio State University Communications Photo Service; p. 360: © PhotoDisc; p. 361: © CORBIS website; p. 364: © Vol. 180/CORBIS; p. 366: Courtesy of California Strawberry Commission

Chapter 11

Opener: © Vol. 82/PhotoDisc; p. 385: © Vol. 45/PhotoDisc; p. 386: © Vol. 51/PhotoDisc; p. 389: © Vol. 164/CORBIS; p. 390: © David R. Frazier/Photo Library, Inc.; p. 394: © Vol. 20/CORBIS; p. 395: © James Mulligan; p. 396: Shore Grilled® Shrimp. Courtesy of Fisheries Products International, Danvers, MA; p. 399: © Gordon Wardlaw; p. 402: © Vol. 103/CORBIS; p. 411: © Vol. 20/CORBIS

Chapter 12

Opener: © Vol. 59/PhotoDisc; 12.1: © Bill Hall; p. 420: © Vol. 75/CORBIS; p. 421: © PhotoDisc; 12.3: © David Frazier Photo Library; p. 423 & 426: © PhotoDisc website; 12.5: © James Mulligan; p. 428: © PhotoDisc website; 12.7: © Paul Casamassimo, DDS, MS; p. 430: © Vol. 83/PhotoDisc; p. 433: © PhotoDisc website; p. 435: © PhotoDisc; 12.9a: © Culver Pictures; 12.9b: © Kobal Collection; 12.9c: © Gilles Caron/Getty Images; 12.9d: © Daniel Simon/Getty Images; p. 442: © Gordon Wardlaw

Chapter 13

Opener : © Vol. 46/PhotoDisc; p. 445: © Vol. 19/CORBIS; p. 447: © Vol. 67/PhotoDisc;
13.3: © Gordon Wardlaw, photographer Greg Wolff; p. 450: © Gordon Wardlaw;
p. 452: © Vol. 15/PhotoDisc; p. 454 and 455: © CORBIS website; p. 457:
© PhotoDisc website; p. 458: © Joanne Scott; p. 459: © Vol. 83/CORBIS; p. 461:
© CORBIS website

Chapter 14

Opener: © Vol. 124/CORBIS; p. 477 (top): © Vol. 180/CORBIS; p. 477 (bottom):
© Joanne Scott; p. 479: © Vol. 19/CORBIS; p. 480: © PhotoDisc; p. 481: © Vol.
135/CORBIS; p. 484: © Vol. 9/CORBIS; p. 485: © Vol. 58/PhotoDisc; p. 486: © Vol.
26/CORBIS; 14.3: © Paul Casamassimo, DDS, MS; p. 489: © Gordon Wardlaw;
p. 493: © Joanne Scott; p. 495: USDA; p. 498: © Vol. 124/CORBIS; p. 500: © Vol.
124/CORBIS; p. 501: © Vol. 24/PhotoDisc; p. 502: © Vol. 19/CORBIS; p. 503: © Vol.
51/PhotoDisc; p. 504: © PhotoDisc website; p. 510: © Greg Kidd and Joanne Scott

Chapter 15

Opener: © Vol. 49/PhotoDisc; p. 515: © Vol. 141/CORBIS; p. 516: © David Craddock;
p. 517: © Vol. 83/PhotoDisc; p. 519: © Vol. 36/CORBIS; p. 520: © Gordon Wardlaw;
p. 522: © Vol. 81/CORBIS; p. 523: © Vol. 81/CORBIS; p. 526: Courtesy of St. Louis
District Dairy Council; p. 533 and 536: © Gordon Wardlaw

Chapter 16

Opener: © Vol. 67/PhotoDisc; p. 542: © Vol. 12/CORBIS; p. 547: USDA; p. 548 (top):
© Gregg Wolff; p. 548 (bottom): © Vol. 48/PhotoDisc; p. 550: © The Ohio State
University Communications Photo Service; p. 552: © Greg Kidd and Joanne Scott;
16.2 (left & right): © Gordon Wardlaw; p. 554 (top): © Vol. 83/CORBIS; p. 554
(bottom): © Object Series 36/PhotoDisc; p. 555: © Vol. 12/PhotoDisc; p. 557: © The
Ohio State University Communications Photo Service; p. 563: © The Ohio State
University Communications Photo Service, Lloyd Lemmermann; p. 565 (top):
© PhotoDisc website; p. 565 (bottom): © Vol. 130/CORBIS; p. 566: © Object Series
Vol. 49/PhotoDisc

Chapter 17

Opener: © Vol. 111/CORBIS; p. 569: © CORBIS website; 17.1 (all): © AP/Wide World
Photos; p. 573 (top & bottom): © The Ohio State University Communications Photo
Service; p. 578: © Vol. 25/PhotoDisc; p. 580 (top): © David R. Frasier, Photolibrary;
p. 580 (bottom): © PhotoDisc website; p. 582: © CORBIS website; p. 586: © CORBIS
website; p. 589: © Vol. 25/CORBIS; p. 590: © The Ohio State University
Communications Photo Service; p. 592: © PhotoDisc website; p. 596: © The Ohio
State University Communications Photo Service, Ken Chamberlain; p. 597 (top):
© The Ohio State University Communications Photo Service, Jodi Miller; p. 597
(bottom): © Vol. 12/PhotoDisc

Appendix

Appendix C.1 (all): © Greg Kidd and Joanne Scott

Index

Page numbers followed by f and t indicate figures and tables, respectively.

Estimated minimum sodium, chloride, and potassium
requirements for healthy persons

Age	Weight (kg)	Sodium (mg)*†	Chloride (mg)*†	Potassium (mg)‡
Months				
0–5	4.5	120	180	500
6–11	8.9	200	300	700
Years				
1	11	225	350	1000
2–5	16	300	500	1400
6–9	25	400	600	1600
10–18	50	500	750	2000
>18§	70	500	750	2000

*No allowance has been included for large, prolonged losses from the skin
through sweat.

†There is no evidence that higher intakes confer any additional health benefit.

‡Desirable intakes of potassium may considerably exceed these values
(~3500 mg for adults).

§No allowance has been included for growth. Values given for people under
18 years of age assume a growth rate corresponding to the
50th percentile reported by the National Center for Health Statistics
and averaged for males and females.

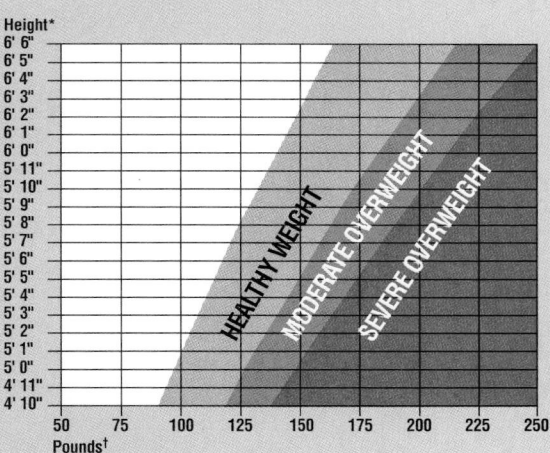

* Without shoes.
† Without clothes. The higher weights apply
  to people with more muscle and bone,
  such as many men.

Dietary Reference Intakes (DRIs): Tolerable Upper Intake Levels (UL[a]), Vitamins
Food and Nutrition Board, Institute of Medicine, National Academies

Life Stage Group	Vitamin A (μg/d)[b]	Vitamin C (mg/d)	Vitamin D (μg/d)	Vitamin E (mg/d)[c,d]	Vitamin K	Thiamin	Riboflavin	Niacin (mg/d)[d]	Vitamin B6 (mg/d)	Folate (μg/d)[d]	Vitamin B12	Pantothenic Acid	Biotin	Choline (g/d)	Carotenoids[e]
Infants															
0–6 mo	600	ND[f]	25	ND	ND	ND	ND	ND	ND	ND	ND	ND	ND	ND	ND
7–12 mo	600	ND	25	ND	ND	ND	ND	ND	ND	ND	ND	ND	ND	ND	ND
Children															
1–3 y	600	400	50	200	ND	ND	ND	10	30	300	ND	ND	ND	1.0	ND
4–8 y	900	650	50	300	ND	ND	ND	15	40	400	ND	ND	ND	1.0	ND
Males, Females															
9–13 y	1,700	1,200	50	600	ND	ND	ND	20	60	600	ND	ND	ND	2.0	ND
14–18 y	2,800	1,800	50	800	ND	ND	ND	30	80	800	ND	ND	ND	3.0	ND
19–70 y	3,000	2,000	50	1,000	ND	ND	ND	35	100	1,000	ND	ND	ND	3.5	ND
>70 y	3,000	2,000	50	1,000	ND	ND	ND	35	100	1,000	ND	ND	ND	3.5	ND
Pregnancy															
≤18 y	2,800	1,800	50	800	ND	ND	ND	30	80	800	ND	ND	ND	3.0	ND
19–50 y	3,000	2,000	50	1,000	ND	ND	ND	35	100	1,000	ND	ND	ND	3.5	ND
Lactation															
≤18 y	2,800	1,800	50	800	ND	ND	ND	30	80	800	ND	ND	ND	3.0	ND
19–50 y	3,000	2,000	50	1,000	ND	ND	ND	35	100	1,000	ND	ND	ND	3.5	ND

[a] UL = The maximum level of daily nutrient intake that is likely to pose no risk of adverse effects. Unless otherwise specified, the UL represents total intake from food, water, and supplements. Due to lack of suitable data, ULs could not be established for vitamin K, thiamin, riboflavin, vitamin B12, pantothenic acid, biotin, or carotenoids. In the absence of ULs, extra caution may be warranted in consuming levels above recommended intakes.

[b] As preformed vitamin A only.

[c] As α-tocopherol; applies to any form of supplemental α-tocopherol.

[d] The ULs for vitamin E, niacin, and folate apply to synthetic forms obtained from supplements, fortified foods, or a combination of the two.

[e] β-Carotene supplements are advised only to serve as a provitamin A source for individuals at risk of vitamin A deficiency.

[f] ND = Not determinable due to lack of data of adverse effects in this age group and concern with regard to lack of ability to handle excess amounts. Source of intake should be from food only to prevent high levels of intake.

SOURCES: *Dietary Reference Intakes for Calcium, Phosphorous, Magnesium, Vitamin D, and Fluoride* (1997); *Dietary Reference Intakes for Thiamin, Riboflavin, Niacin, Vitamin B6, Folate, Vitamin B12, Pantothenic Acid, Biotin, and Choline* (1998); *Dietary Reference Intakes for Vitamin C, Vitamine E, Selenium, and Carotenoids* (2000); and *Dietary Reference Intakes for Vitamin A, Vitamin K, Arsenic, Boron, Chromium, Copper, Iodine, Iron, Manganese, Molybdenum, Nickel, Silicon, Vanadium, and Zinc* (2001). These reports may be accessed via www.nap.edu.